PHARMACOLOGY
for PHARMACY TECHNICIANS

FOURTH EDITION

PHARMACOLOGY

for PHARMACY TECHNICIANS

Kathy Moscou, PhD

Interim Dean, Faculty of Design
Associate Professor
OCAD University
Toronto, Ontario, Canada
Adjunct Professor, Faculty of Applied Health Sciences
Brock University
St Catharines, Ontario, Canada

Karen R. Snipe, CPhT, MAEd

Pharmacy Technician Clinical Coordinator (Ret.)
Trident Technical College
Charleston, South Carolina

ELSEVIER

Elsevier
3251 Riverport Lane
St. Louis, Missouri 63043

PHARMACOLOGY FOR PHARMACY TECHNICIANS, FOURTH EDITION

ISBN: 978-0-323-83211-3

Notice

Practitioners and researchers must always rely on their own experience and knowledge in evaluating and using any information, methods, compounds or experiments described herein. Because of rapid advances in the medical sciences, in particular, independent verification of diagnoses and drug dosages should be made. To the fullest extent of the law, no responsibility is assumed by Elsevier, authors, editors or contributors for any injury and/or damage to persons or property as a matter of products liability, negligence or otherwise, or from any use or operation of any methods, products, instructions, or ideas contained in the material herein.

Previous editions copyrighted 2019, 2013, and 2009.

Senior Content Strategist: Luke E. Held
Senior Content Development Specialist: Vasowati Shome
Publishing Services Manager: Deepthi Unni
Project Manager: Thoufiq Mohammed
Design Direction: Patrick Ferguson

Printed in India

Last digit is the print number: 9   8   7   6   5   4   3   2   1

Reviewers

Technical Reviewer

Ashlee Mattingly, PharmD
Abilities Lab Pharmacist and Technician Training Coordinator
Department of Pharmacy Practice and Science
University of Maryland School of Pharmacy
Baltimore, Maryland

Reviewers

Melissa Ballard, CPhT
Assistant Professor, Pharmacy Technology
Mountwest Community and Technical College
Huntington, West Virginia

Katrina Brasuell, BS, CPhT, Ph TR
Pharmacy Technician Coordinator/Instructor
Vernon College
Wichita Falls, Texas

Thera Celestine, AS
Pharmacy Technology Program Director
Health Science and Workforce Division
Lamar State College – Orange
Orange, Texas

Mary Leigh Curtis, PharmD
Health Technology
Germanna Community College
Fredericksburg, Virginia

Lindsay Elcure, CLS, CPhT
Secondary Health Science Educator
Career and Technology Education – Health Science
Clear Creek High School
League City, Texas

Anthony Guerra, MHCI, PharmD, RPh
Professor, Chemistry/Pharmacology
Des Moines Area Community College
Ankeny, Iowa

Adam R. Hasty, BS, CPhT
Program Director/Instructor
Pharmacy Technician Program
Tennessee College of Applied Technology – Murfreesboro
Murfreesboro, Tennessee

Elena Bablenis Haveles, BS Pharmacy, PharmD, RPh
Adjunct Associate Professor of Pharmacology
Old Dominion University, Schools of Dental Hygiene and
    Nursing
Norfolk, Virginia
Adjunct Professor of Pharmacology
Stratford University, Health Sciences
Virginia Beach, Virginia

Lisa R. Jones, EdS, MHA, BSHCS, AAT, CPhT
Pharmacy Technician Academic Program Coordinator
Allied Health Sciences
Aiken Technical College
Graniteville, South Carolina

Joshua J. Neumiller, PharmD, CDE, FASCP
Vice-Chair and Associate Professor, Department of
    Pharmacotherapy
Director of Experiential Services
Editor-in-Chief, *Diabetes Spectrum*
Washington State University, College of Pharmacy
Pullman, Washington

Bobbi Steelman, CPhT, BSEd, MAEd
Director of Education, Pharmacy Technician Program Director
Academics
Daymar College
Bowling Green, Kentucky

Meera Brown, PharmD, MBA
Senior Manager, Omnichannel Strategy
CVS Health
Austin, TX

Workbook Exercises Reviewer

Brandon Brooks, BS, CPhT
Field Experience and Internship Coordinator
Athens State University
Athens, Alabama

Preface

The pharmacy technician profession has been growing by leaps and bounds because of the increase in the number of prescriptions written, the aging of the population, and the increasing number of new pharmacies. The role of the pharmacy technician has expanded to address the growing need for pharmaceutical services, coupled with increasing requirements for pharmacists to provide cognitive services and direct patient care. It does not matter in which type of pharmacy setting one is employed; a basic understanding of pharmacology is needed to assist the pharmacist effectively in the dispensing of medications and education of the clients of the pharmacy. To this end, *Pharmacology for Pharmacy Technicians* seeks to provide a body of knowledge that will enable the pharmacy technician to understand the principles of pharmacology and apply them to the daily activities and challenges presented in all pharmacy practice settings.

Background

This book was conceived and developed by both a pharmacist and pharmacy technician who saw the need for a comprehensive pharmacology text that would provide knowledge and applications for students in the field of pharmacy practice. The authors have extensive experience training pharmacy technicians and more than 60 years combined experience working with pharmacy technicians in community pharmacy and hospital practice settings in the United States and Canada.

Who Will Benefit From This Book?

Pharmacology for Pharmacy Technicians provides students with comprehensive coverage of pharmacology and gives the instructor the tools necessary to present this information effectively. Today's pharmacy technicians are increasingly called on to perform highly technical tasks that were previously the responsibility of the pharmacist. In all practice settings, pharmacy technicians are required to perform their duties and maintain accuracy and professionalism. Knowledge of pharmacology will increase the pharmacy technician's brand and generic name recognition. Moreover, the study of pharmacology will help pharmacy technicians identify duplicate drugs and speed the process of identifying the drug requested for refill when the patient can't remember the drug name. Given the volume of medication doses currently dispensed, pharmacy technicians need to understand the general principles of pharmacology to be able to assist the pharmacist in spotting medication errors and drug interactions.

Why Is This Book Important to the Profession?

In addition to basic pharmacology, this textbook provides current drug information, tools to enhance learning, and Tech Alerts and Tech Notes that are important aids for pharmacy technicians and other health professionals to prevent medication errors. The material is presented in a format and language that are easily understood and grasped by the reader.

Organization

Pharmacology for Pharmacy Technicians provides an integrated approach to the understanding of pharmacology and pharmacotherapy. Unit I contains content about pharmaceutics, pharmacokinetics, and pharmacodynamics. The unit provides a foundation for understanding pharmacology. Unit II through Unit XI are organized according to body systems—the nervous system, musculoskeletal system, ophthalmic and otic systems, cardiovascular system, gastrointestinal system, respiratory system, reproductive system, endocrine system, and integumentary system. An overview of common disorders of each body system is described, including symptoms. This will help students understand why a given medication is useful for treatment of the condition. The mechanism of action for drugs is also presented. It builds on basic information presented in Unit I and aids in understanding pharmacotherapeutics. Duplicate entries of some drugs are found throughout the text for those that are prescribed for the treatment of more than one medical condition because the rationale for usage may differ according to the medical condition being treated. Each chapter contains a list of basic terminology, key points, review questions, and critical thinking exercises. Common endings of drug classifications are provided to aid in memorizing drugs and their use.

Distinctive Features

Pharmacology for Pharmacy Technicians makes extensive use of tables and figures to enhance learning. U.S. and Canadian brand names are provided for each generic name product. Available strengths and dosage forms are placed in tables along with photographs of many of the top 200 selling drugs to aid in product identification.

Additional unique features include common endings of drug classifications, warning labels for every drug, Tech Alerts for drug look-alike and sound-alike issues, and Tech Notes for important information and precautions. As compared with other pharmacology texts, *Pharmacology for Pharmacy Technicians* is comprehensive and contains descriptions of hundreds of pharmaceuticals.

Learning Aids

A variety of pedagogical features are included in the book to aid in learning:
- **Learning Objectives**. These are listed at the beginning of each chapter and clearly outline what students are expected to learn from the chapter materials.

- A list of **Key Terms** follows the Learning Objectives; the list comprises new terminology and makes it easier for students to learn the new vocabulary. Learning this new terminology is vital to success on the job.
- **Tech Alerts** are found throughout the text and alert the student to drug look-alike and sound-alike issues.
- Helpful **Tech Notes** are presented throughout the chapters and provide critical, need-to-know information regarding dispensing concerns and interesting points about pharmacology.
- **Mini drug monographs** with pill photos are provided for each body system and in every drug classification chapter. These include generic and trade names, strength of medication, route of administration, dosage form, dosing schedule, and warning labels.
- **Key Points** are found at the end of each chapter that summarize the key concepts of the chapter.
- **Review Questions** further enhance student review and retention of chapter content by testing students on the key content within the chapter.
- The **Technician's Corner** provides critical thinking exercises that help students prepare for on-the-job experiences by challenging them to pull together a collection of facts and information to reach a conclusion.
- The **Bibliography** provides a list of sources that students and instructors can use for additional information on the chapter's topic.
- **Appendix:** Workbook exercises include fill-in-the-blank exercises, multiple-choice questions, matching questions, case studies, and true-false questions to reinforce the concepts presented in the textbook.

Ancillaries

For the Instructor

Evolve

We are offering several assets on Evolve (http://evolve.elsevier.com/Moscou/pharmacology) to aid instructors:

- **Test Bank:** An ExamView test bank of more than 1000 questions that features rationales, learning objectives, cognitive levels, and page number references to the text. This can be used as a review in class or for test development.
- **PowerPoint Presentations:** One PowerPoint presentation per chapter. These can be used as is or as a template to prepare lectures.
- **Image Collection:** All the images from the book are available in JPEG format and can be downloaded into PowerPoint presentations. These can be used during lectures to illustrate important concepts.

- **Text Answer Key:** All the answers to the Review Questions and Technician's Corner questions from the text.
- **Workbook Exercises Answer Key:** All the answers to the Workbook exercises.
- **TEACH:** Provides instructors with customizable lesson plans based on learning objectives. With these valuable resources, instructors will save valuable preparation time and can create a learning environment that fully engages students in classroom preparation. The lesson plans are keyed chapter by chapter and are divided into logical lessons to aid in classroom planning.

For the Student

Student Workbook Exercises

The student workbook exercises include:

- Fill-in-the-blank exercises, multiple-choice questions, matching questions, and true-false questions that reinforce the concepts presented in the textbook.
- Research activities and Case Studies that teach students how to keep current with an ever-changing industry.
- Critical thinking exercises that help students apply the knowledge that they learn in class to real-life scenarios, including testing their knowledge of pharmacy calculations.

Evolve

The student resources on Evolve include:

- Two comprehensive practice exams, which include more than 200 questions, to check students' knowledge and comprehension.
- Access to *Clinical Pharmacology*.

Note to the Student

Pharmacology for Pharmacy Technicians was created to provide pharmacy technicians with a strong foundation in pharmacology. As you proceed through this text, you will notice that key concepts are repeated to reinforce learning. Review the key terms before you begin to read the chapter; this will help you understand the chapter better. The chapter summary provides a synopsis of key concepts in each chapter. You will want to refer often to the tables of brand and generic names because this knowledge of brand and generic names is critical for your profession. The drug photos will help you learn to identify commonly prescribed medicines; familiarity with product appearance helps reduce medication errors. You may also find this text useful in other pharmacy technician courses.

Acknowledgments and Dedication

The education of pharmacy technicians to assume ever-expanding professional responsibilities has been the focus of much of my professional career. This book is dedicated to my former students at North Seattle College (formerly North Seattle Community College) and Humber College (Toronto, Canada), whom I have challenged and hopefully inspired to achieve their best, for themselves and the profession. The book is also dedicated to all the pharmacy technicians whom I worked with and learned from during my 40-year career as a pharmacist. I would also like to acknowledge my husband, Gervan Fearon, who has supported me throughout the arduous process of writing this textbook, and my children, Gyasi and Chi Moscou-Jackson, who have started their own professional careers. Finally, I would like to thank the Pharmacy Technician Educators Council and other organizations for encouraging the development of instructional materials for pharmacy technicians.

— Kathy Moscou

The pharmacy technician's role in pharmacy practice has evolved to a point where the knowledge and understanding of pharmacology are vital to patient care. Students will be challenged when learning about all the aspects of pharmacology and its role in healthcare. Being a pharmacy technician for 25 years has shown me that our role is ever expanding, and pharmacists have come to appreciate our knowledge of pharmaceuticals. I would like to thank my family, especially my husband Roy; without their continuous support, I would not have pursued this project. And I'd like to say thank you to my writing partner, Kathy, whose encouragement and support were priceless throughout this project. I dedicate this text to my pharmacy technician students who have inspired me to write teaching materials that are relevant and pertinent to their training.

— Karen Snipe

Contents

Introduction to Pharmacology

The aim of drug therapy is to diagnose, treat, cure, or lessen the symptoms of disease. The study of pharmacology applies knowledge of properties of drugs, mechanism of drug action, anatomy and physiology, and pathology. It is essential to the accurate, effective, and efficient performance of the duties of pharmacy technicians, who, possessing a substantial knowledge of pharmacology, are able to reduce dispensing errors associated with look-alike or sound-alike drugs, as well as recognize drug interactions, incorrect drugs and strengths, incorrect dosage form, improper dosing schedule, therapeutic duplication and drug interactions, and excessive drug alerts screened by the computer before dispensing to patients and hospital medical personnel. Medication errors can be avoided by becoming familiar with trade and generic drug names, their strengths, dosage forms, and dosing frequencies. Pharmacy technicians can also assist patients who do not remember drug names.

In Unit I, pharmacology, pharmacokinetics, and pharmacodynamics of medicines are described. Pharmacokinetics (drug movement) involves four phases: *absorption, distribution, metabolism*, and *elimination* (ADME). These pharmacokinetic phases control the intensity of the drug's effect and the duration of the drug action. Pharmacodynamics looks at patient-related factors that affect how the body responds to drugs that are administered. Age, gender, disease, pregnancy, weight, and genetics are patient-related factors that influence drug response. Psychological factors can also affect drug response, and adherence to drug therapy is influenced by patient belief that the therapy will be beneficial. In Unit I, drug classifications, such as legend (requiring a prescription) or OTC (over the counter), are introduced. Product formulations for administration by mouth (enteral) or injection (parenteral), such as intramuscularly, intravenously, or subcutaneously, inhalation, or topical application are described.

Pharmacy technicians who understand the aspects of pharmacology, pharmacokinetics, pharmacodynamics, the mechanisms of drug action, and strategies to reduce medication errors will be of great benefit to both pharmacists and the patients they serve.

1

Fundamentals of Pharmacology

LEARNING OBJECTIVES

1. Explain why the study of pharmacology is necessary for pharmacy technicians.
2. Illustrate global contributions to the knowledge of pharmaceuticals.
3. Identify key legislation responsible for protecting public health and regulating drug distribution.
4. Describe the drug approval process.
5. Describe commonly dispensed dosage forms.
6. Compare and contrast routes of drug administration.
7. Learn the terminology associated with the fundamentals of pharmacology.

KEY TERMS

Bioavailability The portion of the administered drug dose that enters the systemic circulation and is available to produce drug effect.

Biopharmaceuticals Pharmaceuticals derived from biological sources (e.g., proteins, gene sequences) and manufactured using biotechnology methods such as recombinant DNA technology.

Controlled substance Drug whose possession and distribution is restricted because of its potential for abuse as determined by federal or state law. Controlled substances are placed in schedules according to their abuse potential and effects if abused.

Dosage form Drug formulation (e.g., capsule, tablet, solution).

Dose Amount of a drug required for one application or administration.

Dosing schedule How frequently a drug dose is administered (e.g., "four times a day").

Drug Substance used to diagnose, treat, cure, prevent, or mitigate disease in humans or other animals.

Drug delivery system Dosage form or device designed to release a specific amount of drug.

Enteral Drug dosage form that is administered orally that passes through the gastrointestinal tract.

Homeopathic medicine Drugs that are administered in minute quantities to stimulate natural body healing systems.

Legend drug A drug that is required by state or federal law to be dispensed by a prescription only. Prescriptions must be written for a legitimate medical condition and issued by a practitioner authorized to prescribe.

Over-the-counter (OTC) drug A drug that may be obtained without a prescription.

Parenteral Drug dosage form that is administered by injection or infusion.

Pharmacognosy Science dealing with the biological, biochemical features of natural drugs and their constituents. It is the study of drugs of plant and animal origins.

Pharmacology Study of drugs and their interactions with living systems, including chemical and physical properties, toxicology, and therapeutics.

Pharmacotherapy Use of drugs in the treatment of disease.

Precision medicine Approach to disease treatment and prevention that considers an individual's genetics, environment, and lifestyle when selecting treatment options.

Toxicology Science dealing with the study of poisons.

Pharmacology

Pharmacology is the study of drugs and their interactions with living systems, including chemical and physical properties, *toxicology*, and therapeutics. Knowledge of *pharmacology* is essential to the accurate, effective, and efficient performance of the responsibilities of pharmacy technicians. Pharmacy technicians educated in pharmacology have the skills to properly identify the drug from a patient's profile when a refill is requested and the patient does not remember the drug name. Less time is spent searching for drugs when pharmacy technicians have good brand and generic name recognition. Pharmacy technicians possessing substantial knowledge of pharmacology may be able to reduce dispensing errors associated with look-alike or sound-alike drugs, incorrect drug or strength, incorrect dosage form, and improper dosing schedule. Knowledge of pharmacology facilitates the selection of warning labels for dispensed drugs. Pharmacy technicians who possess a good knowledge of pharmacology understand the importance of recognizing drug interactions, therapeutic duplication, and excessive dose alerts screened by the computer. Overall, pharmacy technicians who have a working knowledge of pharmacology can perform duties within their scope of practice with greater independence.

History of Medicines and Their Use

Plants have been collected, cultivated, and harvested for their healing properties and used in the treatment of illness for centuries. Contributors to the current knowledge about drugs span the globe. Records dating as early as 3000 BC document the pharmacological knowledge by the people of ancient Egypt, Mesopotamia, India, and China. Papyrus Ebers (1550 BC), which was found in Egypt and describes more than 700 medical compounds and lists more than 811 prescriptions, is thought to be a copy of an ancient manuscript that dates to 3000 BC. More than 800 clay tablets have been unearthed describing more than 500 remedies in Mesopotamia (Persian Gulf 2500 BC), and Emperor Shen Nung is credited with writing the *Pen T'sao Ching* (2750 BC) in which more than 1000 medicinal compounds are described and 11,000 prescription remedies are listed. The *Dravyaguna* (2500 BC) is an ancient Ayurvedic manuscript (India) of **materia medica** (medicinal materials) and includes sources, descriptions, criteria for identification, properties, methods for preparation, and therapeutic uses of hundreds of medicinal herbs. Some of the medicinal compounds described in these ancient manuscripts are still used today for essentially the same purposes. For example, castor oil and tincture opii were described in Papyrus Ebers.

Theophrastus (300 BC) was a Greek physician known for his accurate observation of medicinal plants. By the first century, Dioscorides, another Greek physician, described approximately 600 medicinal plants in *De Materia Medica*. Aloe, belladonna, ergot, and opium are a few of the medicines described in the manuscript that are still in use today. Indigenous peoples of the Americas identified the medicinal properties of chinchona bark as a source of quinine to treat malaria. The medicinal properties of willow bark and leaves for treating fever and pain were described by Indigenous peoples in North America, Africa, and China. Willow is a natural source of aspirin.

Since the 20th century, research into medicines and the introduction of new drugs and vaccines have grown exponentially. Antiinfective agents, the discovery of insulin and its use for the treatment of diabetes, and antiretroviral drugs for the treatment of HIV/AIDS have all been discovered since the 1930s. The Human Genome Project, a study of HeLa cells named after Henrietta Lacks, has provided data useful in understanding diseases that are caused by genetic defects or linked to heredity. The study of genes has enabled scientists to develop new genetically modified drugs, such as human insulin. Bioengineering is the process used to produce *biopharmaceuticals*.

A pharmacology timeline is shown in Box 1.1.

Origin of Drugs

Pharmacognosy, a term derived from the Greek words *pharmakon* ("drug") and *gnosis* ("knowledge"), is the branch of science dealing with the study of the natural origin of drugs. Pharmacognosy is the study of the constituents of natural drugs that are responsible for their effects. A *drug* is a substance that affects the normal function or structure of humans or animals and may be used to diagnose, treat, mitigate, cure, or prevent disease. Drugs may come from natural or synthetic origins. Natural drugs may be derived from plants (e.g., digitalis, quinine), animals (e.g., thyroid USP, pepsin), or minerals (e.g., silver nitrate). Some natural drugs are administered in their crude form; however, most frequently, the chief active ingredient(s) are extracted from the crude source.

> ● *Tech Note!*
>
> Some common beverages and foods are natural drugs. Coffee and tea contain the drug caffeine. Ginger and peppermint contain ingredients that can reduce nausea.

Synthetic drugs may be a chemical modification of a natural drug or manufactured entirely from chemical ingredients unrelated to the natural drug. The synthetic drug may be equally potent or more potent. Fentanyl is a synthetically manufactured analgesic that is more potent than the natural drug, morphine (a naturally occurring analgesic derived from the opium poppy). Drugs may also be produced via the process of bioengineering. Erythropoietin and human insulin are examples of biopharmaceuticals. Table 1.1 details common origins of selected drugs.

TABLE 1.1	Drugs and Their Sources		
Classification	Source	Generic Name	Use
Plant	Foxglove	Digitalis	Heart failure (CHF)
	Cinchona	Quinine	Malaria
	Opium poppy	Morphine	Pain
Animal	Thyroid gland	Thyroid USP	Hypothyroidism
	Pancreas	Pancreatin	Digestive aid
Mineral	Silver	Silver sulfadiazine	Burns (antiinfective)
	Gold	Auranofin	Arthritis
Synthetic	Synthetic opioid	Fentanyl	Pain
	Red azo dye	Sulfonamides	Infection
Bioengineering (recombinant DNA and mRNA technology)	Isolated DNA + *Escherichia coli* bacteria	Hepatitis B vaccine*	Hepatitis B prevention
		Human insulin†	Diabetes mellitus
	mRNA	SARS-CoV-2 vaccine	COVID-19 prevention

*Source of hepatitis B vaccine is viral DNA copied into a yeast cell.
†Source of human insulin is isolated DNA + *Escherichia coli* bacteria.

• BOX 1.1   Pharmacology Timeline

3000 BC: Imhotep, Egyptian god of medicine

2750 BC: Emperor Shen Nung (China) was credited with writing the *Pen T'sao Ching*. More than 1000 medicinal compounds were described, and 11,000 prescription remedies were listed.

2500 BC: The *Dravyaguna*, an ancient Ayurvedic manuscript of medicinal materials, sources, descriptions, criteria for identification, properties, methods for preparation, and therapeutic uses of hundreds of medicinal herbs, was written in India.

1550 BC: *Papyrus Ebers*, thought to be a copy of an ancient Egyptian manuscript that dates to 3000 BC, described more than 700 medical compounds and listed more than 811 prescriptions.

1000 BC: Charaka described more than 2000 medicinal substances (including mercury compounds, e.g., merthiolate), methods to improve palatability, and metrology (measurements and dosages).

400 BC: Hippocrates, the "father of medicine"

300 BC: Theophrastus, a Greek physician known for his accurate observation of medicinal plants

AD *100*: Dioscorides, a botanist and pharmacologist, authored *Dioscorides Herbal*.

AD *120 to 200*: Galen, promoted Humoral theory, the dominant theory of disease and treatment for more than 1500 years. This theory states that illness is caused by an imbalance of "humors" and is treated with Simples, Composites, and Entities.

AD *1000*: Avicenna Ibn Sina, known as the "Persian Galen," whose writings unified pharmaceutical and medicinal knowledge of his time and whose teachings were accepted in the West until the 17th century

AD *1500s*: Paracelsus, promoted the concept that disease is a chemical abnormality treated with chemicals. Introduced laudanum, a drug derived from opium that deadens pain.

Indigenous peoples of the Americas had pharmacological knowledge of up to 1200 plants, including:
- West Indies: guaiacum (evergreen tree)
- South America: cocaine (cocoa leaves), curare
- Mexico: jalap (laxative)
- Peru: quinine (cinchona)
- Brazil: balsam Tolu (expectorant)

AD *1700s*: William Withering (United Kingdom) isolated digitalis from foxglove.

Edward Jenner (United Kingdom) developed the vaccine against cowpox. His research led to the development of the smallpox vaccine.

Bernard Courtois (France) discovered iodine, used to treat goiter and to decrease mucus (mucolytic).

Joseph Caventou and Pierre Pelletier (France) discovered quinine, which is used to treat malaria.

Johannes Buchner (Germany) identified salicin from willow bark (ASA) and nicotine in tobacco (niacin).

Emil von Behring (Germany) worked with antitoxins, resulting in diphtheria and tetanus vaccine.

Gregor Mendel (Austria), a famous scientist and monk, discovered the basis of genetics and how genes are woven into heredity.

1800s: *Friedrich Sertürner (Germany) extracted morphine from opium.*

Louis Pasteur's experiments showing that microorganisms can cause disease and heat can kill them became the basis of "germ theory."

1900s: Frederick Banting and Charles Best (Canada) discovered that insulin lowers blood sugar levels and can be used to treat diabetes.

Gerhardt Domagk (Germany) introduced the sulfonamide Prontosil, the first antiinfective agent.

Marie Curie (Poland/France) won the Nobel Prize in recognition of her work in radioactivity and therapeutic effects of radium.

Alexander Fleming (United States) discovered penicillin, a chemical produced by a fungus.

Beyer (United States) was instrumental in the development of thiazide diuretics, derivatives of sulfonamides, and other drugs.

2000s: With the mapping of the human genome and new gene-editing technology, *precision medicine* therapies have been developed such as *ivacaftor* (Kalydeco), a new therapy for the treatment of cystic fibrosis (CF) that was approved for use in patients who have a specific mutation in the CF gene.

Immunobiologic therapies such as monoclonal antibody immunomodulators, monoclonals (e.g., basiliximab, daclizumab, and muromonab), and mTor inhibitors (e.g., everolimus and sirolimus) were introduced.

Vaccines to prevent human papillomavirus (e.g., Gardasil®), new highly active antiretroviral therapy for the treatment of HIV/AIDS (e.g., Triumeq®—abacavir, dolutegravir, lamivudine), and new antiviral therapy for hepatitis C (e.g., Harvoni®—ledipasvir/sofosbuvir) were introduced.

New mechanisms of action for antiviral therapy such as nonstructural protein 5A (NS5A) replication complex inhibitors were introduced (e.g., Daklinza—daclatasvir).

New advances have been made in cellular and gene therapies (e.g., Hemacord—HPC cord blood).

2020s: Dr. Kizzmekia Corbett, lead scientist in developing mRNA SARS-CoV-2 vaccines for the prevention of COVID-19 viral infection

What Is Pharmacology?

Pharmacognosy and pharmacology are both sciences that involve the study of medicinal substances. However, the science of pharmacology involves the action of drugs on humans and animals. The aim of drug therapy is to diagnose, treat, cure, or lessen the symptoms of disease. The study of pharmacology applies knowledge of properties of drugs, mechanism of drug action, anatomy and physiology, and pathology. Selection of the appropriate drug for a patient in the proper ***dose*** and ***dosage form***, administered at an appropriate dosing schedule, requires knowledge of pharmacology. The drug dose is the amount of drug units given for a single administration (e.g., two tablets, one teaspoonful). The ***dosing schedule*** is the number of times the drug dose is administered per day.

What Is Pharmacotherapy?

Pharmacotherapy is defined as the use of drugs in the treatment of disease. Contrasting philosophies about pharmacotherapy exist. Allopathic medicine, sometimes called Western medicine, is a system of medical practice in which the goal of pharmacotherapy is to fight disease by using drugs or surgery that produces effects different from or incompatible with those produced by the disease being treated. In ***homeopathic medicine*** drugs are administered in minute quantities to produce effects similar to the disease in healthy persons yet stimulate the body's natural healing systems in individuals with disease.

Research and Development

In 1906, the Pure Food and Drug Act was passed to protect the public from ineffective and harmful drugs. This act was expanded in 1938, and standards for allowing new drugs onto the market were set. Today, it can take several years to move a new drug from the idea phase to making it available to the public. An expedited, conditional approval process may be used to make select drugs and vaccines available more quickly, as occurred with the approval of COVID-19 vaccines.

There are many steps in the drug development process (Fig. 1.1). The steps from the test tube to production and distribution of a new drug involve preclinical research, clinical studies, the new drug application process, and review. Thousands of chemical compounds may be tested before one is discovered that can produce the desired effects with a minimal level of adverse effects. Manufacturers of new drugs must submit data showing that their drug is reasonably safe before a preliminary small-scale clinical study is approved. Preclinical research is conducted to determine a pharmacological profile for the drug and acute toxicity of the drug in at least two species of animals. Upon completion of the preclinical phase, drug manufacturers file an Investigational New Drug (IND) application. Only approved INDs move to the clinical study phase.

There are three clinical study phases (Fig. 1.2). In phase 1 clinical trials, the drug is administered to a small number of healthy volunteers who are enrolled in the clinical study. Preliminary information about the drug's pharmacology, mechanism of

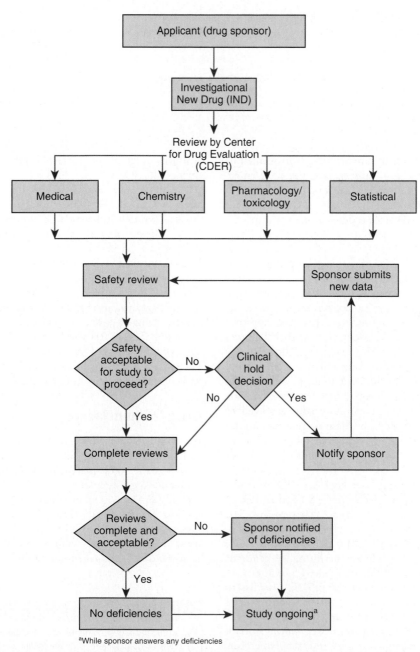

aWhile sponsor answers any deficiencies

• **Fig. 1.1** The Investigational New Drug process.

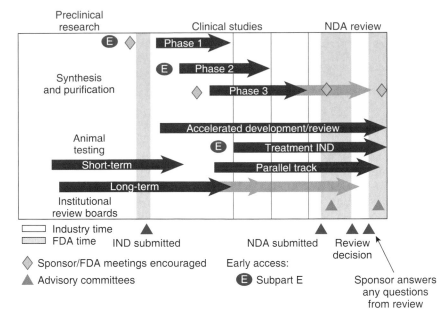

• **Fig. 1.2** The preclinical and clinical phases of the new drug development process. *FDA*, US Food and Drug Administration; *IND*, Investigational New Drug. (From The New Drug Development Process, Food and Drug Administration: New drug development and review process [http://www.fda.gov/Drugs/ DevelopmentApprovalProcess/SmallBusinessAssistance/ucm053131.htm]).

action, and efficacy (effectiveness in humans in a controlled clinical trial) is gathered in phase 1. If appropriate, the drug enters phase 2 clinical studies. Phase 2 studies are controlled trials with a limited number of patients with the condition to be treated. During this phase, data are collected to determine the drug's efficacy and the drug's side effects in patients with the disease. Phase 3 clinical studies involve hundreds to a few thousand patients. Drug safety is evaluated, and the benefit of taking the drug is compared with the risks associated with taking the drug. If safety and efficacy are shown, the drug begins the new drug application process and then moves on to review. An accelerated process exists to speed drug and vaccine development, review, and approval when the drug provides significant benefit over existing therapies or the drug will be used to treat a life-threatening illness or the vaccine will reduce the risk for contracting a life-threatening viral infection, such as COVID-19. In the United States and Canada, additional safety information is required to be collected in the postmarketing phase when a drug is conditionally approved or approved under an expedited process. Phase 4 trials are studies that are conducted after the drug is marketed to the public to determine safety and effectiveness when the drug is used in "real-world" conditions.

In 1992, the Prescription Drug User Fees Act (PDUFA) was passed to allow companies to pay a fee to the US Food and Drug Administration (FDA) in return for a faster review period. The PDUFA was renewed in July 2012 (PDUFA V) and again in August 2017 (PDUFA VI). PDUFA VII was approved in 2022 and is effective until 2027. PDUFA sets performance goals for the speed in which new drug and biologic license applications are reviewed. The FDA Amendments Act permits PDUFA user fees to be used for risk management and communication, increasing the FDA's responsibility to adopt a more proactive approach to pharmacovigilance, and set guidelines for postmarket clinical studies. Congress passed the 21st Century Cures Act in 2016, which further regulates medical product development and innovations, and

advances to speed the process to get them to patients who need them.

Drug approval and marketing of new drugs are also regulated in Canada. Preclinical and phase I to IV clinical studies are also required in Canada. A Notice of Compliance (NOC) or NOC/c (approval with conditions) must be issued before a new drug can be marketed in Canada. Prescription drugs are issued a Drug Identification Number (DIN). The Pharmaceutical Drugs Directorate (PDD) reviews scientific information on safety and efficacy of drugs, premarket clinical trial and investigational testing applications, and emerging drug safety issues by monitoring adverse drug reactions of premarketed drugs. The information that the PDD gathers will be reviewed in determining whether a drug will be approved in Canada. The Marketed Health Products Directorate is responsible for monitoring postmarket drug safety and communicating risks to the public.

Drug Nomenclature

All drugs are identified by a generic name, a chemical name, and a proprietary name. In the United States, the name of a new drug is made according to standards set by the Center for Drug Evaluation and Research (CDER). The standards published in the CDER Data Standards Manual (DSM) are used by the Drug Product Reference File (DPRF) and the Drug Registration and Listing System (DRLS). (The CDER DSM is available at https:// www.fda.gov/drugs/electronic-regulatory-submission-and-review/ data-standards-manual-monographs.)

> ● *Tech Note!*
>
> Every drug has a generic name; however, the drug cannot be manufactured by a generic manufacturer until the patent expires.

TABLE 1.2	Examples of Common Endings to Official Drug Names	
Classification	Common Ending	Prototypical Drug
Benzodiazepine	-zepam -zolam	Diazepam Alprazolam
Corticosteroid	-sone -lone	Prednisone Prednisolone
Nonsteroidal antiinflammatory drug (NSAID)	-profen -olac	Ibuprofen Ketorolac
β-Adrenergic blocking drug (β-blocker)	-olol	Propranolol
H_2 receptor antagonist	-tidine	Cimetidine
Proton pump inhibitor	-prazole	Omeprazole
Calcium channel blockers (dihydropyridines)	-dipine	Nifedipine
Macrolide antiinfective	-thromycin	Erythromycin

TABLE 1.3	Examples of Chemical, Generic, and Proprietary Names	
Generic Name	Chemical Name	Brand Name
Fluoxetine HCl	N-Methyl-3-phenyl-3-[4-(trifluoromethyl)phenoxy] propan-1-amine	Prozac
Acetaminophen	N-(4-Hydroxyphenyl)acetamide	Tylenol
Ibuprofen	2-[4-(2-methylpropyl)phenyl] propanoic acid	Motrin

Official drug names are nonproprietary names that are selected by the US Adopted Name (USAN) Council and must be approved by the FDA. The USAN and International Nonproprietary Name (INN) designated by the World Health Organization is usually identical. The drug name that is published in an official compendium like the US Pharmacopeia is the official name. If a drug contains more than one active ingredient, all official drug names must be listed. The ending of the official name of many drugs indicates the pharmacological class to which the drug belongs (Table 1.2). For example, many local anesthetics have the common ending "-caine."

The generic name is the official or unofficial nonproprietary name commonly used to designate the drug. The chemical name describes the molecular structure of the drug. The chemical structure of the drug determines its activity and side effects.

The proprietary name, or brand name, is assigned by the drug manufacturer according to nomenclature guidelines and must be approved by the CDER. Factors considered when selecting a suitable proprietary name are risk for medication errors caused by existing look-alike and sound-alike names and ease of association with the generic name or active ingredient name (Table 1.3).

Tech Note!

Brand name or proprietary drugs are commonly written beginning with a capital letter, whereas generic or nonproprietary drugs begin with a lowercase letter.

Comparisons Between Brand Name Drugs and Generic Drugs and Biosimilars

The innovator of a new drug may apply for patent protection. If awarded, the manufacturer is given up to 20 years' exclusive rights to manufacture and distribute the new drug. The manufacturer selects a brand name for the drug according to CDER recommendations. When the drug is off patent, other drug companies may manufacture a generic equivalent. Generic drugs contain the same active ingredient as the original manufacturer's drug in the same strength and in the same dosage form. Generic drugs may contain

different inactive ingredients. Occasionally, these inactive ingredients result in slight differences between brand name and generic products that affect how much of the drug is available to produce drug action or how quickly drug effect is produced. Generic drugs that are not significantly different from the innovator's product receive an "A" rating from the FDA and may be substituted for the brand name product according to state and federal product substitution laws.

Generic drugs are always less expensive than brand name drugs. In many states and provinces, pharmacists routinely dispense generic drugs. Most prescription drug insurance plans require that generic drugs be dispensed; brand name drugs are dispensed only when the prescriber insists that a brand name drug is necessary.

A biosimilar is a biopharmaceutical or biologic that is designed to have active properties similar to a biologic that has previously been approved. An example is infliximab (Remicade®), a biologic used to treat Crohn's disease, ulcerative colitis, and psoriatic arthritis. Infliximab-DYYB (Inflectra®), infliximab-QBTX (Ixifi®), and infliximab-ABDA (Renflexis®) are examples of biosimilars.

Tech Note!

Technicians must concentrate on memorizing each drug's generic name and brand name. Medication errors can be avoided by arranging drugs on the pharmacy shelves according to the generic names.

Tech Note!

Many drug names look and sound alike. Technicians should become familiar with the Institute for Safe Medication Practices' (ISMP) list of look-alike and sound-alike drug names. See list at https://www.ismp.org/recommendations/confused-drug-names-list.

Drug Legislation

The Pure Food and Drug Act (1906) was the first significant legislation passed to protect the public from harmful and ineffective drugs in the United States. Over the years, many more laws have been passed that regulate drug manufacturing and distribution. The Durham-Humphrey Amendment (1951) established the distinction between *legend drugs* and drugs that could safely be used by the public without supervision by a health care provider. Legend drugs can be obtained only by prescription. "Rx only" (United States) or "Pr" (Canada) must be printed on the manufacturer's product label for all legend drugs (prescription only). *Over-the-counter (OTC) drugs* do not require a prescription.

TABLE 1.4   Controlled Substances (United States): Schedules, Classification, Dispensing Rules, and Examples

Schedule	Classification	Dispensing Rules	Examples
C-I	The drug has a high potential for abuse. The drug has no currently accepted medical use in treatment in the United States.	Only with approved protocol or investigational use	Ecstasy, heroin, LSD, marijuana, PCP
C-II	The drug has a high potential for abuse. Abuse of the drug may lead to severe psychological or physical dependence. The drug has an accepted medical use in treatment in the United States.	Written prescription (except emergency situations) No refills allowed	Methylphenidate, codeine, meperidine, oxycodone, secobarbital, hydromorphone, amphetamine
C-III	The drug has a potential for abuse less than that of C-II drugs. Abuse may lead to moderate or low physical dependence or high psychological dependence. The drug has an accepted medical use in treatment in the United States.	Written, oral, or faxed prescription Prescriptions expire within 6 months Refillable (no more than five refills within 6 months)	Codeine with acetaminophen, hydrocodone with acetaminophen, methyltestosterone, phendimetrazine, buprenorphine
C-IV	The drug has a potential for abuse less than that of C-III drugs. Abuse may lead to limited physical dependence or psychological dependence relative to the C-III drugs. The drug has an accepted medical use in treatment in the United States.	Written, oral, or faxed prescription Prescriptions expire within 6 months Refillable (no more than five refills within 6 months)	Alprazolam, butorphanol, diazepam, diethylpropion, pentazocine plus naloxone, phentermine, triazolam, carisoprodol
C-V	The drug has a potential for abuse less than that of C-IV drugs. Abuse may lead to limited physical dependence or psychological dependence relative to C-IV drugs. The drug has an accepted medical use in treatment in the United States.	*Prescription:* May be dispensed only for a medical purpose *OTC:* Rules vary for each state	Diphenoxylate plus atropine, lacosamide

LSD, Lysergic acid diethylamide; *OTC,* over the counter; *PCP,* phencyclidine.

The Kefauver-Harris Amendment (1962) requires drugs to be safe and effective before they are made available to the public. INDs (Investigational New Drugs) are limited to drug study participants until clinical studies have shown them to be safe and effective. The Drug Price Competition Act and Patent Restoration Act (1984) encouraged the creation of generic drugs by streamlining the drug approval process for drugs no longer patented. A patent gives exclusive production rights to manufacturers of proprietary drugs for up to 20 years. When a patent has expired, manufacturers of generic drugs may produce and market the drug. Generic manufacturers are not required to conduct additional studies to prove safety and effectiveness but instead are permitted to rely on safety data submitted by the manufacturer of the proprietary drug. There is a transitional status between Rx only and OTC drugs known as behind-the-counter (BTC) drugs in the United States and Canada. BTC drugs are classified in National Association of Pharmacy Regulatory Authority (NAPRA) Schedule II in Canada. BTC drugs may be sold without prescription, but access is restricted, and pharmacist intervention is required to ensure safe, appropriate use and to monitor misuse, abuse, chronic use, and the need for physician referral. Examples of BTC Schedule II drugs include iron supplements, insulin, aspirin for pediatric use, nitroglycerin, and exempt narcotics (e.g., Tylenol with codeine 8 mg) and pseudoephedrine.

In the United States, the Combat Methamphetamine Epidemic Act of 2005 (CMEA) was passed to curb the illegal manufacture and use of "crystal meth." The CMEA was signed into law on March 6, 2006, to regulate, among other things, retail OTC sales of ephedrine, pseudoephedrine, and phenylpropanolamine products used to manufacture crystal meth. Purchase limits, placement of the product out of direct customer access, sales logbooks, customer identification verification, employee training, and self-certification of regulated sellers are required provisions of the CMEA.

The Comprehensive Drug Abuse Prevention and Control Act, also known as the Controlled Substance Act (CSA), was passed by Congress in 1970. It regulates drugs that have a history for abuse in the United States. Access to **controlled substances** is more restrictive than access to legend drugs. Controlled substances are placed in Schedule C-I, C-II, C-III, C-IV, or C-V categories according to their abuse potential and effects if abused (Table 1.4). Controlled substance schedules are determined by federal and state laws.

Legislation limits access to drugs with a potential for abuse in Canada, too. Narcotics, controlled drugs, and benzodiazepines and targeted substances are regulated by the Controlled Drug and Substances Act. Controlled drugs are identified by a ◈ symbol on the product label. Narcotic drugs are identified by a Ⓝ symbol on the product label, and the symbol used to identify benzodiazepines and targeted substances is ▨. Examples of narcotics, controlled substances, and benzodiazepines are given in Table 1.5.

> ● **Tech Note!**
>
> It is important to know the drug schedule and dispensing requirements for prescription and BTC drugs.

TABLE 1.5	Examples of Narcotics, Controlled Substances, and Benzodiazepines and Targeted Substances (Canada)	
	Examples	**Dispensing Rules**
Narcotics	Codeine, meperidine, hydromorphone, morphine, oxycodone	Written, faxed, or electronic prescription only No refills permitted Part fills allowed No transfers
Verbal narcotics	Narcotic preparations containing two or more non-narcotic ingredients (e.g., codeine + acetaminophen and caffeine)	Written, faxed, electronic, or verbal prescription No refills permitted Part fills allowed No transfers
Controlled substances	Amphetamines (e.g., Dexedrine), methylphenidate (part I, schedule G), barbiturates (e.g., secobarbital) (part II), anabolic steroids (e.g., testosterone) (part III)	Written, faxed, or verbal prescription Refills permitted for part I controlled substances only when written on prescription Verbal refills permitted on part II and III controlled substances Part fills allowed
Benzodiazepines and targeted substances	Diazepam, clonazepam	Written, faxed, or verbal prescription Refills may be dispensed when authorized if <1 year has elapsed since the original prescription was issued

Drug Dosage Forms and Delivery Systems

Drugs are formulated for delivery by mouth (oral), injection (parenteral), inhalation, or topical application to skin or a mucous membrane. Factors influencing the choice for drug formulation are chemical properties of the drug and human physiology. Chemical properties of the drug influence the absorption, distribution, metabolism, and elimination of the drug in the body. Normal physiological processes can affect the effectiveness of the drug. For example, drugs formulated for transdermal administration must have sufficient lipid solubility to enable the drug to pass through the cell membranes of skin and get to the site of action. Insulin is formulated for subcutaneous injection because it is composed of two amino acid strands and, if formulated for oral delivery, would be destroyed by the digestive enzymes that break down protein foods.

> ● *Tech Note!*
>
> The Latin abbreviation for "by mouth" is PO (per os). It can be easily remembered as "per oral."

Dosage Forms for Oral (Enteral) Administration

Oral administration is safe, easy, and generally more economical than parenteral administration. Common oral formulations include tablets, capsules, solutions, emulsions, syrups, suspensions, and elixirs.

Tablets

Tablets are solid dosage forms containing one or more active ingredients plus binders and fillers. Binders are added to aid in compressing the drug into a tablet shape. Fillers make up the required bulk and help bind the tablet. Binders and fillers are inactive ingredients but may influence the rate of drug absorption. Tablets are formulated to deliver their contents immediately or over time. Types of tablets are listed "below."

Repeat-action tablets are layered. The outer layer rapidly disintegrates in the stomach, and the inner layer dissolves in the small intestine.

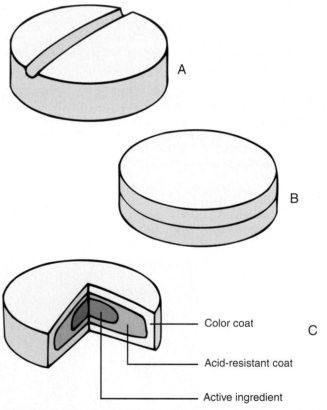

• **Fig. 1.3** Enteric-coated tablets. **A**, Scored side. **B**, Unscored side. **C**, Interior of tablet. (From Clayton BD, Willihnganz MJ: *Basic pharmacology for nurses*, ed 17, St Louis, 2017, Elsevier.)

Delayed-action tablets slow the release of the drug to avoid stomach upset, improve absorption, or prevent drug destruction in the stomach.

Enteric-coated tablets are a type of delayed-action tablet (Fig. 1.3). Enteric-coated tablets do not dissolve in the stomach. They release their contents in the small intestine.

Sustained-release and *time-release tablets* deliver their contents over time. Some drugs are formulated to deliver their contents over

24 hours and need to be taken only once a day. Sustained-release drugs should be swallowed whole; crushing may cause the contents to be released immediately. Sustained release and time release are patented processes.

Film coating and *sugar coating* tablets make them easier to swallow and improves taste.

Chewable tablets are formulated for people who have difficulty swallowing pills. Many children's medicines are available in a chewable dosage form.

Sublingual tablets and *buccal tablets* dissolve in the mouth. Sublingual tablets are dissolved under the tongue, and buccal tablets are dissolved in the cheek pouch. Many blood vessels are located in the mouth. Drugs that are destroyed by stomach acids or need to get into the bloodstream rapidly (e.g., nitroglycerin) may be formulated for sublingual or buccal administration.

Oral disintegrating tablets or *orodispersible tablets* (both abbreviated as *ODT*) are similar to sublingual tablets, but they disintegrate more rapidly (in <60 seconds) when placed on the tongue.

Pastilles are solid medicated preparations designed to dissolve slowly in the mouth. They are softer than lozenges, and their bases are either glycerol and gelatin or acacia and sugar.

Troches and *lozenges* are dissolved in the mouth. Troches may also be chewed.

Thin film tablets have a thin layer of film that disintegrates or dissolves to release the drug. The film may be applied to sublingual tablets (dissolve on the tongue), buccal tablets (absorption in the mouth), and extended-release tablets.

> ● **Tech Note!**
>
> Pharmacy technicians must carefully read the labels of medications available for immediate release, sustained release, and delayed release to avoid errors. Many are available in the same strength.

Capsules

Capsules are solid dosage forms containing one or more active ingredients plus binders and fillers (Fig. 1.4). Capsules are formulated to deliver their contents immediately or over time. An osmotic controlled-release capsule delivers the drug through a rigid water-permeable membrane with one or more small holes. As the capsule passes through the body, the osmotic pressure of water entering the capsule pushes the active drug through the opening in the capsule.

Oral Liquids

Oral liquids include suspensions, solutions, syrups, elixirs, tinctures, and emulsions (explained below). Typically, they are water based. Drugs formulated in liquids are easy to swallow. Liquid medicines work more rapidly than tablets or capsules.

Suspensions contain small drug particles (solute) suspended in a solvent (Fig. 1.5). Drug particles settle to the bottom of the bottle when suspensions are left standing. Suspensions may be administered orally, topically, or rectally. *Solutions* are dosage forms in which drug particles completely dissolve in the liquid. Solutions remain clear.

Syrups contain a high concentration of sucrose or other sugar.

Elixirs contain between 5% and 40% alcohol.

Tinctures may contain as little as 17% alcohol or as much as 80% alcohol.

Emulsions are similar to suspensions. Drugs suspended in oil may be dispersed in water (O/W), or drugs suspended in water may be dispersed in oil (W/O).

> ● **Tech Note!**
>
> When suspensions are dispensed, a SHAKE WELL auxiliary label should be placed on the prescription bottle.

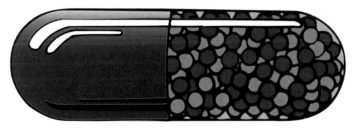

• **Fig. 1.4** Capsules. (From Clayton BD, Willihnganz MJ: *Basic pharmacology for nurses*, ed 17, St Louis, 2017, Elsevier.)

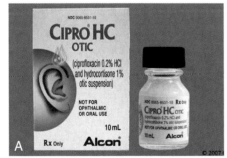
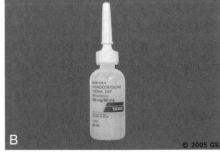
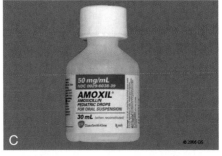

• **Fig. 1.5** Suspensions. **A**, Otic suspensions. **B**, Rectal suspension. **C**, Oral suspension. (Copyright © Gold Standard, Inc., 2007.)

Dosage Forms for Topical Administration

Solutions, suspensions, and emulsions are also formulated for topical application to the skin, eye, ear, and mucous membranes of the rectum and vagina. Topical dosage forms not previously described include ointments, creams, and suppositories.

> **● Tech Note!**
>
> Eye drops (sterile) may be placed in the ear, but ear drops (nonsterile) should not be used in the eye.

Dusting powders are free-flowing very fine powders for external use.
Ointments are semisolid preparations containing petrolatum or another oily base (lanolin, wool fat). They soften dry, scaly skin and protect the skin by forming a barrier between the skin and harmful substances.
Creams are semisolid emulsions. Vanishing creams have high water content and are O/W emulsions; cold cream is a W/O emulsion.
Hydrogels contain up to 99% water and are a controlled-release **drug delivery system**. They are used in transdermal implants (e.g., histrelin) and wound dressings (e.g., Tegaderm™ hydrogel wound filler).
Suppositories are solid or semisolid dosage forms intended to be inserted into a body orifice. They are shaped for vaginal, urethral, or rectal insertion. Suppositories melt at body temperature, dispersing the medicine (Fig. 1.6).

> **● Tech Note!**
>
> The auxiliary label FOR TOPICAL USE ONLY should be applied to topical products that are dispensed.

> **● Tech Note!**
>
> Patients should be advised to remove the foil or outer wrapper from the suppository before inserting it into the rectum or vagina.

Transdermal Drug Delivery Systems (Patches)

Transdermal patches are controlled-release devices that deliver medication across skin membranes into the general circulation (Fig. 1.7). They produce systemic effects (throughout the body) in addition to local effects. Medicines formulated for transdermal application are used to treat angina (e.g., nitroglycerin), male hypogonadism (e.g., testosterone), menopause (e.g., estrogen), pain (e.g., fentanyl), Attention-Deficit/Hyperactivity Disorder (methylphenidate), and Alzheimer disease (rivastigmine).

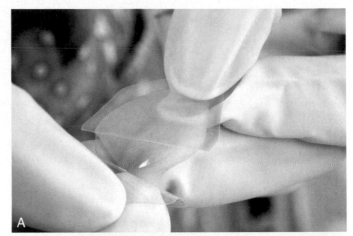

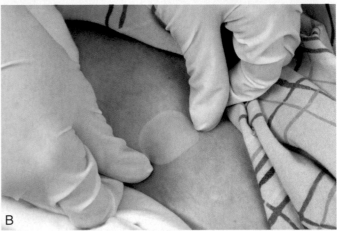

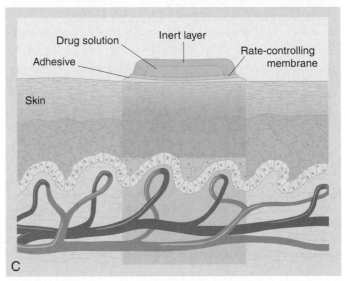

• **Fig. 1.7** Transdermal patches. **A** and **B**, Examples of transdermal patches. **C**, Distribution of drug applied as a transdermal patch across skin membranes to blood vessels. (A and B, Courtesy Rick Brady Riva, MD. From Lilley LL, Collins SR, Snyder JS: *Pharmacology and the nursing process*, ed 8, St Louis, 2017, Elsevier. C, From Page C, Hoffman B, Curtis M, et al: *Integrated pharmacology*, ed 3, Philadelphia, 2006, Mosby.)

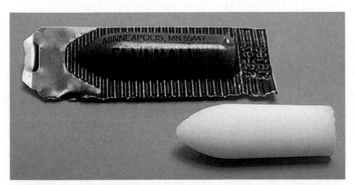

• **Fig. 1.6** Typical shapes of suppositories. (From Clayton BD, Willihnganz MJ: *Basic pharmacology for nurses*, ed 17, St Louis, 2017, Elsevier.)

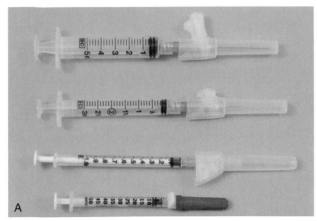 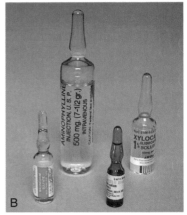 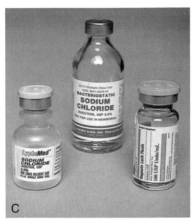

• **Fig. 1.8** Typical containers for parenteral medications. **A**, Syringes. **B**, Ampules. **C**, Vials. (From Potter PA, et al: *Essentials for nursing practice*, ed 8, St Louis, 2015, Elsevier.)

Dosage Forms for Parenteral Administration

Parenteral drugs are injected or infused (slowly injected) directly into a blood vessel, muscle, skin, or joint (Fig. 1.8). Parenterally administered drugs enter the bloodstream, often producing rapid action. In the bloodstream, the side effects cannot be easily stopped. To avoid introducing contaminants that are harmful into a patient, pharmacy technicians must prepare parenterally administered drugs using aseptic technique in a sterile environment. The following are examples of parenteral drugs:

Intravenous (IV) solutions are injected or infused directly into a vein and go immediately into the bloodstream.

Intramuscular (IM) solutions and suspensions are injected deep into a skeletal muscle.

Subcutaneous (subcut) solutions and suspensions are injected just beneath the skin.

Intraarticular solutions are injected directly into a joint.

Intradermal solutions are injected into the dermal layer (allergy tests or tuberculosis vaccinations).

Intrathecal solutions are injected directly into the cerebrospinal fluid.

> ● *Tech Note!*
>
> To avoid drug contamination, aseptic technique must always be followed when preparing drugs for parenteral administration.

Dosage Forms for Respiratory Tract Administration

Solutions and suspensions are applied to mucous membranes of the nose as sprays or drops. Microfine powders, solutions, and gaseous drugs are inhaled into the lungs using a metered-dose aerosol inhaler (Fig. 1.9) or a nebulizer. A nebulizer is a device that turns solutions into vapors that can be inhaled.

Routes of Administration

The formulation of a drug is largely controlled by the chemical properties of the drug and human physiology. The method of drug administration is determined by drug dosage form. When a drug is available for administration via more than one route,

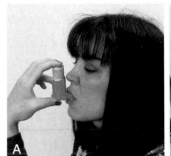 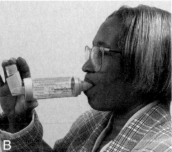

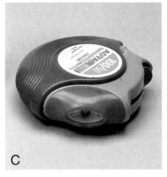

• **Fig. 1.9** **A**, Proper use of an inhaler. **B**, Inhaler with spacer (also known as an aerochamber). **C**, Accuhaler. (A and B, From Potter PA, Perry AG, Stockert P, Hall A: *Fundamentals of nursing*, ed 9, St Louis, 2017, Elsevier. C, From Clayton BD, Willihnganz MJ: *Basic pharmacology for nurses*, ed 17, St Louis, 2017, Elsevier.)

the selection of one route of administration over another is made according to the properties of the drug (e.g., lipid solubility, ionization), ease of administration, pathophysiology (e.g., kidney or liver disease), and therapeutic objectives (e.g., need for rapid onset or long duration of action).

The major routes of drug administration are ***enteral*** (oral), ***parenteral*** (IV, IM, subcut), inhalation, and topical. Enteral, parenteral, and inhalation routes typically produce systemic effects. Systemic effects extend beyond the area of drug application or administration. Drugs that are applied topically usually produce a local effect. Local effects occur predominantly at or near the site of application. These are general rules. Some drugs that are administered orally produce a local effect (e.g., antacids, neomycin), and some drugs administered by injection produce a local effect (e.g., local anesthetics). Transdermal patches produce systemic effects.

Enteral Drug Administration

Oral administration is safe and easy compared with parenteral administration. No special techniques are required for administration, and if needed, the drug can be removed from the body via vomiting (emesis) or binding with activated charcoal. Drugs available for oral administration are generally less expensive than their parenteral dosage form. All orally administered drugs must disintegrate and dissolve into solution before they can be absorbed and distributed. This process is the pharmaceutical phase of drug disposition. Tablets and capsules contain binders and fillers that can influence the rate and extent of disintegration and dissolution.

Disadvantages of oral administration are variable absorption and decreased bioavailability. ***Bioavailability*** is the fraction of the administered drug dose that enters the systemic circulation and is available to produce drug effect. The extent to which a drug is absorbed and distributed to the site of action may be influenced by the presence of food in the stomach, which can delay the absorption of some drugs and aid the absorption of others. The first-pass effect, a process whereby the liver metabolizes a fraction of an administered dose of drug before it passes into the general circulation, also reduces bioavailability (see Chapter 2).

> **● Tech Note!**
> It is important to apply warning labels to medications that inform the patient to TAKE WITH FOOD or TAKE ON AN EMPTY STOMACH.

There are other disadvantages to oral administration. Drugs that are swallowed must pass through the gastrointestinal (GI) tract. Stomach contents contain powerful acids and digestive enzymes. These acids and enzymes can significantly decrease the amount of drug to be absorbed or inactivate some drugs (e.g., penicillin G, insulin).

Parenteral Drug Administration

Parenteral administration is preferred when the patient is unable to swallow (e.g., unconscious) or is experiencing nausea and vomiting or the drug is poorly absorbed via an oral route. Medicines that are administered parenterally bypass the GI tract. Drugs administered parenterally directly enter the general circulation and therefore are not subject to degradation by GI and liver enzymes. The bioavailability of parenterally administered drugs is greater than that of orally administered drugs. An advantage of parenteral administration is the rapid onset of action. The amount of drug delivered parenterally can be carefully controlled by managing flow rates. The exact amount of drug circulating throughout the body cannot be controlled when drugs are administered orally. There are disadvantages to parenteral administration of drugs. Aseptic technique must be used when preparing drugs for parenteral administration to avoid introducing life-threatening contaminants into the patient's bloodstream. After a drug has been administered parenterally, it cannot be recalled through vomiting. Table 1.6 compares the advantages and disadvantages of oral and parenteral administration.

TABLE 1.6	Summary of Potential Advantages and Disadvantages of Oral Versus Parenteral Administration	
Oral	**Intravascular**
Self-administration easy	Self-administration difficult
Safer; recall by emesis	No recall
Absorption slower	Absorption faster
Less expensive	Relatively expensive
Bioavailability lower	Bioavailability higher
Degraded by gastrointestinal enzymes	Not degraded by gastrointestinal enzymes
Subject to the "first-pass effect"	Not subject to the "first-pass effect"
Sterile preparation not critical	Aseptic product preparation critical

> **● Tech Note!**
> Pharmacy technicians must carefully read the labels of medications to avoid dispensing errors. Many parenteral drugs are available for immediate release and slow depot release. Many are available in the same strength.

Parenteral drugs must be administered using specialized techniques. Proper injection procedures must be followed to avoid harm to the patient (Fig. 1.10). When a large volume of a drug is to be administered intravenously (injected into a vein), it must be injected slowly to avoid the destruction of red blood cells (hemolysis). Drugs formulated for IM administration (injected into a muscle) may produce a rapid onset or a slow onset of action. Rapid-onset formulations are typically prepared in water-soluble solutions. Slow-onset, prolonged duration-of-action formulations are suspended in oil or other nonaqueous vehicles (solvent). The drug is slowly released from the muscle depot into which it was injected and then becomes available to produce its effects. Drugs intended for subcutaneous injection pose fewer risks than intravascular administration; however, aseptic technique must still be followed, and the site of injection must be rotated to avoid complications.

> **● Tech Note!**
> Make sure to double-check your calculations for parenteral medications. After being administered, the drug cannot be recalled from the body.

Inhalation

Inhalation is one of the most effective ways to rapidly deliver drugs locally to cells of the respiratory tract and into the general circulation. Absorption problems that are encountered with oral administration are avoided. Some of the side effects associated with oral or parenteral administration are minimized. Inhalation is an effective method for the delivery of medications used to treat asthma and other respiratory disorders. Some medicines used to produce general anesthesia are administered by inhalation.

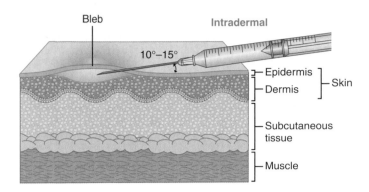

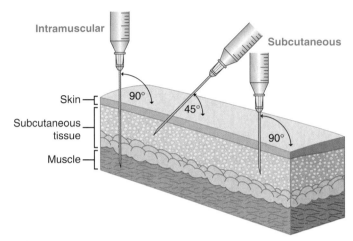

• **Fig. 1.10** Forms of injection: intradermal injection, subcutaneous injection, and intramuscular injection. (From McCuistion LE, DiMaggio K, Winton MB, et al: *Pharmacology: a patient-centered nursing process approach*, ed 9, St Louis, 2018, Elsevier.)

Transdermal Drug Administration

Drugs that are formulated for transdermal administration are applied to the skin to produce systemic effects. Drugs such as nitroglycerin, estrogen, testosterone, methylphenidate, nicotine, and scopolamine are available for transdermal administration. Patients may experience systemic side effects and local side effects from drugs applied as transdermal patches. Local side effects such as skin irritation are often associated with the adhesives used to affix the patch to the skin and can be minimized by rotating the site where the patch is applied.

Topical

Topically administered drugs typically produce a local effect. For example, hydrocortisone cream applied to the skin will reduce itchiness and redness associated with rashes without the systemic side effects associated with oral administration of the drug unless the drug is applied to a large percentage of body surface area. Side effects associated with topical administration are usually localized to the site of application. Topical administration is not exclusively used to produce a local effect. Nitroglycerin cream, a drug used for the treatment of angina, is an example of a topically administered drug used for its systemic effects.

TECHNICIAN'S CORNER

1. The Kefauver-Harris Amendment (1962) requires all drugs to be safe and effective before they are made available to the public. Exactly what is involved in making a drug "safe and effective" for public use?
2. A customer comes to the pharmacy and requests only brand name drugs because they heard "brand" is better. How would you explain that generic drugs are therapeutically equivalent?

Key Points

- Knowledge of pharmacology is essential to the accurate, effective, and efficient performance of pharmacy technician responsibilities.
- Pharmacy technicians possessing a substantial knowledge of pharmacology may be able to reduce dispensing errors.
- Less time is spent searching for drugs when pharmacy technicians have good brand and generic name recognition and can perform their duties with greater independence.
- Knowledge of pharmacology facilitates selection of warning labels for drugs dispensed.
- Pharmacy technicians who possess a good understanding of pharmacology understand the importance of recognizing drug interactions, therapeutic duplication, and excessive dose alerts screened by the computer.
- People from around the globe have contributed to the knowledge of drugs.
- Drugs may come from natural or synthetic origins.
- Plants have been collected, cultivated, and harvested for their healing properties and used in the treatment of illness for centuries.
- Pharmacognosy is the study of the constituents of natural drugs that are responsible for their effects.
- Natural drugs may be derived from plants, animals, or minerals.

- Synthetic drugs may be a chemical modification of a natural drug or manufactured entirely from chemical ingredients unrelated to the natural drug.
- Drugs may also be produced by the process of bioengineering. Drugs produced by bioengineering are called *biopharmaceuticals*.
- Pharmacology is the study of the action of drugs on humans and animals.
- The new drug application process takes years to complete and includes preclinical research; clinical studies; phase 1, phase 2, and phase 3 drug trials; and phase 4 postmarket studies.
- The Food and Drug Administration regulates the new drug and Investigational New Drug process in the United States. The Pharmaceutical Drugs Directorate and the Marketed Health Products Directorate regulate new drugs in Canada.
- The name of a new drug is made according to standards set by the Center for Drug Evaluation and Research.
- The generic name is the nonproprietary drug name.
- The chemical name describes the molecular structure of the drug.
- The proprietary name, or brand name, is assigned by the drug manufacturer. Factors considered when selecting a suitable proprietary name are existing look-alike and sound-alike

names and ease of association with the generic name or active ingredient name.

- Generic drugs contain the same active ingredient as the original manufacturer's drug in the same strength and in the same dosage form but may contain different inactive ingredients.
- The Durham-Humphrey Amendment established the distinction between legend drugs and OTC drugs.
- The Kefauver-Harris Amendment requires all drugs be safe and effective before they are made available to the public.
- The Drug Price Competition Act and Patent Restoration Act encouraged the creation of generic drugs.
- Access to controlled substances is more restrictive than access to legend drugs because controlled substances may cause physical or psychological dependence.
- BTC drugs may be sold without a prescription, but access is restricted and pharmacist intervention is required.
- Drugs are formulated for delivery by mouth, injection, inhalation, or topical application to skin or a mucous membrane. Factors influencing the choice for drug formulation are chemical properties of the drug and human physiology.
- When a drug is available for administration by more than one route, the selection of one route of administration over another is made according to the properties of the drug, ease of administration, therapeutic objectives, and whether the patient has a preexisting disease.
- The major routes of drug administration are enteral (oral), parenteral (IV, IM, subcut), inhalation, and topical.
- The enteral, parenteral, and inhalation routes typically produce systemic effects.
- Topical administration may produce local effects or systemic effects depending on the drug.
- Drugs such as nitroglycerin, estrogen, and testosterone are formulated for transdermal administration but produce systemic effects.

- Orally administered drugs must disintegrate and dissolve into solution before they can be absorbed and distributed. This process is called the pharmaceutical phase.
- Drugs that are swallowed must pass through the gastrointestinal tract. Acids in the stomach and digestive enzymes can inactivate some drugs (e.g., penicillin G).
- Medicines that are administered parenterally bypass the gastrointestinal tract. Drugs administered parenterally directly enter the general circulation and therefore are not subject to the degradation by gastrointestinal and liver enzymes.
- An advantage to parenteral administration is the rapid onset of action.
- Aseptic technique must be used when preparing drugs for parenteral administration to avoid introducing life-threatening contaminants into the patient's bloodstream.
- When a large volume of a drug is to be administered intravenously (injected into a vein), it must be injected slowly to avoid destruction of red blood cells (hemolysis).
- Drugs formulated for intramuscular administration (injected into a muscle) may produce a rapid onset or a slow onset of action. Rapid-onset formulations are typically prepared in water-soluble solutions, and slow-onset, prolonged duration-of-action formulations are suspended in oil or other nonaqueous vehicles (solvent).
- Inhalation is one of the most effective ways to rapidly deliver drugs locally to cells of the respiratory tract and into the general circulation. Inhalation is an effective method for delivery of medications used to treat asthma, other respiratory disorders, and general anesthetics.
- Transdermal patches may cause skin irritation, which is associated with the adhesive. Rotating the site of patch application can reduce risk of skin irritation.

Review Questions

1. Enteral drugs are administered by:
   a. mouth
   b. inhalation
   c. injection
   d. application to the skin
2. What is the study of the constituents of natural drugs that are responsible for their effects?
   a. pharmacology
   b. pharmacogenomics
   c. pharmacognosy
   d. pharmacokinetics
3. In 1906, what law was passed to protect the public from ineffective and harmful drugs?
   a. Pure Food and Drug Act
   b. Harrison Narcotic Act
   c. Pure Food Drug and Cosmetic Act
   d. None of the above
4. Which of the following drugs is *not* made from a plant?
   a. morphine
   b. fentanyl
   c. quinine
   d. digitalis

5. The study of pharmacology applies knowledge of:
   a. properties of drugs
   b. mechanism of drug action
   c. anatomy, physiology, and pathology
   d. all of the above
6. Which of the following is *not* a step in developing and receiving approval for a new drug?
   a. preclinical research
   b. clinical studies
   c. marketing
   d. new drug application process and review
7. The official, nonproprietary name of the drug is the:
   a. generic name
   b. trade name
   c. brand name
   d. chemical name
8. Which drugs can be obtained *only* by prescription?
   a. herbal remedies
   b. legend
   c. compounded
   d. all of the above

9. Which of the following is **not** an oral formulation?
   a. tablet
   b. capsule
   c. suspension
   d. suppository

10. Parenterally administered drugs must be prepared using:
   a. aseptic technique in sterile environment
   b. countertops cleaned with alcohol
   c. patient carts in nursing units
   d. none of the above

Bibliography

Basch E, Ulbricht C. *Natural standard herb & supplement handbook: the clinical bottom line*. St Louis: Mosby; 2005.

Food and Drug Administration (2017). CDER data standards manual. Retrieved September 9, 2022, from https://www.fda.gov/Drugs/DevelopmentApprovalProcess/FormsSubmissionRequirements/ElectronicSubmissions/DataStandardsManualmonographs/ucm071748.htm

Food and Drug Administration (2015). PDUFA legislation and background. Retrieved September 15, 2022, from https://www.fda.gov/ForIndustry/UserFees/PrescriptionDrugUserFee/ucm144411.htm

Food and Drug Administration (2017). Development & approval process (Drugs). Retrieved September 15, 2022, from https://www.fda.gov/Drugs/DevelopmentApprovalProcess/default.htm

Food and Drug Administration (2017). Drugs@FDA glossary of terms. Retrieved September 15, 2022, from http://www.fda.gov/Drugs/InformationOnDrugs/ucm079436.htm

Goodman L, Gilman A. *The pharmacological basis of therapeutics*. ed 5. New York: Macmillan; 1975:1–8.

Haas LF. Neurological stamp: Papyrus of Ebers and Smith. *J Neurol Neurosurg Psychiatry*. 1999;67:578.

Le J. (2017). The Merck manual consumer version. Introduction to administration and kinetics of drugs. Retrieved September 15, 2022, from http://www.merck.com/mmhe/sec02/ch010/ch010a.html

National Human Genome Research Institute (2019). Retrieved June 14, 2022, from https://www.genome.gov/sites/default/files/media/files/2019-07/hela_timeline.pdf

National Library of Medicine, History of Medicine Division: Classics of traditional Chinese medicine. Retrieved September 15, 2022, from https://www.nlm.nih.gov/exhibition/chinesemedicine/emperors.html

National Library of Medicine, Medline Plus. What is precision medicine? Retrieved June 14, 2022, from https://medlineplus.gov/genetics/understanding/precisionmedicine/definition/

Shargel L, Mutnick A, Souney P, eds. *Comprehensive pharmacy review*. ed 4. Philadelphia: Lippincott Williams & Wilkins; 2001:28–66.

Tyler V, Brady L, Robbers J, eds. *Pharmacognosy*. ed 9. Philadelphia: Lea & Febiger; 1988:1–6.

United States Drug Enforcement Administration: Title 21: food and drugs, chapter 13: drug abuse prevention and control. Retrieved July 5, 2023, from https://www.govinfo.gov/content/pkg/USCODE-2014-title21/html/USCODE-2014-title21-chap13-subchapI.htm

Wiktorowicz ME, Lexchin J, Moscou K, et al. *Keeping an eye on prescription drugs, keeping Canadians safe. Active monitoring systems for drug safety and effectiveness in Canada and internationally*. Toronto: Health Council of Canada; 2010. Retrieved September 15, 2022, from https://publications.gc.ca/collections/collection_2011/ccs-hcc/H174-21-2010-eng.pdf

2

Principles of Pharmacology

LEARNING OBJECTIVES

1. Give a definition for each pharmacokinetic phase.
2. Describe factors that influence each pharmacokinetic phase.
3. Explain the importance of the first-pass effect.
4. Describe the function of the blood-brain barrier.
5. List major routes of drug elimination.
6. Describe elimination half-life.
7. Explain the importance of bioavailability to generic drug substitution.
8. Learn the terminology associated with the principles of pharmacology.

KEY TERMS

Absorption Process involving the movement of drug molecules from the site of administration into the circulatory system.

Anion Negatively charged particle.

Bicarbonate Substance used as a buffer to maintain the normal levels of acidity (pH) in blood and other fluids in the body.

Bioavailability The fraction of an administered dose that enters the systemic circulation in an unchanged form and is available to produce its effects.

Bioequivalent drug Drug that shows no statistical differences in the rate and extent of absorption when it is administered in the same strength, dosage form, and route of administration as the brand name product.

Biotransformation Process of drug metabolism in the body that transforms a drug to a more active, equally active, or inactive metabolite.

Colloids Proteins or other large molecules that remain suspended in the blood for a long period and are too large to cross membranes.

Crystalloids Intravenous solutions that contain electrolytes in concentrations similar to those of plasma.

Diffusion Passive movement of molecules across cell membranes from an area of high drug concentration to lower concentration.

Distribution Process of movement of the drug from the circulatory system across barrier membranes to the site of drug action.

Duration of action Time between the onset of action and discontinuation of drug action.

Electrolytes Small charged molecules essential for homeostasis that play an important role in body chemistry.

Elimination Process that results in the removal of a drug from the body.

Enzyme Protein capable of causing a chemical reaction. Enzymes are involved in the metabolism of some drugs.

First-pass effect Process whereby only a fraction of an orally administered drug reaches systemic circulation because much of the drug is metabolized in the liver to an inactive metabolite before entering the general circulation.

Half-life (t½) Length of time it takes for the plasma concentration of an administered drug to be reduced by half.

Hydrophilic Having a strong affinity for water; water loving. Able to dissolve in and absorb water.

Hydrophobic Lacking an affinity for water; water hating. Resistant to wetting.

Ionization Chemical process involving the gain or release of a proton (H^+). Ionized drug molecules may have a positive or negative charge.

Lipid Fatlike substance.

Lipophilic Having an affinity for lipids; lipid loving.

Metabolism Biochemical process involving transformation of active drugs to a compound that can be easily eliminated, or the conversion of prodrugs to active drugs.

Metabolite Product of drug metabolism. Metabolites may be inactivated drugs or active drugs with equal or greater activity than the parent drug.

Microvilli Brushlike structures on each villus in the small intestine that increase the surface area for absorption.

Onset of action Time it takes for drug action to begin.

Osmosis The movement of water across a semipermeable membrane from a higher to lower concentration.

Peak effect Maximum drug effect produced by a given dose of drug after the drug has reached its maximum concentration in the body.

Pharmaceutical alternative Drug that contains the same active ingredient as the brand name drug; however, the strength and dosage form may be different.

Pharmaceutical equivalent Drug that contains identical amount of active ingredient as brand name drug but may have different inactive ingredients, be manufactured in a different dosage form, and exhibit different rates of absorption.

Pharmacokinetics Science dealing with the movement of an administered drug within the body that includes the study of absorption, distribution, metabolism, and elimination.

Prodrug Drug administered in an inactive form that is metabolized in the body to an active form.

Therapeutic alternative Drug that contains different active ingredient(s) than the brand name drug yet produces the same desired therapeutic outcome.

Pharmacokinetics

The word ***pharmacokinetics*** is derived from the Greek words *pharmaco* ("drug") and *kinesis* ("movement"). There are four pharmacokinetic phases: absorption, distribution, metabolism, and elimination (ADME). Drugs that are administered must be absorbed into the bloodstream and distributed to their site of action before they can begin to produce their effect. The body metabolizes the drug, and then it is eliminated. As a drug moves throughout the body, it undergoes changes that may increase or decrease its absorption, distribution, metabolism, or elimination. These pharmacokinetic phases control the intensity of the drug's effect and the duration of the drug action (Fig. 2.1).

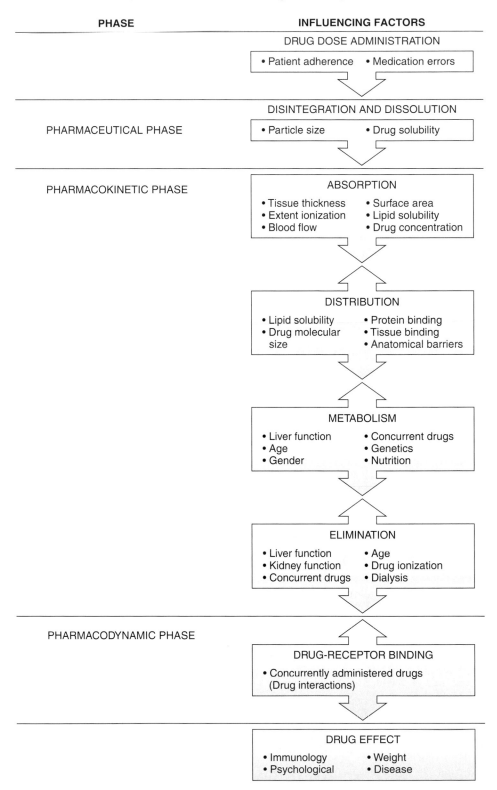

PHASE	INFLUENCING FACTORS
	DRUG DOSE ADMINISTRATION
	• Patient adherence • Medication errors
	DISINTEGRATION AND DISSOLUTION
PHARMACEUTICAL PHASE	• Particle size • Drug solubility
PHARMACOKINETIC PHASE	**ABSORPTION**
	• Tissue thickness • Surface area
	• Extent ionization • Lipid solubility
	• Blood flow • Drug concentration
	DISTRIBUTION
	• Lipid solubility • Protein binding
	• Drug molecular • Tissue binding
	size • Anatomical barriers
	METABOLISM
	• Liver function • Concurrent drugs
	• Age • Genetics
	• Gender • Nutrition
	ELIMINATION
	• Liver function • Age
	• Kidney function • Drug ionization
	• Concurrent drugs • Dialysis
PHARMACODYNAMIC PHASE	**DRUG-RECEPTOR BINDING**
	• Concurrently administered drugs (Drug interactions)
	DRUG EFFECT
	• Immunology • Weight
	• Psychological • Disease

• **Fig. 2.1** Phases of drug distribution.

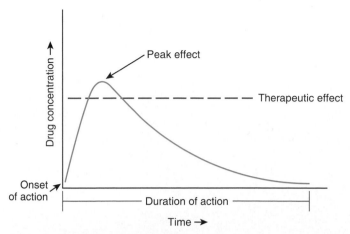

• **Fig. 2.2** Onset of action, peak effect, duration of action, and therapeutic effect.

> ### ● *Tech Note!*
>
> A good way to remember the order of the pharmacokinetic phases is to use the acronym ADME.

The length of time it takes for drug action to begin after a dose is administered is called the **onset of action**. The onset of action is not achieved until the drug reaches the minimum concentration in the body needed to produce drug action. The maximum drug effect, or **peak effect**, occurs after the maximum drug concentration of the drug is reached in the body. The **duration of action** is the time between the onset of action and discontinuation of drug action. The duration of action is the amount of time the drug concentration remains within the therapeutic range (Fig. 2.2).

Pharmacokinetic Phases

Absorption

Absorption is the first pharmacokinetic phase. Absorption is the process that involves the movement of drug molecules from the site of administration, across cell membranes, and into the circulatory system of the body (blood or lymphatic system). Absorption may occur across the skin or cells that line blood vessels. How quickly or slowly a drug is absorbed is determined by the characteristics of the drug, the drug dosage form, the route of administration, human anatomy, and physiology. The amount of drug absorbed is also influenced by many factors. Absorption of tablets and capsules that have been swallowed does not begin until after the drug goes into solution, so factors affecting disintegration or dissolution of the drug (pharmaceutical phase) can decrease absorption (see Chapter 1). Absorption of drugs taken by mouth may also be delayed when food is present in the stomach. The ease with which the drug is able to cross cell membranes is a factor with how readily the drug is absorbed via oral, rectal, vaginal, and other routes of administration.

Cell Membrane

Drug movement from the site of administration into the circulatory system depends on the ability of the drug to move across cell membranes. The cell membrane is a complex structure of **lipids**, protein, and water-filled channels (Fig. 2.3). Movement across the cell membrane is restricted unless the drug can pass through the lipid layers of the cell membrane or is small enough to pass

through the small water-filled (aqueous) channels. A lipid-soluble drug can move easily across the cell membrane. Caffeine, vitamin C (ascorbic acid), vitamin B_3 (niacin), and ephedrine are examples of drugs that pass through aqueous channels in the cell membrane.

Drug Transport Mechanisms

Passive Transport

Drug absorption across the cell membrane may occur via passive or active transport mechanisms. Drugs that are absorbed by passive diffusion move from a region of greater concentration to a region of lesser concentration. When the drug first enters the body, the concentration at the administration site is greater than in the bloodstream. Lipid-soluble drugs readily diffuse across the cell membrane of the blood vessel into the bloodstream. Lipid-soluble drugs are **lipophilic** (lipid loving) and **hydrophobic** (water hating). Water-soluble drugs are **hydrophilic** (water loving) and move through the small water channels in the cell membrane. Most drugs are transported via passive transport.

Active Transport

Active transport mechanisms permit the drug to move across cell membranes without regard to concentration. A drug can move from an area where drug concentration is low to an area where the concentration is high. Active transport takes energy and requires special carrier proteins or pumps to "carry the drug" across the cell membrane.

Factors Influencing Absorption

Effect of pH on Drug Absorption

Most drugs are either weak acids or weak bases. In solution, weak acids and weak bases exist between the ionized and the nonionized state. In solution, weak acids (HA) disassociate, releasing a proton (H^+) and negatively charged **anion** (A^-).

$$HA \rightleftharpoons H^+ + A^-$$

Weak bases also release a proton when they are in solution; however, when the proton is released, the resulting drug molecule is nonionized (uncharged).

$$B^+H \rightleftharpoons B + H^+$$

Weakly acidic drugs are more ionized when they are in basic solutions. When the drugs are in an acidic solution, they are less ionized. Weakly basic drugs are more ionized when they are in acidic solution and less ionized in basic solution. This is important because as the drug travels throughout the body, it passes through acidic solutions (e.g., in the stomach) and basic solutions (e.g., in the small intestine). The ability of a drug to diffuse across the cell membrane depends on properties of the drug and the pH of the body fluid in which it is dissolved. The pH is a measure of how acidic or alkaline (basic) a solution is. A pH of 1 is very acidic (e.g., stomach acids [HCl]). A pH of 7 is neutral. Plasma has a pH between the range of 7.35 and 7.45. A pH of greater than 7 is alkaline. Intravenous solutions that contain **electrolytes** in concentrations similar to those of plasma are called **crystalloids**.

Diffusion across the cell membrane is greatest when the drug is lipid soluble and nonionized. When a weakly acidic drug such as phenobarbital is in the stomach, it is less ionized and can readily cross the cell membranes. Absorption is high. When the drug moves into the small intestine, ionization increases and absorption is reduced. **Osmosis** is the movement of water across a

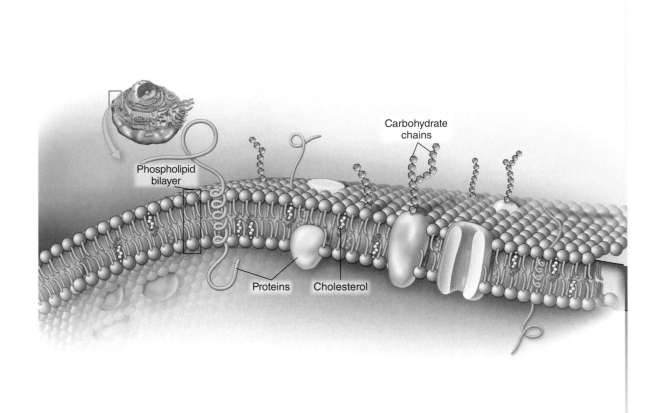

• **Fig. 2.3** Plasma membrane. (From Patton KT, Thibodeau GA: *The human body in health and disease,* ed 7, St Louis, 2018, Elsevier.)

semipermeable membrane from a higher to lower concentration. Electrolytes are more concentrated inside than outside the cells, and the water outside the cells is less concentrated, or diluted, because it contains fewer electrolytes.

Effect of Blood Flow on Drug Absorption

Absorption is greatest in areas of the body that have a good blood supply. Medications administered sublingually have good absorption because many blood vessels are located under the tongue. Absorption of orally administered drugs is greatest in the small intestine. The structure of the intestine is designed to perform the specialized job of absorption. Thousands of **microvilli** line the walls of the small intestine. The microvilli are filled with blood vessels. As the drug passes through the cell membrane of the microvilli, it is quickly absorbed into the bloodstream. Absorption of drugs that are injected intramuscularly or subcutaneously is increased when the patient applies heat to the muscle, exercises, or does some other activity to stimulate blood flow to the site of administration.

Effect of Surface Area on Drug Absorption

Microvilli also increase the surface area of the small intestine, making it the largest absorbing surface in the body (Fig. 2.4). The area for absorption in the small intestine is approximately 1000 times greater than in the stomach.

Effect of Contact Time at the Absorption Surface

Drug absorption increases the longer the drug is in contact with the absorbing surface. Drug absorption is decreased if the patient has diarrhea because of the rapid passage of contents through the gastrointestinal (GI) tract. Absorption of delayed-release drugs can be increased when a drug is taken with food because of delayed gastric emptying.

Effect of Tissue Thickness on Absorption

Drug absorption is greater across single cell membranes than multiple cell layers because some drugs may become trapped in cell layers. As tissue thickness increases, the portion of the drug trapped in the cell layers increases.

Distribution

Distribution is the process of movement of the drug from the circulatory system across barrier membranes to the site of drug action (Fig. 2.5). It is the second pharmacokinetic phase. The volume of drug that is distributed is influenced by the properties of the drug, the extent of drug binding to blood proteins or tissue, the blood supply to the region, and the ability of the drug to cross natural body barriers. The drug may be distributed to water compartments of the body or to fat cells or proteins. Water compartments include plasma, extracellular fluid, and total body water.

Body Fluid Compartments and Electrolytes

Extracellular fluid consists mainly of the plasma found in the blood vessels and the interstitial fluid that surrounds the cells. Intracellular fluid refers to the water inside the cells.

Sodium, potassium, and chloride are major electrolytes found in the body. Sodium is the major positive ion in extracellular fluid.

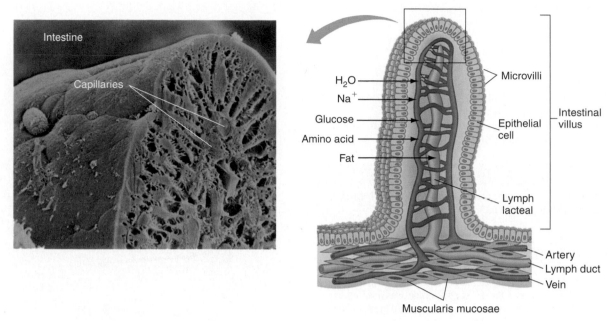

• **Fig. 2.4** Intestinal villi showing absorbing surfaces. (From Patton KT, Thibodeau GA: *Anatomy and physiology*, ed 9, St Louis, 2016, Elsevier.)

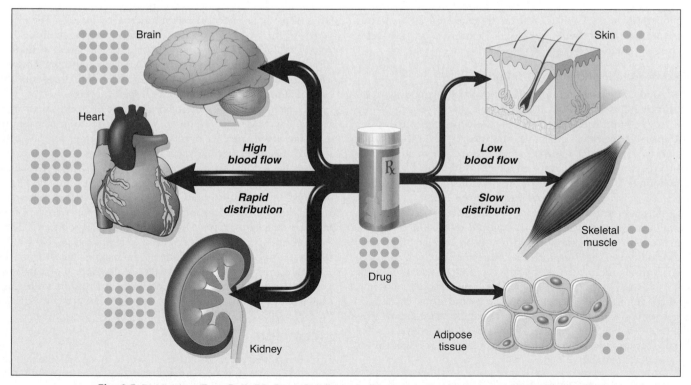

• **Fig. 2.5** Distribution. (From Raffa RB, Rawls SM, Beyzarov EP: *Netter's illustrated pharmacology*, Philadelphia, 2005, WB Saunders.)

Sodium regulates the total amount of water in the body and the transmission of sodium into and out of individual cells. It plays a role in critical processes in the brain, nervous system, and muscles that require electrical signals for communication.

Potassium is the other major cation found inside of cells. The proper level of potassium is essential for normal cell function. Regulation of the heartbeat and muscle contraction are two important functions of potassium.

Chloride is the major anion (negatively charged ion) found in the fluid outside of cells and in blood.

> **● Tech Note!**
>
> 0.9% Sodium chloride (NaCl) is also known as normal saline (NS) because it is the same concentration (isotonic) as in the body.

> **● Tech Note!**
>
> Water follows sodium ions when they are moved through the cell membrane. Lots of sodium in the body means that water stays inside (instead of leaving through kidney cells and then the bladder), which means that there is more blood volume and blood pressure is higher.

Factors Influencing Distribution

Effect of Drug Properties on Distribution

The distribution of a drug across the blood vessel cell membrane and transport to its site of action are influenced by the chemical nature of the drug, such as lipid solubility. Drugs that are lipid soluble, nonionized, or a size small enough to pass through slit junctions in the capillary wall are readily distributed. Slit junctions vary in size. Slit junctions in the capillaries of the brain are so tight that drugs cannot pass through them. On the other hand, slit junctions in the capillaries of the liver and spleen are larger; therefore the size of the drug molecule is less of a limiting factor to drug distribution.

Effect of Protein Binding on Distribution

The blood contains albumin, a plasma protein. Many drugs have an affinity for albumin and bind (reversible) to the protein. When the drug is bound to plasma proteins, it is unable to move out of the blood vessels to get to the site of drug action. **Colloids**, proteins, or other large molecules that are too large to cross membranes remain suspended in the blood for a long time. Plasma proteins act like a drug reservoir for the bound drug trapped within the blood vessels. As the concentration of the unbound or "free" drug decreases in the bloodstream, the drug that is bound to the plasma protein is released and transported to the site of action. When two drugs are administered that both have an affinity for plasma albumin, the drug with the greatest affinity will competitively bind to the protein. Albumin has the greatest affinity for weak acids and hydrophobic drugs. This competition for albumin binding can result in the release of the bound drug, enabling it to get to its site of action. Severe burns can decrease plasma protein levels (hypoalbuminemia), which may alter the level of "free drug." Competitive protein binding represents a mechanism for drug interactions (Fig. 2.6).

Anatomic Barriers to Distribution

Natural body barriers may limit access to the site of drug action. The anatomic structures that selectively limit drug access are the

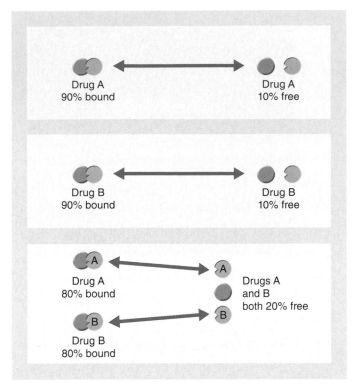

● **Fig. 2.6** Protein binding and free fraction of drugs. (From Page C, Hoffman B, Curtis M, et al: *Integrated pharmacology*, ed 3, Philadelphia, 2006, Mosby.)

blood-brain barrier, blood-placenta barrier, and blood-testicular barrier.

The blood-brain barrier is composed of cells lining the capillaries of the brain that form tight junctions (Fig. 2.7). The blood vessels in the brain are also surrounded by fatty structures called *glial feet* (also known as *astrocyte foot processes*). These structures limit the passage of ions between the capillaries and brain tissue. They permit passage of lipid-soluble, hydrophobic drugs into the brain and limit access of ionized hydrophilic drugs.

The blood-placenta barrier limits access of drugs taken by a pregnant woman to the fetus; however, many drugs are able to cross the blood-placenta barrier, so it is important for pregnant women to ask their physicians or pharmacists about potential safety issues before taking a drug. Before 2015, drugs were classified in five pregnancy safety categories (A, B, C, D, and X). Drugs classified in pregnancy safety category A were shown to be safe when taken during pregnancy. Fetal abnormalities were reported in drugs listed in category X. In 2015, the US Food and Drug Administration replaced this system of classification. New rules require manufacturers to include a summary of the drug's risks if taken during pregnancy and lactation, description of data supporting the drug summary, and information to aid in counseling of pregnant women and the health care provider prescribing.

Metabolism

Few drugs that are administered are eliminated unchanged. Most drugs are transformed by **enzymes** to a **metabolite(s)**. **Biotransformation** is the process of drug metabolism in the body that transforms a drug to a more active, equally active, or inactive metabolite. The primary site of biotransformation is the liver;

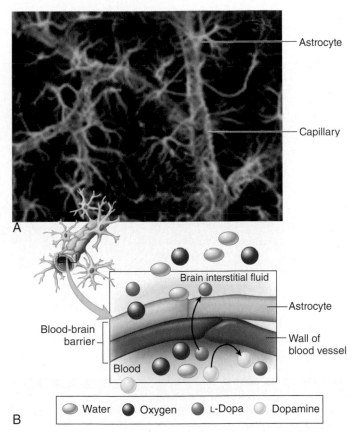

TABLE 2.1   **Products of Metabolism**

Parent Drug	Example	Metabolite	Example
Active drug	6-Mercaptopurine	Inactive drug	6-Mercapturic acid
Active drug	Prednisolone Imipramine	Equally active drug	Prednisone Desipramine
Active drug	Diazepam Codeine	More active drug	Oxazepam Morphine
Inactive drug	Fosamprenavir Levodopa Fosinopril	Active drug	Amprenavir Dopamine Fosinoprilat

• **Fig. 2.7** Barriers. (**A**, Courtesy Marie Simar Couldwell, MD, and Maiken Nedergaard. In Patton KT, Thibodeau GA: *Anatomy of physiology*, ed 9, St Louis, 2016, Elsevier. **B** and **C**, From Patton KT, Thibodeau GA: *Anatomy and physiology*, ed 9, St Louis, 2016, Elsevier.)

however, *metabolism* may occur in the intestines, lung, kidney, or other cells in the body. Microsomal enzymes in the liver are responsible for transforming lipophilic drugs to compounds that can be more easily eliminated by the kidney. The cytochrome P-450 (CYP450) system is frequently involved in this process. Drugs that interfere with the enzymes of the CYP450 system can enhance or inhibit the metabolism of other drugs that are taken concurrently. Phenobarbital, a drug used in the treatment of epilepsy, increases metabolic enzyme activity of other antiseizure medications (phenytoin, valproic acid), resulting in increased elimination of the drugs. This decreases their effectiveness. CYP450 activity is also found in the mucous membranes of the nose. Metabolic enzymes are found in saliva and are secreted by bacteria in the intestines.

Not all drugs are metabolized to inactive metabolites. Table 2.1 shows the potential products of metabolism.

Latanoprost is a drug that is used to treat glaucoma. It is an example of a drug that is metabolized in the eye rather than in the liver. It is also a good example of a prodrug. *Prodrugs* are drugs that are administered in an inactive form and must be metabolized to their active form. Drugs may be formulated as prodrugs to avoid side effects or to increase distribution to the site of action. Levodopa is a prodrug that is metabolized to dopamine in the brain. The drug is used to treat Parkinson disease. Levodopa is able to cross the blood-brain barrier better than dopamine. Administration of the prodrug increases the volume of drug distributed into the brain. Adding the drug carbidopa to levodopa further increases the amount of drug that is converted

to dopamine because carbidopa interrupts levodopa metabolism outside the brain.

"First-Pass Effect"

Orally administered drugs must pass into the hepatoportal circulation (liver) before entering the general circulation. The *first-pass effect* is a process whereby only a fraction of an orally administered drug reaches systemic circulation. Much of the drug is metabolized in the liver to an inactive metabolite before passing into the general circulation (Fig. 2.8). Orally administered nitroglycerin is approximately 90% cleared during a single pass through the liver. Sublingual administration avoids the first-pass effect because drugs administered by this route can pass directly into the general circulation, through the many blood vessels located under the tongue, before passing through the liver. Morphine is also subject to the first-pass effect.

Factors Influencing Metabolism

When metabolism is increased, the duration of effect of many drugs is reduced except prodrugs, for which the onset of drug action begins with metabolism.

Effect of Liver Function on Metabolism

The liver is the primary site for metabolism. If the liver is functioning below capacity, metabolism is decreased. Drug doses are often reduced in the presence of liver dysfunction.

Effect of Disease on Metabolism

Diseases such as hepatitis decrease the metabolic capacity of the liver. Lung disease and kidney disease can also reduce the ability of the body to metabolize drugs. Heart failure decreases blood flow to the liver, altering the extent of drug metabolism.

Effect of Age on Metabolism

Metabolism in the liver is decreased in elderly adults and infants. Age-related changes in the liver decrease metabolic enzyme function in elderly adults. Metabolizing enzyme systems (CYP450) are not fully developed in infants; therefore their ability to metabolize drugs is decreased. Infants and elderly adults generally require lower doses of drug to produce therapeutic effects.

Effect of Concurrent Administration of Drugs (Interactions)

Administration of two or more drugs that both use the same metabolic pathways can alter the metabolism of each other. CYP450 isoform substrates are a large group of metabolic enzymes.

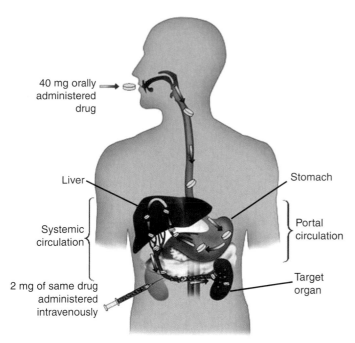

40 mg orally administered drug

Liver

Stomach

Systemic circulation

Portal circulation

2 mg of same drug administered intravenously

Target organ

• **Fig. 2.8** The first-pass effect. (From Lilley LL, Aucker RS: *Pharmacology and the nursing process*, ed 3, St Louis, 2001, Mosby.)

TABLE 2.2	Routes of Drug Elimination
Routes	**Eliminated in**
Major	
Kidney	Urine
Lung	Expired air
Bowel	Feces
Minor	
Liver	Bile
Skin	Sweat
Eyes	Tears
Mouth	Saliva
Nose	Mucus
Penis	Semen
Breast	Breast milk

The metabolism of many drugs is altered by the coadministration of CYP450 substrate inducers or inhibitors. Enzyme inducer–substrate binding increases metabolic enzyme activity, and enzyme inhibitor–substrate binding decreases metabolic enzyme activity. For example, the metabolism of phenytoin is decreased when administered concurrently with the antifungal agents ketoconazole and fluconazole because they are metabolic enzyme inducers.

Cigarette smoke contains ingredients that can stimulate the activity of metabolic enzymes. These enzymes increase the metabolism and clearance of theophylline, a drug used to treat asthma.

Effect of Genetics on Metabolism

A genetic deficiency of a metabolic enzyme can reduce the body's ability to metabolize drugs that use the enzyme. NutraSweet (aspartame) is a common sweetener found in diet foods and beverages. It is a derivative of the amino acid phenylalanine. People diagnosed with the disorder phenylketonuria lack the enzyme needed to metabolize the amino acid phenylalanine to tyrosine. If they consume products containing aspartame, then they may build up toxic levels of phenylalanine.

Effect of Nutrition on Metabolism

Metabolism is decreased when nutritional status is severely depressed, as in starvation. Low-protein diets and diets deficient in essential fatty acids can reduce the synthesis of drug-metabolizing enzymes and decrease metabolism. Deficiencies of vitamins and minerals can affect metabolism because they catalyze biochemical reactions in the body. For example, vitamin B_2 catalyzes oxidation-reduction reactions. Oxidation and reduction are metabolic processes that result in drug inactivation.

Foods can influence metabolism of drugs. Many drug interactions are linked to consumption of grapefruit juice. Grapefruit juice is an inhibitor of metabolic enzyme CYP3A4. When drugs that have a CYP3A4 substrate, such as the anticholesterol drug

lovastatin and the antiretroviral drug saquinavir, are taken with grapefruit juice, metabolism is reduced and blood levels of the drugs can increase, along with drug effects.

> **Tech Note!**
>
> Be sure to apply the warning label stating "DO NOT TAKE WITH GRAPEFRUIT JUICE" when appropriate.

Effect of Gender on Metabolism

The rate of metabolism of some drugs varies between men and women, suggesting the sex hormones may influence metabolism. Men metabolize propranolol (a heart drug) faster than do women. Women metabolize acetaminophen (an analgesic) slightly faster than do men.

Elimination

Elimination is the final pharmacokinetic phase. Elimination results in removal of the drug from the body and discontinuation of drug action. The three major routes of drug elimination are the kidney, lung, and bowel (Table 2.2).

The normal function of the kidney is to filter the blood and remove things that are foreign or harmful. This job is done by the nephrons of the kidney (Fig. 2.9). Free drug (not bound to albumin) is transported to Bowman capsule, where it is filtered by the glomerulus. As the drug moves through the nephron to the distal convoluted tubule, its concentration increases. If the drug is nonionized, it may diffuse out of the nephron back into the systemic circulation and continue to produce drug action. When the drug is ionized, elimination in the urine is increased.

Factors Influencing Elimination

Effect of Kidney Function on Elimination

Kidney dysfunction can have a profound effect on elimination of drugs from the body. Poor kidney function decreases the extent of drug cleared and the rate of clearance. This can cause a buildup of drug in the body and produce toxic drug effects. Drugs that are highly eliminated via the kidneys require a reduction in dose to avoid toxicity when kidney function is impaired. When kidney

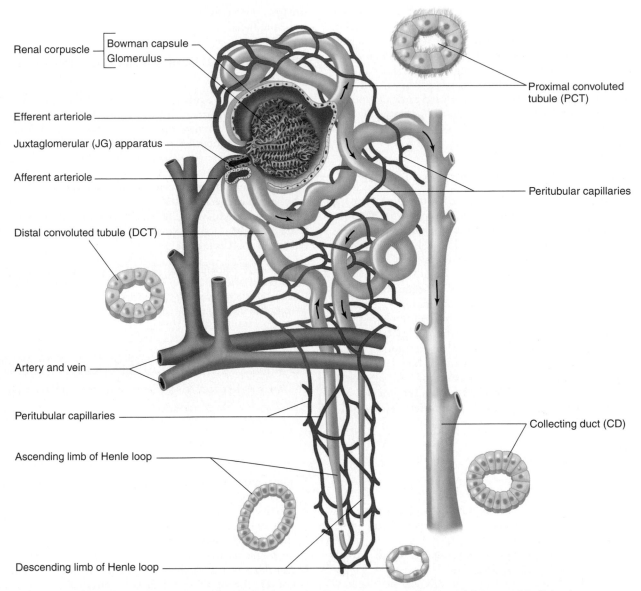

Renal corpuscle
— Bowman capsule
— Glomerulus

Efferent arteriole

Juxtaglomerular (JG) apparatus

Afferent arteriole

Distal convoluted tubule (DCT)

Artery and vein

Peritubular capillaries

Ascending limb of Henle loop

Descending limb of Henle loop

Proximal convoluted tubule (PCT)

Peritubular capillaries

Collecting duct (CD)

• **Fig. 2.9** Nephron. (From Patton KT, Thibodeau GA: *The human body in health and disease*, ed 7, St Louis, 2018, Elsevier.)

function is critically impaired, dialysis is needed. Dialysis mechanically filters the blood and can increase drug elimination.

Effect of Drug Ionization on Elimination

Changes in the acidity of the urine can influence the rate in which a drug is cleared from the body. Weakly acidic drugs are less ionized in acidic urine. As the pH of the urine becomes more basic, the *ionization* of acidic drugs increases. Weak bases are more ionized when the urine is acidic and less ionized when the urine is basic. Drugs that are ionized are eliminated in the urine. Nonionized drugs are reabsorbed back into the circulatory system to continue their drug action.

Effect of Disease on Elimination

Lung, kidney, and bowel disease decrease the body's capacity to eliminate drugs and their metabolites. Bowel disease may increase or decrease elimination. Crohn's disease causes excessive diarrhea, which speeds the elimination of drugs. When movement of

contents of the bowel is slowed, drug elimination is delayed. Lung diseases such as chronic obstructive pulmonary disease decrease elimination in expired air.

Effect of Concurrent Administration of Drugs (Interactions)

Drug interactions can result in increased or decreased elimination of drugs. Pharmacists and health care providers may purposefully recommend concurrent administration of two drugs to delay elimination and prolong drug action or to speed elimination. Urinary buffers may be administered to adjust the level of acidity in the urine to influence the degree of ionization. Urinary acidifiers (e.g., vitamin C) decrease the elimination of acidic drugs. Urinary alkalinizers (e.g., *bicarbonate*) decrease the elimination of basic drugs.

Elimination Half-Life ($t^{1/2}$)

Elimination *half-life ($t^{1/2}$)* refers to the time it takes for 50% of a drug to be cleared from the bloodstream. It takes approximately eight half-lives to entirely eliminate a drug from the body. Every drug has a unique half-life that is dependent on characteristics of the drug (e.g., active metabolites). Knowledge of elimination half-life is important; it is an indicator of how long a drug will produce effects in the body. The half-life of a drug can be as short as a few minutes (e.g., drugs used to produce general anesthesia) or as long as several days (e.g., levothyroxine, a drug used to treat hypothyroidism). Drugs with long half-lives are dosed less frequently than are drugs with very short half-lives.

Bioavailability and Bioequivalence of Drugs

Bioavailability is defined as the rate and extent to which the active ingredient of an administered drug enters the systemic circulation, reaches the site of action, and is available to produce its effect. The bioavailability of a drug is influenced by drug absorption, the first-pass effect, and distribution to the site of action. The bioavailability of generic drugs is compared with the innovator's product to determine whether the generic is bioequivalent. Tests are conducted to measure maximum concentration (C_{max}) of the drug in the bloodstream after a single dose is administered. The time it takes to reach maximum concentration (T_{max}) is also measured. Bioavailability tests are conducted to determine whether the generic drug achieves the same maximum blood concentration in the same time as the brand name drug. The generic is bioequivalent if no statistical differences are found in the rate and extent of absorption when the drug is administered in the same

strength, dosage form, and route of administration as the brand name product.

Pharmaceutical Equivalents and Pharmaceutical Alternatives

Pharmaceutical equivalents differ from bioequivalents. *Bioequivalent drugs* and pharmaceutical equivalent drugs both contain the same active ingredient in the same strength as the innovator's drug (brand name). *Pharmaceutical equivalents* may have different inactive ingredients, be manufactured in a different dosage form, and exhibit different rates of absorption than the brand name. *Pharmaceutical alternatives* contain the same active ingredient as the brand name product; however, the strength and dosage form may be different. A *therapeutic alternative* may contain different active ingredients yet produce the same desired therapeutic outcome.

> ### ● *Tech Note!*
> Product substitution laws regulate the dispensing of generic drugs. Only generics that are bioequivalent can be substituted and dispensed when brand name drugs are prescribed.

TECHNICIAN'S CORNER

1. What is the difference between bioavailability and bioequivalence?

Key Points

- There are four pharmacokinetic phases: absorption, distribution, metabolism, and elimination.
- As a drug moves throughout the body, it undergoes changes that may increase or decrease its absorption, distribution, metabolism, or elimination.
- Pharmacokinetic phases control the intensity of the drug's effect and the duration of the drug action.
- The onset of drug action begins once the drug reaches the minimum concentration necessary to produce a therapeutic effect.
- The peak effect occurs when the maximum concentration of the drug is reached in the body.
- Duration of action is the time between the onset of action and discontinuation of drug action.
- The pharmaceutical phase of drug disposition involves drug disintegration and dissolution.
- Drugs administered parenterally directly enter the general circulation; therefore they are not subject to the first-pass effect and are not degraded by GI enzymes.
- The bioavailability of parenterally administered drugs is greater than orally administered drugs.
- Absorption is the process that involves the movement of drug molecules from the site of administration, across cell membranes, into the circulatory system of the body (blood or lymphatic system).
- Drugs are absorbed across cell membranes via active and passive transport mechanisms.
- Factors influencing absorption are chemical nature of the drug, pH, blood flow, surface area, and tissue thickness.

- Distribution is the process of movement of the drug from the circulatory system across barrier membranes to the site of drug action.
- Factors influencing distribution are the chemical nature of the drug, protein and tissue binding, and ability to move across anatomic barriers.
- Metabolism is a biochemical process involving enzymes that convert the administered drug to metabolites that are more active or less active than the original drug.
- Drugs that interfere with the enzymes of the CYP450 can enhance or inhibit the metabolism of other drugs that are taken concurrently.
- First-pass metabolism describes a process whereby only a fraction of an orally administered drug reaches systemic circulation because the drug is metabolized in the liver to an inactive metabolite before passing into the general circulation.
- Factors influencing metabolism are liver function, disease, age, drug interactions, genetics, nutrition, and gender.
- Elimination results in removal of the drug from the body and discontinuation of drug action.
- Factors influencing elimination are kidney function, disease, drug ionization, and drug interactions.
- Elimination half-life ($t^{1/2}$) refers to the time it takes for 50% of a drug to be cleared from the bloodstream. It takes approximately eight half-lives to eliminate a drug from the body.
- Bioavailability is the rate and extent to which the active ingredient of an administered drug enters the systemic circulation, reaches the site of action, and is available to produce its effect.

- A generic drug is bioequivalent if no statistical differences are found in the rate and extent of absorption when the drug is administered in the same strength, dosage form, and route of administration as the brand name product.
- Pharmaceutical equivalents may have different inactive ingredients, be manufactured in a different dosage form, and exhibit different rates of absorption than the brand name.
- Pharmaceutical alternatives contain the same active ingredient as the brand name drug; however, the strength and dosage form may be different.
- A therapeutic alternative may contain different active ingredients yet produce the same desired therapeutic outcome.

Review Questions

1. Name the four phases of pharmacokinetics.
   a. absorption, dissolution, catabolism, elimination
   b. absorption, distribution, metabolism, elimination
   c. assimilation, dissolution, metabolism, excretion
   d. assimilation, distribution, anabolism, excretion
2. Lipid-soluble drugs are _____.
   a. hydrophobic
   b. lipophobic
   c. lipophilic
   d. a and c
3. A process whereby the liver clears a portion of an administered dose of drug before it passes into the general circulation is known as the:
   a. first-pass effect
   b. dissolution effect
   c. metabolite effect
   d. liver-pass effect
4. A drug that contains different active ingredient(s) than the brand name drug yet produces the same desired therapeutic outcome is called a therapeutic _____.
   a. equivalent
   b. alternative
   c. substitution
   d. replacement
5. The process that involves the movement of drug molecules from the site of administration, across cell membranes, into the circulatory system of the body is known as:
   a. distribution
   b. metabolism
   c. absorption
   d. elimination
6. Which factors might the pharmacist NOT consider when counseling a woman about the risks and benefits of taking a drug during pregnancy?
   a. The summary of drug risks described in the product packaging
   b. Data supporting the summary of potential risks listed in the package insert
   c. Anecdotal stories provided by friends, family, or found on websites
   d. Peer-reviewed literature (journal articles)
7. The metabolism of drugs via biochemical processes involving enzymes to metabolites is termed:
   a. bioequivalence
   b. biotransformation
   c. bioavailability
   d. bioeffect
8. A drug that is administered in an inactive form and must be metabolized to its active form is called a(an):
   a. investigational drug
   b. metabolite
   c. prodrug
   d. none of the above
9. Which body organ serves as the primary site of the metabolism of drugs?
   a. kidney
   b. lungs
   c. stomach
   d. liver
10. The time it takes for 50% of the drug to be cleared from the bloodstream is termed the:
    a. distribution half-life ($t^{1/2}$)
    b. elimination half-life ($t^{1/2}$)
    c. metabolism half-life ($t^{1/2}$)
    d. absorption half-life ($t^{1/2}$)

Bibliography

DiPiro JT, Talbert RL, Yee GC, et al. *Pharmacotherapy: A pathophysiologic approach*. ed 9. McGraw Hill; 2014.
Fulcher E, Soto C, Fulcher R. *Pharmacology: Principles and applications. A worktext for allied health professionals*. Philadelphia: WB Saunders; 2003:21–22 60–65, 83.
Indiana University School of Medicine: Flockhart Table ™ - Cytochrome P450 Drug Interaction Table, 2016. Retrieved September 20, 2022, from http://medicine.iupui.edu/clinpharm/ddis/main-table.
Page CP, Hoffman BB, Curtis MJ, et al. *Integrated pharmacology*. Philadelphia: Elsevier Mosby; 2005:57–70.
Raffa RB, Rawls SM, Beyzarov EP. *Netter's illustrated pharmacology*. Philadelphia: WB Saunders; 2005:10–11 25–27.
Shargel L, Mutnick A, Souney P, et al. *Comprehensive pharmacy review*. ed 4. Baltimore: Lippincott Williams & Wilkins; 2001:42–65 78–84, 131–132.

3

Pharmacodynamics

LEARNING OBJECTIVES

1. Explain the drug-receptor theory.
2. Compare and contrast agonists, antagonists, and partial agonists.
3. Illustrate the relationship between drug effectiveness and potency.
4. Discuss the importance of pharmacodynamics to drug action.
5. Discuss the factors influencing patient response to drug therapy.
6. List ways to improve patient adherence to drug therapy.
7. Learn terminology associated with pharmacodynamics and drug action.

KEY TERMS

Affinity Attraction that the receptor site has for the drug.

Agonist Drug that binds to its receptor site and stimulates a cellular response.

Antagonist Drug that binds to the receptor site and does not produce an action. An antagonist prevents another drug or natural body chemical from binding and activating the receptor site.

Efficacy Measure of a drug's effectiveness.

Idiosyncratic reaction Unexpected drug reaction.

Inverse agonist Drug that has affinity and activity at the receptor site. The drug can turn "off" a receptor that is activated or turn "on" a receptor that is not currently active.

Mechanism of action Manner in which a drug produces its effect.

Noncompetitive antagonist Drug that binds to an alternative receptor site that prevents the agonist from binding to and producing its desired action.

Partial agonist Drug that behaves like an agonist under some conditions and acts like an antagonist under different conditions.

Pharmacodynamics Study of drugs and their action on the living organism.

Pharmacotherapeutics Use of drugs in the treatment of disease and drug effects. It is the study of factors that influence patient response to drugs.

Potency Measure of the amount of drug required to produce a response. It is the effective dose concentration.

Receptor site Location of drug-cell binding.

Therapeutic index (TI) Ratio of the effective dose to the lethal dose.

Pharmacodynamics

The previous chapter looked at how a drug is altered as it travels throughout the compartments of the body. *Pharmacodynamics* is the study of drugs and their action on a living organism. Pharmacodynamics looks at how the body responds to drugs that are administered. The *mechanism of action* (MOA) describes how the drug produces its effect. An understanding of pathophysiology and a drug's MOA can aid decision making about the best drug to treat a patient's medical condition. Pathophysiology is the study of disease in the body.

Drug-Receptor Interactions

According to *drug-receptor theory*, drugs interact or bind with targeted cells in the body to produce pharmacologic action. Most drugs bind with specific proteins in the body; however, they may also bind to carbohydrates, lipids, or enzymes. The location of drug-cell binding is called the *receptor site*. Drug-receptor binding is similar to the action of a lock and key (Fig. 3.1). The drug is the key, and the receptor site is the lock. The more similar the drug is to the shape of the receptor site, the greater the *affinity*, or attraction, that the receptor site has for the drug. When two or more drugs are administered, the receptor site will preferentially bind with the drug for which it has the greatest affinity (the drug that best fits the lock). Drug binding to the receptor is usually reversible. Most drugs spontaneously bind and disassociate with the receptor site.

Some drugs do not produce their actions by directly binding to a receptor site on the cell. They are able to produce a change in cell membrane stability or excitability through nonspecific mechanisms. Some general anesthetic gases produce their effects via nonspecific interactions.

Second Messengers

Drug response does not always occur by stimulation of the primary drug receptor. In some cases, stimulation of the primary receptor causes a second receptor to be activated, and it is only after the release of the second messenger that the desired drug effect is produced.

Types of Drug-Receptor Interactions

A drug may be classified as an agonist, partial agonist, antagonist, inverse agonist, competitive antagonist, or noncompetitive antagonist based on its effect at the receptor site (Table 3.1).

Agonists

An *agonist* is a drug that binds to and activates the receptor site, eliciting a cellular response (Fig. 3.2). Agonist binding may activate a receptor that was resting or turn off a receptor that was activated. *Inverse agonists* are drugs that have affinity at the receptor site but produce opposite actions (turn "off" a receptor that is activated or turn "on" a receptor that is not currently active). When two or more agonists are administered together, a competition for drug-receptor binding sites occurs. The drug with the greatest affinity will bind to the receptor site. The result of agonist binding may mimic the effects produced by binding of normal body chemicals to their target receptor. An example is the binding of barbiturates to their drug-receptor site. Binding mimics the effects produced by the neurotransmitter γ-aminobutyric acid (GABA), a chemical messenger of the nervous system. Drug-receptor binding may also stimulate the release of a normal biologic chemical. For example, when the drug amantadine is administered, it stimulates the release of the neurotransmitter dopamine. An increase in dopamine levels reduces the symptoms associated with Parkinson disease. It is not necessary for all drug-receptor sites to be occupied before the maximum drug effect is achieved.

Antagonists

Antagonists bind to the receptor site and do not activate the receptor. They prevent another drug or natural body chemical from binding by occupying or inactivating the receptor site.

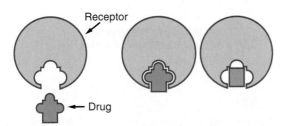

• **Fig. 3.1** Drug-receptor interactions. (From Clayton BD, Willihnganz MJ: *Basic pharmacology for nurses*, ed 17, St Louis, 2017, Elsevier.)

Antagonists block the actions of agonists, inverse agonists, and partial agonists.

Naloxone is an example of a pure antagonist. Administration reverses the effects of opioids (e.g., fentanyl) by occupying the receptor site and preventing the fentanyl from binding.

Noncompetitive antagonists bind to an alternative site than the agonist to prevent the agonist from binding the receptor. Noncompetitive antagonist binding results in inactivation of the receptor site.

Partial Agonists

A *partial agonist* behaves like an agonist under some conditions and acts like an antagonist under different conditions. Buprenorphine is an example of a partial agonist. It behaves like an antagonist in patients who are under the influence of a high concentration of an opioid agonist or when administered after recent exposure to high concentrations of an opioid agonist. It acts like an agonist in opioid-naïve patients who have not had any recent exposure to opioids.

TABLE 3.1	Summary of Effects of Drug-Receptor Binding
Interaction Term	**Definition**
Agonist	Drug binds to a receptor, and there is a response.
Partial agonist	Drug binds to a receptor, and there is a diminished response compared with that elicited by the agonist.
Antagonist	Drug binds to receptor, but there is no response. Drug prevents binding of agonists.
Competitive antagonist	Drug competes with the agonist for binding to receptor. If it binds, there is no response.
Noncompetitive antagonist	Drug combines with different parts of receptor and inactivates it, so agonist has no effect.

From Lilley LL, Collins SR, Snyder JS: *Pharmacology and the nursing process*, ed 8, St Louis, 2017, Elsevier.

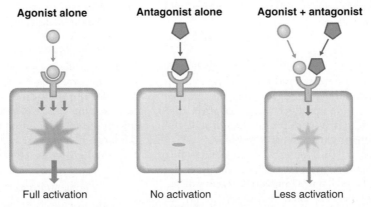

• **Fig. 3.2** Effect of agonist and antagonist binding. Agonists are drugs that occupy receptors and activate them. Antagonists are drugs that occupy receptors but do not activate them. Antagonists block receptor activation by agonists.

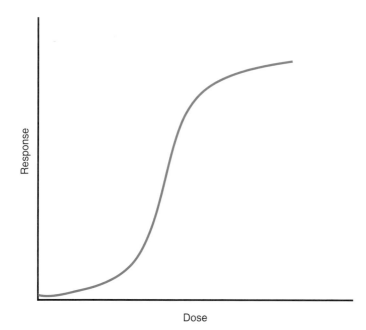

• **Fig. 3.3** Dose-response curve.

Dose-Response Relationship

Typically, increasing the drug dose will increase the cellular response and a drug's effect. Other factors that may influence the strength of the response to a dose of administered drug are pharmacokinetic factors (absorption, distribution, metabolism, and elimination) and individual properties of a drug. A dose-response curve shows the relationship between the effect(s) of a drug and the administered dose. The effects produced by a given drug dose can be quantified and graphed. The graph is called a dose-response curve. The dose-response curve shows the drug's relative efficacy and potency (Fig. 3.3). A steep dose-response curve indicates that a small change in drug dose will produce a large change in the drug response. A flatter dose-response curve shows that a large increase in the dose of the drug administered is needed to produce a greater drug response.

Efficacy

Efficacy is a measure of the drug's effectiveness under controlled conditions, as opposed to real-world conditions (Fig. 3.4). The efficacy of an antagonist is measured by the extent to which it interferes with the effect of an agonist. Efficacy can be measured for each effect produced by a drug.

Potency

Efficacy and **potency** are related. Drugs that have a high efficacy at a low dose are very potent. In other words, only a small dose is required to produce the maximum drug effect. Drugs that must be administered in very high doses to produce a minimal effect have low potency. In Fig. 3.5, drug A is more potent than drug B and drug C because a lower dose produces an equal response.

Efficacy is more important than potency when determining usefulness of a drug, unless the dose that is required to produce the therapeutic effect is so large that it is impractical to administer. When choosing between two equally effective drugs, pharmacokinetic factors, the disease, and the ability of the patient to tolerate the side effects of the drug become more important than the dose that is required to produce an effect.

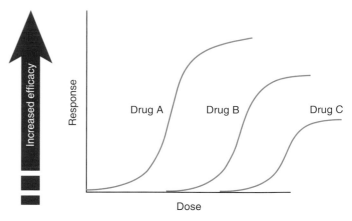

• **Fig. 3.4** Efficacy.

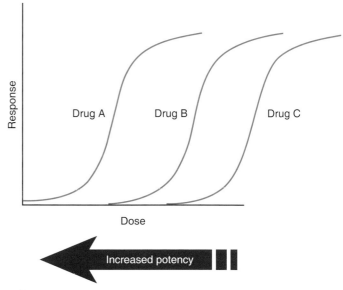

• **Fig. 3.5** Potency.

Ceiling Effect

In Fig. 3.3 the dose-response curve shows that as the drug dose increases, the drug effect increases. Drug effects increase up to a ceiling. This ceiling effect may be reached when all drug receptors are saturated or when the maximum possible effect that could be produced is reached. For example, the ceiling effect for opioid analgesics is reached at the point when no more pain relief is achieved even if additional opioid is administered.

Therapeutic Index

All drugs produce toxic effects that can lead to death. When the lethal dose of a drug is close to the effective dose, the drug is not very safe. The safest drugs have a wide margin between the lethal dose and the effective dose. The **therapeutic index (TI)** is the ratio of the effective dose to the lethal dose; the formula is shown as follows. ED_{50} represents the effective dose for 50% of a population, and LD_{50} is the lethal dose for 50% of a population.

$$\text{Therapeutic index (TI)} = \frac{\text{Lethal dose}(LD_{50})}{\text{Effective dose}(ED_{50})}$$

Digoxin, a drug used to treat heart disease, has a narrow TI. The drug dose needed to increase the force of heart contractions is similar to the drug dose that can cause the heart to stop beating. Another drug with a small TI is warfarin. The dose required to prolong blood clotting time is near the dose that causes hemorrhage and death. Patients respond differently to different doses of drug. Variation in patient response to a drug can become critical when the TI is narrow.

● Tech Note!

The pharmacy should consider the therapeutic index when making product substitution decisions, especially for drugs with a narrow therapeutic index (e.g., digoxin) or bioequivalency problems (e.g., phenytoin).

Factors Influencing Pharmacotherapeutics

Pharmacotherapeutics is the process of using drugs for the treatment of disease. Factors that influence patient response to drugs range from pharmacokinetics to patient-specific factors. A variety of patient-related factors ranging from the presence of chronic disease, drug allergies, age, obesity, or gender to the patient's belief that the therapy will be beneficial can affect the success of pharmacotherapy. Drug response is heightened if the patient has had a previous exposure to the drug that produced an allergic reaction and decreased if the patient has developed tolerance to the effects of the drug. The patient's response to a drug is not always predictable. Drug doses and dosing schedules should be modified to control for known factors that influence patient drug response.

Patient Physiologic Factors

Humans are unique, and individual variability influences the outcome of drug therapy. Physiologic factors that may affect drug response are described in this section. Desired therapeutic effects are achieved when optimum drug doses are administered. Doses that are too low result in subtherapeutic effects. Doses that are too high result in toxic effects.

Age

The human body undergoes physiologic and hormonal changes between birth and death. Age-related changes influence how effectively the body is able to handle drugs. Neonates and infants have an underdeveloped capacity to absorb, distribute, metabolize, and eliminate drugs. The ability of the lungs, liver, and kidneys to process and eliminate drugs declines as humans age. Elderly adults and infants require lower drug doses.

Weight

Drug doses for children are often calculated according to the child's weight; however, dose calculations based on body surface area are more accurate than those based on weight. Dose adjustments may need to be considered for obese or severely underweight adults. Drug doses must be increased in obese patients to produce therapeutic effects. Doses are decreased in severely underweight or emaciated adults and children to avoid toxic side effects.

Gender

Gender may influence drug distribution and metabolism. The fat-to-muscle ratio varies between women and men and may influence the volume of drug distribution. In addition, the rate of metabolism of some drugs varies between men and women, suggesting the sex hormones may influence metabolism.

Genetics

Genetics influences enzyme and protein production in the body. Absence of certain enzymes can produce deadly side effects in people who take drugs that require the enzyme for metabolism and elimination.

Disease

The presence of disease can significantly influence pharmacotherapeutics. More severe drug reactions can occur in patients with kidney disease, liver disease, or lung disease because their ability to distribute, metabolize, and eliminate drugs may be compromised. The effects of a drug may diminish because the disease itself becomes more debilitating over time. Parkinson disease is linked to progressive destruction of dopamine-releasing nerve cells in the body. The ability of anti–Parkinson disease drugs to improve patient symptoms decreases as the disease progresses.

Pregnancy

Drug response may be altered during pregnancy because of pregnancy-related physiologic changes. Gastrointestinal motility slows, which can increase drug absorption and drug effects. Pregnancy increases in blood volume, urination, and vomiting may alter drug absorption, distribution, and elimination, resulting in decreased drug response.

Immunologic Factors

Hypersensitivity reactions are extreme allergic reactions and can occur after a single dose of the drug or after multiple exposures to the drug. The reaction occurs because the patient develops antibodies to the drug. The presence of antibodies causes the release of histamine and other body chemicals that produce allergic symptoms. Symptoms may range from a mild rash to anaphylactic shock.

Desensitization

Repeated exposures to a drug may result in a decreased drug response. Desensitization is caused by changes to drug receptors (especially proteins) that decrease drug-receptor binding or reduce receptor site activation when binding occurs. When desensitization occurs, the effects can be limited to a single receptor or may influence multiple receptors. When drug-receptor binding involves a second messenger, the result may be desensitization to the effects that would have been produced by binding to multiple receptors (i.e., all of the receptors normally activated by binding of the drug to its primary receptor). Desensitization may be used therapeutically to minimize allergic reactions (e.g., allergy shots).

Idiosyncratic Reactions

Sometimes the response to a drug cannot be predicted. Unexpected drug reactions are known as *idiosyncratic reactions*.

Psychological Factors

Drug therapy is influenced by the patient's belief that the therapy will be beneficial. Studies have shown that sugar pills can produce the desired effect if the patient believes they will be effective. This is known as the placebo effect. Double-blind clinical studies are conducted to control for the placebo effect. In a double-blind study, some of the people in the study receive a drug containing active ingredients, and others receive a drug look-alike that does not contain active ingredients. Neither the people taking the drug nor their care providers know who is receiving the real drug. This reduces the risk that drug effects reported are caused by placebo effect. This also decreases the likelihood that care providers will treat their patient differently because they know they are receiving the active drug. Increased attention can also improve patient outcomes.

Adverse Drug Reactions

Few drugs are so specific that they produce only their desired therapeutic effect. Drugs may additionally produce undesired effects. An adverse drug reaction (ADR) is an undesired side effect of a drug. An ADR may be mild (e.g., sedation and nausea) or severe (e.g., hepatotoxicity and seizures). Approximately 10% of people who receive health care in industrialized countries will experience a preventable ADR.

ADRs have an impact on patients, family members, employers, pharmacies, health care facilities, and society. ADRs can cause or prolong hospitalization, missed school or work, and even death. ADRs are estimated to cost more than $30.1 billion annually in the United States and nearly $49 million annually in Canada. Nearly 80% of drug-related costs are due to hospitalization.

Some populations are at greater risk for ADRs than others. The elderly are at increased risk for ADRs because they are more likely to be on multiple-drug therapy, and their capacity to metabolize and eliminate drugs is less than that of younger adults. Multiple-drug therapy (polypharmacy) is also a risk factor for hospitalized patients. The average patient in the hospital is prescribed up to 10 drugs. The risk for drug side effects and drug interactions increases with the number of medications a person is administered.

ADRs may be localized and occur only at the site where the drug was administered. Other adverse reactions are widespread and occur throughout the body. Adverse effects may cause minor discomfort such as a rash, or they may be life-threatening (e.g., coma and death).

Common adverse effects that occur in the central nervous system are drowsiness, dizziness, stimulation, or confusion. Life-threatening central nervous system effects include respiratory depression, coma, and death. Hepatotoxicity is a toxic adverse reaction that occurs in the liver. Some common drugs that can produce hepatotoxicity are acetaminophen and isoniazid (a drug used to treat tuberculosis). Nephrotoxicity is a serious adverse effect that occurs in the kidney. Nonsteroidal antiinflammatory drugs such as ibuprofen and naproxen can produce nephrotoxicity.

ADRs also occur as a result of nonsterile drug preparation. Intravenous fluids and other parenterals must be prepared using aseptic technique. Failure to use aseptic technique can result in the introduction of contaminants, pathogens, and fever-causing agents into the solution. Prolonged illness or death may occur if the contaminated solution is injected into a patient.

> ### ● Tech Note!
>
> USP 797 established standards to reduce contamination when compounding sterile products. USP Chapter 800 standards increased protections for personnel and other health care workers who compound hazardous drugs, including all the antineoplastic and other hazardous drugs on the National Institute for Occupational Safety and Health (NIOSH) list.

Teratogenicity

Drugs that produce harm to a developing fetus are called teratogens. To reduce possible harm to the fetus, pregnant women and their health care providers must weigh the risks versus the benefit of taking drugs during pregnancy. To assist in their decision making, the US Food and Drug Administration (FDA) requires manufacturers to include a summary of the drug's risks if taken during pregnancy and lactation and a description of data supporting the drug summary in drug product package labeling.

Carcinogenicity

Drugs and natural products that stimulate the growth of cancers are classified as carcinogens. Carcinogenic drugs interact with DNA and produce permanent genetic mutations. Many of the drugs used to treat one type of cancer are capable of producing cancers in other areas. Drugs used to treat ovarian cancer, such as melphalan, increase the risk for acute nonlymphocytic leukemia (ANLL). The synthetic estrogen diethylstilbestrol (DES) is no longer prescribed to women to prevent miscarriage because it increases the risks for breast and uterine cancer. The drug is still prescribed for the treatment of prostate cancer. Sassafras tea was widely used as a cleansing tea or tonic until it was discovered to be carcinogenic in the 1960s.

Dependence and Tolerance

Patients taking controlled substances may develop dependence or tolerance to the drug's effects. Drugs are placed in controlled substance schedules according to their likelihood to produce physiologic or psychological dependence. Patients who have developed dependence to a drug continue to take the drug to prevent the onset of withdrawal symptoms. Once tolerance to a drug has developed, the patient must take increasing doses of the drug to produce the same effects as were previously produced by a lower dose. Tolerance may occur to the therapeutic effect or side effects. Tolerance develops to the sedation produced by some antiseizure drugs such as clonazepam before tolerance develops to the desired antiseizure effects.

Improving Adherence to Drug Therapy

Drug therapy is strongly influenced by whether the patient takes the medication as prescribed or whether medication is taken at all. Adherence to drug therapy is defined as taking the prescribed medication in the correct dose, at the right time, and without missed doses. It is currently recognized that patients and their caregivers must be actively involved in making decisions about drug therapy. Patients who recognize the importance of the drug therapy and are involved in decisions regarding therapeutic options are more likely to adhere to therapy.

Factors Influencing Adherence to Drug Therapy

Lack of adherence to drug therapy is associated with poor health outcomes. Understanding why medications are not taken as prescribed is important for the design of strategies to improve adherence. Strategies for improving adherence must be targeted at patients, caregivers, pharmacists, pharmacy technicians, clinicians, and other health care providers.

Belief That Therapy Is Beneficial

Adherence to the prescribed drug therapy is increased when patients believe therapy is beneficial. This is particularly important when the medication has substantial adverse effects. Hypertension is known as the silent killer because often no symptoms are present. Medications to treat hypertension may cause dizziness, upset stomach, impotence, or even depression, causing many patients to discontinue drug therapy. Adherence to drug therapy can avoid many of the complications associated with untreated hypertension.

Adverse Drug Reactions

ADRs are a principal cause of discontinuation of drug therapy. Even fear of potential adverse reactions is a sufficient disincentive for some patients to avoid taking their medications. Many drug formulations have been developed to minimize drug side effects. Enteric-coated formulations reduce the risk of stomach upset. Gastrointestinal side effects are avoided by use of drugs formulated for transdermal application.

Pharmacy technicians can assist pharmacists in reducing patients' anxiety about adverse reactions by alerting the pharmacists when patients have questions about their drug therapy and making certain patients receive pharmacist counseling for new medicines. Pharmacy technicians can also play a key role in helping patients limit adverse reactions by distributing patient drug information leaflets and affixing warning labels, also called auxiliary labels, to prescription vials, which are intended to ensure that the maximum benefits of drug therapy are achieved with minimum side effects. For example, taking medication with food or a glass of water can decrease the risk for upset stomach. Acting within their scope of practice, pharmacy technicians can assist pharmacists in providing drug information that may reduce the risk for drug side effects and increase adherence to prescribed drug therapy.

> ### ● Tech Note!
> Many pharmacy computer systems now print auxiliary labels directly onto prescription labels using a different color for identification purposes.

Lack of A Medication Administration Routine

Adherence is improved when patients develop a regular routine for taking medicine. The pharmacist and pharmacy technician can work with patients to develop a routine for taking medications that fits the patient's lifestyle. Some pharmacies sell devices that prompt the patient to remember to take medicines.

Understanding Dosing Schedule

Dosing schedules must be convenient and understandable if patients are to avoid missed doses or taking double doses. Adherence to drug therapy becomes more difficult as the number of medications prescribed increases. Selection of drug formulations that are taken once a day may improve adherence. The pharmacy may also dispense the medicine in compliance blister packs.

> ### ● Tech Note!
> Extended-release (ER) medications promote patient adherence. Instead of taking medications three or four times a day, an ER, sustained-release (SR), or controlled-dose (CD) tablet may be taken once daily.

Ability to Afford Drug Therapy

People with low socioeconomic status are at increased risk for low adherence. Poverty decreases the ability to afford medications and decreases access to health care when adverse events are experienced. When drug therapy is expensive, prescriptions may not be filled. When prescriptions are filled, patients may take less than the dose prescribed to make the prescription last longer. Pharmacy personnel can work with prescribers to ensure that effective and affordable drugs (e.g., generics) are prescribed and dispensed when appropriate. Pharmacy technicians can also contact insurance companies to obtain approval for nonformulary medicines.

Reporting Adverse Drug Reactions

ADRs are reported to the FDA by drug manufacturers, health care professionals, and consumers using the Medwatch FDA Voluntary Reporting Form 3500 (Fig. 3.6). The ADR reports are compiled into a computerized information database called the Adverse Event Reporting System (AERS). Vaccine adverse events are reported to the Vaccine Event Reporting System (VAERS). The reports are analyzed and mined for signals of safety issues. The information is used to issue safety alerts for drugs, biologics, devices, and dietary supplements; update product labeling; send out a "Dear Health Care Professional" letter; or even reevaluate the drug approval decision. If reevaluation results in a decision to withdraw drug approval, then a recall will be issued. Patient and consumer information sheets are also available from the FDA. In Canada, ADRs are also reported by drug manufacturers, consumers, and health professionals. ADRs are reported to the Canada Vigilance Program. ADR reporting forms can be obtained from the MedEffect Canada website (http://www.hc-sc.gc.ca/dhp-mps/medeff/report-declaration/index-eng.php).

> ### TECHNICIAN'S CORNER
> 1. How can pharmacy technicians assist patients in reducing anxiety about adverse reactions?
> 2. Explain how people with low socioeconomic status are at an increased risk for adverse reactions.

U.S. Department of Health and Human Services

MEDWATCH

The FDA Safety Information and
Adverse Event Reporting Program

For VOLUNTARY reporting of
adverse events, product problems and
product use errors

Form Approved: OMB No. 0910-0291, Expires: 9/30/2018
See PRA statement on reverse.

FDA USE ONLY

Triage unit
sequence #

FDA Rec. Date

Note: For date prompts of "dd-mmm-yyyy" please use 2-digit day, 3-letter month abbreviation, and 4-digit year; for example, 01-Jul-2015.

A. PATIENT INFORMATION

1. **Patient Identifier**

2. **Age**
   - ☐ Year(s) ☐ Month(s)
   - ☐ Week(s) ☐ Days(s)
   - _____ or Date of Birth (e.g., 08 Feb 1925)
   - __ __ – __ __ __ – __ __ __ __

In Confidence

3. **Sex**
   - ☐ Female
   - ☐ Male

4. **Weight**
   - ☐ lb
   - ☐ kg

5.a. **Ethnicity** (Check single best answer)
   - ☐ Hispanic/Latino
   - ☐ Not Hispanic/Latino

5.b. **Race** (Check all that apply)
   - ☐ Asian   ☐ American Indian or Alaskan Native
   - ☐ Black or African American   ☐ White
   - ☐ Native Hawaiian or Other Pacific Islander

B. ADVERSE EVENT, PRODUCT PROBLEM

1. **Check all that apply**
   - ☐ Adverse Event   ☐ Product Problem (e.g., defects/malfunctions)
   - ☐ Product Use Error   ☐ Problem with Different Manufacturer of Same Medicine

2. **Outcome Attributed to Adverse Event** (Check all that apply)
   - ☐ Death   Include date (dd-mmm-yyyy): __ __ – __ __ __ – __ __ __ __
   - ☐ Life-threatening   ☐ Disability or Permanent Damage
   - ☐ Hospitalization – initial or prolonged   ☐ Congenital Anomaly/Birth Defects
   - ☐ Other Serious (Important Medical Events)
   - ☐ Required Intervention to Prevent Permanent Impairment/Damage (Devices)

3. **Date of Event** (dd-mmm-yyyy)
   __ __ – __ __ __ – __ __ __ __

4. **Date of this Report** (dd-mmm-yyyy)
   __ __ – __ __ __ – __ __ __ __

5. **Describe Event, Problem or Product Use Error**

6. **Relevant Tests/Laboratory Data, Including Dates**

7. **Other Relevant History, Including Preexisting Medical Conditions** (e.g., allergies, pregnancy, smoking and alcohol use, liver/kidney problems, etc.)

C. PRODUCT AVAILABILITY

2. **Product Available for Evaluation?** (Do not send product to FDA)
   - ☐ Yes   ☐ No   ☐ Returned to Manufacturer on (dd-mmm-yyyy)
   __ __ – __ __ __ – __ __ __ __

D. SUSPECT PRODUCTS

1. **Name, Manufacturer/Compounder, Strength** (from product label)

#1 – Name and Strength	#1 – NDC # or Unique ID
#1 – Manufacturer/Compounder	#1 – Lot #
#2 – Name and Strength	#2 – NDC # or Unique ID
#2 – Manufacturer/Compounder	#2 – Lot #

3.

	Dose or Amount	Frequency	Route
#1			
#2			

4. **Dates of Use** (From/To for each) (If unknown, give duration, or best estimate) (dd-mmm-yyyy)
   #1
   #2

5. **Diagnosis or Reason for Use** (indication)
   #1
   #2

6. **Is the Product Compounded?**
   - #1 ☐ Yes ☐ No
   - #2 ☐ Yes ☐ No

7. **Is the Product Over-the-Counter?**
   - #1 ☐ Yes ☐ No
   - #2 ☐ Yes ☐ No

8. **Expiration Date** (dd-mmm-yyyy)
   #1 __ __ – __ __ __ – __ __ __ __   #2 __ __ – __ __ __ – __ __ __ __

9. **Event Abated After Use Stopped or Dose Reduced?**
   - #1 ☐ Yes ☐ No ☐ Doesn't apply
   - #2 ☐ Yes ☐ No ☐ Doesn't apply

10. **Event Reappeared After Reintroduction?**
   - #1 ☐ Yes ☐ No ☐ Doesn't apply
   - #2 ☐ Yes ☐ No ☐ Doesn't apply

E. SUSPECT MEDICAL DEVICE

1. **Brand Name**

2. **Common Device Name**   2b. **Procode**

3. **Manufacturer Name, City and State**

4. **Model #**   **Lot #**   5. **Operator of Device**
   ☐ Health Professional

Catalog #   **Expiration Date** (dd-mmm-yyyy)   ☐ Lay User/Patient
   __ __ – __ __ __ – __ __ __ __   ☐ Other

Serial #   **Unique Identifier (UDI) #**

6. **If Implanted, Give Date** (dd-mmm-yyyy)   7. **If Explanted, Give Date** (dd-mmm-yyyy)
   __ __ – __ __ __ – __ __ __ __   __ __ – __ __ __ – __ __ __ __

8. **Is this a single-use device that was reprocessed and reused on a patient?**   ☐ Yes   ☐ No

9. **If Yes to Item 8, Enter Name and Address of Reprocessor**

F. OTHER (CONCOMITANT) MEDICAL PRODUCTS

Product names and therapy dates (Exclude treatment of event)

G. REPORTER (See confidentiality section on back)

1. **Name and Address**

Last Name:	First Name:
Address:	
City:	State/Province/Region:
Country:	ZIP/Postal Code:
Phone #:	Email:

2. **Health Professional?**
   ☐ Yes ☐ No

3. **Occupation**

4. **Also Reported to:**
   - ☐ Manufacturer/Compounder
   - ☐ User Facility
   - ☐ Distributor/Importer

5. **If you do NOT want your identity disclosed to the manufacturer, please mark this box:** ☐

PLEASE TYPE OR USE BLACK INK

FORM FDA 3500 (10/15)   Submission of a report does not constitute an admission that medical personnel or the product caused or contributed to the event.

• **Fig. 3.6** Food and Drug Administration voluntary reporting form 3500. (Courtesy US Food and Drug Administration, Rockville, MD.)

Key Points

- Pharmacodynamics looks at how the body responds to drugs that are administered.
- Drugs interact or bind with targeted cells in the body to produce pharmacological action.
- Drug-receptor binding is similar to a lock and key. The more similar the drug is to the shape of the receptor site, the greater is the affinity the receptor site has for the drug.
- Drug-receptor binding enhances or inhibits normal biologic processes.
- An agonist (e.g., fentanyl) is a drug that binds to its receptor site and stimulates a cellular response. Agonist binding may activate a receptor that was resting or turn off a receptor that was activated.
- Antagonists (e.g., naloxone) bind to the receptor site and prevent an agonist from activating the receptor. They prevent another drug or natural body chemical from binding by occupying or inactivating the receptor site. Binding may reverse the action of a currently administered drug.
- Partial agonists (e.g., Suboxone®) behave like antagonists in the presence of a high concentration of a full agonist or when administered after recent exposure to high concentrations of an agonist.
- Efficacy is a measure of the drug's effectiveness under controlled conditions rather than "real-world" conditions.
- Drugs that are administered in very low doses yet produce a maximum effect have high potency.
- The dose-response curve shows a drug's relative efficacy and potency. A steep dose-response curve indicates that a small change in drug dose will produce a big change in the drug response.
- The TI is the ratio of the effective dose to the lethal dose. Safe drugs have a wide margin between the lethal dose and the effective dose.

- Successful drug therapy is influenced by a variety of factors. The patient's response to a drug is not always predictable.
- Age, gender, disease, pregnancy, weight, and genetics are patient-related factors that influence drug response.
- Drug allergies cause a heightened response to drugs and can occur after one or more exposures to a drug.
- Patients may become desensitized to the effects of drugs.
- Idiosyncratic reactions are unpredictable.
- Psychological factors can influence drug response. The placebo effect demonstrates that patients can experience drug effects even when no active drug has been administered.
- Drugs produce desired effects (therapeutic effects) and undesired effects. Undesired effects are called adverse reactions.
- Multiple-drug therapy increases risks for ADRs. Elderly adults have increased risks for ADRs because they typically take several drugs.
- ADRs can be mild or severe. Effects range from rash, upset stomach, and sedation to hepatotoxicity, teratogenicity, and anaphylactic shock.
- Dependence and tolerance are adverse reactions associated with controlled substances. When tolerance develops, the patient must take increasing doses of the drug to get the desired effect. When dependence has developed, patients continue to take the drug to prevent withdrawal symptoms.
- Patients, caregivers, pharmacists, pharmacy technicians, clinicians, and other health care providers must work as a team to improve adherence to drug therapy.
- Many factors influence patient adherence to drug therapy including patient belief that the therapy will be beneficial.
- Selection of effective, affordable medicines that have few side effects and that are dosed in convenient schedules improves adherence to drug therapy.

Review Questions

1. An _____ is a drug that binds to a receptor site and elicits cellular response.
   a. agonist
   b. antagonist
   c. alternative
   d. antimetabolite

2. All drugs produce toxic effects that can lead to death. The therapeutic _____ is the ratio of the effective dose to the lethal dose.
   a. equivalence
   b. derivative
   c. index
   d. window

3. The process of using drugs in the treatment of disease is called _____.
   a. pharmacodynamics
   b. pharmacotherapeutics
   c. pharmacokinetics
   d. pharmacognosy

4. What is the measure of a drug's effectiveness called?
   a. availability
   b. bioequivalence
   c. efficacy
   d. potency

5. Humans are unique, and individual variability influences the outcome of drug therapy. Name some physiologic factors that influence drug therapy.
   a. age, weight, and gender
   b. genetics, disease, and pregnancy
   c. allergies, hypersensitivities, and desensitization
   d. both a and b

6. Toxic adverse reactions that cause hepatotoxicity occur in the _____, and toxic adverse reactions that cause nephrotoxicity occur in the _____.
   a. liver, lungs
   b. liver, kidneys
   c. kidneys, bladder
   d. kidneys, nephrons

7. _____ and _____ are associated with the use of controlled substances.
   a. Hypersensitivities and dependence
   b. Tolerance and toxicity
   c. Dependence and tolerance
   d. Toxicity and anaphylaxis

8. To which government agency are adverse reactions reported in the United States?
   a. DEA
   b. TJC
   c. CMS
   d. FDA
9. An adverse effect produced by drugs on fetuses is called _____.
   a. carcinogenic
   b. teratogenic

   c. pathogenic
   d. toxic
10. One drug that has a narrow therapeutic index is _____.
    a. acetaminophen
    b. penicillin
    c. digoxin
    d. melphalan

Bibliography

Adverse Drug Reaction Canada: What Are Adverse Drug Reactions and How Can They Be Prevented? July 9, 2021. Retrieved June 20, 2022, from adrcanada.org/2021/07/09/featured-content/.

Baker GR, Norton PG, Flintolf V, et al. The Canadian Adverse Events Study: the incidence of adverse events among hospital patients in Canada. *Can Med Assoc J*. 2004;170:1678–1686.

Canadian Institutes for Health Information: Adverse Drug Reaction–Related Hospitalizations Among Seniors, 2006 to 2011, 2013. Retrieved September 5, 2017, from www.cihi.ca.

DiPiro JT, Talbert R, Yee CG, et al. *Pharmacotherapy: a pathophysiologic approach*. ed 9. New York: McGraw Hill; 2014.

Edwards IR. The WHO World Alliance for Patient Safety: a new challenge or an old one neglected? *Drug Saf*. 2005;28:379–386.

Page C, Curtis M, Sutter M, et al. *Integrated pharmacology*. Philadelphia: Elsevier Mosby; 2005:57–70, 314.

Passarelli M, Jacob-Filho W, Figueras A. Adverse drug reactions in an elderly hospitalised population: inappropriate prescription is a leading cause. *Drugs Aging*. 2005;22:767–777.

Raffa RB, Rawls SM, Beyzarov EP. *Netter's illustrated pharmacology*. Philadelphia: WB Saunders; 2005:10–11, 21–23.

Ratajczak H. Drug-induced hypersensitivity: role in drug development. *Toxicol Rev*. 2004;23:265–280.

Sorensen L, Stokes J, Purdie D, et al. Medication management at home: medication-related risk factors associated with poor health outcomes. *Age Ageing*. 2005;34:626–632.

Sultana J, Cutroneo P, Trifirò G. Clinical and economic burden of adverse drug reactions. *J Pharmacol Pharmacother*. 2013;4(Suppl 1):S72–S77.

Tyler V, Brady L, Robbers J. *Pharmacognosy*. ed 9. Philadelphia: Lea & Febiger; 1988:486.

U.S. Food and Drug Administration: Adverse Event Reporting System. Retrieved June 20, 2022, from https://www.fda.gov/drugs/drug-approvals-and-databases/fda-adverse-event-reporting-system-faers.

U.S. Food and Drug Administration: Pregnancy and Lactation Labeling (Drugs) Final Rule. Retrieved June 20, 2022, from https://www.fda.gov/drugs/labeling-information-drug-products/pregnancy-and-lactation-labeling-drugs-final-rule

USP: FAQs: <800> Hazardous Drugs—Handling in Healthcare Settings, August 18, 2017. Retrieved June 20, 2022, from http://www.usp.org/frequently-asked-questions/hazardous-drugs-handling-healthcare-settings.

Wu WK, Pantaleo N. Evaluation of outpatient adverse drug reactions leading to hospitalization. *Am J Health Syst Pharm*. 2003;60:253–259.

4

Drug Interactions and Medication Errors

LEARNING OBJECTIVES

1. Learn the terminology associated with drug interactions and medication errors.
2. Give examples of drug-drug interactions, drug-food interactions, and drug-disease contraindications.
3. Describe several mechanisms for drug interactions.
4. List ways to avoid drug interactions.
5. Categorize medication errors.
6. Identify medication errors made by pharmacists and pharmacy technicians.
7. Describe techniques used to avoid medication errors in the pharmacy.

KEY TERMS

Additive effect Concurrent administration of two drugs enhances the effects produced by the individual drugs.

Antagonism A drug-drug interaction or drug-food interaction that decreases or blocks the effect of another drug.

Drug-disease contraindication Drug administration should be avoided because it may worsen the patient's medical condition.

Drug-drug interaction Effect that occurs when two or more drugs are administered at the same time.

Drug-food interaction Altered drug response that occurs when a drug is administered with certain foods.

Medication error An error made in the process of prescribing, preparing, dispensing, or administering drug therapy.

Potentiation Process where one drug, acting at a separate site or via a different mechanism of action, increases the effect of another drug. The drug produces no effect when administered alone. Food can also potentiate the effects of a drug.

Synergistic effects Drug-drug or drug-food interaction that produces an effect that is greater than would be produced if either drug were administered alone.

Therapeutic duplication Administration of two drugs that produce similar effects and side effects. These drugs may belong to the same therapeutic class.

Drug Interactions

Drug effects are influenced by concurrent administration with foods and other drugs. The more drugs that are administered to a patient, the more likely it is that interactions will occur. Drug-drug interactions and drug-food interactions can increase or decrease the intended drug effects. They may also increase or decrease drug side effects. Drug interactions may produce life-threatening or minor undesired effects, or they may enhance the desired drug effect. Low doses of antidepressant drugs such as amitriptyline are administered along with pain medications such as hydrocodone to enhance pain relief. By administering these two drugs together, less hydrocodone is needed, and the patient's risk for development of tolerance and dependence from the hydrocodone is reduced. The study of pharmacology is important because it helps healthcare providers predict if a drug interaction may occur.

Drug-Drug Interactions

An interaction that occurs between two or more drugs administered at the same time is called a ***drug-drug interaction***. Drug-drug interactions may increase or decrease the effect or side effects of the drug. Tetracycline and penicillin both treat infections.

If the drugs are administered together, the infection-fighting ability of penicillin is reduced by the tetracycline. The antifungal action of ketoconazole is reduced if the drug is taken with antacids. Antiulcer drugs such as cimetidine increase the effects of alcohol. Amoxicillin reduces the effectiveness of oral contraceptives.

> ● **Tech Note!**
>
> The pharmacy technician should alert the pharmacist to drug interactions that are identified by prescription-filling software when they are inputting new or refill prescription data.

Drug-Food Interactions

Foods may contain enzymes, vitamins, or minerals that enhance or interfere with drug effects. An interaction between an administered drug and food(s) consumed at the same time is called a ***drug-food interaction***. The interaction may influence side effects too. A classic example is the interaction between dairy products and the antiinfective tetracycline. Tetracycline binds with the calcium in milk or cheese, decreasing the drug's effectiveness. The effectiveness of levothyroxine, a synthetic thyroid hormone, is decreased when iron supplements are taken concurrently. Grapefruit juice inhibits the metabolism of the cholesterol-lowering drug atorvastatin, thereby increasing the drug's effects and side effects.

Additive Effects

Additive effects may occur when two drugs are administered concurrently. The increased effect is equal to the sum of the individual effects produced by each of the drugs alone. Many drug interactions produce additive effects. The sleeping pill temazepam is administered to promote drowsiness. Alcoholic beverages also cause drowsiness. When alcoholic beverages are consumed together with temazepam, the sedation caused by temazepam adds to the sedation caused by alcohol.

Additive effects can be described using the equation

$$1+1=2$$

Synergistic Effects

Drug-drug interactions and drug-food interactions may produce synergistic effects. **Synergistic effects** result when two drugs administered together produce effects that are greater than would be produced if either drug were administered alone or would be seen with additive effects. Bleeding is a potential side effect of warfarin and aspirin. When warfarin and aspirin are administered together, excessive bleeding may occur.

Synergistic effects can be described using the equation

$$1+1=3$$

Potentiation

The process whereby one drug, or a food, increases the effects of another drug, yet does not produce any effect when administered alone, is called **potentiation**. Carbidopa exhibits no anti–Parkinson disease activity when administered alone but can increase the anti–Parkinson disease effects of levodopa. Carbidopa decreases the destruction of levodopa in the gastrointestinal tract, thereby increasing the amount of levodopa that can get to its site of action in the brain. Grapefruit juice increases the effects of some antihypertensive drugs (e.g., diltiazem) because it inhibits metabolic enzymes. The action of the antifungal griseofulvin is increased when it is taken with fatty foods because food increases the absorption of the drug.

Potentiation can be described using the equation:

$$1+0=2$$

Antagonism

Antagonism is a drug-drug interaction or drug-food interaction that blocks drug effects. Naloxone is administered to block the respiratory depression produced by opioids (e.g., fentanyl, morphine, and heroin). Vitamin K is an antidote for the drug warfarin. It is administered to stop bleeding caused by an excessive dose of warfarin.

Antagonism can be described using the equation:

$$1+1=0$$

Mechanisms of Drug Interactions

Drug-drug interactions and drug-food interactions occur via many different mechanisms. Coadministration of drugs or drugs with food can increase absorption, distribution, metabolism, or elimination and result in increased or decreased drug action or side effects. Epinephrine is added to local anesthetics to constrict blood vessels at the site of injection and thereby augment the local anesthetic effects at the injection site. Absorption of a drug can also be increased by administration of a second drug that speeds or slows movement within the gastrointestinal system. Prokinetic drugs such as metoclopramide stimulate movement through the stomach and increase the absorption of drugs that are primarily absorbed in the small intestine and decrease absorption of drugs that are absorbed in the stomach. Drugs that decrease the rate of gastric emptying or movement through the intestines, such as codeine and loperamide, can increase the absorption and effects of drugs (Fig. 4.1).

Drugs that are weak acids and weak bases are involved in many drug interactions. The absorption of cimetidine (H2 receptor antagonist) is decreased when taken with antacids because antacids make the pH more alkaline and cimetidine is a weak acid. Absorption of cimetidine is greatest in an acidic pH. Intravenous solutions of acids and bases are incompatible and, when combined,

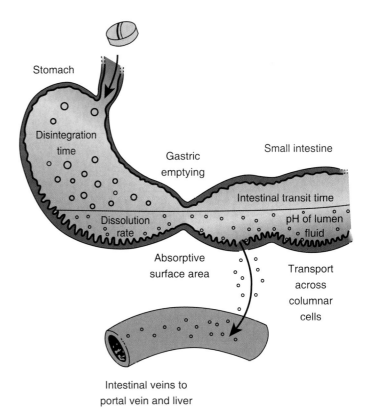

• **Fig. 4.1** Factors involved in gastrointestinal drug interactions. (From Kalant H, Grant DM, Mitchell J: *Principles of medical pharmacology*, ed 7, Philadelphia, 2007, Elsevier.)

form solid particles (precipitate). For example, if calcium gluconate is added to a solution of floxacillin sodium 2g in normal saline, thick white clumps form. The resulting intravenous solution is not usable.

Displacement from protein binding sites is a mechanism for drug interactions that influences the distribution of a drug. Displacement increases the amount of drug that is free to get to its site of action and produce effects (see also Chapter 2, Fig. 2.6). Warfarin is a drug that is highly protein bound. Even a small change in the percentage of "free" drug, drug not bound to protein and able to get to the binding site, can increase warfarin's effects and risk for hemorrhage. Sulfonamides are a class of antiinfective agents that are also strongly protein bound. When a sulfonamide and warfarin are both administered, displacement occurs.

Interactions that alter the rate of drug metabolism are caused by induction or inhibition of metabolic enzymes. Barbiturates such as phenobarbital stimulate metabolic enzymes of other antiseizure medications (phenytoin, valproic acid). Grapefruit juice is a powerful inhibitor of metabolic enzyme CYP3A4 and potentiates the effect of anticholesterol drugs such as atorvastatin. H2 receptor antagonists alter the metabolism of alcohol. When drugs such as cimetidine and ranitidine are taken with alcohol, the effects of alcohol may be increased and may last longer.

Some drug interactions influence elimination of drugs. Altering the pH of the urine can increase the elimination of a drug or enhance its reabsorption. Elimination of acidic drugs is increased when drugs that make the urine alkaline are administered. Elimination of alkaline drugs is increased when drugs that make the urine more acidic are administered.

Drug interactions that involve competition for a common transport system in the kidney can affect the elimination of some drugs. This describes the drug-drug interaction between penicillin and probenecid. When the drugs are administered together, elimination of penicillin is decreased.

Avoiding Undesired Drug Interactions

Studies indicate that between 7% and 22% of adverse drug reactions (ADRs) are caused by drug-drug interactions. Drug interactions that produce undesired effects should be avoided because undesired drug interactions can cancel the desired drug effect or reduced drug effect. At the opposite extreme, a drug interaction can produce toxic or harmful effects (Table 4.1). Failure to recognize drug interactions can harm the patient or prolong patient illness. It is the responsibility of pharmacists and pharmacy technicians to screen all prescriptions for potential drug interactions before dispensing the medication. Pharmacy technicians play a significant role in the screening process.

Pharmacy technicians play a key role in entering patient data into the pharmacy's prescription-filling software. Data entered into the computer must be complete and accurate if screening for drug interactions is to be effective. ***Drug-disease contraindications*** can be avoided by maintaining an up-to-date patient history of chronic and acute medical conditions. Computers prospectively screen for drug interactions so that adjustments can be made to the patient drug therapy before the drug is dispensed. When a drug-disease contradiction is identified by computer software, the pharmacy technician must alert the pharmacist so the significance of the computer-screened drug-disease contraindication can be evaluated. Drug-drug interactions can also be avoided by maintenance of an up-to-date patient profile. Pharmacy technicians and pharmacists should query patients about current nonprescription

TABLE 4.1	Summary of Selected Drug and Food Interactions		
Drug	**Effects or Side Effects Are Increased by:**	**Effects or Side Effects Are Decreased by:**
tetracycline		penicillin antacids dairy products
ketoconazole		antacids
alcoholic beverage (ethanol)	cimetidine	
oral contraceptives		amoxicillin
levothyroxine		iron supplements
triazolam	alcoholic beverages	
warfarin	NSAIDS (e.g., aspirin, ibuprofen)	vitamin K
levodopa	carbidopa	
verapamil	grapefruit juice	
griseofulvin	fatty foods	
morphine		naloxone
lidocaine	epinephrine	
cimetidine		antacids
phenobarbital		phenytoin sodium bicarbonate
penicillin	probenecid	

drug use, as well as prescription drug use. Information about prescriptions filled at other pharmacies should be obtained, if possible, and entered into the pharmacy's computer system.

> ### Tech Note!
> When taking a patient's medication history, ask the following: "Are you taking any over-the-counter medications? Are you taking any herbal supplements or vitamins? What other prescription drugs are you taking?"

Pharmacy technicians must also be knowledgeable of intravenous drug incompatibilities. Combining acidic intravenous solutions and alkaline solutions causes precipitation of the drug out of the solution. Intravenous solutions that contain precipitates cannot be used and must be destroyed.

Drug-food interactions can be avoided by counseling patients to avoid consuming foods that interact with their medications. Spacing the time between food consumption and medication administration is often sufficient to avoid an undesired interaction. Pharmacy technicians can play an active role in ensuring that appropriate warning labels are affixed to prescription containers when this task is within their scope of practice.

Medication Errors

The National Coordinating Council for Medication Error Reporting and Prevention defines a ***medication error*** as "any preventable event that may cause or lead to inappropriate medication use or patient harm while the medication is in the control of the health care professional, patient, or consumer. Such events may be related to professional practice, health care products, procedures, and systems, including prescribing; communicating drug orders; product labeling, packaging, and nomenclature; compounding; dispensing; distribution; administration; education; monitoring; and use." Medication errors harm approximately 1.3 million people in the United States annually and cause at least one death each day. Medication mishaps in prescribing, repackaging, dispensing, administering, or monitoring can occur anywhere in the distribution system. Common causes of such errors include poor communication, inappropriate directions for medication use, look-alike and sound-alike product names, medical abbreviations, and poor handwriting by prescribers. Directions for use of medications can be confusing, leading to misuse by patients. Poor aseptic technique and procedures for medication preparation can also contribute to the problem. In addition to the previous points, job stress, a lack of knowledge and training in the use or preparation of products, and similar labeling or packaging of a product may be the cause of, or contribute to, actual or potential errors.

Medication errors are made by physicians, pharmacists, nurses, and pharmacy technicians in the health care setting. Medication errors typically occur in the process of ordering, transcribing, dispensing, and administering medications. Adverse drug events result from prescribing inappropriate medicines for patients, translating prescription orders, improper preparation or selection of drug to dispense, and improper drug administration. Medication errors may also be made by patients. Patient errors typically involve taking the wrong dose or forgetting to take a dose.

Medication Errors Made by Health Care Providers Who Prescribe Medication

Medication errors that are made by health care providers in hospital and ambulatory care settings account for 70% of all medication errors. They can be harmful to patients. As many as 4 in 1000 prescription errors are made when medications are ordered by physicians, nurse practitioners, pharmacists, dentists, and other health professionals legally able to prescribe medicines. Medication errors associated with prescribers are often a result of miscommunication or misinformation.

Miscommunication

Miscommunication of the drug ordered may involve poor handwriting, confusion between drugs with similar names, misuse of zeros and decimal points, confusion of metric and other dosing units, or inappropriate abbreviations.

Poor Handwriting

Many jokes have been made about physicians' poor handwriting (often called "chicken scratch"); however, medication errors that are made because prescriptions were not decipherable are no laughing matter. When prescriptions are illegible, there may be confusion between drugs with similar names. Electronic prescribing has been shown to eliminate medication errors caused by illegible handwriting and results in a sevenfold decrease in overall medication errors compared with handwritten prescriptions.

Confusion Between Drugs With Similar Names

Although the Center for Disease Evaluation and Research (CDER) tries to avoid assigning names to new drugs that are similar to existing drugs, sometimes this happens. Drugs with similar looking or sounding names are referred to as "look-alike" and "sound-alike" drugs. According to the US Food and Drug Administration (FDA) MedWatch, medication errors have been made involving ZyrTEC and Zantac, VinCRIStine and VinBLAStine, GlipiZIDE and GlyBURIDE, LamMICtal and LamISIL, and Zyprexa and CeleXA. When prescribers fail to write legibly, confusion about the drug to dispense arises (Table 4.2).

Misuse of Zeroes and Decimal Points

Orders for medication may be incorrect because the strength is written incorrectly or is illegible. Haloperidol is a drug used to treat schizophrenia. It is available as a 0.5-mg tablet and as a 5-mg tablet. If the decimal point to the left is illegible or the zero is omitted, there may be confusion about which strength to dispense. On the other hand, if the 5-mg tablet was ordered and the prescription was written as 5.0 mg, it could be confused with 50 mg. In both cases, if the error is not caught, the patient receives 10 times the desired dose (Fig. 4.2).

> ● *Tech Note!*
>
> To avoid medication errors, always place a zero in front of the decimal when calculating and recording doses that are less than 1 mL or 1 mg.

Confusion of Metric and Other Dosing Units or Inappropriate Abbreviations

Prescriptions may be written using metric units or apothecary units. Medication errors have been caused by improper conversion between the two systems of measurement. For example, the apothecary symbol for 1 dram (3i) has been interpreted as 3 mL, 4 mL, and 5 mL. Most pharmacists and pharmacy technicians interpret 3i = 5 mL = 1 teaspoonful. Prescribers unfamiliar with apothecary symbols may confuse the symbol for ounce (3) and dram (3), causing toxic or subtherapeutic effects.

Misinformation

Medication errors made by prescribers may also occur because of lack of information or misinformation. Studies have shown that more than 25% of the prescribing errors made in hospitals are associated with incomplete medication histories being obtained at the time of admission. A complete history is needed of patients' allergies, other medicines they are taking, previous diagnoses, and laboratory results to prevent medication errors.

Errors of Omission

An error of omission occurs when information is not collected or recorded in the patient's medical history. Studies have shown a 67% error rate in obtaining prescription medication histories. Medication histories taken by physicians were less accurate than histories taken by pharmacists. An incomplete drug history may be a cause for prescribing a drug similar to one currently being administered. This is called ***therapeutic duplication***. Therapeutic duplication may increase or decrease desired effects. If both drugs compete for the same drug-receptor binding sites or the same transport systems, the drug with the greatest affinity will bind. If the drug bound to the receptor is less potent, it decreases the

TABLE 4.2 Selected FDA, ISMP, and The Joint Commission List of Confused Drug Names

Drug Name	Confused With Drug Name
acetaZOLAMIDE	acetoHEXAMIDE
ALPRAZolam	LORazepam cloazePAM
aMILoride	amLODIPine
ARIPiprazole	RABEprazole
AVINza	INVanz
azaCITIDine	azaTHIOprine
buPROPion	busPIRone
carBAMazepine	OXcarbazepine
CARBOplatin	CISplatin
ceFAZolin	cefoTEtan cefOXitin cefTAZidime cefTRIAXone
CeleBREX	CeleXA, Cerebyx
chlorproMAZINE	chlorproPAMIDE chlodiazePOXIDE
clomiPHENE	clomiPRAMINE
clonazePAM	cloNIDine cloZAPine cloBAZam LORazepam
cyclosPORINE	cycloSERINE
DAPTOmycin	DACTINomycin
DAUNOrubicin	DOXOrubicin
DEPO-Medrol	SOLU-Medrol
diazePAM	dilTIAZem
dimenhydrinate	diphenhydrAMINE
DOBUTamine	DOPamine
DOCEtaxel	PACLitaxel
DOXOrubicin	IDArubicin
Effexor	Effexor XR
ePHEDrine	EPINEPHrine
fentaNYL	SUFentanil
FLUoxetine	DULoxetine PARoxetine
fluvoxaMINE	FluPHENAzine flavoxATE
glyBURIDE	glipiZIDE
guaiFENesin	guanFACINE
HumaLOG	HumuLIN
hydrALAZINE	hydrOXYzine hydroCHLOROthiazide
HYDROmorphone	morphine oxyMORphone
inFLIXimab	riTUXimab

TABLE 4.2 Selected FDA, ISMP, and The Joint Commission List of Confused Drug Names —cont'd

Drug Name	Confused With Drug Name
ISOtretinoin	tretinoin
LaMICtal	LamISIL
lamiVUDine	lamoTRIgine
levETIRAcetam	levOCARNitine levoFLOXacin
LEVOleucovprin	leucovorin
medroxyPROGESTERone	methylPREDNISolone methylTESTOSTERone HYDROXYprogesterone
methazolAMIDE	methIMAzole metOLazole
miFEPRIStone	miSOPROStol
mitomycin	mitoXANTRONE
NIFEdipine	niCARdipine niMODipine
NovoLOG	NovoLIN, HumaLOG
OLANZapine	QUEtiapine
oxyCODONE	HYDROcodone OxyCONTIN oxyMORphone
PAZOPanib	PONATinib
penicillamine	penicillin
PENTobarbital	PHENobarbital
predniSONE	prednisoLONE
quiNIDine	quiNINE
ranitidine	reMANTAdine
risperiDONE	rOPINIRole RisperDAL
sAXagliptin	SITagliptin SUMAtriptan
SEROquel	SINEquan
sulfADIAZINE	sulfiSOXAZOLE
Retrovir	ritonavir
Tobrex	Tobradex
TOLAZamide	TOLBUTamide
traMADol	traZODone
valacyclovir	valGANciclovir
vinBLAStine	vinCRIStine
Wellbutrin SR	Wellbutrin XL
ZyrPREXA	ZyrTEC

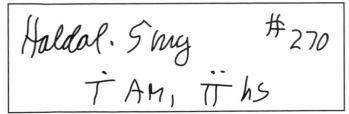

• **Fig. 4.2** Decimal point error example.

desired drug effect. Therapeutic duplication may increase adverse reactions. Omission of drug allergy information could result in a prescription written and filled for a medicine that may cause extreme harm to the patient. Prescriptions written for drugs that are contraindicated often occur because a patient's disease state or allergies have not been recorded in the patient profile. An example of a drug-disease contraindication is the administration of the antidepressant bupropion to patients with a history of seizures. Patients can reduce their risk for drug interactions caused by errors of omission by filling all prescriptions at a single pharmacy that has the patient's complete medication history. Patients should also provide the pharmacy with a list of all regularly taken nonprescription drugs such as aspirin.

> ● **Tech Note!**
>
> Pharmacy technicians may encounter the abbreviations NKDA (no known drug allergies) or NDA (no drug allergies).

Errors of Commission

Commission errors result when a previously discontinued drug is accidentally restarted or a nonprescribed drug is accidentally added to the patient's medication history. This can occur when inaccurate drug histories are collected from caregivers (when the patient is too ill to provide their own drug history) or because of patient confusion. When this occurs, unneeded drugs are taken, and the patient is at risk for adverse reactions.

Prescriptions written for the wrong strength or wrong dosing schedule are medication errors that are not specifically errors of omission or commission but do involve prescribers. This type of error occurs when the prescriber lacks familiarity with the drug that is being prescribed. The error may occur when drug dose and dosing frequency are determined according to patient weight and inaccurate weight information is given in the medical history.

Medication Errors Made by Health Care Providers Who Dispense Medication

Pharmacists, pharmacy technicians, and pharmacy assistants make preventable medication errors too! Medication errors made by pharmacy personnel usually involve transcribing errors, incorrect interpretation of prescription contents, improper product preparation, lack of prescription monitoring, product labeling, and inaccurate dispensing. Some dispensing errors are caused by distractions in the pharmacy. The pharmacist or pharmacy technician filling a medication order may become distracted when their workflow is interrupted by the telephone ringing or by questions from a patient at the pharmacy counter.

> ● **Tech Note!**
>
> Always check the original prescription against the prescription label and the NDC number or DIN on the stock bottle to ensure accuracy.

Confusing or Inappropriate Abbreviations

Serious medication errors have been caused by confusing abbreviations. This problem is so serious that The Joint Commission and the National Coordinating Council for Medication Error Reporting and Prevention have recommended abolishment of the use of certain abbreviations (Table 4.3).

> ● **Tech Note!**
>
> When in doubt about what is written on a prescription, always get a second opinion. Never guess at what the medication might be. Ask for help to verify the drug in question.

Inaccurate Transcribing

Poor handwriting is responsible for many transcription errors. Medication orders received by the pharmacy must be translated and entered into the computer. If the order is illegible, the pharmacy must verify the order to prevent incorrect selection of the drug and strength ordered. Medication orders received by telephone or left on a computer messaging system are also subject to transcription errors. Verbal medication orders must be written down accurately, or medication errors may result.

Insufficient Monitoring of Drug Therapy

Medication errors occur when a pharmacy fails to carefully monitor drug therapy. An important role of the pharmacist is to monitor the appropriateness of drug therapy. Pharmacy technicians assist the pharmacist with this task. Together they review each prescription to determine whether the medication ordered, dose, and dosing frequency are appropriate for the patient. Pharmacy technicians also help the pharmacist screen for drug interactions, drug-disease contraindications, and drug allergies. Monitoring drug therapy also reduces therapeutic duplication. Pharmacy technicians and pharmacists work together to alert the prescriber when they see that two therapeutically equivalent drugs are ordered for the patient. Monitoring also prevents refills of discontinued medication.

Improper Medication Preparation

Another medication error made by pharmacy staff is improper sterile and nonsterile compounding. Medications for parenteral administration must be prepared using aseptic technique. Medication errors associated with incorrect calculations also occur. Combining incompatible drugs is another source of medication errors.

> ● **Tech Note!**
>
> It is vitally important to adopt an "aseptic attitude" when preparing parenteral medications. Handwashing, hood cleaning, dose calculating, and proper aseptic technique ensure that the sterile products are not contaminated or inaccurate.

Improper Labeling

Medication errors can involve several types of improper labeling of drugs to be dispensed. A labeling error has occurred when the correct drug is selected but the container is labeled with the wrong drug name, dosage form, strength, or quantity. Putting the wrong

TABLE 4.3	Dangerous Abbreviations*		
Do Not Use	**Potential Problem**		**Use Instead**
AU, AS, AD	Misinterpreted as "OU" (both eyes), "OS" (left eye), "OD" (right eye or once daily)		Write "both ears", "left ear", "right ear"
OU, OS, OD	Misinterpreted as "AU" (both ears), "AS" (left ear), "AD" (right ear)		Write "both eyes", "left eye", "right eye"
U (unit)	Mistaken for "0" (zero), the number "4" (four), or "cc"		Write "unit"
IU (International Unit)	Mistaken for IV (intravenous) or the number 10 (ten)		Write "International Unit"
μg	Mistaken for mg (milligrams) resulting in 1000-fold overdose		Write "mcg" or "micrograms"
Q.D., QD, q.d., qd, (Latin abbreviation for every day)	Period after the Q mistaken for "I" and misinterpreted as QID (four times a day). In Canada, once daily is abbreviated OD which may be misinterpreted as every other day or right eye.		Write "daily"
Q.O.D., QOD, q.o.d, qod (Latin abbreviation for every other day)	Period after the Q mistaken for "I" and the "O" mistaken for "I". Misinterpreted as once daily or four times a day.		Write "every other day"
SC or SQ	Mistaken as SL (sublingual)		Write subcutaneous
TIW	Misinterpreted as three times a day or twice a week		Write as three times a week
D/C	Patient's medications have been prematurely discontinued because D/C can be interpreted as either discharge or discontinue		Do not abbreviate
Cc	Mistaken for U (units) when poorly written		Write "mL" or "milliliters"
HS	Latin for hour of sleep, the abbreviation may be misinterpreted as half-strength		Do not abbreviate
MS, MSO₄, and MgSO₄	Can mean morphine sulfate or magnesium sulfate; confused for one another		Write "morphine sulfate"
Trailing zero (X.0 mg)ᵃ	Decimal point is missed		Write X mg
Lack of leading zero (.X mg)	Decimal point is missed		Write 0.X mg
Additional Abbreviations, Acronyms, and Symbols to Consider Avoiding			
< (greater than) and > (less than)	Misinterpreted as the number "7" (seven) or the letter "L"; confused for each other		Write "greater than" and "less than"
Apothecary units	Unfamiliar to many practitioners; confused with metric units		Use metric units
@	Mistaken for the number "2" (two)		Write "at"

*Applies to all orders and all medication-related documentation that is handwritten (including free-text computer entry) or on preprinted forms.
ᵃException: A "trailing zero" may be used only when required to demonstrate the level of precision of the value being reported, such as for laboratory results, imaging studies that report size of lesions, or catheter or tube sizes. It may not be used in medication orders or other medication-related documentation.
Adapted from National Coordinating Council for Medication Error Reporting and Prevention (2017) and Dangerous Abbreviations and The Joint Commission (2017). Facts about the Official "Do Not Use" List of Abbreviations.

patient's name on the label and incorrect or incomplete directions typed on the label are other preventable label errors.

Product Selection Errors

Selection of the wrong drug to dispense is a preventable error. This type of error most often occurs when drugs have similar names or similar packaging (Fig. 4.3). Other product selection errors include dispensing the wrong strength or wrong dosage form.

Bagging Errors

Placing the correct prescription in the wrong patient's bag is a bagging error. Placing additional prescriptions into a patient's bag or omitting a prescription from the bag are also bagging errors.

Miscellaneous Dispensing Errors

A properly filled prescription that is dispensed to the wrong patient is a medication error. This may occur when two customers have similar names. The pharmacy staff may incorrectly hear the name of the person who wants to pick up their prescription. The patient may incorrectly hear the name of the person the pharmacy staff has announced. This error is preventable. Always verify the name and identification of the person picking up a prescription.

Medication Errors Made by Health Care Providers Who Administer Medication

Medication errors are made by health care providers and caregivers who administer medications. One example of an error is administering a drug to the wrong patient. Sometimes the correct drug is given to the right patient, but the drug strength, dosing frequency, or dosage form is incorrect. These are all examples of medication errors.

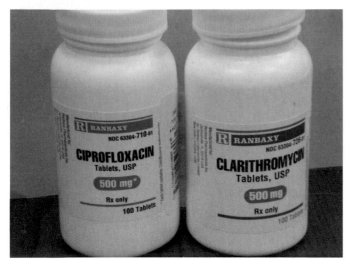

• **Fig. 4.3** Example of look-alike packaging. (Courtesy Institute for Safe Medication Practices [ISMP]).

Medication Errors Made by Patients

Medication errors are made by patients too! Pharmacists, pharmacy technicians, and other health care providers can help patients prevent medication errors. Patients are often confused by generic and trade names. Their medicines may be labeled using the generic name in the hospital. The community pharmacy may label the same drug with the brand name. The patient may not realize the drugs are the same and take a double dose. A similar situation occurs when two similar medicines are prescribed by different physicians. The patient is unaware that taking both medicines is therapeutic duplication. Confusion is one reason why patients refill medications that have been discontinued by their health care provider.

Two other medication errors are important to note. They are (1) taking too much medicine and (2) taking too little medicine. Some patients believe the saying, "If one pill is good, then two pills are better." Others do not realize the importance of taking medicines without missing doses. They do not realize that a chronic illness becomes worse or drug resistance can develop when doses are skipped. For some patients, the medication is too expensive, and they take less than the prescribed dose to try to "stretch"

the prescription and make it last longer. Regardless of the reason, taking too little or too much medicine can negatively influence drug therapy outcomes.

Avoiding Medication Errors

Pharmacy technicians can play an important role in preventing medication errors. Some tips for preventing medication errors are:
- Always verify prescriptions with similar drug names. Verify spelling and strength.
- Always verify unfamiliar abbreviations or abbreviations published in The Joint Commission's "do not use" list or the National Coordinating Council for Medication Error Reporting and Prevention dangerous abbreviation list.
- Always confirm the drug name, strength, and dosing schedule when prescriptions are written and the handwriting is illegible. Never guess.
- Avoid product selection errors by using the pull–dispense–review (PDR) system. Verify the drug name and NDC number or DIN when selecting (pulling) the drug from the shelf. Check the drug name, strength, and dosage form against the medication order. Confirm the drug a third time when returning the medicine to the shelf.
- Become familiar with the brand and generic names of commonly dispensed drugs.
- Become familiar with the strengths, dosage forms, and dosing frequencies of commonly dispensed drugs.
- Alert the pharmacist of all drug interactions and therapeutic duplications.
- Develop a routine to avoid errors associated with distractions.
- Check the identification of each person picking up prescriptions.
- Dispense patient information sheets as required.
- Affix warning labels to prescription vials as required.
- Verify all calculations.
- Check all labels for accuracy.

TECHNICIAN'S CORNER

1. Look-alike and sound-alike drugs are responsible for dispensing errors. How might dispensing errors be avoided?
2. What should a pharmacy technician do if they are unsure about the name of a medication handwritten on a prescription?

Key Points

- Drug-drug interactions and drug-food interactions can increase or decrease intended drug effects.
- The more drugs that are administered to a patient, the more likely it is that interactions will occur.
- Drug-drug interactions may increase or decrease side effects of drugs.
- Foods may contain enzymes, vitamins, or minerals that enhance or interfere with drug effects.
- Additive effects are said to occur when the coadministration of two drugs results in increased side effects.
- Synergistic effects result when two drugs administered together produce effects that are greater than would be produced if either drug were administered alone.

- The process during which one drug or a food increases the effects of another drug yet does not produce any effect when administered alone is called potentiation.
- Antagonism is a drug-drug interaction or drug-food interaction that causes decreased drug effects.
- Interactions that are caused by induction or inhibition of metabolic enzymes can alter the rate of drug metabolism.
- Interactions that involve competition for a common transport system in the kidney can affect the elimination of some drugs.
- It is the responsibility of the pharmacy technician to alert the pharmacist when the pharmacy software identifies a potential drug interaction.

- Drug-disease contradictions and drug-drug interactions can be avoided by maintaining an up-to-date history of each patient's chronic and acute medical conditions.
- Pharmacy technicians must be knowledgeable of intravenous drug incompatibilities. Combining acidic intravenous solutions and alkaline solutions causes the precipitation of the drug out of the solution.
- Medication errors in the health care setting typically occur in the process of ordering, transcribing, dispensing, and administering medications.
- Poor handwriting is responsible for many medication errors. When prescriptions are illegible, there may be confusion between drugs with similar names.
- Medication errors occur because of misplacement of zeros and decimal points.
- Medication errors have been caused by improper conversion between systems of measurement.
- Medication errors occur when pharmacists, pharmacy technicians, physicians, and other health care workers lack familiarity with the drug that is being prescribed.

- Medication errors made by pharmacy personnel usually involve transcribing errors, incorrect interpretation of prescription contents, improper product preparation, lack of prescription monitoring, product labeling, and inaccurate dispensing.
- Some dispensing errors are caused by distractions in the pharmacy.
- Medication errors made by patients can be minimized by proper education.
- Medication errors can be avoided by verifying prescriptions with similar drug names and unfamiliar abbreviations.
- Avoid product selection errors by using the PDR system and checking all labels for accuracy.
- Prevent medication errors by becoming familiar with brand and generic names and the strengths, dosage forms, and dosing frequencies of commonly dispensed drugs.
- Medication errors can be minimized by verifying all calculations.

Review Questions

1. Indicate whether the following statement is true or false: Drug-drug interactions may increase or decrease the effect or side effects of the drug.
   a. true
   b. false
2. When the coadministration of two drugs results in increased side effects, the interaction is described as _____.
   a. antagonistic
   b. additive
   c. adverse
   d. absorption
3. When warfarin and aspirin are administered together, excessive bleeding occurs. This type of effect is _____.
   a. antagonistic
   b. idiosyncratic
   c. both a and b
   d. synergistic
4. Whose responsibility is it to watch for potential drug interactions during the prescription filling process?
   a. pharmacist
   b. technician
   c. pharmacist and technician
   d. pharmacy manager
5. Medication errors made by pharmacy personnel typically occur in the process of:
   a. prescribing medications
   b. transcribing medications
   c. administering medications
   d. a, b, and c
6. Orders for medication may be incorrect because the strength is written incorrectly or is illegible. Which of the following is the correct way of writing the dose for digoxin?
   a. digoxin 0.25 mg
   b. digoxin 25 mg
   c. digoxin .25 mg
   d. digoxin 025 mg

7. All of the following are "checks" to ensure that the right medication is pulled from the pharmacy shelf when preparing a prescription EXCEPT_____.
   a. Compare the NDC number or DIN on the bottle with the computer-generated pharmacy label.
   b. Check with the pharmacy assistant every time a prescription is filled.
   c. Check the drug name against the medication order.
   d. Check the drug strength and dosage form against the medication order.
8. To which federal agency should medication errors be reported to using the MedWatch program?
   a. DEA (Drug Enforcement Agency)
   b. FDA (Food and Drug Administration)
   c. TJC (The Joint Commission)
   d. ISMP (Institute for Safe Medication Practices Canada)
9. Which agency developed a "do not use" abbreviation list to avoid medication errors?
   a. Food and Drug Administration
   b. Drug Enforcement Agency
   c. Health Canada
   d. The Joint Commission
10. Dispensing errors can be avoided by _____.
   a. verifying the name of the person picking up the medication
   b. verifying that the medication is placed in the correct patient's bag
   c. being alert for patients with similar names
   d. all of the above

Bibliography

Adubofour K, Keenan C, Daftary A, et al. Strategies to reduce medication errors in ambulatory practice. *J Natl Med Assoc.* 2004;96:1558.

Corbett AH, Dana WJ, Fuller MA, et al. *Drug information handbook.* ed 24. Hudson, OH: APhA Lexi-Comp; 2015.

Institute for Safe Medication Practices. (2016). FDA and ISMP Lists of Look-Alike Drug Names with Recommended Tall Man Letters. Retrieved June 24, 2022, from https://www.ismp.org/recommendations/tall-man-letters-list.

Institute for Safe Medication Practices. (2019). List of Confused Drugs. Retrieved June 24, 2022, from https://www.ismp.org/tools/confused-drugnames.pdf.

National Coordinating Council for Medication Error Reporting and Prevention. (2022). Dangerous Abbreviations. Retrieved June 24, 2022, from http://nccmerp.org/dangerous-abbreviations.

Page C, Curtis M, Sutter M, et al. *Integrated pharmacology.* Philadelphia: Elsevier Mosby; 2005:57–70.

Passarelli M, Jacob-Filho W, Figueras A. Adverse drug reactions in an elderly hospitalised population: inappropriate prescription is a leading cause. *Drugs Aging.* 2005;22:767–777.

Shargel L, Mutnick A, Souney P, et al. *Comprehensive pharmacy review.* ed 4. Baltimore: Lippincott Williams & Wilkins; 2001:42–65 78–84, 131–132.

Tam V, Knowles S, Cornish P, et al. Frequency, type and clinical importance of medication history errors at admission to hospital: a systematic review. *CMAJ.* 2005;173(5).

The Joint Commission. (2022). Facts about the Official "Do Not Use" List of Abbreviations. Retrieved June 24, 2022, from https://www.jointcommission.org/facts_about_do_not_use_list/.

U.S. Food and Drug Administration. (2022). Medication Errors Related to Drugs. Retrieved June 24, 2022, from https://www.fda.gov/drugs/drugsafety/medicationerrors/default.htm.

U.S. Food and Drug Administration. (2019). Strategies to Reduce Medication Errors: Working to Improve Medication Safety. Retrieved June 24, 2022, from https://www.fda.gov/drugs/resourcesforyou/consumers/ucm143553.htm.

Velo GP, Minuz P. Medication errors: prescribing faults and prescription errors. *Br J Clin Pharmacol.* 2009;67(6):624–628.

Drugs Affecting the Autonomic Nervous System and Central Nervous System

The nervous system is made up of the central nervous system (CNS; brain and spinal cord) and the peripheral nervous system (PNS). The central nervous system integrates sensory input and motor output. The peripheral nervous system comprises the autonomic and somatic systems. The autonomic nervous system (ANS) is divided into the parasympathetic and sympathetic systems. The parasympathetic nervous system regulates involuntary actions such as the heartbeat, smooth muscle contraction, and glandular secretions. The sympathetic nervous system predominates whenever the body is undergoing physical or psychological stress initiating a "fight or flight" response. The nervous system transmits information very rapidly by nerve impulses conducted from one area of the body to another, communicating changes in the body's internal and external environment, and responding by initiating changes in muscles and glands. A healthy nervous system is vitally important for normal physiologic function. There are more than 600 diseases of the nervous system. Many of the drugs that act on the brain and nervous system relieve symptoms such as pain, insomnia, and anxiety or treat mood disorders.

In Unit II, the pharmacotherapy for anxiety, depression, psychosis (e.g., schizophrenia), Parkinson disease, Huntington disease, seizures, pain, migraine headache, Alzheimer disease, sleep disorders, and attention-deficit/hyperactivity disorder (ADHD) is described. A brief description of each disorder is provided, followed by a description of the drugs indicated for treatment that includes mechanisms of action, adverse reactions, strength(s), and dosage forms.

5

Treatment of Anxiety

LEARNING OBJECTIVES

1. Learn the terminology associated with anxiety and its treatment.
2. List and describe the function of neurotransmitters associated with symptoms of anxiety.
3. Classify medications used to treat anxiety.
4. Describe the mechanism of action for each class of drugs used to treat anxiety.
5. Identify significant drug look-alike or sound-alike issues.
6. Identify warning labels and precautionary messages associated with medications used to treat anxiety.

KEY TERMS

Anxiety Condition associated with tension, apprehension, fear, or panic.

Anxiolytic Drug used to treat anxiety.

Drug dependence Person taking the drug must continue to take the drug to avoid the onset of physical or psychological withdrawal symptoms (or both).

Generalized anxiety disorder Condition that is associated with excessive worrying and tension that is experienced daily for more than 6 months.

Obsessive-compulsive disorder A condition associated with an inability to control or stop repeated unwanted thoughts or behaviors.

Panic disorder Condition associated with repeated sudden onset of feelings of terror.

Phobia Irrational fear of things or situations that produce symptoms of intense anxiety.

Posttraumatic stress disorder Stress disorder that develops in persons who have participated in, witnessed, or been a victim of a terrifying event.

Social anxiety disorder A chronic mental health condition in which social interactions cause irrational anxiety.

Tolerance Increasing doses of a drug are required to achieve the same effects as were achieved previously at lower doses.

Overview

Anxiety disorder is the leading mental health illness and affects more than 40 million US adults, according to Anxiety & Depression Association of America. In any 12-month period, approximately 19.1% of US adults have excessive anxiety. In 2019, more than 4.4 million Canadians 14 years of age and older (11.6% of the population) reported having a mood or anxiety disorder, according to Statistics Canada. In both the United States and Canada, the prevalence of anxiety has increased during the COVID-19 pandemic. The cause of anxiety disorders may be environmental, biologic, developmental, associated with socioeconomic conditions, or a combination of several of these individual factors. Anxiety disorders can interfere with routine daily activities, work, school, and social relationships.

The major types of anxiety disorders are generalized anxiety disorder (GAD), panic disorder, obsessive-compulsive disorder (OCD), social anxiety disorder (SAD), posttraumatic stress disorder (PTSD), and separation anxiety disorder. Individuals diagnosed with anxiety disorders experience intense fear, apprehension, tension, or panic out of proportion to the actual threat or danger.

Certain physiologic symptoms are diagnostic for individual anxiety disorders; however, some symptoms are common to all anxiety disorders. Common physiologic symptoms include increased heart rate, palpitations, shortness of breath, rapid breathing, nausea, sweating, and dry mouth. All of these symptoms are associated with hyperactivity of the autonomic nervous system. More specifically, the physiologic symptoms produced by anxiety are related to stimulation of the sympathetic nervous system and the parasympathetic nervous system.

Generalized Anxiety Disorder

Although most adults will experience anxiety at one point in their lives, excessive worrying and tension that are experienced daily for longer than 6 months is an indication of *generalized anxiety disorder*. It may produce restlessness, difficulty concentrating, sleep problems, and irritability. It is the most common type of anxiety disorder. In any given year, 6.8 million Americans (3.1% of the adult population) are affected, according to Anxiety & Depression Association of America. GAD affects approximately 3% of the Canadian adult population in any given year. Women are more likely to have GAD than are men, according to Statistics Canada (2019).

Panic Disorder

Panic disorder affects approximately 6 million American adults in any given year. The 12-month prevalence in Canada is 1.6% of the adult population. It occurs twice as frequently in women than in men. It may be accompanied by major depression. Signs and symptoms of panic disorder include a sudden onset of terror, shortness of breath, increased heart rate, trembling, and nausea. The person may feel paralyzed by fear and unable to perform routine daily activities. Most symptoms of panic disorder last for only a few minutes.

Panic attacks may be triggered by a phobia. A *phobia* is an irrational fear of things or situations that produce symptoms of intense anxiety. Phobias cause the person to try to avoid the thing that is feared. Agoraphobia is a condition in which people become so fearful of situations that may produce "panicky feelings" that they isolate themselves or severely restrict their activities. Other common phobias are claustrophobia (fear of being in confined spaces), aviophobia (fear of flying), and acrophobia (fear of heights). More than 19 million Americans are affected by social phobias. In any given year, 6.7% of Canadian adults experience a social phobia. Approximately 8% of the populations of the United States and Canada have some type of phobia.

Obsessive-Compulsive Disorder

Obsessive-compulsive disorder is a condition associated with an inability to control or stop repeated unwanted thoughts or behaviors. Individuals create rituals, which they perform repeatedly, to lessen anxieties about the things they fear. A person who fears germs may wash their hands excessively. Approximately 1% of the Canadian population between the ages of 15 and 64 years has been diagnosed with OCD. More than 2 million Americans (1% of the adult population) are affected by OCD in any given year. The lifetime incidence of OCD worldwide is 1.7% to 4%.

Posttraumatic Stress Disorder

Posttraumatic stress disorder may develop in persons who have participated in, witnessed, or been a victim of a terrifying event. According to National Institutes of Mental Health, nearly 3.5% of the adult population in the United States have experienced PTSD. PTSD may occur in soldiers who have committed atrocities or witnessed horrific events during wartime. Up to 67% of the people exposed to mass violence develop PTSD. Women, men, and children who have been sexually assaulted may develop PTSD. Up to 65% of men and 45.9% of women who have been sexually assaulted have PTSD. PTSD is likely to develop at some point in the lifetimes of children who have been sexually abused. Some people develop PTSD after a natural disaster such as an earthquake, flood, or human disasters such as an airplane crash. Depression, substance abuse, and anxiety disorders may accompany PTSD.

Social Anxiety Disorder

Social anxiety disorder (social phobia) is an anxiety disorder that causes affected individuals to shy away from everyday social situations where they fear embarrassment or humiliation. Fear of public speaking or asking questions in a public forum is often associated with a social phobia. SAD affects 15 million adults or 6.8% of the US population. Women are twice as likely to be affected as men.

Neurochemistry of Anxiety

There are four major classes of medicines used for the treatment of anxiety. They are selective serotonin reuptake inhibitors (SSRIs) (e.g., citalopram, fluoxetine, and sertraline), serotonin-norepinephrine reuptake inhibitors (SNRIs) (e.g., venlafaxine and duloxetine), tricyclic antidepressants (TCAs) (e.g., amitriptyline and nortriptyline), and benzodiazepines (e.g., alprazolam and lorazepam). The drugs act on the neurotransmitters γ-aminobutyric acid (GABA), serotonin (5-hydroxytryptamine [5-HT]), and norepinephrine (NE).

Role of γ-Aminobutyric Acid

The mechanism of action for most drugs used to treat anxiety is to potentiate the effects of GABA, a neurotransmitter. GABA decreases neuronal excitability and nerve impulse transmission.

Role of Serotonin

5-HT is another neurotransmitter that plays a role in the treatment of anxiety. Numerous 5-HT receptors have been identified. Most are located in the pons and midbrain. Activation of the 5-HT$_{1A}$ autoreceptors in the raphe region of the brain decreases firing of serotonergic neurons that are linked to anxiety-like behavior.

Role of Norepinephrine

NE is an important neurotransmitter for the sympathetic nervous system. It is responsible for mediating some of the adrenergic-related symptoms of anxiety (e.g., increased heart rate).

Drugs Used to Treat Anxiety

Anxiety disorder is treated by the administration of anxiolytics and psychotherapy, including cognitive behavioral therapy. An *anxiolytic* is a drug that reduces symptoms of anxiety.

Benzodiazepines

Benzodiazepines are indicated for short-term treatment of anxiety (Table 5.1). They reduce anxiety even when taken in low doses. Other indications for benzodiazepines are panic attack, insomnia, seizure disorder, and muscle relaxation. These additional indications are listed under the description of individual benzodiazepines.

> **● *Tech Note!***
>
> Two common endings for drugs that are classified as benzodiazepines are -*epam* and -*olam*.

Mechanism of Action

Benzodiazepines bind to receptor sites on the GABA$_A$ complex. They promote relaxation and reduce physical symptoms of anxiety, including muscular tension (Fig. 5.1).

Pharmacokinetics

Benzodiazepines readily cross the blood-brain barrier. The duration of action varies from one benzodiazepine to another and may influence the selection of one benzodiazepine over another.

TABLE 5.1	Benzodiazepines Used in the Treatment of Anxiety	
Generic Name	**US Brand Name(s)** / **Canadian Brand(s)**	**Dosage Forms and Strengths**
alprazolam[a]	Xanax, Xanax XR / Generics	Solution (concentrate)[c]: 1 mg/mL Tablets (Xanax): 0.25 mg, 0.5 mg, 1 mg, 2 mg Tablets, triscored (TS)[b]: 2 mg Tablets, extended release (Xanax XR)[c]: 0.5 mg, 1 mg, 2 mg, 3 mg Tablets, disintegrating[c]: 0.25 mg, 0.5 mg, 1 mg, 2 mg
clonazepam[a]	Klonopin / Generics	Tablets: 0.5 mg, 1 mg, 2 mg Tablets, disintegrating[c]: 0.125 mg, 0.25 mg, 0.5 mg, 1 mg, 2 mg
clorazepate[a]	Tranxene / Generics	Tablets: 3.75 mg, 7.5 mg, 15 mg
diazepam[a]	Diastat, Diastat Acudial, Diazepam Intensol, Valium, Valtoco[d] / Diastat, Valium	Rectal gel (Diastat): 2.5 mg/0.5 mL[c], 5 mg/mL, 10 mg/2 mL[b], 15 mg/3 mL[b] and 20 mg/4 mL[c] prefilled syringes Injection, IM: 5 mg/mL Nasal Spray (Valtoco)[c]: 5 mg/spray, 7.5 mg/spray, 10 mg/spray Oral, solution[c]: 1 mg/1 mL Oral concentrate (Diazepam Intensol)[c]: 5 mg/mL Tablets (Valium): 2 mg, 5 mg, 10 mg
lorazepam[a]	Ativan, Loreev XR / Ativan	Capsule, extended release (Loreev XR)[c]: 1 mg, 1.5 mg, 2 mg, 3 mg Injection, solution (Ativan): 2 mg/mL[c], 4 mg/mL Solution, oral concentrate[c]: 2 mg/mL Tablets (Ativan): 0.5 mg, 1 mg, 2 mg Tablets, sublingual[b]: 0.5 mg, 1 mg, 2 mg
midazolam[a]	Nayzilam[d], Seizalam[d] / Generic	Injection, solution: 1 mg/mL and 5 mg/mL Injection, intramuscular (Seizalam)[c]: 5 mg/mL Nasal spray (Nayzilam)[c]: 5 mg/spray Syrup[c]: 2 mg/mL
oxazepam[a]	Generic / Generic	Capsules[c]: 10 mg, 15 mg, 30 mg Tablets[b]: 10 mg, 15 mg, 30 mg

[a]Generic available.
[b]Available in Canada only.
[c]Available in the United States only.
[d]for treatment of acute intermittent seizures (e.g., Cluster seizures).
IM, Intramuscular.

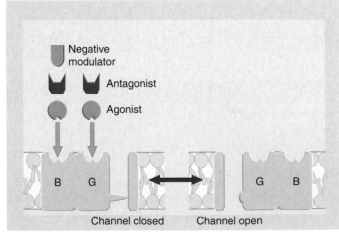

Mechanism of action of

G = GABA receptor site
B = benzodiazepine binding site

• **Fig. 5.1** Anxiolytic agents. (From Page C, Curtis M, Sutter M, et al. *Integrated pharmacology,* ed 3, Philadelphia, 2006, Mosby.)

A benzodiazepine that has a long duration of action may have long-lasting, unwanted side effects. The effects of some benzodiazepines may persist for up to 3 days.

The benzodiazepines are fully metabolized, and some agents are metabolized to active metabolites (see Chapter 2). The half-life ($t^{1/2}$) of the active metabolites can be several days, which accounts for the long duration of action of some anxiolytics such as diazepam.

Adverse Reactions

Certain side effects are common to all benzodiazepines, but others are drug specific. All benzodiazepines produce some degree of sedation, ataxia, confusion, and reduced motor performance. Benzodiazepines can also interfere with cognitive functions and memory because they produce a type of amnesia. This side effect is sometimes used purposefully, such as when benzodiazepines are used to reduce anxiety associated with dental or medical procedures. The person receiving the drug "forgets" the procedure, so anxiety associated with future procedures is reduced. Adverse reactions are dose dependent, and side effects increase as the dose increases. The therapeutic index for benzodiazepines is high. The lethal dose is approximately 1000 times greater than the typical therapeutic dose.

Tolerance and Dependence

All benzodiazepines are capable of producing tolerance and dependence, which is why they are classified as class IV controlled substances in the United States. Benzodiazepines are categorized as a targeted substance in Canada and listed in Schedule IV of the Canadian Controlled Drugs and Substances Act.

Tolerance to a drug is said to have developed when the patient must take increasing doses to achieve the same effects as were achieved previously at lower doses. Tolerance to benzodiazepines can develop in as little as 14 days. Benzodiazepines are also known to produce *drug dependence*. When drug dependence has developed, the person taking the drug must continue to take the drug to avoid the onset of physical or psychological withdrawal symptoms (or both). Sudden cessation of benzodiazepines can bring on the onset of withdrawal symptoms such as tremors, anxiety, insomnia, agitation, and confusion. Onset of withdrawal symptoms is drug specific. Withdrawal symptoms develop soon after discontinuation of benzodiazepines with short half-lives. The onset of withdrawal symptoms is delayed after abrupt discontinuation of benzodiazepines that have long half-lives. The risk of developing withdrawal symptoms is minimized when benzodiazepines are discontinued slowly.

> **● Tech Note!**
>
> Class IV drugs produce less risk for physical and psychological addiction than do class I, II, and III drugs.

Precautions

Benzodiazepines potentiate the sedative effects of other central nervous system (CNS) depressants. They also should be used cautiously in patients who have liver disease. When midazolam is administered, respiratory resuscitation equipment should be readily available. There is a drug interaction between midazolam and cimetidine that results in increased midazolam levels.

> **● Tech Note!**
>
> ALPRAZolam, LORazepam, and clonazePAM have look-alike/sound-alike issues.

> **❶ Tech Alert!**
>
> ClomiPRAMINE and clomiPHENE have look-alike/sound-alike issues.

> **❶ Tech Alert!**
>
> Diazepam oral solution and oral concentrate have look-alike/sound-alike issues.

> **❶ Tech Alert!**
>
> Lorazepam and alprazolam have look-alike/sound-alike issues. Ativan and Atarax have look-alike/sound-alike issues.

Azapirones

Buspirone is the only azapirone approved in Canada and the United States. Azapirones are effective in management of anxiety disorders (Table 5.2) and have a benefit over benzodiazepines because they do not produce tolerance or dependence.

TABLE 5.2 Azapirones Used in the Treatment of Anxiety

Generic Name	US Brand Name(s) / Canadian Brand(s)	Dosage Forms and Strengths
buspirone[a]	Generics / Generics	**Tablets:** 5 mg[b], 7.5 mg[b], 10 mg, 15 mg[b], 30 mg[b]

[a]Generic available.
[b]Available in the United States only.

Mechanism of Action

The action produced by azapirones is believed to be caused by binding at dopamine (DA2) and 5-HT (5-HT$_{1A}$) receptors. Azapirones are partial agonists at the 5-HT$_{1A}$ receptors. Azapirones have no effect on GABA receptors and lack CNS depressant activity.

Pharmacokinetics

The onset of action of buspirone is slow, and maximum therapeutic effects are achieved 3 to 6 weeks after therapy has been initiated. Buspirone is metabolized in the liver and eliminated in urine. The elimination half-life is between 2 and 3 hours. Food increases the bioavailability of buspirone.

Adverse Reactions

The most common adverse effects associated with buspirone therapy are dizziness, restlessness, headache, nausea, diarrhea, and insomnia. Buspirone produces only minimal sedation.

Precautions

Buspirone should be used with caution in patients with liver or kidney disease.

> **❶ Tech Alert!**
>
> BusPIRone and buPROPion have look-alike/sound-alike issues.

Miscellaneous Anxiolytic Agents

Hydroxyzine

Hydroxyzine is an antihistamine (see Chapter 24) that is also approved for the treatment of GADs. It is a histamine-1 receptor antagonist. Hydroxyzine may be used in children and adults to reduce anxiety associated with dental and minor medical procedures. It produces a fair bit of sedation but, similar to buspirone, does not produce tolerance or dependence. Other side effects are dizziness, headache, dry mucous membranes, and urinary retention.

Men with prostate disease and lactating women should avoid hydroxyzine because the antihistamine decreases urine flow and breast milk. Sedation is increased when the drug is taken with other CNS depressants or alcohol (Table 5.3).

> **❶ Tech Alert!**
>
> HydrOXYzine HCl and hydrOXYzine pamoate have look-alike/sound-alike issues. Verify all prescriptions when the strength and dosage form have been omitted.

❶ Tech Alert!

HydrOXYzine, hydrALAZINE, and HYDROmorphone have look-alike/sound-alike issues.

TABLE 5.3   Miscellaneous Drugs Used in the Treatment of Anxiety

Generic Name	US Brand Name(s) / Canadian Brand(s)	Dosage Forms and Strengths
hydroxyzine HCl[a]	Generics	**Capsules**[b]: 10 mg, 25 mg, 50 mg
	Atarax	**Injection, solution:** 25 mg/mL[c], 50 mg/mL
		Syrup: 10 mg/5 mL (2 mg/mL)
		Tablets[c]: 10 mg, 25 mg, 50 mg
hydroxyzine pamoate[a]	Vistaril	**Capsules**[c]: 25 mg, 50 mg, 100 mg
	Not available	

[a]Generic available.
[b]Available in Canada only.
[c]Available in the United States only.

Antidepressants

Anxiety and depression often are seen in the same patient. Some agents are effective in treating both conditions. Citalopram, escitalopram, fluoxetine, fluvoxamine, paroxetine, and sertraline are SSRIs used in the treatment of anxiety disorders. Duloxetine and paroxetine (SNRIs), clomipramine (TCA), and monoamine oxidase inhibitors (MAOIs) are antidepressants prescribed for the treatment of anxiety disorders (see Chapter 6) (Table 5.4). Fluoxetine and sertraline are indicated for OCD. Sertraline is also labeled for use in the treatment of panic disorder, social phobia, and PTSD. Venlafaxine is an SNRI and is used in the management of GADs. Clomipramine, a TCA, is indicated for the treatment of OCD.

Treatment of OCD with antidepressants requires higher doses than the treatment of depression, and it takes a longer time for maximum benefits to be achieved. For example, clomipramine may take up to 6 weeks for full effects to be noticed. Maximum benefits of fluoxetine and sertraline are achieved in 1 to 3 weeks.

Mechanism of Action

SSRIs inhibit 5-HT reuptake into the presynaptic neuron, increasing 5-HT availability at postsynaptic receptor sites. SNRIs and TCAs inhibit the reuptake of 5-HT and noradrenaline. MAOI binding increases synaptic availability of 5-HT, noradrenaline, and dopamine.

Adverse Reactions

Some adverse reactions are common to all the antidepressants used in the treatment of anxiety. Others are drug specific. Clomipramine

TABLE 5.4   Antidepressants Used in the Treatment of Anxiety

Generic Name	US Brand Name(s) / Canadian Brand(s)	Dosage Forms and Strengths
clomipramine[a]	Anafranil	**Capsules:** 25 mg[b], 50 mg, 75 mg
	Anafranil	**Tablets**[c]: 10 mg, 25 mg, 50 mg
duloxetine[a]	Cymbalta, Drizalma Sprinkle	**Capsules delayed release:** 20 mg[b], 30 mg, 60 mg
	Cymbalta	**Capsule (Drizalma Sprinkle)**[b]: 20 mg, 30 mg, 40 mg, 60 mg
escitalopram[a]	Lexapro	**Oral solution**[b]: 5 mg/5 mL
	Cipralex	**Tablets:** 5 mg[b], 10 mg, 20 mg
fluoxetine[a]	Prozac	**Capsule (Prozac):** 10 mg, 20 mg, 40 mg, 60 mg[c]
	Prozac	**Capsule, delayed release:** 90 mg
		Oral solution: 20 mg/5 mL
		Tablets[b]: 10 mg, 20 mg
paroxetine[a]	Brisdelle, Paxil, Paxil CR, Pexeva	**Capsule, as mesylate (Brisdelle):** 7.5 mg
	Paxil, Paxil CR	**Suspension, oral (Paxil)**[b]: 10 mg/5 mL
		Tablet, as HCl (Paxil): 10 mg, 20 mg, 30 mg, 40 mg[b]
		Tablets, controlled release (Paxil CR): 12.5 mg, 25 mg, 37.5 mg[b]
sertraline[a]	Zoloft	**Capsules**[c]: 25 mg, 50 mg, 100 mg
	Zoloft	**Solution, oral concentrate**[b]: 20 mg/mL
		Tablets[b]: 25 mg, 50 mg, 100 mg
venlafaxine[a]	Effexor XR	**Capsules, extended release (Effexor XR):** 37.5 mg, 75 mg, 150 mg
	Effexor XR	**Tablets**[b]: 25 mg, 37.5 mg, 50 mg, 75 mg, 100 mg
		Tablets, extended release[b]: 37.5 mg, 75 mg, 150 mg, 225 mg
		Tablets, extended release as besylate[b]: 112.5 mg

[a]Generic available.
[b]Available in the United States only.
[c]Available in Canada only.

may produce sedation or decreased alertness; fluoxetine, paroxetine, and sertraline may cause insomnia, decreased appetite, dry mouth, dizziness, and agitation or tremor; and paroxetine may also produce headache, nausea, diarrhea, and sexual dysfunction.

No tolerance or dependence is associated with any of the antidepressants. However, some serious side effects are possible. Clomipramine may produce seizures. Serotonin syndrome is a serious condition associated with the use of drugs such as sertraline and fluoxetine. Serotonin syndrome is potentially fatal and produces symptoms of confusion, agitation, diarrhea, tremors, increased blood pressure, and seizures. A detailed description of specific mechanisms of action and pharmacokinetics of these drugs will be discussed in Chapter 6.

❶ Tech Alert!

ClonazePAM, cloNIDine, and clozapine have look-alike/sound-alike issues.

❶ Tech Alert!

FLUoxetine, DULoxetine, PARoxetine, and fluvoxaMINE have look-alike/sound-alike issues.

Beta-Adrenergic Antagonists

Rapid heart rate is a common symptom of anxiety. Beta-adrenergic antagonists, also known as β-blockers, are administered to reduce palpitations. Beta-adrenergic antagonists are not approved by the US Food and Drug Administration (FDA) for the treatment of anxiety; however, the β-blockers (e.g., propranolol and nadolol) may be prescribed to control the symptoms that accompany anxiety and to prevent stage fright. Propranolol diminishes sympathetic activity in the brain. Recent studies suggest that propranolol may weaken the formation of stressful memories, making it useful in the treatment of PTSD; however, it is not yet approved by the FDA for this use.

TECHNICIAN'S CORNER

1. What happens if a patient stops using benzodiazepines abruptly?
2. What is the difference between tolerance and dependence on a drug?
3. What is social anxiety disorder?

Summary of Drugs Used in the Treatment of Anxiety Disorders

	Generic Name	US Brand Name	Usual Adult Oral Dose and Dosing Schedule	Warning Labels
Benzodiazepines				
	alprazolam	Xanax	**Generalized anxiety disorder:** immediate release 0.25–4 mg daily (in 2–3 divided doses) **Panic disorder:** 1–10 mg/day in 3 divided doses (immediate release); 0.5–6 mg once daily (extended release) **Anxiety associated with depression:** 2.5–3 mg/day in divided doses)	MAY CAUSE DROWSINESS; MAY IMPAIR ABILITY TO DRIVE. AVOID ALCOHOL. MAY BE HABIT FORMING. DO NOT CRUSH, BREAK, OR CHEW (extended release).
	clonazepam	Klonopin	**Panic disorder:** 0.25–1 mg twice a day (maximum, 4 mg/day)	
	clorazepate	Tranxene	**Generalized anxiety disorder:** 7.5–15 mg 2–4 times/day (immediate release); 11.25–22.5 mg once daily (sustained release) **Ethanol withdrawal:** 30 mg 2–4 times/day; increase up to maximum of 90 mg/day (reduce gradually)	
	diazepam	Valium, Diastat	**Anxiety disorder:** 2–10 mg 2–4 times/day (oral); 2–10 mg every 3–4 hours (IM, IV) **Ethanol withdrawal:** 5–10 mg IV every 3–4 hours as needed	
	lorazepam	Ativan	**Anxiety and sedation:** Oral 1–10 mg daily in 2–3 divided doses **Preprocedure sedation:** 0.05 mg/kg IM (maximum, 4 mg/dose) or 0.044 mg/kg IV (maximum, 2 mg/dose)	

Continued

Summary of Drugs Used in the Treatment of Anxiety Disorders—cont'd

	Generic Name	US Brand Name	Usual Adult Oral Dose and Dosing Schedule	Warning Labels
	midazolam	generic	**Conscious sedation for preoperative procedures:** 0.5–2 mg slow IV every 2–3 min (maximum, 2.5–5 mg)	MAY CAUSE DIZZINESS AND DISORIENTATION. MAY CAUSE PAIN, SWELLING, OR REDNESS AT INJECTION SITE.
	oxazepam	generic	**Anxiety:** 10–30 mg 3–4 times a day	MAY CAUSE DROWSINESS; MAY IMPAIR ABILITY TO DRIVE. AVOID ALCOHOL. MAY BE HABIT FORMING. DO NOT CRUSH, BREAK, OR CHEW (extended release).
			Ethanol withdrawal: 15–30 mg 3–4 times a day	
Azapirones				
	buspirone	generic	7.5–15 mg twice daily (maximum dose, 60 mg/day)	MAY CAUSE DROWSINESS; MAY IMPAIR ABILITY TO DRIVE. TAKE WITH FOOD.
Miscellaneous Anxiolytics				
	hydroxyzine HCl	Atarax	**Anxiety:** 25–100 mg 4 times a day (maximum dose, 400 mg/day) **Ethanol withdrawal:** 50–100 mg IM 4 times a day	MAY CAUSE DROWSINESS; AVOID ALCOHOL, MAY INTENSIFY THIS EFFECT.
	hydroxyzine pamoate	Vistaril	**Anxiety:** 50–100 mg IM 4 times a day	MAY IMPAIR ABILITY TO DRIVE.
			Preoperative sedation: 50–100 mg as a single dose (oral); 25–100 mg (IM)	
Antidepressants Used in the Treatment of Anxiety Disorders				
	clomipramine	Anafranil	**Obsessive-compulsive disorder:** 25–100 mg/day in divided doses (maximum, 250 mg/day)	MAY CAUSE DIZZINESS OR DROWSINESS; ALCOHOL MAY INTENSIFY THIS EFFECT.
	duloxetine	Cymbalta	**Generalized anxiety disorder:** 60 mg PO once daily	MAY IMPAIR ABILITY TO DRIVE. SWALLOW WHOLE; DO NOT CRUSH OR CHEW (delayed and extended release—Cymbalta, Prozac weekly, Paxil CR, Effexor XR). DO NOT DISCONTINUE WITHOUT MEDICAL SUPERVISION.
	escitalopram	Lexapro, Cipralex[a]	**Generalized anxiety disorder:** 10–20 mg once daily	
	fluoxetine	Prozac	**Obsessive-compulsive disorder:** 20–80 mg/day	
			Panic disorder: 20 mg/day (maximum, 60 mg/day)	
	paroxetine	Paxil	**Generalized anxiety disorder:** 20–50 mg/day	
			Obsessive-compulsive disorder: 20–60 mg/day	
			Panic disorder: 10–60 mg/day (Paxil, Pexeva) or 12.5–75 mg/day (Paxil CR)	
			Posttraumatic stress disorder: 12.5–25 mg daily (Paxil CR) 20 mg/day (immediate release)	
			Social phobias: 20 mg/day (Paxil) or 12.5–37.5 mg/day (Paxil CR)	
	sertraline	Zoloft	**Obsessive-compulsive disorder:** 50 mg/day (maximum 400 mg/day)	
			Panic disorder, posttraumatic stress disorder, and social phobias: 50 mg/day (up to 200 mg/day)	
	venlafaxine	Effexor XR	**Generalized anxiety disorder, panic disorder, and social phobias:** 37.5–75 mg once daily (maximum 225 mg/day); increase by 37.5 mg every 4–7 days	

[a]Available in Canada only. *IM,* Intramuscular; *IV,* intravenous; *PO,* oral.

Key Points

- Anxiety disorders are the leading mental health illness.
- The cause of anxiety disorders may be environmental, biologic, or developmental; associated with socioeconomic conditions; or a combination of several of these individual factors.
- The four major types of anxiety disorders are generalized anxiety disorder, panic disorder, obsessive-compulsive disorder, and posttraumatic stress disorder.
- Common physiologic symptoms include increased heart rate, palpitations, shortness of breath, rapid breathing, nausea, sweating, and dry mouth. All of these symptoms are associated with hyperactivity of the autonomic nervous system.
- Generalized anxiety disorder is associated with excessive worry and tension that are experienced daily for longer than 6 months.
- Obsessive-compulsive disorder is a condition associated with an inability to control or stop repeated unwanted thoughts or behaviors.
- Panic disorder is a condition associated with repeated sudden onset of feelings of terror.
- A phobia is an irrational fear of things or situations that produce symptoms of intense anxiety.
- Social phobias cause affected individuals to shy away from social situations where they fear embarrassment or humiliation. Fear of public speaking is an example of a social phobia.
- Posttraumatic stress disorder is a stress disorder that develops in persons who have participated in, witnessed, or been a victim of a terrifying event.
- Anxiety disorder is treated by the administration of anxiolytics and psychotherapy, including cognitive behavioral therapy.
- The mechanism of action for most anxiolytics is to enhance binding of the neurotransmitter GABA to receptors.
- Benzodiazepines are used in the treatment of anxiety.
- Benzodiazepines may have a long-acting, intermediate-acting, or short-acting duration of action.
- Benzodiazepines can produce a type of amnesia that causes the person receiving the drug to "forget," reducing anxiety associated with future dental or medical procedures.
- All benzodiazepines are capable of producing tolerance and dependence.
- When tolerance develops, increasing doses of a drug are required to achieve the same effects as were achieved previously at lower doses. When drug dependence has developed, the person taking the drug must continue to take the drug to avoid the onset of physiologic or psychological withdrawal symptoms (or both).
- All benzodiazepines are scheduled class IV controlled substances in the United States and are targeted substances in Canada.
- Withdrawal symptoms develop soon after discontinuation of benzodiazepines with short half-lives and are delayed after abrupt discontinuation of benzodiazepines that have long half-lives.
- Buspirone is an azapirone that is used to treat anxiety.
- Buspirone does not produce tolerance or dependence. Abrupt discontinuation does not produce withdrawal symptoms.
- Hydroxyzine is an antihistamine that is indicated for the treatment of anxiety. It is used in children and adults to reduce anxiety associated with dental and minor medical procedures.
- TCAs, SSRIs, and MAOIs are antidepressants prescribed for the treatment of anxiety disorders.
- Serotonin syndrome is a potentially life-threatening adverse drug reaction caused by excessive 5-HT that produces symptoms of confusion, agitation, diarrhea, tremors, increased blood pressure, and seizures.
- Beta-adrenergic antagonists are administered to reduce the palpitations associated with anxiety and are also useful for the management of stage fright.

Review Questions

1. Is the following statement true or false? "Women are twice as likely as men to be diagnosed with generalized anxiety disorder."
   a. true
   b. false
2. The_____ treatment of anxiety is associated with increases in drug-receptor binding to the neurotransmitters γ-aminobutyric acid, serotonin, and norepinephrine.
   a. therapeutic
   b. psychological
   c. pharmacologic
   d. physiologic
3. Anxiety disorder is treated by the administration of _____ and psychotherapy.
   a. analgesics
   b. anxiolytics
   c. antiinflammatories
   d. antipsychotics
4. Benzodiazepines are indicated for _____ treatment of anxiety.
   a. short-term
   b. long-term

5. _____ to a drug is said to have developed when the patient must take increasing doses to achieve the same effects as were achieved previously at lower doses.
   a. Dependence
   b. Addiction
   c. Tolerance
   d. none of the above
6. Which of the following benzodiazepines is indicated for the treatment of anxiety disorders, ethanol withdrawal, skeletal muscle relaxation, and seizure disorders?
   a. Alprazolam
   b. Clonazepam
   c. Lorazepam
   d. Diazepam
7. Buspirone is the only drug in this class.
   a. Azapirone
   b. Antihistamine
   c. Amiodarone
   d. a and c

8. _____ is an antihistamine that is indicated for the treatment of anxiety.
   a. Promethazine
   b. Hydroxyzine
   c. Apresoline
   d. none of the above
9. Clomipramine, fluoxetine, and sertraline are antidepressants that are indicated for the treatment of
   a. panic disorders
   b. social phobias
   c. obsessive-compulsive disorder
   d. posttraumatic stress disorder
10. Rapid heart rate is a common symptom of anxiety. Beta-adrenergic antagonists are administered to reduce the palpitations. One example is:
   a. Propranolol
   b. Diazepam
   c. Escitalopram
   d. Hydroxyzine

Bibliography

Anxiety & Depression Association of America. (2022). Anxiety Disorders – Facts & Statistics. Retrieved June 25, 2022, from https://adaa.org/understanding-anxiety/facts-statistics.

Anxiety & Depression Association of America: Generalized Anxiety Disorder (GAD). Retrieved June 25, 2022, from https://www.adaa.org/understanding-anxiety/generalized-anxiety-disorder-gad.

Bourin M. Serotoninergic systems in anxiety. *JSM Anxiety Depress.* 2016;1(2):1007.

Health Canada. (2022). Drug Product Database. Retrieved July 9, 2022, from https://health-products.canada.ca/dpd-bdpp/index-eng.jsp.

Greenberg W, Aronson S. Obsessive-compulsive disorder, eMedicine 2016. Retrieved June 25, 2022, from http://emedicine.medscape.com/article/1934139-overview.

Institute for Safe Medication Practices. (2016). FDA and ISMP Lists of Look-Alike Drug Names with Recommended Tall Man Letters. Retrieved June 24, 2022, from https://www.ismp.org/recommendations/tall-man-letters-list.

Institute for Safe Medication Practices. (2019). List of Confused Drugs. Retrieved June 24, 2022, from https://www.ismp.org/tools/confused-drugnames.pdf.

National Institute of Mental Health: Generalized Anxiety Disorders: When worry gets out of control. U.S. Department of Health and Human Services NIH publication no. QF 16-4677, Bethesda, MD, 2016.

National Institute of Mental Health: Panic Disorder: When fear overwhelms. U.S. Department of Health and Human Services NIH publication no. QF 16-4679, Bethesda, MD.

National Institute of Mental Health, National Institutes of Health: Anxiety Disorders, 2016. Retrieved June 25, 2022, from https://www.nimh.nih.gov/health/topics/anxiety-disorders.

Osland S, Arnold PD, Pringsheim T. The prevalence of diagnosed obsessive compulsive disorder and associated comorbidities: a population-based Canadian study. *Psychiatry Res.* 2018;268:137–142.

Page C, Curtis M, Sutter M, et al. *Integrated pharmacology.* Philadelphia: Elsevier Mosby; 2005:239–241.

Public Health Agency of Canada: Mood and Anxiety Disorders in Canada, 2014. Retrieved June 26, 2022, from http://healthycanadians.gc.ca/publications/diseases-conditions-maladies-affections/mental-mood-anxiety-anxieux-humeur/alt/mental-mood-anxiety-anxieux-humeur-eng.pdf.

Raffa R, Rawls S, Beyzarov E. *Netter's illustrated pharmacology, Philadelphia.* WB. Saunders; 2005:65–66.

Ravindran L, Stein MB. The pharmacologic treatment of anxiety disorders: a review of progress. *J Clin Psychiatry.* 2010;71(7):839–854.

Statistics Canada. (2020). Canadian Community Health Survey, 2019. Understanding the perceived mental health of Canadians prior to the COVID-19 pandemic. Retrieved June 25, 2022, from https://www150.statcan.gc.ca/n1/daily-quotidien/200806/dq200806a-eng.htm.

U.S. Food and Drug Administration. (nd). Drugs@FDA: FDA Approved Drugs. Retrieved July 9, 2022. from https://www.accessdata.fda.gov/scripts/cder/daf/index.cfm.

6

Treatment of Depression

LEARNING OBJECTIVES

1. Learn the terminology associated with depression and its treatment.
2. List and describe the function of neurotransmitters associated with symptoms of depression.
3. Classify medications used to treat depression.
4. Describe mechanism of action for each class of drugs used to treat depression.
5. Identify significant drug look-alike and sound-alike issues.
6. Identify warning labels and precautionary messages associated with medications used to treat depression.

KEY TERMS

Adjunct drug therapy Initiated to complement the effects of another drug.

Bipolar affective disorder Mental health illness associated with repeated episodes of mood swings between depression and periods of mania, racing thoughts, distractibility, and increased goal-directed behavior.

Enuresis Bedwetting or uncontrollable urination during sleep.

Major depressive disorder Mental health illness associated with persistent feelings of intense sadness and loss of interest in activities that were previously enjoyable.

Monoamine oxidase Enzyme found in the liver, intestine, and terminal neuron, responsible for degradation of monoamine neurotransmitters and dietary amines.

Serotonin syndrome Potentially life-threatening adverse drug reaction that produces symptoms of confusion, agitation, diarrhea, tremors, and increased blood pressure and is caused by excessive serotonin.

Overview

In 2020, an estimated 21 million Americans over the age of 18 years experienced a major depressive episode according to the National Institute of Mental Health. The prevalence was highest in young adults between the ages of 18 and 25 years. At some time in their lives, 1 in 5 Canadian adults will experience a mood disorder such as depression. Major depression affects approximately 5.4% of Canadian adults. Depression affects men, women, and children. Depressive disorder may be precipitated by hormonal changes (premenstrual syndrome, pregnancy, postpartum), substance abuse (alcohol and other drugs), or illness such as Parkinson disease, heart attack, or thyroid dysfunction. It is also associated with social determinants of health such as racism, poverty, homelessness, discrimination, and unemployment. Heredity plays a role as well, particularly in bipolar disorder because children born to a parent with bipolar disorder are at increased risk for the illness.

Depressive illness influences most aspects of a person's life and lifestyle. It affects self-esteem, mood, thoughts, eating, and sleeping. Depression reduces the ability to think and concentrate. Feelings of worthlessness or guilt often accompany depressive episodes. As many as 12% of depressed patients contemplate or attempt suicide. Without treatment, symptoms of depression can persist for a few weeks to years.

The three primary types of depressive disorders are major depression, bipolar disorder, and dysthymia. *Major depressive disorder* (MDD) is also called *clinical depression* and is associated with feelings of intense sadness. These feelings persist for several weeks and are usually accompanied by a lack of interest in activities that were previously thought to be enjoyable, fatigue, irritability, and insomnia or hypersomnia. Sometimes the depression manifests itself in other physical ailments for which no treatments are able to cure or reduce symptoms. *Bipolar disorder*, formerly called *manic-depressive disorder*, is associated with sudden swings in mood between depression and periods of mania. Mania is associated with hyperactivity, racing thoughts, insomnia, distractibility, and increased goal-directed behavior. Manic periods can last for 1 or more weeks, during which time the person may sleep little and produce a prolific amount of work. Several well-known people such as Vincent Van Gogh are believed to have had bipolar disorder. *Dysthymia* produces symptoms that are similar to major depression, but the symptoms are less severe. People diagnosed with dysthymia have symptoms that are chronic and, although not typically debilitating, keep the person from functioning well and feeling good.

The causes of depression are not completely known, but a deficiency of certain neurotransmitters is involved. This explains why people with depression cannot "pull themselves together" to get better. Drug treatment is aimed at restoring depleted neurotransmitters to normal levels.

Neurochemistry of Depression

Biogenic Amine Theory

According to the biogenic amine hypothesis, major depression results from a decrease in monoamine neurotransmitters in the brain. This hypothesis was made upon the discovery that patients treated with drugs that deplete monoamine neurotransmitter stores in the neuron develop depression. Neurotransmitter binding sites are also less sensitive in depressed persons.

In contrast, if depletion of monoamine neurotransmitters causes depression, what is the effect of excessive levels of these neurotransmitters? Bipolar affective disorder (BPAD) is believed to be associated with increased levels of monoamine neurotransmitters (Fig. 6.1). The complete neurochemistry of BPAD is unclear.

The monoamine neurotransmitters that are thought to be involved in depression and BPAD are norepinephrine (NE), serotonin (5-HT), and dopamine (DA).

Role of Norepinephrine

The neurotransmitter NE plays an important role in the treatment of depression. It is widely distributed in the brain and in the periphery. Decreased levels in the brain are responsible for depression, and increased levels in the periphery can cause serious effects such as hypertension.

Role of Serotonin

5-HT plays an important role in the treatment of depression. 5-HT is an excitatory neurotransmitter. More than nine 5-HT receptors have been identified. 5-HT receptors that have been well studied are 5-HT_{1A}, 5-HT_{2A}, 5-HT_{2C}, and 5-HT_3. Drugs that antagonize 5-HT_{2A} and 5-HT_{2C} receptors are used in the treatment of depression and negative-symptom schizophrenia. Drugs that antagonize 5-HT_3 receptors are used to treat nausea. In addition to improved mood, 5-HT is involved in regulation of the sleep-wake cycle and pain perception.

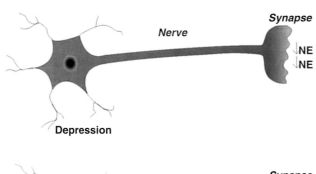

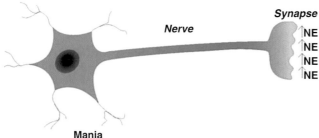

• **Fig. 6.1** Biogenic amine hypothesis. (From Lilley LL, Collins S, Snyder JS. *Pharmacology and the nursing process*, ed 8, St Louis, 2017, Elsevier.)

Role of Dopamine

There are five types of DA receptors. Binding to D2, D3, and D4 receptors is inhibitory, and binding to D1 and D5 is excitatory. DA binding plays less of a role in the treatment and management of depression compared with the neurotransmitters NE and 5-HT. Drugs that are used in the treatment of Parkinson disease and schizophrenia potentiate the activity of DA (see Chapter 8).

Drugs Used to Treat Depression

Antidepressants are categorized according to the method that they use to potentiate the actions of NE, 5-HT, and DA. Nonspecific antidepressants increase the binding of more than one monoamine neurotransmitter. There are two primary mechanisms of action (MOAs) of marketed antidepressants (Fig. 6.2). One MOA is inhibition of the reuptake of one or more of the monoamine neurotransmitters involved in depression. The other MOA is to block the degradation of monoamine neurotransmitters. The MOAs for drugs used to treat depression may differ, but all antidepressants are equally effective. Selection of one antidepressant over another is based on the patient's ability to tolerate drug side effects. The effects of antidepressants are not immediate and increase over time.

Tricyclic Antidepressants

The tricyclic antidepressants (TCAs) are the oldest class of medication used in the treatment of depression. The effectiveness of newer agents is compared with that of TCAs. The TCAs are used for the treatment and management of several medical conditions in addition to depression. They are also prescribed for *enuresis*, commonly known as bedwetting (imipramine and nortriptyline). They are prescribed for the treatment of obsessive-compulsive disorder (clomipramine) and as *adjunct drug therapy* in the management of chronic pain (amitriptyline, nortriptyline). Doxepin is prescribed for sleep disorders in lower doses than used for depression. Doxepin is also prescribed as a cream for itching.

Mechanism of Action

In depression, sufficient neurotransmitters may be released into the synaptic cleft; however, the neurotransmitters may be returned to the neuron before binding occurs. The TCAs work by producing a nonspecific blockade of the reuptake of monoamine neurotransmitters. The TCAs block the reuptake of NE and 5-HT in the presynaptic neuron and in postsynaptic receptors. When the reuptake of NE and 5-HT into the neuron is blocked, the neurotransmitters remain in the synaptic cleft longer. The longer the neurotransmitter remains in the synaptic cleft, the greater the opportunity for binding to receptor sites (Fig. 6.3). The TCAs also have some affinity for adrenergic, cholinergic (muscarinic), and histaminic postsynaptic receptors.

Pharmacokinetics

The TCAs are readily absorbed when administered orally. They are lipophilic, so they are widely distributed within the central nervous system. The onset of action, duration of action, and half-life ($t^{1/2}$) vary among agents. The $t^{1/2}$ of the TCAs can be as short as 4 hours (imipramine) and as long as 96 hours (nortriptyline). Their long half-lives are associated with their high degree of lipid solubility.

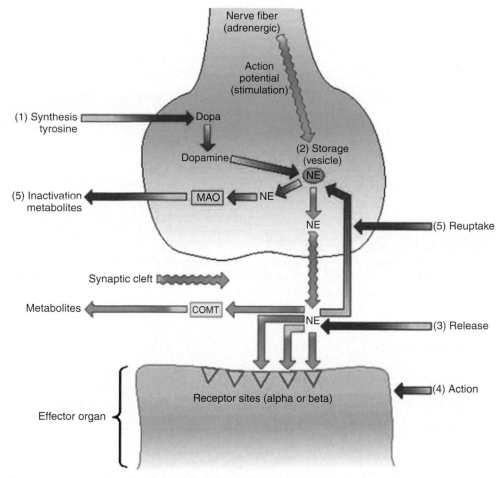

• **Fig. 6.2** Site of neurotransmitter synthesis, storage, release, action, and inactivation. (From Lilley LL, Harrington S, Snyder JS. *Pharmacology and the nursing process*, ed 5, St Louis, 2007, Mosby.)

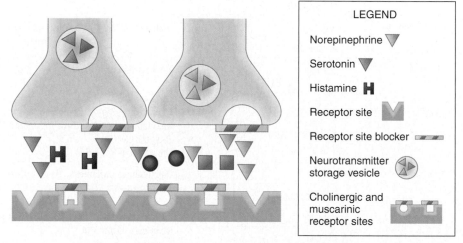

LEGEND

Norepinephrine ▼

Serotonin ▼

Histamine **H**

Receptor site

Receptor site blocker

Neurotransmitter storage vesicle

Cholinergic and muscarinic receptor sites

• **Fig. 6.3** Mechanism of action for tricyclic antidepressants.

The long duration of action of these agents permits once-daily dosing.

The TCAs are metabolized by microsomal enzymes in the liver. Several of the TCAs are metabolized to active metabolites. Amitriptyline is metabolized to nortriptyline, and desipramine is a metabolite of imipramine. They are ultimately eliminated in the urine.

Although the onset of action may be relatively short, maximum antidepressant benefit may take up to 6 weeks to be achieved.

Tech Note!

Dry mouth is a side effect of TCAs. It can be relieved by sucking on sugarless candy. TCAs can also increase cravings for sweets!

Adverse Reactions

The TCAs all have a similar structure, so the side effects of the drugs are similar. What varies is the degree to which a particular

TCA will produce the side effect. For example, all TCAs can produce sedation, but some TCAs, such as amitriptyline, have high sedative activity, whereas other TCAs, such as desipramine, have low sedative activity.

TCA adverse reactions are related to effects produced by increased binding to adrenergic, cholinergic, serotonergic, and histaminic receptors. Increased cardiovascular activity is caused by the rise in NE levels. Hypotension and reflex tachycardia are caused by postsynaptic adrenergic blockade. Sedation, weight gain, and hypotension are produced by histaminic receptor blockade. Blockade of cholinergic (muscarinic) receptors can lead to blurred vision, dry mouth, constipation, urinary retention, confusion, and delirium. The TCAs may also produce photosensitivity.

> ● **Tech Note!**
>
> Prescriptions for small quantities of the TCAs may be written for patients with depression who are believed to be suicidal.

Precautions

Hypotension produced by the TCAs is a problem for elderly adults because they are at increased risk for fainting or falling. The TCAs have a narrow therapeutic index and can produce cardiotoxicity at doses that are six to eight times higher than the therapeutic dose.

> ● **Tech Alert!**
>
> The TCAs should not be discontinued abruptly; patients should be gradually weaned off the drug.

Selective Serotonin Reuptake Inhibitors

Citalopram (Celexa), escitalopram (Cipralex), fluoxetine (Prozac), fluvoxamine (Luvox), paroxetine (Paxil), sertraline (Zoloft), vilazodone (Viibryd), and vortioxetine (Trintellix) are selective serotonin reuptake inhibitors (SSRIs). The SSRIs are the most widely prescribed antidepressants. They are categorized by their MOAs rather than by their chemical structure. The SSRIs are also

Tricyclic Antidepressants

	Generic Name	US Brand Name(s) / Canadian Brand(s)	Dosage Forms and Strengths
	amitriptyline[a]	Generics Elavil	**Tablets:** 10 mg, 25 mg, 50 mg, 75 mg, 100 mg, 150 mg[b]
	amoxapine[a]	Generics Not available	**Tablets:** 25 mg, 50 mg, 100 mg, 150 mg
	clomipramine[a]	Anafranil Anafranil	**Capsules:** 10 mg[d], 25 mg, 50 mg, 75 mg[b]
	desipramine[a]	Norpramin Generic only	**Tablets:** 10 mg, 25 mg, 50 mg, 75 mg, 100 mg, 150 mg[b]
	doxepin[a]	Silenor, Zonalon[c] Sinequan, Silenor	**Capsules:** 10 mg, 25 mg, 50 mg, 75 mg, 100 mg **Solution, oral concentrate**[b]: 10 mg/mL **Tablet:** 3 mg, 6 mg **Cream (Zonalon)**[b]: 5%
	imipramine[a]	Tofranil Generics only	**Capsules, as pamoate**[b]: 75 mg, 100 mg, 125 mg, 150 mg **Tablets, as HCl:** 10 mg, 25 mg, 50 mg, 75 mg[d]
	nortriptyline[a]	Pamelor Aventyl	**Capsules:** 10 mg, 25 mg, 50 mg[b], 75 mg[b] **Solution**[b]: 10 mg/5 mL
	protriptyline[a]	Generics only Not available	**Tablets:** 5 mg, 10 mg
	trimipramine[a]	Generics only Generics only	**Capsules:** 25 mg[b], 50 mg[b], 75 mg[d], 100 mg[b] **Tablets**[d]: 12.5 mg, 25 mg, 50 mg

[a]Generic available.
[b]Available in the United States only.
[c]Zonalon is a cream that is used for the treatment of itching.
[d]Available in Canada only.

used in treating obsessive-compulsive disorder, premenstrual dysphoric disorder, and panic disorder. Fluoxetine is also indicated for treatment of anorexia and bulimia.

Mechanism of Action

The SSRIs are potent inhibitors of 5-HT, yet they have little action on the reuptake of NE or DA. They produce a selective blockade of the reuptake of 5-HT at the synaptic cleft. The SSRIs are equally effective as TCAs, yet they lack the cardiotoxic effects associated with the TCAs. This makes them the drugs of choice when heart disease is present.

Pharmacokinetics

The SSRIs are well absorbed from the gastrointestinal tract. Some, such as fluoxetine, are metabolized to an active metabolite producing a long duration of action. There are many drug interactions involving SSRIs because they are extensively metabolized via the cytochrome P-450 (CYP450) isoenzyme system in the liver and are also highly protein bound. Drug interactions may interfere with the rate of drug clearance of either the SSRI or drug that is administered with it. Therefore the effects and/or side effects of drugs coadministered with SSRIs may be increased.

Adverse Reactions

Insomnia is one of the more common side effects of SSRI administration. Fluoxetine and other SSRIs are dosed once daily in the morning to minimize nighttime sleeplessness. Other side effects include decreased appetite, nausea, agitation or anxiety, and diarrhea. Sexual dysfunction may also occur. The most serious side effects are serotonin syndrome and suicidal ideation. Suicidal ideation is characterized by persistent thoughts of suicide. Symptoms of *serotonin syndrome* are confusion, agitation, diarrhea, tremors, increased blood pressure, and seizures. Both conditions are potentially fatal.

● Tech Note!

Patients should be advised to suck sugarless candy to control the dry mouth caused by fluvoxamine.

Precautions

The SSRIs are fairly well tolerated, but to avoid adverse reactions, the dose should be increased gradually to desired levels, and the dose should be tapered to discontinue the drug. Serotonin syndrome can result from coadministration with monoamine oxidase inhibitors (MAOIs). The SSRIs should be used cautiously in patients with liver disease.

● Tech Note!

Doxepin oral concentrate should not be diluted in carbonated beverages.

Monoamine Oxidase Inhibitors

MAOIs are used to treat depression and Parkinson disease. *Monoamine oxidase* is an enzyme. The enzyme inactivates neurotransmitters that have been released so they do not accumulate when no longer needed. There are two forms of MAO: subtype A (MAO_A) and subtype B (MAO_B). MAO_A is found in the terminal neuron, liver, and intestines, and MAO_B is predominantly found in the brain.

Selective Serotonin Reuptake Inhibitors

Generic Name	US Brand Name(s) / Canadian Brand(s)	Dosage Forms and Strengths
citalopram[a]	Celexa	**Solution, oral[b]:** 10 mg/5 mL
	Celexa	**Tablet:** 10 mg, 20 mg, 30 mg[c], 40 mg **Tablet, disintegrating:** 40 mg[b]
escitalopram[a]	Lexapro	**Solution, oral[b]:** 1 mg/mL (240 mL)
	Cipralex	**Tablet:** 5 mg[b], 10 mg, 20 mg **Tablet, disintegrating:** 10 mg, 20 mg[c]
fluoxetine[a]	Prozac	**Capsule:** 10 mg, 20 mg, 40 mg[b], 60 mg[c]
	Prozac	**Capsule, delayed release (Prozac Weekly)[b]:** 90 mg **Solution, oral:** 20 mg/5 mL **Tablet[b]:** 10 mg, 20 mg
fluoxetine + olanzapine	Symbyax	**Capsules:**
	Not available	fluoxetine 25 mg + olanzapine 3 mg fluoxetine 25 mg + olanzapine 6 mg fluoxetine 25 mg + olanzapine 12 mg fluoxetine 50 mg + olanzapine 6 mg fluoxetine 50 mg + olanzapine 12 mg
fluvoxamine[a]	Luvox	**Capsule, extended release[b]:** 100 mg, 150 mg
	Luvox	**Tablet:** 25 mg[b], 50 mg, 100 mg

Continued

Selective Serotonin Reuptake Inhibitors—cont'd

Generic Name	US Brand Name(s) Canadian Brand(s)	Dosage Forms and Strengths
paroxetine[a]	Brisdelle, Paxil, Paxil CR, Pexeva Paxil, Paxil CR	**Capsule, as mesylate (Brisdelle)**[b]: 7.5 mg **Suspension, oral**[b]: 10 mg/5 mL **Tablets, as HCl (Paxil):** 10 mg, 20 mg, 30 mg, 40 mg[b] **Tablets, as controlled release (Paxil CR):** 12.5 mg, 25 mg, 37.5 mg[b] **Tablets, as mesylate (Pexeva)**[b]: 10 mg, 20 mg, 30 mg, 40 mg
sertraline[a]	Zoloft Zoloft	**Capsules:** 25 mg, 50 mg, 100 mg **Solution, oral concentrate:** 20 mg/mL[b] **Tablets**[b]: 25 mg, 50 mg, 100 mg
vilazodone[a,b]	Viibryd Viibryd	**Tablets:** 10 mg, 20 mg, 40 mg
vortioxetine	Trintellix Trintellix	**Tablet:** 5 mg, 10 mg, 20 mg

[a]Generic available.
[b]Available in the United States only.

Mechanism of Action

The MAOIs interfere with the breakdown of monoamine neurotransmitters and dietary amines (e.g., tyramine) (Fig. 6.4). The MAOIs that are used in the treatment of major depression primarily interfere with the action of MAO_A. Drugs that preferentially interfere with MAO_B are used in the treatment of Parkinson disease.

Pharmacokinetics

The MAOIs are readily absorbed when taken orally, but elimination is slow. The drugs are categorized as reversible or irreversible inhibitors of MAO according to the time it takes for enzyme levels to return to normal when the drug is discontinued. It takes approximately 3 to 5 days for MAO levels to return to normal after discontinuation of reversible MAOIs. Recovery takes up to 2 weeks when irreversible MAOIs are administered.

Adverse Reactions

The MAOIs were first discovered in the 1950s, but the risk for serious side effects has limited their widespread use. Mild adverse reactions include sedation, dry mouth, urinary retention, constipation, orthostatic hypotension, impotence, and weight gain. The severity of these side effects is equal to or less than that of most TCAs. The most serious adverse reaction is hypertensive crisis.

Hypertensive crisis can be fatal and is caused by drug-drug and drug-food interactions with MAOIs. When MAOIs are administered, their effect on MAO in the liver is to block the breakdown of dietary amines (e.g., tyramine). As tyramine levels increase in the general circulation, the tyramine travels to peripheral sympathetic nerve terminals, where it promotes the release of NE stores. Excess circulating NE causes blood pressure to rise to dangerously high levels and produces excessive stimulation of the heart.

● Tech Note!

Symptoms of hypertensive crisis are throbbing headache, neck stiffness, and palpitations.

Precautions

To avoid the risk of hypertensive crisis, patients taking MAOIs are advised to avoid eating certain foods and beverages containing high amounts of tyramine (Table 6.1).

Serotonin-Noradrenaline Reuptake Inhibitors

Duloxetine (Cymbalta), desvenlafaxine (Pristiq), levomilnacipran (Fatzima), and venlafaxine (Effexor) are serotonin-noradrenaline reuptake inhibitors (SNRIs). They inhibit the reuptake of 5-HT and NE. Dual inhibition of 5-HT and NE is more effective than inhibition of either 5-HT or NE alone.

Adverse Reactions

Their side effects are similar to SSRIs, but, unlike the SSRIs, the SNRIs produce anticholinergic side effects, a modest increase in blood pressure, and may cause hepatotoxicity. Common side effects of venlafaxine, desvenlafaxine, and duloxetine are nausea,

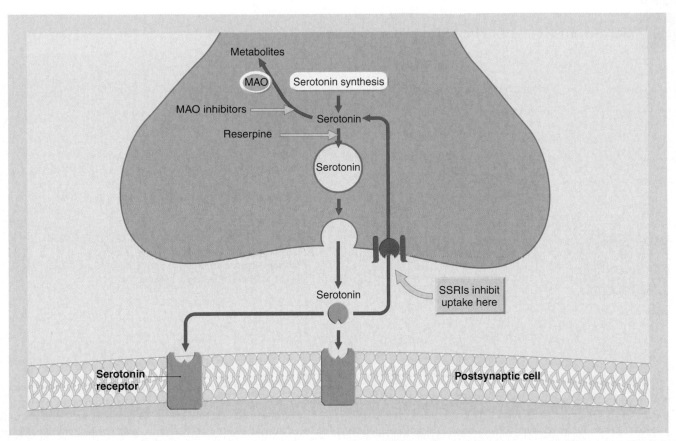

• **Fig. 6.4** Mechanism of action of monoamine oxidase inhibitors. (From Page CP, Hoffman B, Curtis MJ, et al: *Integrated pharmacology*, ed 3, Philadelphia, 2006, Mosby.)

Monoamine Oxidase Inhibitors

Generic Name	US Brand Name(s) Canadian Brand(s)	Dosage Forms and Strengths
isocarboxazid	Marplan	**Tablets:** 10 mg
	Not available	
moclobemide[a,b]	Not available	**Tablets:** 100 mg, 150 mg, 300 mg
	Manerix	
phenelzine[c]	Nardil	**Tablets:** 15 mg
	Nardil	
selegiline[c]	Emsam	**Transdermal patch:** 6 mg/24 h, 9 mg/24 h, 12 mg/24 h
	Patch not available	
tranylcypromine[a,c]	Parnate	**Tablets:** 10 mg
	Parnate	

[a]Generic available.
[b]Reversible MAOI.
[c]Irreversible MAOI.

TABLE 6.1	Foods and Beverages to Avoid While Taking Monoamine Oxidase Inhibitors
Beverages	Chianti, other red wines, alcohol-free beer, caffeine
Food	Cheeses (especially strong, aged, or processed varieties), sauerkraut, yogurt, raisins, bananas, sour cream, pickled herring, liver (especially chicken liver), dry sausage (including hard salami and pepperoni), canned figs, avocados, turkey, yeast extracts, fava beans, broad bean pods, chocolate
Seasonings	Soy sauce, papaya products (including certain meat tenderizers)

● **Tech Note!**

Patients taking MAOIs should be given a list of tyramine-containing foods and a list of drugs to avoid.

Atypical Antidepressants

Bupropion, mirtazapine, nefazodone, trazodone, and brexpiprazole are atypical antidepressants. In addition to depression, bupropion is used to treat seasonal affective disorder and smoking cessation. Contrave® is a combination drug containing bupropion and naltrexone that is used to treat obesity. Schizophrenia is the primary indication for Rexulti® (brexpiprazole); however, the drug is also used as an adjunct to antidepressants for the treatment of major depressive disorder (see Chapter 7).

headache, dry mouth, and dizziness. Sedation is common with venlafaxine and desvenlafaxine. Duloxetine may cause asthenia (weakness).

Serotonin-Noradrenaline Reuptake Inhibitors

Generic Name	US Brand Name(s) Canadian Brand(s)	Dosage Forms and Strengths
desvenlafaxine[a]	Pristiq	Tablets, extended release: 25 mg[b] 50 mg, 100 mg
	Pristiq	
duloxetine[a]	Cymbalta, Drizalma Sprinkle	Capsules, delayed release: 20 mg[b], 30 mg, 60 mg
	Cymbalta	Capsule (Drizalma Sprinkle)[b]: 20 mg, 30 mg, 40 mg, 60 mg
levomilnacipran	Fetzima	Capsule, extended release: 20 mg, 40 mg, 80 mg, 120 mg
	Fetzima	
venlafaxine[a]	Effexor-XR	Capsules, as extended release (Effexor-XR): 37.5 mg, 75 mg, 150 mg
	Effexor-XR	Tablets[b]: 25 mg, 37.5 mg, 50 mg, 75 mg, 100 mg
		Tablets, extended release[b]: 37.5 mg, 75 mg, 150 mg, 225 mg
		Tablet, extended release, as besylate: 112.5 mg

[a]Generic available.
[b]Available in the United States only.

Mechanism of Action

Bupropion is a noradrenaline-DA inhibitor. Mirtazapine affects NE and 5-HT levels. It is metabolized by hepatic microsomal enzymes and is subject to drug interactions involving activation and inhibition of CYP450 isozymes. Trazodone is a weak inhibitor of 5-HT.

> **Tech Note!**
>
> Contents of Effexor-XR capsules and Drizalma Sprinkle can be sprinkled onto food.

Adverse Reactions

Although it is well tolerated, bupropion in doses greater than 450 mg/day or 150 mg/dose increases the risk for seizures in people with seizure disorders. Mirtazapine may cause drowsiness or dizziness, dry mouth, constipation, blurred vision, diabetes, and suicide ideation. Nefazodone and trazodone produce low to moderate sedation, but they may negatively affect cardiac stimulation. Side effects of trazodone are sedation, hypotension, nausea, and priapism (painful persistent erection). The most common side effect of vortioxetine is nausea (21% to 32%). It may also produce serotonin syndrome (hyperreflexia, nausea/vomiting, sedation, dizziness, sweating, facial flush, restlessness, shivering, and elevated blood pressure).

> **Tech Note!**
>
> Patients should be advised to avoid discontinuing antidepressants abruptly.

Drugs Used to Treat Bipolar Disorder

Mood stabilizers are used in the treatment of bipolar disorder. Lithium is the oldest of these agents, introduced more than 50 years ago. Several medications used in the treatment of seizures have been discovered to also effectively treat bipolar disorder.

Lithium is administered to reduce current symptoms of mania and depression, as well as to prevent recurrence of future episodes.

Lithium is rapidly absorbed from the gastrointestinal tract, which accounts for its rapid onset of action. The drug has a long half-life (24 hours), which increases the longer the patient is on lithium therapy. The half-life can double over the course of 1 year of continuous therapy. Lithium is not metabolized and is eliminated unchanged in the urine. Lithium has a narrow therapeutic index. A competitive interaction may occur between lithium and sodium in the kidneys that can result in lithium toxicity. Increased sodium intake can decrease lithium reabsorption. Dehydration can increase lithium reabsorption. Plasma lithium levels and renal function should be monitored regularly to avoid the development of lithium toxicity.

Early-onset side effects associated with lithium carbonate are sedation, nausea, increased urination, dry mouth, difficulty concentrating, and tremors. Adverse reactions associated with long-term use include weight gain, acne, impotence, hypothyroidism, rash, and hair loss. Lithium is contraindicated in pregnancy.

Valproic acid, carbamazepine, and lamotrigine are antiseizure drugs with demonstrated efficacy in the treatment of bipolar disorder. They are indicated as an adjunct to lithium therapy or when lithium administration has not produced desired results. Side effects of valproic acid and its salts, divalproex sodium and sodium valproate, include sedation, nausea, ataxia, and liver dysfunction. The side effects of carbamazepine include sedation, dizziness, ataxia, and visual disturbances. Lamotrigine is used in the treatment of bipolar disorder and seizures, and side effects include sedation, nausea, ataxia, blurred vision, double vision, and rash. The use of valproic acid, carbamazepine, and lamotrigine in the treatment of seizure disorder is described in Chapter 9.

Atypical Antidepressants

Generic Name	US Brand Name(s) / Canadian Brand(s)	Dosage Forms and Strengths
brexpiprazole	Rexulti	**Tablet:** 0.25 mg, 0.5 mg, 1 mg, 2 mg, 3 mg, 4 mg
	Rexulti	
bupropion[a]	Aplenzin, Forfivo XL, Wellbutrin SR, Wellbutrin XL	**Tablets, as HCl:** 75 mg, 100 mg
		Tablets, as HCl, extended release 24-hour: 150 mg (Zyban), 150 mg, 300 mg (Wellbutrin XL), 450 mg (Forfivo XL)[c]
	Wellbutrin SR, Wellbutrin XL, Zyban[b]	**Tablets, as hydrobromide, extended release (Aplenzin)[c]:** 174 mg, 348 mg, 522 mg
		Tablets, as sustained release 12-hour (Wellbutrin SR): 100 mg, 150 mg, 200 mg[c]
bupropion + naltrexone	Contrave[d]	**Tablet:** 90 mg bupropion + 8 mg naltrexone
	Contrave[d]	
mirtazapine[a]	Remeron, Remeron SolTab	**Tablets:** 15 mg, 30 mg, 45 mg
	Remeron, Remeron RD	**Tablets, orally disintegrating (Remeron SolTab, Remeron RD):** 15 mg, 30 mg, 45 mg
nefazodone	Generics only	**Tablets:** 50 mg, 100 mg, 150 mg, 200 mg, 250 mg
	Not available	
trazodone[a]	Generics only	**Tablets:** 50 mg, 75 mg[e], 100 mg, 150 mg, 300 mg[c]
	Generics only	

[a]Generic available.
[b]Zyban is indicated for smoking cessation.
[c]Available in the United States only.
[d]Contrave is indicated for weight management.
[e]Available in Canada only.

⚠ Tech Alert!

The following drugs have look-alike/sound-alike issues:
Wellbutrin SR and Wellbutrin XL;
buPROPion and busPIRone;
Remeron and Remeron SolTab

⚠ Tech Alert!

The following drugs have look-alike/sound-alike issues:
Lithium carbonate immediate release and lithium carbonate extended release (both are available in a 300-mg strength)

● Tech Note!

Pharmacy technicians can assist the pharmacist in ensuring optimal drug therapy by alerting the pharmacist when they detect or suspect nonadherence. The pharmacist will determine whether intervention is necessary.

TECHNICIAN'S CORNER

1. For patients taking MAOI antidepressants, what kinds of foods should they avoid?
2. What is the difference between "feeling blue" and major depression?

Drugs Used in the Treatment of Bipolar Disorder

Generic Name	US Brand Name(s) / Canadian Brand(s)	Dosage Forms and Strengths
lithium carbonate[a] lithium citrate[a]	Lithobid / Carbolith, Lithane, Lithmax	**Capsules (Carbolith, Lithane):** 150 mg, 300 mg, 600 mg **Syrup, as citrate:** 300 mg/5 mL[b] (8 mmol/5 mL)[c] **Tablets:** 300 mg **Tablets, extended release (Lithobid, Lithmax):** 300 mg, 450 mg[b]
divalproex sodium[a]	Depakote, Depakote ER / Epival	**Capsules, delayed release[b] pellets (Depakote):** 125 mg **Tablets, delayed release (Depakote, Epival):** 125 mg, 250 mg, 500 mg **Tablets, extended release (Depakote ER)[b]:** 250 mg, 500 mg
carbamazepine[a]	Carbatrol, Equetro, Epitol, Tegretol, Tegretol-XR, Teril / Tegretol, Tegretol CR	**Capsules, extended release (Carbatrol, Equetro):** 100 mg, 200 mg, 300 mg[b] **Suspension (Tegretol, Teril):** 100 mg/5 mL **Tablets, chewable:** 100 mg, 200 mg[c] **Tablets (Epitol, Tegretol):** 100 mg, 200 mg, 300 mg, 400 mg **Tablets, extended release (Tegretol-XR, Tegretol CR):** 100 mg[b], 200 mg, 400 mg
lamotrigine[a]	Lamictal, Lamictal CD, Lamictal ODT, Lamictal XR / Lamictal	**Tablets:** 25 mg, 100 mg, 150 mg, 200 mg[b] **Tablets, as dispersible for suspension (Lamictal CD):** 2 mg, 5 mg, 25 mg[b] **Tablets, extended release (Lamictal XR)[b]:** 25 mg, 50 mg, 100 mg, 200 mg, 250 mg, 300 mg **Tablets, orally disintegrating (Lamictal ODT)[b]:** 25 mg, 50 mg, 100 mg, 200 mg

[a]Generic available.
[b]Available in the United States only.
[c]Available in Canada only.

Summary of Drugs Used in the Treatment of Depression*

Generic Name	US Brand Name	Usual Adult Oral Dose and Dosing Schedule	Warning Labels
Tricyclic Antidepressants			
amitriptyline	Generic	75–100 mg daily in 1–3 divided doses (maximum 300 mg/day) (oral)	MAY CAUSE DROWSINESS; ALCOHOL MAY INTENSIFY THIS EFFECT. MAY IMPAIR ABILITY TO DRIVE. DO NOT DISCONTINUE WITHOUT MEDICAL SUPERVISION. AVOID PROLONGED EXPOSURE TO SUNLIGHT. MAY DISCOLOR URINE (BLUE-GREEN)— amitriptyline. TAKE WITH FOOD— clomipramine.
clomipramine	Anafranil	25–100 mg daily, as tolerated, during the first 2 weeks. May increase gradually up to 250 mg daily.	
desipramine	Norpramin	100–200 mg/day (maximum dose, 300 mg/day in a single or divided doses)	
doxepin	Sinequan	Initiate with 50–150 mg/day and gradually increase to 300 mg/day	
imipramine	Tofranil	Start with 25 mg 3–4 times a day (maximum dose, 300 mg/day)	
nortriptyline	Pamelor	25 mg 3–4 times per day up to 150 mg/day	
protriptyline	Generics	15–60 mg daily in 3–4 divided doses	
trimipramine	Generics	75–200 mg/day in 1–3 divided doses	

Summary of Drugs Used in the Treatment of Depression*—cont'd

	Generic Name	US Brand Name	Usual Adult Oral Dose and Dosing Schedule	Warning Labels
Selective Serotonin Reuptake Inhibitors				
	citalopram	Celexa	20–40 mg/day (maximum, 40 mg/day)	MAY IMPAIR ABILITY TO DRIVE.
	escitalopram	Lexapro	10–20 mg/day	AVOID ALCOHOL.
	fluoxetine	Prozac	20–60 mg/day (maximum 80 mg/day) or 90 mg/week (Prozac Weekly)	MAY CAUSE DIZZINESS. SWALLOW WHOLE; DO NOT CRUSH OR CHEW (delayed release).
	fluvoxamine	Luvox	100–300 mg daily (divide into 2 doses with larger dose at bedtime)	DO NOT DISCONTINUE WITHOUT MEDICAL SUPERVISION.
	paroxetine	Paxil Paxil CR	20 mg/day (Paxil) Maximum dose: 50 mg/day 25 mg once daily (Paxil CR) Maximum dose: 62.5 mg/day	
	sertraline	Zoloft	50–200 mg/day	
	vortioxetine	Trintellix	10–20 mg once daily	
	fluoxetine + olanzapine	Symbyax	25 mg fluoxetine/6 mg olanzapine every evening. May increase to 75 mg/18 mg.	MAY CAUSE DIZZINESS. MAY IMPAIR ABILITY TO DRIVE. AVOID ALCOHOL.
Monoamine Oxidase Inhibitors				
	isocarboxazid	Marplan	10 mg twice daily increasing gradually to a maximum of 60 mg/day	TAKE WITH FOOD— moclobemide. AVOID ALCOHOL.
	moclobemide	Manerix (Canada)	300–600 mg/day divided into 2 doses per day	MAY CAUSE DIZZINESS OR DROWSINESS.
	phenelzine	Nardil	15 mg 3 times a day (maximum 90 mg/day)	DO NOT DISCONTINUE WITHOUT MEDICAL SUPERVISION.
	selegine patch	Emsam	Apply and rotate one 6-mg patch every 24 hours. May increase dose to maximum 12 mg/24 h.	AVOID TYRAMINE-RICH FOODS AND BEVERAGES.
	tranylcypromine	Parnate	30 mg/day in divided dose (maximum dose, 60 mg/day)	ROTATE APPLICATION SITE— Emsam.
Serotonin-Noradrenaline Reuptake Inhibitors				
	desvenlafaxine[a]	Pristiq	50 mg once daily	MAY CAUSE DIZZINESS OR DROWSINESS.
	duloxetine	Cymbalta	40–60 mg/day	MAY IMPAIR ABILITY TO DRIVE.
	venlafaxine	Effexor	75–375 mg/day in 2–3 divided doses (immediate release) or 75–225 mg/day (extended release)	AVOID ALCOHOL. TAKE WITH FOOD— venlafaxine. SWALLOW WHOLE; DO NOT CRUSH OR CHEW (extended and sustained release). DO NOT DISCONTINUE WITHOUT MEDICAL SUPERVISION.

Continued

Summary of Drugs Used in the Treatment of Depression*—cont'd

	Generic Name	US Brand Name	Usual Adult Oral Dose and Dosing Schedule	Warning Labels
Atypical Antidepressants				
	brexpiprazole	Rexulti	MDD: 0.5–1 mg/day, maximum 3 mg/day	MAY CAUSE DIZZINESS OR DROWSINESS. MAY IMPAIR ABILITY TO DRIVE. AVOID ALCOHOL. TAKE WITH FOOD— nefazodone, trazodone
	bupropion	Wellbutrin	For depression: 100 mg 2–3 times a day (immediate release); 150 mg twice a day (sustained release); 300 mg once daily (extended release)	
	mirtazapine	Remeron	15–45 mg/day (dosed at bedtime)	
	nefazodone	Generics	200–600 mg/day in 2 divided doses	
	trazodone	Generics	150 mg daily in 2–3 divided doses (maximum dose, 600 mg/day)	
	vilazodone	Viibryd	40 mg once daily	

*Psychiatric drug dosing can vary considerably.
ªGeneric available.
MDD, Major depressive disorder.

Summary of Drugs Used in the Treatment of Bipolar Affective Disorder*

Generic Name	US Brand Name	Usual Adult Oral Dose and Dosing Schedule	Warning Labels
lithium	Lithonate, Lithobid	900–1800 mg/day in 3–4 divided doses (immediate release) or 900–1200 mg/day in 2 divided doses (sustained release)	MAY CAUSE DIZZINESS OR DROWSINESS; MAY IMPAIR ABILITY TO DRIVE. AVOID ALCOHOL. TAKE WITH FOOD. DRINK PLENTY OF WATER—lithium, Symbyax. SWALLOW WHOLE; DO NOT CRUSH OR CHEW (controlled or slow release). AVOID PREGNANCY—divalproex, carbamazepine, lithium. DO NOT DISCONTINUE WITHOUT MEDICAL SUPERVISION.
divalproex sodium	Depakote	750–1500 mg/day in divided doses	
carbamazepine	Tegretol	400 mg/day in 2 divided doses (maximum, 1600 mg/day)	
lamotrigine	Lamictal	100 mg–200 mg/day	

*Psychiatric drug dosing can vary considerably.

Key Points

- Depressive disorders affect more than 21 million Americans in a given year, and at some time in their lives, 5.4% Canadians will be affected.
- Depression affects self-esteem, moods, thoughts, eating, and sleeping and produces feelings of worthlessness or guilt. It also reduces the ability to think and concentrate.
- Major depression is associated with persistent feelings of sadness, emptiness, or hopelessness.
- Bipolar disorder is associated with sudden swings in mood between depression and periods of mania.
- Dysthymia produces symptoms that are chronic and keep the person from functioning well.

- According to the biogenic amine theory, major depression results from a decrease in monoamine neurotransmitters in the brain.
- Bipolar affective disorder (mania) is believed to be associated with increased levels of monoamine neurotransmitters.
- Monoamine neurotransmitters associated with depression and bipolar disorder are norepinephrine (NE), serotonin (5-HT), and dopamine (DA).
- The mechanisms of action for drugs used to treat depression may differ; however, all antidepressants are equally effective.
- Inhibition of the reuptake of specific monoamine neurotransmitters is one of the ways antidepressants produce their effects. The other mechanism of action is to block the degradation of monoamine neurotransmitters.
- Selection of one antidepressant over another is based on the patient's ability to tolerate drug side effects.
- Tricyclic antidepressants (TCAs) are the oldest class of medication used in the treatment of depression.
- The TCAs are nonspecific reuptake inhibitors of monoamine neurotransmitters.

- The selective serotonin reuptake inhibitors (SSRIs) work by producing selective blockade of the reuptake of 5-HT at the synaptic cleft.
- The SSRIs are equally effective as the TCAs yet lack the cardiotoxic effects associated with TCAs.
- The monoamine oxidase inhibitors (MAOIs) interfere with the degradation of monoamine neurotransmitters and dietary amines (e.g., tyramine).
- Hypertensive crisis is a life-threatening adverse reaction caused by drug-drug and drug-food interactions with MAOIs.
- Lithium is administered to treat bipolar disorder. It reduces current symptoms of mania and depression and prevents recurrence of future episodes.
- Lithium has a narrow therapeutic index.
- Many drugs used to treat seizure disorders (e.g., divalproex sodium and carbamazepine) are also used for the treatment of bipolar disorder.

Review Questions

1. A mental health illness that persists for several weeks and is associated with persistent feelings of sadness, emptiness, or hopelessness is _____.
   a. bipolar disorder
   b. obsessive-compulsive disorder
   c. major depressive disorder
   d. schizophrenia
2. Wellbutrin is a _____.
   a. noradrenaline-dopamine inhibitor
   b. monoamine oxidase inhibitor
   c. selective serotonin reuptake inhibitor
   d. tricyclic antidepressant
3. Select the antidepressant that is available as an orally disintegrating tablet.
   a. Pristiq
   b. Fetzima
   c. Remeron
   d. Cymbalta
4. The most widely prescribed class of antidepressants is:
   a. TCAs
   b. SSRIs
   c. MAOIs
   d. PPIs
5. The brand name for citalopram is:
   a. Celexa
   b. Celebrex
   c. Cerebryx
   d. none of the above
6. You receive a prescription for desvenlafaxine 37.5 mg with directions to take one capsule two to three times a day. You consult the pharmacist because:
   a. the usual dosing schedule for desvenlafaxine is once daily
   b. desvenlafaxine is not available in 37.5 mg
   c. both a & b
   d. none of the above

7. To avoid the risk of hypertensive crisis, patients taking _____ are advised to avoid eating certain foods containing tyramine.
   a. SSRIs
   b. TCAs
   c. MAOIs
   d. a and b
8. _____ is an example of an atypical antidepressant.
   a. Fluoxetine
   b. Tranylcypromine
   c. Imipramine
   d. Mirtazapine
9. Bupropion is indicated for the treatment of depression and smoking cessation.
   a. true
   b. false
10. An example of a 5-HT–noradrenaline reuptake inhibitor is:
    a. fluoxetine
    b. sertraline
    c. venlafaxine
    d. nortriptyline
11. Valproic acid, carbamazepine, and lamotrigine are _____ drugs with demonstrated efficacy in the treatment of bipolar disorder.
    a. antiseizure
    b. antidepressant
    c. antimania
    d. antianxiety
12. The oldest drug used to treat bipolar disorder is _____.
    a. fluoxetine
    b. tranylcypromine
    c. lithium
    d. escitalopram

Bibliography

Anxiety & Depression Association of America. (2016). What Is Depression? Retrieved January 15, 2017, from https://www.adaa.org/understanding-anxiety/depression.

Canadian Mental Health Association. (2021). Fast Facts about Mental Health and Mental Illness. Retrieved July 9, 2022, from https://cmha.ca/brochure/fast-facts-about-mental-illness/.

Health Canada. (2022). Drug Product Database. Retrieved July 10, 2022, from https://health-products.canada.ca/dpd-bdpp/index-eng.jsp.

Institute for Safe Medication Practices. (2016). FDA and ISMP Lists of Look-Alike Drug Names with Recommended Tall Man Letters. Retrieved June 24, 2022, from https://www.ismp.org/recommendations/tall-man-letters-list.

Institute for Safe Medication Practices. (2019). List of Confused Drugs. Retrieved June 24, 2022, from https://www.ismp.org/tools/confused-drugnames.pdf.

Kalant H, Grant D, Mitchell J. *Principles of medical pharmacology.* ed 7. Toronto: Elsevier Canada, A Division of Reed Elsevier Canada; 2007:316–333.

Lance L, Lacy C, Armstrong L, et al. *Drug information handbook for the allied health professional.* ed 12. Hudson, OH: APhA Lexi-Comp; 2005.

Neurological protein may hold the key to new treatments for depression—Press release, Toronto, 2010, Centre for Addiction and Mental Health.

National Institute of Mental Health. (2022). Major Depression: Definitions. Retrieved July 9, 2022, from https://www.nimh.nih.gov/health/statistics/major-depression.

Page C, Curtis M, Sutter M, et al. *Integrated pharmacology.* Philadelphia: Elsevier Mosby; 2005:239–241.

Public Health Agency of Canada. (2016). What Is Depression? Retrieved September 15, 2022, from http://www.phac-aspc.gc.ca/cd-mc/mi-mm/depression-eng.php.

Statistics Canada. (2020). Trends in the Prevalence of Depression and Anxiety Disorders among Working-Age Canadian Adults between 2000 and 2016. Retrieved July 9, 2022, from https://www.doi.org/10.25318/82-003-x202001200002-eng.

U.S. Department of Health and Human Services, National Institutes of Health, National Institute of Mental Health. *Depression (NIH Publication No. 15-3561).* Bethesda, MD: U.S. Government Printing Office; 2015.

U.S. Food and Drug Administration. (nd). Drugs@FDA: FDA Approved Drug Products. Retrieved July 10, 2022, from https://www.accessdata.fda.gov/scripts/cder/daf/index.cfm.

7

Treatment of Schizophrenia and Psychoses

LEARNING OBJECTIVES

1. Learn the terminology associated with schizophrenia.
2. Describe the symptoms of schizophrenia.
3. List and describe the function of neurotransmitters associated with the symptoms of schizophrenia and psychoses.
4. Classify medications used to treat schizophrenia and psychoses.
5. Describe the mechanism of action for each class of drugs used to treat schizophrenia and psychoses.
6. Identify warning labels and precautionary messages associated with medications used to treat schizophrenia and psychoses.
7. Identify significant drug look-alike and sound-alike issues.

KEY TERMS

Catatonia Symptom of schizophrenia associated with unresponsiveness and immobility.

Delusion Irrational thoughts or false beliefs that dominate a person's behavior and viewpoint and do not change even when evidence is provided that beliefs are not valid.

Extrapyramidal symptoms Excessive muscle movement (motor activity) associated with use of neuroleptics that includes muscular rigidity, tremor, bradykinesia (slow movement), and difficulty in walking.

Hallucination Visions or voices that exist only in the mind and cannot be seen or heard by others.

Negative symptoms Sign of schizophrenia that is associated with decreased ability to think, plan, or express emotion.

Neuroleptic (antipsychotic) Drug used to treat schizophrenia and psychoses.

Neuroleptic malignant syndrome Potentially fatal reaction to administration of neuroleptic medications. Symptoms include stupor, muscle rigidity, and high temperature.

Positive symptoms Hallucinations, delusions, or other unusual thoughts or perceptions that are symptoms of schizophrenia.

Postural hypotension Drop in blood pressure caused by a change in posture.

Pseudoparkinsonism A reversible condition that resembles parkinsonism resulting from an adverse reaction to the administration of antipsychotic drugs.

Psychosis Mental state characterized by disorganized behavior and thought, delusions, hallucinations, and a loss of touch with reality.

Schizophrenia Type of psychosis characterized by delusions of thought, visual or auditory hallucinations (or both), and speech disturbances. Paranoid schizophrenia is characterized by delusions of persecution.

Tardive dyskinesia Inappropriate postures of the neck, trunk, and limbs accompanied by involuntary thrusting of the tongue.

Overview

Schizophrenia is a chronic and major *psychosis* that is characterized by delusions of thought, visual or auditory hallucinations (or both), and speech disturbances. Persons diagnosed with schizophrenia often see visions or hear voices that cannot be seen or heard by others. It is a long-term mental disorder that involves a breakdown between thought, emotion, and behavior.

Paranoid schizophrenia is characterized by delusions of persecution. Paranoid schizophrenia is particularly challenging because the patient may believe that the health care team is prescribing medicines and therapies intended to cause harm.

Schizophrenia affects more than 24 million people worldwide according to the World Health Organization. The onset typically occurs in the late teens, after puberty begins, to the mid-20s; the onset in men is slightly earlier than in women, who may not develop symptoms until the mid-20s to the early 30s. The onset of symptoms after age 45 years is rare.

Heredity, environmental factors, and brain structure and function may increase the risk of developing schizophrenia. Schizophrenia runs in families; however, having a family member with schizophrenia does not mean other family members will develop the condition. Exposure to viruses, fetal malnutrition, and substance abuse are also thought to influence the development of schizophrenia.

People diagnosed with schizophrenia often exhibit negative symptoms, positive symptoms, and cognitive symptoms. People who exhibit **negative symptoms** may not show visible signs of emotion or facial expressions or interact socially with others. Speech is monotonous. **Positive symptoms** may appear as bizarre behavior. People with schizophrenia may have delusions. **Delusions** are irrational thoughts or false beliefs that dominate a person's behavior. The person's viewpoint is unlikely to change, even when evidence is provided that the beliefs are not valid. An example of a delusion is the belief that television characters are broadcasting personal messages to the person with schizophrenia. People with schizophrenia may also have visual or auditory **hallucinations**. They respond to visions and voices that only they can see. They may talk to themselves or, when speaking to others, may fail to complete sentences (their thoughts may be finished in their mind). Their thoughts are often disorganized. Schizophrenia may interfere with the performance of routine activities of daily living. Memory loss may impede the person's ability to function on a job. Schizophrenia may also decrease the person's capacity to interpret information and make decisions.

Schizophrenia also produces physical symptoms. The person may be clumsy and appear catatonic or make repetitive movements. People who exhibit symptoms of **catatonia** are unresponsive and immobile. Five Facts You Should Know About Schizophrenia:

1. Schizophrenia literally means a "split mind".
2. There are "positive" and "negative" symptoms of schizophrenia.
3. Schizophrenia has genetic and environmental causes.
4. The first signs of schizophrenia usually appear at adolescence.
5. Schizophrenia is rare.

Neurochemistry of Schizophrenia and Psychoses

Interactions between brain chemicals (e.g., dopamine and serotonin) play a role in schizophrenia. Drugs that block dopamine signals are used in the treatment of schizophrenia. Dopamine pathways project to various emotional areas of the brain involved in cognition and regulation of motivation and emotion. Pathways in the midbrain control muscle movement, and treatments for schizophrenia can produce **pseudoparkinsonism**, Parkinson disease–like symptoms (e.g., tremor and bradykinesia), as a side effect.

Other neurotransmitters that have been identified as playing a role in symptoms of schizophrenia include serotonin, cholecystokinin (CCK), neurotensin, γ-aminobutyric acid (GABA), and glutamate (Fig. 7.1).

Drugs Used to Treat Schizophrenia and Psychosis

Neuroleptics (antipsychotics) are classified by structure and function. Functionally, all antipsychotics fall into two classes based on their affinity for dopamine receptors. Dopamine (D_2) is considered the most important neurotransmitter involved in the treatment and symptoms of schizophrenia. High-potency neuroleptics have a strong affinity for dopamine receptors. "Atypical" and low-potency antipsychotics have a weaker affinity for dopamine receptors and produce fewer side effects associated with blockade. Dopamine receptor blockade in the nigrostriatal tract produces Parkinson disease–like symptoms (pseudoparkinsonism). Some antipsychotic drugs block serotonin (5-hydroxytryptamine [5-HT]) receptors. They are useful in the treatment of negative symptoms of schizophrenia and protect against long-term motor effects associated with some drugs used to treat psychosis. CCK and neurotensin are peptide neurotransmitters. CCK is thought to be associated with the auditory hallucinations of schizophrenia. Drugs that increase neurotensin levels improve negative symptoms of schizophrenia. Abnormalities of the GABA system are believed to be associated with working memory deficits in schizophrenia. Glutamate is an amino acid that acts as an excitatory neurotransmitter in the central nervous system. Drugs that interfere with glutamate signaling in the brain are thought to decrease psychosis.

All antipsychotic agents are equally effective. The selection of agents to treat schizophrenia is based on a balance between the achievement of the desired response and the patient's ability to tolerate drug side effects.

First-Generation Antipsychotics (neuroleptics) and Second-Generation Antipsychotics

Phenothiazines, butyrophenones, and thioxanthenes are categorized as first-generation antipsychotics. They are classified as

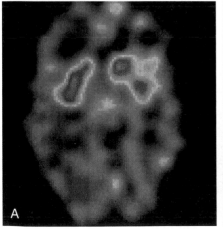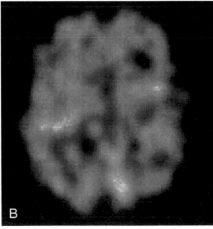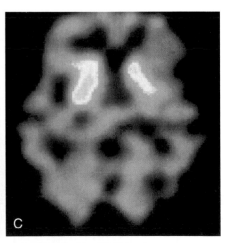

• **Fig. 7.1** The cerebral distribution of dopamine receptors in treated and untreated schizophrenia. (A) Striatal dopamine receptors in untreated schizophrenia. (B) Complete blockade of receptors with typical neuroleptic. (C) Partial blockade of receptors with equally effective dose of clozapine. (From Page CP, Hoffman BB, Curtis MJ, et al. *Integrated pharmacology*, ed 3, Philadelphia, 2006, Mosby.)

low, medium, and high potency. The prototype for low-potency antipsychotics is chlorpromazine; medium potency, fluphenazine; and high potency, haloperidol. All other types of antipsychotics are categorized as second-generation antipsychotics. Clozapine (thienobenzodiazepines), risperidone (benzixasoles), and aripiprazole (quinolinones) are examples of atypical antipsychotics.

> **❶ Tech Alert!**
>
> The following drugs have look-alike/sound-alike issues:
>
> chlorproMAZINE, clomiPRAMINE, and chlorproPAMIDE;
> fluPHENAZine and fluvoxaMINE;
> SEROquel and SINEquan

> **◼ Tech Note!**
>
> Phenothiazines are also prescribed for the treatment of nausea and vomiting (chlorpromazine, perphenazine, promethazine).

Mechanism of Action

First-generation antipsychotics block dopamine at postsynaptic receptor sites in the brain. They have a strong alpha-adrenergic blocking action that accounts for the hypotension produced by first-generation antipsychotics (Fig. 7.2). Atypical antipsychotics such as clozapine show strong affinity for serotonin receptors in addition to the dopaminergic receptor blockade.

> **❶ Tech Alert!**
>
> The FDA requires a boxed warning be included in the labeling of all neuroleptics, stating that the treatment of behavioral disorders in elderly patients with dementia with atypical and conventional antipsychotics is associated with increased mortality.

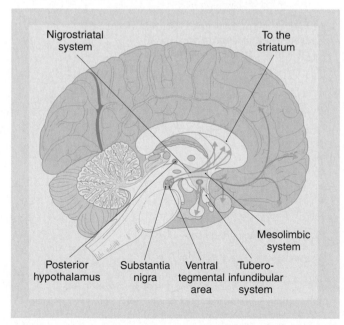

• **Fig. 7.2** Dopamine pathways. (From Page CP, Hoffman BB, Curtis MJ, et al. *Integrated pharmacology*, ed 3, Philadelphia, 2006, Mosby.)

> **❶ Tech Alert!**
>
> The FDA requires a boxed warning be included in the labeling of all atypical neuroleptics, stating the agents are associated with hyperglycemia and the onset of diabetes.

Pharmacokinetics

First-generation antipsychotics are well absorbed orally, rectally, and parenterally. They readily cross the blood-brain barrier because of their lipid solubility. They are up to 90% bound to plasma proteins. They are also rapidly metabolized in the liver, and some produce active metabolites. For example, paliperidone is the active metabolite of risperidone. Antipsychotics are eliminated in the urine.

Several antipsychotics are available in slow-release depot formulations for intramuscular injection. The therapeutic effects of slow-release dosage forms (e.g., Invega Sustenna, Haldol deconoate) persist for up to 4 weeks after injection, and one injection of Invega Hafyera persists for 6 months. Atypical antipsychotics are also available in oral dosage forms designed for rapid action (e.g., Zyprexa Zydis oral disintegrating tablets), and once daily dosing with extended-release tablets (e.g., Seroquel XR) and parental dosage forms for extended action (e.g., Invega Trinza every 3 months intramuscular injection).

Adverse Reactions

Up to 80% of the people who are prescribed antipsychotics will experience adverse reactions. Most adverse reactions are predictable and associated with dopaminergic, serotonergic, cholinergic, alpha-adrenergic, or histaminergic blockade (H1). Adverse effects are classified as central nervous system effects and peripheral nervous system effects. Sedation (histamine blockade), confusion, decreased ability to regulate body temperature, weight gain, increased appetite, and increased release of some endocrine hormones are central nervous system effects. Peripheral nervous system adverse effects include blurred vision, dry mouth, and urinary retention (cholinergic blockade). Alpha-adrenergic blockade can cause **postural hypotension**—a drop in blood pressure caused by a change in posture.

Extrapyramidal effects and tardive dyskinesia are associated with dopaminergic blockade and occur more frequently in elderly patients. **Extrapyramidal symptoms** are exhibited as excessive muscle movement. **Tardive dyskinesia** causes inappropriate postures of the neck, trunk, and limbs, and is accompanied by involuntary thrusting of the tongue and lip smacking. There is no effective prevention or treatment for tardive dyskinesia.

Other adverse effects are hepatotoxicity and jaundice, bone marrow depression, photosensitivity, and failure to ejaculate. Increased release of prolactin can produce pseudopregnancy-type symptoms. Phenothiazines may also increase vitamin B_2 requirements.

> **❶ Tech Alert!**
>
> Chlorpromazine oral concentrate and thioridazine oral concentrate are incompatible in enteral formulas (tube feeding).

Phenothiazines

Generic Name	US Brand Name(s) Canadian Brand(s)	Dosage Forms and Strengths
chlorpromazine[a]	Generic only Generic only	**Injection, solution**[b]: 25 mg/mL **Tablets**: 10 mg[b], 25 mg, 50 mg, 100 mg, 200 mg[b]
fluphenazine[a]	Generic only Generic only	**Elixir, as hydrochloride**[b]: 2.5 mg/5 mL **Injection, hydrochloride solution**[b]: 2.5 mg/mL **Solution, oral concentrate**[b]: 5 mg/mL **Tablets**: 1 mg, 2 mg[c], 2.5 mg[b], 5 mg, 10 mg[b]
methotrimeprazine	Not available Nozinan	**Solution, for injection (Nozinan)**: 25 mg/mL **Tablet (generics)**: 2 mg, 5 mg, 25 mg, 50 mg
perphenazine[a]	Generic only Generic only	**Tablets**: 2 mg, 4 mg, 8 mg, 16 mg
thioridazine[a]	Generic only Not available	**Tablets**: 10 mg, 25 mg, 50 mg, 100 mg
trifluoperazine[a]	Generic only Generic only	**Tablets**: 1 mg[b], 2mg[b], 5 mg, 10 mg, 20 mg

[a]Generic available.
[b]Available in the United States only.
[c]Available in Canada only.

Butyrophenones

Generic Name	US Brand Name(s) Canadian Brand(s)	Dosage Forms and Strengths
haloperidol[a]	Haldol Generic only	**Injection, oil, as deconoate**: 50 mg/mL[b]; 100 mg/mL **Injection, intramuscular**[c]: 5 mg/mL **Tablets**: 0.5 mg, 1 mg, 2 mg, 5 mg, 10 mg, 20 mg[b]

[a]Generic available.
[b]Available in the United States only.
[c]Available in Canada only.

Thioxanthenes

Generic Name	US Brand Name(s) Canadian Brand(s)	Dosage Forms and Strengths
thiothixene[a]	Generic only Not Available	**Capsules**: 1 mg, 2 mg, 5 mg, 10 mg
zuclopenthixol	Not Available Clopixol, Clopixol Acuphase, Clopixol Depot	**Intramuscular injection, as acetate (Clopixol Acuphase)**: 50 mg/mL **Intramuscular injection, as deconoate (Clopixol Depot)**: 200 mg/mL **Tablets**: 10 mg, 25 mg

[a]Generic available.

First-Generation Neuroleptics

> **● Tech Note!**
>
> Do not mix haloperidol oral concentrate with coffee or tea.

Second-Generation Neuroleptics

Second-generation antipsychotics that are used in the treatment and management of schizophrenia are aripiprazole, asenapine, brexpiprazole, cariprazine, clozapine, iloperidone, lurasidone, olanzapine, paliperidone, quetiapine, risperidone, and ziprasidone. In addition to treating schizophrenia, some antipsychotic drugs are used to treat bipolar disorder. The drugs that are used for bipolar disorder are olanzapine, risperidone, ziprasidone, and quetiapine.

Mechanisms of Action

Second-generation antipsychotics act by several mechanisms of action. Some act to stabilize the dopamine system. Some are partial agonists of dopamine (e.g., aripiprazole), and others produce mixed effects on dopamine and serotonin (asenapine). Risperidone, paliperidone, and iloperidone are classified as benzisoxazoles. Loxapine is an atypical antipsychotic drug that is structurally similar to the antidepressant amoxapine. Lurasidone and ziprasidone are classified as benzisothiazol derivatives. Quetiapine is classified as a dibenzothiazepine.

> **● Tech Note!**
>
> Patients, prescribers, and pharmacists must be enrolled in a registry to dispense clozapine.

Second-Generation Neuroleptics

Generic Name	US Brand Name(s) / Canadian Brand(s)	Dosage Forms and Strengths
aripiprazole[a]	Abilify, Abilify Maintena Abilify Mycite Kit, Aristada, Aristada Initio Kit	**Powder for injection (Abilify Maintena)**: 300 mg/vial, 400 mg/vial **Solution, oral**[b]: 1 mg/mL **Tablets (Abilify, Abilify Mycite Kit)**: 2 mg, 5 mg, 10 mg, 15 mg, 20 mg, 30 mg **Tablet, oral disintegrating**[b]: 10 mg, 15 mg **Tablet**: 2 mg, 5 mg, 10 mg, 15 mg, 20 mg, 30 mg **Injectable IM suspension, as aripiprazole lauroxil (Aristada Maintena)**[b]: 441 mg/1.6 mL, 662 mg/2.4 mL, 882 mg/3.2 mL, 1064 mg/3.9 mL
	Abilify	
asenapine[a,b]	Saphris	**Tablets, sublingual**: 2.5 mg[b], 5 mg, 10 mg **Transdermal patch (Secuado)**: 3.8 mg/24 h, 5.7 mg/24 h, 7.6 mg/24 h
	Secuado	
	Saphris	
brexpiprazole	Rexulti	**Tablet**: 0.25 mg, 0.5 mg, 1 mg, 2 mg, 3 mg, 4 mg
	Rexulti	
cariprazine	Vraylar	**Capsule**: 1.5 mg, 3 mg, 4.5 mg, 6 mg
	Vraylar	
clozapine[a]	Clozaril, Versacloz	**Suspension, oral**[b]: 50 mg/mL **Tablets**: 12.5 mg[b], 25 mg, 50 mg, 100 mg, 200 mg **Tablets, oral disintegrating**[b]: 12.5 mg, 25 mg, 100 mg, 150 mg, 200 mg
	Clozaril	
iloperidone[a]	Fanapt	**Tablets**: 1 mg, 2 mg, 4 mg, 6 mg, 8 mg, 10 mg, 12 mg
	Not available	
loxapine[a]	Adasuve	**Capsules (Xylac)**[b]: 2.5 mg, 10 mg, 25 mg **Injection (Loxapac IM)**[c]: 50 mg/mL **Powder, for inhalation (Adasuve)**[b]: 10 mg **Tablets**[c]: 2.5 mg, 5 mg, 10 mg, 25 mg, 50 mg
	Loxapac IM, Xylac	
lurasidone[a]	Latuda	**Tablets**: 20 mg, 40 mg, 60 mg, 80 mg, 120 mg
	Latuda	
olanzapine[a]	Zyprexa, Zyprexa Relprevv, Zyprexa Zydis	**Injection IM, powder for reconstitution**: 10 mg/vial **Injection, extended-release powder (Zyprexa Relprevv)**[b]: 210 mg, 300 mg, 405 mg/vial **Tablets**: 2.5 mg, 5 mg, 7.5 mg, 10 mg, 15 mg, 20 mg **Tablets, oral disintegrating (Zyprexa Zydis)**: 5 mg, 10 mg, 15 mg, 20 mg
	Zyprexa, Zyprexa Zydis	

Continued

Second-Generation Neuroleptics —cont'd

Generic Name	US Brand Name(s) / Canadian Brand(s)	Dosage Forms and Strengths
paliperidone[a][b]	Invega, Invega Hafyera, Invega Sustenna, Invega Trinza	**Suspension, for extended-release IM injection (Invega Hafyera):** 1.092 g/3.5 mL, 1.560 g/5 mL **Suspension, for extended-release IM injection (Invega Sustenna):** In United States: 39 mg/0.25 mL, 78 mg/0.5 mL, 117 mg/0.75 mL, 156 mg/1 mL, 234 mg/1.5 mL **In Canada:** 50 mg/0.5 mL, 75 mg/0.75 mL, 100 mg/1 mL, 150 mg/1.5 mL **Suspension, for extended-release IM prefilled syringe (Invega Trinza):** In United States: 273 mg/0.875 mL, 410 mg/1.315 mL, 546 mg/1.75 mL, 819 mg/2.625 mL **In Canada:** 175 mg/0.875 mL, 350 mg/1.75 mL, 525 mg/2.625 mL **Tablet, extended release (Invega):** 1.5 mg[b], 3 mg, 6 mg, 9 mg
	Invega, Invega Sustenna, Invega Trinza	
quetiapine[a]	Seroquel, Seroquel XR	**Tablets:** 25 mg, 50 mg[b], 100 mg, 200 mg, 300 mg, 400 mg[b] **Tablets, extended release (Seroquel XR):** 50 mg, 150 mg, 200 mg, 300 mg, 400 mg
	Seroquel, Seroquel XR	
risperidone[a]	Perseris Kit, Risperdal, Risperdal Consta	**Injection (Risperdal Consta):** 12.5 mg, 25 mg, 37.5 mg, 50 mg (vials and prefilled syringes) **Solution, oral:** 1 mg/mL **Suspension, extended release IM injection (Perseris Kit)[b]:** 90 mg, 120 mg **Tablets:** 0.25 mg, 0.5 mg, 1 mg, 2 mg, 3 mg, 4 mg **Tablet, oral disintegrating[b]:** 0.5 mg, 1 mg, 2 mg, 3 mg, 4 mg
	Risperdal, Risperdal Consta	
ziprasidone[a]	Geodon	**Capsule:** 20 mg, 40 mg, 60 mg, 80 mg **Injection, powder for reconstitution:[b]** 20 mg
	Zeldox	

[a]Generic available
[b]Available in the United States only.
[c]Available in Canada only.

❶ Tech Alert!

ZyPREXA and ZyrTEC have look-alike/sound-alike issues.

● Tech Note!

Risperidone oral solution should not be diluted with cola or tea.

● Tech Note!

Dispense haloperidol, loxapine, risperidone, and aripiprazole oral solutions with the measuring device provided with packaging.

Adverse Reactions

Common side effects of atypical antipsychotics are dizziness, drowsiness, hypotension, headache, confusion, nausea, weight gain, increased urination or urinary retention, thirst, dry mouth, and sexual dysfunction (aripiprazole, asenapine, clozapine, lurasidone, ziprasidone, iloperidone, paliperidone, quetiapine, and risperidone). Aripiprazole may cause insomnia. Newer atypical antipsychotics such as ziprasidone and olanzapine have less risk for extrapyramidal symptoms, but they are associated with hyperglycemia and the onset of diabetes. The atypical antipsychotics are also associated with an increased risk for cardiovascular morbidity and mortality. Aripiprazole and asenapine can cause QT interval prolongation, so they should be used cautiously in patients with heart disease.

Precautions

Neuroleptic malignant syndrome is a life-threatening side effect of neuroleptic administration. It produces symptoms of muscle rigidity, increased body temperature (hyperthermia), fluctuating consciousness, and renal failure. Clozapine use is restricted because it can produce a fatal drop in white blood cells (agranulocytosis). Patients on clozapine therapy are required to have white blood cell levels monitored weekly while taking the medication. Antipsychotic agents should be used cautiously in patients with seizure disorders. Low-potency agents and clozapine are most likely to induce seizures. All of the second-generation neuroleptic drugs have a boxed warning: Elderly patients with dementia-related psychosis treated with antipsychotic drugs are at an increased risk of death. Mortality most commonly occurs due to sudden heart failure, sudden death, or infection. Aripiprazole and asenapine may produce suicidal thoughts.

Summary of Drugs Used in the Treatment of Psychosis

	Generic Name	US Brand Name	Usual Adult Oral Dose and Dosing Schedule	Warning Labels
Phenothiazines				
	chlorpromazine	Generics	25–2000 mg/day in 3–4 divided doses (oral) or 300 mg–800 mg/day IM or IV (maintenance dose)	MAY CAUSE DROWSINESS; MAY IMPAIR ABILITY TO DRIVE; AVOID ALCOHOL. MAINTAIN ADEQUATE HYDRATION. AVOID PROLONGED EXPOSURE TO SUNLIGHT. DO NOT DISCONTINUE WITHOUT MEDICAL SUPERVISION. DILUTE ORAL CONCENTRATE BEFORE ADMINISTERING—chlorpromazine, fluphenazine. MAY DISCOLOR URINE (PINK-REDDISH BROWN)—thioridazine. MAY CAUSE DRY MOUTH. CHEWING GUM OR SUCKING SUGARLESS CANDY MAY IMPROVE SYMPTOMS.
	fluphenazine	Generics	**Oral:** 2.5–10 mg/day dosed every 6–8 h (maximum, 20 mg/day) **IM (as HCl):** 2.5 mg–10 mg/day or IM (as deconoate) 12.5 mg every 3 weeks	
	methotrimeprazine	Generics	**Oral:** 50–200 mg/day in 2–3 divided doses **IM:** 75–100 mg given as 3–4 injections/day	
	perphenazine	Generics	4–16 mg 2–4 times a day (maximum, 64 mg/day)	
	thioridazine	Generics	50–100 mg 3 times a day up to 800 mg/day divided in 2–4 doses	
	trifluoperazine	Generics	**Oral:** 2–5 mg twice daily (maximum, 100 mg) **IM:** 1–2 mg every 4–6 h (maximum, 6 mg/24 h)	
Butyrophenones				
	haloperidol	Generics	**Oral:** 0.5–5 mg 2–3 times/day (maximum, 100 mg/day) **IM (lactate):** 2–5 mg every 4–8 h **IM (deconoate):** 10–20 times oral dose (up to 300 mg) once every 4 weeks.	MAY CAUSE DROWSINESS; MAY IMPAIR ABILITY TO DRIVE; AVOID ALCOHOL. DO NOT DISCONTINUE WITHOUT MEDICAL SUPERVISION. DILUTE ORAL CONCENTRATE BEFORE ADMINISTRATION. MAINTAIN ADEQUATE HYDRATION. AVOID PROLONGED EXPOSURE TO SUNLIGHT.
Thioxanthenes				
	thiothixene	Generics	2 mg 3 times a day (maximum, 60 mg/day)	MAY CAUSE DROWSINESS; MAY IMPAIR ABILITY TO DRIVE; AVOID ALCOHOL. DO NOT DISCONTINUE WITHOUT MEDICAL SUPERVISION. MAINTAIN ADEQUATE HYDRATION. AVOID PROLONGED EXPOSURE TO SUNLIGHT.
	zuclopenthixol	Clopixol	**Injection, as acetate:** 50–150 mg IM every 2–3 days **Injection, as deconoate:** 150–300 mg IM every 2–4 weeks **Tablets:** 10–50 mg/day in 2–3 divided doses	

Continued

Summary of Drugs Used in the Treatment of Psychosis—cont'd

Generic Name	US Brand Name	Usual Adult Oral Dose and Dosing Schedule	Warning Labels
Atypical Antipsychotics			
aripiprazole	Abilify	**Oral Solution and Tablet, oral disintegrating**: 10–15 mg once daily Inject 441–882 mg IM monthly (Aristada Maintena); inject 300–400 mg in the buttocks monthly (Abilify Maintena)	MAY CAUSE DIZZINESS OR DROWSINESS—aripiprazole, asenapine, brexpiprazole, clozapine, iloperidone, loxapine, lurasidone, olanzapine, paliperidone, quetiapine, risperidone, ziprasidone MAY IMPAIR ABILITY TO DRIVE—aripiprazole, asenapine, clozapine, loxapine, lurasidone, olanzapine, quetiapine, ziprasidone AVOID ALCOHOL—aripiprazole, asenapine, clozapine, iloperidone, loxapine, lurasidone, olanzapine, quetiapine, ziprasidone MAINTAIN ADEQUATE HYDRATION—asenapine, clozapine, loxapine lurasidone, olanzapine, quetiapine, ziprasidone DO NOT DISCONTINUE WITHOUT MEDICAL SUPERVISION—aripiprazole, asenapine, clozapine, olanzapine, iloperidone, loxapine, lurasidone, quetiapine, ziprasidone ORAL SOLUTION MAY BE MIXED IN MILK, JUICE, WATER, OR COFFEE; AVOID CARBONATED BEVERAGES AND TEA—risperidone SWALLOW WHOLE; DON'T CRUSH OR CHEW—all extended release ROTATE SITE OF APPLICATION—Secuado RECONSTITUTE WITH STERILE WATER FOR INJECTION—Abilify Maintena
asenapine	Saphris Secuado	Dissolve sublingually 5 mg twice daily Apply 1 patch every 24 h (Secuado)	
brexpiprazole	Rexulti	For depression: Start 0.5–1 mg once daily, increase to 2 mg daily; max 3 mg/day	
clozapine	Clozaril	Begin 12.5 mg 1–2 times a day; increase to 300–450 mg/day (maximum, 900 mg/day)	
iloperidone	Fanapt	Start 1 mg twice daily; increase to 2 mg twice daily on day 2; then increase by 2 mg twice daily up to 12 mg twice daily (day 7)	
loxapine	Adasuve	**Inhaler (Adasuve):** Inhale 10 mg once per 24 h **Oral (Xylac):** 20–100 mg/day divided into 2–4 doses per day **IM:** Inject 12.5–50 mg IM every 4-6 h	
lurasidone	Latuda	40–160 mg once daily	
olanzapine	Zyprexa	5–10 mg/day (maximum, 20 mg/day)	

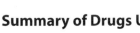

Summary of Drugs Used in the Treatment of Psychosis—cont'd

Generic Name	US Brand Name	Usual Adult Oral Dose and Dosing Schedule	Warning Labels
paliperidone	Invega	**Oral:** 6 mg once daily in the morning (maximum, 12 mg/day) **IM, extended release (Invega Sustenna):** Inject 39–234 mg IM once monthly (United States package labeling); 50–150 mg IM once monthly (Canada package labeling) **IM, extended release (Invega Trinza):** 273–819 mg IM once every 3 months (United States package labeling); 175–525 mg IM once every 3 months (Canada package labeling) **IM, extended release (Invega Hafyera):** 1092–1560 mg IM once every 6 months	
risperidone	Risperdal	2–8 mg/day (oral) or 25 mg every 2 weeks (IM) or every 4 weeks (Risperdal Consta) Inject 90–120 mg subcutaneous abdominal monthly (Perseris Kit)	
quetiapine	Seroquel, Seroquel XR	Start with 25 mg twice a day; increase to 300–800 mg/day dosed 2–3 times a day **Extended release:** 400–800 mg once daily; start with 50 mg once every evening and increase by 50 mg once daily	
ziprasidone	Geodon	**Oral:** 20 mg twice daily (maximum, 80 mg twice daily) **IM:** 10 mg every 2 h (maximum, 40 mg/day)	

TECHNICIAN'S CORNER

1. New dosage forms for antipsychotic medications are administered monthly, every 3 months, or every 6 months. Why might a long-acting medication be useful in the treatment of schizophrenia?
2. Compare and contrast negative symptoms and positive symptoms of schizophrenia.

Key Points

- Schizophrenia is a chronic and major psychosis characterized by delusions of thought, visual or auditory hallucinations (or both), and speech disturbances.
- Schizophrenia affects about 1% of the population worldwide.
- The onset typically occurs in the late teens after puberty begins to the mid-20s.
- Symptoms of schizophrenia in women may not develop until the mid-20s to early 30s.
- Neurotransmitters that have been identified as playing a role in schizophrenia are dopamine, serotonin, CCK, neurotensin, GABA, and glutamate.
- Dopamine receptor blockade treats symptoms of schizophrenia but may produce Parkinson disease–like symptoms (pseudoparkinsonism).
- Neuroleptics (antipsychotics) are classified by structure and function.
- Functional classifications for antipsychotics are based on their affinity for dopamine receptors. High-potency antipsychotics have a strong affinity for dopamine receptors. Atypical neuroleptics such as clozapine show strong affinity for serotonin receptors in addition to dopaminergic receptor blockade.
- Atypical neuroleptics are associated with the onset of diabetes.

- Atypical neuroleptics are associated with increased mortality in elderly patients with dementia-related psychosis.
- First-generation antipsychotics are well absorbed orally, rectally, and parenterally.
- Typical and atypical neuroleptics are available in slow-release depot formulations for intramuscular injection, and the therapeutic effects persist for up to 4 weeks after injection.
- Up to 80% of the people who are prescribed antipsychotic medications will experience adverse reactions.

- Extrapyramidal effects and tardive dyskinesia are associated with dopaminergic blockade and occur more frequently in elderly patients.
- Neuroleptic malignant syndrome is a life-threatening side effect of antipsychotic drugs.
- Clozapine use is restricted because it can produce a fatal drop in white blood cell levels (agranulocytosis).

Review Questions

1. Schizophrenia runs in families.
   a. true
   b. false
2. Select the drug that is marketed as a oral disintegrating tablet.
   a. Invega
   b. Seroquel
   c. Saphris
   d. Latuda
3. Select the drug that is marketed as a extended release tablet/capsule.
   a. Abilify
   b. Seroquel
   c. Risperdal
   d. Zyprexa
4. Phenothiazines, butyrophenones, and thioxanthines are categorized as _____ neuroleptics.
   a. first-generation (typical)
   b. second-generation (atypical)
5. What causes inappropriate postures of the neck, trunk, and limbs, accompanied by involuntary thrusting of the tongue and lip smacking?
   a. extrapyramidal symptoms
   b. tardive dyskinesia
   c. hyperkinesia
   d. catatonia

6. The use of _____ is restricted because it can produce a fatal drop in white blood cells (agranulocytosis).
   a. quetiapine
   b. clozapine
   c. olanzapine
   d. nifedipine
7. Select the drug that is marketed as a 6-month extended duration intramuscular injection.
   a. Invega Hafyera
   b. Invega Sustenna
   c. Clozaril
   d. Invega Trinza
8. Hallucinations, delusions, or other unusual thoughts or perceptions are _____ symptoms of schizophrenia.
   a. positive
   b. negative
9. Selection of schizophrenia agents is based on a balance between achievement of desired response to the drug and the patient's ability to tolerate drug side effects.
   a. true
   b. false
10. Risperidone is available in which dosage forms?
    a. oral solution
    b. injection
    c. tablet
    d. a, b, and c

Bibliography

Health Canada. (2022). Drug Product Database. Retrieved July 11, 2022, from https://health-products.canada.ca/dpd-bdpp/index-eng.jsp.

Institute for Safe Medication Practices. (2016). FDA and ISMP Lists of Look-Alike Drug Names with Recommended Tall Man Letters. Retrieved July 11, 2022, from https://www.ismp.org/recommendations/tall-man-letters-list.

Institute for Safe Medication Practices. (2019). List of Confused Drugs. Retrieved July 11, 2022, from https://www.ismp.org/tools/confused-drugnames.pdf.

Kalant H, Grant D, Mitchell J. *Principles of medical pharmacology.* ed 7. Toronto: Elsevier Canada, A Division of Reed Elsevier Canada; 2007:303–315.

Keating D, McWilliams S, Schneider I, et al. Pharmacological guidelines for schizophrenia: a systematic review and comparison of recommendations for the first episode. *BMJ Open.* 2017;7:e013881.

Lance L, Lacy C, Armstrong L, et al. *Drug information handbook for the allied health professional.* ed 12. Hudson, OH: APhA Lexi-Comp; 2005.

Miyamoto S, Miyake N, Jarskog L, et al. Pharmacological treatment of schizophrenia: a critical review of the pharmacology and clinical effects of current and future therapeutic agents. *Mol Psychiatry.* 2012;17:1206–1227.

National Institutes of Mental Health: *Schizophrenia.* NIH Publication No. 21-MH-8082, Bethesda, 2021, US Department of Health and Human Services. Retrieved July 11, 2022, from: https://www.nimh.nih.gov/health/publications/schizophrenia.

Page C, Curtis M, Sutter M, et al. *Integrated pharmacology.* Philadelphia: Elsevier Mosby; 2005:242–247.

U.S. Food and Drug Administration. (nd). Drugs@FDA: FDA Approved Drug Products. Retrieved July 11, 2022, from https://www.accessdata.fda.gov/scripts/cder/daf/index.cfm.

8

Treatment of Alzheimer, Huntington, and Parkinson Disease

LEARNING OBJECTIVES

1. Learn the terminology associated with the treatment of Alzheimer, Huntington, and Parkinson disease.
2. Describe the etiology of Alzheimer, Huntington, and Parkinson disease.
3. Classify medications used in the treatment of Alzheimer, Huntington, and Parkinson disease.
4. Describe the mechanism of action for each class of drugs used to treat Alzheimer, Huntington, and Parkinson disease.
5. Identify significant drug look-alike and sound-alike issues.
6. Identify warning labels and precautionary messages associated with medications used to treat Alzheimer, Huntington, and Parkinson disease.

KEY TERMS

Acetylcholinesterase Enzyme that degrades the neurotransmitter acetylcholine.

Alzheimer disease Neurodegenerative disease that causes memory loss and behavioral changes.

ApoE4 allele Defective form of apolipoprotein E that is associated with Alzheimer disease.

Bradykinesia Slowness in initiating and carrying out voluntary movements.

Cognitive functions The ability to take in information via the senses, process the details, commit the information to memory, and recall it when necessary.

Dementia Condition associated with a loss of memory and cognition.

Huntington disease Progressive and degenerative disease of neurons that affects muscle movement, cognitive functions, and emotions.

Neurodegeneration Destruction of nerve cells.

Neuroprotective Protects nerve cells from damage.

Parkinson disease Progressive disorder of the nervous system involving degeneration of dopaminergic neurons and causing impaired muscle movement.

Plaques Substances composed of a protein called beta amyloid that fill the spaces between neurons and interfere with the transmission of signals between neurons.

Pseudoparkinsonism Drug-induced condition that resembles Parkinson disease.

Tangles Twisted fibers made up of clumps of a protein called tau that interfere with nerve signal transmission.

Alzheimer Disease

Alzheimer disease is a neurodegenerative disease that causes memory loss and behavioral changes. According to the National Institutes of Health National Institute on Aging, up to 5.8 million Americans have Alzheimer disease. More than 747,000 Canadians have Alzheimer disease or a related dementia. It is not fully known why someone will develop Alzheimer disease; however, several risk factors are believed to be involved. They are age, having a family member with Alzheimer disease, genetics, environmental factors (e.g., air pollution), cardiovascular disease, cerebrovascular disease, and traumatic brain injury. Conditions that cause long-term cognitive impairment, such as long COVID or its treatment with mechanical ventilation, are increasingly being recognized as a potential risk for Alzheimer disease.

The most important risk for Alzheimer disease is age. The risk increases with age. In fact, nearly 5% of the adult population 65 years of age will have Alzheimer disease. That percentage doubles by age 70 years, and by age 85 years, it is estimated that 33% of Americans and 1 in 4 Canadians will have the disease. Although advancing age is an important risk factor for the development of Alzheimer disease, *dementia* is not a normal part of the aging process. Less than 5% of the people have familial Alzheimer disease (FAD); however, having a family member with Alzheimer disease is a risk factor of developing the disease. There is a 50% chance of children inheriting the gene that causes Alzheimer disease. Late-onset Alzheimer disease is linked to several nonhereditary genes. Apolipoprotein E (ApoE) helps carry cholesterol in the blood. Approximately 40% of people with Alzheimer disease have a defective form of ApoE, although not everyone with a defective

ApoE4 allele will develop the disease. Only 15% of people with the defective *ApoE4 allele* will develop Alzheimer disease. Other factors that may play a role in Alzheimer disease are inflammation, oxidative damage, iron deregulation, and cholesterol metabolism blood-brain barrier dysfunction.

The most commonly reported symptom of Alzheimer disease is forgetfulness. Mild cognitive impairment (MCI) is often an early stage of Alzheimer disease (Box 8.1). MCI is a decline in cognitive abilities such as language, memory reasoning, judgment, or perception that is not caused by normal aging. The person may not recall recent events or names of familiar people or things. This increases as the disease progresses and may interfere with the performance of activities of daily living such as personal hygiene. In the mid to late stages of Alzheimer disease, the person may have difficulty reading, speaking, writing, and walking. The person may become anxious, angry, and aggressive. In addition, the person may be confused and wander, unable to find the way back to where they started. Many people confuse the differences between the normal aging process and Alzheimer disease. Table 8.1 shows some comparisons between the disease and normal aging.

Pathophysiology of Alzheimer Disease

Alzheimer disease causes damage to the part of the brain that is involved in memory. The disease causes cholinergic nerve cells in the brain to die. The cerebral cortex shrinks in size, and the ability to think and function diminishes. Abnormal structures, called plaques and tangles, develop in the brain (Fig. 8.1). *Plaques* are dense substances composed of a protein called beta amyloid. The plaques fill the spaces between neurons in the brain and interfere with the transmission of signals between the neurons. *Tangles* look like twisted fibers and are made up of clumps of a protein called tau. Tangles are also thought to block the transmission of messages between neurons. The accumulation of plaques and tangles also produces inflammation, which further damages neurons.

Comorbid conditions such as cerebrovascular disease, high blood pressure, diabetes, sleep apnea, and Parkinson disease are believed to speed the progression of Alzheimer disease. Lewy bodies, abnormal clumps of protein, found in people with Alzheimer disease are also associated with Parkinson disease. Sleep deprivation can increase beta amyloid deposits. Microvascular infarcts and inflammation, which block blood supply and nourishment to the brain, are common in patients with cerebrovascular disease, diabetes, and Alzheimer disease.

Role of Neurotransmitters

Several neurotransmitters play a significant role in Alzheimer disease. The most significant is acetylcholine (ACh). ACh levels gradually decline as the disease progresses, producing the symptoms associated with Alzheimer disease. Glutamate also plays a role in the development of Alzheimer disease. Glutamate is an excitatory amino acid that is involved in memory formation and learning. There are three classes of glutamatergic receptors. The most important is *N*-methyl-D-aspartate (NMDA). NMDA is believed to contribute to the process of *neurodegeneration*.

Other neurotransmitters that are believed to play a part in Alzheimer disease are dopamine, norepinephrine, and serotonin. Reduced nicotinic receptor function is also correlated to impaired memory.

Drug Treatment for Alzheimer Disease

Drugs that increase ACh levels at the synapse are used to treat Alzheimer disease. Three of the six drugs currently approved for the treatment of Alzheimer disease are *acetylcholinesterase* (AChE) inhibitors. AChE is an enzyme that degrades ACh. AChE inhibitors increase levels of ACh. AChE-R appears to protect against the degeneration of cholinergic neurons. *Neuroprotective* agents protect nerve cells from damage. The AChE inhibitors are typically prescribed for the treatment of mild to moderate disease.

Drugs that block glutamate activity are also used in the treatment of Alzheimer disease. Mematine is glutamate regulator that acts at the NMDA receptor site. It improves memory, attention, reason, language, and the ability to perform simple tasks. It is prescribed for moderate to severe disease. Aducanumab and lecanemab-IRMB (Leqembi) are monoclonal antibodies that are used to treat Alzheimer disease. Aducanumab was approved in 2021 and lecanemab-IRMB was approved in 2023. All other drugs target Alzheimer symptoms.

TABLE 8.1	Comparisons Between Alzheimer Disease and Normal Aging
Alzheimer Disease	**Normal Aging**
Making poor judgments and decisions a lot of the time	Making a bad decision once in a while
Problems taking care of monthly bills	Missing a monthly payment
Losing track of the date or time of year	Forgetting which day it is and remembering it later
Trouble having a conversation	Sometimes forgetting which word to use
Misplacing things often and being unable to find them	Losing things from time to time

Courtesy of the National Institute on Aging, Understanding Alzheimer's disease: what you need to know (https://www.nia.nih.gov/alzheimers/publication/understanding-alzheimers-disease/introduction).

• BOX 8.1 Stages of Alzheimer Disease

Mild Dementia
1. Memory loss of recent events
2. Difficulty with problem solving, complex tasks, and sound judgments
3. Changes in personality
4. Difficulty organizing and expressing thoughts
5. Getting lost or misplacing belongings

Moderate Dementia
1. Show increasing poor judgment and deepening confusion
2. Experiencing greater memory loss
3. Need help with daily activities
4. Undergo significant changes in personal behavior

Severe Dementia
1. Experience a decline in physical abilities
2. Lose the ability to communicate coherently
3. Require daily assistance with personal care

Source: Adapted from Mayo Clinic Alheimer's stages: How the disease progresses (https://www.mayoclinic.org/diseases-conditions/alzheimers-disease/in-depth/alzheimers-stages/art-20048448)

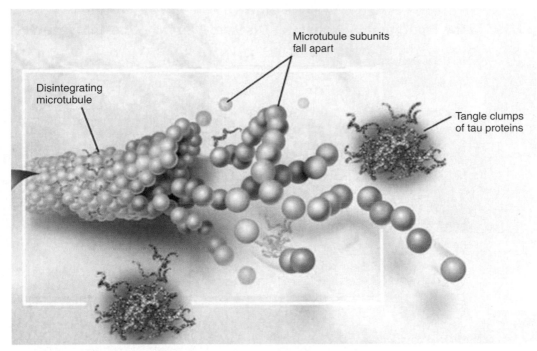

• Fig. 8.1 Disintegrating neurons and tangles. (Courtesy The Alzheimer's Disease Education and Referral Center, National Institute on Aging, Bethesda, MD.)

Mechanism of Action and Pharmacokinetics

Donepezil (Aricept), rivastigmine (Exelon), and galantamine (Razadyne, Reminyl) are AChE inhibitors. In addition to AChE inhibition, galantamine slightly increases glutamate activity.

Donepezil is highly protein bound and metabolized by cytochrome P-450 (CYP450) isoenzymes and thus subject to drug interactions with drugs that are similarly protein bound and metabolized by enzymes in the liver. Donepezil is available as a swallowable tablet and an oral disintegrating tablet. Its bioavailability is not diminished by food; therefore it may be taken without regard to meals. In contrast, the bioavailability of galantamine is delayed by food; however, the drug is nearly 90% bioavailable, and protein binding and CYP450 metabolism are minimal. Rivastigmine readily crosses the blood-brain barrier, where it is metabolized at central nervous system receptor sites. Cholinesterase inhibition lasts up to 10 hours. Over a 24-hour period, 50% of the drug is released from rivastigmine transdermal patches.

Memantine (Namenda) blocks the actions of glutamate at NMDA receptor sites. This mechanism of action is theorized to protect the neuron from further damage. All dosage forms of memantine exhibit 100% bioavailability. The drug is minimally subject to drug interactions involving CYP450 isozymes; however, alkaline urine can decrease drug clearance by as much as 80%. Food has little effect on absorption, and memantine may be taken without regard to meals.

Aducanumab and lecanemab-IRMB are monoclonal antibody (IgG1). Their effects on reducing amyloid beta plaques increase as the antibody dose increases.

> **● Tech Note!**
>
> In the United States, galantamine was formerly marketed under the brand name Reminyl but is now marketed as Razadyne.

> **● Tech Note!**
>
> Rivastimine premixed solution must be consumed within 4 hours of mixing.

Adverse Reactions

Donepezil, galantamine, rivastigmine, and memantine can all produce abdominal pain and cramping, dizziness, diarrhea, nausea, and urinary incontinence. In some patients, donepezil and rivastigmine may increase urinary frequency. Tremor has been reported in all agents except donepezil. Pseudoparkinsonism has been reported with the use of rivastigmine and memantine. Myocardial infarction, erectile dysfunction, and suicide ideation have been reported with memantine. Side effects of Aduhelm (aducanumab) and Leqembi (lecanemab-IRMB) include headache, dizziness, falls, nausea, confusion, and vision changes. ARIA is a serious side effect of aducanumab and lecanenumab that casues temporary swelling in areas of the brain.

> **● Tech Note!**
>
> Dispense Razadyne solution with manufacturer's calibrated syringe.

Nonpharmacological Measures to Reduce Risks for Alzheimer Disease

Head injury protection and adoption of a healthy lifestyle that includes reduction in cholesterol, adequate intellectual stimulation, and decreased obesity are modifiable factors that may reduce the risk for Alzheimer disease. Social interaction keeps the brain stimulated. Some studies have shown that aerobic exercise can reduce risks for obesity, improve cognition, and reduce plaque formation. A diet that includes vegetables, legumes, fruits, cereals, olive oil, decreased saturated fats, dairy products, fish, lean meat,

Drugs Used in the Treatment of Alzheimer Disease: Acetylcholinesterase Inhibitors

Generic Name	US Brand Name(s) / Canadian Brand(s)	Dosage Forms and Strengths
donepezil[a]	Adlarity, Aricept	**Tablets:** 5 mg, 10 mg, 23 mg[b]
	Aricept, Aricept RDT	**Tablets, oral disintegrating (Aricept RDT):** 5 mg, 10 mg **Transdermal patch (Adlarity)**[b]**:** 5 mg/day, 10 mg/day
donepezil + memantine[a]	Namzaric	**Capsule, extended release**[b]**:** 10 mg donepezil + 7 mg memantine; 10 mg donepezil + 14 mg memantine; 10 mg donepezil + 21 mg memantine; 10 mg donepezil + 28 mg memantine
	Not available	
galantamine[a]	Razadyne ER	**Tablets**[b]**:** 4 mg, 8 mg, 12 mg
	Generics	**Tablets, extended release (Razadyne ER):** 8 mg, 16 mg, 24 mg
rivastigmine[a]	Exelon	**Capsules:** 1.5 mg, 3 mg, 4.5 mg, 6 mg **Solution, oral**[c]**:** 2 mg/mL
	Exelon, Exelon patch-5, Exelon patch-10, Exelon patch-15	**Transdermal patch:** 4.6 mg/24 h, 9.5 mg/24 h, 13.3 mg/24 h

[a]Generic available.
[b]Available in the United States only.
[c]Available in Canada only.

Drugs Used in the Treatment of Alzheimer Disease: N-Methyl-D-Aspartate Receptor Inhibitor

Generic Name	US Brand Name(s) / Canadian Brand(s)	Dosage Forms and Strengths
memantine[a,b]	Namenda, Namenda XR	**Solution, oral:** 2 mg/ mL[b]
	Ebixa	**Tablets:** 5 mg, 10 mg **Capsule (Namenda XR)**[b]**:** 7 mg, 14 mg, 21 mg, 28 mg

[a]Generic available
[b]Available in the United States only.

Drugs Used to Reduce Beta-Amyloid Plaques

Generic Name	US Brand Name(s) / Canadian Brand(s)	Dosage Forms and Strengths
aducanumab	Aduhelm	Solution, for injection: 170 mg/1.7 mL, 300 mg/3 mL
	Not available	
lecanenumab	Leqembi	Solution, for infusion 100 mg/mL(in 2 mL and 5 mL single use vials)
	Not available	

poultry, and antioxidants can reduce vascular disease, a comorbid condition linked to increasing the progression of Alzheimer disease. Vitamin E, folate, selenium, and other antioxidants are being studied for their possible benefit in preventing Alzheimer disease.

Parkinson Disease

Parkinson disease is a progressive disorder of the nervous system involving degeneration of dopaminergic neurons in the basal ganglia and nigrostriatal pathways in the brain. The basal ganglia are part of the extrapyramidal system that initiates, controls, and modulates movement and posture.

Loss of dopaminergic neurons results in reduction of available dopamine. Symptoms of Parkinson disease are a result of an imbalance between dopamine and ACh (Fig. 8.2). As the loss of dopaminergic neurons progresses, voluntary muscle movement diminishes.

Approximately 1 million people in the United States have Parkinson disease. Nearly 1 in 500 people are living with Parkinson disease in Canada. The disease disproportionately affects elderly men, and they are 1.5 times more likely to have Parkinson disease than women. The average age at onset of Parkinson disease is 60 years. The prevalence and incidence (number of new cases) increase with age. The onset of Parkinson disease in persons younger than 40 years old is rare and has been associated with ingestion of illicit drugs contaminated with MPTP (1-methyl-4-phenyl-1,2,3,6-tetrahydropyridine).

The etiology of Parkinson disease is thought to be related to environmental and genetic factors. Recent studies with twins have shown a familial inheritance of the chromosome 4 gene. Environmental causes are associated with pesticide exposure and exposure to drugs that destroy dopaminergic neurons in nigrostriatal pathways. Exposure to pesticides may increase the long-term risk for development of Parkinson disease from 3% to 5%, according to a cohort study that reviewed surveys of 143,000 participants in the United States, the "Cancer Prevention Study II Nutrition Cohort" begun in 1982. The risks appear to be greater in men than in women. Other environmental toxins that may cause development of Parkinson disease are carbon monoxide poisoning and heavy metal poisoning (mercury). Infectious diseases such as viral encephalitis are thought to be possible triggers for Parkinson disease.

Pseudoparkinsonism is a drug-induced condition that resembles Parkinson disease. It is caused by administration of drugs

Summary of Drugs Used in the Treatment of Alzheimer Disease

Generic Name	US Brand Name	Usual Adult Oral Dose and Dosing Schedule	Warning Labels
aducanumab	Aduhelm	10 mg/kg infused over 1 h every 4 weeks	MAY CAUSE DIZZINESS OR DROWSINESS— donepezil, galantamine, rivastigmine, memantine, aducanumab.
donepezil	Aricept	**Tablets/ODT:** 5–23 mg once daily at bedtime	TAKE WITH FOOD—galantamine, rivastigmine.
donepezil + memantine	Namzaric	**Tablet:** 1 tablet once daily	DISSOLVE IN MOUTH—donepezil ODT. DO NOT DISCONTINUE WITHOUT MEDICAL SUPERVISION.
galantamine	Reminyl	**Tablets:** 4–12 mg twice a day **Extended release tablets:** 8–24 mg once daily	REMOVE OLD PATCH AND ROTATE SITE OF APPLICATION—donepezil, rivastigmine
rivastigmine	Exelon	**Capsules/solution:** 1.5–6 mg twice a day **Transdermal patch:** Apply one patch daily 4.6–13.3 mg once daily	MAINTAIN ADEQUATE HYDRATION—galantamine. SWALLOW WHOLE; DO NOT CRUSH OR CHEW— donepezil + memantine, galantamine ER, memantine XR.
memantine	Namenda	**Tablets:** 5–10 mg twice a day **Capsules XR:** 7–28 mg once daily	MAY MIX SOLUTION WITH WATER, JUICE, OR SODA ONLY—rivastigmine. CAPSULES MAY BE SPRINKLED ON APPLESAUCE— memantine XR.
lecanenumab	leqembi	Infuse 10 mg/kg over 1 hour every 2 weeks	STORE IN FRIDGE; DON'T FREEZE (2°C to 8°C or 36°F to 46°F). —aducanumab, lecanenumab. PROTECT FROM LIGHT—aducanumab, lecanenumab. DILUTE WITH 0.9% NS BEFORE USE—aducanumab, lecanenumab.

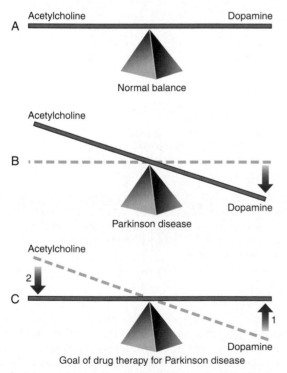

A. Normal balance of acetylcholine and dopamine in the CNS.
B. In Parkinson disease, a decrease in dopamine results in an imbalance.
C. Drug therapy in Parkinson disease is aimed at correcting the imbalance between acetylcholine and dopamine. This can be accomplished by either
1. increasing the supply of dopamine, or
2. blocking or lowering acetylcholine levels.

• **Fig. 8.2** Balance of acetylcholine and dopamine versus Parkinson disease. *CNS*, Central nervous system. (From Lilley LL, Harrington S, Snyder JS. *Pharmacology and the nursing process*, ed 5, St Louis, 2007, Mosby.)

that block dopaminergic receptors in the basal ganglia in the brain. Examples of drugs that produce pseudoparkinsonism are neuroleptics (e.g., phenothiazines), administered to treat schizophrenia, and reserpine, a drug that is used to treat hypertension.

Characteristic signs of Parkinson disease are **bradykinesia** and slowness in initiating and carrying out voluntary movements accompanied by muscle rigidity and tremors. When a person wishes to move their arm, the onset of movement is often delayed. When the forward motion begins, movements will be slow, rigid, and tremulous. Tremors are usually present at rest and may reduce the person's ability to perform skilled tasks. Postural and gait abnormalities are also typically present. The person walks with a characteristic shuffle. Other visible signs of Parkinson disease are a blank facial expression, drooling, and speech impairment.

Cognitive functions and motor functions may be impaired. Parkinson disease can cause memory loss, and affected persons may exhibit signs of dementia. Parkinson disease can also cause depression.

Parkinson disease is treated by the administration of pharmaceuticals, exercise, and nutritional support.

Drugs Used to Treat Parkinson Disease

The strategy for treatment of Parkinson disease is to restore the balance between dopamine and ACh. The amount of dopamine available for release diminishes as Parkinson disease progresses because degeneration of dopaminergic neurons increases. This results in unopposed cholinergic excitation and produces the tremors, muscle rigidity, and immobility associated with Parkinson disease. Dopamine agonist drugs increase dopamine by promoting the release of existing stores of dopamine, directly stimulating dopamine receptors, or inhibiting the degradation of dopamine in the terminal neuron (Fig. 8.3). Dopamine regulates direct and indirect extrapyramidal pathways. Apomorphine, bromocriptine, pramipexole, ropinirole, and rotigotine are dopamine agonists. Apomorphine and opicapone are newer agents that are indicated

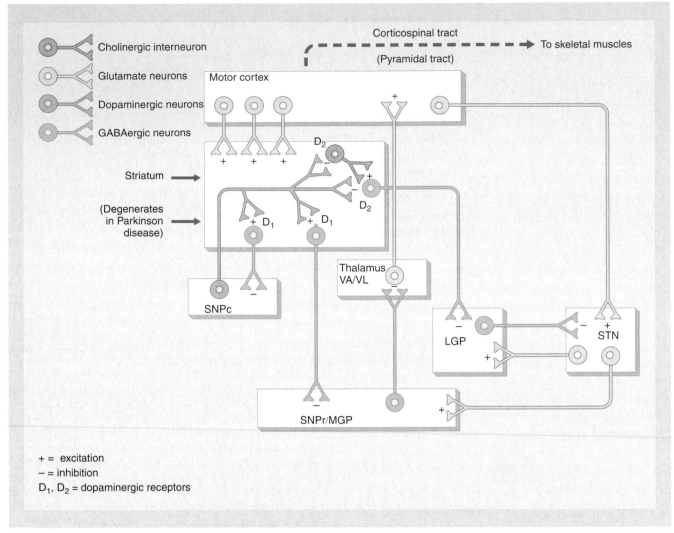

• **Fig. 8.3** Summary of basal ganglia systems involved in Parkinson disease. *LGP*, Lateral globus pallidus; *SNPc*, substantia nigra pars compacta; *SNPr/MGP*, substantia nigra pars reticula/medial globus pallidus; *STN*, subthalamic nucleus; *VA/VL*, ventroanterior/ventrolateral thalamic nuclei. (From Page C, Curtis M, Sutter M, et al. *Integrated pharmacology*, ed 3, Philadelphia, 2006, Mosby.)

for the acute, intermittent treatment of "off" episodes in patients with Parkinson disease.

Mechanism of Action

Stimulation of GABAergic neurons by dopamine (D_2) sends inhibitory feedback to the motor cortex via the indirect pathway. This results in impaired voluntary muscle movement. Anticholinergics may be administered to decrease ACh levels because excessive stimulation of cholinergic neurons causes symptoms of immobility in Parkinson disease.

There is a decrease in the effectiveness of most anti-Parkinson drugs over time because of the disease's progressive neurodegeneration. The efficacy of levodopa and amantadine also declines with long-term therapy because of desensitization of dopamine receptors.

> **Tech Note!**
>
> In addition to the treatment of Parkinson disease, bromocriptine 0.8 mg (Cylcoset) is indicated as adjunct therapy for the treatment of type 2 diabetes mellitus.

> **Tech Note!**
>
> Carbidopa/levodopa (Duopa, Duodopa) is also marketed for infusion in an intestinal pump. It is indicated for the treatment of advanced levodopa-responsive Parkinson disease.

Pharmacokinetics

The absorption, distribution, metabolism, and elimination of drugs used to treat Parkinson disease vary. Levodopa is a prodrug and a dopamine precursor. It is administered rather than dopamine (which is available for use as a cardiac stimulant) because dopamine does not cross the blood-brain barrier. Although levodopa readily crosses the blood-brain barrier, much of the orally administered drug is metabolized in the gastrointestinal tract and in peripheral tissues (see Fig. 8.3). Only a small percentage actually reaches the neuron to be converted to dopamine. Sustained-release preparations of levodopa can further reduce the bioavailability of levodopa by as much as 30%.

Carbidopa and benserazide are adjuvants that boost the effectiveness of levodopa. Carbidopa and benserazide inhibit the metabolism (decarboxylation) of levodopa in the gastrointestinal tract and peripheral tissues. The bioavailability of levodopa is increased by 75% when combined with carbidopa. Catechol-*O*-methyltransferase (COMT) is the enzyme responsible for peripheral and central metabolism of catecholamines that also metabolizes levodopa. Entacapone, opicapone, and tolcapone are COMT inhibitors that can boost the bioavailability of levodopa by up to 50%.

> ❶ **Tech Alert!**
>
> The following drugs have look-alike/sound-alike issues:
>
> ReQuip and ReQuip XL;
> riMANTAdine and raNITIdine;
> Sinemet and Sinemet CR;
> selegiline and sertraline

Common Adverse Reactions

Gastrointestinal distress such as nausea, vomiting, and decreased appetite are common side effects of most of the drugs used to treat Parkinson disease. Other common side effects are dizziness or lightheadedness, insomnia, and confusion. Apomorphine and opicapone can also cause hallucinations or delusions. Hypotension is also associated with most of the drugs used to treat Parkinson disease. Many of the anti-Parkinson drugs that increase dopamine also produce dry mouth and constipation. Drugs that treat Parkinson disease can produce auditory and visual hallucinations. People older than the age of 65 years are most susceptible.

> ● **Tech Note!**
>
> High-protein diets and iron supplements may decrease the absorption of Parkinson drugs containing levodopa.

Precautions

Selegiline and rasagiline are monoamine oxidase type B ($MAOI_B$) inhibitors that can increase the risk for hypertensive crisis. Patients taking Prolopa (levodopa plus benserazide) may experience sudden drowsiness without warning and should be cautioned about risks for driving accidents. It is recommended that patients with diabetes test their blood glucose levels more frequently when taking Prolopa.

> ● **Tech Note!**
>
> Selegiline and rasagiline are MAOIs. Dispense with a list of tyramine-containing foods and beverages to avoid. Dietary restrictions are not required for selegiline patches.

> ● **Tech Note!**
>
> Do not take Kynmobi if you are taking medicines to treat nausea called 5-HT3 antagonists, including ondansetron, granisetron, dolasetron, palosetron, and alosetron.

Drugs That Reduce Cholinergic Activity

Anticholinergics are administered as adjunctive treatment of Parkinson disease and to lessen drug-induced extrapyramidal symptoms. Side effects are dizziness, sedation, confusion, dry mouth, blurred vision, constipation, urinary retention, heat intolerance, hypotension, and hallucinations.

Huntington Disease

Huntington disease is another progressive and degenerative disease of neurons that affects muscle movement, cognitive functions, and emotions. Huntington disease is similar to Parkinson disease in that it is associated with defects in the basal ganglia. Unlike Parkinson disease, it produces excessive, abnormal muscle movement rather than immobility.

Huntington disease is a hereditary disorder. It affects approximately one person in every 10,000. Children born to a parent

Drugs That Enhance Dopaminergic Activity

Generic Name	US Brand Name(s) / Canadian Brand(s)	Dosage Forms and Strengths
amantadine[a]	Gocovri Osmolex ER	**Capsules:** 100 mg
	Generics	**Capsule, extended release (Gocovri, Osmolex ER):** 68.5 mg, 137 mg Gocovri; 129 mg, 193 mg (Osmolex ER)
		Syrup, oral: 50 mg/5 mL
		Tablets: 100 mg[b]
apomorphine	Kynmobi, Apokyn	**Solution, for injection (Apokyn, Movapo)**[a]**:** 10 mg/mL
	Kynmobi, Movapo	**Sublingual film Kynmobi:** 10 mg, 15 mg, 20 mg, 25 mg, 30 mg
bromocriptine[a]	Parlodel	**Capsules:** 5 mg
	Generics	**Tablets:** 2.5 mg
carbidopa[a]	Lodosyn	**Tablets:** 25 mg
	Not available	
entacapone[a]	Comtan	**Tablets:** 200 mg
	Comtan	

Continued

Drugs That Enhance Dopaminergic Activity—cont'd

Generic Name	US Brand Name(s) / Canadian Brand(s)	Dosage Forms and Strengths
levodopa and carbidopa[a]	Dhivy, Duopa, Rytary, Sinemet, Sinemet CR Duodopa	**Capsule, extended release (Rytary):** 23.75 mg carbidopa + 95 mg levodopa; 36.25 mg carbidopa + 145 mg levodopa; 48.75 mg carbidopa + 195 mg levodopa; 61.25 mg carbidopa + 245 mg levodopa **Gel, intestinal (Duodopa):** 5 mg carbidopa + 20 mg levodopa per 1 mL **Suspension, enteral (Duopa):** 4.63 mg carbidopa + 20 mg levodopa per 1 mL **Tablets, extended release (Sinemet CR):** 25 mg carbidopa + 100 mg levodopa; 50 mg carbidopa + 200 mg levodopa **Tablets, immediate release (Dhivy, Sinemet):** 10 mg carbidopa + 100 mg levodopa; 25 mg carbidopa + 100 mg levodopa; 25 mg carbidopa + 250 mg levodopa **Tablets, immediate oral disintegrating:** 10 mg carbidopa + 100 mg levodopa; 25 mg carbidopa + 100 mg levodopa; 25 mg carbidopa + 250 mg levodopa
levodopa and benserazide	Not available Prolopa	**Capsules:** 50 mg levodopa + 12.5 mg benserazide; 100 mg levodopa + 25 mg benserazide; 200 mg levodopa + 50 mg benserazide
levodopa, carbidopa, and entacapone	Stalevo Stalevo	**Tablets:** carbidopa 12.5 mg + levodopa 50 mg + entacapone 200 mg; carbidopa 18.75 mg + levodopa 75 mg + entacapone 200 mg; carbidopa 25 mg + levodopa 100 mg + entacapone 200 mg; carbidopa 31.5 mg + levodopa 125 mg + entacapone 200 mg; carbidopa 37.5 mg + levodopa 150 mg + entacapone 200 mg; carbidopa 50 mg + levodopa 200 mg + entacapone 200 mg
opicapone	Ongentys Not Available	**Capsule:** 25 mg, 50 mg
pramipexole[a]	Mirapex ER Mirapex	**Tablets:** 0.125 mg, 0.25 mg, 0.5 mg, 1 mg, 1.25 mg, 1.5 mg **Tablets, extended release (Mirapex ER)[b]:** 0.375 mg, 0.75 mg, 1.5 mg, 2.25 mg, 3 mg, 3.75 mg, 4.5 mg
rasagiline[a]	Azilect Azilect	**Tablets:** 0.5 mg, 1 mg
ropinirole[a]	Generics Generics	**Tablets:** 0.25 mg, 0.5 mg[b], 1 mg, 2 mg, 3 mg[b], 4 mg[b], 5 mg **Tablets, extended release[b]:** 2 mg, 4 mg, 6 mg, 8 mg, 12 mg
rotigotine	Neupro Neupro	**Transdermal film:** 1 mg/24 h, 2 mg/24 h, 3 mg/24 h, 4 mg/24 h, 6 mg/24 h, 8 mg/24 h
selegiline[a] (L-deprenyl)	Eldepryl, Zelapar Emsam Generics	**Capsules[b]:** 5 mg **Tablets:** 5 mg **Tablets, oral disintegrating (Zelapar)[b]:** 1.25 mg **Transdermal patch (Emsam)[b]:** 6 mg/24 h, 9 mg/24 h, 12 mg/24 h
tolcapone[a]	Tasmar Not available	**Tablets:** 100 mg

[a]Generic available.
[b]Available in the United States only.

who has Huntington disease have a 50% chance of inheriting the gene for the disease. If the gene is inherited, the child will develop Huntington disease at some point. The onset of Huntington disease typically occurs in middle age (30 to 50 years); symptoms rarely occur after age 55. Juvenile onset is associated with rapid progression of symptoms and shorter life expectancy. Patients may live with the illness for 10 to 30 years.

Characteristic symptoms of Huntington disease are tremors, rhythmic oscillations or circular movements around the ankles or wrists, and sudden abnormal movements. Movements are typically repetitive. Choreiform movements, unpredictable, irregular, and jerking motions, are also signs of the disease. The person may also have speech impairment and difficulty swallowing and may exhibit facial grimaces.

Huntington disease also causes emotional and intellectual changes. The person has difficulty concentrating, which worsens as the disease progresses. Irritability, mood swings, and depression are other symptoms of the disease. Cognitive impairment 0may appear as fixation on an idea, slowed thinking and responses, memory problems, and difficulty sequencing activities.

Neurochemistry of Huntington Disease

Huntington disease causes defects in the basal ganglia that result in increased concentrations of dopamine and decreased activity of the enzymes that synthesize GABA and ACh. Deficient levels of ACh and GABA lead to hyperactivity of dopaminergic neurons in nigrostriatal pathways. The balance between GABA, ACh, and dopamine is upset, and this produces the excessive muscle movement associated with Huntington disease.

Drugs Used to Treat Huntington Disease

Deutetrabenazine (Austedo) and tetrabenzine (Xenazine) are the only two drugs approved by the US Food and Drug Administration (FDA) for the treatment of Huntington disease.

Drugs That Reduce Cholinergic Activity

Generic Name	US Brand Name(s)	Dosage Forms and Strengths
	Canadian Brand(s)	
benztropine[a]	Generics	**Injection:** 1 mg/mL
	Generics	**Tablets:** 0.5 mg[b], 1 mg, 2 mg[b]
trihexyphenidyl[a]	Generic only	**Elixir**[b]**:** 2 mg/5 mL
	Generic only	**Tablets:** 2 mg, 5 mg

[a]Generic available.
[b]Available in the United States only

Summary of Drugs Used in the Treatment of Parkinson Disease

Generic Name	US Brand Name	Usual Adult Oral Dose and Dosing Schedule	Warning Labels
Drugs That Increase Dopamine Levels			
amantadine	Generics	100 mg twice a day up to 300–400 mg/day	MAY CAUSE DIZZINESS; MAY IMPAIR ABILITY TO DRIVE—all.
apomorphine	Apokyn, Kynmobi	Inject 0.2 mL (2 mg) - 0.6 mL (6 mg) subcutaneously up to a maximum of 5 doses per day or 2 mL (Apokyn).	AVOID ALCOHOL. DO NOT DISCONTINUE WITHOUT MEDICAL SUPERVISION. KEEP IN THE FOIL POUCH UNTIL READY TO USE—apomorphine.
bromocriptine	Parlodel	Start 1.25 mg twice/day; increase to 40–100 mg/day	AVOID IRON SUPPLEMENTS WITHIN 2 HOURS OF DOSE—levodopa/carbidopa, levodopa, carbidopa and entacapone, levodopa and benserazide.
entacapone	Comtan	200 mg up to 8 times a day (only effective in combination with levodopa/carbidopa)	
levodopa and carbidopa	Sinemet	**Immediate release:** carbidopa 25 mg/levodopa 100 mg 3–4 times a day (maximum, carbidopa 200 mg/levodopa 2000 mg) **Sustained release:** carbidopa 50 mg/levodopa 200 mg 2 times a day (maximum, carbidopa 400 mg/levodopa 1600 mg)	MAY CAUSE SUDDEN, EXCESSIVE DROWSINESS—Prolopa. SWALLOW WHOLE; DO NOT CRUSH OR CHEW (sustained release, Prolopa).
levodopa and benserazide	Prolopa	Initiate 1 capsule Prolopa (100 mg levodopa + 25 mg benserazide) 1–2 times a day; increase to 4–8 capsules daily in 4–6 divided doses	
levodopa, carbidopa, and entacapone	Stalevo	Individualized (maximum, 1600 mg/day)	

Continued

Summary of Drugs Used in the Treatment of Parkinson Disease—cont'd

Generic Name	US Brand Name	Usual Adult Oral Dose and Dosing Schedule	Warning Labels
opicapone	Ongentys	50 mg once daily at bedtime	TAKE WITH FOOD—bromocriptine, Prolopa. AVOID FOODS HIGH IN TYRAMINE—rasagiline, selegiline. MAY DISCOLOR URINE—Stavelo, tolcapone, entacapone, Sinemet. SWALLOW WHOLE; DO NOT CRUSH OR CHEW—extended release.
pramipexole	Mirapex	Start 0.125 mg/day in 3 divided doses; increase to 1.5–4.5 mg/day	
rasagiline	Azilect	0.5–1 mg once daily	
ropinerole	ReQuip	Start 0.25 mg 3 times/day; increase weekly to a maximum 24 mg/day	
selegiline	Generics	5 mg twice a day or 10 mg once daily	
tolcapone	Tasmar	100 mg 3 times a day	
Anticholinergics			
benztropine	Cogentin	0.5–6 mg/day (usual dose 1–2 mg at bedtime)	MAY CAUSE DROWSINESS; MAY IMPAIR ABILITY TO DRIVE. AVOID ALCOHOL. MAINTAIN ADEQUATE HYDRATION. DO NOT DISCONTINUE WITHOUT MEDICAL SUPERVISION.
trihexyphenidyl	Generics	5–15 mg/day in 3–4 divided doses	

Drugs That Deplete Stores of Dopamine

Generic Name	US Brand Name(s) / Canadian Brand(s)	Dosage Forms and Strengths
deutetrabenzine	Austedo	**Tablets:** 6 mg, 9 mg, 12 mg
	Not Available	
tetrabenazine[a]	Xenazine	**Tablets:** 12.5 mg[b], 25 mg
	Nitoman	

[a]Generic available.
[b]Strength available in the United States only.

Mechanism of Action

Deutetrabenzine and tetrabenzine decrease excessive dopaminergic activity. This is accomplished by depleting stores of dopamine in the neuron. Drugs that block dopamine receptors may also be administered.

Common Side Effects

Side effects of deutetrabenazine and tetrabenazine are hypotension, sedation, constipation, dizziness, depression, suicide ideation, and pseudoparkinsonism.

Drugs That Block Dopamine Receptors

Neuroleptics (e.g., haloperidol, fluphenazine, risperidone, and olanzapine) have been administered to control choreiform movements but are not approved by the FDA for this purpose. Side effects include sedation, confusion, weight gain, increased appetite, blurred vision, dry mouth, urinary retention, constipation, postural hypotension, pseudoparkinsonism, extrapyramidal symptoms, tardive dyskinesia, photosensitivity, and sexual dysfunction.

Summary of Drugs Used in the Treatment of Huntington Disease

Generic Name	US Brand Name	Usual Adult Oral Dose and Dosing Schedule	Warning Labels
Drugs That Decrease Dopamine Levels			
deutetrabenazine	Austedo	Start with 6 mg once daily; may increase up to 48 mg daily; daily doses of 12 mg or more should be given in 2 divided doses	SWALLOW WHOLE; DO NOT CRUSH OR CHEW—deutetrabenazine. TAKE WITH FOOD—deutetrabenazine.
tetrabenazine	Xenazine, Nitoman (Canada)	25–37.5 mg 2–3 times/day (maximum, 50 mg/day)	MAY CAUSE DROWSINESS; MAY IMPAIR ABILITY TO DRIVE; LIMIT ALCOHOL. DO NOT DISCONTINUE WITH MEDICAL SUPERVISION. DILUTE ORAL CONCENTRATE BEFORE ADMINISTRATION—haloperidol. MAINTAIN ADEQUATE HYDRATION—haloperidol. AVOID PROLONGED EXPOSURE TO SUNLIGHT—haloperidol.

TECHNICIAN'S CORNER

1. According to the most current research, a brain-healthy diet is one that reduces the risk of heart disease and diabetes, encourages good blood flow to the brain, and is low in fat and cholesterol. What sort of physical, mental, and social activities can be added to daily living to delay the onset of Alzheimer disease?
2. What are public health strategies to reduce the risk of Parkinson disease in young persons exposed to (1) street drugs or (2) environmental toxins?

Key Points

- Cognitive impairment and memory loss are symptoms of Alzheimer, Huntington, and Parkinson disease.
- Risks for Alzheimer disease are age, heredity, and environmental factors.
- Abnormal structures called plaques and tangles form and interfere with the transmission of messages between neurons.
- Alzheimer disease causes cholinergic nerve cells in the brain to die.
- Alzheimer disease is treated with drugs that increase acetylcholine levels or drugs that block glutamate activity.
- AChE is an enzyme that degrades ACh. AChE inhibitors increase levels of ACh.
- Three of the drugs approved for the treatment of Alzheimer disease are AChE inhibitors. They are donepezil (Aricept), rivastigmine (Exelon), and galantamine (Reminyl).
- Memantine (Namenda) blocks the actions of glutamate at the NMDA receptor.
- Parkinson disease is a progressive disorder of the nervous system involving degeneration of dopaminergic neurons in the basal ganglia of the brain.
- Symptoms of Parkinson disease are caused by an imbalance between dopamine and acetylcholine.
- The average age at onset of Parkinson disease is 60 years. Men are more often affected than women.
- Environmental factors (e.g., exposure to pesticides, carbon monoxide poisoning) and infectious diseases (e.g., viral encephalitis and syphilis) can increase the risk for Parkinson disease.
- Antipsychotic drugs can cause pseudoparkinsonism, a drug-induced condition that resembles Parkinson disease.
- Physical signs of Parkinson disease are bradykinesia, muscle rigidity, tremors, postural and gait abnormalities, and walking with a characteristic shuffle. Other visible signs of Parkinson disease are a blank facial expression, drooling, and speech impairment.
- Aducanymab and lecanenumab are monoclonal antibodies used to treat Alzheimer Disease.
- Levodopa is a prodrug and is a dopamine precursor.
- Benserazide, carbidopa, and tolcapone are combined with levodopa to inhibit levodopa's metabolism and increase its effects.
- Dizziness, hypotension, confusion, and gastrointestinal distress are common side effects of most of the drugs used to treat Parkinson disease. People older than the age of 65 years are most susceptible to side effects of anti-Parkinson drugs.
- Side effects of anticholinergic drugs are dry mouth, blurred vision, constipation, and urinary retention.
- The effectiveness of anti-Parkinson drugs declines over time because of the progressive nature of the disease. The efficacy of levodopa and amantadine also declines with long-term therapy because of desensitization of dopamine receptors.
- Selegiline and rasagiline are $MAOI_B$ and are associated with a risk for hypertensive crisis.
- Huntington disease is a progressive and degenerative disease of neurons that affects muscle movement, cognitive functions, and emotions.
- Huntington disease is a hereditary disorder.
- Characteristic symptoms of Huntington disease are choreiform movements (e.g., unpredictable, irregular, and jerking tremors), rhythmic oscillations or circular movements around the ankles or wrists, and sudden abnormal movements.
- In Huntington disease, the balance between GABA, acetylcholine, and dopamine is upset, which produces the excessive muscle movement associated with Huntington disease.
- Huntington disease is primarily treated with drugs that decrease excessive dopaminergic activity.

Review Questions

1. Parkinson disease is a progressive disorder of the nervous system that is associated with an imbalance between _____ and _____.
   a. epinephrine, dopamine
   b. dopamine, serotonin
   c. acetylcholine, norepinephrine
   d. dopamine, acetylcholine

2. The most commonly reported symptom of Alzheimer disease is _____.
   a. pain
   b. forgetfulness
   c. heart problems
   d. incontinence

3. Drugs that increase _____ levels at the synapse are used to treat Alzheimer disease.
   a. dopamine
   b. acetylcholine
   c. serotonin
   d. glutamate

4. Which drug is marketed in foil packaging to protect it from moisture?
   a. Ongentys
   b. Mirapex ER
   c. Sinemet
   d. Kynmobi
   e. Duopa/Duodopa

5. The warning label MAY CAUSE DIZZINESS should be placed on prescriptions dispensed for Aricept and Namenda.
   a. true
   b. false

6. _____ is a prodrug and is a dopamine precursor.
   a. Levodopa
   b. Carbidopa
   c. Cogentin
   d. ReQuip

7. The effects of levodopa are increased by combining the drug with all of the following EXCEPT:
   a. tolcapone
   b. carbidopa
   c. selegiline
   d. benserazide

8. _____ is a common side effect of most of the drugs used to treat Parkinson disease.
   a. Headache
   b. Gastrointestinal distress
   c. Muscle spasms
   d. Flu-like symptoms

9. You receive a prescription for Ongentys 50 mg take one tablet QID for Parkinson disease. You consult the pharmacist because _____.
   a. Ongentys is not available in 50 mg
   b. the usual dosing schedule for Ongentys is once daily
   c. Ongentys is not used for the treatment of Parkinson disease
   d. none of the above

10. Huntington disease is treated with drugs that _____ excessive dopaminergic activity.
    a. increase
    b. decrease

Bibliography

Alzhcimer's Association: 2022 Alzheimer's disease facts and figures, *Alzheimers Dement* 18, 2022.

Ascherio A, Chen H, Weisskopf MG, et al. Pesticide exposure and risk for Parkinson's disease. *Ann Neurol.* 2006;60:197–203.

Bourne C, Clayton C, Murch A, et al. Cognitive impairment and behavioural difficulties in patients with Huntington's disease. *Nurs Stand.* 2006;20:41–44.

Canadian Institute for Health Information. Dementia in Canada: Summary [Report]. Retrieved September 18, 2022, from https://www.cihi.ca/en/dementia-in-canada/dementia-in-canada-summary.

Geerts H. Pharmacology of acetylcholinesterase inhibitors and *N*-methyl-d-aspartate receptors for the combination therapy in the treatment of Alzheimer's disease. *J Clin Pharmacol.* 2006;46:8S–16S.

Health Canada. (2022). Drug Product Database. Retrieved July 11, 2022, from https://health-products.canada.ca/dpd-bdpp/index-eng.jsp.

Institute for Safe Medication Practices. (2016). FDA and ISMP Lists of Look-Alike Drug Names with Recommended Tall Man Letters. Retrieved July 11, 2022, from https://www.ismp.org/recommendations/tall-man-letters-list.

Institute for Safe Medication Practices. (2019). List of Confused Drugs. Retrieved July 11, 2022, from https://www.ismp.org/tools/confused-drugnames.pdf.

Mao Q, Qin W, Zhang A, Ye N. Recent advances in dopaminergic strategies for the treatment of Parkinson's disease. *Acta Pharmacol Sin.* 2020;41:471–482.

Nance MA, Paulsen JS, Rosenblatt A, et al. A Physician's Guide to the Management of Huntington Disease, 2013. M. Meijer & C. M. Forsyth (Eds). Retrieved July 15, 2022, from http://www.huntingtonsociety.ca/wp-content/uploads/2013/10/PhysGuide2013_WebsiteCopy_Reduced1.pdf.

National Institute on Aging: Basics of Alzheimer's Disease and Dementia—What Is Alzheimer's Disease? Department of Health and Human Services. Retrieved July 15, 2022 from https://www.nia.nih.gov/health/what-alzheimers-disease.

National Institute of Neurological Disorders and Stroke National Institutes of Health: Parkinson's Disease—*Hope through research*, 2015. Bethesda, MD: US Department of Health and Human Services. NINDS, Publication date December 2014. NIH Publication No. 15-139.

Nordberg A. Mechanisms behind the neuroprotective actions of cholinesterase inhibitors in Alzheimer's disease. *Alzheimer Dis Assoc Disord.* 2006;20(Suppl 1):S12–S18.

Page C, Curtis M, Sutter M, et al. *Integrated pharmacology.* Philadelphia: Mosby; 2005:242–247 261–262.

Public Health Agency of Canada. (2020). A Dementia Strategy for Canada: Annual Report. Cat.: HP22-1E-PDF ISSN: 2562-7805 Pub.: 200079. Retrieved July 15, 2022, from https://www.canada.ca/en/public-health/services/publications/diseases-conditions/dementia-strategy-annual-report-parliament-2021.html.

Raffa R, Rawls S, Beyzarov E. *Netter's illustrated pharmacology.* Philadelphia: WB Saunders; 2005:77–78 80–82.

Smetanin P, Kobak P, Briante C, et al. *Rising Tide: the impact of dementia on Canadian society.* Toronto, ON: Alzheimer's Society of Canada; 2010.

Tarsy D. Patient Education: Parkinson disease treatment option—education, support, and therapy (Beyond the Basics), 2016. UptoDate, Inc., Wolters Kluwer.

U.S. Food and Drug Administration. (nd). Drugs@FDA: FDA Approved Drug Products. Retrieved July 11, 2022, from https://www.accessdata.fda.gov/scripts/cder/daf/index.cfm.

USP Center for Advancement of Patient Safety: Use caution–avoid confusion, USP Quality Review No. 79, Rockville, MD, April 2004, USP Center for Advancement of Patient Safety.

9
Treatment of Seizure Disorders

LEARNING OBJECTIVES

1. Learn the terminology associated with seizures.
2. Describe the etiology of seizure disorders.
3. Compare and contrast the function of neurotransmitters associated with symptoms of seizure disorders.
4. Classify medications used in the treatment of seizure disorders.
5. Identify significant drug look-alike and sound-alike issues.
6. Describe mechanism of action for each class of drugs used to treat seizure disorders.
7. Identify significant drug interactions.
8. Identify warning labels and precautionary messages associated with medications used to treat seizure disorders.

KEY TERMS

Absence seizure A seizure in which the person experiences a brief period of unconsciousness and stares vacantly into space.

Anoxia Lack of oxygen to the brain.

Aura Unusual sensation, auditory, visual, or olfactory hallucination that is experienced just before the onset of a seizure.

Complex focal seizures Seizure disorder that produces a blank stare, disorientation, repetitive actions, and memory loss.

Convulsions Sudden contraction of muscles that is caused by seizures.

Eclampsia A life-threatening condition that can develop in pregnant women that causes high blood pressure and seizures.

Epilepsy A chronic noncommunicable disease of the brain characterized by a sudden, excessive, disorderly discharge of cerebral neurons.

Febrile seizure A seizure associated with a sudden spike in body temperature.

Generalized seizure A seizure that spreads across both cerebral hemispheres. Includes tonic-clonic, myoclonic, and absence seizures.

Generalized tonic-clonic seizure A seizure that causes stiffening of the limbs, difficulty breathing, and jerking movements and is followed by disorientation and limbs that become limp.

Gingival hyperplasia Excess growth of gum tissue that may overgrow the teeth.

Hirsutism Excessive growth of body hair (especially in women).

Myoclonic seizure A seizure that is characterized by jerking muscle movements and is caused by contraction of major muscle groups.

Seizure threshold A person's susceptibility to seizures.

Simple focal seizure A seizure that affects only one part of the brain and causes the person to experience unusual sensations or feelings.

Status epilepticus Medical emergency that is characterized by repeated generalized seizures that can deprive the brain of oxygen.

Overview

Epilepsy is one of the oldest known brain disorders and was described as early as 3000 years ago in ancient Babylon. The word *epilepsy* is derived from the Greek word for "attack" because the ancient Greeks believed a person having a seizure was being attacked by demons. The World Health Organization estimates that 50 million people worldwide have epilepsy. Approximately 3.4 million people in the United States (Centers for Disease Control and Prevention) and 300,000 Canadians (Public Health Agency of Canada) are living with epilepsy. The seizure risk increases with age. By 75 years, 3% of the population will have had a seizure caused by age-related cerebrovascular disease that deprives the brain of oxygen. Epilepsy is a type of seizure disorder that is associated with having experienced two or more seizures. Seizures are characterized by a sudden, excessive, disorderly discharge of cerebral neurons. Seizures may also be caused by conditions that range from injury to illness. Half of all seizures have no known cause. When the cause is known, the origin may be birth defects, infection (meningitis, HIV), perinatal injury, malignant tumors, lead poisoning, head trauma, or *eclampsia* (a life-threatening condition that can develop in pregnant women). Wearing seat belts, motorcycle helmets, and bike helmets can reduce the risk for seizures that are caused by head injury. Other causes of seizures include metabolic disturbance, hypoglycemia, electrolyte imbalance, drug and alcohol withdrawal, and use of drugs that lower the *seizure threshold*. Stroke and heart attack can cause seizures because the brain becomes deprived of oxygen (*anoxia*).

The onset of a seizure may be preceded by an aura. An *aura* is an unusual sensation, auditory, visual, or olfactory hallucination that is experienced just before the onset of a seizure. In other words, the person may hear, see, or smell something distinctive immediately before the seizure activity begins. These signs of an upcoming seizure are important because they indicate the location of abnormal neuronal firing in the cerebrum.

Febrile seizures in children are associated with an infection causing a sudden spike in temperature; aggressive treatment with fever reducers is indicated to prevent more seizures. Most children who have febrile seizures will not develop epilepsy.

Seizure Classifications

There are two major seizure classifications (Fig. 9.1): generalized seizures and focal or partial seizures. *Generalized seizures* spread across both of the cerebral hemispheres, whereas partial seizures are confined to a single hemisphere. Tonic-clonic (Fig. 9.2), myoclonic, and absence seizures are generalized seizures. Tonic-clonic and *myoclonic seizures* start with a stiffening of the limbs and difficulty breathing, are followed by jerking movements and loss of bladder and bowel control, and conclude with a postictal phase whereby the limbs become limp and the person may be disoriented. The jerking muscle movement associated with *generalized tonic-clonic* seizures is sometimes referred to as a *convulsion*.

Petit mal seizures are also called *absence seizures*. This type of seizure is associated with a characteristic vacant or absent stare during the seizure. Absence seizures occur more commonly in children. They are barely noticeable to onlookers because no major muscle twitching is exhibited. *Status epilepticus* is a medical emergency that is characterized by repeated, generalized seizures that deprive the brain of oxygen. Antiseizure medicines must be administered intravenously to persons with status epilepticus.

Approximately 60% of people with epilepsy have focal seizures. Focal (partial) seizures involve only one cerebral hemisphere. Focal seizures are classified as simple or complex. *Simple focal seizures* may cause the arms, face, or legs to twitch, and visual, olfactory, or auditory hallucinations may occur. *Complex focal seizures* often begin with a blank stare. The person becomes disoriented and engages in repetitive actions during the seizure. When the seizure is over, the person does not have any memory of the seizure. Psychomotor and temporal lobe seizures are complex partial seizures.

Neurochemistry of Seizures

When there is an abnormality in nerve signaling by neurotransmitters, seizures result. People with epilepsy have an abnormally high level of excitatory neurotransmitters coupled with a low level of inhibitory neurotransmitters. This accounts for the excess neuronal firing that occurs with seizure disorders. γ-Aminobutyric acid (GABA) is an inhibitory neurotransmitter that plays an important role in epilepsy. An excitatory neurotransmitter that plays a role in epilepsy is the amino acid glutamate. Some seizures are linked to a defect in the genes that control the ion channels that open and close to regulate the influx of chloride, sodium, and calcium into the neuron.

Drugs Used to Treat Seizure Disorders

The goal for the treatment of epilepsy and other seizure disorders is to reduce the incidence of seizures by suppressing seizure activity. Successful achievement of this therapeutic goal is dependent

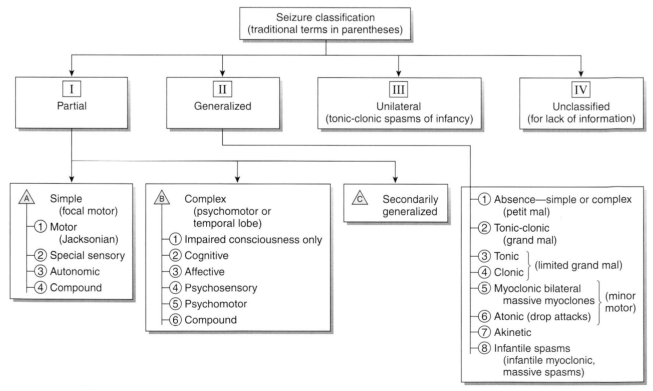

• **Fig. 9.1** Classifications of seizures. (From Clayton BD, Stock YN. *Basic pharmacology for nurses*, ed 12, St Louis, 1997, Mosby.)

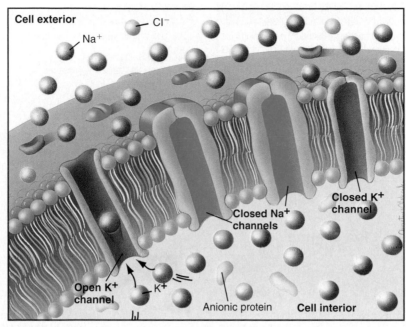

• **Fig. 9.2** Role of ion channels. (From Patton KT, Thibodeau GA. *Anatomy and physiology*, ed 9, St Louis, 2016, Elsevier.)

on correctly classifying the seizure type and selecting an appropriate drug for seizure type, with optimal drug administration and serum monitoring. Monodrug therapy is preferred to lower the incidence of adverse effects, reduce the incidence of drug interactions, improve adherence to drug therapy, and lower medication costs.

Drugs That Modulate Ion Channels

The aim of pharmaceutical treatment of seizures is to suppress seizure activity. This is accomplished by control of ion channels. Neuronal firing is inhibited by drugs that delay the inflow of sodium, potassium, and calcium ions. Drugs that act on ion channels are phenytoin, carbamazepine, oxcarbazepine, eslicarbazine, lamotrigine, gabapentin, pregablin, zonisamide, lacosamide, and ethosuximide. The mechanism of action for levetiracetam is unknown. Studies have shown that it may inhibit calcium ion channels and GABA. Gabapentin and pregabalin are structurally similar to GABA; however, they do not produce their effects by binding to GABA$_A$ receptors. Instead, they both act on ion channels. Gabapentin acts on sodium channels, and pregabalin acts on calcium channels. They are effective in treating partial and generalized seizures. Fosphenytoin is used to treat status epilepticus and seizures occurring during neurosurgery. Carbamazepine and oxcarbazepine are used to treat generalized and complex focal seizures. Ethosuximide and methsuximide are two of only a few drugs that target absence seizures. Carbamazepine and gabapentin are also used in the management of neuropathic pain (see Chapter 10) and bipolar disorder (see Chapter 6).

Pharmacokinetics

The absorption of phenytoin and carbamazepine is variable and is influenced by particle size as well as by inactive ingredients in manufacturers' formulations. This influences bioavailability. Erratic serum blood levels can lead to poor seizure control; therefore switching between different manufacturers' formulations should be avoided, if possible. Ninety percent of phenytoin is

protein bound, so drug interactions involving protein binding are common. Patients taking phenytoin must periodically have their blood levels monitored. Phenytoin can alter the rate of metabolism of other coadministered drugs that use the same metabolic system. For example, phenytoin can reduce the effectiveness of oral contraceptives and other antiseizure drugs.

Fosphenytoin is converted to phenytoin by enzymes in the blood (phosphatases). It has a short half-life of approximately 8 minutes. Unlike phenytoin, which can be administered orally or parenterally, fosphenytoin is available only for parenteral use and is administered intravenously or intramuscularly. It is 100% bioavailable.

Lamotrigine and levetiracetam are rapidly absorbed orally. Oral absorption of zonisamide is slow to moderate. All three drugs have greater than 95% bioavailability. Protein binding is less than 50%, so there are fewer drug interactions than with some of the other antiseizure medications. Lower doses of lamotrigine are required when taken with valproic acid. Higher doses are required when taken with enzyme-inducing drugs.

Common Adverse Reactions

Sedation, dizziness, ataxia, and nausea are common side effects of all of the drugs. Several agents have drug-specific side effects. Phenytoin and fosphenytoin may cause ***hirsutism*** (excessive growth of body hair, especially in women) and ***gingival hyperplasia*** (excessive growth of gum tissue). Infants born to women who take phenytoin during pregnancy may be born with cleft palate. Phenytoin may also decrease folic acid, calcium, and vitamin D absorption; vitamin supplements may be recommended. Carbamazepine and oxcarbazepine may cause double vision (diplopia), bruising, and jaundice. Zonisamide may produce kidney stones.

Precautions

Phenytoin and fosphenytoin are known teratogens, and prenatal exposure may increase risk for congenital malformations. Carbamazepine should be protected from light and moisture. Moisture can decrease the potency by as much as 30%.

■ Tech Note!

Therapeutic blood levels for phenytoin are best maintained by dispensing the same manufacturer's formulation every time a prescription is filled. Avoid switching if possible.

■ Tech Note!

Dilantin is compatible in normal saline. Intravenous solution is stable for 14 hours at room temperature when diluted to 2 mg/mL. Dilantin chewable tablets should be followed by a glass of water.

---

❶ Tech alert!

The following drugs have look-alike/sound-alike issues:

TEGretol XR, TEGretol
OXcarbazepine and carBAMazepine;
LaMICtal and LamISIL;
lamoTRIgine and lamiVUDine

■ Tech Note!

Pregabalin (Lyrica) is a C-V controlled substance in the United States.

Drugs That Inhibit Ion Channels

Generic Name	US Brand Name(s) / Canadian Brand(s)	Dosage Forms and Strengths
carbamazepine[a]	Carbatrol, Equetro, Epitol, Tegretol, Tegretol-XR, Teril Tegretol, Tegretol CR	**Capsules, extended release (Carbatrol, Equetro)[b]:** 100 mg, 200 mg, 300 mg **Suspension (Tegretol, Teril):** 100 mg/5 mL **Tablets, chewable:** 100 mg, 200 mg **Tablets (Epitol, Tegretol):** 200 mg **Tablets, extended release (Tegretol-XR):** 100 mg[b], 200 mg, 400 mg
eslicarbazepine[a b]	Aptiom Aptiom	**Tablets:** 200 mg, 400 mg, 600 mg, 800 mg
ethosuximide[a]	Zarontin Zarontin	**Capsules (Zarontin):** 250 mg **Syrup (Zarontin):** 250 mg/5 mL
fosphenytoin[a]	Cerebyx Cerebyx	**Injection, solution:** 50 mg/mL phenytoin sodium equivalents (PE)
gabapentin[a]	Gralise, Horizant, Neurontin Neurontin	**Capsules:** 100 mg, 300 mg, 400 mg **Solution, oral[b]:** 250 mg/5 mL **Tablets:** 300 mg[b], 600 mg, 800 mg **Tablets, extended release (Horizant)[b]:** 300 mg, 600 mg
lacosamide[a]	Vimpat Vimpat	**Injection, solution:** 10 mg/mL **Solution, oral[b]:** 10 mg/mL **Tablets, oral:** 50 mg, 100 mg, 150 mg, 200 mg
lamotrigine[a]	Lamictal, Lamictal CD, Lamictal ODT kit, Lamictal XR Lamictal	**Tablets (Lamictal):** 25 mg, 100 mg, 150 mg, 200 mg[b] **Tablets, dispersible (Lamictal CD):** 2 mg, 5 mg, 25 mg[b] **Tablets, extended release (Lamictal XR)[b]:** 25 mg, 50 mg, 100 mg, 200 mg, 250 mg, 300 mg **Tablets, oral disintegrating (Lamictal ODT)[b]:** 25 mg, 50 mg, 100 mg, 200 mg
levetiracetam[a]	Elepsia XR, Keppra, Keppra XR, Spritam Keppra	**Injection, solution:** 5 mg/mL[b], 10 mg/mL[b], 15 mg/mL[b], 100 mg/1 mL **Solution, oral[b]:** 100 mg/mL **Tablet, for oral suspension (Spritam)[b]:** 250 mg, 500 mg, 750 mg, 1000 mg **Tablets:** 250 mg, 500 mg, 750 mg, 1000 mg **Tablets, extended release (Keppra XR, Elepsia XR)[b]:** 500 mg, 750 mg, 1 g, 1.5 g

Drugs That Inhibit Ion Channels—cont'd

Generic Name	US Brand Name(s) / Canadian Brand(s)	Dosage Forms and Strengths
methsuximide	Celontin	**Capsules:** 300 mg
	Not Available	
oxcarbazepine[a]	Oxtellar XR, Trileptal	**Suspension:** 60 mg/mL
	Trileptal	**Tablets:** 150 mg, 300 mg, 600 mg **Tablets, extended release**[b]: 150 mg, 300 mg, 600 mg
phenytoin[a]	Dilantin, Phenytek	**Capsule, extended release:** 30 mg, 100 mg, 200 mg[b], 300 mg[b]
	Dilantin, Dilantin Infatab	**Injection, solution:** 50 mg/mL **Suspension:** 30 mg/5 mL[c], 125 mg/5 mL **Tablets, chewable (Dilantin Infatab):** 50 mg
pregabalin[a]	Lyrica, Lyrica CR	**Solution, oral**[b]: 20 mg/mL
	Lyrica	**Tablet, extended release (Lyrica CR):** 82.5 mg, 165 mg, 330 mg **Capsules:** 25 mg, 50 mg, 75 mg, 100 mg[b], 150 mg, 200 mg[b], 225 mg, 300 mg
rufinamide[a b]	Banzel	**Suspension, oral**[b]: 40 mg/mL
	Banzel	**Tablets:** 100 mg[c], 200 mg, 400 mg
zonisamide[a]	Zonegran, Zonisade	**Capsules:** 25 mg, 50 mg, 100 mg
	Not available	**Suspension:** 100 mg/5 mL

[a]Generic available.
[b]Available in the United States only.
[c]Available in Canada only.

Drugs That Potentiate GABA

GABA is an inhibitory neurotransmitter. The GABA receptor regulates the movement of chloride ions into the neuron. Chloride ions are negatively charged. The influx of chloride ions inhibits formation of action potentials suppressing neuronal hyperactivity and seizures.

Valproates, barbiturates (e.g., phenobarbital), and benzodiazepines (e.g., clonazepam) are classifications of drugs that potentiate GABA. Other drugs that produce this effect are ritagabine, tiagabine, topiramate, felbamate, cenobamate, and vigabatrin. Topiramate and felbamate also inhibit ion channels. Phenobarbital was the first drug used to treat seizures. It is indicated in the treatment of generalized tonic-clonic seizures and partial seizures and is administered to children to control febrile seizures. Valproates are described as "broad-spectrum" antiseizure drugs because they are effective in treating all types of seizures. They are one of the few antiseizure drugs indicated for the treatment of absence seizures. Benzodiazepines are indicated for the treatment of status epilepticus (intravenous diazepam), absence seizures and myoclonic seizures (clonazepam), and partial seizures (clorazepate). The mechanism of action and pharmacokinetics of benzodiazepines are discussed in detail in Chapter 5.

Mechanism of Action

One of the mechanisms of action for valproates and their derivatives is to enhance the inhibitory actions of GABA. Other mechanisms of action may be involved, including actions on potassium channels that result in membrane stabilization. Tiagabine blocks the reuptake of GABA in the synapse, and vigabatrin enhances GABA activity by binding to GABA transaminase (GABA-T), the enzyme that inactivates GABA. In addition to GABA potentiation, felbamate is an N-methyl-D-aspartate antagonist and inhibits calcium and sodium channels.

Pharmacokinetics

The effectiveness of all valproic acid derivatives is expressed as valproic acid activity. All valproates are rapidly absorbed when administered orally and have 100% bioavailability. Up to 10% of the drug is passed in breast milk, limiting the use of valproates during lactation. Valproates are up to 95% protein bound, so drug interactions involving protein binding must be considered when dispensing other drugs with them, including other antiseizure medicines such as phenobarbital and phenytoin. The oral absorption of tiagabine is rapid. It is nearly 95% protein bound (i.e., making it susceptible to drug interactions involving protein binding). Vigabatrin has a short half-life, but its effects persist even after blood levels of the drug decline. Antacids decrease the absorption of gabapentin by 20%. The absorption of tiagabine is reduced by foods that have a high fat content. Primidone is a barbiturate used to treat seizures. Primidone is metabolized to phenobarbital. Phenobarbital is capable of self-inducing the enzymes that metabolize it and many other drugs such as phenytoin and valproic acid. It is implicated in many drug interactions involving enzyme induction. The absorption of phenobarbital is moderately slow; however, the drug is readily distributed throughout the central nervous system because of its high degree of lipid solubility. Bioavailability is 100%. Cenobamate has a long half-life (50 to 60 hours). The drug is extensively metabolized in the liver and eliminated in urine. Cenobamate interacts with drugs. Drug-drug interactions with antiseizure drugs may increase blood levels (phenytoin, phenobarbital, clozabam) or decrease blood levels (lamotrigine, carbamazepine).

Common Adverse Reactions

Common adverse reactions of divalproex, phenobarbital, primidone, and tiagabine are dizziness, confusion, drowsiness, unsteadiness, and nausea. Phenobarbital may produce hyperactivity, rather than sedation, in children. Divalproex and cenobamate may cause diplopia (double vision), and vigabatrin can cause irreversible tunnel vision. Other adverse effects for divalproex are bruising or weight gain, hair loss, tremors, and irregular menstruation. Phenobarbital, diazepam, cenobamate, and clonazepam may cause tolerance and dependence. Respiratory depression is a serious side effect of phenobarbital and intravenous diazepam. Diazepam and clonazepam may impair learning.

❶ Tech alert!

The following drugs have look-alike/sound-alike issues:
Cerebyx, CeleBREX, and CeleXA;
DepaKOTE and Depakote ER

❶ Tech alert!

Phenobarbital is a controlled drug (C2) in Canada. Diazepam, clobazam, and clonazepam are controlled substances (C-IV) in the United States and targeted substances in Canada.

● Tech Note!

Depakote sprinkles may be mixed into soft foods.

● Tech Note!

Diazepam for injection is stable for 24 hours at room temperature in concentrations of 0.1 mg or less with normal saline, D5W, or lactated Ringer solution in glass containers.

Drugs That Potentiate GABA

Generic Name	US Brand Name(s) / Canadian Brand(s)	Dosage Forms and Strengths
cenobamate	Xcopri / Not Available	**Tablets:** 12.5 mg, 25 mg, 50 mg, 100 mg, 150 mg, 200 mg
clobazam[a]	Onfi, Sympazan / Generics	**Film, oral (Sympazan):** 5 mg, 10 mg, 20 mg **Suspension, oral (Onfi)[b]:** 2.5 mg/mL **Tablets (Onfi):** 10 mg, 20 mg[b]
clonazepam[a]	Klonopin / Rivotril	**Tablets (Klonopin, Rivotril):** 0.25 mg[c], 0.5 mg, 1 mg, 2 mg
diazepam[a]	Diastat, Diastat AcuDial, Valium, Valtoco / Diastat, Valium	**Injection, solution:** 5 mg/mL **Solution, oral:** 1 mg/mL, 5 mg/mL[b] **Nasal spray (Valtoco):** 5 mg, 7.5 mg, 10 mg/spray **Rectal gel (Diastat):** 5 mg/mL (2.5 mg[b], 5 mg[c], 10 mg, 15 mg[c] and 20[b] mg prefilled syringes) **Tablets:** 2 mg, 5 mg, 10 mg
divalproex sodium[a] valproic acid[a]	Depakote Delayed Release, Depakote ER / Depakene, Epival	**Capsules, as valproic acid (Depakene):** 250 mg **Capsules, delayed release pellets (Depakote)[b]:** 125 mg **Syrup, as valproic acid (Depakene):** 250 mg/5 mL **Tablets, as divalproex sodium delayed release (Depakote, Epival):** 125 mg, 250 mg, 500 mg **Tablets, as divalproex sodium extended release (Depakote ER):** 250 mg, 500 mg
felbamate[a]	Felbatol / Not available	**Suspension, oral:** 600 mg/5 mL **Tablets:** 400 mg, 600 mg
phenobarbital[a]	Not Available / Generics	**Elixir:** 5 mg/mL **Injection, solution:** 30 mg/mL, 120 mg/mL **Tablets:** 15 mg, 30 mg, 60 mg, 100 mg

Drugs That Potentiate GABA —cont'd

Generic Name	US Brand Name(s) / Canadian Brand(s)	Dosage Forms and Strengths
primidone[a]	Mysoline	**Tablets:** 50 mg[b], 125 mg[c], 250 mg
	Generics	
tiagabine[a]	Gabatril	**Tablets:** 2 mg, 4 mg, 12 mg, 16 mg
	Not available	
topiramate[a]	Eprontia, Qudexy XR, Topamax, Trokendi XR	**Capsules, sprinkle:** 15 mg, 25 mg **Capsules, extended release (Qudexy XR, Trokendi XR)[b]:** 25 mg, 50 mg, 100 mg, 150 mg, 200 mg **Solution, oral (Eprontia):** 25 mg/mL **Tablets:** 25 mg, 50 mg[b], 100 mg, 200 mg
	Topamax	
vigabatrin[a,b]	Sabril, Viagdrone	**Powder for oral suspension:** 500 mg packets **Tablets:** 500 mg
	Sabril	

[a]Generic available.
[b]Available in the United States only.
[c]Available in Canada only.

Drugs That Inhibit Glutamate

Perampenal is a glutamate antagonist that is used to treat partial-onset seizures with or without secondary generalized seizures. It is the only drug in its class. Perampenal inhibits glutamate, the primary excitatory neurotransmitter in the central nervous system. This reduces the generation and spread of seizures.

Pharmacokinetics

Perampenal is rapidly absorbed when taken orally. The rate of absorption is reduced if it is taken with food, but the extent of absorption is not affected.

Common Adverse Reactions

Dizziness (36%), somnolence (16%), fatigue (10%), irritability (9%), falls (7%), nausea (7%), ataxia (5%), balance disorder (4%), gait disturbance (4%), vertigo (4%), and weight gain (4%) are the most common side effects. Less common side effects are serious or life-threatening psychiatric and behavioral changes such as aggression, hostility, or homicidal thoughts. The US Food and Drug Administration requires a box warning in the product label.

Miscellaneous

The precise mechanism of action for brivaracetam (Briviact, Brivlera) is unknown. The drug is used to treat partial-onset

Glutamate Receptor Antagonist

Generic Name	US Brand Name(s) / Canadian Brand(s)	Dosage Forms and Strengths
perampanel	Fycompa	**Suspension, oral:** 0.5 mg/mL **Tablet:** 2 mg, 4 mg, 6 mg, 8 mg, 10 mg, 12 mg
	Fycompa	

Miscellaneous

Generic Name	US Brand Name(s) / Canadian Brand(s)	Dosage Forms and Strengths
brivaracetam[a]	Briviact	**Solution, intravenous:** 10 mg/mL **Solution, oral:** 10 mg/mL **Tablet:** 10 mg, 25 mg, 50 mg, 75 mg, 100 mg
	Brivlera	
cannabidiol	Epidiolex	**Solution, oral:** 100 mg/mL
	Not available	

[a]Generic Available in the United States.

seizures. The most common side effects of brivaracetam and cannabidiol are drowsiness, dizziness, and upset stomach. Cannabidiol can also produce suicide ideation.

Summary of Drugs Used for the Treatment of Seizures*

	Generic Name	Brand Name	Usual Adult Oral Dose and Dosing Schedule	Warning Labels
Drugs That Inhibit Ion Channels				
	carbamazepine[a]	Tegretol	800–1200 mg/day in 2 divided doses (XR) or 3–4 divided doses other formulations	MAY CAUSE DROWSINESS; MAY IMPAIR ABILITY TO DRIVE—all.
	eslicarbazepine	Aptiom	800–1600 mg once daily	AVOID ALCOHOL—all.
	ethosuximide[a]	Zarontin	Start 250 mg twice a day; increase up to 1500 mg/day	DO NOT DISCONTINUE WITHOUT MEDICAL SUPERVISION—all.
	fosphenytoin[a]	Cerebyx	**Status epilepticus:** IV loading dose: 15–20 mg/kg (PE) administered at rate of 100–150 mg/min **Nonemergent maintenance dose:** 10–20 mg/kg (PE)/day administered IM or IV	SWALLOW WHOLE; DO NOT CRUSH OR CHEW—extended release.
	gabapentin[a]	Neurontin	300–600 mg 3 times/day	TAKE WITH FOOD—carbamazepine, ethosuximide, gabapentin, methsuximide, oxcarbazepine, phenytoin, pregabalin, rufinamide.
	lacosamide[a]	Vimpat	Start 50 mg twice daily; increase up to 400 mg/day in 2 divided doses	AVOID ANTACIDS—gabapentin, phenytoin.
	lamotrigine[a]	Lamictal	100–500 mg/day in 1–2 divided doses	SHAKE WELL—suspension. TAKE WITH A FULL GLASS OF WATER—chewable tablets. MAY BE HABIT FORMING—pregabalin.
	levetiracetam[a]	Keppra	1000–3000 mg/day in 2 divided doses	STORE AT ROOM TEMPERATURE; DISCARD UNUSED.
	methsuximide	Celontin	300–1200 mg/day in 1–2 divided doses	PORTION 7 WEEKS AFTER OPENING—lacosamide oral solution.
	oxcarbazepine	Trileptal	600–2400 mg/day in 2 divided doses	
	phenytoin	Dilantin	100 mg 3–4 times a day	
	pregabalin[a]	Lyrica	150–600 mg dosed 2–3 times a day	
	rufinamide	Banzel	400–3200 mg/day in 2 divided doses	
	zonisamide	Zonegran	100–600 mg/day in 1 or 2 divided doses	
Drugs That Potentiate GABA				
	cenobamate	Xcopri	12.5 mg once daily; may increase up to 200 mg daily; maximum 400 mg daily	MAY CAUSE DROWSINESS; MAY IMPAIR ABILITY TO DRIVE—clobazam, clonazepam, diazepam, divalproex Na+, phenobarbital, tiagabine, topiramate, vigabatrin.
	clobazam[a]	Onfi (Frisium)	5–15 mg/day (up to 80 mg as necessary) in 1–2 divided doses	AVOID ALCOHOL—clobazam, clonazepam, diazepam, divalproex Na+, phenobarbital, tiagabine, topiramate, vigabatrin.
	clonazepam[a]	Klonopin (Rivatril)	1.5–20 mg/day in 3 divided doses	DO NOT DISCONTINUE WITHOUT MEDICAL SUPERVISION—all.
	diazepam[a]	Valium	**Oral:** 2–10 mg/day in 2–4 divided doses **Nasal spray:** 1–2 sprays (5–20 mg) in one nostril (maximum 1 episode per 5 days or 5 episodes per month) **Rectal gel:** 0.2–0.5 mg/kg/day	SWALLOW WHOLE; DO NOT CRUSH OR CHEW—extended release, cenobamate.
	divalproex sodium[a] valproic acid[a]	Depakote	10–60 mg/kg/day in 2–3 divided doses (delayed release) or once daily (extended release)	APPLY TO THE TOP OF THE TONGUE—Sympazan.
	felbamate	Felbatol	1200–3600 mg/day in 3–4 divided doses	TAKE WITH FOOD—divalproex Na+, tiagabine, vigabatrin.
	phenobarbital[a]	Generics	50–100 mg 2–3 times a day	SHAKE WELL—suspension (vigabatrin).
	primidone[a]	Mysoline	Start 100–125 mg at bedtime; increase to 250 mg 3–4 times/day	TAKE WITH A FULL GLASS OF WATER—chewable tablets.
	tiagabine[a]	Gabatril	Start 4 mg once daily; increase up to 56 mg/day in 2–4 divided doses	MAY BE HABIT FORMING—phenobarbital, clonazepam, diazepam.
	topiramate[a]	Topamax	200–400 mg/day in 2 divided doses (maximum 1600 mg/day) (extended release tablets dosed once daily)	
	vigabatrin	Sabril	500–1500 mg twice per day	

Summary of Drugs Used for the Treatment of Seizures*—cont'd

	Generic Name	Brand Name	Usual Adult Oral Dose and Dosing Schedule	Warning Labels
Drugs That Inhibit Glutamate				
	perampanel	Fycompa	Start 2 mg; maintenance 8–12 mg once daily	MAY CAUSE DROWSINESS; MAY IMPAIR ABILITY TO DRIVE. AVOID ALCOHOL. DO NOT DISCONTINUE WITHOUT MEDICAL SUPERVISION.
Miscellaneous				
	brivaracetam	Briviact, Brivlera	25–100 mg twice daily	MAY CAUSE DIZZINESS OR DROWSINESS; DO NOT DRIVE.
	cannabidiol	Epidiolex	2.5 mg/kg twice daily	STORE ORAL SOLUTION AT ROOM TEMPERATURE.

*Doses of medications used to treat seizures can vary considerably from patient to patient and depending on the specific condition being treated.
ªGeneric available.

TECHNICIAN'S CORNER

1. If you see someone experiencing a seizure, what would you do?
2. What would be the best advice you can give a patient with epilepsy about their medication?

Key Points

- Epilepsy is a type of seizure disorder that is characterized by a sudden, excessive, disorderly discharge of cerebral neurons.
- People with epilepsy have an abnormally high level of excitatory neurotransmitters, coupled with a low level of inhibitory neurotransmitters.
- Half of all seizures have no known cause.
- Known causes of seizures include birth defects, infection (meningitis, AIDS), tumors, head trauma, high fevers, hypoglycemia, drug and alcohol withdrawal, and cerebrovascular disease.
- Wearing seat belts, motorcycle helmets, and bike helmets can reduce head injury and injury-related seizures.
- Status epilepticus is a medical emergency that is characterized by repeated generalized seizures that deprive the brain of oxygen.
- Status epilepticus is treated with intravenous medications.
- Seizures are treated with drugs that modulate ion channels, potentiate GABA, and/or inhibit glutamate.

- The goal of treatment of epilepsy and other seizure disorders is to reduce the incidence of seizures by suppressing seizure activity.
- Therapeutic blood levels for phenytoin are best maintained by dispensing the same manufacturer's formulation each time a prescription is filled.
- Carbamazepine should be protected from light and moisture. Moisture can decrease the potency by as much as 30%.
- Antacids decrease the absorption of gabapentin by 20%. The absorption of tiagabine is reduced by foods that have a high fat content.
- Phenobarbital is a controlled substance in Canada.
- Benzodiazepines used in the treatment of seizures are controlled substances in the United States and targeted substances in Canada.
- Drug therapy with antiepileptic drugs increases the risk for suicide ideation and behavior.

Review Questions

1. All of the following drugs are controlled or targeted substances in Canada and/or the United States EXCEPT _____.
   a. clonazepam
   b. diazepam
   c. phenytoin
   d. pregabalin

2. Febrile seizures in children are associated with an _____, causing a sudden spike in temperature.
   a. injury
   b. injection
   c. infection
   d. a, b, and c

3. The only major seizure classification is generalized seizures.
   a. true
   b. false
4. A medical emergency that is characterized by repeated generalized seizures and deprives the brain of oxygen is called _____.
   a. status epilepticus
   b. myoclonic epilepticus
   c. absence epilepticus
   d. tonic-clonic status
5. The goal of treatment of epilepsy and other seizure disorders is to reduce the incidence of seizures by _____ seizure activity.
   a. stopping
   b. sedating
   c. suppressing
   d. shocking
6. _____ is administered IV in the management of status epilepticus and seizures after neurosurgery.
   a. Tiagabine
   b. Carbamazepine
   c. Valproic acid
   d. Fosphenytoin
7. You receive a prescription for Topamax 100 mg 1 tablet QID. You consult with the pharmacist because Topamax is _____.
   a. not prescribed 100 mg per dose
   b. not dosed QID
   c. not marketed as 100 mg tablets
   d. a capsule
8. You receive a prescription for gabapentin 500 mg 1 tablet TID. You consult with the pharmacist because gabapentin is _____.
   a. not prescribed in a dose greater than 100 mg
   b. not prescribed TID
   c. not marketed as 500 mg tablets
   d. not prescribed for seizures
9. Phenytoin was the first drug that was used to treat seizures.
   a. true
   b. false
10. An unusual sensation or auditory, visual, or olfactory hallucination that is experienced just before the onset of a seizure is called a(n) _____.
   a. halo
   b. aura
   c. vision
   d. hallucination

Bibliography

Glauser T, Shinnar S, Gloss D, et al. Evidence-based guideline: treatment of convulsive status epilepticus in children and adults: Report of the Guideline Committee of the American Epilepsy Society. *Epilepsy Curr.* 2016;16(1):48–61.

Health Canada. (2022). Drug Product Database. Retrieved July 20, 2022, from https://health-products.canada.ca/dpd-bdpp/index-eng.jsp.

Institute for Safe Medication Practices. (2016). FDA and ISMP Lists of Look-Alike Drug Names with Recommended Tall Man Letters. Retrieved July 20, 2022, from https://www.ismp.org/recommendations/tall-man-letters-list.

Institute for Safe Medication Practices. (2019). List of Confused Drugs. Retrieved July 20, 2022, from https://www.ismp.org/tools/confused-drugnames.pdf.

Kalant H, Grant D, Mitchell J. *Principles of medical pharmacology.* ed 7. Toronto: Elsevier Canada, A Division of Reed Elsevier Canada; 2007:223–235.

National Institute of Neurological Disorders and Stroke National Institutes of Health: *Hope through research: the epilepsies and seizures,* NIH Publication No. 15-156. Bethesda, 2015, National Institutes of Health.

Page C, Curtis M, Sutter M, et al. *Integrated pharmacology.* Philadelphia: Elsevier Mosby; 2005:257–259.

Patsalos PN. The clinical pharmacology profile of the new antiepileptic drug perampanel: a novel noncompetitive AMPA receptor antagonist. *Epilepsia.* 2015;56:12–27.

PHAC. (2019). Epilepsy in Canada. Retrieved July 20, 2022, from https://www.canada.ca/en/public-health/services/publications/diseases-conditions/epilepsy.html.

Raffa RB, Rawls SM, Beyzarov EP. *Netter's illustrated pharmacology.* Philadelphia: WB Saunders; 2005:67–70.

Schmidt D, Schachter SC. Drug treatment of epilepsy in adults. *BMJ.* 2014;348:g2546.

U.S. Centers for Disease Control and Prevention. (2022). Epilepsy data and statistics. Retrieved July 20, 2022, from https://www.cdc.gov/epilepsy/data/index.html.

U.S. Food and Drug Administration. (nd). Drugs@FDA: FDA Approved Drug Products. Retrieved July 20, 2022 from https://www.accessdata.fda.gov/scripts/cder/daf/index.cfm.

USP Center for Advancement of Patient Safety: *Use caution: avoid confusion,* USP Quality Review No. 79. Rockville, MD, 2004, USP Center for Advancement of Patient Safety.

World Health Organization. (2022). Epilepsy. Retrieved July 20, 2022 from https://www.who.int/news-room/fact-sheets/detail/epilepsy.

10

Treatment of Pain and Migraine Headache

LEARNING OBJECTIVES

1. Learn the terminology associated with the treatment of pain and migraine headaches.
2. Describe the etiology of pain and migraine headaches.
3. Compare and contrast the treatment of nociceptive pain and neuropathic pain.
4. Compare and contrast the function of neurotransmitters associated with pain and migraine headache symptoms.
5. Classify medications used in the treatment of pain and migraine headaches.
6. Describe mechanisms of action for each class of drugs used to treat pain and migraine headaches.
7. Identify significant drug look-alike and sound-alike issues.
8. Identify warning labels and precautionary messages associated with medications used to treat pain and migraine headaches.
9. Identify significant drug interactions.

KEY TERMS

Acute pain Sudden pain that results from injury or inflammation and is usually self-limiting.

Acupuncture Nonpharmacologic treatment for pain that involves the application of needles to precise points on the body.

Analgesic Drug that reduces pain.

Arthritis Condition that is associated with joint pain.

Biofeedback Nonpharmacologic treatment for pain that involves relaxation techniques and gaining self-control over muscle tension, heart rate, and skin temperature.

Breakthrough pain Pain that occurs in between scheduled doses of analgesics.

Cephalgia Head pain.

Chronic pain Pain that persists for a long period that is worsened by psychological factors and is resistant to many medical treatments.

Cluster headache Intensely painful vascular headache that occurs in groups and produces pain on one side of the head.

Diabetic neuropathy Peripheral nerve disorder caused by diabetes that produces numbness, pain, or tingling in the feet or legs.

Dysphoria Feeling of emotional or mental discomfort, restlessness, and depression; the opposite of euphoria.

Endorphins, enkephalins, and dynorphin Substances released by the body in response to painful stimuli that act as natural painkillers.

Euphoria State of intense happiness or well-being; the opposite of dysphoria.

Fibromyalgia A condition that causes pain all over the body, sleep problems, fatigue, and emotional and mental distress.

Hyperalgesia Heightened sensitivity to pain that can result from treatment of chronic pain with high-dose opioids.

Inflammation A response to tissue irritation or injury that is marked by signs of redness, swelling, heat, and pain.

Migraine Vascular headache that is often accompanied by nausea and visual disturbances.

Neuropathic pain Type of pain associated with nerve injury caused by trauma, infection, or chronic diseases such as diabetes.

Nociceptors Thin nerve fibers in skin, muscle, and other body tissues that carry pain signals.

NSAID Nonsteroidal antiinflammatory drug.

Opiate naïve No current exposure to opioids.

Opioid Naturally occurring or synthetically derived analgesic with properties similar to those of morphine.

Shingles Reoccurring and painful skin rash caused by the herpes zoster virus.

Substance P Peptide that is involved in the production of pain sensations and controls pain perception.

Trigeminal neuralgia Painful condition that produces intense, stabbing pain in areas of the face innervated by branches of the trigeminal nerve.

Overview

Most people will experience some type of physical pain in their lifetime. *Acute pain* is triggered by an injury, burn, infection, or some other stimuli and is self-limiting. *Chronic pain* may persist for years and is often inadequately controlled by pharmaceuticals or other pain management therapies. There is a strong psychological component to pain that is frequently underestimated. Psychological factors can influence a person's tolerance for pain and can determine whether the outcome of treatment is successful. To reduce anxieties associated with pain and the need for higher doses of pain medications, hospitalized patients may be permitted to control the frequency of administration of their doses of pain medications. Patient-controlled analgesia (PCA) is done using a device that is connected to the patient's intravenous line. The patient pushes a button to deliver a measured dose of pain medication.

Pain is often categorized by its origin. *Neuropathic pain* is associated with a nerve injury caused by trauma, infection, or chronic disease such as diabetes. Chronic pain is often of neuropathic origin. Central pain syndrome is a condition that may be caused by stroke, multiple sclerosis (Chapter 12), tumors, epilepsy (Chapter 9), brain or spinal cord trauma, or Parkinson disease (Chapter 8). It is a neurologic condition that can cause chronic pain. Complex regional pain syndrome is characterized by prolonged pain and inflammation after a serious injury to an arm or leg. It may be accompanied by changes in skin color, temperature, or swelling in the area below where the injury occurred.

Nociceptive pain is caused by stimulation of nociceptors in viscera (lungs, gastrointestinal [GI], heart) or skin, muscle, soft tissue, or bone (somatic). *Nociceptors* are thin nerve fibers located in the skin, muscle, and other body tissues that carry pain signals. The division of pain into distinct categories is somewhat simplistic because multiple pathophysiologic mechanisms are probably involved. A multimodal approach to pain management is recommended because untreated pain can affect all body systems. It may produce increased heart rate, anxiety, and muscle spasms and/or decreased immune response and intestinal motility.

Conditions That Produce Pain

Inflammation

Inflammation is an important source of pain. *Inflammation* is a response to tissue irritation or injury that is marked by signs of redness, swelling, heat, and pain. Sport injuries, *arthritis*, sprains, fractures, burns, cuts, bruises, and trauma caused by motor vehicle, workplace, or home accidents may all produce inflammation. Infection can also produce painful inflammation.

Low Back Pain

Up to 84% of adults in the United States and 80% of Canadian adults will experience low back pain at some point in their lives. Nearly 40% of Americans reported low back pain in the previous 3 months on the National Health Survey in the United States (2019). Low back pain is the ranked leading cause of disability globally. Acute low back pain produces symptoms that last less than 6 weeks. Chronic low back pain can persist indefinitely and may produce leg pain or widespread body pain or restrict spinal movement.

Burns

Severe burns can produce excruciating pain. Third-degree burns are the most severe because the skin has been destroyed. First-degree burns are less severe than second- or third-degree burns.

Diabetic Neuropathy

Uncontrolled diabetes can lead to damage to peripheral nerves. Nerve damage results in numbness, pain, or tingling of the feet or legs. Symptoms of *diabetic neuropathy* become more severe as the disease progresses.

Phantom Limb

Pain may be referred. This means that the place where pain symptoms are most strongly felt may be different than the actual origin of the painful stimuli. Patients who have had a limb amputated may describe pain in the area where the limb was removed. It is believed that although the limb is no longer present, the nerves that innervated the limb are remapped or rewired, permitting nerve messages to continue to be received. The ability of the brain to restructure itself and adapt to injury is called plasticity.

Shingles

Shingles produces a reoccurring and painful skin rash and is caused by the herpes zoster virus. The herpes zoster virus, which causes chicken pox, lays dormant in nerve endings until activated. Shingles cannot be cured.

Trigeminal Neuralgia

Trigeminal neuralgia produces headache and intense stabbing pain in areas of the face innervated by branches of the trigeminal nerve (lips, eyes, nose, scalp, forehead, upper jaw, and lower jaw). Approximately 1% to 2% of persons with multiple sclerosis develop trigeminal neuralgia.

Pain Signal Transmission

The pain message begins with stimulation of nociceptors in peripheral tissues. The signal is converted to an electrical impulse (transduction) that then travels to the dorsal horn of the spinal cord (transmission), where it is augmented or diminished by the release of neurotransmitters, amino acids, and neuropeptides (modulation) and then carried to the brain where the pain message is interpreted (perception) (Fig. 10.1).

When an injury occurs, proteins (cytokines) are released that produce painful inflammation. Prostaglandins, important mediators of pain, are also synthesized. Histamine, bradykinin, and serotonin (5-hydroxytryptamine [5-HT]) are also released in response to tissue injury and are part of the immune system response. They produce inflammation, vasodilation, and pain. Glutamate is an amino acid neurotransmitter that enhances the response to painful stimuli. *Substance P* and neurokinin A are peptides that are involved in the modulation of pain sensations that are transmitted to the brain and control how pain is perceived. *Endorphins, enkephalins, and dynorphins* are opioid peptides that bind to opioid receptors in the brain and spinal cord and block or dull the pain sensations by inhibiting the release of substance P and glutamate. They act like natural painkillers (Fig. 10.2).

Drugs Used to Treat Pain

Opioids

Opiates are naturally occurring substances that are derived from the opium poppy and have been used for more than 2000 years to induce sleep and *euphoria* and to relieve diarrhea. Morphine and heroin are examples of opiates. *Opioid* is a term used to describe a drug that acts like morphine, whether naturally occurring or synthetically derived. Opiates and opioid drugs produce analgesia. *Analgesics* are drugs that reduce pain sensations and alter pain perception. Opioid analgesics are less effective in treating neuropathic pain.

Some opioid analgesics are also used to treat opioid dependence. When detoxification is achieved, a maintenance dose is continued. Methadone and buprenorphine are examples of opioid

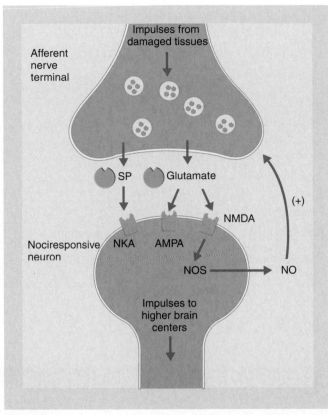

SP = substance P
NO = nitric oxide
NKA = neurokinin A

• **Fig. 10.1** Mechanism of pain perception. (From Page C, Curtis M, Sutter M, et al. *Integrated pharmacology*, ed 3, Philadelphia, 2006, Mosby.)

agonists that are administered for management of drug dependence. Opioid antagonists such as naltrexone are also used to treat drug and alcohol dependence.

Mechanism of Action

Opioids bind to opioid receptors located in the dorsal route of the spinal cord, brainstem, thalamus, hypothalamus, and limbic system to decrease painful sensations and raise the pain threshold.

There are several types of opioid receptors. The effects and adverse reactions produced by opioid drugs are related to the receptors that are stimulated by the drugs. Mu (μ) receptor stimulation produces analgesia, euphoria, respiratory depression, pupillary constriction, decreased GI motility, and physical dependence. Kappa (κ) receptor binding produces analgesia, sedation, pupillary constriction, *dysphoria*, and hallucinations. Delta (δ) receptor stimulation produces analgesia and decreases contractions of smooth muscle.

Classification of Opioids

Agonists

Opioids are categorized according to their action at the opioid receptor. Opioid agonists (e.g., codeine, morphine, and oxycodone) produce analgesia and other adverse effects associated with stimulation of the specific opioid receptor. Partial agonists produce incomplete activation of the opioid receptor, producing less than maximum response.

Antagonists

Antagonists (e.g., naloxone) bind to the opioid receptor but do not activate it. They interfere with agonist binding. Antagonists are administered when reversal of the action of an opioid agonist is desired.

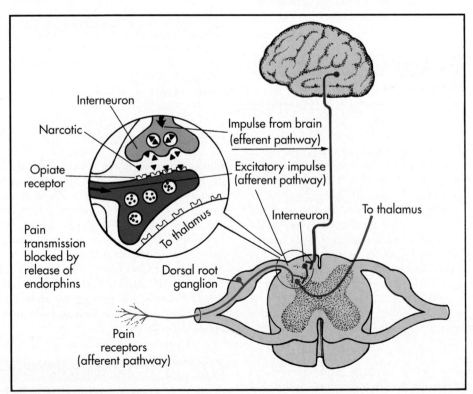

• **Fig. 10.2** Descending pathway and endorphin response. The biologic receptors of the enkephalins and endorphins are located close to known pain receptors in the periphery and ascending and descending pain pathways. (From McCance KL, Huether SE. *Pathophysiology*, ed 7, St Louis, 2014, Elsevier.)

Mixed Agonist/Antagonists

The response produced by some opioids is mixed. Sometimes the opioid behaves like an agonist, and sometimes it behaves like an antagonist (e.g., buprenorphine, butorphanol, and nalbuphine). Agonist activity is exhibited if the patient has had no recent exposure to an opioid agonist *(opiate naïve)*. If the patient is currently taking an opioid agonist, the mixed agonist/antagonist exhibits antagonist activity.

Pharmacokinetics

The analgesic effect produced by opioid agonists is often compared with morphine. When switching between agents or dosage forms, the equivalent analgesic dose must be calculated to achieve the same level of pain relief. Oral absorption of opioid agonists, partial agonists, and mixed agonist/antagonist is varied. Many orally administered opioids exhibit significant first-pass metabolism. The average onset of action of orally administered opioids is approximately 30 minutes after administration. The onset of action of most parenterally administered opioids occurs within 10 to 15 minutes. A few opioids (meperidine, pentazocine, and butorphanol) begin working in less than 5 minutes. Peak effects are achieved between 30 minutes and 2 hours. The duration of action for immediate-release opioids ranges between 2 and 6 hours. The duration of action for controlled-release opioid analgesics may last for up to 72 hours (e.g., fentanyl patches). Fentanyl is 100 times more potent than morphine. Patients who have been prescribed long-acting opioid dosage forms may also be prescribed short-acting opioids to control **breakthrough pain** that may occur between scheduled doses of the long-acting analgesic.

> ● **Tech Note!**
>
> Butorphanol is often prescribed for migraine headache pain.

> ● **Tech Note!**
>
> Immediate-release opioids are used to manage breakthrough pain.

Adverse Reactions

Adverse effects of opioid agonists, partial agonists, and mixed agonist/antagonists are determined by the extent to which they bind to specific opioid receptors. Common side effects caused by acute use are sedation, constipation, and GI upset (Table 10.1). Opioid agonists and partial agonists may produce tolerance and dependence. Tolerance requires increasing doses to produce the same effects. Dependence causes users to continue taking opioids to avoid withdrawal symptoms. Dependence may be physical or psychological. Overdose may lead to respiratory depression and death. Chronic use may additionally produce **hyperalgesia** (a heightened sensitivity to pain that can result from treatment of chronic pain with high-dose opioids), sexual dysfunction, and decreased immune response.

Precautions

Access to opioid agonists, partial agonists, and most mixed agonist/antagonists is restricted in the United States (schedule C-I through C-V) and Canada (straight and verbal narcotics) because they produce tolerance and dependence.

TABLE 10.1	Opioid-Induced Side Effects and Adverse Effects by Body System
Body System	**Side Effect or Adverse Effect**
Central nervous system	Sedation, disorientation, euphoria, light-headedness, dysphoria, lowered seizure threshold, and tremors
Cardiovascular system	Hypotension, palpitations, and flushing
Respiratory tract	Respiratory depression and aggravation of asthma
Gastrointestinal tract	Nausea, vomiting, constipation, and biliary tract spasm
Genitourinary tract	Urinary retention
Other	Itching, rash, and wheal information

From Lilley LL, Harrington S, Snyder JS. *Pharmacology and the nursing process*, ed 5, St Louis, 2007, Mosby.

> ❶ **Tech Alert!**
>
> The following drugs have look-alike/sound-alike issues:
> oxyCODONE and oxyCONTIN;
> HYDROcodone, HYDROmorphone, and oxycodone;
> morphine and oxyMORphone;
> morphine nonconcentrated oral liquid and morphine concentrated oral liquid

> ● **Tech Note!**
>
> Fentanyl transdermal patches are worn for 72 hours and should be dispensed with instructions on proper storage and disposal to prevent accidental overdose or poisoning.

Opioid Antagonists

Opioid antagonists are indicated for the reversal of respiratory depression caused by opioid use. Respiratory depression may be produced by drugs administered during surgery for general anesthesia, may occur in infants born to opioid-dependent women, and occur in opioid overdose. The opioid antagonist naltrexone is indicated for the treatment of opioid overdose and the management of drug and alcohol dependence. Naltrexone may produce drowsiness. The warning labels MAY CAUSE DROWSINESS, MAY IMPAIR ABILITY TO DRIVE, and AVOID ALCOHOL should be applied to prescription vials. Both naltrexone and naloxone can precipitate withdrawal symptoms in patients who are opioid dependent.

> ❶ **Tech Alert!**
>
> Naloxone and naltrexone have look-alike/sound-alike issues.

Tech Note!

Buprenorphine tablets may be prescribed only for the treatment of opioid dependency. Valid prescriptions are written by prescribers who have a Drug Enforcement Administration (DEA) No. specifically for buprenorphine.

Tech Note!

Buprenorphine extended release subcutaneous injection was approved in 2023. It is available in 8 mg, 16 mg, 24 mg, 32 mg, 64 mg, 96 mg, and 128 mg strengths.

Tech Note!

US pharmacies must be enrolled in the Transmucosal Immediate Release Fentanyl Risk Evaluation and Mitigation Strategy (TIRF REMS) Access Program to dispense or distribute transmucosal immediate release fentanyl products (e.g., Actiq, Fentora, Lazanda, and Subsys).

Opioid Overdose: A Public Health Issue

Opioid use and opioid overdose are epidemic in the United States and Canada. The number of Americans who died from an opioid overdose exceeded 105,000 annually in 2022. Opioid-related deaths were up 28.5% from 2020, according to the US Centers for Disease Control and Prevention (CDC). In Canada, 29,052 died of an apparent opioid overdose between 2016 and 2021, according to Government of Canada statistics. In 2922 alone 7328 people died from an opioid overdose. Naloxone is an opioid antagonist available for emergency use to reduce death caused by opioid overdose. Forty-six states have laws that address access to naloxone for opioid overdose. As many as 40 states allow pharmacists to dispense naloxone to the general public without a physician prescription. In Canada and in the United States, pharmacists may dispense intranasal and injectable kits of naloxone. The kits are publicly funded in Canada and may be dispensed free of charge. Naloxone is marketed as a nasal spray (2 mg and 4 mg per spray) and an injectable kit for use by the general public.

Opioid Agonists

Generic Name	US Brand Name(s) Canadian Brand Name(s)	Dosage Forms and Strengths	Controlled Substance Schedule
codeine[a]	Generics Codeine Contin	**Injection**[b]: 30 mg/mL **Syrup, oral**[b]: 5 mg/mL, 10 mg/5 mL **Tablets, controlled release (Codeine Contin)**[b]: 50 mg, 100 mg, 150 mg, 200 mg **Tablets, as phosphate**[b]: 15 mg, 30 mg **Tablets, as sulfate**[c]: 15 mg, 30 mg, 60 mg	**C-II** (US) **Straight narcotic** (Canada)
codeine and acetaminophen (APAP)[a]	generics LENOLTEC No. 1, LENOLTEC No. 2, LENOLTEC No. 3, LENOLTEC No. 4	**Elixir/Suspension**: 120 mg APAP + 12 mg codeine **Tablets**: 300 mg APAP + 8 mg codeine + 15 mg caffeine[b] **Tablets**[b]: 300 mg APAP + 15 mg codeine + 15 mg caffeine; 300 mg APAP + 30 mg codeine + 15 mg caffeine **Tablets**[c]: 300 mg APAP + 15 mg codeine, 300 mg APAP + 30 mg codeine; APAP 300 mg and codeine 60 mg[b c]	**In the US:** APAP + codeine Elixir (**C-V**), tablets (**C-III**) **In Canada:** APAP + caffeine + codeine 8 mg (**Schedule II, exempt narcotic**); tablets containing APAP, caffeine + 15 mg or 30 mg codeine (**Verbal narcotic**); tablets containing APAP + codeine 60 mg (**Straight narcotic**)
fentanyl[a]	Actiq, Fentora, Lazanda, Sublimaze, Subsys Fentora	**Injection, solution (Sublimaze)**: 50 mcg/mL **Lozenge (Actiq)**[c]: 200 mcg, 400 mcg, 600 mcg, 800 mcg, 1200 mcg, 1600 mcg **Nasal spray (Lazanda)**[c]: 100 mcg, 400 mcg **Sublingual spray (Subsys)**: 100 mcg, 200 mcg, 400 mcg, 600 mcg, 800 mcg, 1200 mcg, 1600 mcg **Tablets, buccal (Fentora)**: 100 mcg, 200 mcg, 400 mcg, 600 mcg, 800 mcg **Transdermal**: 12 mcg, 25 mcg, 37.5 mcg[c], 50 mcg, 62.5 mcg[c], 75 mcg, 87.5 mcg[c], 100 mcg	**C-II** (All dosage forms in the US) **Straight narcotic** (All dosage forms in Canada)
hydrocodone[a]	Hysingla ER Generics	**Capsule, extended release**: 10 mg, 15 mg, 20 mg, 30 mg, 40 mg, 50 mg **Syrup**[b]: 1 mg/mL **Tablet, extended release**: 20 mg, 30 mg, 40 mg, 60 mg, 80 mg, 100 mg, 120 mg (Hysingla ER)	**C-II** (All dosage forms in the US) **Straight narcotic** (All dosage forms in Canada)

Continued

Opioid Agonists—cont'd

Generic Name	US Brand Name(s) / Canadian Brand Name(s)	Dosage Forms and Strengths	Controlled Substance Schedule
hydrocodone and acetaminophen[a]	Anexsia 5/325, Anexsia 7.5/325 Not available	**Solution:** 7.5 mg hydrocodone and 325 mg APAP/15 mL; 10 mg hydrocodone and 300 mg APAP/15 mL **Tablets:** 5 mg hydrocodone + 325 mg APAP; 7.5 mg hydrocodone + 325 mg APAP; 10 mg hydrocodone + 325 mg APAP	**C-II** (All dosage forms in the US)
hydrocodone and ibuprofen[a]	Generics Not available	**Tablets:** 5 mg/200 mg, 7.5 mg/200 mg, 10 mg/200 mg	**C-III**
hydromorphone[a]	Dilaudid, Dilaudid, Hydromorph Contin	**Capsules, controlled release (Hydromorph Contin):** 3 mg, 4.5 mg, 6 mg, 9 mg, 12 mg, 18 mg, 24 mg, 30 mg **Injection, powder for reconstitution:** 250 mg per vial **Injection, solution:** 0.2 mg/mL, 1 mg/mL, 2 mg/mL, 10 mg/mL, 20 mg/mL, 50 mg/mL, 100 mg/mL **Liquid, oral:** 1 mg/mL **Tablets, extended release:** 4 mg[b], 8 mg, 12 mg, 16 mg, 32 mg **Tablets, immediate release:** 1 mg[b], 2 mg, 4 mg, 8 mg	**C-II** (US) **Straight narcotic** (Canada)
levorphanol[a]	Generics Not available	**Tablets:** 1 mg, 2 mg, 3 mg	**C-II** (US)
meperidine[a]	Demerol Generics	**Injection, solution (vials and prefilled syringe):** 25 mg/mL[c], 50 mg/mL, 75 mg/mL[c], 100 mg/mL[c] **Solution, oral**[c]: 50 mg/5 mL **Tablets:** 50 mg, 100 mg[c]	**C-II** (US) **Straight narcotic** (Canada)
methadone[a]	Methadose Metadol, Metadol-D Methadose	**Injection, solution**[c]: 10 mg/mL **Solution, oral:** 1 mg/mL, 10 mg/5 mL[c] **Solution, oral concentrate:** 10 mg/mL **Tablets:** 1 mg[b], 5 mg, 10 mg, 25 mg[b] **Tablets, dispersible for oral solution:** 40 mg	**C-II** (US) **Straight narcotic** (Canada)
apomorphine	Apokyn, Kynmobi Kynmobi, Movapo	**Solution, for injection (Apokyn, Movapo):** 10 mg/mL **Sublingual film (Kynmobi):** 10 mg, 15 mg, 20 mg, 25 mg, 30 mg	**C-II** (US) **Straight narcotic** (Canada)
morphine[a]	Duramorph PF, Infumorph, Mitigo, MS Contin Doloral, Kadian, M-Eslon, MS Contin, MS IR, Statex	**Capsules, extended release (M-Eslon):** 10 mg, 15 mg, 30 mg, 60 mg, 100 mg, 200 mg **Capsules, sustained release (Kadian):** 10 mg, 20 mg, 30 mg[c], 50 mg, 60 mg[c], 80 mg[c], 100 mg, 120 mg[c] **Injection, extended release for epidural:** 10 mg/mL **Injection, epidural, intrathecal (Duramorph, Infumorph):** 0.5 mg/mL, 1 mg/mL, 10 mg/mL, 25 mg/mL **Injection, solution:** 2 mg/mL, 4 mg/mL[c], 5 mg/mL, 8 mg/mL[c], 10 mg/mL, 15 mg/mL, 25 mg/mL, 50 mg/mL[b] **Solution, oral (Doloral):** 20 mg/mL, 1 mg/mL[b], 5 mg/mL[b], 10 mg/mL[b], 10 mg/5 mL[c], 20 mg/5 mL[c], 100 mg/5 mL[c]	

Opioid Agonists—cont'd

Generic Name	US Brand Name(s) / Canadian Brand Name(s)	Dosage Forms and Strengths	Controlled Substance Schedule
		Solution, oral drops (Statex): 20 mg/mL, 50 mg/mL **Syrup:** 1 mg/mL, 5 mg/mL, 10 mg/mL **Suppositories:** 5 mg, 10 mg, 20 mg, 30 mg **Tablets, controlled release (MS Contin):** 15 mg, 30 mg, 60 mg, 100 mg, 200 mg **Tablets, immediate release (MS IR):** 5 mg, 10 mg, 20 mg, 30 mg; (Statex): 5 mg, 10 mg, 25 mg, 50 mg **Tablets, sustained release (Oramorph SR):** 15 mg, 30 mg, 60 mg, 100 mg	
oxycodone[a]	Oxaydo, OxyContin, Roxicodone, Roxybond, Xtampza ER OxyNEO, Oxy IR, Supeudol	**Capsule, extended release (Xtampza ER)[c]:** 9 mg, 13.5 mg, 18 mg, 27 mg, 36 mg **Capsules, immediate release:** 5 mg **Solution, oral:** 5 mg/5 mL **Solution, oral concentrate:** 20 mg/mL **Tablets, immediate release (Oxy IR, Oxaydo, Supeudol):** 5 mg, 7.5 mg, 10 mg, 15 mg[c], 20 mg, 30 mg[c] **Tablets, extended release (OxyContin, OxyNEO):** 5 mg[b], 10 mg, 15 mg, 20 mg, 30 mg, 40 mg, 60 mg, 80 mg	**C-II** **Straight narcotic** (Canada)
oxycodone and acetaminophen[a]	Percocet Generics	**Tablets (Percocet):** 2.5 mg/325 mg, 5 mg/325 mg, 7.5 mg/325 mg, 10 mg/325 mg	**C-II** (US) **Straight narcotic** (Canada)
oxycodone and aspirin	Percodan Generics	**Tablets:** 5 mg oxycodone/325 mg aspirin	**C-II** (US) **Straight narcotic** (Canada)
oxymorphone[a]	Generics Not available	**Tablets:** 5 mg, 10 mg **Tablets, extended release:** 5 mg, 7.5 mg, 10 mg, 15 mg, 20 mg, 30 mg, 40 mg	**C-II**

[a]Generic available.
[b]Available in Canada only.
[c]Available in the United States only.

Mixed Agonist/Antagonists

Generic Name	US Brand Name(s) / Canadian Brand(s)	Dosage Forms and Strengths	Controlled Substance Schedule (C-I, C-II, C-III, C-IV, C-V)
buprenorphine	Belbuca, Brixadi, Buprenex, Butrans, Sublocade Butrans, Sublocade	**Film, buccal (Belbuca):** 0.075 mg, 0.15 mg, 0.3 mg, 0.45 mg, 0.6 mg[c], 0.75 mg[c], 0.9 mg[c] **Injection, solution (Buprenex):** 0.3 mg/mL **Solution, extended release for injection (Sublocade):** 100 mg/0.5 mL, 300 mg/1.5 mL **Tablets, sublingual (Subutex):** 2 mg, 8 mg **Transdermal, weekly patch (Butrans):** 5 mcg/h, 7.5 mg/h[c], 10 mcg/h, 15 mg/h, 20 mcg/h **Solution, subcutaneous extended release (Brixadi):** 8 mg/0.16 mL, 16 mg/0.32 mL, 24 mg/0.48 mL, 32 mg/0.64 mL, 64 mg/ 0.18 mL, 96 mg/0.27 mL, 128 mg/0.36 mL	**C-III** (US) **Straight narcotic** (Canada)

Continued

Mixed Agonist/Antagonists —cont'd

Generic Name	US Brand Name(s) / Canadian Brand(s)	Dosage Forms and Strengths	Controlled Substance Schedule (C-I, C-II, C-III, C-IV, C-V)
buprenorphine and naloxone[a]	Suboxone, Zubsolv / Suboxone	**Film, buccal:** 2 mg buprenorphine and 0.5 mg naloxone, 4 mg buprenorphine and 1 mg naloxone, 8 mg buprenorphine and 2 mg naloxone **Tablets, sublingual (Zubsolv):** 0.7 mg buprenorphine and 0.18 mg naloxone, 1.4 mg buprenorphine and 0.36 mg naloxone, 2.9 mg buprenorphine and 0.71 mg naloxone, 5.7 mg buprenorphine and 1.4 mg naloxone, 8.6 mg buprenorphine and 2.1 mg naloxone, 11.4 mg buprenorphine and 2.9 mg naloxone **Tablets, sublingual (Suboxone):** 2 mg buprenorphine and 0.5 mg naloxone, 4 mg buprenorphine and 1 mg naloxone, 8 mg buprenorphine and 2 mg naloxone, 12 mg buprenorphine and 3 mg naloxone, 16 mg buprenorphine and 4 mg naloxone	**C-III** (US) **Straight narcotic** (Canada)
butorphanol[a]	Generics / Generics	**Injection**[b]**:** 1 mg/mL, 2 mg/mL **Intranasal solution:** 10 mg/mL (1 mg/spray)	**C-IV** (US) **Straight narcotic** (Canada)
nalbuphine[a]	Generics / Nubain	**Injection, solution:** 10 mg/mL, 20 mg/mL[b]	**Schedule G Controlled (Canada)**
oxycodone and naloxone	Not available / Targin	**Tablets:** 5 mg oxycodone and 2.5 mg naloxone, 10 mg oxycodone and 5 mg naloxone, 20 mg oxycodone and 10 mg naloxone, 40 mg oxycodone and 20 mg naloxone	**Straight narcotic (Canada)**
pentazocine and naloxone	Generics / Not available	**Tablets:** 50 mg pentazocine + 0.5 mg naloxone	**C-IV**.

[a]Generic available.
[b]Strength available in the United States only.
[c]Strength available in Canada only.

Opioid agonist therapy (OAT) is an effective treatment for opioid use disorder involving opioid drugs such as heroin, oxycodone, hydromorphone, fentanyl, and Percocet. Therapy involves taking an opioid agonist such as methadone (Methadose) or a mixed agonist such as buprenorphine (Suboxone).

> **⊘ Tech Alert!**
>
> Fentanyl SL spray (Subsys®) is not bioequivalent to other fentanyl dosage forms so is not substituted on a microgram-per-microgram basis.

> **⊘ Tech Alert!**
>
> Product selection errors are common because of many strength combinations for hydrocodone and acetaminophen.

> **● Tech Note!**
>
> M-Eslon capsules may be opened and the contents sprinkled on food or in liquid. The sprinkles may be given by gastric tube.

Nonopioid Analgesics
Nonsteroidal Antiinflammatory Drugs, Salicylates, and Acetaminophen

NSAIDs, salicylates (aspirin), and acetaminophen are widely used in the treatment of pain with or without inflammation. NSAIDs and aspirin have analgesic, antiinflammatory, and antipyretic properties. An antipyretic is a drug that can reduce fever. NSAID action and effectiveness are similar to aspirin (ASA).

Mechanism of Action

NSAIDs decrease prostaglandin synthesis by inhibiting the action of cyclooxygenase-1 (COX-1) and cyclooxygenase-2 (COX-2) like aspirin. Most NSAIDs are not selective. COX-1 is expressed continuously and is found throughout the body. It is important for regulation of platelet aggregation and the biosynthesis of prostaglandins that protect the gastric mucosa. COX-2 is formed in selected cells as part of the immune response. COX-2 is involved in the biosynthesis of prostaglandins responsible for pain and inflammation. The analgesic effect of acetaminophen is thought to additionally be caused by inhibition of COX-3 in the brain.

Opioid Antagonists

Generic Name	US Brand Name(s) / Canadian Brand(s)	Dosage Forms and Strengths	Usual Adult Dose
naloxone[a]	Narcan, Kloxxado, Zimhi Narcan	**Injection, solution:** 0.4 mg/mL, 1 mg/mL **Nasal spray (Narcan):** 4 mg/spray **Injection, solution:** 5 mg/0.5 mL (Zimhi) **Nasal spray:** 4 mg/spray (Narcan), 8 mg/spray (Kloxxado)	0.4–2 mg IV every 2–3 min; repeat every 20–60 min Nasal spray: 1 spray in one nostril, repeat in 2–3 minutes as necessary
methylnaltrexone	Relistor Relistor	**Solution, for injection:** 8 mg/0.4 mL[b], 12 mg/0.6 mL **Tablet**[b]**:** 150 mg	450 mg orally or 12 mg subcutaneously once daily for opioid-induced constipation
naltrexone[a]	Vivitrol ReVia	**Powder, for injection (Vivitrol)**[b]**:** 380 mg per vial **Tablets (ReVia):** 50 mg	Tablets: Start 25 mg; 50 mg/day or 100–150 mg 3 times a week (up to 800 mg/day) Injection: 380 mg IM every 4 weeks (Vivitrol)

[a]Generic available.
[b]Available in the United States only.

Summary of Drugs Used to Manage Drug Dependence or Reverse Effects of Opioids

Generic Name	Dose	Onset[a] (min)	Duration[a] (min/h)	Route
buprenorphine	Opioid dependence	30–60 PO	12 h (2 mg) up to 72 h (>16 mg)	IV, PO
buprenorphine and naloxone	Opioid dependence			
methadone	Opioid dependence	30	24–36 h	PO
naloxone	Reverse opioid-induced respiratory depression of overdose	2	30 min	IM, IV, subcutaneous, nasal spray
naltrexone	Alcohol dependence	15–30	50 mg (24 h) 100 mg (48 h) 150 mg (72 h)	PO

[a]Varies according to dose and route of administration.

Pharmacokinetics

Aspirin and NSAIDs are well absorbed orally. Aspirin is a weak acid (acetylsalicylic acid), and the rate of absorption varies according to the pH of the stomach, small intestine, and urine. Enteric-coated aspirin is released in the pH of the intestine rather than in the stomach. Aspirin is eliminated in the urine. Acidification of the urine with vitamin C can increase rate of reabsorption, and sodium bicarbonate enhances elimination (see Chapter 2).

NSAIDs are structurally dissimilar; however, they are biologically similar. Oral absorption is good, and bioavailability ranges between 80% and 99%. They are all highly protein bound, more than 97%, and they all are primarily eliminated in the urine.

Adverse Reactions

All of the NSAIDs and aspirin can produce nausea, GI bleeding, and ulceration. NSAIDs can cause fluid retention, leading to increased blood pressure. Some NSAIDs can produce dizziness. Serious side effects include salicylism (aspirin), hepatotoxicity (ketorolac), and agranulocytosis (indomethacin, flurbiprofen). Celecoxib (Celebrex) remains the only selective COX-2 inhibitor currently in use. Acetaminophen can cause hepatotoxicity.

> **❶ Tech Alert!**
>
> The maximum daily adult dose for acetaminophen and aspirin is 4 g.

> **❶ Tech Alert!**
>
> Acetaminophen doses for children are calculated based on body weight. Consumers should measure the dose using the calibrated device that is supplied with the product.

Summary of Opioid Analgesics

	Generic Name	US Brand Name	Usual Adult Oral Dose and Dosing Schedule	Warning Labels
Opioid Agonists				
	codeine	Generics	**Immediate release, IM and subcut injection**: 15–60 mg every 4–6 h (up to 360 mg/day) **Controlled release**: 50–300 mg every 12 h	MAY CAUSE DROWSINESS; MAY IMPAIR ABILITY TO DRIVE. AVOID ALCOHOL. TAKE WITH FOOD. MAY BE HABIT FORMING. TAKE EACH DOSE WITH A FULL GLASS OF WATER. SWALLOW WHOLE; DO NOT CRUSH OR CHEW—controlled release and delayed release. ROTATE SITE OF APPLICATION—transdermal. PROTECT FROM MOISTURE—Actiq, Belbuca, Fentora, Kynmobi. DO NOT REMOVE FROM FOIL WRAPPER UNTIL READY FOR USE—Actiq, Belbuca, Fentora, Kynmobi.
	codeine and acetaminophen	Tylenol with Codeine #3	1–2 tablets every 4 h (maximum, 4 g daily)	
	fentanyl	Fentora, Subsys	**Transdermal:** Apply one 25–100 mcg/h patch (up to 300 mcg for severe chronic pain) every 72 h **Buccal:** Place one Fentora tablet between the upper cheek and gum for 14–25 minutes; may swallow if not fully disintegrated after 30 minutes **Lozenge (Actiq):** Suck one lozenge in mouth for 15 minutes; may repeat dose if breakthrough pain not relieved **Sublingual (Subsys):** Spray a 100–1600 mcg dose under the tongue; may repeat once after 30 minutes (Subsys®); separate treatments by at least 4 hours	
	hydrocodone and acetaminophen	Anexsia 5/325, Anexsia 7.5/325	1–2 tablets every 4–6 h (maximum dose, hydrocodone 60 mg and APAP 4 g/day)	
	hydrocodone and ibuprofen	Generics	1 tablets every 4–6 h	
	hydromorphone	Dilaudid	**IM/subcut:** 1–2 mg every 2–3 h prn **IV:** 0.2–1 mg every 2–3 h **PCA:** 0.2 mg/mL (range, 0.05–0.4 mg) **Capsule, controlled release (Hydromorph Contin):** 3–30 mg every 12 h **Tablet, controlled release:** 8–32 mg once daily **Oral (immediate release):** 2–8 mg every 3–4 h	
	levorphanol	Generics	**Tablet:** 2–4 mg every 6–8 h (maximum 12 mg daily)	
	meperidine	Demerol	**Oral, IM, and subcut:** 50–150 mg every 3–4 h	
	methadone	Methadose	**For pain (opiate naïve):** **Oral:** 2.5–10 mg every 8–12 h **IV, IM, subcut:** 2.5–10 mg every 8–12 h **Detoxification (oral):** 20–40 mg/day; maintenance dose 80–120 mg/day	

Summary of Opioid Analgesics—cont'd

Generic Name	US Brand Name	Usual Adult Oral Dose and Dosing Schedule	Warning Labels
morphine	MS Contin, Kynmobi	**For pain (opiate naïve):** **Oral (prompt release):** 10–30 mg every 3–4 h **Oral (extended release and sustained release capsules, e.g., M-Eslon):** usual dose 30 mg every 12 h **Sublingual (Kynmobi):** 10–30 mg every 2 h (max 5 doses per day) **Controlled release (tablet, e.g., MS Contin):** Individualized every 8–12 h **PCA:** 0.5–2.5 mg, lockout interval: 5–10 min **IM, subcut:** 5–20 mg every 4 h as needed	
oxycodone	OxyContin, OxyNEO	**Immediate release, tablet (e.g., Oxy IR, Oxaydo):** 5–10 mg every 6 h **Controlled release (capsule, e.g., Xtampza ER):** Individualized; initiate 9 mg every 12 h **Controlled release (tablet, e.g., OxyContin, OxyNeo):** 10–40 mg every 12 h	
oxycodone and acetaminophen	Percocet	1–2 tablets every 4–6 h (maximum, 4 g APAP daily)	
oxymorphone	Generics	**Oral tablet (immediate release):** 10–20 mg every 4–6 h **Oral tablet (extended release):** 5–10 mg every 12 h	

Mixed Agonist/Antagonists

Generic Name	US Brand Name	Usual Adult Oral Dose and Dosing Schedule	Warning Labels
buprenorphine	Belbuca, Buprenex, Butrans	**Belbuca:** Wet the inside of the cheek and place one film twice daily (usual dose 75–150 mcg twice daily) **Buprenex (opiate naïve): IM, IV:** 0.3 mg every 6–8 h **Butrans:** Apply 1 patch every 7 days	MAY CAUSE DROWSINESS; MAY IMPAIR ABILITY TO DRIVE. AVOID ALCOHOL. MAY BE HABIT FORMING.
buprenorphine and naloxone	Suboxone	**Opioid dependence:** 4–24 mg/day titrated according to avoid withdrawal symptoms	
butorphanol	Generics	**Acute pain (IM, IV):** 1–4 mg every 3–4 h **Labor pain:** 1–2 mg within 4 h of anticipated delivery	

Commonly Used Nonopioid Analgesics

Generic Name	Brand Name	Usual Adult Dose	Side Effects	Warning Labels
Salicylates				
aspirin	Ecotrin, Bayer, Anacin	325–650 mg every 4–6 h (maximum, 4 g/day)	GI upset, bleeding, tinnitus, salicylism	TAKE WITH FOOD.
diflunisal	Generics	250–500 mg twice a day	GI upset, rash, drowsiness, jaundice	TAKE WITH FOOD. MAY CAUSE DIZZINESS OR DROWSINESS. AVOID ASPIRIN AND RELATED DRUGS.
***p*-Aminophenol**				
acetaminophen	Tylenol	325–650 mg every 4–6 h (maximum, 4 g/day)	Skin, liver toxicity, kidney toxicity	

Continued

Commonly Used Nonopioid Analgesics—cont'd

	Generic Name	Brand Name	Usual Adult Dose	Side Effects	Warning Labels
Indoles					
	indomethacin	Indocin	25–50 mg 2–3 times a day	GI upset, headache, dizziness (drowsiness—sulindac), tinnitus, agranulocytosis (fatigue, apnea—indomethacin)	TAKE WITH FOOD. MAY CAUSE DIZZINESS OR DROWSINESS. AVOID ASPIRIN AND RELATED DRUGS.
	sulindac	Generics	150–200 mg twice a day maximum, 400 mg/day		
	etodolac	Generics	200–400 mg every 6–8 h		
Phenylpropionic Acid					
	flurbiprofen	Generics	200–300 mg/day in 2–4 divided doses	GI upset, headache, tinnitus, dizziness, kidney toxicity (ibuprofen)	TAKE WITH FOOD. MAY CAUSE DIZZINESS OR DROWSINESS. AVOID ASPIRIN AND RELATED DRUGS.
	ibuprofen	Motrin	200–800 mg every 4–8 h (maximum, 3200 mg/day)		
	ketoprofen	Generics	50–75 mg 3–4 times a day		
		Generics (extended release)	200 mg once a day		
	oxaprozin	Daypro	1200 mg once a day		
Naphthylpropionic Acids					
	naproxen	Naprosyn Naprosyn DS Napralen	**Immediate release:** Start 500 mg (Naproxen[a]), 550 mg (Anaprox); then 250–275 mg every 6–12 h	GI upset, headache, tinnitus, rash, dizziness	TAKE WITH FOOD. MAY CAUSE DIZZINESS OR DROWSINESS. AVOID ASPIRIN AND RELATED DRUGS.
	naproxen sodium	Aleve (OTC) Anaprox Anaprox DS	**Delayed release** (EC Naprosyn): 375–500 mg twice daily **Controlled release** (Napralen): 750–1500 mg once daily (maximum 1500 mg/day)		
Naphthyalkanones					
	nabumetone	Generics	1000–2000 mg/day dosed 1–2 times/day	GI upset, dizziness, agranulocytosis	TAKE WITH FOOD. MAY CAUSE DIZZINESS OR DROWSINESS. AVOID ASPIRIN AND RELATED DRUGS.
Anthranilic Acids					
	meclofenamate	Generics	50–100 mg every 4–6 h (maximum, 400 mg/day)	GI upset, headache, dizziness, increased urination	TAKE WITH FOOD. MAY CAUSE DIZZINESS OR DROWSINESS. AVOID ASPIRIN AND RELATED DRUGS.
Pyrrole Acetic Acid					
	ketorolac	Toradol, Sprix	**Nasal Spray:** Inhale 1 spray in each nostril every 6–8 hours **PO:** 10 mg every 4–6 h (maximum, 40 mg/day) **IM:** Inject 10–30 mg IM every 4–6 h	GI upset, headache, dizziness, rash, liver toxicity (ketorolac), palpitations (tolmetin)	

Commonly Used Nonopioid Analgesics—cont'd

	Generic Name	Brand Name	Usual Adult Dose	Side Effects	Warning Labels
Phenylacetic Acid					
	diclofenac epolamine	Flector, Licart,	**Transdermal patch:** Apply 1 patch twice daily	Systemic administration: GI upset, nausea and vomiting, ulceration	ROTATE SITE OF APPLICATION—Flector, Licart.
	diclofenac sodium	Pennsaid, Voltaren, Voltaren- XR, Voltaren Rapide (Canada)	**Solution (Pennsaid):** Apply 40 mg (2 pumps) twice daily **Immediate release:** 50 mg 2–4 times a day (oral) **Controlled release:** 100 mg once daily (maximum 200 mg/day)	Topical: Local irritation	TAKE WITH FOOD. MAY CAUSE DIZZINESS OR DROWSINESS. AVOID ASPIRIN AND RELATED DRUGS. SWALLOW WHOLE; DO NOT CRUSH OR CHEW. — extended release SHAKE WELL—Cambia.
	diclofenac potassium	Cambia, Zipsor	**Capsule:** 25 mg 4 times a day **Powder, for suspension (Cambia):** Mix 1 packet in 1–2 ounces of water and drink		
	diclofenac + misoprostol	Arthrotec-50, Arthrotec-75	100–150 mg diclofenac tablet 2–3 times per day		
Oxicams					
	meloxicam	Anjesca Mobic	**IV (Anjesco):** 30 mg once daily by bolus **Tablet (Mobic):** 7.5–15 mg once a day	GI upset, constipation or diarrhea, gas, dizziness, edema, GI bleeding, hypertension	TAKE WITH FOOD. MAY CAUSE DIZZINESS OR DROWSINESS. AVOID ASPIRIN AND RELATED DRUGS. SWALLOW WHOLE; DO NOT CRUSH OR CHEW.
	piroxicam	Feldene	20 mg once a day		
COX-2 Inhibitors					
	celecoxib	Celebrex, Elyxyb	100–200 mg twice a day Solution (Elyxyb): 120 mg daily	GI upset, GI ulceration, heart attack, stroke	TAKE WITH FOOD. MAY CAUSE DIZZINESS OR DROWSINESS. AVOID ASPIRIN AND RELATED DRUGS.

a550 mg naproxen Na = (500 mg naproxen base).

Drug Treatment for Neuropathic Pain

Neuropathic pain is associated with nerve injury caused by trauma, infection, or chronic diseases such as uncontrolled diabetes. It is often treated with different drugs than are used to treat pain of nociceptive origin. Neuropathic pain is unique because pain sensations can be felt even after the injury is healed. When nerves are damaged, the body may make adaptations to compensate for the nerve damage. Nerve damage can result in a reorganization of nerves. The rewiring sometimes goes haywire, causing painful sensations even after limbs have been amputated. The threshold for neuron firing (action potential) can increase the response to stimuli. Changes in the sodium and calcium ion channels may increase or decrease levels of ions involved in neuronal firing. Adaptive changes can lead to persistent nerve pain. Nerve injuries can also cause a loss of inhibitory pathways such as the γ-aminobutyric acid (GABA) pathways (described in Chapter 8).

Drugs used in the treatment of neuropathic pain include antidepressants (amitriptyline, duloxetine), antiseizure drugs (gabapentin, lamotrigine), local anesthetics (lidocaine, mexiletine), and capsaicin. The tricyclic antidepressants are often used as first-line agents for the treatment of neuropathic pain. They inhibit the reuptake of neurotransmitters (e.g., norepinephrine and 5-HT) at receptor sites in the spinal cord that are responsible for modulating pain sensation. Duloxetine is a 5-HT–noradrenaline reuptake inhibitor that has been shown to be effective in reducing pain caused by **fibromyalgia** and diabetic neuropathy. There is little evidence to support the use of selective 5-HT reuptake inhibitors for the management of neuropathic pain.

Gabapentin, pregabalin, and carbamazepine are antiseizure drugs that are used for the treatment of diabetic neuropathy, nerve pain caused by herpes virus infection, and trigeminal neuralgia. Topiramate enhances inhibitory effects of GABA in addition to its action on voltage-dependent sodium channels. These drugs are discussed in detail in Chapter 9.

Lidocaine is a local anesthetic used in the treatment of neuropathic pain. Lidocaine blocks sodium channels and may be administered intravenously or topically. Lidocaine patches are indicated for the treatment of nerve pain caused by herpes infection (shingles). Capsaicin is derived from chili peppers. It is applied topically, and it depletes substance P from nerve terminals. It is indicated for the treatment of diabetic neuropathy and shingles.

> ● **Tech Note!**
>
> Pregabalin (Lyrica) is a class V (C-V) controlled substance.

Nondrug Treatment of Pain

The treatment of pain, especially chronic pain, requires a multimodal approach that includes drug therapy and nondrug therapy. Nondrug therapies that may be supportive are education, physical therapy, occupational therapy, **biofeedback**, cognitive behavioral therapy (counseling), **acupuncture**, chiropractic medicine, and transcutaneous electrical stimulation (TENS) (Fig. 10.3). The TENS device delivers electrical impulses through the skin that cause contraction and numbness. This blocks the transmission of pain messages to the spinal cord by peripheral nerves. Cryotherapy (cold packs) and heat packs can reduce swelling, which can also decrease pain.

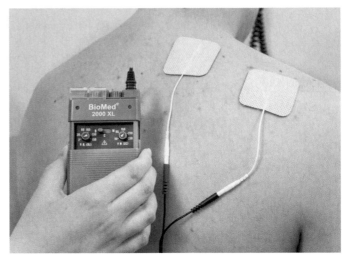

● **Fig. 10.3** Transcutaneous nerve stimulation unit. (From Proctor D, Niedzwiecki B, et al. *Kinn's the medical assistant*, ed 13, St Louis, 2017, Elsevier.)

Commonly Used to Treat Neuropathic Pain

	Generic Name	Brand Name	Usual Adult Dose	Side Effects	Warning Labels
Antidepressants					
	amitriptyline	Generics	25–100 mg at bedtime	Sedation, dry mouth, urinary retention, nausea, blurred vision, photosensitivity	MAY CAUSE DROWSINESS; ALCOHOL MAY INTENSIFY THIS EFFECT. MAY IMPAIR ABILITY TO DRIVE. DO NOT DISCONTINUE WITHOUT MEDICAL SUPERVISION. MAY DISCOLOR URINE (BLUE-GREEN). AVOID PROLONGED EXPOSURE TO SUNLIGHT.
	desipramine	Norpramin	25–150 mg/day in 1–2 doses		
	imipramine	Tofranil	25–150 mg daily in 1–2 divided doses		
Antiseizure Drugs					
	gabapentin	Neurontin Gralise	1200–3600 mg in 3 divided doses	Dizziness, confusion, fatigue, ataxia and nausea, double vision, blurred vision, dry mouth, and constipation	MAY CAUSE DROWSINESS; MAY IMPAIR ABILITY TO DRIVE. AVOID ALCOHOL. TAKE WITH FOOD. DO NOT DISCONTINUE WITHOUT MEDICAL SUPERVISION. SHAKE WELL. SWALLOW WHOLE; DO NOT CRUSH OR CHEW— controlled release. AVOID ANTACIDS WITHIN 2 HOURS OF DOSE— gabapentin, phenytoin. AVOID PREGNANCY— phenytoin.
	pregabalin	Lyrica, Lyrica CR	50–100 mg 3 times a day Extended release: initial, 165 mg orally once daily after an evening meal; increase to 330 mg once daily within 1 week		
	carbamazepine	Tegretol	400–800 mg twice a day (maximum 1200 mg/day)	Nausea, vomiting, sedation, dizziness, ataxia, bruising, jaundice, and visual disturbances	

Commonly Used to Treat Neuropathic Pain—cont'd

	Generic Name	Brand Name	Usual Adult Dose	Side Effects	Warning Labels
Topicals					
	lidocaine	Lidoderm	1–3 patches up to 12 h/day	Numbness, local irritation	ROTATE SITE OF APPLICATION—Lidoderm, Qutenza.
	capsaicin	Zostrix, Qutenza	**Cream**: Apply 3–4 times a day **Patch (Qutenza)**: 1–4 patches once every 3 months	Burning, stinging	WASH HANDS AFTER USE—capsaicin. REMOVE PATCH AFTER 60 MINUTES.

^aNot FDA approved.

Headache

International Headache Society (IHS) classifications for primary headaches include migraine headache, tension-type headache, cluster headache, and trigeminal *cephalgia*. Tension headache is the most common of the primary headaches. It produces bilateral pain, affecting both sides of the head, is mild to moderate in intensity, and is described as having a pressing or tightening quality. Left untreated, tension headaches may last for 30 minutes to up to 7 days. A *cluster headache* is a frequently reoccurring headache that produces severe pain on one side of the head. Cluster headaches may last 15 to 90 minutes and occur more frequently in men.

Migraine Headache

Migraine headaches disproportionately affect women. According to the CDC, approximately 20% of women and 10% of men in 2018 reported having a severe headache or migraine in the past 3 months. Women were twice as likely to experience migraine headache in all age groups in the United States. Up to 24% of Canadians will experience a migraine headache in their lifetime. Migraine headaches occur infrequently in children younger than 10 years of age; the onset is typically between 10 and 29 years old. The prevalence is greatest between 18 and 44 years old and tapers after 60 years old. The probability of developing migraines may be as high as 70% if both parents get migraine headaches.

Once thought to be a vascular headache, it is now believed that migraine pain occurs as a result of biochemical and hormonal changes involving serotonergic and adrenergic pain modulating systems. 5-HT is most commonly implicated; however, prostaglandins, catecholamines, histamine, substance P, and neuroexcitatory amino acids are also thought to play a role.

Migraine headaches are typically unilateral, affecting only one side of the head; however, the headache can spread to the opposite side. IHS classifications include migraine with aura, migraine without aura, menstrual migraine, and chronic migraine. Chronic migraine can occur from overuse of medicines used in the treatment of migraines. An aura is an unusual sensation that is experienced just before the onset of the migraine headache. An aura may present as a temporary flashing light, blind spots, double vision, a smell, paresthesia, weakness, or aphagia (loss of language).

Severe throbbing pain, nausea, photophobia (eyes are sensitive to the light), and phonophobia (sensitivity to noise) are characteristic symptoms of migraine headaches. Resting in a quiet area with the lights off can sometimes improve migraine symptoms. Physical activity worsens migraine symptoms. Acute migraine attacks can last between 4 and 72 hours; the average is 29 hours.

Pathophysiology of Migraine Headaches

Migraine headaches are triggered by numerous events, including stress, insufficient sleep, red wine, caffeine, strong odors, smoke, changes in the weather, physical exhaustion, menstruation, hormonal changes, and exposure to bright or flashing lights. The trigger sets off a series of events that starts with the release of vasoactive neuropeptides that cause blood vessels in the brain to first constrict and then dilate. The trigger produces vasospasms, which reduce blood flow to the brain. Platelets in the blood clump together and cause the release of 5-HT, which further constricts blood vessels. This triggers afferent signals via the trigeminal nerve to release prostaglandins and other neurochemicals that dilate blood vessels, produce inflammation, and stimulate nociceptors. This causes the throbbing head pain characteristic of migraine headaches.

Drug Treatment for Migraine Headache

Treatment of migraines is aimed at stopping the current migraine attack (abortive therapy) and preventing future migraines. Simple analgesics, combination analgesics, 5-HT agonists (including ditans), ergot alkaloids, antidepressants (tricyclic antidepressants, selective 5-HT reuptake inhibitors, and monoamine oxidase inhibitors), calcitonin gene-related peptide antagonists, β-blockers, and antiseizure drugs are used in the treatment and/or prevention of migraine headaches. The overall goal of therapy is to treat attacks rapidly and consistently with minimal adverse effects; decrease the frequency, intensity, and duration of headaches; restore the patient's ability to function; and minimize the use of rescue and backup medications (Table 10.2).

> **● Tech Note!**
>
> *Triptan* is a common ending for drugs used in the treatment of migraine headaches.

TABLE 10.2	Quality of Evidence for Drugs Used in the Acute Treatment of Migraine Headache[a,b]		
Drug Category	Drug	Established Efficacy	Probably Effective
Simple analgesics	aspirin	A	
	celecoxib	A	
	diclofenac	A	
	ibuprofen	A	
	naproxen Na[+]	A	
Combination analgesics	aspirin + acetaminophen + caffeine	A	
	aspirin + butalbital + caffeine		X
Ergotamine and ergotamine combinations	Ergotamine		X
	ergotamine + caffeine		X
	dihydroergotamine nasal spray	A	
	dihydroergotamine subcut, IM, IV		X
Triptans	almotriptan, eletriptan, frovatriptan, naratriptan, rizatriptan, sumatriptan, zolmitriptan	A	
GCRP blockers	rimegepant, ubrogepant	A	
Ditans	lasmitidtan	A	
Opioid analgesics	butorphanol nasal spray codeine + acetaminophen	A	

[a]US Headache Consortium (nd) and American Headache Society Consensus Statement 2021.
[b]Quality of the evidence (A, multiple well-designed randomized, clinical trials directly relevant to the recommendation.

Treatment of Acute Migraine Headache

Simple Analgesics and Combination Analgesics

Simple analgesics (aspirin, acetaminophen, ibuprofen, and naproxen) are often effective in stopping mild to moderate migraine headaches if taken early and in high doses. The effective dose of aspirin or acetaminophen used to treat migraine headaches (up to 1000 mg per dose) is higher than the usual dose recommended for the treatment of mild to moderate tension headaches (325 to 650 mg per dose). Codeine, caffeine, and butalbital may be added to aspirin and acetaminophen to form combination analgesics. Simple analgesics and combined analgesics (aspirin and NSAIDs) reduce pain and decrease inflammation associated with migraine headaches.

Triptans

The triptans are the most widely prescribed drugs for the treatment of migraine headaches. They are administered during an acute attack to lessen symptoms and to stop the headache from progressing to more severe migraine symptoms. They are administered at the first sign of an impending migraine (aura).

> **⊘ Tech Alert!**
> The following drugs have look-alike/sound-alike issues:
> SUMAtriptan and ZOLMitriptan

Mechanism of Action

The triptans are selective 5-HT receptor agonists. They have a high affinity for 5-HT_{1B} and 5-HT_{1D} receptors, which stimulate vasoconstriction (Fig. 10.4).

Pharmacokinetics

The triptans are available for administration via mouth, in the nose, and by injection. Subcutaneous injection produces the most rapid response and is the most effective route of administration; however, intranasal administration is also rapid and has fewer adverse reactions. Oral formulations have slower onsets of action. The half-life of the triptans ranges between 2 hours and 25 hours. Triptans that have a long half-life, such as frovatriptan (24 hours) and naratriptan (8 hours), are more effective in reducing headache reoccurrence.

Adverse Reactions

The vasoconstriction caused by triptans is responsible for their therapeutic effects but can result in serious cardiac side effects, including arrhythmia, angina, coronary vasospasm, and myocardial infarction (heart attack). Vasoconstriction can also cause high blood pressure and stroke. Less serious and more common side effects are pain, tightness, and burning at the site of injection; dizziness; nausea; hot flashes; dry mouth; and fatigue.

Precautions

Overuse of triptans should be avoided. Nearly all triptans are restricted to two doses per 24 hours. Frovatriptan is restricted to three doses per 24 hours. The safety of treating more than four migraines per month has not been established for most of the triptans.

> **⊘ Tech Note!**
> Maxalt-MLT contains phenylalanine.

> **⊘ Tech Note!**
> Review sumatriptan nasal directions carefully—only one spray in one nostril is indicated.

Miscellaneous

Several new agents have been approved since 2018 for the treatment of acute migraines. They work by varied mechanisms of action to effect calcium gene receptor peptide release or binding.

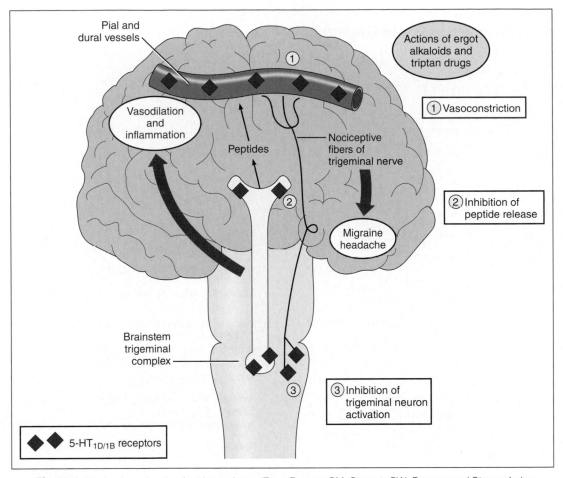

• **Fig. 10.4** Mechanism of action for triptan drugs. (From Brenner GM, Stevens CW. *Brenner and Stevens' pharmacology*, ed 5, Philadelphia, 2018, Elsevier.)

Comparison of Triptans

Generic Name (Brand Name)	Onset (min)	Repeat Time (h)	Route	Headache[a] Effectiveness (%)	Dose (mg)[b]
almotriptan (generic)	30	2	PO, tablet	57–68	25
eletriptan (Relpax)	30	2	PO, tablet	54–65	40
				68–77	80
frovatriptan (Frova)	30	2	PO, tablet	40	2.5
naratriptan (Amerge)	30	4	PO, tablet	48	2.5
rizatriptan (Maxalt, Maxalt-MLT)	30	2	PO, tablet	73	10
		2	Wafer		
sumatriptan (Imitrex)	10–15	1	Subcut	80–85	6
	15	2	Nasal	60–86	20
	30	2	PO, tablet	51–61	50
zolmitriptan (Zomig)	30	2	PO, tablet	59–69	2.5
		2	Wafer		
	10–15		Nasal	24–61	5

[a]Percentage of patients reporting pain relief at 2 hours after dosing.
[b]Dose associated with headache effectiveness (%).

Triptans Dosage Forms and Strength

Generic Name	US Brand Name(s) / Canadian Brand(s)	Dosage Forms and Strengths
almotriptan[a]	Generics	**Tablets:** 6.25 mg, 12.5 mg
	Generics	
eletriptan[a]	Relpax	**Tablets:** 20 mg, 40 mg
	Relpax	
frovatriptan[a]	Frova	**Tablets:** 2.5 mg
	Frova	
naratriptan[a]	Amerge	**Tablets:** 1 mg, 2.5 mg
	Amerge	
rizatriptan[a]	Maxalt, Maxalt-MLT	**Tablets (Maxalt):** 5 mg, 10 mg **Tablets, disintegrating (Maxalt-MLT, Maxalt-RPD):** 5 mg, 10 mg
	Maxalt, Maxalt-RPD	
sumatriptan[a]	Imitrex, Onzetra Xsail, Tosymra, Zembrace Symtouch	**Injection, as solution (Imitrex, Zembrace):** 3 mg/0.5 mL[b], 4 mg/0.5 mL[b], 6 mg/0.5 mL **Intranasal solution:** 5 mg, 20 mg/spray (Imitrex); 10 mg/spray (Tosymra) **Powder, for nasal inhalation (Onzetra Xsail)[b]:** 11 mg **Tablets:** 25 mg, 50 mg, 100 mg
	Imitrex	
zolmitriptan[a]	Zomig, Zomig-ZMT	**Nasal solution:** 2.5 mg/spray, 5 mg/spray **Tablets:** 2.5 mg, 5 mg[b] **Tablets, disintegrating (Zomig-ZMT, Zomig-Rapimelt):** 2.5 mg, 5 mg[b]
	Zomig, Zomig-Rapimelt	
sumatriptan + naproxen Na⁺[a]	Treximet	**Tablets:** 500 mg naproxen Na⁺ + 85 mg sumatriptan
	Suvexx	

[a]Generic available.
[b]Available in the United States only.

Lasmiditan is classified as a "ditan." Ditans bind to serotonin (5-HT) receptors like triptans. They differ from the triptans because they selectively bind to the 5-HT$_F$ receptor. Binding inhibits the release of calcitonin gene-related peptide (CGRP). In contrast, rimegepant and ubrogepant bind to the CGRP receptor (where they act as an antagonist). The CGRP antagonists (rimegepant and ubrogepant) are metabolized in the liver and then eliminated. Therefore drugs that reduce metabolism or speed up metabolism interact with CGRP antagonists. Coadministration with the CYP3A4 inhibitors ketoconazole, itraconazole, and clarithromycin is contraindicated because of their effect on increasing exposure of ubrogepant and rimegepant. The drugs are also highly protein bound, therefore are subject to drug interactions that affect protein binding. The absorption of ubrogepant and rimegepant is delayed when taken with a high-fat meal.

● *Tech Note!*
Ubrogepant should not be taken with grapefruit juice.

● *Tech Note!*
Protect Emgality from direct sunlight. Apply the warning label STORE IN THE REFRIGERATOR; DO NOT FREEZE when Emgality is dispensed.

Miscellaneous Antimigraine Agents

Generic Name	US Brand Name(s) / Canadian Brand(s)	Dosage Forms and Strengths
lasmiditan	Reyvow	**Tablets:** 50 mg, 100 mg, 200 mg
	Not available	
rimegepant	Nurtec ODT	**Tablets, oral disintegrating:** 75 mg
	Not available	
ubrogepant	Ubrelvy	**Tablet:** 50 mg, 100 mg
	Not available	

Adverse Reactions

The most common adverse reactions reported with lasmiditan and ubrogepant are drowsiness or dizziness. Nausea is a common side effect of rimegepant and ubrogepant. Ubrogepant can also produce dry mouth.

Other Acute Treatments for Acute Migraine Headaches
Ergot alkaloids and 5-HT agonists are also prescribed as migraine abortive therapy. Information about these agents is found in

Summary of Drugs Used in the Treatment of Acute Migraine Headaches

Generic Name	US Brand Name	Usual Adult Oral Dose and Dosing Schedule	Warning Labels
Triptans			
almotriptan	Generics	**Oral:** 6.25–12.5 mg as a single dose; repeat dose in 2 h if needed (maximum, 25 mg in 24 h)	DO NOT EXCEED RECOMMENDED DOSAGE. IF NO IMPROVEMENT AFTER FIRST DOSE, DO NOT TAKE A SECOND DOSE.
eletriptan	Relpax	**Oral:** 20–40 mg as a single dose; repeat dose in 2 h if needed (maximum, 80 mg in 24 h)	
frovatriptan	Frova	**Oral:** 2.5 mg as a single dose; repeat dose in 2 h if needed (maximum, 7.5 mg in 24 h)	
naratriptan	Amerge	**Oral:** 1–2.5 mg as a single dose; repeat dose in 4 h if needed (maximum, 5 mg in 24 h)	
rizatriptan	Maxalt	**Oral:** 5–10 mg as a single dose; repeat dose in 2 h if needed (maximum, 30 mg [15 mg if also receiving propranolol] in 24 h)	
sumatriptan	Imitrex	**Oral:** 25 mg, 50 mg, or 100 mg as a single dose; repeat dose in 2 h if needed (maximum, 200 mg in 24 h) **Nasal powder:** Inhale 22 mg (2 nose pieces) in one nostril; repeat dose in 2 h if needed (maximum, 44 mg in 24 h) **Nasal spray:** 1–2 sprays (5 mg, 10 mg), or 1 spray (20 mg) in one nostril; repeat dose in 2 h if needed (maximum, 40 mg in 24 h) **Subcut injection:** 6 mg as a single injection; repeat dose in 1 h if needed	DO NOT INJECT MORE THAN 2 DOSES (6 MG) IN 24 HOURS. USE SPRAY IN ONE NOSTRIL ONLY. IF NO IMPROVEMENT AFTER FIRST DOSE, DO NOT TAKE A SECOND DOSE.
zolmitriptan	Zomig	**Oral:** 2.5–5 mg as a single dose; repeat dose in 2 h if needed (maximum, 10 mg in 24 h) **Nasal solution:** 1 spray as a single dose; repeat dose in 2 h if needed	IF NO IMPROVEMENT AFTER FIRST DOSE, DO NOT TAKE A SECOND DOSE.
sumatriptan + naproxen sodium	Treximet	Take 1 tablet for migraine; may repeat dose in 2 h if needed	DO NOT EXCEED 2 DOSES PER 24 HOURS. MAY CAUSE DIZZINESS OR DROWSINESS. SWALLOW WHOLE; DO NOT CUT, CRUSH, OR CHEW. TAKE WITH A FULL GLASS OF WATER.
Ditans			
lasmiditan	Reyvow	Take 1 tablet if needed for migraine; no more than 1 dose per 24 h	MAY CAUSE DIZZINESS OR DROWSINESS. AVOID ALCOHOL.
GCRP blockers			
rimegepant	Nurtec-ODT	Dissolve 1 tablet on the tongue if needed for migraine; maximum 75 mg/day or 15 migraines per 30 days	IF NO IMPROVEMENT AFTER FIRST DOSE, DO NOT TAKE A SECOND DOSE. DO NOT OPEN FOIL PACK UNTIL READY TO USE. PROTECT FROM SUNLIGHT.
ubrogepant	Ubrelvy	50–100 mg at onset of migraine; may take a second dose after 2 h; max 200 mg in 24 h	AVOID GRAPEFRUIT JUICE.

the **Summary of Nontriptan Drugs Used to Treat Migraine Headaches** table.

Migraine Preventive Agents

Migraine preventive therapy is offered to persons who use abortive medication more than twice per week or when acute-acting agents are contraindicated or have failed to relieve the headache. They are also offered to people who experience six or more migraine headaches per month. They may be offered to people experiencing only three to four migraines if the migraine produces moderate to severe impairment (requires bed rest). Beta blockers (see Chapter 22), tricyclic antidepressants (see Chapter 6), onabotulinumtoxinA (a neuromuscular blocker), neuromuscular blocking agents (see Chapter 13), and antiseizure drugs (see Chapter 9) are all prescribed for prophylaxis (prevention) of migraine headaches. Galcanezumab-GNLM (Emgality) is a humanized monoclonal antibody. When it binds to CGRP ligand, binding to the CGRP receptor is blocked. Emgality is used to prevent migraine headaches. It is injected subcutaneously once monthly.

Summary of Nontriptan Drugs Used to Treat Migraine Headaches

Generic Name	Brand Name	Usual Adult Dose	Side Effects	Warning Labels
dihydroergotamine mesylate	D.H.E. 45	1 mg IM, IV, or SC; repeat in 1 h if needed (maximum, 6 mg/week)	Numbness	DO NOT EXCEED RECOMMENDED DOSAGE.
	Migranal	1 spray in each nostril; repeat after 15 min if needed (maximum, 8 sprays/week)		DO NOT ASSEMBLE SPRAYER UNTIL READY TO USE.
	Trudhesa	1 spray (0.725 mg) in each nostril; may repeat dose in 1 h if needed (maximum, 2 doses/24 h)	Runny nose, drowsiness, nausea, irritated throat	STORE AT ROOM TEMPERATURE; DISCARD OPEN CONTAINERS AFTER 8 HOURS.
ergotamine tartrate	Ergomar	2 mg every 30 min until relief (maximum, 6 mg/day or 10 mg/week)	Nausea, vomiting, numbness, chest pain, abdominal pain	DO NOT EXCEED RECOMMENDED DOSAGE.
butorphanol	Generics	1 spray in one nostril; may repeat in 60–90 min if needed (maximum, 4 doses/day)	Drowsiness, dizziness, nausea, constipation, dry mouth	MAY CAUSE DROWSINESS; MAY IMPAIR ABILITY TO DRIVE. AVOID ALCOHOL.
codeine 30 mg + acetaminophen	Tylenol #3	1–2 tablets every 4 h (maximum, 4 g daily)	Drowsiness, dizziness, nausea, constipation	TAKE WITH FOOD. MAY BE HABIT FORMING.

IM, intramuscularly; *IV*, intravenously; *SC*, subcutaneously.

Drugs Used for the Prevention of Migraine Headaches

Generic Name	US Brand Name(s) / Canadian Brand(s)	Dosage Forms and Strengths
β-Blockers		
propranolol[a]	Inderal LA	**Tablets:** 10 mg, 20 mg, 40 mg, 60 mg, 80 mg
	Generics	**Tablets, extended release (Inderal LA):** 60 mg, 80 mg, 120 mg, 160 mg
Antiepileptic Drugs		
divalproex sodium	Depakote	**Tablets:** 250 mg, 500 mg
	Epival	
topiramate	Topamax, Qudexy XR, Trokendi XR	**Capsule (Topamax):** 15 mg, 25 mg
	Topamax	**Capsule, extended release (Qudexy XR, Trokendi XR):** 25 mg, 50 mg, 100 mg, 150 mg, 200 mg
		Solution, oral (Eprontia): 25 mg/mL
		Tablets (Topamax): 25 mg, 50 mg, 100 mg, 200 mg, 300 mg, 400 mg
Tricyclic Antidepressants		
amitriptyline	Generics	**Tablets:** 10 mg, 25 mg, 50 mg, 75 mg, 100 mg, 150 mg[b]
	Elavil	
Neuromuscular Blockers		
onabotulinumtoxinA	Botox	**Powder for injection:** 50 units[b], 100 units, 200 units[b]
	Botox	

Drugs Used for the Prevention of Migraine Headaches—cont'd

Generic Name	US Brand Name(s) / Canadian Brand(s)	Dosage Forms and Strengths
Monoclonal Antibody		
galcanezumab-GNLM	Emgality / Emgality	**Solution, for SC injection:** 100 mg/mLª, 120 mg/mL prefilled syringes
Miscellaneous		
flunarizine	Not Available / Generics	**Capsule:** 5 mg

ªGeneric available.
ᵇStrength available in the United States only.
SC, subcutaneously.

Summary of Drugs Used for the Prevention of Migraine Headaches

	Generic Name	Brand Name	Usual Adult Dose	Side Effects	Warning Labels
β-Blockers	propranolol	Inderal, Inderal-LA	80–240 mg/day every 6–8 h or 80–240 mg/day (long acting)	Hypotension, lethargy	MAY CAUSE DIZZINESS OR DROWSINESS AND IMPAIR ABILITY TO DRIVE.
Antiepileptic Drugs	topiramate	Topamax, Qudexy XR, Trokendi XR	100 mg/day in 1–2 divided doses		MAY CAUSE DROWSINESS AND IMPAIR ABILITY TO DRIVE. AVOID ALCOHOL. TAKE WITH FOOD.
	divalproex Na⁺	Depakote	250 mg twice daily up to 1000 mg/day	Sedation, nausea, ataxia, and liver dysfunction	
Tricyclic Antidepressants	amitriptyline	generics, Elavil	10–150 mg/day (start at 25 mg/day, increase by 25 mg/week)		MAY CAUSE DROWSINESS AND IMPAIR ABILITY TO DRIVE. AVOID ALCOHOL. TAKE WITH FOOD.
Neuromuscular Blockers	onabotulinumtoxinA	Botox	155 Units administered IM as 5 Units/injection divided across 31 injection sites within 7 specific head and neck muscle areas	Neck pain, stiffness, myasthenia, myalgia, muscle pain, pain at injection site, botulism, blpharedema	
Monoclonal Antibody	galcanezumab-GNLM	Emgality	Inject 240 mg (two 120 mg doses) SC as a loading dose followed by monthly 120 mg doses	Irritation at the injection site	REFRIGERATE; DO NOT FREEZE; PROTECT FROM SUNLIGHT.
Miscellaneous	flunarizine	Generics	10 mg at bedtime		MAY CAUSE DROWSINESS.

IM, intramuscularly; *SC*, subcutaneously.

Key Points

- Acute pain may be triggered by an injury, burn, infection, or some other stimuli and be self-limiting.
- Chronic pain may persist for years and is often inadequately controlled by pharmaceuticals.
- Psychological factors can influence a person's tolerance for pain and can determine whether the outcome of treatment is successful.
- Patient-controlled analgesia (PCA) permits patients to control the frequency of administration of their dose of pain medications.
- Neuropathic pain is associated with nerve injury caused by trauma, infection, or chronic diseases such as uncontrolled diabetes and is often treated with different drugs than other types of pain.
- Osteoarthritis, gout, burns, trauma, and low back pain are examples of pain with a nociceptor origin.
- Painful stimuli trigger the release of neurotransmitters, amino acids, and peptides that carry signals to increase sensitivity to the pain or to dull the painful sensations.
- Histamine, bradykinins, serotonin, prostaglandins, glutamate, and substance P are involved in the transmission of signals for pain sensation and pain perception.
- Endorphins, enkephalin, and dynorphin are the body's natural painkillers and bind to opioid receptors.
- Opioids are naturally occurring or synthetically derived drugs that act like morphine and are used to treat pain.
- Opioid receptors are mu (μ), kappa (κ), and delta (δ), and stimulation produces analgesia. The euphoria, dysphoria, respiratory depression, pupillary constriction, decreased GI motility, and physical dependence associated with opioid use are linked to specific receptors.
- Opioid agonists activate μ, κ, or δ receptors.
- Antagonists bind to the opioid receptor but do not activate it.
- Mixed agonist/antagonists behave like an agonist when the patient has had no recent exposure to an opioid agonist (opiate naïve).
- Equianalgesic doses of opioids produce equivalent pain relief regardless of dosage form.
- Opioid agonists, partial agonists, and most mixed agonist/antagonists are restricted substances because they produce tolerance and dependence.
- Opioid antagonists and some mixed agonist/antagonists are used to treat opioid use disorder and opioid-induced respiratory depression.

- Nonsteroidal antiinflammatory drugs (NSAIDs), acetaminophen, and aspirin are widely used in the treatment of pain with or without inflammation.
- NSAIDs and aspirin have analgesic, antiinflammatory, and antipyretic properties.
- Acetaminophen does not reduce inflammation.
- Aspirin and NSAIDs decrease prostaglandin synthesis by inhibiting the action of cyclooxygenase (COX), an enzyme involved in the biosynthesis of prostaglandins. Prostaglandins are important mediators of pain.
- NSAIDs and aspirin can produce nausea, GI bleeding, and GI ulceration.
- Enteric-coated aspirin is released in the pH of the intestine rather than in the stomach.
- Migraine headaches are triggered by numerous events, including stress, consumption of certain foods, red wine, caffeinated beverages, and exposure to bright or flashing lights.
- During a migraine, blood vessels in the brain dilate, produce inflammation, and stimulate nociceptors, causing the throbbing head pain characteristic of migraine headaches.
- Treatment of migraines is aimed at stopping the current migraine attack and preventing future migraines.
- Simple and combined analgesics, serotonin agonists (including ditans), calcitonin gene-related peptide (CGRP) antagonists, and ergot alkaloids are used in the treatment of acute migraine headaches.
- Galcanezumab-GNLM (Emgality), tricyclic antidepressants, selective serotonin reuptake inhibitors, monoamine oxidase inhibitors, β-blockers, neuromuscular blocking agents, and antiseizure drugs can be used in the prevention of migraine headaches.
- Triptans are selective serotonin receptor agonists and are the most widely prescribed drugs for the treatment of acute migraine headaches.
- Triptans that have long half-lives, frovatriptan and naratriptan, are more effective in preventing headache reoccurrence.
- The use of triptans is restricted to a maximum of two or three doses per 24 hours. The safety of treating more than four migraines per month has not been established for most of the triptans.
- The vasoconstriction caused by triptans is partially responsible for their therapeutic effects but can result in serious effects, including arrhythmia, angina, myocardial infarction, and stroke.

Review Questions

1. _____ pain may be triggered by an injury, burn, infection, or some other stimuli and be self-limiting.
   a. Chronic
   b. Dull
   c. Acute
   d. Nerve

2. The most common of all arthritic conditions is _____.
   a. gout
   b. osteoarthritis
   c. rheumatoid arthritis
   d. ankylosis

3. _____ are hormones that trigger pain response from peripheral nociceptors.
   a. Histamines
   b. Serotonins
   c. Prostaglandins
   d. Norepinephrines

4. Select the drug that is NOT an opioid analgesic.
   a. naloxone
   b. codeine
   c. fentanyl
   d. morphine

5. What US controlled substance schedule does oxycodone fall into?
   a. C-II
   b. C-III
   c. C-IV
   d. C-V

6. Naloxone (Narcan), which is indicated for reversal of respiratory depression caused by opioid use and opioid overdose, is an example of an
   a. agonist
   b. antagonist

7. NSAIDs have analgesic, antiinflammatory, and antipyretic properties.
   a. true
   b. false

8. Select the drug that is used for migraine prevention.
   a. Sumatriptan (Imitrex®)
   b. Lasmiditan (Reyvow®)
   c. Ubrogepant (Ubrelvy®)
   d. galcanezumab-GNLM (Emgality®)

9. Migraine headaches are triggered by numerous events, including _____.
   a. stress or consumption of certain foods
   b. red wine or caffeinated beverages
   c. exposure to bright or flashing lights
   d. all of the above

10. _____ are the most widely prescribed drugs for the treatment of migraine headaches.
    a. Ergot alkaloids
    b. Antiseizures
    c. Antidepressants
    d. Triptans

Bibliography

Adelman J, Lewit E. Comparative aspects of triptans in treating migraine. *Clin Cornerstone*. 2001;4:1–19.

Ailani J, Burch RC, Robbins MS. The Board of Directors of the American Headache Society: The American Headache Society Consensus Statement: Update on integrating new migraine treatments into clinical practice. *Headache*. 2021;61:1021–1039.

Bennett M, Smith S, Torrance N, et al. Can pain be more or less neuropathic? Comparison of symptom assessment tools with ratings of certainty by clinicians, International Association for the Study of Pain. *Pain*. 2006;122:289–294.

DeMaagd G. The pharmacological management of migraine, part 1 overview and abortive therapy. *P T*. 2008;33(7).

Gawel M, Aschoff J, May A, et al. Zolmitriptan 5 mg nasal spray: efficacy and onset of action in the acute treatment of migraine—Results from Phase I of the REALIZE study. *Headache*. 2005:7–16.

Government of Canada. (2022). Opioid- and Stimulant-related Harms in Canada—Public

Health Infobase. Public Health Agency of Canada. Retrieved August 12, 2022, from https://health-infobase.canada.ca/substance-related-harms/opioids-stimulants/.

Health Canada. (2022). Drug Product Database. Retrieved July 20, 2022, from https://health-products.canada.ca/dpd-bdpp/index-eng.jsp.

Institute for Safe Medication Practices. (2016). FDA and ISMP Lists of Look-Alike Drug Names with Recommended Tall Man Letters. Retrieved July 20, 2022, from https://www.ismp.org/recommendations/tall-man-letters-list.

Institute for Safe Medication Practices. (2019). List of Confused Drugs. Retrieved July 20, 2022, from https://www.ismp.org/tools/confused-drugnames.pdf.

Kalant H, Grant D, Mitchell J. *Principles of medical pharmacology*, ed 7, Toronto, Elsevier Canada, A Division of Reed Elsevier Canada, pp 236–251.

Kampman K, Jarvis M. National practice guideline for the use of medications in the treatment of addiction involving opioid use: American Society of Addiction Medicine. *J Addict Med*. 2015;9(5):358–367.

Kelmann L. *Pain characteristics of acute migraine attack, headache*. Ames, IA: Blackwell Publishing; 2006.

Kidd B. Osteoarthritis and joint pain: topical review, International Association for the Study of Pain. *Pain*. 2006;123:6–9.

Lipton RB, Bigal ME, Diamond M, et al. Migraine prevalence, disease burden, and the need for preventive therapy. *Neurology*. 2007;68:343–349.

Macfarlane G, Jones G, Hannaford P. Managing low back pain presenting in primary care: where do we go from here? International Association for the Study of Pain. *Pain*. 2006;122:219–222.

Marcus D. Treatment of nonmalignant chronic pain. *Am Fam Physician*. 2000;61:1–8.

National Institute of Neurological Disorders and Stroke. (2014). *Chronic pain: Hope through research*, Bethesda, MD, NINDS, National Institutes of Health, U.S. Department of Health and Human Services, NIH Publication No. 14-2406.

Page C, Curtis M, Sutter M, et al. *Integrated pharmacology*. Philadelphia: Elsevier Mosby; 2005:272–274.

Raffa RB, Rawls SM, Beyzarov EP. *Netter's illustrated pharmacology*. Philadelphia: Saunders; 2005:85.

QuickStats: Percentage of adults who had a severe headache or migraine in the past 3 months, by sex and age group—National Health Interview Survey, United States, 2018. *MMWR Morb Mortal Wkly Rep*. 2020;69:359.

Silberstein SD, Holland S, Freitag F, et al. Evidence-based guideline update: pharmacologic treatment for episodic migraine prevention in adults: report of the Quality Standards Subcommittee of the American Academy of Neurology and the American Headache Society. *Neurology*. 2012;78:1337–1345.

Sun-Edelstein C, Rapoport AM. Update on the pharmacological treatment of chronic migraine. *Curr Pain Headache Rep*. 2016;20(6).

Teng J, Mekhail N. Neuropathic pain: mechanisms and treatment options, World Institute of Pain. *Pain Pract*. 2003;3:8–21.

U.S. Food and Drug Administration. (nd). Drugs@FDA: FDA Approved Drug Products. Retrieved July 20, 2022, from https://www.accessdata.fda.gov/scripts/cder/daf/index.cfm.

Wootton RJ, Kissoon NR. (2021). *Patient education: migraines in adults (beyond the basics)*. UpToDate. Retrieved August 12, 2022, from https://www.uptodate.com/contents/migraines-in-adults-beyond-the-basics.

Zobeh F, ben Kraiem A, Attwood M, et al. Pharmacological treatment of migraine: Drug classes, mechanisms of action, clinical trials and new treatments. *Br J Pharmacol*. 2021;178:4588–4607.

11

Treatment of Sleep Disorders and Attention-Deficit/Hyperactivity Disorder

LEARNING OBJECTIVES

1. Learn the terminology associated with sleep disorders and attention-deficit/hyperactivity disorder (ADHD).
2. Discuss the reasons why sleep is necessary.
3. Describe the phases of a normal sleep cycle.
4. Describe symptoms associated with sleep deprivation.
5. Describe the types of sleep disorders.
6. Describe the function of neurotransmitters associated with symptoms of sleep.
7. Classify medications used in the treatment of sleep disorders.
8. Describe mechanism of action for each class of drugs used to treat sleep disorders.
9. Identify warning labels and precautionary messages associated with medications used to treat sleep disorders.
10. Describe the etiology of ADHD.
11. Classify medications used in the treatment of ADHD.
12. Describe mechanism of action for each class of drugs used to treat ADHD.
13. Identify warning labels and precautionary messages associated with medications used to treat ADHD.
14. Identify significant drug look-alike and sound-alike issues.

KEY TERMS

Insomnia Condition characterized by difficulty falling asleep, staying asleep, or both.
Melatonin Hormone that is released by the pineal gland that makes a person feel drowsy.
Non-REM sleep Stages 1 through 4 of the sleep cycle.
Rapid eye movement (REM) sleep The stage of sleep when dreaming occurs.
Rebound hypersomnia Condition associated with excessive sleep that follows long-term insomnia or the use of drugs that depress REM and non-REM sleep.

Sedative-hypnotic Drug that causes relaxation and promotes drowsiness.
Sleep apnea A potentially serious sleep disorder in which breathing repeatedly stops and starts.
Stimulant Drug that increases activity in the brain and is used to treat ADHD and narcolepsy.

Overview

Sleep is a necessary biological function for the growth and maintenance of a healthy body. Sleep is needed for a healthy immune system and nervous system. Our physical and mental agility, memory, and emotional and social functioning are also improved when we get sufficient sleep.

The body's sleep cycle is influenced by circadian rhythms. Circadian rhythms are biological changes that occur according to time cycles. The human body operates on a 24-hour clock; however, this clock can be manipulated by external time cues. Sunlight is the primary external time cue. Changes in sunlight and darkness are picked up by the retina in the back of the eye. The retina sends signals to the pineal gland in the brain. The pineal gland controls the release of *melatonin*, a hormone that makes people feel drowsy in addition to regulating body temperature and hormone secretion. The fact that

our normal sleep–wake cycle is linked to sunlight explains why people who work the night shift may feel uncontrollably drowsy in the middle of the night, and it explains why workplace accidents occur more frequently in the middle of the night than during the day.

The amount of time a person needs to sleep ranges between 5 and 16 hours per day. The amount of sleep needed can vary according to age. Infants may sleep up to 16 hours per day, teenagers require as much as 9 hours, and adults need as little as 5 to 8 hours. The patterns of sleep change as people age. Elderly adults often sleep for shorter time spans, sleep more lightly, and dream less than they did as young adults, although their overall sleep requirement may not change.

The normal sleep pattern involves five stages of sleep (Fig. 11.1). In *Stage 1*, the person sleeps lightly and can be awakened easily. Sudden muscle contractions of the limbs may occur, similar to when a person is startled while awake, and the eyes move slowly back and forth. In *Stage 2*, sleep eye movements stop, and

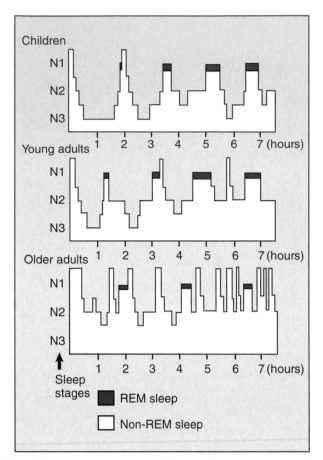

• **Fig. 11.1** Normal sleep cycle. *REM,* Rapid eye movement. (From McCance KL, Huether SE. *Pathophysiology*, ed 7, St Louis, 2014, Elsevier.)

brain activity decreases. *Stage 3* and *Stage 4* sleep are deep sleep. Brain activity slows (delta waves). It is difficult to wake someone from stage 3 or stage 4 sleep; if awakened, the person feels disoriented. *Stage 5* sleep is known as ***rapid eye movement (REM) sleep*** because of the characteristic eye movements that occur. This is the sleep cycle where dreaming occurs, and it lasts between 90 minutes and 110 minutes. REM sleep is crucial to normal emotional and physical functioning. Approximately 2 hours per night is spent in REM sleep. The thalamus and cerebral cortex actively communicate with each other during REM sleep. The cortex is the region of the brain involved in learning and interpretation of information.

Signs of sleep deprivation are a drowsy feeling during the day with or without microsleeps and falling asleep within 5 minutes of lying down. Insufficient sleep can interfere with concentration, affecting work and school. The National Highway Traffic Safety Administration reported that in 2017, nearly 91,000 crashes involved drowsy driving. Government of Canada Motor Vehicle Traffic Statistics (2020) reveal that 2.5% of fatal traffic accidents were attributed to fatigue.

The rate for sleep deprivation–related motor vehicle accidents is similar to driving under the influence of alcohol. Sleep deprivation can also trigger seizures, paranoia, and hallucinations.

Factors that contribute to the inability to get adequate sleep are numerous and include ***sleep apnea***, restless legs syndrome, consumption of caffeinated beverages and foods near bedtime, use of prescription and nonprescription drugs, psychiatric disorders, substance abuse, and chronic illness. Chronic illnesses that can interfere with sleep are gastroesophageal reflux disorder, cardiovascular disease, diabetes, and chronic pain, among others.

Sleep Disorders

Nearly one in three adults in the United States and Canada report that they get insufficient sleep. ***Insomnia*** is a sleep disorder that is categorized according to the length of time the symptoms persist. Acute insomnia typically has a sudden onset and lasts less than 3 months. Patients may have difficulty initiating sleep, maintaining sleep, poor sleep quality, and/or a short duration of sleep. Chronic insomnia lasts longer than 3 months for at least 3 nights per week. It may be associated with a psychiatric or medical condition such as pain.

Restless legs syndrome (RLS) is reported by up to 7% to 10% of the American population. Nearly 80% complain about periodic leg movements during sleep. RLS is more common in elderly adults. Diabetes, pregnancy, and anemia can also cause RLS. Sleep apnea is a sleep disorder that affects up to 26% of people in the United States. Approximately 1 in 4 Canadian adults are at high risk for developing sleep apnea, according to Stats Canada. The condition is associated with an interruption in the supply of oxygen during sleep, which causes the person to awaken. Sleep apnea can increase the risk for cardiovascular disorders such as hypertension, myocardial infarction, and stroke. People with sleep apnea also have an increased risk for arrhythmias, heart failure, diabetes, and obesity. Rarely, sleep apnea is fatal. Sudden death occurs from respiratory arrest during sleep.

Narcolepsy is the least common of the sleep disorders. It affects approximately 1 in 2000 people. It is characterized by falling asleep suddenly and without warning. Attacks may last between a few seconds and 30 minutes. In most cases the cause is unknown; however, some patients with narcolepsy have low levels of the brain chemical that controls wakefulness and arousal (hypocretin). The disorder is not usually hereditary, although it may run in some families.

Treatment of Sleep Disorders

Insomnia

Pharmacologic treatments for insomnia are recommended only for short-term use. Prescription drugs, nonprescription drugs, and natural remedies are commercially available, and all produce drowsiness that enables the person to drift off to sleep (improve sleep latency) and stay asleep (improve sleep maintenance). Prescription drugs that are used to treat insomnia are benzodiazepines, benzodiazepine receptor agonists, melatonin, and orexin receptor antagonists. It is important to note that drugs that promote sleep do not result in a normal pattern of sleep. They alter ***non-REM*** and REM sleep. This can result in ***rebound hypersomnia*** and increased dreaming once the drugs are discontinued. Guidelines recommend prescribing the lowest effective dose and close monitoring of ***sedative-hypnotics*** (drugs that induce relaxation and drowsiness) that are habit forming (e.g., benzodiazepines).

Benzodiazepines and Benzodiazepine Receptor Agonists

Benzodiazepines (e.g., temazepam) and benzodiazepine receptor agonists (e.g., zopiclone, zaleplon, and zolpidem) are prescribed for the short-term treatment of insomnia.

Mechanism of Action and Pharmacokinetics. Benzodiazepines decrease neuronal excitability by opening Cl^- channels. The mechanism of action, pharmacokinetics, and adverse reactions of benzodiazepines were discussed in detail in Chapter 5.

The mechanism of action of benzodiazepine receptor agonists is similar to the benzodiazepines. Zaleplon, zolpidem, eszopiclone, and zopiclone act on benzodiazepine receptors with varying affinity for α-1, α-2, and α-3 subunits. They modulate the GABA-A receptor chloride channel to reduce neuronal excitability. Zolpidem is available as an immediate-release tablet, controlled-release tablet, lingual spray, and sublingual tablet. Peak effects vary according to dosage form administered (≈50 minutes for the oral spray to 90 minutes for the oral tablet). Zolpidem is a biphasic controlled-release formulation. Food reduces absorption, so zolpidem should be taken on an empty stomach.

Adverse Drug Effects. Nearly all of the benzodiazepine and benzodiazepine receptor agonists are controlled substances and can produce tolerance and dependence. Sedation, dizziness, and headache are other side effects common to all. Zaleplon may also produce photosensitivity, and eszopiclone and zopiclone can produce a bitter or metallic taste. Driving, preparing food, and engaging in other activities while asleep, with no recollection of the behaviors, have been reported with zolpidem.

Miscellaneous Drugs Used for the Treatment of Insomnia

Doxepin (Silenor) is an antidepressant (see Chapter 6) that is marketed as a low dose (3 mg and 6 mg) for sleep disorders. Insomnia may also be treated with the selective melatonin receptor agonist ramelteon (Rozerem) or the orexin receptor antagonist suvorexant (Belsomra). Melatonin is a hormone that regulates the circadian rhythm sleep–wake cycle.

Ramelteon is indicated for insomnia caused by difficulty falling asleep. Suvorexant treats insomnia related to difficulty falling asleep and difficulty staying asleep. Doxepin improves sleep maintenance (difficulty staying asleep).

Adverse Drug Effects. Ramelteon may cause headache, dizziness, and gastrointestinal (GI) upset. It may also cause temporary memory loss and sleep walking. Doxepin may increase drowsiness, and it may produce nausea. Sleepiness is the most common side effect of suvorexant; however, headache and worsening depression

Benzodiazepines and Benzodiazepine Receptor Agonists Used in the Treatment of Insomnia

Generic Name	US Brand Name(s) / Canadian Brand(s)	Dosage Forms and Strengths
Benzodiazepines		
estazolam[a]	Generics	**Tablets:** 1 mg, 2 mg
	Not available	
flurazepam[a]	Generics only	**Capsules:** 15 mg, 30 mg
	Generics only	
quazepam	Doral	**Tablets:** 15 mg
	Not available	
temazepam[a]	Restoril	**Capsules:** 7.5 mg[b], 15 mg, 22.5 mg[b], 30 mg
	Restoril	
triazolam[a]	Halcion	**Tablet:** 0.125 mg[b], 0.25 mg
	Generics only	
Benzodiazepine Receptor Agonists		
eszopiclone[a]	Lunesta	**Tablets:** 1 mg, 2 mg, 3 mg
	Lunesta	
zaleplon[a]	Sonata	**Capsules:** 5 mg, 10 mg
	Not available	
zolpidem[a]	Ambien, Ambien CR, Edluar, Zolpimist	**Oromucosal spray (Zolpimist)[b]:** 5 mg **Tablets (Ambien)[b]:** 5 mg, 10 mg **Tablets, controlled release (Ambien CR)[b]:** 6.25 mg, 12.5 mg **Tablets, sublingual[b]:** 1.75 mg, 3.5 mg (generics), 5 mg, 10 mg (Edluar, Sublinox)
	Sublinox	
zopiclone[a]	Not available	**Tablets:** 5 mg, 7.5 mg
	Imovane	

[a]Generic available.
[b]Available in the United States only.
[c]Available in Canada only.

are other side effects. Suvorexant is metabolized by liver enzyme CYP3A, so drug interactions may occur.

Over-the-Counter and Natural Remedies for Insomnia

Several natural remedies have proven effectiveness for promoting sleep; they are melatonin and valerian root. Melatonin is a hormone that is produced by the pineal gland; it is sensitive to light changes and tells the body it is time to sleep. Doses of 3 mg to 5 mg have been used for treatment of short-term insomnia and enhancement of sleep. The greatest evidence for efficacy of melatonin is in preventing jet lag. The use of valerian root dates back more than 2000 years. Galen recommended it for the treatment of insomnia. A dose of 600 mg aqueous extract, taken 1 hour before bedtime, has been shown to be effective. Diphenhydramine and doxylamine are over-the-counter (OTC) drugs that are used for short-term relief of insomnia.

Miscellaneous Drugs Used for the Treatment of Insomnia

| Generic Name | US Brand Name(s) | Dosage Forms and Strengths |
	Canadian Brand(s)	
doxepin[a]	Silenor	**Tablets:** 3 mg, 6 mg
	Silenor	
ramelteon[a]	Rozerem	**Tablets:** 8 mg
	Not available	
suvorexant	Belsomra	**Tablets:** 5 mg, 10 mg, 15 mg, 20 mg
	Not available	

[a]Generic available.

Adverse Drug Effects.   Diphenhydramine and doxylamine should be avoided in men who have benign prostatic hypertrophy because they cause urinary retention. The antihistamines may also reduce the milk supply of breastfeeding women.

Nonpharmacologic Treatments

It is best to avoid the things that can cause sleeplessness when possible. Insomnia prevention tips include the following:

- Avoid stimulants close to bedtime. Caffeinated beverages such as colas, tea, chocolate, fortified water, OTC decongestants, and ephedra-containing herbals are ***stimulants*** and can cause insomnia if consumed near bedtime.
- Adopt a regular sleeping schedule. A routine sleep schedule provides a cue that sleep time is approaching.
- Avoid daytime naps. Naps disrupt the normal sleep cycle.
- Create a safe, comfortable sleeping environment, if possible. Fears about safety and extremes in temperature can prevent sleep.
- Do not go to bed hungry, if possible. Hunger can prevent sleep.
- Exercise 20 to 30 minutes each day (not at bedtime). Maximum benefits are achieved if exercise is performed 5 to 6 hours before bedtime. Exercise before bedtime can interfere with sleep.
- Avoid ambient lighting produced by electronic devices such as cell phones, tablets, laptops, and televisions. Turn off devices before bedtime.
- Do not lie in bed awake. If you do not fall asleep, get up and engage in a nonstimulating activity such as reading. Try to go to sleep again in about 10 minutes.

Numerous apps are marketed for treatment of insomnia that range from white noise and soothing sounds to internet-based cognitive behavioral therapy (Somryst), which is approved by the US Food and Drug Administration (FDA) and requires a prescription.

Narcolepsy

Narcolepsy is a relatively rare condition in which a person suddenly falls asleep, often in response to an emotional stimulus such

Over-the-Counter Medications and Herbals Used in the Treatment of Insomnia

| Generic Name | US Brand Name(s) | Dosage Forms and Strengths |
	Canadian Brand(s)	
diphenhydramine[a]	Nytol Quickcaps, Unisom SleepMelts, Unisom SleepGels, Sominex, ZzzQuil Nighttime	**Capsules:** 25 mg, 50 mg **Solution, oral:** 6.25 mg/5 mL[b], 12.5 mg/5 mL, 25 mg/5 mL **Tablets:** 25 mg, 50 mg **Tablets, ODT (Unisom SleepMelts):** 25 mg
	Extra Strength Nytol Quickgels, Extra Strength Nytol tabs, Sleep-Eze Gelcaps, Sleep-Eze Melts, Unisom Extra Strength	
doxylamine[a]	Unisom SleepTabs, ZzzQuil Ultra	**Solution, oral:** 2.5 mg/2.5 mL **Suspension, oral:** 2.5 mg/2.5 mL **Tablets:** 25 mg **Tablets, chewable:** 5 mg
	Generics	
melatonin[a]	ZzzQuil Pure Zzzs	**Capsules:** 2.5 mg **Capsules, extended release:** 10 mg **Tablet:** 1 mg, 3 mg, 5 mg
	ZzzQuil Pure Zzzs	
valerian[a]	Generics	**Capsule:** 400 mg, 500 mg, 530 mg **Extract:** 50 mg, 250 mg
	Generics	

[a]Generic available.
[b]Available in Canada only.

Summary of Drugs Used in the Treatment of Insomnia

	Generic Name	US Brand Name	Usual Adult Oral Dose and Dosing Schedule	Controlled Substance Schedule (United States)	NAPRA[a] Schedule (Canada)	Warning Labels
Benzodiazepine and Benzodiazepine Receptor Agonists						
	eszopiclone	Lunesta	1–3 mg at bedtime	C-IV		MAY CAUSE DROWSINESS; MAY IMPAIR THE ABILITY TO DRIVE. AVOID ALCOHOL. MAY BE HABIT FORMING. TAKE 30 MINUTES BEFORE BEDTIME.
	estazolam	Generics	1–2 mg at bedtime	C-IV		
	flurazepam	Dalmane	15–30 mg at bedtime	C-IV	TS[b]	
	quazepam	Doral	7.5–15 mg at bedtime	C-IV		
	temazepam	Restoril	7.5–30 mg at bedtime	C-IV	TS	
	triazolam	Halcion	0.125–0.25 mg at bedtime	C-IV	TS	
	zaleplon	Sonata	5–20 mg at bedtime	C-IV		
	zolpidem	Ambien	Sublingual: Dissolve 1 tab under tongue each night (1.75 mg–10 mg) Tablet: Take before bedtime (immediate release 5–10 mg, controlled release 6.25–12 mg)	C-IV		
	zopiclone	Imovane	3.75–7.5 mg at bedtime			
Miscellaneous						
	doxepin	Silenor	3–6 mg 30 min before bedtime			MAY CAUSE DROWSINESS; MAY IMPAIR THE ABILITY TO DRIVE—all. AVOID TAKING AFTER EATING A HIGH-FAT MEAL—ramelteon. AVOID ALCOHOL—all. SWALLOW WHOLE; DO NOT CRUSH OR CHEW—extended release. DISSOLVE SUBLINGUALLY— Edluar, Sublinox. MAY BE HABIT FORMING—all targeted and controlled substances.
	ramelteon	Rozerem	8 mg at bedtime			
	suvorexant	Belsomra	10 mg 30 min before bedtime (maximum 20 mg once daily)	C-IV		

[a]NAPRA, National Association of Pharmacy Regulatory Authorities.
[b]TS, Targeted substance.

as laughter or fear. The primary treatment for narcolepsy is the administration of stimulants. Stimulants used in the treatment of narcolepsy include amphetamine, methylphenidate, modafinil, and armodafinil. Modafinil and armodafinil are nonamphetamine stimulants. It is not fully known how the drugs work, but it is believed they stimulate α_1-adrenergic receptor sites. Modafinil and armodafinil are also prescribed for the treatment of sleep apnea. Pitolisant (Wakix) is a histamine-3 receptor antagonist/inverse agonist that is used to treat daytime sleepiness.

Amphetamine and methylphenidate are stimulants that are classified as sympathomimetics. A sympathomimetic is a drug that mimics the effects produced by stimulation of the sympathetic nervous system. A detailed discussion of amphetamine and methylphenidate is described in the section on treatment for ADHD.

Side Effects and Precautions

The most common adverse effects produced by armodafinil, modafinil, and pitolisant are headache, nausea, insomnia, and dizziness. The drugs may produce tolerance and dependence and are C-IV controlled substances in the United States. Stevens-Johnson syndrome, a fatal drug rash, has been linked to modafinil use. Armodafinil, modafinil, and pitolisant may decrease the effect of hormonal contraceptives.

● Tech Note!

Warning labels that should be affixed to prescription vials for modafinil are:
AVOID ALCOHOL.
MAY DECREASE THE EFFECT OF ORAL CONTRACEPTIVES.
MAY BE HABIT FORMING.

● Tech Note!

Modafinil should be taken in the morning to avoid insomnia.

● Tech Note!

Pitolisant (Wakix) should be taken with food. Wakix may decrease the effectiveness of hormonal contraceptives.

Attention-Deficit/Hyperactivity Disorder

ADHD is the most common childhood neurodevelopmental disorder. In the United States, the Centers for Disease Control and Prevention (CDC) reports that 6 million children ages 3 to 17 years are diagnosed with ADHD. ADHD is more prevalent in children 12 to 17 years (13%) than children 3 to 5 years (2%) and more common in boys (13%) than girls (6%). In Canada, the prevalence of ADHD ranges between 5% and 12%.

Although most statistics are gathered about children, ADHD affects approximately 3% of adults. Symptoms of ADHD are also commonly observed in children without ADHD, making diagnosis challenging (Fig. 11.2). These symptoms are hyperactivity,

---

Look for signs of ADHD.

Put a check mark next to each one that sounds like your child. ☑

My child often…
☐ is moving something—fingers, hands, arms, feet, or legs.
☐ walks, runs, or climbs around when others are seated.
☐ has trouble waiting in line or taking turns.
☐ doesn't finish things.
☐ gets bored after just a short while.
☐ daydreams or seems to be in another world.
☐ talks when other people are talking.
☐ gets frustrated with schoolwork or homework.
☐ acts quickly without thinking first.
☐ is sidetracked by what is going on around him or her.

• **Fig. 11.2** Checklist for signs of attention-deficit/hyperactivity disorder (ADHD). (Courtesy National Institute of Mental Health, Bethesda, MD.)

Drugs Used for the Treatment of Narcolepsy

Generic Name	US Brand Name(s) / Canadian Brand(s)	Dosage Forms and Strengths	Usual Adult Dose	US Controlled Substance Schedule
armodafinil[a]	Nuvigil	**Tablets:** 50 mg, 150 mg, 200 mg, 250 mg	150–250 mg every morning	C-IV
	Not available			
modafinil[a]	Provigil	**Tablets:** 100 mg, 200 mg[b]	200–400 mg once daily	C-IV
	Alertec			
pitolisant	Wakix	Tablets[b]: 4.45 mg, 17.8 mg	Start with 8.9 mg and may increase up to 35.6 mg; maximum benefit may require up to 8 weeks of pharmacotherapy; maximum dose 40 mg/day	
	Wakix	Tablets: 5 mg, 20 mg		

[a]Generic available.
[b]Available in the United States only.

restlessness, an inability to sit still when required, impulsiveness, inattention, distractibility, forgetfulness, and an inability to complete tasks. All children sometimes exhibit these behaviors. A diagnosis of ADHD should be made only when these behaviors occur more frequently than would be expected for the child's age and if the behavior interferes with two or more areas of the child's life. These areas are defined as school, playground, home, community, and social relationships.

ADHD is characterized by a pattern of symptoms that include inattention, hyperactivity, and impulsivity. It is important to note that individuals primarily experience inattentive symptoms, whereas others mostly experience hyperactivity and impulsiveness. Learning disorders such as dyslexia occur in approximately 20% to 30% of children with ADHD.

There is no single cause for ADHD. Genetics is most strongly linked to ADHD. Up to 40% of children who have a parent, sibling, or other close family relative with ADHD also have ADHD.

Exposure to environmental agents such as cigarette smoke and alcohol during pregnancy has shown to increase the risk for ADHD. Exposure to high levels of lead-based paint also increases the risk. This is an important risk factor for children who live in older urban cities and attend school in old buildings that were painted with lead-based paint before it was banned. There is also an increased risk of ADHD in children who live in countries that use leaded gasoline.

Some people believe that consumption of food additives and sugar can make ADHD worse. When placed on a diet that restricted these food additives, approximately 5% of children with ADHD showed improvement in symptoms.

Treatments for Attention-Deficit/Hyperactivity Disorder

A variety of drug treatments are available for treating patients with ADHD; however, medications cannot cure ADHD. They only control symptoms. The most effective therapy for ADHD involves pharmacotherapy with behavioral therapy. The goal of behavioral therapy is to decrease anxiety and improve relationships and social skills.

ADHD is thought to be linked to a deficit of norepineph-rinergic activity in the prefrontal cortex. Treatment is aimed at increasing levels of the neurotransmitters dopamine and norepinephrine. Pharmaceutical treatment of ADHD is achieved with the administration of amphetamine and nonamphetamine stimulants. Amphetamines behave differently in people who have ADHD than they do in people without ADHD. Individuals with ADHD experience decreased hyperactivity and improved focus. Amphetamines produce hyperactivity and a lack of focused behavior when taken by individuals who do not have ADHD.

> **❶ Tech Alert!**
>
> The following drugs have look-alike/sound-alike issues:
>
> Ritalin, Ritalin SR, and Ritalin LA

Mechanism of Action and Pharmacokinetics

Amphetamines are sympathomimetics structurally similar to norepinephrine. They work via three primary mechanisms: they stimulate the release of norepinephrine, block monoamine oxidase (further increasing catecholamine levels), and stimulate the release of dopamine. Increased stimulation of adrenergic receptors by norepinephrine is responsible for the increased alertness, responsiveness, wakefulness, and reduced awareness of fatigue.

Amphetamines are well absorbed from the GI tract, and their lipid solubility enables them to cross the blood-brain barrier. They are metabolized in the liver and eliminated in the urine. Lisdexamfetamine is a prodrug that is metabolized to dextro-amphetamine. Amphetamines are manufactured in immediate-release, sustained-release, and extended-release dosage forms. The duration of action varies according to the dosage form administered. Atomoxetine and viloxazine are nonamphetamine stimulants. Atomoxetine inhibits the reuptake of norepinephrine. Viloxazine (Qelbree™) is a selective noradrenaline reuptake inhibitor. It is an antidepressant that is effective in treating ADHD in children aged 6 to 17 years old.

> **● Tech Note!**
>
> Stimulants should be taken in the morning to avoid insomnia.

> **● Tech Note!**
>
> Metadate CD and Ritalin LA capsules may be opened and the contents sprinkled on cold applesauce.

Adverse Reactions

The most common side effects produced by amphetamines are decreased appetite, nausea, stomachache, anxiety, and irritability. They can also cause insomnia. Insomnia can be minimized if the last dose is taken before 6 PM. Sympathetic nervous system stimulation produced by amphetamines is responsible for the drugs' cardiovascular effects. Amphetamines can cause increased heart rate, palpitations, and arrhythmia. Other side effects produced by amphetamines are dizziness and tremors. Doses greater than therapeutic doses can produce amphetamine syndrome, a type of drug-induced psychosis. The most common side effects of atomoxetine and viloxazine are sleepiness or fatigue, decreased appetite, abdominal pain, and nausea. Viloxazine and atomoxetine may increase suicide risk.

> **● Tech Note!**
>
> The following warning labels should be affixed to prescription vials for amphetamines:
> TAKE WITH FOOD.
> MAY BE HABIT FORMING.
> SWALLOW WHOLE; DO NOT CRUSH OR CHEW (sustained-release and extended-release).
> ROTATE SITE OF APPLICATION (transdermal systems).

Precautions

Amphetamines have a high abuse potential. They are all Schedule C-II controlled substances in the United States. They are also controlled in Canada (National Association of Pharmacy Regulatory Authorities Schedule C1). Atomoxetine is not a controlled substance.

> **● Tech Note!**
>
> The methylphenidate transdermal patch (Daytrana) should be worn for only 9 hours each day and then removed.

Drugs Used for the Treatment of Attention-Deficit/Hyperactivity Disorder

Generic Name	US Brand Name(s) / Canadian Brand(s)	Dosage Forms and Strengths
amphetamine	Adzenys XR-ODT, Evekeo, Evekeo ODT / Not available	**Suspension, oral:** 1.25 mg/mL, 2.5 mg/mL **Tablet:** 5 mg, 10 mg **Tablets, extended release, disintegrating: (Adzenys XR-ODT):** 3.1 mg, 6.3 mg, 9.4 mg, 12.5 mg, 15.7 mg, 18.8 mg
amphetamine + dextroamphetamine[a]	Adderall XR, Dynanavel XR / Adderall XR	**Capsules, extended release (Adderall XR):** 5 mg, 10 mg, 15 mg, 20 mg, 25 mg, 30 mg **Suspension:** 2 mg/0.5 mg/mL **Tablet, extended release:** 5 mg, 10 mg, 15 mg, 20 mg
dextroamphetamine[a]	Dexedrine / Dexedrine, Dexedrine Spansule	**Capsules, extended release (Dexedrine spansule):** 5 mg[b], 10 mg, 15 mg **Tablets, immediate release (Dexedrine):** 5 mg, 10 mg[b]
dexmethylphenidate[a]	Focalin, Focalin XR / Not available	**Capsule, extended release:** 5 mg, 10 mg, 15 mg, 20 mg, 25 mg, 30 mg, 35 mg, 40 mg **Tablets:** 2.5 mg, 5 mg, 10 mg
dexmethylphenidate; serdexmethylphenidate	Azstarys / Not available	**Capsule:** 5.2 mg dexmethylphenidate + 26.1 mg serdexmethylphenidate, 7.8 mg dexmethylphenidate + 39.2 mg serdexmethylphenidate, 10.4 mg dexmethylphenidate + 52.3 mg serdexmethylphenidate
lisdexamfetamine	Vyvanse / Vyvanse	**Capsules:** 10 mg, 20 mg, 30 mg, 40 mg, 50 mg, 60 mg, 70 mg **Tablet, chewable:** 10 mg, 20 mg, 30 mg, 40 mg[b], 50 mg[b], 60 mg[b]
methylphenidate[a]	Aptensio XR, Cotempla XR-ODT, Concerta, Daytrana, Jornay PM, Metadate CD, Methylin, Methylin ER, Quillichew ER, Quillivant XR, Relexxii Ritalin, Ritalin LA / Biphentin, Concerta, Foquest	**Capsules, biphasic extended release (Aptensio XR, Biphentin, Metadate CD, Ritalin LA):** 10 mg, 20 mg, 30 mg, 40 mg, 50 mg, 60 mg, 15 mg (Aptensio XR, Biphentin), and 80 mg (Biphentin only) **Capsule, controlled release (Foquest)[c]:** 25 mg, 35 mg, 45 mg, 55 mg, 70 mg, 85 mg, 100 mg **Capsule, extended release (Journay PM):** 20 mg, 40 mg, 60 mg, 80 mg, 100 mg **Capsule, for suspension (Qullivant XR):** 5 mg/mL **Solution, oral (Methylin):** 2 mg/mL, 1 mg/mL **Tablets, chewable:** 2.5 mg, 5 mg, 10 mg **Tablets, chewable extended release (Quillichew):** 20 mg, 30 mg, 40 mg **Tablets, extended release (Concerta, Relexxii):** 18 mg, 27 mg, 36 mg, 54 mg, 63 mg, 72 mg **Tablets, extended release (Methylin ER):** 10 mg, 20 mg **Tablets, immediate release (Ritalin):** 5 mg[b], 10 mg, 20 mg **Tablet, oral disintegrating (Cotempla XR-ODT):** 8.6 mg, 17.3 mg, 25.9 mg **Tablets, sustained release (Ritalin SR):** 20 mg **Transdermal patch (Daytrana):** 10 mg/9 h, 15 mg/9 h, 20 mg/9 h, 30 mg/9 h
atomoxetine[a]	Strattera / Strattera	**Capsules:** 5 mg[b], 10 mg, 18 mg, 25 mg, 40 mg, 60 mg, 80 mg, 100 mg
viloxazine	Qelbree / Not available	**Capsule:** 100 mg, 150 mg, 200 mg

[a]Generic available.
[b]Available in the United States only.
[c]Available in Canada only.

Summary of Drugs Used in the Treatment of Attention-Deficit/Hyperactivity Disorder

	Generic Name	Brand Name	Usual Child Dosage	Controlled Substance Schedule (Canada)
Amphetamines				
	amphetamine + dextroamphetamine (immediate release)	Adderall	2.5–40 mg/day (1–2 doses/day)	C-II (CDSA I)
	amphetamine + dextroamphetamine (extended release)	Adderall XR	5–30 mg every morning	C-II (CDSA I)
	dextroamphetamine (immediate release)	Dexedrine, Dextrostat	2.5–40 mg 1–2 doses per day	C-II (CDSA I)
	dexmethylphenidate	Focalin	2.5–20 mg/day given as 2 doses/day	C-II (CDSA III)
	lisdexamfetamine	Vyvanse	30–70 mg once daily	C-II (CDSA III)
	methylphenidate (immediate release)	Ritalin	10–20 mg twice a day up to 60 mg/day	C-II (CDSA III)
	methylphenidate (extended release)	Concerta	18–72 mg once daily	C-II (CDSA III)
		Ritalin LA	20 mg once a day up to 60 mg/day	C-II (CDSA III)
		Metadate CD	20 mg once a day up to 60 mg/day	C-II (CDSA III)
		Cotempla XR-ODT	17.3–51.8 mg/day	C-II
		Metadate ER	May replace methylphenidate immediate release (IR) when 8-h dosage of methylphenidate ER corresponds to the titrated 8-h dosage of methylphenidate IR (maximum 60 mg/day)	C-II (CDSA III)
	methylphenidate (sustained release)	Ritalin SR	20–30 mg daily (may replace immediate release tablets when 8-h dosage of methylphenidate SR corresponds to the titrated 8-h dosage of methylphenidate IR; not to exceed 60 mg/day)	C-II (CDSA III)
	methylphenidate (transdermal patch)	Daytrana	1 patch worn for 9 h/day	C-II (CDSA III)
Nonamphetamine				
	atomoxetine	Strattera	40–80 mg/day in 1–2 divided doses (maximum 100 mg/day)	Not controlled
	viloxazine	Quelbree	100–400 mg once daily	Not controlled

TECHNICIAN'S CORNER

1. What do you suppose is the rationale for the large variety of dosage form options for drugs used to treat ADHD?
2. What would you recommend to someone with a sleep disorder who does not want to take any sleep aids?

Key Points

- Sleep is needed for a healthy immune system and nervous system, healthy emotional and social functioning, as well as physical and mental agility.
- The pineal gland controls the release of melatonin, a hormone that makes people feel drowsy.
- Infants may sleep up to 16 hours per day, teenagers require as much as 9 hours, and adults need as little as 5 to 8 hours. Patterns of sleep change as people age.
- There are five stages of sleep (four non–REM stages and REM).
- Dreaming occurs during REM sleep and is crucial to normal emotional and physical functioning.
- Sleep apnea can increase the risk for hypertension, myocardial infarction, and stroke, and is linked to arrhythmias, heart failure, diabetes, and obesity.
- Sleep apnea, restless legs syndrome, consumption of caffeinated beverages and foods, use of prescription and nonprescription drugs, and chronic illness can cause insomnia.
- Pharmacologic treatment for insomnia is recommended for short-term use.
- Prescription drugs, nonprescription drugs, and herbal remedies are commercially available, and all produce drowsiness that enables the person to drift off to sleep and stay asleep.
- Prescription drugs used to treat insomnia are benzodiazepines and nonbenzodiazepine sedative-hypnotics.
- Drugs that promote sleep do not result in a normal pattern of sleep. They alter non-REM and REM sleep.
- Rebound hypersomnia and increased dreaming occur after the drugs are discontinued.

- The mechanism of action for zaleplon, zolpidem, eszopiclone, and zopiclone is similar to benzodiazepines.
- Melatonin and valerian root are herbal remedies that have proven effectiveness for promoting sleep.
- Insomnia prevention tips include: (1) avoid stimulants close to bedtime; (2) adopt a regular sleeping schedule; (3) avoid daytime naps; (4) create a safe, comfortable sleeping environment, if possible; (5) do not go to bed hungry, if possible; (6) exercise; and (7) do not lie in bed awake.
- Stimulants are administered for the treatment of narcolepsy.
- ADHD is the most commonly diagnosed childhood neurodevelopmental disorder.
- Symptoms of ADHD are hyperactivity, restlessness, an inability to sit still when required, impulsiveness, inattention, distractibility, forgetfulness, and an inability to complete tasks.
- The most effective therapy for ADHD involves a combination of drug treatments and behavioral therapy.
- Pharmaceutical treatment of ADHD is achieved with the administration of amphetamines and nonamphetamine stimulants.
- The most common side effects produced by amphetamines are decreased appetite, nausea, stomachache, anxiety, insomnia, and irritability.
- Amphetamines have a high abuse potential and are controlled substances in the United States and Canada.
- The methylphenidate patch (Daytrana) should be applied to the hip area. It should not be worn for more than 9 hours per day.

Review Questions

1. Not getting enough sleep does not affect the immune system, nervous system, or emotional and social functioning of the body.
   a. true
   b. false
2. Circadian rhythms are biological changes that occur according to _____ cycles.
   a. growth
   b. age
   c. time
   d. health
3. The pineal gland controls the release of _____, a hormone that makes people feel drowsy in addition to regulating body temperature and hormone secretion.
   a. serotonin
   b. melatonin
   c. dopamine
   d. acetylcholine
4. Select the drug that is NOT a controlled or targeted substance in the United States and Canada.
   a. Adderall
   b. Ritalin
   c. Restoril
   d. Strattera
5. Pharmacologic treatment for insomnia is recommended for long-term use.
   a. True
   b. False

6. You receive a prescription for Concerta 10 mg 1 tablet once daily. You consult with the pharmacist because_____.
   a. methylphenidate is not marketed as 10 mg
   b. Concerta is not available in a 10-mg tablet
   c. Ritalin is not dosed once daily
   d. the dose is too low
7. Zaleplon and zolpidem are benzodiazepines.
   a. True
   b. False
8. The primary treatment for ADHD is administration of stimulants.
   a. True
   b. False
9. Pharmaceutical treatment of insomnia is achieved with the administration of all of the following EXCEPT _____.
   a. methylphenidate
   b. zolpidem
   c. temazepam
   d. doxepin
10. Amphetamines have a high abuse potential and are classified as Schedule _____ controlled substances in the United States.
   a. C-I
   b. C-II
   c. C-IV
   d. C-III

Bibliography

American Academy of Sleep Medicine. Rising prevalence of sleep apnea in U.S. threatens public health. ScienceDaily. Retrieved August 25, 2022, from www.sciencedaily.com/releases/2014/09/140929105443.htm.

Espinet SD, Graziosi G, Toplak ME, Hesson J, Minhas P. A review of Canadian diagnosed ADHD prevalence and incidence estimates published in the past decade. *Brain Sci.* 2022;12:1051. https://doi.org/10.3390/brainsci12081051.

Ford ES, Wheaton AG, Cunningham TJ, et al. Trends in outpatient visits for insomnia, sleep apnea, and prescriptions for sleep medications among US adults: findings from the National Ambulatory Medical Care Survey, 1999–2010. *Sleep.* 2014;37:1283–1293.

Haddad HW, Hankey PB, Ko J, et al. Viloxazine, a non-stimulant norepinephrine reuptake inhibitor, for the treatment of attention deficit hyperactivity disorder: a 3 year update. *Health Psychol Res.* 2022;10(3).

Hassinger AB, Bletnisky N, Dudekula R, El Solh AA. Selecting a pharmacotherapy regimen for patients with chronic insomnia. *Expert Opin Pharmacother* 21(9), 1035–1043.

Health Canada. (2022). Drug Product Database. Retrieved July 20, 2022, from https://health-products.canada.ca/dpd-bdpp/index-eng.jsp.

Institute for Safe Medication Practices. (2016). FDA and ISMP Lists of Look-Alike Drug Names with Recommended Tall Man Letters. Retrieved July 20, 2022, from https://www.ismp.org/recommendations/tall-man-letters-list.

Institute for Safe Medication Practices. (2019). List of Confused Drugs. Retrieved July 20, 2022, from https://www.ismp.org/tools/confused-drugnames.pdf.

Kalant H, Grant D, Mitchell J. *Principles of medical pharmacology.* ed 7. Toronto: Elsevier Canada, A Division of Reed Elsevier Canada; 2007:339–342.

National Institute of Mental Health: *Attention-deficit/hyperactivity disorder*, Bethesda (MD), 2016, National Institute of Mental Health, National Institutes of Health, US Department of Health and Human Services. Retrieved August 25, 2022, from https://www.nimh.nih.gov/health/topics/attention-deficit-hyperactivity-disorder-adhd/index.shtml.

National Highway Traffic Safety Administration. (nd). Drowsy Driving. Retrieved August 25, 2022, from https://www.nhtsa.gov/risky-driving/drowsy-driving.

National Institute of Neurological Disorders and Stroke, National Institute of Health, U.S. Department of Health and Humans Services: Brain basics: understanding sleep, Bethesda, 2017, National Institute of Neurological disorders and stroke. NIH publication No. 17-3440-c.

Neubauer DN, Pandi-Perumal SR, Spence DW, et al. Pharmacotherapy of insomnia. *J Central Nerv Syst Dis.* 2018;10:2018.

Public Health Agency of Canada: Fast Facts from the 2009 Canadian Community Health Survey—Sleep Apnea Rapid Response, 2010. Retrieved March 5, 2011, from http://www.phac-aspc.gc.ca/cd-mc/sleepapnea-apneesommeil/pdf/sleep-apnea.pdf.

Raffa R, Rawls S, Beyzarov E. *Netter's illustrated pharmacology.* Philadelphia: WB Saunders; 2005:80–82.

Santilli M, Manciocchi E, D'Addazio G, et al. Prevalence of obstructive sleep apnea syndrome: a single-center retrospective study. *Int J Environ Res Public Health.* 2021;18:10277.

U.S. Centers for Disease Control and Prevention. 1 in 3 Adults Don't Get Enough Sleep. Retrieved August 25, 2022, from https://www.cdc.gov/media/releases/2016/p0215-enough-sleep.html.

U.S. Centers for Disease Control and Prevention. (2022). Attention-Deficit/Hyperactivity Disorder (ADHD). Retrieved August 25, 2022, from https://www.cdc.gov/ncbddd/adhd/data.html.

U.S. Food and Drug Administration. (nd). Drugs@FDA: FDA Approved Drug Products. Retrieved July 20, 2022, from https://www.accessdata.fda.gov/scripts/cder/daf/index.cfm.

UNIT III

Drugs Affecting the Musculoskeletal System

The proper functioning of the joints of musculoskeletal system is crucial for purposeful movement because it provides form, support, stability, and movement to the body. When body systems fail to support the function of muscle tissues and the proper functioning of the joints of the skeleton, overexertion or trauma may cause muscle strain, muscle pain (myalgia), muscle bruising (contusion), or sprains. Muscle tension in the head and neck can cause tension headaches. Diseases of the musculature may be caused by autoimmune disorders (e.g., multiple sclerosis and rheumatoid arthritis); infection by bacteria, viruses, or parasites that can produce myositis, *tetanus*, or poliomyelitis; and genetics (e.g., muscular dystrophy). Inflammatory disorders (e.g., bursitis and arthritis) affect large weight-bearing joints (e.g., hip, knees) and are characterized by morning stiffness, limited joint motion, and deep, achy pain on movement.

In Unit III, pharmacotherapy for muscle spasms, conditions requiring neuromuscular blockade, gout, rheumatoid arthritis, osteoarthritis, osteoporosis, and Paget disease is described. A brief description of each disorder is provided, followed by a description of the drugs indicated for treatment that includes mechanisms of action, adverse reactions, strength(s), and dosage forms. Musculoskeletal disorders such as inflammation and pain are treated with nonsteroidal antiinflammatory drugs (NSAIDS), locally acting corticosteroids, and skeletal muscle relaxants. Biological response modifiers (e.g., Humira®) are used in the treatment of autoimmune disorders such as rheumatoid arthritis. Nonpharmacologic therapy to prevent injury and wear and tear of the skeletal and muscular systems (e.g., daily exercise) is also discussed.

12

Neuromuscular Blockade and Muscle Spasms

LEARNING OBJECTIVES

1. Learn the terminology associated with neuromuscular blockade and muscle spasms.
2. Discuss the process of neuromuscular transmission.
3. List medical conditions that cause spasticity.
4. List and classify neuromuscular blocking drugs and drugs used to treat muscle spasms.
5. Describe the mechanism of action for peripheral and central-acting skeletal muscle relaxants.
6. List uses for neuromuscular blocking drugs.
7. Describe the mechanism for reversal of neuromuscular blockade.
8. List strategies for safe management of neuromuscular blocking drugs in the pharmacy.
9. Identify significant drug look-alike and sound-alike issues.
10. Identify warning labels and precautionary messages associated with neuromuscular blockers and medications used to treat spasticity.

KEY TERMS

Acetylcholinesterase Enzyme that degrades acetylcholine and reverses acetylcholine-induced depolarization.

Amyotrophic lateral sclerosis (ALS) Degenerative disease that causes muscle wasting and muscle weakness. ALS is also known as Lou Gehrig disease.

Anaphylactic shock Acute, life-threatening allergic reaction that produces peripheral vasodilation, bronchospasm, laryngeal edema, and airway obstruction.

Antispasmodic Drug used specifically to treat muscle spasms, often resulting from muscle strain or low back sprain.

Botulinum toxin Toxin produced by the bacterium *Clostridium botulinum* that causes muscle paralysis.

Central-acting muscle relaxants Drugs that produce relaxation of muscles by blocking nerve transmission between the spinal cord and muscles.

Cerebral palsy Neurologic disorder that affects muscle movement and coordination.

Clonus Involuntary rhythmic muscle contraction that causes the feet and wrists to involuntarily flex and relax.

Depolarizing neuromuscular blockers Drugs that act as agonists at acetylcholine receptor sites and produce sustained depolarization whereby the receptors convert to an inactive state.

Endotracheal intubation Process of inserting a tube into the trachea or windpipe to facilitate mechanical ventilation.

End plate Projection extending off the end of a motor neuron where the neurotransmitter acetylcholine is released.

Multiple sclerosis Autoimmune disease that causes progressive damage to nerves resulting in spasticity, pain, mood changes, and other physical symptoms.

Neuromuscular junction Space between motor neuron end plate and the muscle sole plate that neurotransmitters must cross.

Nondepolarizing competitive blockers Drugs that compete with acetylcholine for binding sites. When acetylcholine binding is inhibited, muscle contraction is blocked.

Peripheral-acting muscle relaxants Drugs that block nerve transmission between the motor end plate and skeletal muscle receptors.

Sarcomere Contracting unit of muscle fibers.

Sole plate Portion of the membrane of muscle cells that receives messages transmitted by motor neurons.

Spasmolytic Drug that specifically treats muscle spasticity.

Spasticity Motor disorder that causes increased muscle tone, exaggerated tendon jerks, and hyperexcitable muscles.

Overview

Skeletal muscles contract as a response to messages transmitted between peripheral nerves and muscles. Acetylcholine (ACh) is the primary neurotransmitter that sends messages between nerve cells and muscle cells. The process begins with the release of ACh from vesicles located in the motor neuron end plate. The **end plate** is a projection extending off the end of one of the branches of the motor neuron. The end of the motor neuron may be divided into as many as 200 branches. The **sole plate** is the portion of the membrane of muscle cells that receives messages transmitted by motor neurons.

Drugs that block nerve transmission between the motor end plate and skeletal muscle receptors are classified as **peripheral-acting muscle relaxants**. Peripheral-acting drugs are further classified according to their mechanism of action. They are classified as **nondepolarizing competitive blockers** and depolarizing blockers. **Central-acting muscle relaxants** are direct-acting agents that bind to and block calcium channels. Skeletal muscle relaxants that work by central nervous system (CNS) depression (i.e., block nerve transmission between the spinal cord and muscles) are examples of central-acting muscle relaxants.

The release of ACh produces skeletal muscle contraction. Calcium increases ACh release. Drugs that decrease the release of ACh or deplete ACh levels in the neuron also cause skeletal muscle relaxation. **Botulinum toxin** and magnesium are examples of drugs that decrease the release of ACh. Black widow spider venom causes a massive release of ACh from vesicles that is independent of calcium. The venom causes muscle contractions and cramping. If untreated, depletion of ACh causes paralysis.

● Tech Note!

The US Food and Drug Administration (FDA) has issued a warning that onabotulinumtoxin type A (Botox) and botulinum toxin rimabotulinumtoxin type B (Myobloc) injections may spread beyond the injection site, and the toxins' effects may produce respiratory failure and death (2010).

Indication

Neuromuscular blocking agents have been used historically by Indigenous peoples of South America. They were first used in surgery in 1942 and continue to be used currently to induce a controlled, temporary state of paralysis. They are most commonly used in general anesthesia for endotracheal intubation to facilitate mechanical ventilation. **Endotracheal intubation** is the process of inserting a tube into the trachea or windpipe. OnabotulinumtoxinA, commonly known as Botox, is a neuromuscular blocking drug that is used in an outpatient setting. Its use is becoming widespread, and it has been approved by the FDA for a variety of conditions, including temporary removal of wrinkles, treatment of excessive sweating, spasticity, uncontrollable blinking, and chronic migraine (headache more than 15 days per month).

Care must be taken when transcribing and filling orders for neuromuscular blocking drugs because they can cause severe injury or death. To prevent possible injury or death, the US Pharmacopoeia (USP) Interdisciplinary Safe Medication Use Expert Committee has compiled a list of recommendations for the safe use of neuromuscular blocking agents. The recommendations listed in Box 12.1 are modified for pharmacy-specific application.

● Tech Alert!

Institute for Safe Medication Practices (ISMP) Canada recommends adoption of the USP standards for drug vials containing neuromuscular blocking agents. The lids of the vials are clearly marked "Paralyzing Agent" or "Warning: Paralyzing Agent" (Fig. 12.1).

Mechanism of Action

Depolarizing neuromuscular blockers are agonists at nicotinic receptors. They bind to ACh receptors, where they produce sustained depolarization. Prolonged depolarization causes receptors to convert to their inactive state. Depolarization is the process whereby the cell undergoes a shift in electric charge. Positive ions enter the cell (e.g., calcium). When the end plate potential exceeds

---

● BOX 12.1 Safe Management of Neuromuscular Blocking Agents: Recommendations for Pharmacy Practice

Product Selection
- Procurement managers should select products that have distinctive names and packaging to avoid sound-alike/look-alike issues.

Product Storage
- Neuromuscular blocking drugs should be stored apart from other drugs.
- Storage of neuromuscular blocking drugs should be confined to primary care areas and pharmacy areas that care for mechanically ventilated patients.
- Storage conditions for undiluted and diluted solutions should be clearly marked.

Limit Access
- Neuromuscular blocking drugs should be kept in sealed "intubation kits" or "anesthesia kits" until use is needed.
- Opened vials should be immediately discarded or returned to the seal kit after use.
- Neuromuscular blocking drugs should NOT be dispensed in unit dose carts or delivered to general nursing units unless in a sealed kit.
- Neuromuscular blocking drugs should be stored in a single access drawer when stored in drug storage devices such as Pyxis and AccuDose-Rx.
- Neuromuscular blocking drugs requiring refrigeration should be stored in a separate area away from other refrigerated drugs.

Auxiliary Labels or Warning Labels
- Neuromuscular blocking drugs should always be dispensed with the auxiliary label "WARNING: Paralyzing agent. (Use requires mechanical ventilatory assistance.)"
- Overwraps should be considered for individual vials of neuromuscular blocking drugs stored outside of pharmacy and anesthesiology areas, especially drugs stored in the refrigerator.
- Affix preprinted syringe labels to syringes filled with neuromuscular blocking drugs at the time the drug is drawn up to avoid risks associated with unlabeled syringes.

Ordering Practices and Dispensing
- Contact prescriber for complete directions when medication orders for neuromuscular blocking agents are written with "as needed" (PRN) directions.
- Verify patient identity and drug identity with barcode readers when available.

Adapted from US Pharmacopoeia Interdisciplinary Safe Medication Use Expert Committee recommendations.

15 mV, an action potential is produced (Fig. 12.2). The receptors become desensitized, and contractions are prevented until the receptors return to their preactivated state.

Succinylcholine is the only depolarizing neuromuscular blocker currently available. Similar to ACh, it is rapidly inactivated by cholinesterase enzymes. Cholinesterase enzymes are synthesized in the liver and are responsible for the breakdown of succinylcholine.

Nondepolarizing Neuromuscular Blockers

Most nondepolarizing neuromuscular blockers are competitive antagonists at prejunctional and postjunctional receptors. At low doses, they produce no effects of their own when they bind to receptor sites; instead, they compete with ACh for binding sites. At high doses, nondepolarizing drugs weaken neuromuscular transmission and reduce the action of *acetylcholinesterase*, the enzyme that reverses ACh-induced depolarization.

> ● **Tech Note!**
>
> "-curonium" and "-curium" are common endings for nondepolarizing neuromuscular blockers.

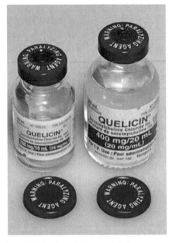

• **Fig. 12.1** Examples of lids for vials containing neuromuscular blocking agents. (Reprinted with permission from ISMP Canada.)

Pharmacokinetics

Most neuromuscular blocking drugs are poorly absorbed from the gastrointestinal tract, so they are administered parenterally. They have low lipid solubility, and they do not easily cross the blood-brain barrier. They are highly water soluble and are primarily eliminated in the urine. Vecuronium is also metabolized in the liver, and its rate of elimination may be decreased if the patient has liver disease. The onset of action is rapid (1 to 4 minutes), and duration of action is short (10 to 90 minutes). This requires a continuous infusion to be administered. An exception is the duration of action for the botulinum toxins, which may last up to 12 weeks. Nondepolarizing neuromuscular blocking drugs have a longer onset and longer duration of action than depolarizing neuromuscular blocking drugs because they are not broken down by the enzyme acetylcholinesterase.

> ● **Tech Note!**
>
> Botox injections are made from a substance derived from the toxin that causes botulism (botulinum toxin).

Adverse Reactions

Common side effects are muscle pain, itching, or burning at the injection site. Hypotension, flushing (vasodilation), tachycardia, or bradycardia may also occur. Allergic reactions that occur may be life-threatening. They may appear as rash and redness on the face and neck or may be serious enough to produce bronchospasm, laryngospasm, and anaphylactic shock. Other life-threatening adverse reactions are respiratory depression, cardiac arrest, and pulmonary edema. Depolarizing neuromuscular blockers (e.g., succinylcholine) cause potassium channels to remain open, producing hyperkalemia. Excess potassium may produce cardiac arrest. OnabotulinumtoxinA injections may produce muscle weakness in the injected muscles. This may cause droopy eyelid muscles *(blepharoptosis)*, headache, nausea, flulike syndrome, redness, and muscle weakness.

> ● **Tech Note!**
>
> *Anaphylactic shock* is an acute, life-threatening allergic reaction that produces peripheral vasodilation, bronchospasm, laryngeal edema, and airway obstruction.

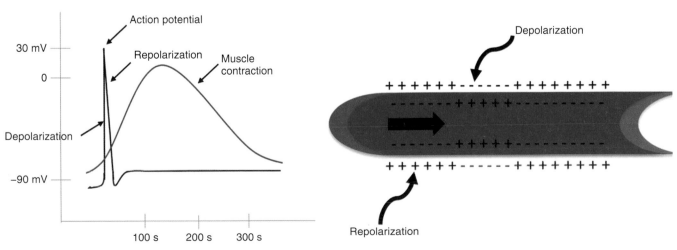

• **Fig. 12.2** Depolarization process.

Neuromuscular Blockers

Generic Name	US Brand Name(s) Canadian Brand(s)	Dosage Forms and Strengths
Depolarizing Neuromuscular Blocking Drugs		
succinylcholine[a]	Anectine, Quelicin	**Injection, solution:** 20 mg/mL
	Quelicin	
Nondepolarizing Neuromuscular Blocking Drugs		
atracurium[a]	Generic	**Injection, solution:** 10 mg/mL
	Not available	
abobotulinumtoxinA	Dysport	**Powder for injection:** 300 units/vial, 500 units/vial
	Dysport	
onabotulinumtoxinA	Botox, Botox Cosmetic	**Powder for injection:** 50 units/vial[b], 100 units/vial, 200 units/vial[b]
	Botox, Botox Cosmetic	
rimabotulinumtoxinB (botulinum toxin type B)	Myobloc	**Injection, solution:** 5000 units/vial
	Not available	
incobotulinumtoxinA	Xeomin	**Powder for injection:** 50 units/vial, 100 units/vial, 200 units/vial[b]
	Xeomin, Xeomin Cosmetic	
cisatracurium[a]	Nimbex	**Injection, solution:** 2 mg/mL, 10 mg/mL[b]
	Generics	
pancuronium[a]	Generics	**Injection, solution:** 1 mg/mL, 2 mg/mL
	Not available	
rocuronium[a]	Generics	**Injection, solution:** 10 mg/mL
	Generics	
vecuronium[a]	Generics	**Powder for injection:** 10 mg/vial, 20 mg/vial
	Not available	

[a]Generic available.
[b]Available in the United States only.

Reversal of Neuromuscular Blockade

Drugs that reverse the effects of neuromuscular blockade must always be readily available any time the drugs are administered. Anticholinesterase drugs inhibit the degradation of ACh by the enzyme acetylcholinesterase at the **neuromuscular junction**. This causes ACh to accumulate. Increasing ACh produces skeletal muscle contraction. Anticholinesterase drugs are most effective after the process of spontaneous recovery from neuromuscular blocking drugs has begun. Neostigmine and pyridostigmine are drugs that reverse neuromuscular blockade.

> ● **Tech Note!**
>
> Tubocurarine, formerly used in anesthesia, is the synthetic version of curare, a natural paralytic drug used by Indigenous South American hunters to immobilize prey.

Adverse Reactions

Pyridostigmine and neostigmine may produce salivation, muscle twitching, muscle weakness, abdominal cramping, nausea, increased bronchial secretions, and difficulty breathing.

Strategies for Safe Use of Neuromuscular Blocking Agents

Neuromuscular blocking drugs are classified "high alert" by the Interdisciplinary Safe Medication Use Expert Committee of the USP because improper use can result in permanent injury, respiratory arrest, and death. Problems associated with neuromuscular blocking drugs have been attributed to improper product selection, improper storage conditions, inappropriate dosing, improper labeling, and inadequate patient monitoring. Improper product selection is caused by similar product packaging and sound-alike drug names. Drug names that sound alike pose

Drugs That Reverse the Effects of Neuromuscular Blockade

Generic Name	US Brand Name(s) / Canadian Brand(s)	Dosage Forms and Strengths
neostigmine[a]	Bloxiverz / Generics	**Injection, solution:** 0.5 mg/mL, 1 mg/mL, 2.5 mg/mL[b]
pyridostigmine[a]	Mestinon, Regonol / Mestinon, Mestinon SR	**Injection, solution (Regonol):** 5 mg/mL[c] **Syrup:** 60 mg/5 mL[c] **Tablets:** 60 mg **Tablets, sustained release (Mestinon SR, Mestinon Timespan):** 180 mg

[a]Generic available.
[b]Available in Canada only.
[c]Available in the United States only.

problems in dispensing regardless of the type of drug. Look-alike packaging is a problem that can be attributed to drug manufacturers, as well as pharmacies dispensing drugs (see Chapter 4). Neuromuscular blocking drugs may be repackaged for unit of use in institutional care settings. Infusion bags and syringes that have been prepared by the pharmacy look alike. Neuromuscular blocking drugs have been administered in place of vaccines, intravenous flush solutions, and antibiotics by mistake. A pharmacy that fails to securely affix the label onto the infusion bag or syringe of a neuromuscular blocking drug is creating a potentially life-threatening situation for a patient. Additional medicine errors occur from inaccurate sterile compounding, dispensing of incorrect drug concentrations, and placing incorrect doses in automated dispensing machines.

Treatment of Muscle Spasms

Overview

Spasticity is a debilitating motor disorder that affects up to 12 million people worldwide. Children and adults are affected. Symptoms of spasticity are increased muscle tone, exaggerated tendon jerks, and hyperexcitability of the stretch reflex. Spasticity can also cause muscle weakness, decreased endurance, and reduction in the capacity to make voluntary muscle movements. It may be accompanied by pain.

Summary of Neuromuscular Blocking Drugs

Generic Name	US Brand Name	Warnings and Storage Conditions
succinylcholine	Quelicin	PARALYZING AGENT. KEEP REFRIGERATED (2°–8°C). PROTECT FROM LIGHT. Multidose vials stable at room temperature for 14 days.
atracurium	Generics	PARALYZING AGENT. KEEP REFRIGERATED (2–8°C). PROTECT FROM LIGHT. Stable at room temperature for 14 days. Infusion solutions should be used within 24 h of preparation.
abobotulinumtoxinA	Dysport	PARALYZING AGENT. KEEP REFRIGERATED (2–8°C). PROTECT FROM LIGHT. After dilution: Refrigerated solutions should be used within 24 h of preparation.
onabotulinumtoxinA	Botox	PARALYZING AGENT. KEEP REFRIGERATED (2–8°C). After dilution: Refrigerated solutions should be used within 24 h of preparation.
incobotulinumtoxinA	Xeomin	PARALYZING AGENT. KEEP REFRIGERATED (2–8°C). After dilution: Refrigerate and use within 24 h; discard unused portion.
rimabotulinumtoxinB	Myobloc	PARALYZING AGENT. KEEP REFRIGERATED; DO NOT FREEZE. After dilution: Use within 4 h and discard unused portion. PROTECT FROM LIGHT.
cisatracurium	Nimbex	PARALYZING AGENT. KEEP REFRIGERATED; DO NOT FREEZE (2–8°C). PROTECT FROM LIGHT. Once warmed to room temperature: Use within 21 days.
pancuronium	Generics	PARALYZING AGENT. KEEP REFRIGERATED (2–8°C). DO NOT STORE IN PLASTIC SYRINGE. Stable for 6 months if stored at room temperature. If mixed, use within 48 hours.

Summary of Neuromuscular Blocking Drugs—cont'd

Generic Name	US Brand Name	Warnings and Storage Conditions
rocuronium	Generics	PARALYZING AGENT. KEEP REFRIGERATED. If unopened, use within 60 days after removal from refrigerator. Once opened, use within 30 days. If mixed, use within 24 h and discard unused portion.
vecuronium	Generics	PARALYZING AGENT. KEEP REFRIGERATED. PROTECT FROM LIGHT. Before dilution: May store at room temperature. After dilution: Refrigerate and use within 24 h if reconstituted with sterile water or use within 5 days if reconstituted with bacteriostatic water.

Summary of Drugs Used to Reverse the Effects of Neuromuscular Blocking Drugs

Generic Name	US Brand Name	Warnings and Storage Conditions
neostigmine	Bloxiverz	STABLE AT ROOM TEMPERATURE. PROTECT FROM LIGHT (injection solution).
pyridostigmine	Mestinon	SWALLOW WHOLE; DO NOT CRUSH OR CHEW—SR tab. PROTECT FROM MOISTURE.

Spasticity may interfere with the normal performance of self-care and activities of daily living, inhibit effective walking, cause fatigue and stiffness, and disturb sleep.

Stroke, spinal cord injury, cerebral palsy, muscle trauma (e.g., whiplash), multiple sclerosis, head injury, and metabolic diseases such as *amyotrophic lateral sclerosis* (Lou Gehrig disease) can all cause spasticity. In fact, 65% to 78% of people with spinal cord injuries and 65% of people who have had a stroke will develop spasticity.

Spasticity can be aggravated by a variety of factors. Fatigue, pain, stress, fever, cold, constipation, immobility, and hormonal changes can all worsen symptoms of spasticity.

Pathophysiology of Spasticity

Any condition that can damage the brain or spinal cord can cause spasticity. Regardless of the cause, the progression to spasticity follows a specific pattern, and the degree of spasticity is related to the duration since the original injury. The four phases are (1) decreased muscle contractility; (2) excessive muscle tone and increased reflex activity lasting from days to years; (3) decreased reflex excitability; and (4) stiff, contracted muscles.

Conditions That Produce Spasticity

Spinal Cord Injury

Spinal cord injury may produce muscle paralysis and loss of tendon reflexes in the region below the level of spinal cord injury immediately after the injury. Within a few weeks, this period of spinal shock ends and is followed by a period of increased muscle tone, exaggerated tendon jerks, and involuntary muscle spasms. It is believed that spasticity develops because the neurons that branch out from the spinal cord to the muscles and tissues of the body (lower motor neurons) grow new synapses that increase response to stretching of the muscle. Normal inhibitory control of sustained neuron firing is lost during the recovery period after spinal cord injury. What follows are unopposed motor neuron excitability. As muscle fibers atrophy, the number of sarcomeres decrease, and connective tissue increases. *Sarcomeres* are units within muscle fibers responsible for muscle contraction.

Spinal cord injury also results in *clonus*, an involuntary rhythmic muscle contraction that produces involuntary flexing and relaxation of the feet and wrists.

Stroke

Stroke can cause a lesion to form in the brain or spinal cord, which results in unopposed motor neuron excitability by normal inhibitory mechanisms.

Cerebral Palsy

Spasticity caused by *cerebral palsy* follows the same pathophysiologic pathway as stroke and spinal cord injury. Treatment is complicated because spasticity impairs effective muscle movement in some people with cerebral palsy and helps maintain posture, making walking easier in other people.

Amyotrophic Lateral Sclerosis

In people who have ALS, upper motor neurons (which carry messages from the brain down to the spinal cord) are damaged. Changes in the presynaptic membrane result in the release of ACh from its storage vesicle. This ultimately causes desensitization of motor nerves, muscle weakness, and cell death.

> **● Tech Note!**
>
> The myelin sheath around neurons acts as an electrical insulator and increases the velocity of impulse transmission.

Multiple Sclerosis

Multiple sclerosis is an autoimmune disease that causes damage to myelinated nerves. Lesions damage nerves in the CNS and cause spasticity, pain, fatigue, dysfunction of the bladder and bowel, impotence, cognitive dysfunction, and changes in mood or depression. Nerve damage and symptoms get progressively worse over time.

Muscle Strain

Muscle strain, sprains, fibromyalgia, tension headaches, low back pain, and neck pain can cause muscle spasms, stiffness, and pain. When spasms are present, they are typically related to local injury or irritation of a specific muscle group.

Neurotransmitters Involved in Spasticity

Spasticity is a symptom of upper motor neuron syndrome. The cause may be excess activity of neurotransmitters that carry excitatory messages, such as ACh and glutamate, or decreased activity or a deficiency of inhibitory transmitters, such as γ-aminobutyric acid (GABA) and glycine. Defective glycine receptors are associated with a rare disease that causes an exaggerated startle reflex called hyperekplexia. This produces intense muscle contractions known as hypertonia. The excitatory actions of glutamate are described in more detail in Chapter 8. The inhibitory action of GABA is described in Chapter 5.

Drugs Used to Treat Spasticity

To manage spasticity, a variety of nonpharmaceutical treatments have been tried. Electrical stimulation, cold packs (cryotherapy), biofeedback, splinting, positioning, and physical therapy have all been proposed. These nondrug therapies may support pharmacologic treatments.

Drugs used in the treatment of spasticity are grouped according to the site of action and are classified as central acting and peripheral acting. They are further classified as **antispasmodics** and **spasmolytic** (antispasticity) agents.

Peripheral-acting antispasticity agents act directly on contractile mechanisms in the muscle or the spinal cord. Central-acting antispasmodic and antispasticity drugs decrease muscle spasms through alterations of CNS conduction. They are classified as benzodiazepines and nonbenzodiazepines according to their mechanism of action. Some drugs are GABAergic. They act on GABA receptors in the CNS. Other agents act at α_2-adrenergic receptor sites.

Peripheral-Acting Drugs

Botulinum Toxins

Botulinum toxin types A and B are used for the treatment of cervical dystonia. Cervical dystonia is a painful condition in which the neck muscles contract involuntarily. The toxins have also been studied in the treatment of poststroke spasticity and cerebral palsy. Only botulinum toxin type A is indicated for the treatment of blepharospasms. The toxin is injected locally to inhibit presynaptic release of ACh at the neuromuscular junction. This causes temporary paralysis in the muscle(s) that have received the injections. The onset of effect begins 3 to 7 days after injections are administered and lasts 3 to 6 months. Resistance develops with repeated use and the frequency of injection should be limited to no sooner than every 3 months.

Dantrolene

Dantrolene is indicated for the treatment of spasticity associated with spinal cord injury, stroke, cerebral palsy, multiple sclerosis, and malignant hyperthermia. Malignant hyperthermia causes severe muscle contractions and fever. Dantrolene reduces spasticity by weakening hyperexcited muscles. It acts directly on contractile mechanisms in skeletal muscle. Dantrolene inhibits calcium-dependent excitation-contraction. The use of dantrolene in the treatment of some spastic conditions is limited because the drug produces muscle weakness. Muscle weakness is undesirable when treating spasticity associated with spinal cord injury or ALS. Other adverse effects produced by dantrolene include sedation, fatigue, diarrhea, and hepatotoxicity. Dalfampridine (Ampyra) is a potassium channel blocker that is used to improve walking in patients with multiple sclerosis. The most common side effects are urinary tract infections, insomnia, headache, dizziness, nausea, and weakness.

Central-Acting Drugs

Central-acting antispasmodics and antispasticity agents decrease muscle spasms by actions on CNS conduction. They bind to receptor sites that control motor movement in the brain and spinal cord. The drugs enhance the actions of GABA, an inhibitory neurotransmitter, or stimulate α_2-adrenergic receptors.

GABAergic Drugs

Drugs That Bind Directly to GABA Receptors. Baclofen is indicated for the treatment of spasticity associated with spinal cord injury and multiple sclerosis. Baclofen is structurally similar to the neurotransmitter GABA and is particularly useful in treatment of spasticity associated with spinal cord injury.

Mechanism of Action and Pharmacokinetics. The site of action for baclofen is the spinal cord, where it acts as an agonist at $GABA_B$ receptor sites. It reduces pain linked to spasticity by inhibiting the release of substance P (see Chapter 10). The ability of baclofen to cross the blood-brain barrier is limited, so its effectiveness is augmented by administering the drug intrathecally. Intrathecal solutions are injected directly into the cerebrospinal fluid (CSF). Surgery is required to implant the intrathecal delivery system. The pump needs to be refilled every 1 to 6 months and must be replaced every 5 to 7 years.

Peripheral-Acting Drugs Used for the Treatment of Spasticity

Generic Name	US Brand Name(s) / Canadian Brand(s)	Dosage Forms and Strengths
dalfampridine	Ampyra	**Tablet, extended release:** 10 mg
	Not available	
dantrolene[a]	Dantrium, Revonto Ryanodex	**Capsules:** 25 mg, 50 mg[b], 100 mg[b]
	Dantrium	**Injection, powder for reconstitution:** 20 mg/vial (Dantirum, Revonto), 250 mg/vial (Ryanodex)[b]

[a]Generic available.
[b]Available in the United States only.

Adverse Reactions.   Adverse reactions include dizziness, drowsiness, headache, nausea, orthostatic hypotension, confusion, and weakness. Sudden discontinuation can cause withdrawal symptoms. Rebound spasticity, hallucinations, itching, hyperthermia, and seizures are signs and symptoms of withdrawal syndrome.

Drugs That Enhance GABA Binding.   Diazepam is classified as a central-acting agent because its site of action: the brainstem and the spinal cord. It is the most commonly used benzodiazepine for the treatment of spasticity, and it is effective in treating hyperactive reflexes and painful muscle spasms. It improves range of motion and decreases anxiety and sleeplessness—both conditions can aggravate spasticity. Diazepam is a C-IV controlled substance in the United States and a targeted substance in Canada. A detailed discussion of the pharmacokinetics and adverse reactions of the benzodiazepines is found in Chapters 5 and 9.

α₂-Adrenergic Drugs.   The α₂-adrenergic agonists (e.g., tizanidine) act like naturally occurring neurotransmitters to screen out unnecessary sensory messages that cause spasticity. They reduce muscle tone and the frequency of muscle spasms in people who have had spinal cord injuries, cerebral palsy, and stroke.

Mechanism of Action and Pharmacokinetics.   Spasticity is reduced when drugs like tizanidine are administered because they prevent the release of excitatory neurotransmitters in the spinal cord and increase the actions of the inhibitory neurotransmitter glycine. Painful muscle spasms are diminished because the drugs interfere with the release of substance P, the neurotransmitter involved in the production of pain sensations and pain perception (see Chapter 10).

Adverse Reactions.   Tizanidine produces sedation, hypotension, and dizziness.

> **⊘ Tech Alert!**
>
> diazePAM and dilTIAZem have look-alike/sound-alike issues.

> **● Tech Note!**
>
> Skeletal muscle relaxants should not be combined with alcohol. Alcohol increases the CNS depression produced by the skeletal muscle relaxants, causing excessive drowsiness and decreased alertness.

Central-Acting Drugs Used for the Treatment of Spasticity (Bind to GABA Receptors)

Generic Name	US Brand Name(s) / Canadian Brand(s)	Dosage Forms and Strengths
baclofen[a]	Fleqsuvy, Gablofen, Lioresal, Livispah, Ozobax Lioresal	**Granules:** 5 mg, 10 mg, 20 mg packets **Solution, intrathecal injection:** 0.05 mg/mL, 0.5 mg/mL, 1 mg/mL[b], 2 mg/mL **Solution:** 5 mg/5 mL **Suspension:** 25 mg/5 mL **Tablets:** 10 mg, 20 mg

[a]Generic available.
[b]Available in the United States only.

> **⊘ Tech Alert!**
>
> Carisoprodol is a C-IV controlled substance in the United States.

Central-Acting Drugs Used for the Treatment of Spasticity (α2-Adrenergic Drugs)

Generic Name	US Brand Name(s) / Canadian Brand(s)	Dosage Forms and Strengths
tizanidine[a]	Zanaflex Generics only	**Capsules**[b]**:** 2 mg, 4 mg, 6 mg **Tablets:** 2 mg[b], 4 mg

[a]Generic available.
[b]Available in the United States only.

Central-Acting Drugs Used for the Treatment of Spasticity (Enhance GABA Binding)

	Generic Name	US Brand Name(s) / Canadian Brand(s)	Dosage Forms and Strengths
	diazepam[a]	Diastat, Diazepam Intensol, Valium, Valtoco Diastat, Valium	**Nasal spray (Valtoco)**[b]**:** 5 mg, 7.5 mg, 10 mg/spray **Rectal gel (Diastat):** 5 mg/mL as 2.5 mg, 10 mg, and 20 mg prefilled syringes **Solution, for injection:** 5 mg/mL **Oral, solution**[b]**:** 1 mg/mL **Oral concentrate (Diazepam Intensol)**[b]**:** 5 mg/mL **Tablets (Valium):** 2 mg, 5 mg, 10 mg

[a]Generic available.
[b]Available in the United States only.

Antispasmodics Used to Treat Muscle Strain

Skeletal muscle relaxants are used to treat muscle stiffness, pain, and spasms associated with muscle tension, strain, sprains, or injury. Drugs in this category include carisoprodol, chlorzoxazone, cyclobenzaprine, metaxalone, methocarbamol, and orphenadrine.

These skeletal muscle relaxants are central acting; however, the mechanism of action is unknown. It is believed their actions may be related to their sedative effects on the CNS.

Common adverse effects are dizziness, drowsiness, and blurred vision. Additional adverse effects are discoloration of urine—chlorzoxazone (orange to reddish purple) and methocarbamol (black, brown, or green).

Skeletal muscle relaxants should be used along with nonpharmaceutical therapies such as rest, exercise, cryotherapy, heat, and physical therapy.

Central-Acting Drugs Used for the Treatment of Muscle Strain

	Generic Name	US Brand Name(s) / Canadian Brand(s)	Dosage Forms and Strengths
	carisoprodol[a]	Soma	**Tablets:** 250 mg, 350 mg
		Not available	
	chlorzoxazone[a]	Generics	**Tablets:** 250 mg, 375 mg, 500 mg, 750 mg
		Not available	
	cyclobenzaprine[a]	Amrix	**Capsules, extended release (Amrix):** 15 mg, 30 mg
		Flexeril	**Tablets:** 5 mg[b], 7.5 mg[b], 10 mg
	metaxalone[a]	Skelaxin	**Tablets:** 400 mg, 800 mg
		Not available	
	methocarbamol[a]	Robaxin	**Tablets:** 500 mg, 750 mg
		Robaxin, Robaxin-750	**Solution, for injection**[b]: 100 mg/mL
	orphenadrine[a]	Generics	**Solution, for injection**[b]: 30 mg/mL (2 mL)
		Generics	**Tablets, extended release:** 100 mg

Combination Products

	Generic Name	Canadian Brand(s)	Dosage Forms and Strengths
	chlorzoxazone + acetaminophen	Not available	**Tablets:** 250 mg chlorzoxazone + 300 mg acetaminophen
		Acetazone Forte, Back Aid Forte[c]	
	chlorzoxazone + acetaminophen + codeine	Not available	**Tablets:** 250 mg chlorzoxazone + 300 mg acetaminophen + 8 mg codeine
		Acetazone Forte C8	
	methocarbamol + aspirin	Not available	**Tablets:** 400 mg methocarbamol + 325 mg aspirin; 400 mg methocarbamol + 500 mg aspirin
		Extra Strength Muscle and Backache Relief with ASA[c], Robaxisal Extra Strength[c]	
	methocarbamol + aspirin + codeine	Not available	**Tablets:** 400 mg methocarbamol + 325 mg aspirin + 16.2 mg codeine; 400 mg methocarbamol + 325 mg aspirin + 32.4 mg codeine
		Robaxisal C¼, Robaxisal C½	
	methocarbamol + acetaminophen	Not available	**Tablets:** 400 mg methocarbamol + 325 mg acetaminophen; 400 mg methocarbamol + 500 mg acetaminophen
		Extra Strength Tylenol Back Pain[c], Extra Strength Tylenol Body Pain Night[c], Robaxacet, Robaxacet Extra Strength[c]	

Central-Acting Drugs Used for the Treatment of Muscle Strain—cont'd

Generic Name	US Brand Name(s) / Canadian Brand(s)	Dosage Forms and Strengths
methocarbamol + acetaminophen + codeine	Not available / Robaxacet-8	400 mg methocarbamol + 325 mg acetaminophen + 8 mg codeine
methocarbamol + ibuprofen	Not available / Motrin Platinum Muscle and Body[c], Robax Platinum[c]	**Tablets:** 500 mg methocarbamol + 200 mg ibuprofen
orphenadrine + caffeine + aspirin	Orphengesic, Orphengesic Forte / Not available	**Tablets:** 25 mg orphenadrine + 30 mg caffeine + 385 mg aspirin; 50 mg orphenadrine + 60 mg caffeine + 770 mg aspirin

[a]Generic available.
[b]Available in the United States only.
[c]Over the counter in Canada.

Summary of Drugs Used in the Treatment of Spasticity

Generic Name	US Brand Name	Usual Adult Oral Dose and Dosing Schedule	Warning Labels
Central-Acting Skeletal Muscle Relaxants			
baclofen	Lioresal	**Oral:** 5 mg 3 times a day (maximum, 80 mg/day)	MAY CAUSE DIZZINESS OR DROWSINESS. MAY IMPAIR ABILITY TO DRIVE. AVOID ALCOHOL. TAKE WITH FOOD—baclofen. MAY DISCOLOR URINE—chlorzoxazone, methocarbamol. MAY BE HABIT FORMING—diazepam. SWALLOW WHOLE; DO NOT CRUSH OR CHEW—cyclobenzaprine, orphenadrine extended release.
carisoprodol	Soma	250–350 mg 4 times a day	
chlorzoxazone	Generics	250–350 mg 3 times a day and at bedtime	
cyclobenzaprine	Generics	5–10 mg 3 times a day (immediate release); 15–30 mg once daily (extended release)	
diazepam	Valium	**Oral:** 2–10 mg 3–4 times a day **IM or IV:** 5–10 mg every 3–4 hours if needed	
metaxalone	Skelaxin	800 mg 3–4 times a day	
methocarbamol	Robaxin	**Oral:** 1.5 g 4 times a day (up to 8 g/day) for 48 h then 750 mg orally every 4 h, 1.5 g 3 times a day, or 1 g 4 times a day	
orphenadrine	Generics	**Oral:** 100 mg twice a day	
tizanidine	Zanaflex	2–4 mg 1–3 times a day (maximum, 36 mg/day)	
Direct-Acting Skeletal Muscle Relaxants			
dantrolene	Dantrium	25–100 mg 3 times a day	MAY CAUSE DIZZINESS OR DROWSINESS. MAY IMPAIR ABILITY TO DRIVE. AVOID ALCOHOL. PROTECT FROM LIGHT AND MOISTURE.

❶ Tech Alert!

Nonprescription skeletal muscle relaxants containing codeine (e.g., Robaxacet-8) are Schedule II, exempt narcotics in Canada. Pharmacist intervention is required to obtain access.

TECHNICIAN'S CORNER

1. Why does the blood-brain barrier prevent some drugs from entering the brain?
2. You are in charge of inventory in the pharmacy and need to alert everyone about the potential of medication errors that can occur with neuromuscular blocking drugs. What medication error prevention strategies would you share with your pharmacy colleagues?

Key Points

- Skeletal muscles contract as a response to messages transmitted between peripheral nerves and muscles by neurotransmitters.
- Acetylcholine (ACh) is the primary neurotransmitter that sends messages between nerve cells and muscle cells.
- The release of ACh produces skeletal muscle contraction. Calcium increases ACh release. Drugs that block nerve transmission between the motor end plate and skeletal muscle receptors are classified as *peripheral-acting muscle relaxants*.
- Skeletal muscle relaxants that work by central nervous system depression (i.e., block nerve transmission between the spinal cord and muscles) are called *central-acting muscle relaxants*.
- Drugs that decrease the release of ACh or deplete ACh levels in the neuron cause skeletal muscle relaxation.
- Anticholinesterase drugs (e.g., neostigmine) reverse the effects of neuromuscular blocking drugs.
- Care must be taken when transcribing and filling orders for neuromuscular blocking drugs because they can cause severe injury or death.
- The vial lids of the neuromuscular blocking drug must be clearly marked "Paralyzing Agent" or "Warning: Paralyzing Agent."
- Neuromuscular blocking drugs are classified "high alert" by the Interdisciplinary Safe Medication Use Expert Committee of the US Pharmacopoeia because improper use can result in permanent injury, respiratory arrest, and death.
- Problems associated with neuromuscular blocking drugs can be avoided by proper product selection, storage conditions, and labeling; appropriate dosing; and patient monitoring.

- Spasticity is a debilitating motor disorder. It interferes with the normal performance of activities of daily living.
- Stroke, spinal cord injury, cerebral palsy, muscle trauma, multiple sclerosis, head injury, and amyotrophic lateral sclerosis can cause spasticity.
- There are four phases to the development of spasticity: (1) decreased muscle contractility; (2) excessive muscle tone and increased reflex activity lasting from days to years; (3) decreased reflex excitability; and (4) stiff, contracted muscles.
- Nonpharmaceutical treatments of spasticity are electrical stimulation, cold packs (cryotherapy), biofeedback, splinting, positioning, and physical therapy.
- Skeletal muscle relaxants are used to treat muscle stiffness, pain, and spasms associated with muscle tension, strain, sprains, or injury.
- Drugs used in the treatment of spasticity are grouped according to the site of action and are classified as central acting and peripheral acting.
- Peripheral-acting drugs act at the neuromuscular junction or directly on contractile mechanisms in the muscle.
- Dantrolene is a peripheral-acting drug that acts directly on contractile mechanisms in skeletal muscle.
- Baclofen is a central-acting drug that looks and acts like GABA, a naturally occurring neurotransmitter.

Review Questions

1. The neurotransmitter that is primarily responsible for transmitting messages between nerve cells and muscle cells is _____.
   a. dopamine
   b. epinephrine
   c. acetylcholine
   d. GABA
2. You prepare a solution of Botox. The solution should be _____.
   a. stored at room temperature until use
   b. stored in the refrigerator until use
   c. discarded if not used within 12 hours
   d. stored in the freezer
3. Botox has not been approved by the FDA for cosmetic use.
   a. true
   b. false

4. Most neuromuscular blocking drugs are poorly absorbed from the gastrointestinal tract so they are administered _____.
   a. topically
   b. enterally
   c. parenterally
   d. transdermally
5. _____ is the most commonly used benzodiazepine for the treatment of spasticity, and it is effective in treating hyperactive reflexes and painful muscle spasms.
   a. Alprazolam
   b. Diazepam
   c. Clonazepam
   d. Lorazepam

6. Neuromuscular blocking drugs are classified "_____" by the Interdisciplinary Safe Medication Use Expert Committee of the USP.
   a. dangerous
   b. high alert
   c. low alert
   d. use with caution
7. Where should most neuromuscular blocking drugs be stored?
   a. in alphabetical order on the shelf
   b. with the oral solutions
   c. with the fast movers
   d. apart from other drugs
8. Neuromuscular blocking drugs should always be dispensed with what auxiliary label?
   a. WARNING: Paralyzing agent. (Use requires mechanical ventilatory assistance.)
   b. WARNING: Allergic reactions possible.
   c. KEEP IN REFRIGERATOR UNTIL READY TO USE.
   d. FOR ONE TIME USE ONLY.

9. The effect of botulinum toxins in reducing spasticity lasts up to _____.
   a. 2 weeks
   b. 4 weeks
   c. 8 weeks
   d. 12 weeks
10. Medication errors can easily happen with nondepolarizing neuromuscular blocking drugs because _____.
   a. all packages look the same
   b. some drugs have look-alike/sound-alike names
   c. doses are all the same
   d. all are made by same manufacturer

Bibliography

Adams MM, Hicks AL. Spasticity after spinal cord injury. *Spinal Cord.* 2005;43:577–586.

Gallichio J. Pharmacologic management of spasticity following stroke. *Phys Ther.* 2004;84:973–981.

Health Canada. (2022). Drug Product Database. Retrieved September 3, 2022, from https://health-products.canada.ca/dpd-bdpp/index-eng.jsp.

Honda M, Sekiguchi Y, Sato N, et al. Involvement of imidazoline receptors in the centrally acting muscle-relaxant effects of tizanidine. *Eur J Pharmacol.* 2002;445:187–193.

Institute for Safe Medication Practices. (2016). FDA and ISMP Lists of Look-Alike Drug Names with Recommended Tall Man Letters. Retrieved July 20, 2022, from https://www.ismp.org/recommendations/tall-man-letters-list.

Institute for Safe Medication Practices. (2019). List of Confused Drugs. Retrieved July 20, 2022, from https://www.ismp.org/tools/confused-drugnames.pdf.

ISMP. Neuromuscular blocking agents: sustaining packaging improvements over time, *ISMP Canada Safety Bull.* 14(7), 2014. Retrieved September 19, 2022, from https://ismpcanada.ca/wp-content/uploads/ISMPCSB2014-7_NeuromuscularBlockingAgents.pdf.

Kalant H, Grant D, Mitchell J. *Principles of medical pharmacology.* ed 7. Toronto: Elsevier Canada, A Division of Reed Elsevier Canada; 2007:176–180.

Lewis C. Botox cosmetic: a look at looking good, U.S. Food and Drug Administration, FDA Consumer Magazine. Retrieved September 19, 2022, from https://permanent.access.gpo.gov/lps1609/www.fda.gov/fdac/features/2002/402_botox.html.

Matthey P, Wang P, Finegan B, et al. Rocuronium anaphylaxis and multiple neuromuscular blocking drug sensitivities. *CJA.* 2000;47(9):890–893.

Mehta S, Burry L, Fischer S, et al. Canadian survey of the use of sedatives, analgesics, and neuromuscular blocking agents in critically ill patients. *Crit Care Med.* 2006;34:374–380.

Ozcakir S, Sivrioglu K. Botulinum toxin in poststroke spasticity. *Clin Med Res.* 2007;5(2):132–138.

Patel D, Soyode O. Pharmacologic interventions for reducing spasticity in cerebral palsy. *Indian J Pediatr.* 2005;72:869–872.

Phillips M, Williams R. Improving the safety of neuromuscular blocking agents: a statement from the USP Safe Medication Use Expert Committee. *Am J Health Syst Pharm.* 2006;63:139–142.

U.S. Food and Drug Administration. (nd). Drugs@FDA: FDA Approved Drug Products. Retrieved September 3, 2022, from https://www.accessdata.fda.gov/scripts/cder/daf/index.cfm.

USP Center for Advancement of Patient Safety: Use caution–avoid confusion, USP Quality Review No. 79, Rockville, MD, April 2004, USP Center for Advancement of Patient Safety.

Witenko C, Moorman-Li R, Motycka C, et al. Considerations for the appropriate use of skeletal muscle relaxants for the management of acute low back pain. *P T.* 2014;39(6):427–435.

Zafonte R, Lombard L, Elovic E. Antispasticity medications: uses and limitations of enteral therapy. *Am J Phys Med Rehabil.* 2004;83(Suppl):S50–S58.

13

Treatment of Gout, Osteoarthritis, and Rheumatoid Arthritis

LEARNING OBJECTIVES

1. Learn the terminology associated with drugs used in the treatment of gout, osteoarthritis, and rheumatoid arthritis.
2. Describe the signs and symptoms of gout, osteoarthritis, and rheumatoid arthritis.
3. List and classify medications used in the treatment of gout, osteoarthritis, and rheumatoid arthritis.
4. Describe the mechanism of action for each class of drugs used in the treatment of gout, osteoarthritis, and rheumatoid arthritis.
5. Identify warning labels and precautionary messages associated with medications used in the treatment of gout, osteoarthritis, and rheumatoid arthritis.

KEY TERMS

Arthritis An inflammatory condition that produces joint pain.
Autoantibody Abnormal antibody that attacks healthy cells and tissue.
Autoimmune disease A disease that occurs when the immune system turns against the parts of the body it is designed to protect.
Gout A disease characterized by deposits of urate crystals in the joints that produces inflammation. It is caused by hyperuricemia.
Hyperuricemia A condition in which urate levels build up in the blood.

Rheumatoid arthritis Chronic disease characterized by inflammation and remodeling of the joints.
Rheumatoid factor Immunoglobulin (antibody) that is present in many people who have rheumatoid arthritis.
Synovium Thin layer of tissue that lines the joint space.
Tumor necrosis factor Inflammatory cytokine released as part of the immune response and found in synovial fluid of people with rheumatoid arthritis.
Urates Product of purine metabolism. Urate crystals may accumulate in joints and produce inflammation and pain.
Uricosuric Drug that increases the renal clearance of urates.

Overview

Gout, also called gouty arthritis, is a disease that is associated with hyperuricemia. *Hyperuricemia* is a condition in which urate levels build up in the blood serum. *Urates* are the product of the metabolism of purines. Population studies show that the prevalence of hyperuricemia in men is greater than in women until menopause; then the rates equalize. Before puberty, boys and girls both have low serum urate levels.

Gout affects approximately 3.9% of the population in the United States and 2.4% of the population in Canada. It is more common in men and older adults. Hyperuricemia and gout are also associated with cardiovascular disease, hyperlipidemia, kidney disease, and hypertension. It is likely that the relationship between hypertension and hyperuricemia is attributable to decreased renal clearance resulting in accumulation of urate. Hyperuricemia increases the risk of coronary heart disease and stroke partly because of its role in producing hyperlipidemia. Hyperlipidemia causes atherosclerosis, a buildup of lipids in arteries that leads to clogged arteries. Hyperuricemia worsens heart failure.

Hyperuricemia is a risk factor for diabetes and is associated with increased insulin resistance. Obesity increases the risk for gout. Weight loss reduces hyperuricemia and insulin resistance. Hyperuricemia can cause kidney disease and make preexisting kidney disease worse. Exposure to lead in the environment can also increase the risk for development of gout.

Pathophysiology of Gout

Gout is characterized by a buildup of urate crystals in joints where they produce inflammation and pain. Deposits of uric acid are called *tophi* (singular, tophus) and look like lumps under the skin around the joints and at the rim of the ear (Fig. 13.1).

The joints most affected are the big toe, foot, ankle, knee, wrist, finger, and elbow. Consumption of foods or beverages high in dietary purines can produce a flare-up of gout symptoms.

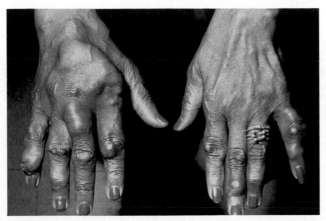

• **Fig. 13.1** Gouty arthritis. (From Swartz MH. *Textbook of physical diagnosis*, ed 7, Philadelphia, 2014, Elsevier.)

Antiinflammatory Drugs Used in the Treatment of Gout

Generic Name	US Brand Name(s) Canadian Brand(s)	Dosage Forms and Strengths
colchicine[a]	Colcrys, Gloperba, Mitigare M infla	**Capsule (Mitigare):** 0.6 mg **Solution, oral (Gloperba):** 0.6 mg/5 mL **Tablets:** 0.6 mg **Tablets, extended release (Myinfla):** 0.5 mg

[a]Generic available.

Uricosurics Used in the Treatment of Gout

Generic Name	US Brand Name(s) Canadian Brand(s)	Dosage Forms and Strengths
probenecid[a]	Generics Not Available	**Tablets:** 500 mg
Combination		
probenecid + colchine[a]	Generics Not available	**Tablets:** 500 mg probenecid + 0.5 mg colchicine

[a]Generic available.

• **BOX 13.1**   **Purine Content of Foods**

Foods considered high in purine content include:
- Alcoholic beverages
- Fish, seafood, and shellfish, including anchovies, sardines, herring, mussels, codfish, scallops, trout, and haddock
- Meats, such as bacon, turkey, veal, and venison, and organ meats such as liver and sweetbreads

Foods considered moderate in purine content include:
- Meats such as beef, chicken, duck, pork, and ham
- Crab, lobster, oysters, and shrimp
- Vegetables and beans such as asparagus, cauliflower, kidney beans, lentils, lima beans, peas, mushrooms, and spinach
- Grains: oatmeal, whole wheat bread, and cereal

Foods considered low in purine content include:
- Dairy products: skim milk and cheese
- Eggs
- Fruit and most vegetables (except those listed above)
- Grains: enriched bread and cereal

For example, beer consumption increases the risk of an acute attack, perhaps because beer contains high levels of purine (Box 13.1).

Some people with gout will experience sharp needlelike painful symptoms, but some people will have no symptoms at all. Acute gout attacks usually resolve spontaneously in 7 to 10 days without treatment; however, people with symptoms may benefit from treatment. Chronic gout is a condition in which there is persistent presence of uric acid crystals in and around the joint. The uric acid crystals may form disfiguring tophi (clumps of uric acid crystals) around the joint. Chronic gout that develops over years may cause permanent joint or kidney damage.

Drugs Used to Treat Gout

Drugs prescribed for the treatment of gout include antiinflammatory and urate-lowering drugs. Urate-lowering therapy includes the administration of uricosurics and inhibitors of uric acid synthesis. Colchicine is an antiinflammatory drug and one of the oldest agents used to treat gout. It is extracted from the autumn crocus plant. It may be used to treat or prevent symptoms. Colchicine penetrates inflammatory cells and inhibits their ability to respond to irritation. Colchicine is most effective if taken at the first signs of an acute gout attack. Common adverse reactions associated with the use of colchicine include nausea, vomiting, and diarrhea. Rare serious adverse reactions are bone marrow suppression and renal failure.

Uricosurics

A *uricosuric* is a drug the increases the renal clearance of urates. Urate-lowering drugs are indicated for patients who experience frequent attacks of gout (more than 2 or 3 attacks per year) to prevent further gout attacks. Probenecid is a uricosuric that inhibits the reabsorption of uric acid in the renal tubules and thereby promotes the elimination of urates. Nausea, vomiting, and worsening of preexisting kidney stones are adverse reactions to probenecid.

> ● *Tech Note!*
>
> Thiazide diuretics (e.g., hydrochlorothiazide) and low-dose aspirin are known to increase urate levels.

Inhibitors of Uric Acid Synthesis
Xanthine Oxidase Inhibitors

Xanthine oxidase inhibitors block the final enzymatic step in the synthesis of uric acid. Allopurinol and febuxostat are xanthine

Inhibitors of Uric Acid Synthesis

Generic Name	US Brand Name(s) Canadian Brand(s)	Dosage Forms and Strengths
allopurinol[a]	Aloprim, Lopurin, Zyloprim Zyloprim	**Injection, powder for reconstitution (Aloprim)**[b]: 500 mg **Tablet (Zyloprim)**: 100 mg, 200 mg[c], 300 mg
febuxostat[a]	Uloric Generics	**Tablets:** 40 mg[b], 80 mg

[a]Generic available.
[b]Available in the United States only.
[c]Available in Canada only.

oxidase inhibitors. Allopurinol is readily absorbed when administered orally and is easily eliminated in the urine. Nausea, drowsiness, headache, diarrhea, and an itchy skin rash are adverse reactions linked to allopurinol use. Febuxostat (Uloric) is more selective than allopurinol. Gout flare-ups have been reported when febuxostat therapy is initiated. Common adverse reactions are nausea, vomiting, headache, diarrhea, and changes in appetite. Serious adverse events that have been reported with febuxostat include myocardial infarction, stroke, and atrial fibrillation. Patients are advised to report muscle pain, an early sign of rhabdomyolysis—a breakdown of muscle tissue that can lead to acute renal failure.

Metabolism of Uric Acid

Recombinant Urate Oxidase Enzymes

Recombinant urate oxidase enzymes lower uric acid levels by metabolizing uric acid to the water-soluble benign purine metabolite allantoin, which is excreted in the urine. Pegloticase (Krystexxa) has been approved by the US Food and Drug Administration (FDA) for patients with chronic gout. Rasburicase (Elitek, Fasturtek) is indicated for the treatment of hyperuricemia in patients receiving chemotherapy who have elevated uric acid. Pegloticase and rasburicase are administered intravenously. Patients may experience infusion reactions such as rash, itching, redness, and anaphylaxis. Additional adverse reactions of pegloticase include nausea and vomiting, constipation or diarrhea, fatigue, arthralgia, upper respiratory infection, fever, heart failure, and hypotension.

Nonpharmacologic Therapy for Gout

Prevention tips include weight loss and consumption of a low purine diet. The purine content of selected food is shown in Box 13.1. Foods high in purines are meat (especially liver), fish (anchovies), dried beans, peas, and gravy. Beer and spirits are also known to increase purine levels. Low-fat dairy products have low purine levels. Rest and applying ice packs for acute attacks are helpful.

Osteoarthritis

Arthritis is a condition that produces joint pain. Inflammation of the fluid that surrounds the joint (synovial fluid) contributes

Recombinant Urate Oxidase Inhibitors

Generic Name	US Brand Name(s) Canadian Brand(s)	Dosage Forms and Strengths
pegloticase	Krystexxa Not available	**Solution, for IV infusion:** 8 mg/mL
rasburicase	Elitek Fasturtek	**Powder, for injection:** 1.5 mg/vial

IV, intravenous.

to the pain associated with osteoarthritis. Osteoarthritis is the most common of all arthritic conditions. It is the leading cause of musculoskeletal pain. Symptoms of osteoarthritis are joint pain, stiffness, swelling, and crepitus (creaking joints). Pain may occur after activity or at rest. Risk factors for osteoarthritis are previous joint injury or surgery, obesity, increasing age, muscle weakness, and occupations that involve excessive joint use.

Acetaminophen, aspirin, and nonsteroidal antiinflammatory drugs (NSAIDs) are used to control pain.

Nonsteroidal Antiinflammatory Drugs

The principal antiinflammatory drugs used for the treatment of acute gout and osteoarthritis are NSAIDs and corticosteroids. The most prescribed NSAID for gout is indomethacin; however, ibuprofen, ketoprofen, and naproxen are also administered. The cyclooxygenase-2 (COX-2) inhibitor celecoxib may also be prescribed for the treatment of acute gout. Celecoxib remains the only COX-2 inhibitor available for sale in the United States and Canada. As per FDA requirements, manufacturers of all NSAIDs must print a boxed warning in the package insert describing the risk for cardiovascular toxicity and gastrointestinal (GI) ulceration. The mechanism of action, pharmacokinetics, and additional adverse reactions for NSAIDS are discussed in Chapter 10.

Usual Dosage and Warnings for Drugs Used in the Treatment of Gout

	Generic Name	US Brand Name	Usual Adult Oral Dose and Dosing Schedule	Warning Labels
Antiinflammatory				
	colchicine	Generics	**Oral, prevention:** 0.6 mg 1–2 times/day, may decrease to 0.6 mg 3 times a week; Extended release: 0.5 mg once daily **Oral, acute attack:** 1.2 mg at first sign of flare-up followed by 0.6 mg in 1 h (maximum, 1.8 mg over 1 h)	AVOID ALCOHOL. TAKE WITH A LOT OF WATER.
Uricosuric				
	probenecid	Generics	250 mg twice daily for 1 week, followed by 500 mg twice daily (maximum 2000 mg/day)	TAKE WITH FOOD. TAKE WITH 8 OZ WATER. AVOID ASPIRIN.
Inhibitors of Uric Acid Synthesis				
	allopurinol	Zyloprim	**Gout:** 200–600 mg/day orally (start 100 mg/day; increase weekly)	TAKE WITH FOOD. AVOID ALCOHOL. MAY CAUSE DIZZINESS OR DROWSINESS. TAKE WITH A LOT OF WATER (10–12 GLASSES/DAY).
	febuxostat	Uloric	**Hyperuricemia, gout:** 40–80 mg/day	TAKE WITH A GLASS OF WATER.
Recombinant Urate Oxidase Enzyme				
	pegloticase	Krystexxa	**Chronic gout:** 8 mg IV over 2 h every 2 weeks	MIX BY GENTLY INVERTING IV BAG; DO NOT SHAKE. REFRIGERATE DILUTED SOLUTION. USE WITHIN 4 HOURS OF RECONSTITUTION—pegloticase.
	rasburicase	Elitek, Fasturtec	**Hyperuricemia (with malignancy):** 0.2 mg/kg as a 30-min infusion once daily for up to 5 days	

IV, intravenous.

Nonsteroidal Antiinflammatory Drugs

Generic Name	US Brand Name Canadian Brands	Dosage Forms and Strengths
celecoxib[a]	Celebrex Celebrex	**Capsule:** 50 mg[b], 100 mg, 200 mg, 400 mg[b]
indomethacin[a]	Indocin Generics	**Capsule:** 25 mg, 50 mg **Powder for injection:** 1 mg base/vial **Suppository:** 50 mg, 100 mg[c] **Suspension, oral use:** 25 mg/5 mL
ibuprofen[a]	Advil, Motrin, Caldolor Advil, Motrin	**Drops**[d]**:** 50 mg/1.25 mL, 100 mg/2.5 mL **Capsule:** 200 mg[d] **Solution, for IV**[b]**:** 4 mg/mL, 100 mg/mL **Suspension, oral**[d]**:** 100 mg/5 mL **Tablets, chewable:** 50 mg 100 mg[b,d] **Tablets:** 100 mg[d], 200 mg[d], 300 mg[e], 400 mg, 600 mg, 800 mg[b]
ketoprofen[a]	Generics Generics	**Capsule:** 50 mg **Capsule, extended release**[b]**:** 200 mg **Tablet, enteric coated**[c]**:** 50 mg, 100 mg **Tablet, extended release**[c]**:** 200 mg

Continued

Nonsteroidal Antiinflammatory Drugs—cont'd

Generic Name	US Brand Name / Canadian Brands	Dosage Forms and Strengths
naproxen[a]	Naprosyn, EC-Naprosyn	**Suspension**: 25 mg/mL[d]
	Naprosyn	**Tablet**: 250 mg, 375 mg, 500 mg
		Tablet, extended release[c]: 750 mg
		Tablet, delayed release (EC-Naprosyn): 375 mg, 500 mg
naproxen Na[+a]	Aleve, Anaprox DS, Naprelen	**Capsule (Liquid gel)**: 220 mg[d]
	Aleve, Aleve Back and Body Pain, Aleve Liquid Gels, Anaprox, Anaprox DS, Maxidol Liquid Gels	**Tablet**: 200 mg[b,d], 220 mg[c,d], 275 mg, 550 mg (Anaprox DS)
		Tablet, extended release (Naprelen): 375 mg, 500 mg, 750 mg

[a]Generic available.
[b]Available in the United States only.
[c]Available in Canada only.
[d]Over the counter.
[e]Over the counter in Canada only.

❶ Tech Alert!

The following drugs have look-alike/sound-alike issues:

CeleBREX, CeleXA, and Cerebyx

Rheumatoid Arthritis

Rheumatoid arthritis (RA) is an *autoimmune disease* that is characterized by inflammation of the lining of the joints. An autoimmune disease occurs when the immune system turns against the parts of the body it is designed to protect. The body attacks its own cells, thinking they are germs or a harmful substance. No one knows exactly why autoimmunity develops. It is believed that several factors may be involved. The trigger may be exposure to a virus, environmental toxins, the sun, drugs, genetics, air pollution, cigarette smoking, diet, obesity, hormonal changes or pregnancy, or some combination of any of these things. What is known is that autoimmunity can affect any organ of the body.

In addition to chronic inflammation, RA produces pain, joint damage, and disability. According to the National Institutes of Health (2021), 1.3 million Americans have RA. One in every 1000 Canadian women and 0.8 per 1000 men is living with RA, according to the Public Health Agency of Canada (2020). Globally, RA is more common in women than in men. Although children have been diagnosed with juvenile RA, the onset of the disease is usually between 30 and 50 years. The rate of development of the condition increases with age.

Most people who have RA have high levels of *rheumatoid factor* (RF), an immunoglobulin (antibody) that regulates other antibodies made by the body. RF is not specific to RA, so its presence is only part of the diagnosis for RA but is not a definitive diagnostic tool. Individuals who have RA may also have high levels of the antibody anti–cyclic citrullinated peptide. It may appear in the blood before RA symptoms develop and thus is an early diagnostic tool.

There are three distinct phases of the disease. In phase 1, the joint lining *(synovium)* or synovial membrane becomes inflamed, causing swelling, pain, and stiffness (Fig. 13.2). In phase 2, rapid cell growth causes the synovium to thicken. In phase 3, inflamed

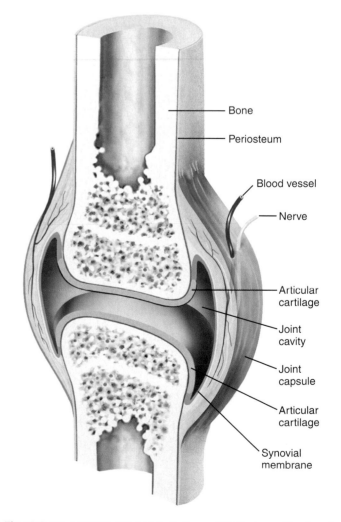

• **Fig. 13.2** Synovial joint. (From Vidic B, Suarez FR. *Photographic atlas of the human body*, St Louis, 1984, Mosby.)

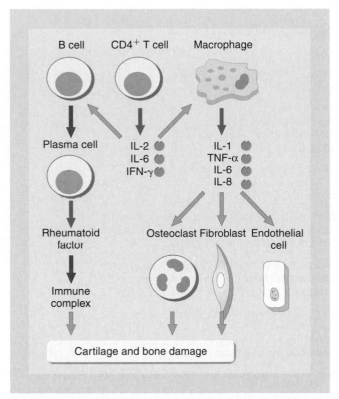

• **Fig. 13.3** Cytokine network in the pathogenesis of rheumatoid arthritis. (From Page C, Curtis M, Sutter M, et al. *Integrated pharmacology*, ed 3, Philadelphia, 2006, Mosby.)

cells in the synovium release enzymes that digest bone and cartilage. Over time, the joint becomes weakened, and ligaments, muscles, and tendons fail to adequately support the affected joint. This results in more pain and disability.

The damaging, chronic cycle of inflammation is stimulated by proinflammatory cytokines (Fig. 13.3) such as interleukins (e.g., IL-1b, IL-6, IL-18, CCL20) and *tumor necrosis factor* (TNF-α). RA causes more than joint problems. Other symptoms of RA are fatigue, weakness, flu-like symptoms, nodules that form under the skin, muscle pain, decreased appetite, depression, and dry mouth.

RA and other autoimmune diseases that affect the musculoskeletal system are treated using pharmacologic and non-pharmacologic therapies. Drug therapy is aimed at suppressing inflammation, pain, and immune system response. Drugs that are used to suppress inflammation and reduce joint swelling and pain include glucocorticosteroids (e.g., dexamethasone and prednisone), NSAIDs (e.g., celecoxib and naproxen), and salicylates (aspirin).

Disease-modifying antirheumatic drugs (DMARDs) are an important group of drugs that slow the progression of RA. Azathioprine and methotrexate (immunosuppressive drugs), hydroxychloroquine (an antimalarial drug), sulfasalazine, and leflunomide are examples of DMARDS. Biologic response modifiers include TNF inhibitors (e.g., adalimumab, certolizumab, etanercept, golimumab, and infliximab), IL antagonists (e.g., anakinra), and the antimalarial drug hydroxychloroquine. Janus kinase inhibitors (e.g., tofacitinib and baricitinib) are prescribed when other therapies have been nonresponsive.

Glucocorticosteroids

Glucocorticosteroids are prescribed to suppress inflammation, reduce flare-ups, and treat pain associated with RA. Oral prednisone and intraarticular injections of corticosteroids may sometimes be given when only one or two joints are involved. Glucocorticosteroids have immunosuppressive actions, and they inhibit the synthesis of antibodies that are responsible for attacking the body's healthy cells. They decrease the accumulation of cells that mobilize to fight when the body believes it is under attack, such as leukocytes and T cells. They interfere with the binding of antibodies to receptor sites on the cell surface. Glucocorticosteroids are potent antiinflammatory drugs too. They decrease the synthesis of proinflammatory substances—prostaglandins (see Chapter 10), leukotrienes, cytokines, arachidonic acid, and macrophages—that are released as part of the inflammatory response and cause swelling, pain, irritation, and other effects. Glucocorticosteroids may also be prescribed for the treatment of ulcerative colitis (Chapter 22), allergic reactions (Chapter 24), cerebral edema, and septic shock or used as a diagnostic agent for endocrine disorders.

Pharmacokinetics

The absorption, distribution, metabolism, and elimination of glucocorticosteroids vary according to the dosage form administered. In general, oral dosage forms are well absorbed in the GI tract and are readily distributed. Metabolism occurs in the liver. Glucocorticosteroids are eliminated in urine.

Adverse Reactions

The adverse effects produced by glucocorticosteroids are numerous and affect all body systems. In the CNS, they cause insomnia and euphoria. In the cardiovascular system, they produce edema and hypertension. In the endocrine system, they may produce hyperglycemia, leading to diabetes. Short-term use of glucocorticosteroids can also cause nausea and weight gain. Other adverse drug effects are osteoporosis, acne, cataracts, poor wound healing, increased risk of infection, and ulceration in the GI tract.

Precautions

Glucocorticosteroids may initially produce muscle weakness. This is a serious problem for people with myasthenia gravis, given that muscle weakness is a symptom of the disease. Glucocorticoid immunosuppressive effects are important to their therapeutic action; however, immunosuppression increases the risk for infections and leads to poor wound healing. Alternate-day therapy can minimize some adverse effects caused by glucocorticosteroids. Long-term use of glucocorticosteroids may increase the need for potassium; vitamins A, B_6, C, and D; folate; calcium; zinc; and phosphorous supplementation.

Disease-Modifying Antirheumatic Drugs

DMARDs slow the disease progression of RA rather than provide symptomatic relief. DMARDs described in this chapter include

Glucocorticosteroids Used in the Treatment of Rheumatoid Arthritis

Generic Name	US Brand Name(s) / Canadian Brand(s)	Dosage Forms and Strengths
dexamethasone[a]	Generics Generics	**Elixir:** 0.5 mg/5 mL **Oral concentrate**[b]: 1 mg/mL **Solution, injection:** 4 mg/mL, 10 mg/mL **Tablet:** 0.5 mg, 0.75 mg, 1 mg[b], 1.5 mg[b], 2 mg, 4 mg, 6 mg[b], 20 mg[b]
hydrocortisone[a]	Cortef, Solu-Cortef Cortef, Solu-Cortef	**Injection, powder for reconstitution (Solu-Cortef):** 100 mg, 250 mg, 500 mg, 1000 mg **Tablets:** 5 mg[b], 10 mg, 20 mg
methylprednisolone[a]	A-Methapred, Depo-Medrol, Medrol, Solu-Medrol Depo-Medrol, Medrol, Solu-Medrol	**Suspension, injection:** 20 mg/mL, 40 mg/mL, 80 mg/mL **Powder, for injection:** 40 mg/vial, 125 mg/vial, 500 mg/vial, 1 g/vial, 2 g/vial[b] **Tablet:** 2 mg[b], 4 mg, 8 mg[b], 16 mg, 32 mg[b]
prednisone[a]	Prednisone Intensol, Rayos Winpred	**Solution, for oral use (Prednisone Intensol):** 5 mg/mL **Tablet, delayed release (Rayos)**[b]: 1 mg, 2 mg, 5 mg **Tablet:** 1 mg, 2.5 mg[b], 5 mg, 10 mg[b], 20 mg[b], 50 mg
prednisolone[a]	Orapred ODT, Pediapred, Prelone Pediapred	**Solution, oral (Pediapred):** 5 mg/5 mL **Syrup (Prelone):** 15 mg/5 mL[b] **Tablet**[b]: 5 mg **Tablet, disintegrating**[b]: 10 mg, 15 mg, 30 mg
triamcinolone[a]	Kenalog-10, Kenalog-40, Kenalog-80, Zilretta Kenalog-10, Kenalog-40	**Suspension, extended release; intraarticular injection (Zilretta)**[b]: 32 mg/vial **Suspension, injectable:** 5 mg/mL[b], 10 mg/mL, 20 mg/mL[b], 40 mg/mL, 80 mg/mL[b]

[a]Generic available.
[b]Available in the United States only.

selected immunosuppressives, TNF inhibitors, IL antagonists, janus kinase (JAK) inhibitors, antimalarials, leflunomide, penicillamine, and sulfasalazine.

Immunosuppressives

Immunosuppressive drugs interfere with the formation of immune cells by damaging RNA and DNA needed for cell replication. They may also block immune system response to autoantibodies. An **autoantibody** is an abnormal antibody that attacks healthy cells and tissue.

Azathioprine, cyclosporine, and methotrexate are immunosuppressive drugs used to treat RA. Methotrexate was one of the first drugs used for the treatment of RA, and it continues to be used as monotherapy or along with other DMARDs. It works by inhibiting the formation of folates that are needed for purine synthesis. Folic acid supplementation is prescribed when methotrexate is administered. Methotrexate also decreases cytokine and immunoglobulin production and COX-2 activity, reducing both inflammation and immune system activity. In addition to RA, methotrexate is prescribed for the treatment of several cancers (Chapter 31) and psoriasis.

Azathioprine blocks purine synthesis to cause DNA damage and suppresses T cell–mediated immune system responses. Cyclosporine is used with azathioprine or glucocorticosteroids to treat severe RA. It selectively interferes with T-cell proliferation and IL production. The result is a decreased immune system response to autoantibodies. Cyclosporine is also prescribed for the prevention of organ transplant rejection and severe psoriasis.

> **❶ Tech Alert!**
>
> The following drugs have look-alike/sound-alike issues:
> cycloSPORINE, cycloSERINE, and cyclophosphamide;
> cycloSPORINE and cycloSPORINE modified

Precautions and Adverse Reactions

Adverse reactions to azathioprine include nausea, vomiting, infections, hepatotoxicity, cytopenia, and myelosuppression. Adverse reactions to cyclosporine include kidney toxicity, infections, nausea, abdominal pain, mouth sores, gingival hyperplasia, headache, hirsutism, weight gain, hepatotoxicity, and hypertension. Methotrexate's side effects include nausea, vomiting, diarrhea, GI ulceration, rash, photosensitivity, hair loss, bone marrow depression, hepatotoxicity, renal toxicity, and stomach pain.

> **● Tech Note!**
>
> Reconstituted solution of azathioprine must be mixed by gently swirling, not shaking.

> **● Tech Note!**
>
> Cyclosporine oral solution must be dispensed in a glass container. Dispense the same manufacturer's product each time (bioavailability issues).

Immunosuppressive Drugs Used in the Treatment of Rheumatoid Arthritis

Generic Name	US Brand Name(s) / Canadian Brand(s)	Dosage Forms and Strengths
azathioprine[a]	Azasan, Imuran / Imuran	**Injection, powder for reconstitution:** 100 mg vial[c] **Tablets:** 25 mg[c], 50 mg, 75 mg[c], and 100 mg[c]
cyclosporine[a]	Gengraf, Neoral, Sandimmune / Neoral, Sandimmune	**Capsules, modified (Gengraf, Neoral):** 10 mg[b], 25 mg, 50 mg[b], 100 mg **Capsules, nonmodified (Sandimmune):** 25 mg, 50 mg, 100 mg **Solution, for injection (Sandimmune)[c]:** 50 mg/mL **Solution, oral:** 100 mg/mL

methotrexate[a]	Otrexup, Rasuvo, Reditrex, Trexall, Xatmep / Metoject Subcutaneous	**Injection, powder for reconstitution:** 1000 mg[c]
		Injection, solution: 25 mg base/mL in 2 mL, 4 mL, 10 mL, and 40 mL vials
		Solution, oral (Xatmep): 2.5 mg/mL (2 mg base)
		Solution, for subcutaneous injection (Otrexup):
		    7.5 mg/0.4 mL, 10 mg/0.4 mL, 12.5 mg/0.4 mL, 15 mg/0.4 mL, 17.5 mg/0.4 mL,
		    20 mg/0.4 mL, 22.5 mg/0.4 mL, 25 mg/0.4 mL
		Solution, for subcutaneous injection (Metoject Subcutaneous, Rasuvo):
		    7.5 mg/0.15 mL[c], 10 mg/0.2 mL, 12.5 mg/0.25 mL, 15 mg/0.3 mL,
		    17.5 mg/0.35 mL, 20 mg/0.4 mL, 22.5 mg/0.45 mL, 25 mg/0.5 mL, 30 mg/0.6 mL
		Solution, for subcutaneous injection (Reditrex): 7.5 mg/0.3 mL, 10 mg/0.4 mL,
		    12.5 mg/0.5 mL[c], 15 mg/0.6 mL, 17.5 mg/0.7 mL[c], 20 mg/0.8 mL, 22.5 mg/mL[c],
		    25 mg/mL
		Solution, for injection (prefilled syringe): 7.5 mg/0.3 mL, 10 mg/0.4 mL,
		    15 mg/0.6 mL, 15 mg/0.15 mL, 20 mg/0.8 mL, 25 mg/mL[b]
		Tablets: 2.5 mg, 10 mg[b]

[a]Generic available.
[b]Available in Canada only.
[c]Available in the United States only.

Antimalarials

Antimalarials have antiinflammatory and analgesic properties that are useful in the management of RA. Although the exact mechanism of action is unknown, antimalarials are known to accumulate inside cell structures, where they raise the pH and interfere with processes that are normally stimulated when the body thinks its own cells are harmful antigens. An antigen is a substance that stimulates an immune response.

Precautions and Adverse Reactions

The most common adverse reaction is GI irritation; however, hydroxychloroquine can cause permanent damage to the retina, resulting in blindness. This adverse reaction is associated with long-term chronic use (greater than 5 years) at doses greater than 6.5 mg/kg per day. Additional adverse reactions include nausea, stomach pain, visual disturbances, and tinnitus.

Janus kinase inhibitors

Baricitinib, tofacitinib, and upadacitinib are JAK inhibitors. Janus kinase is an enzyme. JAK inhibits intracellular factors involved

Antimalarial Drugs Used in the Treatment of Rheumatoid Arthritis

Generic Name	US Brand Name(s) / Canadian Brand(s)	Dosage Forms and Strengths
hydroxychloroquine[a]	Plaquenil / Plaquenil	**Tablets:** 200 mg

[a]Generic available.

in inflammation and the immune response. JAK inhibitors fight inflammation from inside the cell. The package labeling for JAK inhibitors has a boxed warning advising patients older than age 50 years who have at least one cardiovascular risk factor of serious potential cardiovascular adverse effects, including stroke, heart attack, and deep vein thrombosis. Less serious side effects are nausea, vomiting, abdominal pain, dizziness, and headache.

Miscellaneous Disease-Modifying Antirheumatic Drugs

Miscellaneous DMARDs are leflunomide, sulfasalazine, and penicillamine. Leflunomide is a DMARD that is approved for the treatment of RA and selectively blocks the replication of lymphocytes by interfering with pyrimidine synthesis. Sulfasalazine was developed by combining an antiinfective agent (sulfapyridine)

Janus Kinase Inhibitors

Generic Name	US Brand Name(s)	Dosage Forms and Strengths
	Canadian Brand(s)	
baricitinib	Olumiant	**Tablet:** 1 mg[a], 2 mg, 4 mg[a]
	Olumiant	
tofacitinib	Xeljanz, Xeljanz XR	**Tablets:** 5 mg, 10 mg
	Xeljanz, Xekjanz XR	**Tablet, extended release (Xeljanz XR):** 11 mg, 22 mg[a]
upadacitinib	Rinvoq	**Tablet, extended release:** 15 mg, 30 mg, 45 mg[a]
	Rinvoq	

[a]Available in the United States only.

Miscellaneous Disease-Modifying Antirheumatic Drugs

Generic Name	US Brand Name(s)	Dosage Forms and Strengths
	Canadian Brand(s)	
auranofin	Ridaura	**Capsules:** 3 mg
	Ridaura	
leflunomide[a]	Arava	**Tablets:** 10 mg, 20 mg, 100 mg
	Arava	
penicillamine[a]	Cupramine, Depen	**Capsules (Cupramine):** 250 mg
	Cupramine	**Tablets (Depen):** 250 mg
sulfasalazine[a]	Azulfidine, Azulfidine EN-tabs	**Tablets (Azulfidine, Salazopyrin):** 500 mg
	Salazopyrin, Salazopyrin EN-tabs	**Tablets, enteric coated (Azulfidine EN-tab, Salazopyrin EN-tabs):** 500 mg

[a]Generic available.

with an aspirin-like antiinflammatory agent (5-aminosalicylic acid). Sulfasalazine slows the progression of RA but takes approximately 2 to 3 months to produce maximum effects. Penicillamine has antiinflammatory actions and alters the immune system response. This makes it useful in the treatment of RA. It inhibits T-cell function and blocks collagen cross-linking.

Precautions and Adverse Reactions

Common side effects of sulfasalazine are GI upset, increased sensitivity to sunlight, allergy, crystalluria, impaired folic acid absorption, and damage to white blood cells (cytopenia). Leflunomide adverse reactions include nausea, diarrhea, rash, hair loss, liver dysfunction, and fetal toxicity. Adverse reactions to auranofin include itching rash, metallic taste, sore mouth, photosensitivity, cytopenia, interstitial pneumonia, and proteinuria. Penicillamine adverse reactions include rash, GI upset, and nephrotoxicity.

> **⊘ Tech Alert!**
>
> The following drugs have look-alike/sound-alike issues:
> sulfaSALAzine and sulfADIAZINE;
> penicillAMINE and penicillin

Biologic Response Modifiers

Many DMARDs are biologic response modifiers. They interfere with the inflammatory process by reducing mediators of the inflammatory response. They inhibit the release of cells that mobilize to fight what the body believes is a harmful invasion and inhibit the release of substances that produce inflammation. Chronic inflammation can cause degeneration of nerves, bones, and muscles.

Biologic response modifiers interfere with the activity of immune system mediators such as cytokines, leukocytes, B cells, and T cells. TNF is a cytokine that is released by specialized cells to fight what the body believes is a harmful invasion. High levels of TNF are found in the synovial fluid of people with RA, and the factor is responsible for joint-damaging inflammation. TNF-α inhibitors are genetically engineered drugs that block the inflammatory process triggered by high concentrations of TNF. They

prevent cell lysis (destruction) and release of the substances that cause inflammation. Adalimumab, certolizumab, golimumab, and infliximab are monoclonal antibodies that bind to TNF-α to reduce mediators of the inflammatory response. Etanercept and abatacept are fusion proteins that have different mechanisms of action. Etanercept inhibits TNF-α, and abatacept blocks T-cell activation. Rituximab works by depleting circulating B cells. Anakinra is a genetically engineered IL receptor antagonist. Anakinra interferes with the binding of the ILs that promote inflammatory responses. Drug-receptor binding results in fewer lymphocytes and macrophages in synovial fluid. Tocilizumab inhibits IL-6 and may be administered with methotrexate or given as monotherapy.

> **● Tech Note!**
>
> IV bags, tubing, drug vials, and gloves used in preparing cytotoxic drugs like methotrexate and azathioprine are cytotoxic waste and must be properly disposed of in cytotoxic waste containers.

Precautions and Adverse Reactions

Monoclonal antibodies (e.g., adalimumab, infliximab), abatacept, and etanercept increase the risk for opportunistic infections. Tuberculosis and fungal infections are the most commonly reported opportunistic infections. Other common adverse reactions produced by "-mabs" are rash, pruritus, nausea, headache, and injection site redness and itchiness. Redness, itching, and swelling at the injection site are the most common side effects of etanercept. The most common side effects of abatacept are headache, dizziness, nausea, and hypertension. Adverse reactions to anakinra include redness or irritation at the injection site, infections, and bone or muscle weakness. In rare cases, the body recognizes the "mabs" as nonhuman proteins and produces antibodies to the drugs, resulting in allergic and immune system reactions such as anaphylactic

Biologic Response Modifiers Used in the Treatment of Rheumatoid Arthritis

Generic Name	US Brand Name(s) / Canadian Brand(s)	Dosage Forms and Strengths
abatacept	Orencia	**Powder, for IV solution**: 250 mg/vial
	Orencia	**Solution, for subcutaneous injection**[b]: 125 mg/mL
adalimumab adalimumab-AFZB adalimumab-ATTO adalimumab-ADBM adallimumab-BWWD adalimumab-FKJP adalimumab-ADAZ adalimumab-AQVH	Humira Abrilada, Amjevita, Cyltezo Hadlima Hulio Hyrimoz Yusimry Abrilada, Amgevita, Hadlima, Hulio, Humira, Hyrimoz, Idacio, Simlandi, Yuflyma	**Solution, for subcutaneous injection (single-use vial and prefilled syringes)**: 20 mg/0.2 mL (Humira), 20 mg/0.4 mL (Amjevita, Hulio, Hyrimoz), 40 mg/0.8 mL, 40 mg/0.4 mL (Yuflyma), 50 mg/mL (Amgevita), 80 mg/0.8 mL (Simlandi)
anakinra	Kineret	**Injection, solution:** 100 mg/0.67 mL (150 mg/mL prefilled syringe)
	Kineret	
certolizumab pegol	Cimzia	**Powder, for injection solution**: 200 mg/mL
	Cimzia	**Solution, for subcutaneous injection**: 200 mg/mL (single-use vial and prefilled syringe)
etanercept etanercept-SZZS etanercept-YKRO	Enbrel Erelzi Eticovo Brenzys, Enbrel, Erelzi	**Injection, powder for reconstitution (Enbrel, Brenzys)**: 25 mg/vial **Injection, solution (prefilled syringe)**: 25 mg/0.5 mL, 50 mg/mL
golimumab	Simponi, Simponi Aria	**Solution for injection (prefilled syringe)**: 50 mg/0.5 mL, 100 mg/1 mL[b]
	Simponi, Simponi IV	**Solution for IV**: 50 mg/4 mL
infliximab infliximab-AXXQ infliximab- DYYB infliximab-QBTX infliximab-ABDA	Remicade Avsola Inflectra Ixifi Renflexis Avsola Inflectra, Remicade, Remicade SC, Remsima SC, Reflexis	**Injection, powder for reconstitution:** 100 mg vial
rituximab rituximab rituximab-ARRX rituximab-PVVR rituximab-ABBS	Rituxan, Rituxan Hycela Riabni, Ruxience, Truxima Rituxan, Rituxan SC	**Solution, for injection**: 10 mg/mL vial **Subcutaneous injection (rituximab-hyaluronidase human recombinant)**: 1400 mg/11.7 mL, 1600 mg/13.4 mL
tocilizumab	Actemra	**Solution, for injection**: 80 mg/4 mL, 200 mg/10 mL, 400 mg/20 mL
	Actemra	**Subcutaneous injection**: 162 mg/0.9 mL

[a]Generic available.
[b]Available in Canada only.

shock. Abatacept and etanercept may also produce anaphylactic shock. TNF-α inhibitors are associated with the development of secondary cancers. Fatal infusion reactions can occur with rituximab and tocilizumab.

> **● Tech Note!**
>
> "-mab" is the common ending for monoclonal antibody drugs (e.g., TNF-α inhibitors and IL inhibitors).

Dosage and Warnings for Drugs Used in the Treatment of Rheumatoid Arthritis

Generic Name	US Brand Name	Usual Adult Oral Dose and Dosing Schedule	Warning Labels
dexamethasone	Generics	0.75–9 mg/day given in 2–4 divided doses	TAKE WITH FOOD.
hydrocortisone	Cortef	20–240 mg once daily or on alternate days 100–500 mg IV; may repeat IM/IV every 2, 4, or 6 h until stable (up to 48–72 h)	DO NOT DISCONTINUE ABRUPTLY. TAKE AT THE SAME TIME EACH DAY. TAKE WITH A FULL GLASS OF WATER.
methylprednisolone[a]	Medrol	4–48 mg PO daily in 4 divided doses or 10–40 mg IM or IV infused over several minutes	
prednisone	Generics	**Acute:** 5–60 mg PO once daily (may administer twice the daily dose every other day)	

NSAIDS

celecoxib[a]	Celebrex	**Gout, acute:** 800 mg immediately, then 400 mg every 12 hours for 7 days **Osteoarthritis:** 200 mg/day in 1–2 divided doses **RA:** 100–200 mg twice a day	TAKE WITH FOOD. AVOID ASPIRIN AND RELATED PRODUCTS. MAY CAUSE DIZZINESS OR DROWSINESS. SWALLOW WHOLE; DO NOT CRUSH OR CHEW—EC-Naprosyn.
ibuprofen[a]	Motrin	400–800 mg 3–4 times a day (maximum, 3200 mg/day)	
naproxen[a]	Anaprox, Naprosyn	**Gout:** 750 mg, followed by 250 mg every 8 h until attack over **Osteoarthritis/RA:** 500–1000 mg/day in 2 divided doses	

Antimalarial

hydroxychloroquine[a]	Plaquenil	**RA:** 400–600 mg/day; when optimal response is reached (4–12 weeks), reduce dose to 200–400 mg/day	AVOID ANTACIDS (and kaolin products) WITHIN 2 HOURS OF DOSE. TAKE WITH FOOD. AVOID PROLONGED EXPOSURE TO SUNLIGHT.

Immunosuppressive

azathioprine	Imuran	**RA:** 1 mg/kg/day for 6–8 weeks; increase every 4 weeks up to 2.5 mg/kg/day	TAKE WITH FOOD. AVOID PREGNANCY.
cyclosporine	Neoral, Sandimmune	**RA:** 2.5–5 mg/kg/day in 2 divided doses	AVOID ALCOHOL. AVOID GRAPEFRUIT JUICE. AVOID PREGNANCY.
methotrexate	RediTrex, Xatmep	**RA:** 7.5 mg PO or SC once a week or 2.5 mg PO every 12 h for 3 doses/week (maximum, 20 mg/week) **pJIA[a]:** 10 mg/m² once weekly	MAY CAUSE DIZZINESS OR DROWSINESS. AVOID ALCOHOL. AVOID ASPIRIN and NSAIDs. AVOID PROLONGED EXPOSURE TO SUNLIGHT. AVOID PREGNANCY & BREASTFEEDING.

Biologic Response Modifiers

adalimumab[a]	Humira	40 mg SC every other week (if not taking methotrexate may increase to 40 mg/week)	PROTECT FROM LIGHT. REFRIGERATE; DO NOT FREEZE.
certolizumab	Cimzia	400 mg SC, given as two 200-mg SC injections at weeks 0, 2, and 4; then 200 mg SC every other week or 400 mg once every 4 weeks	REFRIGERATE; DO NOT FREEZE. ROTATE SITE OF INJECTION. PROTECT FROM LIGHT.
golimumab	Simponi Aria, Simponi	2 mg/kg IV infusion over 30 minutes at weeks 0 and 4, then every 8 weeks (Simponi Aria); 50 mg SC once monthly (in combination with methotrexate)	ROTATE SITE OF INJECTION. REFRIGERATE; DO NOT FREEZE. PROTECT FROM LIGHT; DO NOT SHAKE.
infliximab	Remicade	3 mg/kg IV infusion at 2 and 6 weeks after first dose; repeat in 8 weeks; maintenance, 3–10 mg/kg at 4- or 8-week intervals (in combination with methotrexate)	REFRIGERATE; DO NOT FREEZE. GENTLY SWIRL RECONSTITUTED PRODUCT; DO NOT SHAKE AFTER MIXING, DISCARD ANY UNUSED PORTION.

Dosage and Warnings for Drugs Used in the Treatment of Rheumatoid Arthritis—cont'd

Generic Name	US Brand Name	Usual Adult Oral Dose and Dosing Schedule	Warning Labels
rituximab	Rituxan	500–1000 mg IV on days 1 and 15; repeat every 16–24 weeks based on clinical evaluation	REFRIGERATE; DO NOT FREEZE. GENTLY INVERT IV BAG TO MIX TO AVOID FOAMING. AFTER MIXING, DISCARD ANY UNUSED PORTION.
tocilizumab	Actemra	**RA:** 4 mg/kg IV every 4 weeks; maximum, 8 mg/kg 162 mg SC every other week or weekly depending on response and weight	REFRIGERATE; DO NOT FREEZE. GENTLY INVERT IV BAG TO MIX TO AVOID FOAMING. AFTER MIXING, DISCARD ANY UNUSED PORTION.
Other Biologic Response Modifiers			
abatacept	Orencia	**Psoriatic arthritis/RA:** 500–1000 mg IV infusion; repeat doses at 2 and 4 weeks after first infusion and every 4 weeks thereafter **RA/Psoriatic arthritis:** 125 mg SC weekly	REFRIGERATE; DO NOT FREEZE. PROTECT FROM LIGHT. USE WITHIN 24 HOURS OF MIXING; DISCARD UNUSED PORTION.
anakinra	Kineret	100 mg SC once daily	ROTATE SITE OF INJECTION. GENTLY SWIRL TO DISSOLVE. REFRIGERATE. PROTECT FROM LIGHT.
etanercept	Enbrel	**Psoriatic arthritis/RA:** 50 mg once weekly	ROTATE SITE OF INJECTION. DO NOT SHAKE. REFRIGERATE. PROTECT FROM LIGHT.
DMARDs			
leflunomide	Arava	Start 100 mg/day for 3 days; decrease to 10–20 mg/day	AVOID PROLONGED EXPOSURE TO SUNLIGHT— auranofin, sulfasalazine.
sulfasalazine	Azulfidine	Start 500–1000 mg/day; increase to 2000–3000 mg/day in 2 divided doses (enteric-coated tablets)	MAINTAIN ADEQUATE HYDRATION— sulfasalazine. MAY DISCOLOR URINE (or skin)—orange-yellow, sulfasalazine.
auranofin	Ridura	6 mg/day in 1–2 divided doses (maximum, 9 mg/day)	
penicillamine	Cupramine	125–250 mg/day (may increase dose every 1–3 months to maximum, 1500 mg/day)	TAKE ON AN EMPTY STOMACH.
JAK Inhibitors			
baricitinib	Olumiant	2 mg once daily	AVOID ASPIRIN AND NSAIDS. SWALLOW WHOLE (Xeljanz XR). AVOID PREGNANCY & BREASTFEEDING.
tofacitinib	Xeljanz	5 mg twice a day or 11 mg extended release tablet once daily	
upadacitinib	Rinvoq	15 mg once daily	

[a]Polyarticular juvenile idiopathic arthritis.
PO, orally; *SC*, subcutaneously.

TECHNICIAN'S CORNER

1. Celebrex is the only prescriptive COX-2 inhibitor left on the market. Discuss the FDA's or Health Canada's role in identifying postmarket drug safety issues.
2. Diets that are low in purine have been recommended to prevent gout attacks. What foods might be recommended to patients with gout?

Key Points

- Gout is the primary disease associated with hyperuricemia, a condition in which urate levels build up in the blood serum.
- The joints most commonly affected by gout are the big toe, foot, ankle, knee, wrist, finger, and elbow. Urate crystals build up in joints and cause inflammation and pain.
- Urate-lowering drugs are prescribed for the treatment of gout.
- Urate-lowering drugs reduce inflammation, dissolve urate crystals, and/or increase urinary elimination of urates.
- A uricosuric is a drug that increases the renal clearance (elimination) of urate crystals.
- Colchicine is the oldest drug used for the treatment of acute gouty arthritis pain.
- Probenecid is a uricosuric used in the treatment of gout.
- Allopurinol, a xanthine oxidase inhibitor, blocks the final enzymatic step in the synthesis of uric acid.
- A low purine diet is recommended to prevent gout attacks.
- Certain meats, fish, and beer increase the risks of an acute gout attack, perhaps because they contain high levels of purines.
- Pegloticase and rasburicase are recombinant urate oxidase enzymes that convert uric acid to a water-soluble purine that is excreted in the urine.
- Nonsteroidal antiinflammatory drugs (NSAIDs) and aspirin are widely used in the treatment of pain and inflammation caused by gout and arthritis.
- Rheumatoid arthritis is an autoimmune disease in which the immune system attacks its own cells. It is characterized by inflammation of the lining of the joints.
- Drug therapy for rheumatoid arthritis is aimed at suppressing inflammation, pain, and immune system response to minimize further joint destruction, preservation of body functions, and prevention of disability.
- Glucocorticosteroids have immunosuppressive actions and are prescribed to suppress inflammation, reduce flare-ups, and treat pain.
- Antimalarial drugs have antiinflammatory and analgesic properties that are useful in the management of rheumatoid arthritis.
- Biologic response modifiers act to inhibit the release of cells that mobilize to fight what the body believes is a harmful invasion and inhibit the release of substances that produce inflammation.
- Immunosuppressive drugs interfere with the formation of immune cells by damaging RNA and DNA needed for cell replication.
- Tumor necrosis factor-α (TNF-α) inhibitors are genetically engineered drugs that block the inflammatory process triggered by high concentrations of TNF.
- Methotrexate blocks purine synthesis needed for lymphocyte cell proliferation, reducing inflammation, and immune system activity.
- Leflunomide interferes with pyrimidine synthesis, and when used along with methotrexate, both pathways in the cell division process for lymphocytes are blocked.
- Sulfasalazine is a combination of an antiinfective agent and an aspirin-like antiinflammatory agent, and it is used to treat RA.
- Penicillamine is used in the treatment of RA because it has antiinflammatory actions and alters immune system response.
- Janus kinase (JAK) inhibitors fight inflammation from inside the cell.

Review Questions

1. _____ is the primary disease associated with hyperuricemia.
   a. Arthritis
   b. Gout
   c. Osteoporosis
   d. Kidney stones
2. All of the listed drugs are prescribed for the treatment of gout EXCEPT _____.
   a. colchicine
   b. clozapine
   c. allopurinol
   d. indomethacin
3. You receive a prescription for rasburicase (Elitek, Fasturtek) 1 mg IM. You consult with the pharmacist about the prescription because _____.
   a. rasburicase is a tablet
   b. rasburicase is an oral solution
   c. rasburicase in administered by IV infusion
   d. is an investigational drug in the United States or Canada
4. You receive a prescription for Uloric 8 mg QID. You consult with the pharmacist because _____.
   a. Uloric is not marketed as 8 mg
   b. Uloric is typically prescribed once daily
   c. Uloric is administered IV
   d. Uloric is an injectable drug

5. Diets _____ in purine have been recommended to prevent gout attacks.
   a. high
   b. low
6. The brand name for allopurinol is _____.
   a. Zyban
   b. Zomig
   c. Zyloprim
   d. Zyrtec
7. A uricosuric is a drug that decreases the renal clearance of urates.
   a. true
   b. false
8. A disease that occurs when the immune system turns against the parts of the body it is designed to protect is called a(n) _____.
   a. autoimmune disease
   b. viral disease
   c. immune disease
   d. bacterial disease

9. Which of the following drugs is indicated for the treatment of active rheumatoid arthritis, ankylosing spondylitis, and chronic plaque psoriasis?
   a. Enbrel
   b. Remicade
   c. Humira
   d. Kineret

10. _____ are prescribed commonly to suppress inflammation, reduce flare-ups, and treat pain associated with multiple sclerosis, myasthenia gravis, systemic erythematosus, myositis, and rheumatoid arthritis.
    a. Mineralocorticoids
    b. Glucocorticosteroids
    c. Anabolic steroids
    d. All of the above

Bibliography

Becker M, Jolly M. Hyperuricemia and associated diseases. *Rheum Dis Clin North Am.* 2006;32:275–293.

FitzGerald JD, Dalbeth N, Mikuls T, et al. 2020 American College of Rheumatology guideline for the management of gout. *Arthritis Care Res (Hoboken).* 2020;72(6):744–760. Errata in *Arthritis Care Res (Hoboken)* 72(8):1187, 2020 and *Arthritis Care Res (Hoboken)* 2021; 73(3):458.

Giannini D, Antonucci M, Petrelli F, et al. One year in review 2020: pathogenesis of rheumatoid arthritis. *Clin Exp Rheumatol.* 2020;38(3):387–397.

Health Canada: Drug Product Database, 2017. Retrieved October 15, 2022, from https://health-products.canada.ca/dpd-bdpp/index-eng.jsp.

Institute for Safe Medication Practices. (2016). FDA and ISMP Lists of Look-Alike Drug Names with Recommended Tall Man Letters. Retrieved July 11, 2022, from https://www.ismp.org/recommendations/tall-man-letters-list.

Institute for Safe Medication Practices. (2019). List of Confused Drugs. Retrieved October 15, 2022, from https://www.ismp.org/tools/confuseddrugnames.pdf.

Kalant H, Grant D, Mitchell J. *Principles of medical pharmacology.* ed 7. Toronto: Elsevier Canada, A Division of Reed Elsevier Canada; 2007:381.

Kwok T, Xu V, Lake S. Gout in Canada. *CMAJ.* 2021;193:E171.

National Institute of Arthritis and Musculoskeletal and Skin Diseases. (2020). *Gout.* Retrieved October 15, 2022, from https://www.niams.nih.gov/Health_Info/Gout/default.asp.

National Institute of Arthritis and Musculoskeletal and Skin Diseases. (2019). *Rheumatoid arthritis*, Bethesda, MD, NIAMS, National Institutes of Health, U.S. Department of Health and Human Services. Retrieved October 15, 2022, from https://www.niams.nih.gov/health-topics/rheumatoid-arthritis#tab-treatment.

Page C, Curtis M, Sutter M, et al. *Integrated pharmacology.* Philadelphia. Mosby; 2005:450–451.

Pohar S, Murphy G. *Febuxostat for prevention of gout attacks* [Issues in emerging health technologies issue 87], Ottawa, 2006, Canadian Agency for Drugs and Technologies in Health.

Public Health Agency of Canada. (2020). Gout and other crystal arthropathies in Canada. Retrieved September 20, 2022, from https://www.canada.ca/en/public-health/services/publications/diseases-conditions/gout-crystal-arthropathies.html.

Public Health Agency of Canada. (2020). Rheumatoid arthritis in Canada. Retrieved October 15, 2022, from https://www.canada.ca/en/public-health/services/publications/diseases-conditions/rheumatoid-arthritis.html.

Robinson PC, Dalbeth N. Advances in pharmacotherapy for the treatment of gout. *Expert Opin Pharmacother.* 2015;16(4):533–546.

Underwood M. Diagnosis and management of gout. *BMJ.* 2006;332:1315–1319.

U.S. Food and Drug Administration. (nd). Drugs@FDA: FDA Approved Drug Products. Retrieved October 15, 2022, from http://www.accessdata.fda.gov/scripts/cder/daf/.

USP Center for Advancement of Patient Safety: Use caution—avoid confusion, USP Quality Review No. 79, Rockville, MD, April 2004, USP Center for Advancement of Patient Safety.

van Delft MAM, Huizinga TWJ. An overview of autoantibodies in rheumatoid arthritis. *J Autoimmun.* 2020;110:102392.

Yip K, Berman J. What is gout? *JAMA.* 2021;326(24):2541.

14

Treatment of Osteoporosis and Paget Disease of the Bone

LEARNING OBJECTIVES

1. Learn the terminology associated with osteoporosis and Paget disease of the bone.
2. Describe the signs and symptoms of osteoporosis.
3. List causes of osteoporosis.
4. Describe the signs and symptoms of Paget disease of the bone.
5. List and classify medications used in the treatment of osteoporosis and Paget disease of the bone.
6. Describe the mechanism of action for each class of drug used in the treatment of osteoporosis and Paget disease of the bone.
7. Identify significant drug look-alike and sound-alike issues.
8. Identify warning labels and precautionary messages associated with medications used to treat osteoporosis and Paget disease of the bone.

KEY TERMS

Bone mineral density Test measurement that is taken to determine the degree of bone loss.
Bone resorption Process during which bone is broken down into mineral ions (e.g., calcium).
Osteoblasts Cells responsible for bone formation, deposit, and mineralization of the collagen matrix of bone.

Osteoclasts Cells responsible for bone resorption.
Osteoporosis Chronic, progressive disease of bone characterized by loss of bone density and bone strength and resulting in increased risk for fractures.
Remodeling Process of continual turnover of bone.

Osteoporosis

An estimated 10.2 million men and women (age 50 years and older) in the United States and 2 million people in Canada have osteoporosis. It is the most common disease of bone and affects women more often than men. *Osteoporosis* is a chronic, progressive disease characterized by loss of bone density and bone strength. It increases the risk for fractures (Fig. 14.1). The risk for osteoporosis increases with age, increasing from 4% of women ages 50 to 59 years up to 52% by age 80 years. The risk is increased in people with low bone mass (decreased *bone mineral density* [BMD]). Fifty-four percent of adults in the United States older than 50 years (43.4 million people) have low bone mass.

In the United States and Canada, one in three women and one in five men with osteoporosis will get a bone fracture during their lifetime. The most common are fractures of the vertebrae of the spine and hips, although fractures of the wrists, feet, toes, and forearm also occur. Fractures caused by osteoporosis are classified according to health outcomes as low-impact or fragility fractures. Low-impact fractures are often caused by falls or another trauma. Fragility fractures may occur in the absence of trauma and can occur from simply coughing or sneezing.

Pathophysiology of Osteoporosis

Primary osteoporosis is associated with the aging process. Up until the age of 30 or 40 years, the percentage of bone formed is greater than the percentage of bone lost. After menopause, women have a dramatic shift in the ratio between bone formation and bone loss, with bone loss exceeding bone formation. In men, this process is more gradual until the age 65 or 70 years; then the rates of bone loss for men and women are approximately equal.

Bone formation and loss is a carefully controlled process and is regulated from birth to death. The process is called *remodeling*. Osteoblasts and osteoclasts are cells that are involved in the bone turnover process. *Osteoblasts* are responsible for bone formation, deposit, and mineralization of the collagen matrix of bone. *Osteoclasts* are responsible for bone resorption. *Bone resorption* is the process whereby bone is broken down into mineral ions (e.g., calcium).

Bone turnover is linked to levels of calcium in the blood. Ninety-nine percent of total body calcium is located in the skeleton. Bones are a reservoir for calcium when serum levels are too low. If serum calcium levels are too low, hormones are released to transfer calcium stored in bones back into serum. When blood calcium levels are too high, hormones are released to reduce serum calcium and deposit excess in bones. The hormones principally responsible for regulation of serum calcium levels are parathyroid hormone (PTH), calcitonin,

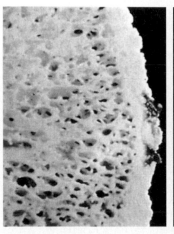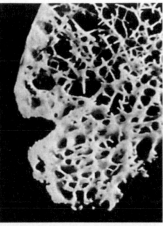

• **Fig. 14.1** Osteoporosis. Normal bone *(left)* versus osteoporotic bone *(right)*. (In Nix S. *Williams' basic nutrition and diet therapy*, ed 15, St Louis, 2017, Elsevier. From Maher AB, Salmond SW, Pellino T. *Orthopaedic nursing*, ed 3, Philadelphia, 2002, Elsevier.)

and vitamin D. PTH is secreted by the parathyroid gland when intestinal absorption of calcium and renal reabsorption of calcium are insufficient to maintain the required calcium balance. Calcitonin reduces serum calcium levels by storing excess in the bone. Vitamin D enhances calcium absorption and is one of the hormones involved in the formation of osteoclasts. PTH and sex hormones are also associated with osteoclast formation. Other hormones linked to the regulation of bone formation and bone loss are estrogen, progesterone, luteinizing hormone, and androgens. Estrogen and progesterone levels are lowered in postmenopausal women, and testosterone levels are reduced in men as part of the normal aging process, which in part explains why osteoporosis increases with age.

Conditions That Produce Osteoporosis

Osteoporosis can be classified as primary or secondary. Secondary osteoporosis may be related to another disease process or can be drug induced. Some of the diseases that can produce secondary osteoporosis include hyperthyroidism, rheumatoid arthritis, inflammatory bowel disease, renal insufficiency, Parkinson disease, multiple sclerosis, chronic obstructive pulmonary disease, and HIV/AIDS. Some of the conditions associated with bone loss are shown in Box 14.1.

Drugs that can induce osteoporosis are administered for a wide variety of diseases. They are used in the treatment of autoimmune diseases of the musculoskeletal system, seizures, prostate cancer, bipolar disorder, hypothyroidism, kidney disease, and other conditions. Alcohol abuse can also produce osteoporosis. Examples of some of the drugs that can produce bone loss leading to osteoporosis are shown in Box 14.2.

Prevention Tips

It is best to lay the foundation for healthy dense bones early in life, although bone health can be improved at any age. Mild weight-bearing exercise, such as walking, climbing stairs, or stretching with elastic exercise bands or weights, along with a diet rich in vitamin D and calcium, is key to strong bones. Lifestyle changes that reduce alcohol consumption and smoking are also important.

Recommended daily allowances (RDAs) for calcium are listed in Table 14.1. The Osteoporosis Society of Canada and the US National Osteoporosis Foundation (NOF) recommend that postmenopausal women and men at risk for fractures ingest 1200 mg of calcium daily. The Canadian guidelines for vitamin D is 800 to 2000 IU daily. The NOF guideline is 800 to 1000 IU daily.

• BOX 14.1   Diseases and Conditions That May Cause Bone Loss

- Chronic obstructive pulmonary disease
- Diabetes
- Eating disorders, especially anorexia nervosa and malnutrition
- Fragility Fracture
- Gastrectomy, including gastrointestinal bypass procedures
- Hyperparathyroidism
- Hyperthyroidism and thyrotoxicosis
- Hypocalcemia and hypophosphatemia
- Kidney disease or liver disease that is chronic and long-lasting
- Malabsorption conditions (e.g., Crohn's disease, ulcerative colitis, celiac disease)
- Malignancies (e.g., multiple myeloma)
- Premature menopause (before 45 years old)
- Rheumatoid arthritis
- Sex hormone deficiency (hypogonadism, premature menopause)
- Smoker

Sources: NIH. (2022). Osteoporosis Retrieved Sept 9, 2023 from https://www.niams.nih.gov/health-topics/osteoporosis, Mayo Clinic. Retrieved Sept 9, 2023 from (2023). Osteoporosis https://www.mayoclinic.org/diseases-conditions/osteoporosis/symptoms-causes/syc-20351968 and Inoue D, Watanabe R, Okazaki R. COPD and osteoporosis: links, risks, and treatment challenges. Int J Chron Obstruct Pulmon Dis. 2016 Mar 29;11:637-48. doi: 10.2147/COPD.S79638. PMID: 27099481; PMCID: PMC4820217 and BC Guidelines. (2012). Osteoporosis: Diagnosis, Treatment and Fracture Prevention retrieved Sept 9, 2023 from https://www2.gov.bc.ca/gov/content/health/practitioner-professional-resources/bc-guidelines/osteoporosis#Step1.

• BOX 14.2   Drugs That Can Produce Bone Loss

- Antidiabetic drugs drugs (e.g., thiazolidinediones)
- Antiseizure drugs (e.g., phenytoin)
- Antirejection/immunosuppressive therapy (e.g., cyclosporine and tacrolimus)
- Breast cancer drugs (e.g., aromatase inhibitors)
- Diuretics (e.g., furosemide)
- Excessive thyroid hormone replacement
- Glucocorticoids (e.g., prednisone)
- "Heartburn" drugs (e.g., proton pump inhibitors)
- Heparin
- Hormone replacement (e.g., progesterone, medroxyprogesterone)
- Mood-altering drugs (e.g., lithium, selective serotonin reuptake inhibitors)
- Prostate cancer drugs (e.g., gonadotropin-releasing hormone agonists like leuprolide)

Sources: Osteoporosis and related fractures in Canada: Report from the Canadian Chronic Disease Surveillance System 2020 https://www.canada.ca/en/public-health/services/publications/diseases-conditions/osteoporosis-related-fractures-2020.html and Honasoge, Mahalakshmi, "Drug-induced Osteoporosis" (2020). Henry Ford Hospital Osteoporosis and Bone & Mineral Disorders Symposium 2020. 4. https://scholarlycommons.henryford.com/obmdsymp2020/4 and Panday K, Gona A, Humphrey MB. Medication-induced osteoporosis: screening and treatment strategies. Ther Adv Musculoskelet Dis. 2014 Oct;6(5):185-202. doi: 10.1177/1759720X14546350. PMID: 25342997; PMCID: PMC4206646.

Milk, leafy green vegetables, and soybeans contain calcium. Vitamin D is produced by the skin upon exposure to sunlight. To find out information about the calcium content of selected foods, visit the Bone Health and Osteoporosis Foundation website at https://www.bonehealthandosteoporosis.org/patients/treatment/calciumvitamin-d/

Calcium can be obtained from calcium supplements in addition to food. Calcium supplements are available as calcium chloride, calcium citrate, calcium carbonate, calcium lactate, and calcium gluconate. The amount of elemental calcium contained in these calcium salts varies. Calcium citrate is most absorbable and easiest to tolerate; however, calcium carbonate provides the greatest

TABLE 14.1 Your Body Needs Calcium and Vitamin D

	If This Is Your Age	You Need This Much Calcium Each Day[a]	If This Is Your Age	You Need This Much Vitamin D
Women	18–50 years	1000 mg	<50 years	400–800 IU
	50+ years	1200 mg	50+ years	800–1000 IU
Men	18–70 years	1000 mg	<50 years	400–800 IU
	71+ years	1200 mg	50+ years	800–1000 IU

[a]From National Institutes of Health Office of Dietary Supplements: Calcium (2022). Retrieved October 11, 2022, from https://ods.od.nih.gov/factsheets/Calcium-HealthProfessional/.

amount of elemental calcium per tablet. Calcium carbonate should be taken on a full stomach. Food increases absorption and decreases upset stomach. Calcium citrate may be taken without regard to food.

> **● Tech Note!**
>
> Aerobic, weight-bearing physical activity (e.g., walking or stairclimbing) up to 20 to 30 minutes daily or 150 minutes per week, plus strength training with weights at least 2 days per week, can improve bone health, but most people are not active enough.

> **● Tech Note!**
>
> Calcium can inhibit absorption of some medicines, such as iron and levothyroxine. Warning labels should instruct patients to avoid calcium within 2 to 4 hours of any other medication taken by mouth.

Paget Disease of Bone

Paget disease is a progressive disease of bone that interferes with your body's normal remodeling process. In Paget disease, new bone is formed quickly and may be larger, misshapen, and/or more prone to fracture. The cause of Paget disease is unknown. It is believed that genetics, viral infection, and environmental factors may be involved. Paget disease is most common in men older than 50 years. Approximately 2% to 3% of Americans and 3% of Canadians have Paget disease.

Pathophysiology of Paget Disease of the Bone

The disease produces excessive bone resorption followed by increased bone formation, resulting in enlarged bones that are structurally weak. Effects of the disease tend to be localized and most commonly affect the pelvis, lumbar sacral spine, skull, femur, or tibia; however, Paget disease may be widespread throughout the body, and the entire skeleton can be affected.

Paget disease causes deformities such as bowed legs, pain, arthritis, deafness, and (rarely) cranial nerve palsies. Pain may be constant or intermittent. Intermittent pain is typically associated with weight-bearing or localized microfractures. Constant pain may even occur at rest.

Calcium Supplements

Generic Name	US Brand Name(s) / Canadian Brand Name(s)	Dosage Forms and Strengths
calcium carbonate[a] (oyster shell calcium)— various manufacturers—some products listed contain vitamin D	Caltrate, Caltrate Soft Chews, Caltrate Minis, TUMS Chewable Ultra Strength, TUMS Chewy Bites, TUMS Smoothies Extra Strength, TUMS Extra Strength, TUMS Ultra 1000, Viactiv + Vit D	**Tablets:** 500 mg, 600 mg, 750 mg, 1000 mg **Chewable tablets:** 500 mg, 600 mg, 750 mg, 1000 mg **Suspension:** 500 mg/5 mL
	Caltrate, Caltrate Select, Caltrate Plus Chewables, TUMS Extra Strength, TUMS Smoothies Extra Strength, TUMS Ultra Strength, Viactiv + Vit D[b]	
calcium citrate[a] (plus vitamin D)	Caltrate + Vit D, Caltrate 600 + D₃, Caltrate Minis, Citracal Gummies with Vit D, Citracal Maximum Plus with Vit D[b]	**Tablet:** 600 mg **Chewable tablets:** 1000 mg
	Caltrate with Vit D₃, Caltrate Soft Chews with Vit D₃, Caltrate Plus, Caltrate Select, Citracal + D	
calcium gluconate[a]	Generics	**Injection:** 100 mg/mL (10%)
	Generics	
calcium chloride[a]	Generics	**Injection:** 100 mg/mL (10%)
	Generics	
calcium phosphate or tricalcium phosphate (plus vitamin D)[a]	Caltrate Gummies	**Chewable gummies:** 110 mg, 250 mg, 500 mg **Tablets:** 600 mg **Suspension:** 500 mg/15 mL
	Caltrate Gummies, L'il Critters Gummies	

[a]Generics available.
[b]Includes vitamin K.

Drugs Used for the Treatment of Osteoporosis and Paget Disease of Bone

Treatment goals for osteoporosis are to increase bone density and reduce risks for future fractures. Pharmacologic agents that are used to treat osteoporosis are categorized as antiresorptive (inhibit bone resorption) or anabolic (promote bone formation). Drug treatment for Paget disease is recommended for patients who have symptoms or are at risk for fractures or deafness.

---

❶ Tech Alert!

The following drugs have look-alike/sound-alike issues:

Actonel and Actos

Antiresorptive Agents

Most of the drugs used to treat osteoporosis and Paget disease are antiresorptive agents. They suppress bone turnover and loss. Bisphosphonates, calcitonin, and estrogens are antiresorptive agents.

Bisphosphonates

Most of the bisphosphonates are used for the treatment of Paget disease and osteoporosis. Bisphosphonates that are marketed in the United States and/or Canada are alendronate, pamidronate, risedronate, tiludronate, and zoledronic acid. Bisphosphonates inhibit bone resorption. Alendronate, ibandronate, and risedronate have been shown to reduce vertebral fractures by up to 40% to 50% and hip fractures by 20% to 50%. Evidence that bisphosphonates reduce fractures and prevent bone deformity in Paget disease of bone is inconclusive for most drugs in the class. However, alendronate, pamidronate, and risedronate are approved by the US Food and Drug Administration (FDA) for Paget disease. Intravenous zoledronic acid is indicated for hypercalcemia caused by malignant tumors rather than osteoporosis and Paget disease.

Mechanism of Action and Pharmacokinetics

Bisphosphonates inhibit bone resorption. Alendronate, ibandronate, pamidronate, and risedronate are nitrogen-containing bisphosphonates. Pamidronate and zoledronic acid are administered by intravenous infusion.

The bisphosphonates are poorly absorbed in the gastrointestinal tract, and food further reduces absorption. All but ibandronate must be taken on an empty stomach at least 30 minutes before the first meal or beverage of the day. Ibandronate must be taken 60 minutes before the first meal. Between 50% and 80% of the drug is eliminated unchanged in the urine within 24 hours of dosing. The remainder permanently binds to bone. Bisphosphonates are available in dosage forms for daily (alendronate, risedronate, ibandronate), weekly (alendronate, risedronate), and monthly (risedronate, ibandronate) dosing. Patient

▌ Bisphosphonates

Generic Name	US Brand Name(s) / Canadian Brand(s)	Dosage Forms and Strengths
alendronate[a]	Binosto, Fosamax / Fosamax	**Effervescent tablet (Binosto)**[b]: 70 mg **Tablets**[c]: 5 mg, 10 mg, 40 mg **Tablets, weekly**: 70 mg
ibandronate[a]	Generics / Not available	**Solution, for injection**: 1 mg/mL **Tablets, monthly**: 150 mg
pamidronate[a]	Aredia / Generics	**Powder, for injection**: 30 mg/vial, 60 mg/vial, 90 mg/vial **Solution, for injection**: 3 mg/mL, 6 mg/mL, 9 mg/mL
risedronate[a]	Actonel, Atelvia / Actonel, Actonel DR	**Tablets**: 5 mg, 30 mg **Tablets weekly**: 35 mg **Tablets, delayed release, weekly**: 35 mg **Tablets, monthly**: 150 mg
zoledronic acid[a]	Reclast, Zometa / Aclasta, Zometa	**Solution, for injection**: 4 mg/5 mL (Zometa), 4 mg/100 mL (Zometa), 5 mg/100 mL (Reclast)
Combinations		
alendronate + cholecalciferol	Fosamax Plus D / Fosavance	**Tablets**: 70 mg alendronate + 2800 IU vitamin D, 70 mg alendronate + 5600 IU vitamin D

[a]Generic available.
[b]Available in the United States only.
[c]Available in Canada only.

Selective Estrogen Receptor Modulators

	Generic Name	US Brand Name(s) Canadian Brand(s)	Dosage Forms and Strengths
	raloxifene[a]	Evista Evista	**Tablets:** 60 mg
	bazedoxifene + conjugated estrogens	Duavee Not Available	**Tablets:** 20 mg bazedoxifene + 0.45 mg conjugated estrogens

[a]Generic available.

Miscellaneous

Generic Name	US Brand Name(s) Canadian Brand(s)	Dosage Forms and Strengths
calcitonin[a]	Miacalcin Generics	**Nasal solution**[b]: 200 units per actuation (spray) **Solution, for injection:** 200 units/mL

[a]Generic available.
[b]Available in the United States only.

adherence is improved when the medication is dosed once weekly or monthly. Zoledronic acid is administered as a single dose annually for osteoporosis treatment or once every 2 years for prevention. It is administered as a single dose to induce remission in Paget disease.

● Tech Note!

An FDA safety announcement warns: "The safety and effectiveness of Reclast for the treatment of osteoporosis is based on clinical data of 3 years' duration. The optimal duration of use has not been determined. Patients should have the need for continued therapy reevaluated on a periodic basis."

Adverse Reactions

Common adverse effects associated with bisphosphonates are painful swallowing, heartburn, diarrhea, nausea, and vomiting. Less common adverse reactions are eye inflammation, musculoskeletal pain, atypical fractures, and osteonecrosis or erosion of the jawbone. Bisphosphonates increase the risk for atypical femoral fracture when used for more than 5 years.

● Tech Note!

An FDA safety alert recommends that bisphosphonates be discontinued in patients experiencing a femoral shaft fracture; otherwise, patients should continue with therapy and report any hip or thigh pain.

Precautions

To prevent injury to the esophagus by bisphosphonates, the patient should sit or stand upright for 30 to 60 minutes (depending on the agent) after taking the medication. Each tablet should be taken with 6 to 8 oz of water. Calcium and vitamin D supplementation is recommended in conjunction with bisphosphonates but should not be administered at the same time. Multivitamins with iron, calcium supplements, and antacids should be avoided within 2 hours of administration of the prescribed bisphosphonate dose.

Selective Estrogen Receptor Modulators

Selective estrogen receptor modulators (SERMs) treat and prevent further destruction of bone architecture. They are indicated for treatment in postmenopausal women.

Mechanism of Action and Pharmacokinetics

Raloxifene (Evista) and bazedoxifene + conjugated estrogens (Duavee, Duavive) are indicated for the treatment and prevention of osteoporosis. They reduce new fractures of the vertebrae by 30% to 50% over 3 years but have no effect on hip fractures. Only 2% of the amount of raloxifene administered is bioavailable. First-pass metabolism and protein binding limit the amount of drug absorbed to produce a therapeutic effect.

Adverse Reactions

Common side effects are hot flashes, leg cramps, peripheral edema, stroke, and venous thromboembolism (VTE). Patients may be instructed to discontinue raloxifene at least 72 hours before and during prolonged immobilization (e.g., bed rest, after surgery) until fully ambulatory again, to prevent VTE.

Calcitonin

Calcitonin is a hormone that is secreted by the thyroid gland and inhibits the rate of bone turnover stimulated by release of PTH. It lowers serum calcium levels by decreasing intestinal absorption of calcium and increasing renal elimination of calcium. These actions make calcitonin useful for the treatment of Paget disease. The effectiveness of calcitonin in the treatment of osteoporosis is related to its ability to increase BMD. It has been shown to reduce vertebral fracture risk by 33% to 36% over 3 years but has not proven effective in decreasing hip fractures.

Hormone Replacement Therapy

Generic Name	US Brand Name(s) Canadian Brand(s)	Dosage Forms and Strengths
estradiol[a]	Climara, Menostar, Vivelle, Vivelle-Dot Climara, Estradot, Oesclim	**Tablets, oral:** 0.5 mg, 1 mg, 2 mg **Transdermal patch, biweekly (Estradot, Oesclim, Vivelle, Vivelle Dot):** 0.025 mg/24 h, 0.0375 mg/24 h, 0.05 mg/24 h, 0.06 mg/24 h[b], 0.075 mg/24 h, 0.1 mg/24 h **Transdermal patch, weekly (Climara):** 0.025 mg/24 h, 0.0375 mg/24 h[b], 0.05 mg/24 h, 0.06 mg/24 h[b], 0.075 mg/24 h, 0.1 mg/24 h and 0.014 mg/24 h (Menostar)[b]
conjugated estrogens[a]	Premarin Premarin	**Tablets:** 0.3 mg, 0.45 mg[b], 0.625 mg, 0.9 mg, 1.25 mg
conjugated estrogens + medroxyprogesterone	Premphase, Prempro Not Available	**Tablets (Premphase 14/14):** conjugated estrogens 0.625 mg (14 maroon tablets) and 0.625 mg conjugated estrogen + 5 mg medroxyprogesterone (14 blue tablets) **Tablets (Prempro):** 0.3 mg conjugated estrogen + 1.5 mg medroxyprogesterone[b]; 0.45 mg conjugated estrogen + 1.5 mg medroxyprogesterone[b]; 0.625 mg conjugated estrogen + 2.5 mg medroxyprogesterone; 0.625 mg conjugated estrogen + 5 mg medroxyprogesterone
conjugated estrogens + bazedoxifene[a]	Duavee Not available	**Tablets:** 45 mg conjugated estrogens + 20 mg bazedoxifene

[a]Generics available.
[b]Available in the United States.

Anabolic Agents

Generic Name	US Brand Name(s) Canadian Brand(s)	Dosage Forms and Strengths
abaloparatide	Tymlos Not available	**Solution, for SC injection:** 3.12 mg/1.56 mL (2 mg/mL)
teriparatide[a]	Bonsity, Forteo Forteo, Osnuvo	**Solution, for injection:** 250 mcg/mL

[a]Generic in Canada only.
SC, subcutaneous.

Monoclonal Antibody

Generic Name	US Brand Name(s) Canadian Brand(s)	Dosage Forms and Strengths
denosumab	Prolia, Xgeva Prolia, Xgeva	**Solution, for injection:** 60 mg/mL (Prolia), 70 mg/mL (120 mg/1.7 mL) (Xgeva)
romosozumab	Evenity Evenity	**Solution, for injection:** 105 mg/1.17 mL

❶ Tech Alert!

Calcitonin and calcitriol have look-alike/sound-alike issues.

Absorption of calcitonin from intramuscular and subcutaneous injection sites is rapid, and the half-life of calcitonin is short (20 minutes). The bioavailability of calcitonin when administered intranasally is 3% to 50%. Local adverse reactions are mainly irritation of the nose or injection site.

Hormone Replacement Therapy

Estrogen deficiency occurs with the onset of menopause and increases osteoclast activity. Osteoclasts are responsible for bone resorption. Hormone replacement restores estrogen levels and

Usual Dosage and Warnings for Drugs Used in the Treatment of Osteoporosis and Paget Disease

	Generic Name	US Brand Name	Usual Adult Oral Dose and Dosing Schedule	Warning Labels
Bisphosphonates				
	alendronate	Fosamax	**Osteoporosis, prevention:** 5 mg once a day or 35 mg once weekly **Osteoporosis, treatment:** 10 mg once a day or 70 mg once weekly **Paget disease:** 40 mg once daily for 6 months	STAND OR SIT UPRIGHT FOR AT LEAST 30 MINUTES AFTER TAKING DOSE; DO NOT LIE DOWN—alendronate, etidronate, risedronate. STAND OR SIT UPRIGHT FOR A LEAST 1 HOUR AFTER TAKING DOSE; DO NOT LIE DOWN—ibandronate. TAKE 30 MINUTES BEFORE THE FIRST MEAL OF THE DAY WITH 6–8 OZ OF WATER. TAKE 1 HOUR BEFORE FIRST MEAL OF THE DAY—ibandronate. AVOID DAIRY PRODUCTS AND ANTACIDS CONTAINING CALCIUM, MAGNESIUM, OR IRON WITHIN 2 HOURS OF DOSE. TAKE ON AN EMPTY STOMACH (TAKE 2 HOURS BEFORE FOOD)—etidronate.
	ibandronate	Boniva	**Osteoporosis:** 150 mg once monthly or administer 3 mg IV bolus every 3 months	
	etidronate	Didronel	**Paget disease:** 5 mg to 10 mg/kg/day for up to 6 months or 11 mg to 20 mg/kg/day up to 3 months; re-treat if needed after a drug-free period of 90 days	
	pamidronate	Aredia	**Paget disease:** 30 mg infused intravenously over 4 h for 3 days in a row	
	risedronate	Actonel	**Osteoporosis:** 5 mg once a day, 35 mg once weekly, 75 mg once daily for 2 days a month, or 150 mg once a month **Paget disease:** 30 mg once a day for 2 months; re-treat if needed after a 2-month drug-free period	
Bisphosphonate Combinations				
	alendronate + cholecalciferol	Fosamax Plus D	1 tablet once weekly	
Selective Estrogen Receptor Modulators				
	raloxifene	Evista	60 mg/day	TAKE WITH OR WITHOUT FOOD.
Hormone Replacement Therapy				
	estradiol	Estrace	**Prevention of osteoporosis:** **Oral:** 0.5 mg/day (3 weeks on and 1 week off) **Transdermal patch, as Climara, Menostar:** 1 patch once weekly **Transdermal patch, as Estraderm, Estradot, Vivelle-Dot:** 1 patch twice weekly	TAKE WITH FOOD. ROTATE SITE OF APPLICATION—patch. STORE IN MANUFACTURER FOIL POUCH AND BLISTER PACKAGE—Duavee. DISCARD 60 DAYS AFTER OPENING POUCH—Duavee.
	conjugated estrogens	Premarin	**Prevention of osteoporosis:** 0.3 mg cyclically or daily	
	conjugated estrogens + bazedoxifene[a]	Duavee	**Prevention of osteoporosis:** Take 1 tablet daily	

Usual Dosage and Warnings for Drugs Used in the Treatment of Osteoporosis and Paget Disease—cont'd

	Generic Name	US Brand Name	Usual Adult Oral Dose and Dosing Schedule	Warning Labels
	estrogens + medroxy-progesterone	Premphase, Prempro	**Prevention of osteoporosis**: **Premphase**: Take maroon tablets on days 1–14 (0.625 mg conjugated estrogen) and blue tablets on days 15–28 (estrogens + 5 mg medroxyprogesterone) **Prempro**: Take 1 tablet daily	
Calcitonin Hormone				
	calcitonin	Miacalcin	**Osteoporosis:** Inject 100 units/day (IM, subcut) or 1 spray in 1 nostril (200 units/day) (intranasal) **Paget disease:** Start 100 units/day (IM, subcut); maintenance 50–100 units every 1–3 days	SPRAY IN ALTERNATE NOSTRILS DAILY.
Monoclonal Antibody				
	denosumab	Prolia, Xgeva	**Osteoporosis:** 60 mg subcut every 6 months	REFRIGERATE. DO NOT SHAKE. PROTECT FROM LIGHT.
	romosozumab	Evenity	Inject 2 separate subcut injections of 210 mg once monthly	
Parathyroid Hormone Analog				
	abaloparatide	Tymlos	Inject 80 mg subcut once daily	REFERIGERATE UNTIL OPENING THEN STORE AT ROOM TEMPERATURE FOR UP TO 30 DAYS.
	teriparatide	Forteo	**Osteoporosis:** 20 mcg subcut once a day Not recommended for use beyond 2 years.	REFRIGERATE; DO NOT FREEZE. DISCARD AFTER 28 DAYS OF OPENING.

FDA, Food and Drug Administration; *IM*, intramuscular; *IV*, intravenous; *subcut*, subcutaneous.

inhibits the effects of estrogen deficiency on bone. Estrogens with or without progestins are indicated for prevention of osteoporosis, decreasing bone turnover, bone loss, and fractures. Hormone replacement therapy (HRT) is not a first-line therapy for the prevention of osteoporosis because of the increased risk for coronary heart disease, stroke, thromboembolism, and breast and uterine cancers. HRT also has beneficial effects on BMD and reduces the relative risk for vertebral and hip fractures up to 34%. Increases in BMD are dose dependent; higher doses produce increased BMD. Increases in BMD occur with oral and transdermal dosage forms.

Estrogens (conjugated estrogens, esterified estrogens, estradiol) with and without progestins (levonorgestrel, medroxyprogesterone, norethindrone, or norgestimate) are prescribed for HRT in the treatment of osteoporosis. HRT is also indicated for the treatment of menopausal symptoms (hot flashes, vaginal dryness and atrophy), postmenopausal urogenital symptoms (urgency, dysuria), abnormal uterine bleeding, hypoestrogenism, and breast and prostate cancer (palliation). These drugs are discussed in detail in Chapter 27. Adverse reactions include headache, nausea, rash at the site of patch application, coronary heart disease, depression, stroke, thromboembolism, and breast and uterine cancers.

❶ Tech Alert!

The following drugs have look-alike/sound-alike issues:

Estratest and Estratest HS

Anabolic Agents

PTH analogs increase the rate of bone remodeling, thicken structural units of bone (ostens), and produce bone architecture that closely resembles normal bone. They decrease osteoblast cell death, allowing the balance between bone formation and bone resorption to shift toward bone formation. This is an improvement over bisphosphonates because alendronate, risedronate, and etidronate only prevent further destruction of bone architecture. They do not restore normal structure. Teriparatide and abaloparatide are a genetically engineered human PTH. They are administered subcutaneously and are injected once daily. They are indicated for postmenopausal women at high risk for fracture. Common adverse reactions are orthostatic hypotension, dizziness, headache, hypercalcemia, leg cramps, nausea, and hyperuricemia. For safety, using longer than 2 years is not recommended.

⊘ Tech Alert!

Because of the potential risk for osteosarcoma, the FDA requires a boxed warning for teriparatide stating that its use is limited to patients for whom the benefit outweighs the risk.

Receptor Activator of Nuclear Factor κB Ligand Inhibitors

Denosumab and romosozumab are monoclonal antibodies that improve bone mass and strength. Romosozumab increases bone formation by osteoclast activation, and both drugs decrease bone resorption. Denosumab is a RANKL (receptor activator of nuclear factor κB ligand) inhibitor, and romosozumab inhibits sclerostin, which regulates bone metabolism. Both drugs are administered subcutaneously. Denosumab is administered twice a year, and romosozumab is injected once a month. Romosozumab has a box warning describing the risk of myocardial infarction, stroke, and cardiovascular death. Adverse reactions include increased risk for infection, hypocalcemia, skin rashes, osteonecrosis of the jaw, and femoral fractures. The anabolic effect of romosozumab decreases after 12 monthly doses of therapy. To prevent BMD loss after discontinuation of denosumab and romosozumab, therapy with antiresorptive agents (e.g., bisphosphonates) is recommended.

TECHNICIAN'S CORNER

1. Mild weight-bearing exercise, along with a diet rich in vitamin D and calcium, is key to strong bones that resist fractures. Come up with a 10-day plan of meals and exercises for a client who is menopausal and overweight.
2. Why are lifestyle changes that reduce alcohol consumption and smoking so important to prevent osteoporosis or Paget disease?

Key Points

- Osteoporosis is a chronic, progressive disease of bone characterized by loss of bone density and bone strength and resulting in increased fracture risk.
- People who have osteoporosis are at risk for fractures.
- Secondary osteoporosis may be caused by diseases or drugs (e.g., prednisone).
- After menopause, women's rate of bone loss exceeds the rate of bone formed. The rate of bone loss for men and women is equal after age 65 to 70 years.
- Ninety-nine percent of total body calcium is located in the skeleton; therefore bones are a reservoir for calcium when serum levels are too low.
- The hormones principally responsible for regulation of serum calcium levels are parathyroid hormone, calcitonin, and vitamin D.
- Other hormones linked to the regulation of bone formation and bone loss are estrogen, progestins, luteinizing hormone, and androgens.
- Paget disease is also a progressive disease of bone.
- Paget disease is characterized by excessive bone resorption in focal areas followed by increased bone formation that results in enlarged bones that are structurally weak.

- Paget disease can cause bone deformities, pain, fractures, and deafness.
- Prevention and treatment of osteoporosis includes lifelong nutritional calcium and vitamin D intake, exercise (weight bearing and strength training), lifestyle changes (e.g., reduce alcohol and smoking), and pharmacotherapy.
- Pharmacologic agents that are used in the treatment of osteoporosis and Paget disease are categorized as antiresorptive (inhibit bone resorption) or anabolic (promote bone formation).
- Bisphosphonates, calcitonin, SERMs, and estrogen are antiresorptive agents.
- Parathyroid hormone analogs are anabolic agents.
- Bisphosphonates must be taken on an empty stomach at least 30 to 60 minutes (depending on the agent) before the first meal or beverage of the day.
- Patients taking oral bisphosphonates must sit upright or stand for at least 30 to 60 minutes after dosing to avoid possible esophageal ulceration.
- Calcium and vitamin D supplementation is recommended in conjunction with bisphosphonate and receptor activator of nuclear factor κB ligand (RANKL) therapy.

Review Questions

1. A chronic, progressive disease of bone characterized by loss of bone density and bone strength and resulting in increased fracture risk is called _____.
   a. rheumatoid arthritis
   b. osteoporosis
   c. brittle bone disease
   d. osteosarcoma
2. Alcohol abuse can also produce osteoporosis.
   a. true
   b. false

3. You receive a prescription for alendronate 70 mg take 1 tablet daily, 30 minutes before meals. You consult the pharmacist because _____.
   a. alendronate 70 mg should be taken with food
   b. alendronate 70 mg should be taken once weekly
   c. alendronate should be taken twice weekly
   d. alendronate should be taken once monthly
4. The goals of osteoporosis treatment are to _____ bone density and to _____ risks for future fractures.
   a. decrease, reduce
   b. increase, reduce
   c. reduce, remove
   d. decrease, increase

5. Most of the drugs used to treat osteoporosis and Paget disease are _____ agents.
   a. absorption
   b. antifracture
   c. antiresorptive
   d. anticalcium

6. Only some of the bisphosphonates are indicated for the treatment of Paget disease.
   a. true
   b. false

7. _____is a selective estrogen receptor modulator (SERM) indicated for the treatment and prevention of osteoporosis in postmenopausal women and prevents further destruction of bone architecture.
   a. Fosamax
   b. Evista
   c. Boniva
   d. Osteo-cal

8. Hormone replacement therapy is the first-line therapy for the prevention of osteoporosis because of the increased risk for coronary heart disease, stroke, thromboembolism, and breast and uterine cancer.
   a. true
   b. false

9. A diet rich in vitamin _____ and _____ is key to strong bones.
   a. C, calcium
   b. D, sodium
   c. D, calcium
   d. B, iron

10. You receive a prescription for Miacalcin, directions 1 spray in each nostril once daily. You consult with the pharmacist because _____.
    a. Miacalcin is not marketed as a nasal spray
    b. Miacalcin is used twice daily
    c. Miacalcin should be used in only one nostril per dose
    d. Miacalcin is a tablet

Bibliography

Alibhai S, Rahman S, Warde P, et al. Prevention and management of osteoporosis in men receiving androgen deprivation therapy: a survey of urologists and radiation oncologists. *Urology.* 2006;68:126–131.

American Pharmacists Association New approaches to the management of osteoporosis. *Pharmacy Today.* 2010;13(1):1–12.

Cosman F, de Beur SJ, LeBoff MS, et al. Clinician's guide to prevention and treatment of osteoporosis. *Osteoporos Int.* 2014;25:2359–2381.

Cranney A, Papaioannou A, Zytaruk N, et al. For the Clinical Guidelines Committee of Osteoporosis Canada: parathyroid hormone for the treatment of osteoporosis: a systematic review. *CMAJ.* 2006;175:52–59.

Drieling RL, LaCroix AZ, Beresford SAA, et al. Long-term oral bisphosphonate therapy and fractures in older women: The Women's Health Initiative. *J Am Geriatr Soc.* 2017;65(9):1924–1931.

Gold D, Alexander I, Ettinger M. How can osteoporosis patients benefit more from their therapy? Adherence issues with bisphosphonate therapy. *Ann Pharmacother.* 2006;40:1143–1150.

Health Canada. (2018). Drug Product Database. Retrieved October 11, 2022, from https://health-products.canada.ca/dpd-bdpp/index-eng.jsp.

Kalant H, Grant D, Mitchell J. *Principles of medical pharmacology.* ed 7. Toronto: Elsevier Canada, A Division of Reed Elsevier Canada; 2007:860–861 878–889.

Mauck K, Clarke B. Diagnosis, screening, prevention, and treatment of osteoporosis. *Mayo Clin Proc.* 2006;81:662–672.

Osteoporosis Canada. (2022). Osteoporosis Facts & Statistics. Retrieved October 11, 2022, from https://osteoporosis.ca/facts-and-stats/.

Osteoporosis Canada. (2022). Calcium. Retrieved October 11, 2022, https://osteoporosis.ca/calcium/.

Ralston SH, Corral-Gudino L, Cooper C, et al. Diagnosis and management of Paget's disease of bone in adults: a clinical guideline. *J Bone Miner Res.* 2019;34(4):579–604.

Reid I, Miller P, Lyles K, et al. Comparison of a single infusion of zoledronic acid with risedronate for Paget's disease. *N Engl J Med.* 2005;353:898–908.

U.S. Department of Health and Human Services. (2004). *The 2004 Surgeon General's Report on bone health and osteoporosis*: what it means to you, Washington, DC, U.S. Department of Health and Human Services, Office of the Surgeon General.

U.S. Food and Drug Administration. (nd). Drugs@FDA: FDA Approved Drug Products: U.S. Department Health and Human Services. Retrieved October 11, 2022, from http://www.accessdata.fda.gov/scripts/cder/daf/.

Walsh J. Paget's disease of bone: clinical update. *MJA.* 2004;181:262–265.

Wright NC, Looker AC, Saag KG, et al. The recent prevalence of osteoporosis and low bone mass in the United States based on bone mineral density at the femoral neck or lumbar spine. *J Bone Miner Res.* 2014;29(11):2520–2526.

UNIT **IV**

Drugs Affecting the Ophthalmic and Otic Systems

The eye and the ear are sense organs that have specialized structures to maintain vision, balance, and hearing. The eyes provide visual input about an ever-changing environment that is important for identifying danger, language, learning, communicating, working, and performing activities of daily living. The ear is divided into three anatomic parts: the external ear, middle ear, and inner ear. The ear has dual sensory functions, hearing and balance (or equilibrium). The stimulation or trigger for hearing and balance is the activation of hair cells, receptors that transmit nerve impulses and are perceived in the brain as sound or balance.

In Unit IV, pharmacotherapy for glaucoma, dry eye, and eye infections is presented. Pharmacotherapy for disorders of the ear, such as Meniere disease, vertigo, and ear infections, is also described. A brief description of each disorder is provided, followed by a description of the drugs indicated for treatment that includes mechanisms of action, adverse reactions, strength(s), and dosage forms. Antibiotics that are used for the treatment of eye and ear infections are discussed in Unit IV chapters. Antibiotics that are used in the treatment of other types of infection are presented in Unit X.

15

Treatment of Diseases of the Eye

LEARNING OBJECTIVES

1. Learn the terminology associated with the eye and the treatment of glaucoma and ophthalmic infections.
2. List and categorize medications used in the treatment of ophthalmic infections and glaucoma.
3. Describe the mechanism of action for each class of drugs used in the treatment of ophthalmic infections and glaucoma.
4. Identify significant drug look-alike and sound-alike issues.
5. Identify warning labels and precautionary messages associated with medications used in the treatment of ophthalmic infections and glaucoma.

KEY TERMS

Angle-closure glaucoma Sudden increase in intraocular pressure caused by obstruction of the drainage portal between the cornea and iris (angle) that can rapidly progress to blindness.

Aqueous humor Fluid made in the front part of the eye.

Blepharitis Chronic disease of the eye that produces distinctive flaky scales that form on the eyelids and eyelashes.

Conjunctivitis (pink eye) Common, self-limiting ailment that causes itching, burning, and teary outflow.

Cytomegalovirus retinitis Viral opportunistic infection of the eye that can cause pain and blindness.

Dry eye disease Occurs when the eye does not produce tears properly or when the tears are not of the correct consistency and evaporate too quickly.

Herpes simplex keratitis Painful eye infection caused by herpes simplex virus that can lead to blindness.

Herpes zoster ophthalmicus Painful eye infection caused by herpes zoster virus that can lead to blindness.

Intraocular pressure Inner pressure of the eye. Normal intraocular pressure ranges from 12 to 22 mm Hg.

Iritis Condition associated with inflammation of the iris.

Keratitis Severe infection of the cornea that may be caused by bacteria or fungi.

Open-angle glaucoma Disorder characterized by gradual increase of pressure in the eye that can damage the optic nerve and lead to permanent blindness.

Peripheral vision Sometimes called "side vision," this is usually the first area of vision to be lost with glaucoma.

Photopsia Condition similar to floaters and associated with flashes of light.

Stye Painful lump located on the eyelid margin caused by an acute self-limiting infection of the oil glands of the eyelid.

Uveitis Serious eye condition that produces inflammation of the uvea and can cause scarring of the eye and blindness if untreated.

Vitreous floaters Particles that float in the vitreous and cast shadows on the retina and appear as spots, cobwebs, or spiders.

Dry Eye Disease

Dry eye occurs when the eye does not produce tears properly or when tears are not of the correct consistency and evaporate too quickly. A common symptom is excessive tearing. Inflammation of the surface of the eye may occur along with dry eye, and if left untreated, this condition can lead to pain, ulcers, or scars on the cornea, and some loss of vision. Permanent loss of vision from dry eye is uncommon.

Dry eye can make it more difficult to perform some activities, such as using a computer or reading for an extended period. It can decrease tolerance for dry environments such as the air inside an airplane. *Dry eye disease* (keratoconjunctivitis sicca) is treated with prescription and over-the-counter (OTC) eye drops. Cyclosporine and lifitegrast ophthalmic drops are prescription products that treat moderate to severe dry eye disease.

Cyclosporine is a calcineurin inhibitor immunosuppressant that increases tear production. Lifitegrast is a lymphocyte function associated antigen-1 antagonist. It is unknown how the drug works in treating dry eye disease, but it is believed to block inflammatory processes.

OTC lubricating eye drops (e.g., TheraTears, Tears Naturale, and Systane) provide relief of mild symptoms.

Bacterial Infections of the Eye

Stye

A *stye* (hordeolum) is a small, painful lump located on the eyelid margin (Fig. 15.1). It is caused by an acute, self-limiting infection of the oil glands of the eyelid and typically resolves on its own in a few days.

Prescription Ophthalmic Eye Drops Used to Treat Dry Eye Disease

Generic Name	US Brand Name(s)	Dosage Forms and Strengths
	Canada Brand Name(s)	
cyclosporine[a]	Cequa, Restasis, Verkazia	**Ophthalmic emulsion:** 0.05% (Restasis), 0.09% (Cequa), 0.1% (Verkazia)
	Cequa, Restasis, Verkzia	
lifitegrast[a]	Xiidra	**Ophthalmic solution:** 5%
	Xiidra	

[a]Generic available in Canada.

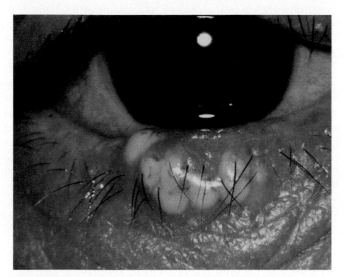

• **Fig. 15.1** Stye. (Courtesy of the Cogan Collection, National Eye Institute/ National Institutes of Health.)

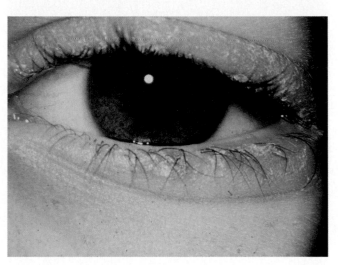

• **Fig. 15.2** Psoriatic blepharitis. (Courtesy of the Cogan Collection, National Eye Institute/National Institutes of Health.)

Blepharitis

Blepharitis is also known as granulated eyelids because of the distinctive flaky scales found on the eyelids and eyelashes produced by the condition. There are two forms of blepharitis: anterior blepharitis and posterior blepharitis. Anterior blepharitis affects the outside of the eyelid where the eyelashes are attached and is caused by bacteria *(Staphylococcus)* and dandruff—a mild, noninflammatory form of seborrheic dermatitis (see Chapter 36). Posterior blepharitis affects the inside of the eyelid and is caused by dysfunction of the oil glands in the eyelid, seborrhea, psoriasis (Fig. 15.2), and acne rosacea. The symptoms of blepharitis are eye pain or burning, excessive tearing, feeling of "something in the eye," light sensitivity, blurred vision, dry eye, and flaky scales on the eyelids and eyelashes.

Blepharitis is self-treated by applying clean warm compresses to the eyelids to loosen the scales followed by cleansing the eyelids with a mild eyelid scrub. Antiinfective ointments, corticosteroid eye drops, and artificial tears may also be used to manage the symptoms of blepharitis. Aminoglycoside antiinfective medications are used in the treatment of blepharitis and include gentamicin, neomycin, and tobramycin.

Conjunctivitis

Conjunctivitis (pink eye) is a common ailment that causes itching, burning, and teary outflow and is caused by allergies, bacteria, or a virus. Viral and allergic conjunctivitis is typically self-limiting and resolves without treatment with antiinfective agents. Conjunctivitis of bacterial origin is contagious and is treated with antibiotic eye drops or orally administered antiinfective medications. Conjunctivitis in newborns may be caused by exposure to a sexually transmitted infection and is treated preventively by administering antibiotic drops at birth. Antibacterial agents that are used in treatment include aminoglycosides, sulfonamides, quinolones, and macrolides. The antiviral trifluridine is used to treat keratoconjunctivitis caused by herpes simplex type 1 virus (Fig. 15.3).

Iritis

Iritis is a condition associated with inflammation of the iris. Most causes of iritis are unknown; known causes are herpes virus, autoimmune disease, eye trauma, infectious disease (histoplasmosis, toxoplasmosis, syphilis, tuberculosis), and juvenile rheumatoid arthritis.

Symptoms of iritis include redness, blurred vision, inflammation, pain, and light sensitivity. Iritis is treated with the administration of corticosteroids (to reduce inflammation) and mydriatics (to reduce painful swelling). Mydriatic medications act on the dilator muscle and arterioles of the conjunctiva to produce vasoconstriction and dilation of the pupil. Antiviral medications are administered when iritis is caused by a viral infection.

Keratitis

Keratitis is a severe infection of the cornea and may be caused by bacteria or fungi. If untreated, the infection can cause permanent loss of vision. The most common causes of microbial keratitis and fungal keratitis are trauma, immunodeficiency, and chronic eye surface disease. Contact lens use can also cause microbial and fungal keratitis. Soft contact lens wearers, especially those who wear their contact lenses overnight, are at greater risk for eye infection. Up to 20 contact lens users out of 10,000 will develop microbial keratitis each year, globally. The incidence of fungal keratitis varies according to geographic region. The incidence is higher in the southern United States (up to 35% of microbial keratitis cases) and lowest in the northeastern United States (up to 2% of microbial keratitis cases).

Uveitis

Uveitis is a serious eye condition that produces inflammation of the uvea and can cause scarring of the eye and blindness if untreated. There are three kinds of uveitis, each associated with a different part of the eye.

Uveitis may be caused by the herpes virus, histoplasmosis (fungus), toxoplasmosis (parasite), or autoimmune disease, but most of the time the cause is unknown. Symptoms of uveitis include redness, blurred vision, pain, inflammation, and light sensitivity. These symptoms may develop suddenly or can develop over a prolonged period.

Uveitis is treated with the administration of corticosteroids (to reduce inflammation), mydriatic medications (to reduce painful swelling), and antiinfective, antiviral, or antifungal drugs as appropriate. Immune modulators such as adalimumab (Humira) have been studied as a treatment because uveitis may occur in patients who have autoimmune conditions (e.g., ulcerative colitis). Immune modulators have not yet been approved by the US Food and Drug Administration (FDA) for the treatment of uveitis.

Most drugs used to treat eye infections are applied topically. Topical agents used in the treatment of eye infections are listed in the drug tables in this chapter.

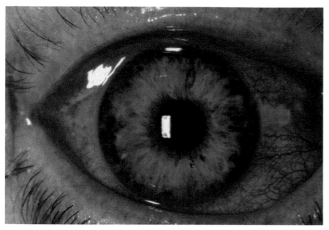

• **Fig. 15.3** Viral conjunctivitis. (Courtesy of the Cogan Collection, National Eye Institute/National Institutes of Health.)

Topical Ophthalmic Medications Used to Treat Bacterial Infections

Generic Name	US Brand Name(s) / Canadian Brand(s)	Dosage Forms and Strengths
Aminoglycosides		
gentamicin[a]	Genoptic	**Solution, ophthalmic:** 0.3%
	Not available	
tobramycin[a]	Tobrex	**Ointment, ophthalmic:** 0.3%
	Tobrex	**Solution, ophthalmic:** 0.3%
neomycin sulfate + polymyxin B sulfate + gramicidin[a]	Neosporin	**Solution, ophthalmic:** 1.75 mg/mL neomycin + 10,000 units/mL polymyxin B + 0.025 mg/mL gramicidin
	Not available	
polymyxin B sulfate + gramacidin[a]	Not available	**Solution, ophthalmic:** 10,000 units polymyxin B + 0.025 mg/mL gramicidin
	Optimyxin Ophthalmic/Otic	
Sulfonamides		
sulfacetamide Na+[a]	Bleph-10	**Ointment, ophthalmic:** 10%
	Not available	**Solution, ophthalmic:** 10%
trimethoprim + polymyxin B sulfate[a]	Polytrim	**Solution, ophthalmic:** 1 mg trimethoprim + 10,000 units polymyxin B/mL
	Polytrim	

Topical Ophthalmic Medications Used to Treat Bacterial Infections—cont'd

Generic Name	US Brand Name(s) Canadian Brand(s)	Dosage Forms and Strengths
Quinolones		
besifloxacin	Besivance Besivance	**Suspension, ophthalmic:** 0.6%
ciprofloxacin[a]	Ciloxan Ciloxan	**Ointment, ophthalmic:** 0.3% **Solution, ophthalmic:** 0.3%
gatifloxacin[a]	Zymar, Zymaxid Zymar	**Solution, ophthalmic:** 0.3% (Zymar), 0.5% (Zymaxid)
levofloxacin[a]	Generics Not available	**Solution, ophthalmic:** 0.5%
moxifloxacin[a]	Moxeza, Vigamox Vigamox	**Solution, ophthalmic:** 0.5%
ofloxacin[a]	Ocuflox Ocuflox	**Solution, ophthalmic:** 0.3%
Macrolides		
azithromycin	AzaSite Not available	**Solution, ophthalmic:** 1%
erythromycin[a]	Generics Generics	**Ointment, ophthalmic:** 0.5%
Antiinfective + Corticosteroid		
neomycin + dexamethasone + polymyxin[a]	Maxitrol Maxitrol	**Suspension, ophthalmic:** 3.5 mg neomycin + 0.1% dexamethasone + 6000 units polymyxin/mL[b]; 3.5 mg/mL neomycin + 0.1% dexamethasone + 10,000 units polymyxin/mL[c] **Ointment, ophthalmic:** 3.5 mg neomycin + 0.1% dexamethasone + 6000 units polymyxin/g[b]; 3.5 mg neomycin + 0.1% dexamethasone + 10,000 units polymyxin/g[c]
gentamicin + prednisolone	Pred-G Not available	**Suspension, ophthalmic:** 0.3% gentamicin + 1% prednisolone **Ointment, ophthalmic:** 0.3% gentamicin + 0.6% prednisolone
sulfacetamide + prednisolone acetate[a]	Blephamide Not available	**Ointment, ophthalmic:** 10% sulfacetamide + 0.2% prednisolone **Solution, ophthalmic:** 10% sulfacetamide + 0.2% prednisolone
tobramycin + dexamethasone	Tobradex, Tobradex ST Tobradex	**Ointment, ophthalmic:** 0.3% tobramycin + 0.1% dexamethasone **Suspension, ophthalmic:** 0.3% tobramycin + 0.1% dexamethasone (Tobradex); 0.3% tobramycin + 0.05% dexamethasone (Tobradex ST)
tobramycin + loteprednol	Zylet Not available	**Suspension, ophthalmic:** 0.3% tobramycin + 0.5% loteprednol

[a]Generic available.
[b]Available in Canada only.
[c]Available in the United States only.

Viral Infections of the Eye

Cytomegalovirus Retinitis

Cytomegalovirus (CMV) retinitis is an opportunistic infection in the eye that occurs in patients who have HIV/AIDS or take immunosuppressive drugs. The most common symptoms of CMV retinitis are decreased vision, eye pain, floaters, and photopsia. If untreated, CMV retinitis can lead to blindness. *Vitreous floaters* are particles that cast shadows on the retina and appear as spots, cobwebs, or spiders. *Photopsia* is a condition similar to floaters and is associated with flashes of light.

CMV retinitis is treated by administration of antiviral agents such as ganciclovir, valganciclovir, foscarnet, and cidofovir.

Herpetic Eye Disease

The herpes virus is the most common cause of blindness globally. The two strains of the virus that cause eye infections are *herpes zoster ophthalmicus* and *herpes simplex keratitis*. Nearly 1.5 million people develop herpes simplex virus (HSV) keratitis annually, leading to up to 40,000 cases of severe visual impairment or blindness. Other common viral infections caused by the herpes virus are chicken pox and shingles *(herpes zoster,* caused by *varicella-zoster virus)* and cold sores on the lips and mouth *(herpes simplex 1).*

Both herpes zoster ophthalmicus and herpes simplex keratitis produce eye pain because the virus lives around nerve fibers that, when activated, produce pain. Symptoms specifically associated with herpes zoster ophthalmicus are swelling and rash or sores around the eye, eyelids, or forehead. Symptoms of HSV keratitis are excessive tearing, decreased vision, a gritty feeling in the eye, and pain when looking at bright light.

Viral infections of the eye are treated with antiviral medications. They may be administered topically in the eye or by mouth or intravenous infusion according to the drug and condition being treated. Antiviral agents that are used in the treatment of herpetic eye disease are listed the following table. A detailed discussion of antiviral drugs is found in Chapter 30.

Corticosteroids may also be prescribed to reduce inflammation of the trabecular meshwork. Inflammation can impede the outflow of eye fluids and lead to increased intraocular pressure (IOP) and pain. The use of corticosteroids must be carefully monitored because the drugs sometimes increase IOP. Mydriatic medications may be administered to maintain the normal flow of eye fluids and prevent buildup of IOP.

> ### ⓘ Tech Alert!
> valGANcyclovir and valACYclovir have look-alike/sound-alike issues.

Fungal Infections of the Eye

Fusarium keratitis is a rare fungal infection of the eye that occasionally occurs in people who wear soft contact lenses. If untreated, it can lead to blindness. See the discussion of keratitis for more information. Fusarium keratitis and other fungal infections of the eye are treated with antifungal drugs such as natamycin.

Ophthalmic Antifungal Medications

Generic Name	US Brand Name(s) / Canadian Brand(s)	Dosage Form and Strength
Natamycin	Natacyn	**Suspension, ophthalmic:** 5%
	Not available	

Drugs Used to Treat Viral Infections in the Eye

Generic Name	US Brand Name(s) / Canadian Brand(s)	Dosage Forms and Strengths
cidofovir[a]	Generics	**Solution for injection:** 75 mg/mL
	Generics	
foscarnet	Foscavir	**Solution, for injection:** 24 mg/mL
	Vocarvi	
ganciclovir[a]	Ganzyk-RTU, Zirgan	**Gel, ophthalmic (Zirgan):** 0.15% **Powder, for injection (Cytovene):** 500 mg per vial **Intravenous solution:** 2 mg/mL (Ganzyk-RTU)
	Cytovene	
trifluridine[a]	Viroptic	**Solution, ophthalmic:** 1%
	Not available	
valganciclovir[a]	Valcyte	**Solution, oral:** 50 mg/mL **Tablet:** 450 mg
	Valcyte	

[a]Generic available.

Parasitic Infections of the Eye

Ocular *toxoplasmosis* is caused by a parasite and is transmitted by handling or eating raw and undercooked meat or by handling cat feces. According to the Centers for Disease Control and Prevention, more than 800,000 persons are infected with toxoplasmosis annually and approximately 3600 will develop ocular toxoplasmosis. Exposure to the protozoa causes the development of antigens that can cause ocular inflammation, vasculitis, uveitis, and retinal edema. Ocular toxoplasmosis can cause blindness. First-line pharmacotherapy for toxoplasmosis in adults, children, and pregnant women beyond 18 weeks' gestation includes pyrimethamine, sulfadiazine (sulfonamides), and folinic acid.

Helminthes are parasitic worms that can cause eye infections and blindness. Three species can cause infection in the human eye. *Onchocerca volvulus* is a roundworm that causes onchocerciasis. Onchocerciasis is also known as river blindness and is the second leading cause of infectious blindness in the world, according to the World Health Organization. *Taenia solium* is a flatworm that causes cysticercosis, an infection caused by eating undercooked pork. Toxocariasis is the fifth leading cause of uveitis worldwide. Dogs, cats, wolves, and foxes are carriers of the worm that causes toxocariasis. Toxocariasis is an infection that is contracted by eating soil that is infested with feces containing worm eggs and is most common in children. Infections can cause loss of vision in the affected eye and strabismus. The dog is also the carrier of another roundworm *(Ancylostoma caninum)* that produces inflammation in the retina that progresses to atrophy of the optic nerve and blindness.

Ivermectin kills the living worms that cause onchocerciasis infection and prevents inflammation and scarring. A single dose of ivermectin is administered yearly. Cysticercosis and toxocariasis are treated by the administration of topical corticosteroids and systemic anthelminthic drugs such as albendazole and thiabendazole. Surgical removal of the living worms may be necessary for cysticercosis to reduce damage to the eye that might occur when drug therapy is used.

> ● *Tech Note!*
>
> Ophthalmic drugs can be used in the ear, but otic drugs cannot be used in the eye. All ophthalmic drugs must be sterile.

Summary of Treatments of Bacterial, Fungal, and Viral Infections of the Eye

Glaucoma

It is estimated that more than 80 million people worldwide have glaucoma. This number is expected to increase to 111 million by 2040, making glaucoma the second leading cause of blindness worldwide. More than 3 million Americans and 728,000 Canadians are living with the disease. The prevalence of glaucoma increases with age, growing steadily after age 60 years. Having a family history for glaucoma also increases the risk. Diabetes, which is discussed in Chapter 26, is a risk factor for neurovascular glaucoma.

Summary of Agents Used to Treat Bacterial, Fungal, and Viral Infections of the Eye

Generic Name	Brand Name	Usual Dosage
Aminoglycosides		
gentamicin 0.3%	Genoptic	Instill 1–2 drops every 4 h while awake until resolved (solution) *or* Apply ½-inch ribbon of ointment 2–3 times a day to eyelid margin
tobramycin 0.3%	Tobrex	Instill 1–2 drops in eye(s) every 4 h *or* Apply ointment 2–3 times a day (every 3–4 h for severe infection)
neomycin + polymyxin B + gramicidin	Neosporin Ophthalmic solution	Instill 1–2 drops in eye(s) every 4 h (or up to 2 drops every hour for severe infection)
Sulfonamides		
sulfacetamide Na+ 10%	Bleph-10	Instill 1–2 drops every 1 h while awake until resolved (solution)
trimethoprim 1 mg + polymyxin B 10,000 units	Polytrim	Instill 1 drop into eye(s) every 3 h up to 6 doses/day for 7–10 days
Quinolones		
besifloxacin	Besivance	Instill 1 drop in the affected eye(s) 3 times daily, 4–12 h apart, for 7 days
ciprofloxacin 0.3%	Ciloxan	Instill 1–2 drops in eye(s) every 2 h while awake for 2 days; then 1–2 drops every 4 h for 5 days *or* Apply ½-inch ribbon to conjunctival sac 3 times a day for 2 days; then twice daily for 5 days

Continued

Summary of Agents Used to Treat Bacterial, Fungal, and Viral Infections of the Eye—cont'd

Generic Name	Brand Name	Usual Dosage
gatifloxacin	Zymaxid, Zymar	On day 1–2, instill 1 drop in each affected eye every 2 h while awake up to 8 times daily; on days thereafter 1 drop in each affected eye 2–4 times daily while awake (3–7 days)
levofloxacin	Generics	Instill 1–2 drops in eye(s) every 2 h while awake days 1–2; then instill every 4 h days 3–7 (up to 4 times a day)
moxifloxacin	Vigamox, Moxeza	Instill 1 drop in affected eye(s) 3 times a day for 7 days (Vigamox); instill 1 drop in affected eye(s) 2 times a day for 7 days (Moxeza)
ofloxacin	Ocuflox	Instill 1 drop in affected eye every 2–4 h for 2 days; then use 1–2 drops 4 times a day for 5 days more
Macrolides		
azithromycin	AzaSite	Instill 1 drop in the affected eye(s) twice daily (8–12 h apart) for the first 2 days followed by 1 drop in the affected eye(s) once daily for the next 5 days
erythromycin	Generics	Apply ½-inch (1.25 cm) 2–6 times a day until resolved
Antiinfective + Corticosteroid		
neomycin + polymyxin B + dexamethasone	Maxitrol	Apply a ½-inch ribbon of ointment 3–4 times a day or at bedtime *or* Instill 1–2 drops into eye(s) every 4–6 h (up to every 1 h if severe disease)
gentamicin + prednisolone	Pred-G	Instill 1 drop into eye(s) 2–4 times a day (up to every 1 h during first 24–48 h) *or* Apply a ½-inch ribbon of ointment 1–3 times a day
sulfacetamide + prednisolone	Blephamide	Apply to lower conjunctival sac up to 6 times a day *or* Instill 2 drops every 4 h during the day and at bedtime
tobramycin + dexamethasone	Tobradex	Instill 1–2 drops in eye(s) every 4–6 h *or* Apply ointment every 6–8 h
tobramycin + loteprednol	Zylet	Instill 1–2 drops into the conjunctival sac of the affected eye(s) every 4–6 h (up to every 1–2 h during first 24–48 h)
Antiviral		
cidofovir	Generics	**CMV:** Infuse 5 mg/kg IV over 1 h once weekly for 2 weeks, then once every other week
ganciclovir	Cytovene, Zirgan Ganzyk-RTU	**CMV retinitis:** Infuse 5 mg/kg IV every 12 h for 14–21 days; then once daily 7 days/week (or 6 mg/kg/day for 5 days/week)
foscarnet	Foscavir, Vocarvi	**CMV retinitis:** Infuse 60 mg/kg/dose every 8 h or 90 mg every 12 h for 14–21 days; then 90–120 mg/kg/day every 24 h
trifluridine	Viroptic	**Herpes simplex keratoconjunctivitis:** Instill 1 drop in eye(s) every 2 h while awake up to 9 drops/day until corneal ulcer heals; then 1 drop every 4 h for 7 days
valganciclovir	Valcyte	**CMV retinitis:** 900 mg twice a day for 21 days; then take once daily thereafter
Antifungal		
natamycin	Natacyn	**Keratitis**: Instill 1 drop into conjunctival sac every 1–2 h for 3–4 days; then 1 drop every 3–4 h for 14–21 days or until resolved. **Blepharitis and conjunctivitis**: 1 drop every 4–6 h until resolved.

CMV, Cytomeglovirus; *IV,* intravenous.

Pathophysiology

There are several types of glaucoma, and all are associated with progressive damage to the structures in the eye responsible for vision. *Peripheral vision* is first to be lost. The person gradually loses the ability to see images from the sides, top, or bottom of the eye(s). Eventually, only central vision remains (Fig. 15.4).

Open-angle glaucoma is the most common and results from abnormal accumulation of *aqueous humor* (Fig. 15.5). This in turn causes excessive *intraocular pressure* that produces degeneration of the optic nerve. Sometimes damage to the optic nerve can occur in the absence of increased IOP. When this happens, low-tension or normal-tension glaucoma is said to be the cause. The unit of measure for IOP is millimeters of mercury (mm Hg).

IOP rises rapidly to dangerously high levels when a person has narrow-angle or *angle-closure glaucoma*. Normally, aqueous fluids drain from the eye through an opening in the eye where the cornea and iris meet. This region is called the angle (see Fig. 15.5). When the angle becomes obstructed, as occurs with inflammation or partial blockage of the trabecular meshwork, aqueous humor drainage is impaired, and there is a sudden increase in eye pressure. Pain and nausea may occur. If untreated, blindness can result in as little as a few days. Children born with defects in the structure of the angle of the eye may develop congenital glaucoma. Children with congenital glaucoma often have cloudy eyes, light sensitivity, and excessive tearing. If treated promptly, impaired vision may be avoided.

Treatment

Drugs used in the treatment of glaucoma can be divided into two main classifications according to their method of action. The drugs lower IOP by decreasing the formation of fluids that build up in the eye, or they promote drainage of fluids that accumulate. This is accomplished by actions on parasympathetic or sympathetic nerves that control secretion of fluids and contraction of muscles that block fluid drainage. More than a single agent may be administered for the treatment of glaucoma. When two drops are administered, the second drop should be placed in the eye at least 5 minutes after the first agent. This will give the first eye drop time to "soak in" and avoid being washed away by the second drop.

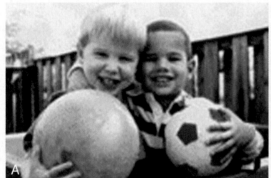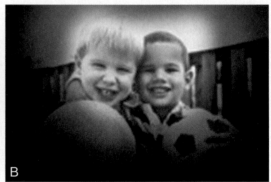

• **Fig. 15.4** Glaucoma. (**A**) Normal vision. (**B**) Glaucoma. (Courtesy of US National Institutes of Health National Eye Institute.)

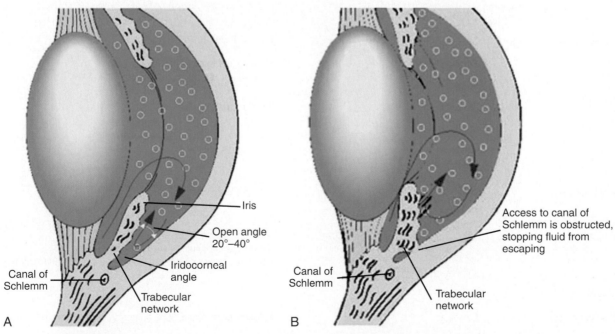

• **Fig. 15.5** (**A**) Aqueous humor: flow. (**B**) Aqueous humor: obstruction. (From Clayton BD, Stock YN, Harroun RD. *Basic pharmacology for nurses*, ed 14, St Louis, 2007, Mosby.)

● **Tech Note!**

-"lol" is a common ending for β-adrenergic antagonists (also known as β-blockers).

Drugs That Decrease Aqueous Humor Formation

Beta-Adrenergic Antagonists

Most drugs used to treat open-angle glaucoma are β-adrenergic antagonists, also called β-blockers. They reduce intraocular hypertension. Stimulation of β-adrenergic receptors on ciliary cells increases secretion of aqueous humor. β-Adrenergic antagonists decrease aqueous humor formation by inhibiting the action of epinephrine and norepinephrine on β-adrenergic receptors located on the muscle and on blood vessels within the ciliary body. Betaxolol is the only β-adrenergic antagonist that is selective for β_1-receptor sites. This means that betaxolol may be safer for use in patients who have asthma, congestive heart failure, or other conditions in which blockade of β_2-receptor sites is undesirable. Adverse reactions produced by betaxolol are blurred vision, light sensitivity (photophobia), dizziness, and nausea. Local adverse reactions to carteolol, levobunolol, and timolol include burning, pain, and itching in addition to blurred vision. Systemic effects are less common and include dizziness, weakness, depression, hypotension, decreased heart rate, and difficulty breathing. Systemic absorption may be reduced by applying finger pressure to the lacrimal sac for 1 to 2 minutes after placing the drops in the eyes.

● **Tech Note!**

To minimize systemic side effects, patients are advised to apply gentle pressure to the lacrimal sac for 1 to 2 minutes after the administration of eye drops.

Alpha-Adrenergic Agonists

The α-adrenergic receptor agonists are used for the prevention and treatment of increased IOP. There are two α-adrenergic receptors in the eye (α_1 and α_2). Administration of α_1-adrenergic receptor agonists reduces blood flow in the ciliary body, and administration of α_2-adrenergic receptor agonists reduces the formation of aqueous humor. Administration of α_2-adrenergic agonists produces effects similar to administration of α-adrenergic antagonists. Adverse reactions produced by apraclonidine and brimonidine may be systemic and local. Local reactions include blurred vision, decreased night and distance vision, dry eyes, and irritated eyelids. Systemic effects are drowsiness and headache.

Carbonic Anhydrase Inhibitors

Carbonic anhydrase inhibitors are indicated for the treatment of open-angle glaucoma. Acetazolamide and methazolamide tablets are also indicated for prevention of secondary acute angle-closure glaucoma, short-term treatment of angle-closure glaucoma when surgery must be delayed, reduction of IOP after cataract surgery, edema, and prevention of altitude sickness. Carbonic anhydrase inhibitors inhibit the enzyme carbonic anhydrase. The enzyme is involved in the process of converting carbon dioxide and water to bicarbonate. The enzyme is found in many parts of the body, including the ciliary structures of the eye. The production of aqueous humor depends on the transport of bicarbonate and sodium ions. Administration of carbonic anhydrase inhibitors decreases the rate of production of aqueous humor, thereby decreasing IOP. Adverse effects of acetazolamide and methazolamide include dizziness, drowsiness, potassium loss, frequent urination, kidney stones, a tingling sensation in the fingers and toes, bitter or metallic taste, nausea, impotence, and depression. Brinzolamide and dorzolamide produce local adverse effects that include blurred vision, a bitter taste in the mouth, and burning or stinging dry eyes. Less common reactions are irritation, discharge from the eyes, soreness, headache, and dizziness.

Beta-Adrenergic Antagonists

Generic Name	US Brand Name(s) Canadian Brand(s)	Dosage Forms and Strengths
betaxolol[a]	Betoptic, Betoptic S	**Solution, ophthalmic (Betoptic):** 0.5%
	Betoptic S	**Suspension, ophthalmic (Betoptic S):** 0.25%
carteolol[a]	Generics	**Solution, ophthalmic:** 1%
	Not available	
levobunolol[a]	Betagan	**Solution, ophthalmic:** 0.5%
	Not available	
timolol hemihydrate[a]	Betimol	**Solution, ophthalmic:** 0.25%, 0.5%
	Not available	
timolol maleate[a]	Istalol, Timoptic, Timoptic in OcuDose, Timoptic XE	**Solution, gel forming (Timoptic XE):** 0.25%, 0.5% **Solution, ophthalmic (Timoptic):** 0.25%, 0.5%
	Timoptic, Timoptic XE	**Solution, preservative free (Timoptic in OcuDose):** 0.25%, 0.5%
Combinations		
timolol + brimonidine[a]	Combigan	**Solution, ophthalmic:** 0.2% brimonidine + 0.5% timolol
	Combigan	

[a]Generic available.

Alpha-Adrenergic Agonists

Generic Name	US Brand Name(s)	Dosage Forms and Strengths
	Canadian Brand(s)	
apraclonidine[a]	Iopidine	**Solution, ophthalmic:** 0.5%, 1%
	Iopidine	
brimonidine[a]	Alphagan P, Lumify, Mirvaso, Qoliana	**Gel, ophthalmic (Mirvaso, Onreltea):** 0.33%
	Alphagan, Alphagan P, Lumify, Onreltea	**Solution, ophthalmic:** 0.1%[b], 0.15% (Alphagan P, Qoliana), 0.2% (Alphagan), 0.025% (Lumify)[c]

[a]Generic available.
[b]Available in the United States only.
[c]Available without a prescription to reduce eye redness.

Carbonic Anhydrase Inhibitors

Generic Name	US Brand Name(s)	Dosage Forms and Strengths
	Canadian Brand(s)	
acetazolamide[a]	Generics	**Capsule, sustained release[b]:** 500 mg[b]
	Generics	**Powder, for IV use:** 500 mg/vial
		Tablets: 125 mg[b], 250 mg
brinzolamide[a, b]	Azopt	**Suspension, ophthalmic:** 1%
	Azopt	
dorzolamide[a]	Trusopt	**Solution, ophthalmic:** 2%
	Trusopt, Trusopt PF	
methazolamide[a]	Generics	**Tablets:** 25 mg[b], 50 mg
	Generics	

Carbonic Anhydrase Inhibitor Combination

brinzolamide + brimonidine	Simbrinza	**Solution, ophthalmic:** 0.2% brimonidine + 1% brinzolamide
	Simbrinza	
brinzolamide + timolol	Not available	**Suspension, ophthalmic:** 1% brinzolamide + 0.5% timolol
	Azarga	
dorzolamide and timolol[a]	Cosopt, Cosopt PF	**Solution, ophthalmic:** 2% dorzolamide and 0.5% timolol
	Cosopt, Cosopt PF	

[a]Generic available.
[b]Available in the United States only.

> ● **Tech Note!**
>
> "-zolamide" is a common ending for carbonic anhydrase inhibitors.

> ● **Tech Note!**
>
> Carbonic anhydrase inhibitors may cause allergic reactions in people who have allergies to sulfonamide antiinfective agents.

Drugs That Increase Aqueous Humor Drainage

Miotics are drugs that promote drainage of the aqueous humor. They produce this effect via a variety of mechanisms of action. Cholinergic agonists, acetylcholinesterase inhibitors, and prostaglandin analogs all promote drainage of accumulated levels of aqueous humor and reduce IOP.

Cholinergic Agonists and Cholinesterase Inhibitors

Cholinergic agonists (pilocarpine, carbachol, and echothiophate) are used to reduce IOP caused by glaucoma and cataract surgery.

Cholinergic Agonists

Generic Name	US Brand Name(s) Canadian Brand(s)	Dosage Forms and Strengths
carbachol	Miostat	**Solution, ophthalmic:** 0.01%
	Miostat	
pilocarpine[a]	Isopto Carpine, Vuity	**Solution, ophthalmic (Isopto Carpine):** 1%[b], 2%, 4%[b], 1.25% (Vuity)
	Generics	
Cholinesterase Inhibitor		
echothiophate iodide	Phospholine iodide	**Powder for reconstitution:** 0.125%
	Not available	

[a]Generic available.
[b]Available in the United States only.

• BOX 15.1   Directions for Preparing Echothiophate Iodide Eye Drops

- Use aseptic technique.
- Tear off aluminum seals and remove and discard rubber plugs from both the drug and diluent containers.
- Pour the diluent into the drug container.
- Remove the dropper assembly from its sterile wrapping. Holding the dropper assembly by the screw cap and WITHOUT COMPRESSING RUBBER BULB, insert it into drug container and screw down tightly.
- Shake for several seconds to ensure mixing.

Cholinergic agonists bind to receptor sites and produce effects that mimic the neurotransmitter acetylcholine. Binding produces parasympathetic nervous system effects in the eye, such as contraction of ciliary muscles, and results in miosis. Pilocarpine is a cholinergic agonist that is used in the treatment of open- and closed-angle glaucoma. Cholinergic agonists also produce dilation of the trabecular meshwork to decrease IOP. Pilocarpine (Salagen) is also used to treat xerostomia (dry mouth).

Echothiophate iodide is a cholinesterase inhibitor. Cholinesterase inhibitors block the enzyme that deactivates acetylcholine (see Chapter 12). This prolongs the effects of acetylcholine and administered cholinergic agonists. Adverse reactions include blurred vision, change in near or distance vision, difficulty in seeing at night or in dim light, headache, twitching of the eyelids, and watering of the eyes. For preparation instructions, see Box 15.1.

Prostaglandin Analogs

Bimatoprost, latanoprost, latanoprostene, and travoprost are prostaglandin analogs that are prodrugs. They mimic the action of prostaglandin F2α and relax the ciliary muscles to permit drainage of aqueous humors. Prostaglandin analogs directly dilate the trabecular meshwork to promote drainage. The use of prostaglandin analogs can cause changes in the color or pigmentation of the eyes and may thicken eyelashes. Latisse (bimatoprost) is marketed as a topical solution to increase the growth of eyelashes in patients who have hypotrichosis, a condition whereby they have no eyelashes.

Prostaglandin Analogs

Generic Name	US Brand Name(s) Canadian Brand(s)	Dosage Forms and Strengths
bimatoprost	Durysta, Latisse, Lumigan	**Implant (Durysta):** 10 mcg
	Latisse, Lumigan RC, Vistitan	**Solution, topical (Latisse):** 0.03% **Solution, ophthalmic:** 0.01%, 0.03%
latanoprostene bunod	Vyzulta	**Solution, ophthalmic:** 0.024%
	Vyzulta	
latanoprost[a]	Xalatan, Xelpros	**Emulsion, ophthalmic (Xelpros):** 0.005%
	Monoprost, Xalatan	**Solution, ophthalmic:** 0.005%
tafluprost[a]	Zioptan	**Solution, ophthalmic:** 0.0015%
	Not available	
travoprost[a]	Travatan Z	**Solution, ophthalmic:** 0.003% (Izba), 0.004% (Travatan Z)
	Izba, Travatan Z	
Combination		
latanoprost + netarsudil	Rocklatan	**Solution, ophthalmic:** 0.005% latanoprost + 0.02% netarsudil
	Not available	
latanoprost + timolol[a]	Not available	**Solution, ophthalmic:** 0.5% timolol + 0.005% latanoprost
	Xalacom	
travoprost + timolol[a]	Not available	**Solution, ophthalmic:** 0.5% timolol + 0.004% travoprost
	DuoTrav PQ	

[a]Generic available.

Bimatoprost, latanoprost, and travoprost may decrease vision and produce eye irritation, eye pain, itchy eyes, redness of eye, dry eyes, sun sensitivity, or watery eyes.

● *Tech Note!*

"-prost" is a common ending for drugs that are prostaglandin analogs.

Rho Kinase Inhibitor

Netarsudil is a Rho kinase inhibitor. Rho kinase inhibitors increase the outflow of aqueous humor through the trabecular meshwork, thereby decreasing IOP. Netarsudil also inhibits the production of aqueous humor by inhibiting norepinephrine transport. This action prolongs the reduction of IOP that occurs by constricting blood vessels in the eye.

Miscellaneous

Medical use of cannabis is legal in many US states, and cannabis possession is legal in Canada. However, the use of cannabis to lower IOP is controversial. Although some studies have shown mild, transient reduction in IOP, studies have shown only short-term effect. Cannabis has not been shown to be as effective as currently available drugs that are indicated for the treatment of glaucoma.

Nondrug Treatment

Laser Surgery

Laser surgery may be performed to reduce IOP. There are three forms of laser surgery for glaucoma. Laser peripheral iridotomy creates a new drainage hole in the iris, permitting fluids to drain out of the eye. Laser trabeculoplasty unblocks existing channels, and laser cyclophotocoagulation, a type of laser surgery that is performed to reduce the amount of fluid entering the eye, is indicated for people who have severe glaucoma and have not responded to standard glaucoma surgery. Laser cyclophotocoagulation partially destroys the tissues that make the fluid in the eye.

Rho Kinase Inhibitor

Generic Name	US Brand Name(s) Canadian Brand(s)	Dosage Forms and Strengths
netarsudil	Rhopressa	**Solution, ophthalmic:** 0.02%
	Not available	

Summary of Drugs Used to Treat Glaucoma

Generic	Brand Name	Usual Dose	Warning Labels
Decrease Aqueous Humor Formation			
Beta-Adrenergic Antagonists			
betaxolol	Betoptic-S	**Open-angle glaucoma:** Instill 1 drop twice a day in affected eye(s)	SHAKE WELL—betaxolol suspension. WASH HANDS BEFORE USE; AVOID CONTAMINATION OF TIP—all.
carteolol	Generics	**Open-angle glaucoma:** Instill 1 drop twice a day in affected eye(s)	REMOVE CONTACT LENSES BEFORE USE; WAIT AT LEAST 15 MIN BEFORE REINSERTING—all.
levobunolol	Betagan	**Open-angle glaucoma:** Instill 1–2 drops in affected eye(s) 2 times a day 0.25% or once daily 0.5%	STORE AT ROOM TEMPERATURE—all. PROTECT FROM LIGHT—all.
timolol maleate	Timoptic, Timoptic XE	**Open-angle glaucoma:** Timoptic: Instill 1 drop twice daily in affected eye(s) Timoptic XE, Istalol: Instill 1 drop daily in the morning	DO NOT DISCONTINUE WITHOUT MEDICAL SUPERVISION—all.
timolol hemihydrate	Betimol	**Open-angle glaucoma:** Instill 1 drop twice daily in affected eye(s)	
Alpha-Adrenergic Agonists			
apraclonidine	Iopidine	Instill 1–2 drops in affected eye(s) 3 times a day	STORE AT ROOM TEMPERATURE—all. PROTECT FROM LIGHT—all.
brimonidine	Alphagan	Instill 1 drop in affected eye(s) 3 times a day	WASH HANDS BEFORE USE; AVOID CONTAMINATION OF TIP—all.
brimonidine + timolol	Combigan	Instill 1 drop in affected eye(s) 2 times a day	REMOVE CONTACT LENSES BEFORE USE; WAIT AT LEAST 15 MIN BEFORE REINSERTING—all. DO NOT DISCONTINUE WITHOUT MEDICAL SUPERVISION—all.

Continued

Summary of Drugs Used to Treat Glaucoma—cont'd

Generic	Brand Name	Usual Dose	Warning Labels
Decrease Aqueous Humor Formation			

Carbonic Anhydrase Inhibitors

Generic	Brand Name	Usual Dose	Warning Labels
acetazolamide	Diamox	**Oral (sustained release):** 500 mg twice daily **Oral (immediate release):** 250 mg 1–4 times a day	TAKE WITH FOOD—acetazolamide, methazolamide. SWALLOW WHOLE; DO NOT CRUSH OR CHEW—sustained-release capsule. MAY CAUSE DIZZINESS OR DROWSINESS—acetazolamide, methazolamide. SHAKE WELL—brinzolamide, brinzolamide + timolol. REMOVE CONTACT LENSES BEFORE USE; WAIT AT LEAST 15 MIN BEFORE REINSERTING—brinzolamide, dorzolamide, dorzolamide + timolol. WASH HANDS BEFORE USE; AVOID CONTAMINATION OF TIP—brinzolamide, dorzolamide, dorzolamide + timolol. STORE AT ROOM TEMPERATURE—brinzolamide, dorzolamide, dorzolamide + timolol. PROTECT FROM LIGHT—brinzolamide, dorzolamide, dorzolamide + timolol. DO NOT DISCONTINUE WITHOUT MEDICAL SUPERVISION—brinzolamide, dorzolamide, dorzolamide + timolol.
brinzolamide	Azopt	Instill 1 drop 3 times a day	
dorzolamide	Trusopt	Instill 1 drop 3 times a day	
brinzolamide + timolol	Azarga	Instill 1 drop 2 times a day	
dorzolamide + timolol	Cosopt	Instill 1 drop twice a day	
methazolamide	Generics	**Oral:** 50–100 mg 2–3 times a day	

Increase Drainage of Aqueous Humor
Cholinergic Agonists

Generic	Brand Name	Usual Dose	Warning Labels
carbachol	Miostat	Instill 1–2 drops up to 3 times a day	WASH HANDS BEFORE USE; AVOID CONTAMINATION OF TIP—all. DO NOT DISCONTINUE WITHOUT MEDICAL SUPERVISION—all. STORE AT ROOM TEMPERATURE—carbachol. DO NOT WEAR CONTACT LENSES—carbachol.
pilocarpine	Isopto Carpine	**Solution:** Instill 1 drop up to 3 times a day	

Cholinesterase Inhibitor

Generic	Brand Name	Usual Dose	Warning Labels
echothiophate	Phospholine Iodide	**Open-angle glaucoma:** Instill 1 drop twice a day	REFRIGERATE OR STORE RECONSTITUTED SOLUTION FOR UP TO 4 WEEKS AT ROOM TEMPERATURE.

Prostaglandin Analogs

Generic	Brand Name	Usual Dose	Warning Labels
bimatoprost	Lumigan	Instill 1 drop once daily in the evening	WASH HANDS BEFORE USE; AVOID CONTAMINATION OF TIP—all. REMOVE CONTACT LENSES BEFORE USE; WAIT AT LEAST 15 MIN BEFORE REINSERTING—all. DO NOT DISCONTINUE WITHOUT MEDICAL SUPERVISION—all. REFRIGERATE; DO NOT FREEZE—latanoprost, latanoprost + timolol. STORE AT ROOM TEMPERATURE—bimatoprost, travoprost, travoprost + timolol.
latanoprost	Xalatan	Instill 1 drop once daily in the evening	
travoprost	Travatan	Instill 1 drop in affected eye(s) once daily in the evening	
latanoprost + timolol	Xalacom	**Open-angle glaucoma:** Instill 1 drop in affected eye(s) once daily	
travoprost + timolol	DuoTrav	**Open-angle glaucoma:** Instill 1 drop in affected eye(s) once daily	

Rho Kinase Inhibitor

Generic	Brand Name	Usual Dose	Warning Labels
netarsudil	Rhopressa	Instill 1 drop in affected eye(s) once daily	REFRIGERATE; DO NOT FREEZE (unopened bottles); may store opened bottles at room temperature. PROTECT FROM LIGHT. DISCARD 6 WEEKS AFTER OPENING.
latanoprost + netarsudil	Rocklatan	Instill 1 drop in affected eye(s) once daily	

TECHNICIAN'S CORNER

1. The prevalence of glaucoma in a person with diabetes is greater than in persons without diabetes. What can be done to help diabetic patients decrease the chance of developing glaucoma?
2. How can contact lens users reduce the risk of eye infections?

Key Points

- Glaucoma is the second leading cause of blindness worldwide.
- The percentage of the population who will develop glaucoma increases with advancing age.
- There are several types of glaucoma: open-angle, angle-closure, low-tension, and secondary glaucoma.
- The most common form of glaucoma is open-angle glaucoma.
- Increased IOP is caused by a buildup of aqueous humor and is a symptom of glaucoma.
- Drugs used in the treatment of glaucoma can be divided into two main classifications according to their method of action: drugs that decrease formation of aqueous humor and drugs that promote drainage of aqueous humor.
- Drug classifications that decrease formation of the aqueous humor are β-blockers, α-adrenergic agonists, and carbonic anhydrase inhibitors.
- Drug classifications that promote drainage of the aqueous humor are cholinergics, cholinesterase inhibitors, and prostaglandin analogs.
- Rho kinase inhibitors (netarsudil) promote drainage of aqueous humor and decrease formation of aqueous humor.
- Miotics are drugs that cause contraction of the pupil. Drugs that promote drainage of the aqueous humor produce miosis.
- Blepharitis is self-treated by applying clean warm compresses. In some cases, antiinfective ointments, corticosteroid eye drops, and artificial tears may be administered to manage the symptoms.
- Conjunctivitis (pink eye) may be caused by a virus or bacteria.
- Uveitis is treated with the administration of corticosteroids (to reduce inflammation), mydriatic agents (to reduce painful swelling), and antiinfective or antiviral medication as appropriate.
- Soft contact lens wearers, especially those who wear their contact lenses overnight, are at risk for fungal keratitis.
- A stye is a small, painful lump on the eyelid that is caused by an acute self-limiting infection of the oil glands of the eyelid.
- CMV retinitis is an opportunistic infection in the eye that occurs in patients who have HIV/AIDS or who take immunosuppressive drugs and if untreated can cause blindness.
- CMV retinitis is treated by administration of antiviral medications such as ganciclovir, valganciclovir, foscarnet, and cidofovir.
- Herpes zoster ophthalmicus and herpes simplex virus keratitis are treated by administering antiviral eye drops, orally administered drugs, or both.
- Toxoplasmosis can cause ocular inflammation, vasculitis, uveitis, and retinal edema and is treated by administering pyrimethamine, sulfadiazine, and folinic acid.
- Onchocerciasis (river blindness) is caused by a roundworm.
- Onchocerciasis is treated by administering a single dose of ivermectin yearly.
- Cysticercosis is treated with praziquantel, corticosteroids, and surgical removal of the living worms.
- Toxocariasis is treated by administering topical corticosteroids and systemic anthelminthic drugs such as thiabendazole.

Review Questions

1. Keratitis is a severe infection of the iris and may be caused by bacteria or fungi.
   a. true
   b. false
2. The medical term for "granulated eyelids" is:
   a. uveitis
   b. keratitis
   c. blepharitis
   d. iritis
3. A stye (hordeolum) is a small, painful lump located on the:
   a. eyelid
   b. iris
   c. conjunctiva
   d. pupil
4. The most common form of glaucoma is _____.
   a. open angle
   b. closed angle
   c. narrow angle
   d. wide angle

5. The mechanism of action of drugs used in the treatment of glaucoma is to _____.
   a. lower intraocular pressure by decreasing the formation of fluids
   b. promote drainage of fluids that accumulate
   c. lower intraocular pressure by increasing the formation of fluids
   d. a and b
6. Lumify is _____.
   a. used to treat glaucoma
   b. an over-the-counter eye drop used to treat red eye
   c. available by prescription only
   d. required to be stored in the refrigerator
7. Miotics are drugs that are used to decrease the drainage of the aqueous humor.
   a. true
   b. false

8. Select the drug that is a β-adrenergic antagonist indicated for the treatment of open-angle glaucoma.
   a. latanoprost
   b. acetazolamide
   c. epinephrine
   d. timolol

9. Select the FALSE statement about latanoprost.
   a. It must be stored in the refrigerator.
   b. It may increase pigmentation in the eye.

c. It must be metabolized to its biologically active form.
d. It must be premixed before use.

10. Laser surgery is not recommended to reduce intraocular pressure.
   a. true
   b. false

Bibliography

Allison K, Patel D, Alabi O. Epidemiology of glaucoma: the past, present, and predictions for the future. *Cureus*. 2020;12(11):e11686.

Ament C, Young L. Ocular manifestations of helminthic infections: onchocerciasis, cysticercosis, toxocariasis, and diffuse unilateral subacute neuroretinitis. *Int Ophthalmol Clin*. 2006;46:1–10.

Bourne R. Worldwide glaucoma through the looking glass. *Br J Ophthalmol*. 2006;90:253–254.

Centers for Disease Control and Prevention: Conjunctivitis treatment, 2019. Retrieved September 4, 2022, from http://www.cdc.gov/conjunctivitis/about/treatment.html.

Centers for Disease Control and Prevention: *Fusarium* keratitis—multiple states, *MMWR Morb Mortal Wkly Rep* 55:1–2, 2006. Retrieved September 3, 2022, from http://www.cdc.gov/mmwr/preview/mmwrhtml/mm55d410a1.htm.

Chabner D. *The language of medicine*. ed 8. Philadelphia: WB Saunders; 2007.

Glaucoma Research Foundation: Glaucoma facts & stats, 2022. Retrieved September 3, 2022, from http://www.glaucoma.org/glaucoma/glaucoma-facts-and-stats.php.

Glaucoma Research Foundation: Glaucoma medications and their side effects, 2016. Last reviewed 2022. Retrieved September 4, 2022, from http://www.glaucoma.org/gleams/glaucoma-medications-and-their-side-effects.php.

Gordon K. (2021). The cost of vision loss and blindness in Canada—summary report. The Canadian Council of the Blind. Retrieved September 9, 2022, from https://www.fightingblindness.ca/wp-content/uploads/2021/05/KG-EN-ACC-Cost-of-Vision-loss-and-Blindness-in-Canada-Final.pdf.

Green L, Pavan-Langston D. Herpes simplex ocular inflammatory disease. *Int Ophthalmol Clin*. 2006;46:27–37.

Hatami H, Ghaffari Jolfayi A, Ebrahimi A, et al. Contact lens associated bacterial keratitis: common organisms, antibiotic therapy, and global resistance trends: a systematic review. *Front Ophthalmol*. 2021;1:759271.

Health Canada. (2022). Drug product database. Retrieved September 9, 2022, from https://health-products.canada.ca/dpd-bdpp/index-eng.jsp.

Institute for Safe Medication Practices. (2016). FDA and ISMP Lists of Look-Alike Drug Names with Recommended Tall Man Letters. Retrieved from July 20, 2022, from https://www.ismp.org/recommendations/tall-man-letters-list.

Institute for Safe Medication Practices. (2019). List of Confused Drugs. Retrieved from July 20, 2022, from https://www.ismp.org/tools/confuseddrugnames.pdf.

Kolko M. Present and new treatment strategies in the management of glaucoma. *Open Ophthalmol J*. 2015;9(Suppl 1):89–100. M5.

Limaye AP, Babu TM, Boeckh M. Progress and challenges in the prevention, diagnosis, and management of cytomegalovirus infection in transplantation. *Clin Microbiol Rev*. 2021;34:e00043–19.

Moshirfar M, Parker L, Birdsong OC, et al. Use of Rho kinase inhibitors in ophthalmology: a review of the literature. *Med Hypothesis Discov Innov Ophthalmol*. 2018;7(3):101–111.

National Eye Institute: Fact about dry eye, 2022. Retrieved September 9, 2022, from https://www.nei.nih.gov/sites/default/files/health-pdfs/factsaboutdrycyc.pdf.

Page C, Curtis M, Sutter M, et al. *Integrated pharmacology*. Philadelphia: Mosby; 2005:523–534.

Patton K. *Survival guide for anatomy and physiology*. St Louis: Mosby; 2006.

Raffa R, Rawls S, Beyzarov E. *Netter's illustrated pharmacology*, Philadelphia, 2005, WB Saunders, p 48.

Thibodeau GA, Patton KT. *Anatomy and physiology*, ed 6, St Louis, 2007, Mosby.

U.S. Food and Drug Administration. (nd). Drugs@FDA: FDA-Approved Drug Products. Retrieved September 9, 2022, from https://www.accessdata.fda.gov/scripts/cder/daf/index.cfm.

16

Treatment of Disorders of the Ear

LEARNING OBJECTIVES

1. Learn the terminology associated with the ear and ear infections.
2. Describe factors that influence the sense of balance.
3. Describe disorders of the ear and ear infections.
4. List and categorize medications used in the treatment of disorders of the ear and ear infections.
5. Identify significant drug look-alike and sound-alike issues.
6. Identify warning labels and precautionary messages associated with medications used in the treatment of disorders of the ear and ear infections.

KEY TERMS

Cerumen Waxlike substance that is secreted by modified sweat glands in the ear.
Emollient A softening agent, such as an ointment or lotion. Used in the ear to soften ear wax.
Equilibrium Steadiness or balance accompanied by a sense of knowing where the body is in relationship to surroundings.
Labyrinth Bony structure in the inner ear consisting of three parts (vestibule, cochlea, and semicircular canals) and involved in balance.
Ménière disease Chronic inner ear disease associated with intermittent buildup of fluid in the inner ear that causes hearing loss and vertigo.

Otitis externa Inflammation of the ear canal or external ear.
Otitis media Inflammation of the middle ear typically caused by viral or bacterial infection.
Tinnitus Intermittent or continuous whistling, crackling, squeaking, or ringing noise in the ears.
Tympanic membrane Eardrum.
Vertigo Feeling of spinning in space (dizziness and loss of balance).

Disorders Affecting Hearing

Hearing loss can be caused by otosclerosis, autoimmune disease, or sudden sensorineural hearing loss (SSHL). Otosclerosis is a disorder that causes destruction of bones in the ear. Hearing loss is typically caused by the immobilization of bones in the ear called stapes (anatomy of the ear is shown in Fig. 16.1). Symptoms such as tinnitus may appear in childhood or early adulthood.

SSHL progresses rapidly (hours to days) and typically causes hearing loss in only one ear. Vertigo and tinnitus are other symptoms. The exact cause of SSHL is unknown. It is believed it may be caused by a viral infection, vascular disorder, tumor, or rupture of the inner ear membrane or may be drug induced. Medications that can cause SSHL include loop diuretics, aminoglycoside antibiotics, and antineoplastic agents. Drug-induced SSHL may disappear when the drug is stopped. SSHL that is not drug induced is treated with vasodilating drugs and plasma expanders (e.g., normal saline, 5% glucose). Symptoms such as mild hearing loss resolve spontaneously without treatment. Moderate hearing loss is commonly treated with glucocorticosteroids; however, a recent

Cochrane review found little evidence to support this practice (see Chapter 13). Patients who have severe hearing loss may have no benefits from the administration of glucocorticosteroids.

Autoimmune diseases such as multiple sclerosis can also cause hearing loss, but sometimes autoimmune hearing loss occurs in the absence of any other disease. Progression occurs over several months, and hearing loss may occur in both ears. Glucocorticosteroids such as prednisone are used in treatment (see Chapter 13).

Disorders Resulting in Impaired Perception of Sound

Tinnitus is a condition that can cause intermittent or continuous whistling, crackling, squeaking, or ringing noise in the ears. Sometimes it is described as ringing in the ear. It may be caused by disease or bilateral hearing loss caused by normal aging, or it may be induced by drugs or noise. Tinnitus may be the first sign of ototoxicity. Alcohol and salicylates (aspirin) are the most common causes of drug-induced tinnitus.

Nonpharmacologic treatment for tinnitus includes masking the noise using a noise generator, stress management, and avoiding alcohol or things that make tinnitus worse. Medications may produce some symptom relief if tinnitus is severe. Numerous classifications of drugs have been used to manage tinnitus; however, none have been approved by the US Food and Drug Administration (FDA) for the condition and use is "off label."

Disorders Resulting in Impaired Perception of Motion

The sense organs involved in balance or *equilibrium* are found in the vestibule and the three semicircular canals of the *labyrinth* (see Fig. 16.1). The sense organs associated with the semicircular canals function in dynamic equilibrium to maintain balance when the head or body itself is rotated or suddenly moved. Fluids in the semicircular canals shift when the body is in motion to inform the direction and speed of rotation. The superior, posterior, and horizontal semicircular canals inform whether movement is up or down and side to side.

Vertigo

Vertigo and other balance disorders produce symptoms of dizziness or spinning, nausea and vomiting, blurred vision, disorientation, and a feeling of falling because of sense of balance being impaired. Our perception of balance and movement is a function of input from our eye, inner ear, and sense receptors on the skin and skeleton. The body integrates the input it gets from these sources and compares it with previous experience. *Vertigo* is caused by a neural mismatch or sensory conflict, infection, and/or inflammation. A sensory conflict occurs when our eyes tell us that our body should be moving yet our body remains still, such as when we watch a movie of a roller coaster. Similarly, when we read a book in a car that is moving, our inner ear and skin receptors tell us we are in motion, yet our eyes are fixed on the book that is not moving. Again, a sensory conflict occurs. Sensory conflicts may also occur from an inner ear infection, especially if only one ear is involved and one ear receives motion signals and the other ear receives none or a different signal. Head trauma, degeneration of otolith organs (benign positional vertigo), inflammation of the vestibular nerve, bacterial infection of the labyrinths, brainstem or cerebral pathology, Ménière disease, or motion sickness may also produce vertigo.

Benign Paroxysmal Positional Vertigo

Benign paroxysmal positional vertigo (BPPV) is the number one cause of vertigo, accounting for approximately 20% of all cases. It can occur after trauma to the inner ear, infection, or normal aging. Dizziness or vertigo occurs when otoliths (calcium carbonate crystals) dislodge and shift in the semicircular canals of the ear with changes in the head's position. Impaired structures in the semicircular canals send misinformation about the head's position, resulting in dizziness.

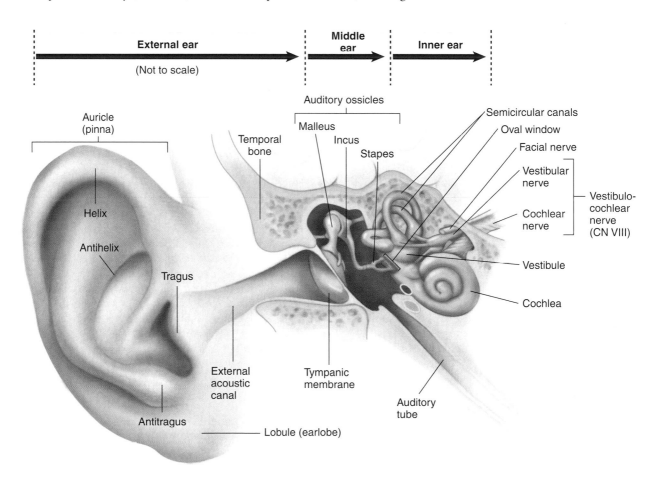

• **Fig. 16.1** The ear. (From Patton KT, Thibodeau GA. *The human body in health and disease*, ed 7, St Louis, 2018, Elsevier.)

Agents Used to Manage Vertigo and Ménière Disease

Generic Name	US Brand Name(s) / Canadian Brand(s)	Dosage Forms and Strengths
betahistine[a]	Not available	Tablets: 8 mg, 16 mg, 24 mg
	Serc	
dimenhydrinate[a]	Dramamine Original (OTC)	Capsule: 50 mg
	Gravol (OTC)	Solution: 15 mg/5 mL (Gravol)
		Suppositories (Gravol): 25 mg, 100 mg
		Tablets: 50 mg
		Tablets, chewable: 15 mg[b], 25 mg[c], 50 mg
		Tablets, combined release: 100 mg[b]
meclizine[a]	Bonine, Dramamine Less Drowsy Formula (OTC)	Tablets: 12.5 mg, 25 mg
	Not available	Tablets, chewable: 25 mg
scopolamine[a]	Transderm Scōp	Transdermal patch: 1 mg/72 h[c]
	Not available	

[a]Generic available.
[b]Available in Canada only.
[c]Available in the United States only.
OTC, Over the counter.

Ménière Disease

Ménière disease is the second most common cause of vertigo. It is a chronic inner ear disease associated with intermittent buildup of fluid in the inner ear. It is characterized by tinnitus, progressive nerve deafness, and vertigo. The cause is unknown. Nonpharmacologic treatment for Ménière disease includes diet and lifestyle changes. Reducing sodium, caffeine, nicotine, and alcohol consumption may be helpful.

Treatment of Disorders of the Ear

Vertigo and Ménière Disease

Many of the treatments for vertigo, Ménière disease, and other balance disorders do not involve drug therapy. Physical therapy is the treatment of choice for BPPV. Physical therapy is used to manipulate the head and shift otoliths that have dislodged. A low-sodium diet and lifestyle changes that restrict alcohol consumption are useful for the treatment of Ménière disease.

When drug therapy is indicated, antihistamines are most widely used and may be prescribed in tablet, transdermal patch, and rectal suppository dosage forms. This is most likely because centrally acting antihistamines have anticholinergic actions that can moderate symptoms of motion sickness. Acetylcholine and histamine are excitatory neurotransmitters involved in the control of vomiting (emesis). Nausea and vomiting are common symptoms of vertigo. Moreover, antihistamines and anticholinergics are vestibular suppressants. Vestibular suppression is useful because it reduces the eye activity responsible for symptoms of vertigo. Administration of vestibular suppressants is not recommended when treatment for vertigo involves physical manipulation of the head and "retraining" of vestibular pathways.

Betahistine, dimenhydrinate, diphenhydramine, and meclizine are antihistamines used to manage vertigo and Ménière disease. Side effects common to all these drugs are sedation, dry mouth, urinary retention, and blurred vision. Transdermal patches may produce local irritation, burning, or pain at the site where the patch is applied. Dry mouth, thickened bronchial secretions, and urinary retention may be produced, limiting their use in patients with prostate disease, asthma, and other conditions. Use should be limited in lactating women because the drugs may reduce the supply of breast milk. Aminoglycoside antiinfective medications such as gentamicin and streptomycin may be prescribed for Ménière disease, but their use is controversial because they can cause ototoxicity. Diuretics may also be prescribed to reduce fluid accumulation in the ear and other body fluids. Diuretics are discussed in Chapter 18.

> **⊘ Tech Alert!**
>
> Dimenhydrinate and diphenhydramine have look-alike/sound-alike issues.

Bacterial Infections of the Ear

Otitis Externa

Otitis externa, also known as swimmer's ear, is an inflammation of the external auditory canal. It may be caused by bacterial infection, fungal infection, seborrheic dermatitis, or psoriasis. The most common cause is bacterial infection. Fungi (*Candida* spp.) account for only 10% of the cases of otitis externa. Risk factors for development of otitis externa are (1) exposure to excessive moisture (swimming, humidity, sweating), (2) high environmental temperature, (3) irritation caused by earwax removal, (4) insertion of objects into the ear, and (5) chronic dermatologic disease.

The most common symptoms of otitis externa are ear discomfort or pain, itchiness, and discharge (otorrhea). Topical and systemic drugs are used to treat and control the symptoms of otitis externa. Antiinfective agents used in treatment are listed in the drug tables in this chapter. Otiprio (ciprofloxacin) is formulated for intratympanic or otic use and is used to treat otitis externa and otitis media.

Usual Dosage and Warning Labels for Agents Used to Treat Vertigo and Ménière Disease

Generic	Brand	Usual Dose	Warning Labels
betahistine	Serc (Canada only)	**Vertigo:** 8–16 mg 3 times a day or 24 mg twice daily	MAY CAUSE DROWSINESS; MAY IMPAIR ABILITY TO DRIVE. AVOID ALCOHOL. MAINTAIN ADEQUATE FLUID INTAKE. OBSERVE GOOD ORAL HYGIENE. ROTATE SITE OF PATCH APPLICATION—scopolamine. TAKE WITH FOOD—betahistine.
dimenhydrinate	Dramamine, Gravol	**Vertigo, motion sickness, nausea, and vomiting:** 50–100 mg every 4–6 h (maximum, 400 mg/day)	
meclizine	Generics	**Motion sickness:** 25–50 mg 1 h before travel; repeat in 12–24 h as needed **Vertigo:** 25–100 mg/day in divided doses	
scopolamine	Transderm Scōp	**Motion sickness:** Place patch behind ear at least 4 hours before it is needed; replace every 72 h as needed	

Treatment of Otitis Externa

Topical Antiinfective Drugs Used to Treat Otitis Externa

Generic Name	US Brand Name(s) Canadian brand name(s)	Usual Dosage
Quinolones		
ciprofloxacin	Cetraxal 0.2%, Otiprio 6% Not available	Instill contents of the single-use container in affected ear twice daily for 7 days (Cetraxal); insert a single dose in the external ear canal(s) or intratympanically (Otiprio)
ofloxacin otic drops 0.3%[a]	Generic Not available	Instill 5–10 drops in affected ear(s) once daily for 7 days
Antiinfective + Corticosteroid		
ciprofloxacin 0.3% + dexamethasone 1%[a]	Ciprodex Ciprodex	Instill 4 drops in ear(s) 2 times a day for 7 days
ciprofloxacin 0.2% + hydrocortisone 1%	Cipro HC otic suspension Not available	Instill 3 drops in affected ear(s) 2 times a day for 7 days
ciprofloxacin 0.3% + fluocinolone 0.025%	Otovel Otixal	Instill contents of single-use vial (0.25 mL) in the affected ear canal every 12 h for 7 days
gramicidin 025 mg + polymyxin B 10,000 units	Not available Polysporin Eye and Ear drops (OTC)	Instill 1–2 drops in affected eye or ear 4 times a day for 7 days
polymyxin B 10,000 units + lidocaine 50 mg	Not available Polysporin + Pain Relief Ear drops (OTC)	Instill 3–4 drops in affected ear(s) 4 times a day for 5–7 days
neomycin 0.35% + polymyxin B 10,000 units + hydrocortisone 1%[a]	Oticair Not available	Instill 4 drops in ear(s) 3–4 times a day

[a]Generic available.
OTC, Over the counter.

---

❶ *Tech Alert!*

Shake Otiprio for 5 to 8 seconds to mix. Keep the vial cold during preparation to prevent gel formation.

Otitis Media

Otitis media is an inflammation in the middle ear. It may accompany an upper respiratory infection. Children are more susceptible to otitis media than are adults because their eustachian tubes are shorter and straighter. When the eustachian tube is blocked

• BOX 16.1 Oral Antiinfective Medications Used as First-Line Treatment for Otitis Media

Penicillins (if no penicillin allergy)

amoxicillin

amoxicillin + clavulanate[a] (Augmentin[b], Clavulin[c])—if initial amoxicillin therapy fails

Cephalosporins (if penicillin allergy not life-threatening)

cefuroxime[a]

cefprozil[a]

ceftriaxone[a]

Macrolides (Alternate antiinfective drugs if first-line therapy fails or is inappropriate for patient)

azithromycin[a] (Zithromax)

clarithromycin[a] (Biaxin)

[a] Generic available.
[b] Available in the United States only.
[c] Available in Canada only.

Pharmacologic Treatments for Miscellaneous Ear Conditions

Generic Name	US Brand Name(s) / Canadian Brand(s)	Dosage Forms and Strengths
Analgesics		
antipyrine and benzocaine[a]	Not available / Auralgan	Solution, otic: antipyrine 5.4% and benzocaine 1.4%

[a] Generic available.

by swelling or mucus from a cold, fluids accumulate and collect in the normally air-filled middle ear. Bacteria may collect in the fluid, along with white blood cells released by the body to fight the infection. Hearing becomes impaired because the eardrum and middle ear bones are unable to move as freely. Pain and pressure builds, and finally, the eardrum may tear to release the pressure.

Historically, otitis media has been treated aggressively with orally administered antiinfective drugs; however, new evidence shows that the infection is self-limiting in many cases and will resolve on its own without treatment. Excessive use of antiinfective agents may increase the risk of the development of bacterial resistance. Watchful waiting (up to 48 to 72 hours to see if symptoms disappear) rather than antimicrobial treatment is endorsed by the American Academy of Pediatrics 2020 guidelines for children ages 6 to 24 months without severe illness.

Evidence shows that prophylactic use of antihistamines and decongestants is ineffective in preventing or treating acute otitis media and can be harmful in children younger than 2 years of age. Oral antiinfective agents used in the treatment of otitis media are listed in Box 16.1. These agents are described fully in Unit 10.

Auralgia

Ear pain, also called auralgia or otalgia, is a symptom of *otitis externa*, *otitis media*, swimmer's ear, and many other disorders, including viral inflammation of the *tympanic membrane*, temporomandibular joint disorders, referred pain from abscessed teeth, and others. It is treated by administration of topical analgesics, local anesthetics, or oral analgesics. Corticosteroids such as hydrocortisone are combined with otic agents to reduce inflammation and pain. Local anesthetics numb or anesthetize the ear canal and tympanic membrane, further reducing pain and irritation.

When the ear is inflamed, otic drops can produce stinging. This can be minimized by administering suspensions rather than solutions containing alcohol if this option is available. Otic drops should also be warmed to room temperature before administering into the ear. Sweet olive oil is a home remedy for ear pain. The oil has no analgesic properties, but the warmed oil may be soothing and dislodge cerumen, which may be the cause of the pain.

Water-Clogged Ears and Swimmer's Ear

Water-clogged ears and swimmer's ear are different conditions that are sometimes confused. Water-clogged ears are caused by fluids that accumulate in the ear after swimming or showering. Swimmer's ear produces inflammation and infection of the external ear after prolonged exposure to water, along with damage to the lining of the ear canal. Damage to the lining typically occurs when the person uses a rigid object to remove water from the ears. Swimmer's ear produces acute pain, itching, and a foul-smelling discharge from the ear.

Both conditions cause earache. Nonprescription drying agents are safe and effective for treatment of water-clogged ears. Alcohol (Auro-Dri) and mild acidic solutions of vinegar (acetic acid) dry excess water and soothe the eardrum. Alcohol-containing eardrops may produce stinging if the ears are inflamed.

• Tech Note!

The pH is a measure of how acidic or alkaline (or basic) a solution is. A pH of 1 indicates that the solution is very acidic (e.g., stomach acids [HCl]). A pH of 7 is neutral. Plasma pH ranges between 7.35 and 7.45. A pH of greater than 7 is considered alkaline.

Cerumen Impaction

Cerumen (earwax) is a normal and necessary substance produced by the ear. It functions to reduce the risk for bacterial infections in the ear because earwax has a pH of 6.5 and is bactericidal. Cerumen repels water and helps keep the ear dry during swimming and bathing. It lubricates the skin of the external ear canal and provides a barrier to entry of airborne substances (dust, insects) into the ear canal.

The healthy ear continuously replaces old cerumen. If cerumen becomes impacted, it can produce hearing loss, pressure, and ear pain. This condition is more common in people who wear hearing aids or regularly place earplugs and earphones in the ear. A cotton-tipped applicator or other small sharp object should never be used to remove earwax. These objects can cause accidental perforation of the eardrum (tympanic membrane).

Agents used to remove excess cerumen are called cerumenolytics. Emollients and carbamide peroxide are the principal ingredients found in cerumenolytics. **Emollients** are used to soften the wax, enabling it to slide out of the ear. Olive oil, mineral oil, and glycerin are emollients found in otic agents for earwax removal.

Peroxide-based products are used to break up the earwax and bubble away the debris. Carbamide peroxide 6.5% (over the counter [OTC]) and triethanolamine polypeptide oleate-condensate (OTC in Canada) are agents available to remove earwax.

After administration of emollients or peroxide-based agents, the affected ear is gently cleansed (irrigated) with warm water to remove dislodged cerumen. Ear irrigation is performed using a bulb syringe.

Treatments for Water-Clogged Ears and Swimmer's Ear

Generic Name	US Brand Name(s) / Canadian Brand Name(s)	Dosage Forms and Strengths
acetic acid solution[a]	Vosol	**Solution, otic:** 2%
	Not available	
Combination Otic Drops		
acetic acid + hydrocortisone solution[a]	Vosol HC	**Solution, otic:** 2% acetic acid + 1% hydrocortisone
	Not available	
isopropyl alcohol + glycerin[a]	Auro-Dri Ear-Water Drying Aid (OTC), Swim-Ear Ear-Water Drying Aid (OTC)	**Solution, otic:** 95% isopropyl alcohol and glycerin 5%
	Auro-Dri Ear-Water Drying Aid (OTC)	

[a]Generic available.
OTC, Over the counter.

Cerumenolytic Agents Used to Aid in Earwax Removal

Generic Name	US Brand Name(s) / Canadian Brand Name(s)	Dosage Forms and Strengths
carbamide peroxide (also known as urea hydrogen peroxide)[a]	Murine EAR Wax Removal System, Debrox (OTC)	**Solution, otic:** 6.5%
	Murine EAR Wax Removal System (OTC)	

[a]Generic available.
OTC, Over the counter.

Summary of Drugs Used to Treat Miscellaneous Conditions of the Ear

Generic	Brand	Usual Dose	Warning Labels
Analgesics			
antipyrine and benzocaine	Auralgan	Instill 1–2 drops in ear canal 3–4 times a day or up to every 1–2 h until pain relieved	FOR THE EAR.
Drying Agents			
acetic acid solution	Generics	Instill 4–6 drops in ear canal. Repeat every 2–3 h as needed.	FOR THE EAR.
isopropyl alcohol and glycerin	Auro-Dri Ear-Water Drying Aid	**Water-clogged ears:** Instill 4–5 drops in affected ear(s)	
Cerumenolytics			
carbamide peroxide	MURINE Ear Wax Removal System (OTC)	**Earwax removal:** Instill 5–10 drops twice daily for up to 4 days	FOR THE EAR.

OTC, Over the counter.

TECHNICIAN'S CORNER

1. How does ear candling work to remove unwanted cerumen or debris from the ear? What risks are associated with this practice?
2. How can putting a baby to bed with a bottle of milk contribute to otitis media?

Key Points

- Perception of balance and movement is a function of input from the eyes, inner ear, and sense receptors on the skin and skeleton.
- The semicircular canals located in the inner ear control the sense of equilibrium or balance.
- Otosclerosis and autoimmune diseases such as multiple sclerosis and sudden sensorineural hearing loss are conditions that can cause hearing loss.
- Otosclerosis also causes ringing in the ears (tinnitus).
- Tinnitus is a condition that produces ringing in the ear.
- Tinnitus may be drug induced. Aspirin and alcohol are common drugs that can cause tinnitus.
- Aminoglycoside antiinfective drugs (gentamicin) and loop diuretics can cause ototoxicity.
- Vertigo is a balance disorder that is caused by a neural mismatch or sensory conflict.
- Vertigo can occur from head trauma or degeneration of otolith organs, inflammation of the vestibular nerve, bacterial infection of the labyrinths, brainstem or cerebral pathology, or Ménière disease.
- Vertigo and other balance disorders produce symptoms of dizziness or spinning, nausea and vomiting, blurred vision, disorientation, and a feeling of falling.
- Treatment of balance disorders may involve physical therapy, diet, and lifestyle changes.
- When drug therapy is indicated, antihistamines are most widely used.
- Antihistamines have anticholinergic actions that can moderate symptoms of motion sickness but produce urinary retention and other side effects that limit their use in patients with prostate disease or asthma or in women who are lactating.
- Other side effects that are common to all antihistamine drugs are sedation, dry mouth, and blurred vision.
- One scopolamine transdermal patch placed behind the ear prevents motion sickness for up to 3 days.

- Ear pain, also called auralgia or otalgia, is a symptom of otitis externa and otitis media.
- Ear pain is treated by administration of topical analgesics, local anesthetics, or oral analgesics.
- When the ear is inflamed, otic suspensions are more soothing than solutions that contain alcohol.
- Water-clogged ears and swimmer's ear are different conditions that are sometimes confused.
- Swimmer's ear produces inflammation and infection of the external ear.
- Nonprescription drying agents are safe and effective for treatment of water-clogged ears.
- Cerumen (earwax) is bactericidal and water repellent, and it provides a barrier to entry of airborne substances and lubricates the skin of the external ear canal.
- A cotton-tipped applicator or other small sharp objects should never be used to remove earwax.
- Emollients and carbamide peroxide are the principal ingredients found in cerumenolytic agents.
- After administration of emollients or peroxide-based agents, the affected ear is gently cleansed (irrigated) with warm water to remove cerumen that has become dislodged.
- Otitis externa is inflammation of the external auditory canal and is most commonly caused by a bacterial infection.
- Risk factors for development of otitis externa are (1) exposure to excessive moisture (swimming, humidity, sweating), (2) high environmental temperature, (3) irritation caused by earwax removal, (4) insertion of objects into the ear, and (5) chronic dermatologic disease.
- Otitis media is an inflammation in the middle ear.
- Excessive use of antiinfective agents to treat otitis media may increase the risk of development of bacterial resistance.
- Decongestants and antihistamines are not recommended for prophylaxis or treatment of otitis media in children.

Review Questions

1. Otitis media is an inflammation in the _____ ear.
   a. inner
   b. outer
   c. middle
   d. cochlea
2. Prophylactic use of _____ is ineffective in preventing otitis media.
   a. antihistamines
   b. decongestants
   c. both a and b
   d. none of the above
3. The most common cause of otitis externa is _____
   a. viral infection
   b. bacterial infection
   c. psoriasis
   d. lupus
4. The most common cause for drug-induced tinnitus is _____.
   a. noise
   b. aspirin
   c. alcohol
   d. b and c

5. Which drug treatment for vertigo is available in a "patch" form?
   a. diphenhydramine
   b. scopolamine
   c. dimenhydrinate
   d. betahistine
6. Corticosteroids such as hydrocortisone are combined with _____ agents to reduce inflammation and pain in the ear.
   a. optic
   b. otic
   c. glaucoma
   d. ocular
7. Swimmer's ear produces inflammation and infection of the _____ ear after prolonged exposure to water, along with damage to the lining of the ear canal.
   a. internal
   b. inner
   c. external
   d. semicircular canals

8. Children are more susceptible to otitis media than are adults because their eustachian tubes are longer and straighter than those of adults.
   a. true
   b. false
9. Olive oil, mineral oil, and glycerin are emollients found in otic agents for removal of _____.
   a. earwax
   b. fluid
   c. bacteria
   d. foreign material
10. Carbamide peroxide 6.5% is an approved agent for _____ removal.
    a. earwax
    b. fluid
    c. bacteria
    d. foreign material

Bibliography

Canadian Paediatric Society. (2016, reaffirmed 2022). Management of acute otitis media in children six months of age or older: Position statement. Retrieved September 15, 2022, from https://cps.ca/en/documents/position/acute-otitis-media.

Hain T, Uddin M. Pharmacological treatment of vertigo. *CNS Drugs*. 2003;17:85–100.

Health Canada. (2022). Drug product database. Retrieved September 22, 2022, from https://health-products.canada.ca/dpd-bdpp/index-eng.jsp.

Hoberman A, Paradise JL, Rockette HE, et al. Treatment of acute otitis media in children under 2 years of age. *N Engl J Med*. 2011;364(2):105–115.

Kim SH, Kim D, Lee JM, et al. Review of pharmacotherapy for tinnitus. *Healthcare (Basel)*. 2021;9(6):779.

Koo L, Young L. Management of ocular toxoplasmosis. *Int Ophthalmol Clin*. 2006;46:183–193.

Mayo Clinic. (2022). Ménière's disease: treatment and drugs. Retrieved September 19, 2022, from http://www.mayoclinic.com/health/menieres-disease/DS00535/DSECTION=treatments-and-drugs.

National Institute on Deafness and Other Communication Disorders. (2018). Balance disorders, Bethesda, MD, NIDCD, National Institutes of Health, US Department of Health and Human Services. Retrieved September 15, 2022, from https://www.nidcd.nih.gov/health/balance-disorders.

National Institute on Deafness and Other Communication Disorders. (2022). NIDCD Fact Sheet: Ear Infections in Children. NIH Publication No.13-4799, Bethesda, MD, NIDCD, National Institutes of Health, US Department of Health and Human Services. Retrieved September 15, 2022, from https://www.nidcd.nih.gov/health/ear-infections-children.

National Library of Medicine. (nd). Tinnitus. Retrieved September 15, 2022, from http://www.nlm.nih.gov/medlineplus/tinnitus.html.

Page C, Curtis M, Sutter M, et al. *Integrated pharmacology*. Philadelphia: Mosby; 2005:539–544.

Patton K. *Survival guide for anatomy and physiology*. St Louis: Mosby; 2006.

Plontke SK, Meisner C, Agrawal S, et al. Intratympanic corticosteroids for sudden sensorineural hearing loss. *Cochrane Database Syst Rev*. 2022;7:CD008080.

Thibodeau GA, Patton KT. *Anatomy and physiology*. ed 6. St Louis: Mosby; 2007.

Uppal S, Bajaj Y, Coatesworth AP. Otosclerosis 2: the medical management of otosclerosis. *Int J Clin Pract*. 2010;64(2):256–265.

U.S. Food and Drug Administration. (nd). Drugs@FDA: FDA Approved Drug Products. Retrieved September 19, 2022, from https://www.accessdata.fda.gov/scripts/cder/daf/index.cfm.

UNIT V

Drugs Affecting the Cardiovascular System

Maintaining the body's internal environment (homeostasis) depends on the continual transport of oxygen, nutrients, and biochemical messengers among the body's cells. Blood is a complex transport medium that performs vital pickup and delivery services for the body. It is the keystone of the body's heat-regulating mechanism and can absorb large quantities of heat without an appreciable increase in its own temperature, transferring it from the body's core to the surface to be dissipated.

Heart health is maintained by lifestyle factors that include healthy eating and moderate to strenuous exercise. When the heart fails, numerous types of drugs are used in the treatment of heart disease. For example, anticoagulants prevent clot formations, β-adrenergic drugs reduce the workload of the heart, calcium channel blockers reduce vascular contractions and improve coronary blood flow, digitalis slows and increases the strength of cardiac contractions, nitroglycerin dilates coronary blood vessels, and tissue plasminogen activator (t-PA) helps dissolve clots.

In Unit V, the pharmacotherapy for diseases of the cardiovascular system is described. Angina, hypertension, arrhythmias, coronary heart disease, and stroke are covered. A brief description of each disorder is provided, followed by a description of the drugs indicated for treatment that includes mechanisms of action, adverse reactions, strength(s), and dosage forms. Lifestyle changes that are important in preventing and managing heart disease are also described in Unit V.

17

Treatment of Angina

LEARNING OBJECTIVES

1. Learn the terminology associated with the treatment of angina.
2. List the symptoms of and risk factors for angina.
3. Explain the role of coronary artery disease in the development of angina.
4. Identify lifestyle changes that reduce the risk for angina.
5. List and categorize medications used to treat angina.
6. Describe mechanism of action for each classification of drugs used to treat angina.
7. Identify significant drug look-alike and sound-alike issues.
8. List common endings for drug classes used in the treatment of angina.
9. Identify warning labels and precautionary messages associated with medications used to treat angina.

KEY TERMS

Angina pectoris Symptomatic manifestation of ischemic heart disease characterized by a severe squeezing or pressure-like chest pain and brought on by exertion or stress.

Arteriosclerosis Thickening and loss of elasticity of arterial walls; sometimes called "hardening of the arteries."

Atheromas Hard plaque formed within an artery.

Atherosclerosis Process in which plaques (atheromas) containing cholesterol, lipid material, and lipophages are formed within arteries.

Coronary artery disease Condition that occurs when the arteries that supply blood to the heart muscle become hardened and narrowed.

Embolus A moving blood clot.

Hyperlipidemia Increased concentration of cholesterol and triglycerides in the blood that is associated with the development of atherosclerosis.

Ischemia Deficient blood supply to an area of the body. Myocardial ischemia results in angina and myocardial infarction.

Ischemic heart disease Any condition in which heart muscle is damaged or works inefficiently because of an absence or relative deficiency of its blood supply.

Necrosis Cell death that may be caused by lack of blood and oxygen to the affected areas.

Myocardial infarction Also referred to as a "heart attack." Results in heart muscle tissue death and is caused by the occlusion (blockage) of a coronary artery.

Thrombus Stationary blood clot.

Vasospasm Spasms that constrict blood vessels and reduce the flow of blood and oxygen.

Overview

The word "angina" is derived from the Latin word *ango*, which means "to choke." *Angina pectoris* occurs when there is an imbalance between the heart's demand for oxygen and the oxygen supply (Fig. 17.1). The symptoms of angina are described as severe squeezing or pressure-like chest pain, sometimes radiating to the arms, shoulders, neck, or jaw. The pain is sometimes described as severe heartburn or indigestion. Angina is a symptom of *ischemic heart disease*. *Ischemia* is caused by loss of blood supply to a region of the body. As many as 10 million people in the United States have angina. People with a history of heart disease, hypertension, and diabetes are at risk for angina.

Lifestyle can also be a risk factor for the condition. In fact, angina is often classified as a chronic disease of lifestyle because many of the risks for developing the condition are related to lifestyle. Risk factors associated with lifestyle include smoking, overeating, a diet high in cholesterol and salt, excessive alcohol consumption, obesity, and lack of exercise. Stress is also a risk factor for angina.

High dietary cholesterol is a contributing factor for the development of *coronary artery disease* (CAD) and myocardial ischemia. Cholesterol, lipid material, and lipophages are deposited within arteries. The lipid streaks harden into plaques (atheromas); this process is called *atherosclerosis*. An *atheroma* can increase in size and reduce blood flow and has the potential to result in

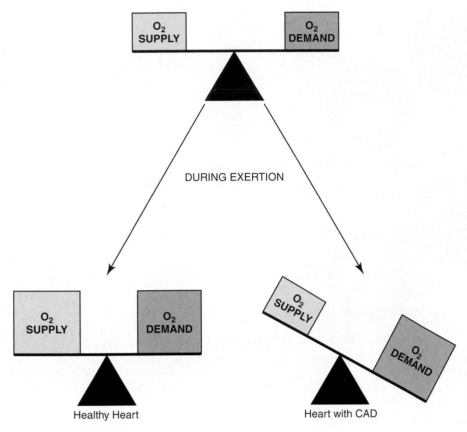

DURING REST
Healthy Heart and Heart with CAD

DURING EXERTION

Healthy Heart

Heart with CAD

• **Fig. 17.1** Effect of exertion on the balance between oxygen supply and oxygen demand in the healthy heart and the heart with coronary artery disease (CAD). (From Burchum JR, Rosenthal LD, Jones BO. *Lehne's pharmacology for nursing care*, ed 9, St Louis, 2016, Elsevier.)

thrombus (blood clot) formation (Fig. 17.2). A thrombus can further occlude the artery in which it was formed. A thrombus that breaks off is called an embolus (moving blood clot); it can travel to a smaller artery, where it completely blocks the blood vessel, causing ischemia (inadequate blood supply.) Prolonged ischemia can result in tissue necrosis (death), leading to *myocardial infarction* (heart attack) or stroke. *Arteriosclerosis*, sometimes called "hardening of the arteries," is a condition in which arterial walls thicken and lose elasticity. Arteriosclerosis may occur as part of the normal aging process. Other risk factors are smoking tobacco, obesity, diabetes, and hypertension. When arteriosclerosis occurs in the coronary arteries, the arteries become less able to dilate and increase the heart's blood supply when needed.

> ● *Tech Note!*
>
> A *thrombus* is a stationary blood clot; an *embolus* is a moving blood clot.

Angina Variants

Angina variants vary in their pattern and ability to be relieved by medication. They are called stable angina, unstable angina, and vasospastic angina (also known as Prinzmetal angina). Angina is characterized by an imbalance between blood supplied to the

heart muscle and the blood and oxygen needed. The symptoms of angina occur when the blood supplied to the heart is insufficient to meet the heart's need for oxygen.

Stable (Exertional) Angina

Symptoms of stable angina are predictable and are typically brought on by physical exertion, smoking, eating heavy meals, exposure to extreme changes in temperature (hot or cold), or emotional stress. Physical exertion is the most common reason for the onset of angina. Although the amount of blood and oxygen that is supplied to the heart meets its needs under typical conditions, it is insufficient during periods of physical exertion. Rest and antianginal medications such as nitroglycerin adequately treat the acute symptoms of stable angina. Symptoms often subside within 5 minutes.

Unstable Angina

Unstable angina is a serious condition requiring evaluation because it may precede a myocardial infarction (heart attack). It may occur at rest without physical exertion and may result when an embolus partially or completely blocks an artery. Myocardial ischemia causes the symptoms of pain and chest pressure. Symptoms are not relieved by rest or antianginal medicine and may last for up to 30 minutes.

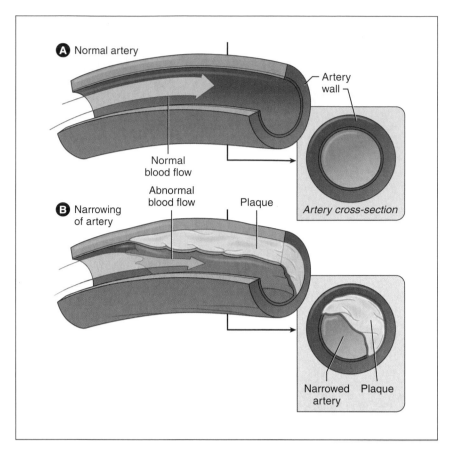

- **Fig. 17.2** Plaque buildup in an artery. (**A**) Normal artery without plaque buildup. (**B**) Narrowed artery with plaque buildup. (Courtesy of National Institutes of Health, Bethesda, MD.)

Variant Angina

Vasospastic angina is caused by **vasospasm** of the coronary arteries. Spasms reduce the opening of the artery, decreasing the blood supply and oxygen to the heart. Angina pains typically occur at rest, during the night or early morning. Unlike unstable angina, symptoms are relieved by medications (e.g., nitrates and calcium channel blockers). Symptoms often persist longer than stable angina and may exceed 5 minutes.

Microvascular Angina

Microvascular angina or cardiac syndrome X is a form of stable angina that may produce greater chest pain and last longer. This type of angina may be a symptom of coronary microvascular disorder that occurs when the tiny blood vessels that nourish the heart do not function well. It differs from other forms of angina because some patients have no CAD risk factors. Microvascular angina most often occurs during exercise but can occur at rest.

Nonpharmacologic Treatment of Angina

Lifestyle Change

Change in modifiable lifestyle practices is an important part of the treatment and prevention of angina and other cardiovascular diseases. Lifestyle changes can reduce the risk for angina, as well as decrease the frequency and severity of symptoms and prevent or slow the progression of angina to myocardial infarction or death.

We may not be able to limit our exposure to stressful situations, but we can control the volume of food we consume and lose weight if necessary. Increasing our level of daily activity, while avoiding overexertion, is another modifiable lifestyle change that we can make. If you smoke, you should quit.

Other lifestyle changes that should be implemented if possible include:
- Taking frequent rest breaks if necessary to avoid angina that is caused by exertion
- Avoiding foods high in salt and cholesterol
- Eating small portions rather than a heavy meal
- Learning techniques to manage stress
- Being an advocate for workplace and community-wide changes that facilitate lifestyle change (e.g., nutritious food choices in school and workplace cafeterias)

Drugs Used in the Treatment of Angina

The primary cause of angina is an imbalance between oxygen supply and oxygen demand in the heart. Drugs used in the treatment of angina are administered to increase the blood and oxygen supply to the heart and/or decrease the heart's demand for oxygen (workload). Nitrates, some β-blockers, calcium channel blockers, and the late sodium current blocker ranolazine are approved as antianginal medications by the US Food and Drug Administration (FDA) and Health Canada. The mechanisms of action of the drugs vary. They produce their effects by dilating blood vessels (veins and arteries), decreasing heart rate, reducing cardiac contractility, or reducing vasospasms.

Treatment of angina is no longer simply focused on prevention of acute symptoms. Current drug therapy also aims to decrease cardiovascular events by treating and preventing the cardiovascular diseases that often accompany angina. Drugs may be administered to persons who have angina to treat comorbid conditions such as hypertension (see Chapter 18), *hyperlipidemia*, atherosclerosis, atherothrombosis, and myocardial infarction. The following drug classes are used to treat angina: nitrates, β-blockers, calcium channel blockers, and late sodium current blockers.

Nitrates

The organic nitrates are the oldest class of drugs used to treat acute symptoms of angina. Nitrates reduce oxygen demand and increase oxygen supply. They dilate blood vessels (arteries and veins) and increase supply of oxygen to the heart. Nitrates that are commonly used for treatment and prevention of angina are nitroglycerin, isosorbide dinitrate, and isosorbide mononitrate. Nitrates are also indicated for the treatment of congestive heart failure, pulmonary hypertension, and hypertensive emergencies.

> ● **Tech Note!**
>
> Sublingual nitroglycerin is packaged by manufacturers in amber glass bottles and should be dispensed in the manufacturer's original container. Dispense nitroglycerin without a safety cap for easy access. It is one of the few drugs exempted from the Poison Prevention Packaging Act. Opened bottles should be replaced within 3-6 months of opening.

Mechanism of Action

Most nitrates are prodrugs that are converted in the body to nitric oxide. Nitric oxide acts at the cellular level to reduce intracellular calcium, block muscle contraction, and relax blood vessels. Nitrates dilate the veins at very low doses and arterioles at higher doses. When nitrates dilate veins, they reduce heart muscle tension and decrease oxygen demand. When nitrates relax and dilate coronary arteries, oxygen is increased to the heart. Nitrate relaxation of smooth muscles in the veins reduces fluid backup in the ventricles and the work needed to pump blood out of the ventricles. In the case of obstruction of a coronary artery, nitrates may cause the dilation of adjacent arteries, shifting blood supply away from the blocked region.

> ● **Tech Note!**
>
> Isosorbide dinitrate is also available in unit dose packaging.

> ● **Tech Note!**
>
> It is important for patients using patches to rotate the sites on the skin to prevent skin irritation.

Pharmacokinetics

Nitrates are formulated for a variety of dosage delivery systems. Nitroglycerin dosage forms include parenteral, sublingual tablets, lingual spray, capsules, ointments, and transdermal patches. Some dosage delivery systems are designed to deliver nitroglycerin quickly and are used to treat acute symptoms. These include

parenteral solution, sublingual tablets, and lingual spray. The other dosage forms of nitroglycerin deliver medication over an extended period (up to 24 hours) and are intended to prevent symptoms of angina. BiDil is a fixed dose combination of isosorbide dinitrate (20 mg) (a vasodilator that affects both arteries and veins) and hydralazine HCl (37.5 mg), a predominantly arterial vasodilator.

Nitroglycerin is lipid soluble and readily crosses cell membranes. It is subject to extensive first-pass metabolism, and only 10% of an oral dose is available to produce effects. This explains why parenteral and sublingual dosage forms produce actions more quickly and are more potent than enteral dosage forms (capsules).

Nitroglycerin is volatile and loses its potency on exposure to air, light, and moisture. Potency can also be lost if it is repackaged in plastic prescription vials. Sublingual nitroglycerin is packaged by manufacturers in amber glass bottles and should be dispensed in the manufacturer's original container.

Isosorbide mononitrate is a long-acting metabolite of isosorbide dinitrate. Isosorbide dinitrate and isosorbide mononitrate are not used to treat acute symptoms. Immediate-release and extended-action tablets are formulated for prevention. Isosorbide dinitrate and isosorbide mononitrate are more stable than nitroglycerin and do not need to be dispensed in the manufacturer's original container.

> ● **Tech Alert!**
>
> A warning label may be placed on prescriptions for sildenafil (Viagra), vardenafil (Cialis), and tadalafil (Levitra) (treatment for erectile dysfunction), warning that use with nitroglycerin may cause a fatal drop in blood pressure.

Adverse Reactions

Some of the adverse reactions to nitrates are dosage form dependent, and other effects are common regardless of the dosage delivery system. Adverse reactions associated with vasodilation are the most common and include hypotension, facial flushing, dizziness, and headache. Nausea and vomiting, weakness, and fatigue are additional side effects produced by nitroglycerin, isosorbide dinitrate, and isosorbide mononitrate. Sublingual dosage forms can cause stinging or burning under the tongue, and adhesives used in patches can produce allergic reactions.

> ● **Tech Note!**
>
> All nitrates have "nitro" or "nitra" in their brand or generic name.

> ● **Tech Note!**
>
> Nitroglycerin ointment is also marketed for the treatment of anal fissure pain. RECTIV nitroglycerin ointment is applied rectally.

Precautions

Patients who use nitrates can develop tolerance to their effects. This means the drug actions are less effective over time. Tolerance is most common with long-acting nitrates. To minimize the risk for development of tolerance, it is important to avoid continuous exposure to the drug. Transdermal patches are designed to deliver their effects for 24 hours; however, the patch should never be worn

Nitrates Used in the Treatment of Angina

Generic Name	US Brand Name(s)	Dosage Forms and Strengths
	Canadian Brand(s)	
isosorbide dinitrate[a]	Isordil	**Tablets, extended release:** 40 mg[b]
	Generics	**Tablets, immediate release (Isordil):** 5 mg[b], 10 mg, 20 mg[b], 30 mg, 40 mg[b]
isosorbide mononitrate[a]	Monoket	**Tablets (Monoket):** 10 mg, 20 mg
	Imdur	**Tablets, extended release (Imdur):** 30 mg[b], 60 mg, 120 mg[b]
isosorbide dinitrate + hydralazine[a]	BiDil	**Tablets:** 20 mg (isosorbide) + 37.5 mg (hydralazine)
	Not available	
nitroglycerin[a]	Nitro-Dur, Nitrolingual pump spray Nitromist, Nitrostat	**Ointment[b]:** 2%, **Solution, for injection (Nitroject):** 50 mg/10 mL **Tablets, sublingual:** 0.3 mg, 0.4 mg, 0.6 mg **Transdermal patch:** 0.1 mg/h (5 cm²)[b], 0.2 mg/h (10 cm²), 0.4 mg/h (20 cm²), 0.6 mg/h, 0.8 mg (40 cm²) **Translingual spray:** 0.4 mg/spray (200 sprays/canister)
	Nitro-Dur, Nitroject, Nitrostat, Nitrolingual, Rho-Nitro Pump spray, Trinipatch	

[a]Generic available.
[b]Available in the United States only.

for the entire 24-hour period. Patients should be instructed to remove the patch after 10 to 12 hours. Patients must be nitrate-free for at least 10 to 12 hours per day.

Late Sodium Channel Current Blockade

Ranexa (ranolazine) is used to treat adult patients with chronic angina. It is classified as a late sodium channel current blocker. It is the only drug in its class. Ranolazine improves coronary blood flow. It works by reducing the sodium-calcium exchange. This decreases calcium ions, thereby decreasing contractility and relaxing heart muscle.

Common side effects of ranolazine are dizziness, headache, nausea, and constipation. Ranolazine may cause serious side effects such as changes in the electrical activity of the heart. It may also cause kidney failure in people with severe kidney problems. Ranexa is an extended-release tablet that must be swallowed whole. It should not be taken with grapefruit juice because this will cause an increase of the drug in the blood. Ranolazine may be used at the same time with β-blockers, calcium channel blockers, nitrates, angiotensin-converting enzyme (ACE) inhibitors, and angiotensin receptor blockers (ARBs).

ⓘ Tech Alert!

The following drugs have look-alike/sound-alike issues: metoprolol succinate and metoprolol tartrate

Sodium Channel Current Blockers

Generic Name	US Brand Name(s)	Dosage Forms and Strengths
	Canadian Brand Name(s)	
ranolazine	Ranexa	**Tablets, extended release:** 500 mg, 1 g extended release
	Corzyna	

Beta-Adrenergic Blockers

The β-adrenergic blockers are administered to reduce the heart's demand for oxygen. This is achieved by decreasing the heart rate and thereby reducing the workload of the heart. There are many β-adrenergic blockers; however, only a few are currently approved for the management of angina. They are acebutolol atenolol, metoprolol, nadolol, and propranolol. β-Adrenergic blockers are also indicated for the management of hypertension and post–myocardial infarction (see Chapters 18 and 19) and for the prevention of migraine headache (see Chapter 10).

Mechanism of Action

The β-adrenergic blockers decrease the frequency and severity of stable (exertional) angina. They bind to β-receptor sites and block activity of the sympathetic nervous system on cardiac muscle. Heart contractility is lessened, and the heart rate is slowed, thereby reducing the workload of the heart. When the heart works less, its need for oxygen and blood supply is reduced.

The β-adrenergic blocking drugs used to treat stable angina include cardioselective β₁-adrenergic blockers and nonselective mixed β₁/β₂-blockers (e.g., propranolol and nadolol). More discussion is found in Chapter 18.

> **● Tech Note!**
>
> The β-adrenergic blockers are easily identified because their generic name ends in "-lol."

Pharmacokinetics

The β-adrenergic blockers are formulated in immediate- and long-acting dosage forms. The elimination half-life varies for specific agents and ranges from as short as 3 to 4 hours (propranolol) to as long as 24 hours (nadolol). Most agents are dosed once or twice a day except short-acting propranolol, which is dosed two to four times a day.

Adverse Reactions

The β-adrenergic blockers can produce dizziness, fatigue, bradycardia, hypotension, impotence, heart block (a heartbeat that is prolonged and the rhythm is too slow), and occasionally insomnia. They should be used cautiously in persons with diabetes because they can decrease heart rate, masking one of the principal signs of hypoglycemia. Patients with diabetes using β-blockers should be educated about other signals of hypoglycemia. β-blockers should be used cautiously in individuals who have asthma because bronchospasm is a side effect. Abrupt discontinuation of β-adrenergic blockers should be avoided because it can produce tachycardia and a sudden increase in the workload of the heart.

> **● Tech Note!**
>
> Hyperlipidemia is a risk factor for angina. Caduet is a combination drug that combines the calcium channel blocker amlodipine with the lipid-lowering drug atorvastatin.

Calcium Channel Blockers

Calcium channel blockers are used in the treatment of variant and stable angina because of their ability to reduce vasospasms that restrict the flow of blood and oxygen. Calcium channel blockers improve exercise tolerance by decreasing the workload of the heart. Calcium channel blockers are effective in the treatment of stable angina alone and in combination with nitrates or β-blockers.

> **❶ Tech Alert!**
>
> The following drugs have look-alike/sound-alike issues:
> Cardizem, Cardizem LA, and Cardizem CD;
> dilTIAZem and diazePAM;
> Tiazac and Ziac;
> niCARDipine, NIFEdipine;
> Procardia, Procardia XL, and Cartia XT

Mechanism of Action

Calcium channel blockers block L-type voltage-dependent calcium channels, suppress depolarization, and reduce contraction of the heart muscle. There are two classes of Ca^{2+} channel blockers: dihydropyridines (amlodipine, nifedipine, nicardipine, nimodipine, nisoldipine) and nondihydropyridines, which

Beta-Adrenergic Blockers

Generic Name	US Brand Name(s) / Canadian Brand(s)	Dosage Forms and Strengths
atenolol[a]	Tenormin / Tenormin	**Tablets:** 25 mg, 50 mg, 100 mg
metoprolol tartrate[a]	Lopressor / Lopressor	**Tablets:** 25 mg, 50 mg, 100 mg
metoprolol succinate ER[a]	Kapspargo Sprinkle, Toprol XL / Not available	**Tablets, extended release:** 25 mg[b], 50 mg[b], 100 mg, 200 mg
nadolol[a]	Corgard / Generics	**Tablets:** 20 mg[b], 40 mg, 80 mg, 160 mg[c]
propranolol[a]	Inderal-LA, InnoPran XL / Generics	**Capsules, extended release (InnoPran XL)**[b]: 80 mg, 120 mg **Capsules, sustained release (Inderal LA)**[b]: 60 mg, 80 mg, 120 mg, 160 mg **Injection, solution (Inderal)**[b]: 1 mg/mL **Solution, oral**[b]: 20 mg/5 mL, 40 mg/5 mL **Tablet:** 10 mg, 20 mg, 40 mg, 60 mg[b], 80 mg

[a]Generic available.
[b]Available in United States only.
[c]Available in Canada only.

include phenylalkylamines (verapamil) and benzothiazepines (diltiazem).

Verapamil and diltiazem reduce heart oxygen consumption during exercise by decreasing heart rate and heart contractions. Amlodipine, nifedipine, nicardipine, nimodipine, and nisoldipine are more selective for blood vessels, so they are able to increase blood and oxygen supply without slowing heart rate or contractions or increasing the risk of heart block.

> ● *Tech Note!*
>
> Calcium channel blockers classified as dihydropyridines are easily identified because their generic name ends in "-dipine."

Adverse Reactions

Some adverse drug reactions are common to all calcium channel blockers; other side effects are specific to drug classification. All calcium channel blockers produce hypotension. The dihydropyridines (e.g., nifedipine) produce vasodilation that can lead to dizziness, flushing, and headache. Peripheral edema is caused by venodilation. Verapamil and diltiazem may produce heart failure, bradycardia, and heart block because they slow conduction through the atrioventricular node.

> ● *Tech Note!*
>
> Grapefruit juice decreases the metabolism of calcium channel blockers. Apply the warning label AVOID GRAPEFRUIT JUICE.

Calcium Channel Blockers

	Generic Name	US Brand Name(s) / Canadian Brand(s)	Dosage Forms and Strengths
	amlodipine[a]	Katerzia, Norvasc, Norliqva — Norvasc	**Solution, oral (Katerzia, Norliqva):** 1 mg/mL **Tablets:** 2.5 mg, 5 mg, 10 mg
	diltiazem[a]	Cardizem, Cardizem CD, Cardizem LA, Cartia XT, Taztia XT, Tiazac — Tiazac, Tiazac XC	**Capsules, extended release:** 120 mg, 180 mg, 240 mg, 300 mg, 360 mg, 420 mg (Tiazac only)[b] **Tablets, immediate release (Cardizem):** 30 mg, 60 mg, 90 mg[b], 120 mg[b] **Tablets, extended release (Cardizem LA, Tiazac XC):** 120 mg, 180 mg, 240 mg, 300 mg, 360 mg, 420 mg[b] (Cardizem LA only)
	nicardipine[a]	Generics only — Not available	**Capsules:** 20 mg, 30 mg
	nifedipine[a]	Procardia, Procardia XL — Adalat XL SRT	**Capsule (Procardia):** 5 mg[c], 10 mg, 20 mg **Tablets, extended release (Adalat XL SRT, Procardia XL):** 30 mg, 60 mg, 90 mg[b]
	verapamil[a]	Verelan, Verelan PM — Isoptin SR	**Capsules, extended release (Verelan PM)[b]:** 100 mg, 200 mg, 300 mg **Capsules, extended release (Verelan)[b]:** 120 mg, 180 mg, 240 mg, 360 mg **Tablets, immediate release (Calan):** 40 mg[b], 80 mg, 120 mg, 160 mg[b] **Tablets, sustained release (Isoptin SR):** 120 mg, 180 mg[c], 240 mg

Calcium Channel Blocker Combinations (Only Combinations Approved for the Treatment of Angina Are Listed)

	amlodipine + atorvastatin[a]	Caduet — Caduet	**Tablets:** amlodipine 2.5 mg + atorvastatin 10 mg[b], amlodipine 2.5 mg + atorvastatin 20 mg[b], amlodipine 2.5 mg + atorvastatin 40 mg[b], amlodipine 5 mg + atorvastatin 10 mg, amlodipine 5 mg + atorvastatin 20 mg, amlodipine 5 mg + atorvastatin 40 mg, amlodipine 5 mg + atorvastatin 80 mg, amlodipine 10 mg + atorvastatin 10 mg, amlodipine 10 mg + atorvastatin 20 mg, amlodipine 10 mg + atorvastatin 40 mg, amlodipine 10 mg + atorvastatin 80 mg

[a]Generic available.
[b]Available in the United States only.
[c]Available in Canada only.

Summary of Drugs Used in the Treatment of Angina

	Generic	Brand	Usual Dose	Warning Labels
Nitrates				
	isosorbide dinitrate	Isordil	**Angina:** 5–40 mg 2–3 times a day or up to 160 mg SR (1–4 capsules) not less than once every 18 hours	TAKE ON AN EMPTY STOMACH—isosorbide dinitrate. SWALLOW WHOLE; DO NOT CRUSH OR CHEW—sustained and extended release. AVOID ALCOHOL.
	isosorbide mononitrate	Imdur	**Angina:** 5–20 mg twice a day (7 h apart), 30–60 mg/day (extended release) up to maximum, 240 mg/day	
	nitroglycerin	Nitrostat	**Oral:** 2.5–6.5 mg 2–4 times a day (maximum, 26 mg 4 times a day) **Ointment:** ½–2 inches (1.25–5.08 cm) of 2% ointment (7.5–30 mg) twice a day (6 h apart) **Powder:** 1–2 packets at onset of symptoms; may take 1 additional packet every 5 minutes until symptoms subside up to a maximum of 15 minutes (3 doses) **Transdermal patch:** Wear 1 patch (0.2–0.8 mg/h) for 12–14 h/day; patch off for 10–12 h/day **Sublingual:** Dissolve 1 tablet sublingually as needed for chest pain; may repeat 1 tablet every 5 min if no relief up to 3 tablets (15 min) or dissolve 1 tablet sublingually 5 min before strenuous activity **Translingual spray:** Place 1–2 sprays in mouth as needed for chest pain; may repeat every 5 min if no relief up to 3 doses (15 min) or use 5–10 min before strenuous activity	STORE IN MANUFACTURER'S ORIGINAL CONTAINER—sublingual, capsules. REPLACE VIALS 3–6 MONTHS AFTER OPENING—sublingual. ROTATE SITE OF APPLICATION—transdermal patch. HOLD SPRAY IN MOUTH FOR UP TO 10 SECONDS BEFORE SWALLOWING—translingual spray. IF NO RELIEF OF SYMPTOMS AFTER 3 DOSES OF SUBLINGUAL TABS OR LINGUAL SPRAY (OR 15 MIN), CALL 911—all immediate-release dosage forms. SWALLOW WHOLE; DO NOT CRUSH OR CHEW—sustained and extended release.
Late Sodium Channel Blocker				
	ranolazine	Ranexa	The initial dose is 500 mg twice a day and may be increased to 1000 mg twice a day if needed	AVOID GRAPEFRUIT JUICE.
Beta-Adrenergic Blockers				
	atenolol	Tenormin	**Angina:** 50 mg/day (may increase to 100–200 mg once daily)	MAY CAUSE DIZZINESS; USE CAUTION WHEN DRIVING OR PERFORMING TASKS REQUIRING ALERTNESS. AVOID ABRUPT DISCONTINUATION. TAKE WITH FOOD—metoprolol (immediate release). SWALLOW WHOLE; DO NOT CRUSH OR CHEW—sustained release.
	metoprolol tartrate	Lopressor	**Angina (immediate release):** Start with 50 mg twice daily increasing to 100–400 mg/day in 2–3 divided doses	
	metoprolol succinate	Toprol XL	**Angina (extended release):** 100–400 mg/day as a single dose	
	nadolol	Corgard	**Angina:** Begin at 40–80 mg/day; increase to 240 mg once daily	
	propranolol	Generics, Inderal LA	**Angina:** 80–320 mg/day in 2–4 divided doses or 80–320 mg once daily (extended release)	

Summary of Drugs Used in the Treatment of Angina

	Generic	Brand	Usual Dose	Warning Labels
Calcium Channel Blockers				
	amlodipine	Norvasc	**Angina:** 5–10 mg once daily	MAY CAUSE DIZZINESS; USE CAUTION WHEN DRIVING OR PERFORMING TASKS REQUIRING ALERTNESS. AVOID ABRUPT DISCONTINUATION. SWALLOW WHOLE; DO NOT CRUSH OR CHEW—extended and sustained release. TAKE WITH FOOD—nicardipine (sustained release).
	diltiazem	Cardizem, Cardizem CD	**Extended release, caps:** 120–180 mg once daily (maximum, 540 mg/day) **Immediate release, tablet:** 30 mg 4 times a day (maximum, 180–360 mg/day)	
	nicardipine	Generics	**Immediate release:** 20–40 mg 3 times a day	
	nifedipine	Procardia, Procardia XL	**Immediate release:** 10–30 mg 3–4 times a day (maximum 180 mg/day) **Sustained release:** 30–60 mg once daily (maximum, 120–180 mg/day)	
	verapamil	Calan SR, Verelan, Isoptin SR	**Extended release:** Begin 180 mg orally once daily at bedtime; may increase up to 480 mg once daily **Immediate release:** Begin 80–120 mg 3 times a day; may increase to 240–480 mg/day	
Calcium Channel Blocker Combinations				
	amlodipine + atorvastatin	Caduet	5–10 mg amlodipine once daily	MAY CAUSE DIZZINESS. AVOID GRAPEFRUIT JUICE.

> **● Tech Note!**
>
> Be careful when retrieving Cardizem and diltiazem from the shelf because of the many types of dosage forms available (Cardizem CD and LA, diltiazem CD, ER, T).

Other Drug Classifications

ACE inhibitors, anticoagulants, antiplatelet drugs, glycoprotein IIb/IIIa drugs, and antihyperlipidemic agents may be administered to patients who have angina, especially when they have comorbid conditions (simultaneous chronic diseases, e.g., angina plus hypertension and dyslipidemia). Drugs used to treat hypertension and dyslipidemia are discussed in Chapters 18 and 19.

TECHNICIAN'S CORNER

1. What is the major difference between arteriosclerosis and atherosclerosis?
2. Both nitroglycerin and sildenafil have vasodilating effects on blood vessels. Why is it so important not to use these drugs at the same time?

Key Points

- Angina is a symptom of ischemic heart disease.
- The symptoms of angina are described as severe squeezing or pressure-like chest pain, sometimes radiating to the arms, shoulders, neck, or jaw.
- Angina pain is sometimes described as severe heartburn or indigestion.
- People with a history of heart disease, hypertension, and diabetes are at risk for angina; however, lifestyle is a significant risk for the condition.
- Lifestyle risk factors are smoking, overeating, a diet high in cholesterol and salt, excessive alcohol consumption, obesity, lack of exercise, and stress.
- Coronary artery disease causes myocardial ischemia.
- Atherosclerosis is a disease of the coronary arteries that results in the buildup of lipid streaks in arteries.
- Atherosclerosis can block the flow of blood through the artery, producing ischemia and cell death (**necrosis**).
- The three angina variants are stable, unstable, and vasospastic.

- In all types of angina there is an imbalance between blood supplied to the heart muscle and the need for blood and oxygen.
- Symptoms of stable angina are typically brought on by physical exertion, smoking, eating heavy meals, exposure to extreme changes in temperature (hot or cold), and emotional stress.
- Unstable angina may occur at rest without physical exertion and results when an embolus partially or completely occludes an artery.
- Symptoms of vasospastic angina are caused by vasospasm of the coronary arteries.
- Lifestyle changes can reduce the risk, frequency, and severity of symptoms and prevent or slow the progression of angina to myocardial infarction or death.
- Recommended lifestyle changes are to (1) take frequent rest breaks, (2) avoid eating foods high in salt and cholesterol, (3) eat smaller portions, and (4) learn techniques to manage stress. Advocating for workplace and community-wide changes can support lifestyle change.
- Drugs used in the treatment of angina are administered to increase the blood and oxygen supply to the heart and to decrease the workload of the heart.
- Drug therapy for angina is focused on treatment and prevention of symptoms and treatment and prevention of cardiovascular diseases that often accompany angina.
- The organic nitrates are the oldest class of drugs used to treat acute symptoms of angina. They dilate blood vessels (arteries and veins) and increase the supply of oxygen to the heart.
- Nitrates that are commonly used in the treatment and prevention of angina are nitroglycerin, isosorbide dinitrate, and isosorbide mononitrate.
- Nitroglycerin is formulated for parenteral, oral, sublingual, and topical use.

- Dosage delivery systems that are designed to deliver nitroglycerin quickly are used to treat acute symptoms; they include sublingual tablets and lingual spray.
- Nitroglycerin extended-release capsules, patches, and ointments deliver medication over an extended period (up to 24 hours) to prevent symptoms of angina.
- Isosorbide dinitrate and isosorbide mononitrate are administered for prevention.
- Adverse reactions of nitrates include hypotension, facial flushing, dizziness, headache, nausea and vomiting, weakness, and fatigue.
- To minimize the risk for development of tolerance to nitrates, it is important to have a 10- to 12-hour drug-free period each day.
- A fatal drop in blood pressure can occur when drugs used to treat erectile dysfunction (sildenafil [Viagra], vardenafil [Cialis], and tadalafil [Levitra]) are administered to patients who are taking nitroglycerin.
- The β-blockers are easily identified because their generic name ends in "-lol."
- The β-blockers decrease the heart rate and workload of the heart, thereby reducing the heart's demand for oxygen.
- The β-blockers decrease the frequency and severity of stable (exertional) angina.
- Adverse reactions of the β-blockers are dizziness, fatigue, bradycardia, hypotension, impotence, heart block, and occasionally insomnia.
- Calcium channel blockers classified as dihydropyridines are easily identified because their generic name ends in "-dipine."
- Calcium channel blockers are used in treatment of vasospastic and stable angina.
- Calcium channel blockers reduce vasospasms and improve exercise tolerance by decreasing the workload of the heart and improving blood flow.

Review Questions

1. Thickening and loss of elasticity of arterial walls that is sometimes called "hardening of the arteries" characterizes _____.
   a. atherosclerosis
   b. arteriosclerosis
   c. angiosclerosis
   d. vasosclerosis
2. People with what kind of health history are at risk for angina?
   a. heart disease
   b. hypertension
   c. diabetes
   d. all of the above
3. You receive a prescription for nitroglycerin 0.4 mg SL #30 1 tablet SL PRN chest pain. Refill X3. After consulting the pharmacist, you _____.
   a. dispense the prescription as written in a plastic prescription vial
   b. place the tablets in a compliance pack (bubble pack) to improve adherence
   c. dispense 100 tablets in the manufacturer's original container
   d. tell the patient that nitroglycerin is not marketed as a sublingual tablet

4. A common drug ending for β-blockers is:
   a. "dipine"
   b. "prolol"
   c. "olol"
   d. "orbide"
5. The organic nitrates are the oldest class of drugs used to treat acute symptoms of angina.
   a. true
   b. false
6. Nitroglycerin is available in all of the dosage forms except?
   a. ointment
   b. transdermal patch
   c. extended-release capsule
   d. sublingual spray
7. Stable angina may occur at rest without physical exertion. It can occur when an embolus partially or completely occludes an artery.
   a. true
   b. false

8. Calcium channel blockers are used in treatment of what types of angina?
   a. vasospastic
   b. stable
   c. unstable
   d. a and b
9. The generic name for Tenormin is _____.
   a. atenolol
   b. nifedipine
   c. nadolol
   d. amlodipine

10. Which drug must be dispensed in the manufacturer's original container?
    a. isosorbide dinitrate
    b. isosorbide mononitrate
    c. sublingual nitroglycerin
    d. diltiazem

Bibliography

Banerjee K, Ghosh RK, Kamatam S, et al. Role of ranolazine in cardiovascular disease and diabetes: exploring beyond angina. *Int J Cardiol*. 2017;227:556–564.

Barton JC, Kaski JC. Ethnic and regional differences in the management of angina: the way forward. *Eur Cardiol*. 2022;17:e07.

Gulati M, Levy P, Mukherjee D, et al. AHA/ACC/ASE/CHEST/SAEM/SCCT/SCMR guideline for the evaluation and diagnosis of chest pain. *J Am Coll Cardiol*. 2021;78(22):e187–e285.

Health Canada. (2018). Drug Product Database. Retrieved October 18, 2022, from https://health-products.canada.ca/dpd-bdpp/index-eng.jsp.

Institute for Safe Medication Practices. (2016). FDA and ISMP Lists of Look-Alike Drug Names with Recommended Tall Man Letters. Retrieved October 18, 2022, from https://www.ismp.org/recommendations/tall-man-letters-list.

Institute for Safe Medication Practices. (2019). List of Confused Drugs. Retrieved October 18, 2022, from https://www.ismp.org/tools/confuseddrugnames.pdf.

Jain A, Elgendy IY, Al-Ani M, et al. Advancements in pharmacotherapy for angina. *Expert Opin Pharmacother*. 2017;18(5):457–469.

Kalant H, Grant D, Mitchell J. *Principles of medical pharmacology*. ed 7. Toronto, Ontario, Canada: Elsevier Canada, A Division of Reed Elsevier Canada; 2007:451–453 458–460.

Kloner RA, Chaitman B. Angina and its management. *J Cardiovasc Pharmacol Ther*. 2017;22(3):199–209.

Manolis AJ, Boden WE, Collins P, et al. State of the art approach to managing angina and ischemia: tailoring treatment to the evidence. *Eur J Intern Med*. 2021;92:40–47.

National Heart, Lung, and Blood Institute. (2022). Angina, Bethesda, MD, National Heart and Blood Institute, National Institutes of Health, US Department of Health and Human Services. Retrieved October 30, 2022, from http://www.nhlbi.nih.gov/health/dci/Diseases/Angina/Angina_All.html.

Page C, Curtis M, Sutter M, et al. *Integrated pharmacology*. Philadelphia: Mosby; 2005:377–383.

Rehan R, Weaver J, Yong A. Coronary vasospastic angina: a review of the pathogenesis, diagnosis, and management. *Life*. 2022;12:1124.

U.S. Food and Drug Administration. (nd). Drugs@FDA: FDA Approved Drug Products. Retrieved October 18, 2022, from http://www.accessdata.fda.gov/scripts/cder/daf/.

18

Treatment of Hypertension

LEARNING OBJECTIVES

1. Learn the terminology associated with the treatment of hypertension.
2. List risk factors for development of hypertension.
3. List complications associated with untreated or poorly controlled hypertension.
4. Explain the role of coronary heart disease in the development of hypertension.
5. Identify lifestyle changes that reduce the risk for hypertension.
6. List and categorize medications used to treat hypertension.
7. Describe mechanism of action for each class of drugs used to treat hypertension.
8. List common endings for drug classes used in the treatment of hypertension.
9. Identify significant drug look-alike and sound-alike issues.
10. Identify warning labels and precautionary messages associated with medications used to treat hypertension.

KEY TERMS

Aldosterone Hormone that promotes sodium and fluid reabsorption.
Angiotensin II Potent vasoconstrictor that is produced when the renin–aldosterone–angiotensin system is activated.
Angiotensin-converting enzyme Enzyme that catalyzes the conversion of angiotensin I to angiotensin II.
Cardiac output Volume of blood ejected from the left ventricle in 1 minute.
Diastolic blood pressure Measure of blood pressure when the heart is at rest (diastole).
Diuretic Drug that produces diuresis (urination).
Hyperkalemia Elevated serum potassium levels.
Hypertension High blood pressure; elevated diastolic blood pressure, systolic blood pressure, or both.
Isolated systolic hypertension Elevated systolic blood pressure only. Diastolic blood pressure is within the normal range.

Metabolic syndrome Important risk factor for hypertension that promotes the development of atherosclerosis and cardiovascular disease.
Orthostatic hypotension Sudden drop in blood pressure that occurs when arising from lying down or sitting to standing.
Peripheral vascular resistance Resistance to the flow of blood in peripheral arterial blood vessels that affects blood vessel diameter, vessel length, and blood viscosity.
Renin–aldosterone–angiotensin system System that is activated when there is a drop in renal blood flow. Activation increases blood volume, blood flow to the kidneys, vasoconstriction, and blood pressure.
Systolic blood pressure Measure of the pressure when the heart's ventricles are contracting (systole).

Blood Pressure

Blood pressure is necessary to circulate blood, oxygen (O_2), and nutrients to body organs and to remove carbon dioxide (CO_2) and waste products. Without blood pressure, circulatory collapse and death would result.

When blood pressure is taken, two pressures are measured. They are the systolic pressure and the diastolic pressure.

$$BP = \frac{Systole}{Diastole}$$

The **systolic blood pressure** (SBP) is a measure of the pressure when the heart's ventricles are contracting (systole). The **diastolic blood pressure** (DBP) is a measure of the heart at rest (diastole).

Average normal blood pressure is

<120 mm Hg (systole)

<80 mm Hg (diastole)

Hypertension

It is estimated that more than one billion adults worldwide have **hypertension**. It is the most diagnosed medical condition in the United States, affecting one in four adult women and four in ten adult men. Nearly one in four Canadian adults 25 years or older have high blood pressure. The Canadian Comprehensive Hypertension (CCH) Guidelines 2020 define hypertension as blood pressure that exceeds 135 to 140 mm Hg/85 to 90 mm Hg, depending on whether an automated office blood pressure was taken. The American College of Cardiologists (ACC) and American Heart Association (AHA) define stage 1 hypertension as 130 to 139 mm Hg/80 to 89 mm Hg. *Isolated systolic hypertension* is a condition in which only the SBP is elevated and DBP is within the normal range.

What Causes Hypertension?

In more than 90% of cases, the actual cause for hypertension is unknown, yet some risk factors for chronic elevated high blood pressure are known. *Metabolic syndrome*, a condition characterized by abdominal obesity, high blood pressure, high blood sugar, and hyperlipidemia, is an important risk factor for hypertension because it promotes the development of atherosclerosis and cardiovascular disease. Diabetes and dyslipidemia (abnormal amounts of lipids in blood) are other risk factors for hypertension. Box 18.1 lists additional risk factors for high blood pressure.

Drugs may also induce high blood pressure (Box 18.2).

Blood Pressure Classifications

Elevated Blood Pressure

Elevated blood pressure is defined as SBP ranging between 120 and 129 mm Hg and DBP less than 80 mm Hg. Reduction of blood pressure to normal levels is beneficial for persons with elevated blood pressure with and without preexisting disease. Lifestyle modification is often sufficient; however, drug therapy

---

• **BOX 18.1** **Hypertension Risk Factors**

- Age (men older than 55 years; women older than 65 years)
- Chronic conditions (e.g., diabetes mellitus, kidney disease, and sleep apnea)
- Family history of heart disease
- Metabolic syndrome
- Obesity
- Tobacco usage or vaping
- Decreased physical activity
- Dyslipidemia
- Diet high in salt and saturated fats
- Excessive alcohol consumption
- Low potassium levels
- Stress
- Pregnancy

• **BOX 18.2** **Select Drugs That Can Increase Blood Pressure**

- Nonsteroidal antiinflammatory drugs (cyclooxygenase-2 inhibitors)
- Cocaine, amphetamines
- Decongestants
- Diet pills
- Oral contraceptives
- Glucocorticosteroids (e.g., prednisone, hydrocortisone, methylprednisolone)
- Mineralocorticoids (aldosterone)
- Cyclosporine and tacrolimus
- Erythropoietin
- Licorice
- Herbals (ma huang, ephedra, bitter orange)

---

should be added to the treatment program for people who have diabetes or kidney disease if lifestyle changes do not bring blood pressure down to the normal range.

Gestational Hypertension

Hypertension during pregnancy is dangerous to the pregnant woman and the fetus. Gestational hypertension typically occurs after 20 weeks of pregnancy in susceptible women.

Masked Hypertension

Patients whose blood pressure is elevated in measurements taken outside of the physician's office but controlled according to measurements taken in the physician's office have "masked hypertension."

White Coat Hypertension

"White coat hypertension" is the opposite of masked hypertension. People who have white coat hypertension have abnormally high blood pressure when the measurement is taken by a health care professional, but blood pressure measurements taken in a nonclinic setting are within normal range (Table 18.1).

Complications Associated With Untreated or Poorly Controlled Hypertension

Hypertension is sometimes called the "silent killer" because it can cause damage to the body without any obvious symptoms. Hypertension can cause damage to the kidneys, heart, brain, arteries, and eyes. Hypertension can weaken arteries and cause aneurysms that can bleed and cause death if they occur in the brain, aorta, or abdomen. When arteries in the brain are narrowed or blocked, it can affect the ability to think and learn or cause vascular dementia. Hypertension can cause blindness when blood

---

TABLE 18.1	Summary of Blood Pressure Classifications and Target Blood Pressure Goals	
	2017 ACC/AHA	**2018 CHEP**
Normal	<120/<80	<120/<80
Elevated blood pressure	120–129/<80	
Hypertension		
Stage 1	130–139/80–89	135/85 AOBP or out of office BP measurement
Stage 2	≥140/≥90	140/90 Non-AOBP
Isolated systolic hypertension	Systolic ≥ 140 Diastolic ≤ 90	Systolic ≥ 140 Diastolic ≤ 90
Diabetes or chronic kidney disease	130/80	130/80

ACC, American College of Cardiology; *AHA*, American Heart Association; *AOBP*, automated office blood pressure (without physician present); *BP*, blood pressure; *CHEP*, Canadian Hypertension Education Program.

vessels to the retina are damaged and scarred. For each 20 mm Hg increase in SBP and 10 mm Hg increase in DBP, there is a twofold increase in risk of death from ischemic heart disease (IHD) and stroke. This is because hypertension can damage arteries and make them stiff and thick.

Nonpharmacological Management of Hypertension

Hypertension poses a serious public health challenge because of the risks for death and long-term disability. It is categorized as a chronic disease of lifestyle because it is associated with obesity, excess dietary sodium intake, physical inactivity, excessive alcohol consumption, and inadequate consumption of fruits and vegetables. As many as one in three adults and one in five children are obese or overweight in the United States, according to CDC data. Fewer than 20% engage in regular physical activity or consume adequate fruits and vegetables (five servings per day).

Lifestyle modification is an important strategy for prevention and management of hypertension and can reduce SBP between 4 and 20 mm Hg. A reduction of as little as 5 mm Hg can lower the risk of death from stroke by 14% and death from coronary heart disease (CHD) by 9%. The US Joint National Committee on the Prevention, Detection, Evaluation, and Treatment of High Blood Pressure recommendations for lifestyle changes are listed in Table 18.2.

The ability to make lifestyle changes is associated with social determinants of health. Some of the social determinants of health that affect hypertension and other cardiovascular diseases are poverty, racism, and housing. Poverty affects the ability to purchase DASH diet healthy foods. Racism has an impact on stress, a risk factor of hypertension. Poverty and racism affect housing. More than 50% of Americans do not live within half a mile of a park or live in neighborhoods without adequate infrastructure to safely engage in exercise. Moreover, 40% of US households live in food deserts or areas that are more than one mile from retailers that sell healthy foods.

TABLE 18.2	Lifestyle Modifications for Management and Prevention of Hypertension
Modification	Recommendation
Weight loss	Maintain normal body weight Body mass index (18.5–24.9 kg/m²)
Diet	Reduce salt (sodium) intake (≤2 g sodium)[a] Increase potassium rich foods (e.g., bananas) Reduce saturated and total fats Eat 5 or more servings of fruits and vegetables/day
Physical activity	Engage in 30–60 min of aerobic physical activity 4–7 days per week
Alcohol consumption	Drink no more than 2 alcoholic beverages[b] per day—men (women and lightweight persons, 1 drink/day)
Tobacco usage	Stop smoking cigarettes and cigars

Adapted from Hypertension Canada's 2018 Guidelines for Diagnosis, Risk Assessment, Prevention, and Treatment of Hypertension in Adults and Children, 2018 American College of Cardiology/American Heart Association Task Force on Clinical Practice Guidelines.
[a]American Heart Association recommends < 1500 mg/day.
[b]Alcoholic beverage = 24 oz of beer, 10 oz of wine, or 3 oz of whiskey (80 proof).

> ● **Tech Note!**
>
> Natural licorice may aggravate hypertension and interfere with the effects of antihypertensive drugs. It increases sodium and water retention and potassium depletion.

> ● **Tech Note!**
>
> Processed foods contain "hidden sodium" and account for nearly 80% of the daily sodium consumed.

Drugs Used in the Treatment of Hypertension

Lifestyle modification is the first step in prevention and management of hypertension in people with normal blood pressure or who have elevated blood pressure; however, most people with hypertension will require drug therapy with one or more drugs and lifestyle modification. Pharmaceutical management of hypertension can be challenging because medications prescribed to reduce blood pressure can sometimes produce more symptoms than the disease, resulting in poor adherence to drug therapy. Drugs used in the treatment of hypertension work at the sites for blood pressure regulation, which are the kidneys, heart, blood vessels, brain, and sympathetic nerves.

Diuretics

The kidneys play a major role in regulating blood pressure. **Diuretics** exert their effects on the kidneys where they increase the elimination of water, sodium, and selected electrolytes (K^+, Cl^-, HCO_3^-). The diuretics lower blood pressure by decreasing blood volume, peripheral resistance in blood vessels, and **cardiac output**. There are several classifications of diuretics. They are thiazide, loop, and potassium (K^+) sparing. **Aldosterone** antagonists are K^+ sparing and are sometimes classified as diuretics because their site of action is the kidney.

Thiazide Diuretics

Thiazide diuretics are a first-line therapy for hypertension. They promote the elimination of water, sodium, potassium, magnesium, and chloride ions. Fluid loss decreases blood volume, yet this is not the primary mechanism of action for their effectiveness in decreasing blood pressure.

Thiazides act at the distal convoluted tubule, where they block the sodium–chloride cotransporter (Fig. 18.1). This interferes with calcium transport into arterioles, decreasing vasoconstriction. Peripheral resistance is lowered along with blood pressure. Thiazides indirectly stimulate aldosterone secretion, causing potassium excretion.

> ● **Tech Note!**
>
> Most thiazide diuretics share the common ending "-thiazide."

> ● **Tech Note!**
>
> Patients taking thiazides may be advised to eat potassium-rich foods to replenish potassium depleted by the diuretics.

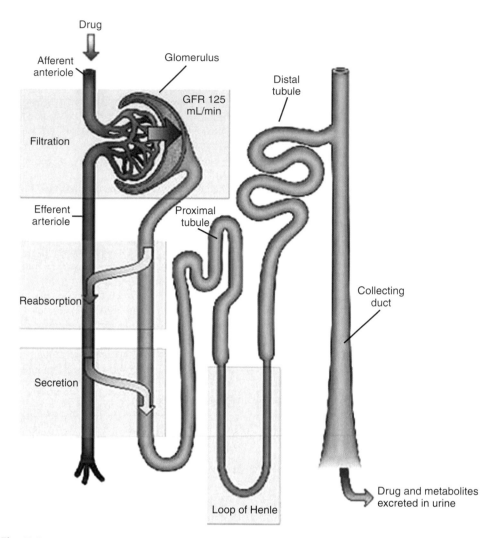

• **Fig. 18.1** Nephron. *GFR*, Glomerular filtration rate. (From Patton KT, Thibodeau GA: *The human body in health and disease*, ed 7, St Louis, 2018, Elsevier.)

> **⬤ *Tech Note!***
>
> Hydrochlorothiazide is commonly abbreviated HCTZ.

Pharmacokinetics

Thiazide diuretics are readily absorbed orally. They are weak acids and are highly protein bound. Their lipid solubility permits reabsorption along the distal nephron. Their duration of effect varies from as little as 6 hours to as long as 48 hours depending on the drug. Most thiazide diuretics are dosed once a day.

Adverse Reactions and Precautions

Thiazide diuretics can cause dehydration, hyponatremia (sodium loss), and electrolyte deficiency including hypokalemia (potassium loss), hypomagnesemia (magnesium loss), and hypochloremia (chloride loss).

The thiazide diuretics can precipitate a flare-up of gout because they can cause hyperuricemia (excess uric acid). They should be used with caution in patients with diabetes because they may produce hyperglycemia and glucose intolerance. The thiazides have direct and indirect effects on insulin release. Other adverse drug reactions are gastrointestinal upset, impotence, and photosensitivity. Diuretics should be taken in the morning to avoid the need to urinate in the middle of the night.

> **⚠ *Tech Alert!***
>
> The following drugs have look-alike/sound-alike issues:
> hydroCHLOROthiazide, hydrOXYzine, and hydrALAZINE;
> metOLazone and methIMAzole

Loop Diuretics

The loop diuretics are the most potent diuretics. They inhibit the reabsorption of 20% to 30% of sodium load; the thiazides inhibit only 5% to 10%, and the potassium-sparing diuretics inhibit only

Thiazide Diuretics

Generic Name	US Brand Name / Canadian Brand(s)	Dosage Forms and Strengths
chlorothiazide[a]	Diuril	Injection, powder for reconstitution[b]: 500 mg vial
	Not available	Suspension, oral: 250 mg/5 mL
chlorthalidone[a]	Generics	Tablets: 25 mg[b], 50 mg
	Generics	
hydrochlorothiazide[a]	Microzide	Capsules (Microzide): 12.5 mg
	Generics	Tablets: 12.5 mg, 25 mg, 50 mg
indapamide[a]	Generics	Tablets: 1.25 mg, 2.5 mg
	Generics	
metolazone[a]	Generics	Tablets, slow acting (Zaroxolyn): 2.5 mg, 5 mg[b], 10 mg[b]
	Zaroxolyn	

[a]Generic available.
[b]Available in the United States only.

1% to 3% of the sodium load. Loop diuretics increase potassium excretion and are often administered with a potassium supplement to reduce the risk of hypokalemia. They also stimulate aldosterone secretion, similar to the thiazides, and increase calcium excretion.

> **① Tech Alert!**
>
> The following drugs have look-alike/sound-alike issues:
> Lasix and Luvox

Pharmacokinetics

The loop diuretics are readily absorbed from the gastrointestinal tract. They are up to 98% protein bound. The site of action of loop diuretics is the ascending limb of the loop of Henle. In contrast, the thiazide diuretics' site of action is at the distal convoluted tubule. Differences among the loop diuretics are associated with their degree of metabolism in the liver and the extent to which they are eliminated unchanged in the urine. Whereas bumetanide is partially metabolized in the liver and 50% is excreted unchanged in the urine, torsemide's metabolism in the liver is greater and 20% is excreted unchanged. Torsemide's long half-life permits once-daily dosing.

Adverse Reactions and Precautions

The loop diuretics can cause dehydration, severe hypotension, hypokalemia, hyperuricemia, and photosensitivity. Deafness has occurred when large doses are infused rapidly. Patients taking loop diuretics should take the last dose of the day in early evening to avoid the need to urinate in the middle of the night.

Potassium Supplements

Potassium supplements may be prescribed to reduce the risk for hypokalemia or to treat hyperkalemia.

Potassium-Sparing Diuretics

The potassium-sparing diuretics inhibit sodium reabsorption while avoiding potassium loss. They are less effective than loop and thiazide diuretics. Combining K+-sparing diuretics with a thiazide diuretic increases their effectiveness. Examples are amiloride–hydrochlorothiazide and triamterene–hydrochlorothiazide.

Triamterene is readily absorbed in the gastrointestinal tract, and amiloride is 50% absorbed. The duration of effect ranges from 7 to 9 hours (triamterene) and 24 hours (amiloride).

Adverse Reactions and Precautions

Hyperkalemia occurs when serum potassium levels are elevated higher than 5.5 mEq/L. It is the most serious adverse reaction of the potassium-sparing diuretics, and the risk is increased if they are prescribed concurrently with angiotensin-converting enzyme (ACE) inhibitors. They may also cause nausea or vomiting. Hyperkalemia may produce cardiac arrhythmias, and the risk is increased in patients with heart failure who take digoxin. Patients should be advised to avoid salt substitutes because they contain potassium chloride (KCl). Strategies to manage hyperkalemia are list in Box 18.3.

Aldosterone Receptor Antagonists

Aldosterone is a hormone that is released when the kidney perceives a decrease in blood flow and blood pressure. Aldosterone causes sodium and water reabsorption to increase blood pressure. Spironolactone is an aldosterone antagonist. Spironolactone is

Loop Diuretics

Generic Name	US Brand Name Canadian Brand(s)	Dosage Forms and Strengths
bumetanide[a,b]	Bumex	**Injection, solution**[b]: 0.25 mg/mL
	Burinex	**Tablets:** 0.5 mg[b], 1 mg, 2 mg[b], 5 mg[c]
furosemide[a]	Furoscix, Lasix	**Injection, solution:** 10 mg/mL, 80 mg/10 mL (Furoscix)[b]
	Lasix, Lasix Special	**Solution, oral:** 10 mg/mL, 40 mg/5 mL[b] **Tablets:** 20 mg, 40 mg, 80 mg, 500 mg (Lasix Special)[c]
torsemide[a]	Soaanz	**Tablets:** 5 mg, 10 mg, 20 mg, 40 mg, 100 mg
	Not available	

[a]Generic available.
[b]Available in the United States only.
[c]Available in Canada only.

Electrolyte Replacement Therapy: Potassium*

Generic Name	US Brand Name(s) Canadian Brand Name(s)	Dosage Forms and Strengths
potassium chloride[a,b]	Klor Con, Klor Con M10, Klor Con M15, Klor Con M20	**Capsule (Klor Con):** 8 mEq, 10 mEq **Tablet, extended release (Klor-Con):** 8 mEq, 10 mEq
	No prescription oral products	**Tablet, microdispersed (Klor Con M):** 10 mEq, 15 mEq, 20 mEq **Solution, oral:** 20 mEq/15 mL, 40 mEq/15 mL **Solution, for intravenous use (in D$_5$W):** 10 mEq (10 mmol), 15 mEq (15 mmol), 20 mEq (20 mml), 30 mEq (30 mmol), 40 mEq (40 mmol)

[a]Available in the United States only.
[b]Generic available.
*Prescription-only products listed.

sometimes classified as a potassium-sparing diuretic because it conserves potassium. In addition to its use in treating hypertension, spironolactone is used to treat primary aldosteronism, hypokalemia, and heart failure. It can take several weeks to see maximal effect, which differs from loop diuretics, which work immediately.

Spironolactone is about as effective as triamterene and amiloride (sodium reabsorption is approximately 1% to 3%). It is readily absorbed orally and is eliminated in urine. It has a long half-life and is dosed once daily. Eplerenone is a selective aldosterone receptor antagonist (SARA). It is indicated for the treatment of hypertension as monotherapy or used with other antihypertensive drugs. It is also indicated for the treatment of heart failure. Eplerenone increases the excretion of renin and aldosterone.

Adverse Reactions and Precautions

Eplerenone and spironolactone may cause hyperkalemia. Other adverse reactions are nausea, an unpleasant aftertaste, gynecomastia (breast enlargement in males), hirsutism (excessive hair growth in women), impotence, and menstrual irregularities. Potassium-containing salt substitutes should be avoided when eplerenone and spironolactone are administered.

Angiotensin-Converting Enzyme Inhibitors

The ACE inhibitors target the *renin–aldosterone–angiotensin system* (RAAS) to lower blood pressure. The RAAS responds to decreased blood flow to the kidneys by activating mediators to increase blood flow. This in turn increases blood pressure.

Potassium-Sparing Diuretics

Generic Name	US Brand Name Canadian Brand(s)	Dosage Forms and Strengths
amiloride[a]	Midamor	Tablet: 5 mg,
	Midamor	
triamterene[a]	Dyrenium	Capsule: 50 mg, 100 mg,
	Not available	

Combination Diuretics

triamterene + HCTZ[a]	Maxzide	Capsule: 25 mg hydrochlorothiazide + 37.5 mg triamterene
	Generics	Tablet: 25 mg hydrochlorothiazide + 50 mg triamterene

Aldosterone Receptor Antagonists

Generic Name	US Brand Name Canadian Brand(s)	Dosage Forms and Strengths
eplerenone[a]	Inspra	Tablets: 25 mg, 50 mg,
	Inspra	
spironolactone[a]	Aldactone, Carospir	Oral suspension (Carospir): 25 mg/5 mL,
	Aldactone	Tablets: 25 mg, 50 mg[b], 100 mg,

Combination Aldosterone Receptor Antagonists

spironolactone + hydrochlorothiazide[a]	Aldactazide	Tablets: 25 mg spironolactone + 25 mg HCTZ
	Aldactazide	50 mg spironolactone + 50 mg HCTZ

[a]Generic available.
[b]Available in the United States only.
HCTZ, Hydrochlorothiazide.

The ACE inhibitors are first-line therapy for treatment of hypertension. They are recommended over other first-line therapies when patients have chronic kidney disease, diabetes, or coronary artery disease, according to Canadian (CCH), American (ACC, AHA), and World Health Organization guidelines.

> **Tech Note!**
>
> The ACE inhibitors share the common ending "-pril."

> **Tech Alert!**
>
> The following drugs have look-alike/sound-alike issues:
> benazepril and Benadryl;
> captopril and carvedilol;

Mechanism of Action

The ACE inhibitors lower blood pressure by blocking the action of the *angiotensin-converting enzyme*. The angiotensin-converting enzyme catalyzes the conversion of angiotensin I to its active metabolite angiotensin II. *Angiotensin II* is a potent vasoconstrictor. It stimulates the release of aldosterone and promotes the release of norepinephrine from sympathetic neurons. The ACE inhibitors also decrease reabsorption of sodium in the renal tubules. In addition, they cause the accumulation of bradykinins (peptides that produce dilation of arteries). This reduces peripheral resistance, further lowering blood pressure.

Pharmacokinetics

The ACE inhibitors differ in activity, metabolism, and elimination, which may influence which ACE is prescribed. For example, enalapril, perindopril, quinapril, ramipril, and trandolapril are prodrugs.

Angiotensin-Converting Enzyme Inhibitors

	Generic Name	US Brand Name / Canadian Brand(s)	Dosage Forms and Strengths
	benazepril[a]	Lotensin Generics	**Tablets:** 5 mg, 10 mg, 20 mg, 40 mg,[b]
	captopril[a]	Generics Generics	**Tablets:** 12.5 mg, 25 mg, 50 mg, 100 mg,
	enalapril maleate[a]	Epaned, Vasotec Vasotec IV	**Injection, solution (as enalaprilat):** 1.25 mg/mL, **Solution, oral (Epaned):** 1 mg/mL, **Tablets:** 2.5 mg, 5 mg, 10 mg, 20 mg,
	enalapril sodium[a]	Not available Vasotec	**Tablets:** 2 mg, 4 mg, 8 mg, 16 mg,
	fosinopril[a]	Generics Generics	**Tablets:** 10 mg, 20 mg, 40 mg,[b]
	lisinopril[a]	Qbrelis, Zestril Zestril	**Solution, oral (Qbrelis):** 1 mg/mL, **Tablets:** 2.5 mg[b], 5 mg, 10 mg, 20 mg, 30 mg[b], 40 mg,[b]
	moexipril[a]	Generic Not available	**Tablet, film-coated:** 7.5 mg, 15 mg,
	perindopril[a]	Generics Coversyl	**Tablets:** 2 mg, 4 mg, 8 mg,
	quinapril[a]	Accupril Accupril	**Tablets:** 5 mg, 10 mg, 20 mg, 40 mg,
	ramipril[a]	Altace Altace	**Capsules:** 1.25 mg, 2.5 mg, 5 mg, 10 mg, 15 mg,[c]
	trandolapril[a]	Generics Mavik	**Tablets:** 0.5 mg[c], 1 mg, 2 mg, 4 mg,

Combination Angiotensin-Converting Enzyme Inhibitors and Diuretics

	Generic Name	US Brand Name / Canadian Brand(s)	Dosage Forms and Strengths
	benazepril + hydrochlorothiazide[a]	Lotensin HCT Not available	**Tablets:** benazepril 10 mg + hydrochlorothiazide 12.5 mg, benazepril 20 mg + hydrochlorothiazide 12.5 mg, benazepril 20 mg + hydrochlorothiazide 25 mg,
	enalapril + hydrochlorothiazide[a]	Vaseretic Vaseretic	**Tablets:** enalapril 5 mg + hydrochlorothiazide 12.5 mg, enalapril 10 mg + hydrochlorothiazide 25 mg, enalapril 8 mg + hydrochlorothiazide 25 mgv,[c]
	fosinopril + hydrochlorothiazide	Generics Not available	**Tablets:** fosinopril 10 mg + hydrochlorothiazide 12.5 mg, fosinopril 20 mg + hydrochlorothiazide 12.5 mg,
	lisinopril + hydrochlorothiazide[a]	Zestoretic Zestoretic	**Tablets:** lisinopril 10 mg + hydrochlorothiazide 12.5 mg, lisinopril 20 mg + hydrochlorothiazide 12.5 mg, lisinopril 20 mg + hydrochlorothiazide 25 mg,

Angiotensin-Converting Enzyme Inhibitors—cont'd

Generic Name	US Brand Name Canadian Brand(s)	Dosage Forms and Strengths
moexipril + hydrochlorothiazide[a]	Generics Not available	**Tablets:** moexipril 7.5 mg + hydrochlorothiazide 12.5 mg, moexipril 15 mg + hydrochlorothiazide 12.5 mg, moexipril 15 mg + hydrochlorothiazide 25 mg,
quinapril + hydrochlorothiazide[a]	Accuretic Accuretic	**Tablets:** quinapril 10 mg + hydrochlorothiazide 12.5 mg, quinapril 20 mg + hydrochlorothiazide 12.5 mg, quinapril 20 mg + hydrochlorothiazide 25 mg,
ramipril + hydrochlorothiazide[a]	Not available Altace HCT	**Tablets:** ramipril 2.5 mg + hydrochlorothiazide 12.5 mg, ramipril 5 mg + hydrochlorothiazide 12.5 mg, ramipril 10 mg + hydrochlorothiazide 12.5 mg, ramipril 5 mg + hydrochlorothiazide 25 mg, ramipril 10 mg + hydrochlorothiazide 25 mg,

Combination Angiotensin-Converting Enzyme Inhibitor and Calcium Channel Blocker

Generic Name	US Brand Name Canadian Brand(s)	Dosage Forms and Strengths
benazepril + amlodipine[a]	Lotrel Not available	**Capsules:** benazepril 10 mg + amlodipine 2.5 mg, benazepril 10 mg + amlodipine 5 mg, benazepril 20 mg + amlodipine 5 mg, benazepril 20 mg + amlodipine 10 mg, benazepril 40 mg + amlodipine 5 mg, benazepril 40 mg + amlodipine 10 mg,
trandolapril + verapamil	Generics Not available	**Tablets, extended release:** trandolapril 1 mg + verapamil 240 mg, trandolapril 2 mg + verapamil 180 mg, trandolapril 2 mg + verapamil 240 mg, trandolapril 4 mg + verapamil 240 mg,

[a]Generic available.
[b]Available in the United States only.
[c]Available in Canada only.

They would not be the first choice of drugs for patients with decreased liver function because prodrugs have limited activity until they undergo metabolism. Enalaprilat, perindoprilat, quinaprilat, ramiprilat, and trandolaprilat are their active metabolites. Captopril and lisinopril are already active compounds. Fosinopril is a good choice for patients with decreased kidney function because 50% is eliminated by the kidney and 50% by the liver. All other ACE inhibitors are 90% eliminated by the kidney and can accumulate if kidney disease is present.

> **● Tech Note!**
>
> The contents of Altace capsules may be sprinkled on food or dissolved in liquid.

Adverse Reactions and Precautions

Dry cough is a characteristic side effect that is caused by the accumulation of bradykinins. Other adverse drug reactions are hyperkalemia, light-headedness, hypotension, diarrhea, and skin rashes. Angioedema is a rare but potentially lethal allergic reaction that can cause swelling of the throat or airways. The ACE inhibitors are contraindicated in pregnancy because they can interfere with fetal development of the kidneys. Fetal death has been reported. Salt substitutes should be avoided to reduce risks for hyperkalemia.

Angiotensin II Receptor Antagonists

The angiotensin II receptor blockers (ARBs) lower blood pressure by competitively binding at the angiotensin II receptor site. They decrease cardiac contractility and inhibit sodium reabsorption and vasoconstriction—the opposite of effects produced by activating angiotensin receptors. ARBs also reduce ventricular and arterial hypertrophy that is associated with chronic hypertension because the drugs inhibit angiotensin II–stimulated growth of smooth muscle.

The ARBs are similar to ACE inhibitors in effectiveness but produce less dry cough, perhaps because they do not increase bradykinin levels like the ACE inhibitors. The ARBs are first-line therapy for treatment of hypertension, especially in patients with diabetes and coronary artery disease who cannot tolerate ACE inhibitors.

> **● Tech Note!**
>
> Angiotensin II antagonists share the common ending "-sartan."

Pharmacokinetics

The plasma half-lives of individual ARBs vary. Losartan, one of the first ARBs to be marketed, has a relatively short half-life (only 2 hours), but it has an active metabolite with a plasma half-life of up to 6 to 9 hours. Losartan has an active metabolite that is 10 to 40 times more potent than the parent compound. The duration of action for irbesartan, candesartan, and telmisartan is longer (12 to 18 hours). The drugs are administered as a single daily dose.

Adverse Reactions and Precautions

Common adverse drug reactions associated with the ARBs are fatigue, headache, abdominal cramps, dizziness, hyperkalemia, diarrhea, impotence, and muscle cramps. The ARBs are contraindicated in the second and third trimesters of pregnancy because they can interfere with fetal development of the kidneys, and fetal death has been reported.

① *Tech Alert!*

The following drugs have look-alike/sound-alike issues:
Cozaar, Colace, and Zocor;
Diovan, Dioval, and Zyban

Beta-Adrenergic Blockers (β-Blockers)

The β-blockers used in the treatment of hypertension block the effect of norepinephrine and epinephrine on the heart and blood vessels to reduce heart rate and blood pressure.

● *Tech Note!*

Blockers share the common ending "-olol."

Angiotensin II Receptor Antagonists

Generic Name	US Brand Name / Canadian Brand(s)	Dosage Forms and Strengths
azilsartan	Edarbi	**Tablet:** 40 mg, 80 mg,
	Edarbi	
candesartan[a]	Atacand	**Tablets:** 4 mg, 8 mg, 16 mg, 32 mg,
	Atacand	
eprosartan	Not available	**Tablets:** 400 mg, 600 mg,
	Teveten	
irbesartan[a]	Avapro	**Tablets:** 75 mg, 150 mg, 300 mg,
	Avapro	
losartan[a]	Cozaar	**Tablets:** 25 mg, 50 mg, 100 mg,
	Cozaar	irbesartan and losartan
olmesartan[a]	Benicar	**Tablets:** 5 mg[b], 20 mg, 40 mg,
	Olmetec	
telmisartan[a]	Micardis	**Tablets:** 20 mg[b], 40 mg, 80 mg,
	Micardis	
valsartan[a]	Diovan	**Tablets:** 40 mg, 80 mg, 160 mg, 320 mg,
	Diovan	

Combination Angiotensin II Receptor Antagonists and Diuretics

azilsartan + chlorthalidone	Edarbyclor	**Tablets:** azilsartan 40 mg + chlorthalidone 12.5 mg,
	Edarbyclor	azilsartan 40 mg + chlorthalidone 25 mg,

Angiotensin II Receptor Antagonists—cont'd

Generic Name	US Brand Name / Canadian Brand(s)	Dosage Forms and Strengths
candesartan + hydrochlorothiazide[a]	Atacand HCT / Atacand Plus	**Tablets:** candesartan 16 mg + hydrochlorothiazide 12.5 mg, candesartan 32 mg + hydrochlorothiazide 12.5 mg, candesartan 32 mg + hydrochlorothiazide 25 mg,
eprosartan + hydrochlorothiazide	Not available / Teveten Plus	**Tablets:** eprosartan 600 mg + hydrochlorothiazide 12.5 mg,
irbesartan + hydrochlorothiazide[a]	Avalide / Avalide	**Tablets:** irbesartan 150 mg + hydrochlorothiazide 12.5 mg, irbesartan 300 mg + hydrochlorothiazide 12.5 mg,
losartan + hydrochlorothiazide[a]	Hyzaar / Hyzaar, Hyzaar DS	**Tablets:** losartan 50 mg + hydrochlorothiazide 12.5 mg, losartan 100 mg + hydrochlorothiazide 12.5 mg, losartan 100 mg + hydrochlorothiazide 25 mg,
olmesartan + hydrochlorothiazide[a]	Benicar HCT / Olmetec Plus	**Tablets:** olmesartan 20 mg + hydrochlorothiazide 12.5 mg, olmesartan 40 mg + hydrochlorothiazide 12.5 mg, olmesartan 40 mg + hydrochlorothiazide 25 mg,
telmisartan + hydrochlorothiazide[a]	Micardis HCT / Micardis Plus	**Tablets:** telmisartan 40 mg + hydrochlorothiazide 12.5 mg,[b] telmisartan 80 mg + hydrochlorothiazide 12.5 mg, telmisartan 80 mg + hydrochlorothiazide 25 mg,
valsartan + hydrochlorothiazide[a]	Diovan HCT / Diovan HCT	**Tablets:** valsartan 80 mg + hydrochlorothiazide 12.5 mg, valsartan 160 mg + hydrochlorothiazide 12.5 mg, valsartan 160 mg + hydrochlorothiazide 25 mg, valsartan 320 mg + hydrochlorothiazide 12.5 mg, valsartan 320 mg + hydrochlorothiazide 25 mg,

[a]Generic available.
[b]Available in the United States only.

Mechanism of Action

The β-adrenergic blockers used in the treatment of hypertension may be selective (β_1) or nonselective (β_1, β_2). β_1-Selective agents are first-line therapy for patients who have hypertension and angina or after myocardial infarction.

All β-blockers decrease blood pressure, reduce the heart rate, and decrease the force of contractions in the heart, which lowers the cardiac output. Chronic use produces vasodilation. This may be caused by decreased renin release. Renin acts to convert the hormone angiotensinogen to angiotensin I, a precursor to angiotensin II, a potent vasoconstrictor.

Adverse Reactions and Precautions

Adverse drug reactions associated with β-adrenergic blockers are dizziness, lethargy, nausea, palpitations, impotence, bradycardia, hypoglycemia, cardiac rhythm disturbance, congestive heart failure, and depression. They may also produce bronchospasm, although selective β_1-adrenergic blockers are less likely to produce this effect.

β-Blockers should not be discontinued abruptly because this may cause the onset of arrhythmias or angina. β-Adrenergic blockers should be used with caution in patients with diabetes because they mask the signs of hypoglycemia.

❶ Tech Alert!

The following drugs have look-alike/sound-alike issues: metoprolol succinate and metoprolol tartrate; carvedilol and captopril

Alpha₁-Adrenergic Antagonists (α_1-Blockers)

The arteries have an abundance of α_1 receptors that mediate vasoconstriction. Administration of α_1-blockers produces vascular relaxation, which reduces *peripheral vascular resistance* and lowers blood pressure (Fig. 18.2). Low-density lipoprotein cholesterol levels are also reduced when α_1-adrenergic blockers are administered, making them useful in the treatment of ischemic heart disease. Doxazosin and terazosin can also reduce urethral resistance and increase urine flow, making them effective in the treatment of benign prostatic hyperplasia.

Adverse Reactions

Adverse drug effects are postural hypotension, dizziness, reflex tachycardia, headache, weakness, and fatigue.

Beta-Adrenergic Blockers

Generic Name	US Brand Name Canadian Brand(s)	Dosage Forms and Strengths
β-Blockers: Nonselective		
nadolol[a]	Corgard	**Tablets:** 20 mg[b], 40 mg, 80 mg, 160 mg,[c]
	Generics	
pindolol[a]	Generics	**Tablets:** 5 mg, 10 mg, 15 mg,[c]
	Visken	
propranolol[a]	Hemangeol*, Inderal LA, InnoPran XL Generics	**Capsules, extended release (InnoPran XL)**[b]: 80 mg, 120 mg, **Capsules, sustained release (Inderal LA)**[b]: 60 mg, 80 mg, 120 mg, 160 mg, **Injection, solution:** 1 mg/mL, **Solution, oral**[b]: 20 mg/5 mL, 40 mg/5 mL, **Tablets:** 10 mg, 20 mg, 40 mg, 60 mg[b], 80 mg,
timolol[a]	Generics	**Tablets:** 5 mg, 10 mg, 20 mg,
	Generics	
β-Blockers: β-1 Selective		
acebutolol[a]	Generics	**Capsulesb:** 200 mg, 400 mg, **Tabletsc:** 100 mg, 200 mg, 400 mg,
	Generics	
atenolol[a]	Tenormin	**Tablets:** 25 mg, 50 mg, 100 mg,
	Tenormin	
betaxolol[a]	Generics	**Tablets:** 10 mg, 20 mg,
	Not available	
bisoprolol[a]	Generics	**Tablets:** 5 mg, 10 mg,
	Generics	
metoprolol[a]	Kapspargo Sprinkle, Lopressor, Toprol XL Generics	**Capsule, extended release (Kapspargo Sprinkle):** 25 mg, 50 mg, 100 mg, 200 mg, **Injection, solution (Lopressor):** 1 mg/mL, **Tablets, immediate release (Lopressor):** 25 mg, 50 mg, 100 mg, **Tablets, extended release (Toprol XL):** 25 mg, 50 mg, 100 mg, 200 mg, **Tablets, extended release:** 100 mg,
nebivolol[a, b]	Bystolic	**Tablet:** 2.5 mg, 5 mg, 10 mg, 20 mg,
	Bystolic	
Combination β-Blockers and Diuretics		
atenolol + chlorthalidone[a]	Tenoretic 50, Tenoretic 100 Generics	**Tablets:** atenolol 50 mg + chlorthalidone 25 mg, atenolol 100 mg + chlorthalidone 25 mg,
bisoprolol + hydrochlorothiazide[a]	Ziac Not available	**Tablets:** bisoprolol 2.5 mg + hydrochlorothiazide 6.25 mg, bisoprolol 5 mg + hydrochlorothiazide 6.25 mg, bisoprolol 10 mg + hydrochlorothiazide 6.25 mg,
metoprolol + hydrochlorothiazide[a]	Lopressor HCT Not available	**Tablets:** metoprolol 50 mg + hydrochlorothiazide 25 mg, metoprolol 100 mg + hydrochlorothiazide 25 mg, metoprolol 100 mg + hydrochlorothiazide 50 mg,
pindolol + hydrochlorothiazide	Not available Viskazide	**Tablets:** pindolol 10 mg + hydrochlorothiazide 25 mg, pindolol 10 mg + hydrochlorothiazide 50 mg,

*Used for the treatment of proliferating infantile hemangioma, a condition causing benign vascular tumors.
[a]Generic available.
[b]Available in the United States only.
[c]Available in Canada only.

Combination β₁- and α₁-Blockers

Generic Name	US Brand Name Canadian Brand(s)	Dosage Forms and Strengths
carvedilol[a]	Coreg, Coreg CR Generics	**Tablets:** 3.125 mg, 6.25 mg, 12.5 mg, 25 mg, **Capsules, extended release (Coreg CR)**[b]: 10 mg, 20 mg, 40 mg, 80 mg,
labetalol[a]	Trandate Trandate	**Injection, solution, and prefilled syringe:** 5 mg/mL, **Tablets:** 100 mg, 200 mg, 300 mg,[b]

[a]Generic available.
[b]Available in the United States only.

α₁-Blockers

Generic Name	US Brand Name Canadian Brand(s)	Dosage Forms and Strengths
doxazosin[a]	Cardura, Cardura XL Generics	**Tablets:** 1 mg, 2 mg, 4 mg, 8 mg,[b] **Tablets, extended release (Cardura XL)**[b]: 4 mg, 8 mg,
prazosin[a]	Minipress Generics	**Capsules**[b]: 1 mg, 2 mg, 5 mg, **Tablet**[c]: 1 mg, 2 mg, 5 mg,
terazosin[a]	Generics Generics	**Capsules**[b]: 1 mg, 2 mg, 5 mg, 10 mg, **Tablets**[c]: 1 mg, 2 mg, 5 mg, 10 mg,

[a]Generic available.
[b]Available in the United States only.
[c]Available in Canada only.

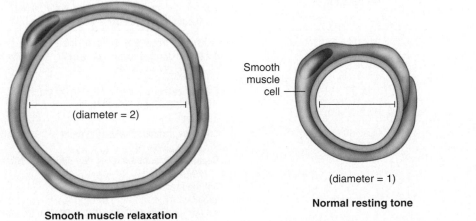

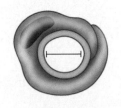

Decreased resistance

(diameter = 2)

Smooth muscle relaxation

Smooth muscle cell

(diameter = 1)

Normal resting tone

Increased resistance

(diameter = 1/2)

Smooth muscle contraction

• **Fig. 18.2** Peripheral vascular resistance. (From Patton KT, Thibodeau GA: *The human body in health and disease*, ed 7, St Louis, 2018, Elsevier.)

Calcium Channel Blockers

There are two classes of calcium channel blockers. The dihydropyridines are selective for blood vessels and are effective at lowering blood pressure because of their ability to relax blood vessels. Examples of drugs in this class are amlodipine, felodipine, isradipine, nicardipine, nifedipine, and nisoldipine. Verapamil and diltiazem are nondihydropyridines. Verapamil is classified as a phenylalkylamine, and diltiazem is classified as a benzothiazepine. Both drugs decrease cardiac workload, heart rate, and heart contractions. Verapamil is more selective for the heart muscle (myocardium) than blood vessels. Diltiazem's action is intermediate between verapamil and dihydropyridines.

Adverse Effects

Dihydropyridines (e.g., nifedipine) may produce dizziness, flushing, and headache. Nondihydropyridines (e.g., diltiazem) can produce bradycardia and constipation. The exact mechanism of action, pharmacokinetics, and more adverse reactions are discussed in Chapter 17.

Calcium Channel Blockers

Generic Name	US Brand Name / Canadian Brand(s)	Dosage Forms and Strengths
amlodipine[a]	Katerzia, Norvasc, Norliqva	**Solution, oral (Norliqva):** 1 mg/mL, **Suspension, oral (Katerzia):** 1 mg/mL, **Tablets:** 2.5 mg, 5 mg, 10 mg,
	Norvasc	
diltiazem[a]	Cardizem, Cardizem CD, Cardizem LA, Cartia XT, Tiazac, Taztia XT	**Capsule, controlled delivery (Cardizem CD):** 120 mg, 180 mg, 240 mg, 300 mg, **Capsules, extended release (Cartia XT, Diltzac, Taztia XT):** 120 mg, 180 mg, 240 mg, 300 mg, 360 mg, 420 mg[b] (Tiazac only)
	Tiazac, Tiazac XC	**Injection, powder for reconstitution[b]:** 100 mg, **Solution for injection:** 5 mg/mL, **Tablets:** 30 mg, 60 mg, 90 mg[b], 120 mg,[b] **Tablets, extended release (Cardizem LA, Tiazac XC):** 120 mg, 180 mg, 240 mg, 300 mg, 360 mg, 420 mg,[b]
felodipine[a]	Generics	**Tablets, extended release:** 2.5 mg, 5 mg, 10 mg
	Plendil	
isradipine[a]	Generics	**Capsules:** 2.5 mg, 5 mg
	Not available	
levamlodipine	Conjupri	**Tablet:** 2.5 mg, 5 mg
	Not available	
nicardipine[a]	Generics	**Capsules:** 20 mg, 30 mg **Solution for injection:** 2.5 mg/mL **Solution for injection, premixed:** mg/mL in NaCl 0.9% 0.2 mg/mL in NaCl 0.9%
	Not available	
nifedipine[a]	Procardia, Procardia XL	**Capsules (Procardia):** 5 mg[c], 10 mg, 20 mg[b] **Tablets, extended release (Adalat XL, Procardia XL):** 30 mg, 60 mg, 90 mg
	Adalat XL	
nisoldipine[a]	Sular ER	**Tablets, extended release:** 8.5 mg, 17 mg, 20 mg, 25.5 mg, 30 mg, 34 mg, 40 mg
	Not available	
verapamil[a]	Calan SR, Verelan	**Capsules, extended release (Verelan):** 120 mg, 180 mg, 240 mg, 360 mg **Capsules, extended release (Verelan PM):** 100 mg, 200 mg, 300 mg **Solution for injection:** 2.5 mg/mL **Tablets:** 40 mg[b], 80 mg, 120 mg, 160 mg **Tablets, extended release (Calan SR, Isoptin SR):** 120 mg, 180 mg, 240 mg,
	Isoptin SR	

Calcium Channel Blockers—cont'd

Generic Name	US Brand Name / Canadian Brand(s)	Dosage Forms and Strengths
Combination Calcium Channel Blocker and ACE Inhibitors		
amlodipine + benazepril[a]	Lotrel / Not available	**Capsules:** amlodipine 2.5 mg + benazepril 10 mg, amlodipine 5 mg + benazepril 10 mg, amlodipine 5 mg + benazepril 20 mg, amlodipine 5 mg + benazepril 40 mg, amlodipine 10 mg + benazepril 20 mg, amlodipine 10 mg + benazepril 40 mg,
amlodipine + perindopril[a, c]	Prestalia / Viacoram	**Tablets:** amlodipine 2.5 mg + perindopril 3.5 mg, amlodipine 5 mg + perindopril 7 mg, amlodipine 10 mg + perindopril 14 mg,
Combination Calcium Channel Blocker and Angiotensin II Receptor Blockers		
amlodipine + olmesartan[a]	Azor / Not available	**Tablets:** amlodipine 5 mg + olmesartan 20 mg, amlodipine 5 mg + olmesartan 40 mg, amlodipine 10 mg + olmesartan 20 mg, amlodipine 10 mg + olmesartan 40 mg,
amlodipine + olmesartan + hydrochlorothiazide[a]	Tribenzor / Not available	**Tablets:** amlodipine 5 mg + olmesartan 20 mg + hydrochlorothiazide 12.5 mg, amlodipine 5 mg + olmesartan 40 mg + ydrochlorothiazide 12.5 mg, amlodipine 5 mg + olmesartan 40 mg + hydrochlorothiazide 25 mg, amlodipine 10 mg + olmesartan 40 mg + hydrochlorothiazide 12.5 mg, amlodipine 10 mg + olmesartan 40 mg + hydrochlorothiazide 25 mg,
amlodipine + telmisartan[a]	Generics / Twynsta	**Tablets:** amlodipine 5 mg + telmisartan 40 mg, amlodipine 5 mg + telmisartan 80 mg, amlodipine 10 mg + telmisartan 40 mg, amlodipine 10 mg + telmisartan 80 mg,
amlodipine + valsartan[a]	Exforge / Not available	**Tablets:** amlodipine 5 mg + valsartan 160 mg, amlodipine 5 mg + valsartan 320 mg, amlodipine 10 mg + valsartan 160 mg, amlodipine 10 mg + valsartan 320 mg,
amlodipine + valsartan + hydrochlorothiazide[a]	Exforge HCT / Not available	**Tablets:** amlodipine 5 mg + valsartan 160 mg + HCTZ 12.5 mg, amlodipine 5 mg + valsartan 160 mg + HCTZ 25 mg, amlodipine 10 mg + valsartan 160 mg + HCTZ 12.5 mg, amlodipine 10 mg + valsartan 160 mg + HCTZ 25 mg, amlodipine 10 mg + valsartan 320 mg + HCTZ 25 mg,
Combination Calcium Channel Blocker + Anticholesterol		
amlodipine + atorvastatin[a]	Caduet / Caduet	**Tablets:** amlodipine 2.5 mg + atorvastatin 10 mg,[b] amlodipine 2.5 mg + atorvastatin 20 mg,[b] amlodipine 2.5 mg + atorvastatin 40 mg,[b] amlodipine 5 mg + atorvastatin 10 mg, amlodipine 5 mg + atorvastatin 20 mg, amlodipine 5 mg + atorvastatin 40 mg, amlodipine 5 mg + atorvastatin 80 mg, amlodipine 10 mg + atorvastatin 10 mg, amlodipine 10 mg + atorvastatin 20 mg, amlodipine 10 mg + atorvastatin 40 mg, amlodipine 10 mg + atorvastatin 80 mg,

[a]Generic available.
[b]Available in the United States only.
[c]Available in Canada only.
ACE, Angiotensin-converting enzyme; *HCTZ*, hydrochlorothiazide.

❗ Tech Alert!

Carvedilol and captopril have look-alike/sound-alike issues.

Central-Acting α₂-Agonists

Blood pressure is controlled by a complex feedback mechanism. Increased adrenergic stimulation in the brain leads to decreased sympathetic nervous system messages flowing from the central nervous system (CNS). Methyldopa is a prodrug that acts like a false neurotransmitter. It is metabolized to α-methylnorepinephrine, which the body thinks is norepinephrine. It is selective in mimicking the autoinhibitory effects of norepinephrine. When methyldopa binds to receptors, efferent sympathetic activity is reduced, blood vessels dilate, and peripheral resistance is decreased. Clonidine inhibits norepinephrine release from the CNS and peripheral sites.

❗ Tech Alert!

The following drugs have look-alike/sound-alike issues:
cloNIDine, cloZAPine, and KlonoPIN;
guanFACINE and guaiFENesin

Adverse Reactions

Common adverse drug effects of centrally acting α₂-agonists are sedation, dry mouth, **orthostatic hypotension**, impotence, and constipation. Methyldopa can also cause depression, nasal stuffiness, and gastrointestinal upset. Methyldopa may produce galactorrhea, hemolytic anemia, and liver dysfunction.

Direct Vasodilators

Hydralazine and minoxidil decrease peripheral resistance and reduce blood pressure by relaxing vascular smooth muscle. Minoxidil works by activating adenosine triphosphate–sensitive K^+ channels, setting in motion a chain of events that decrease calcium influx (through L-type calcium channels) into vascular smooth muscle. This decreases arterial blood vessel contractions.

Neither hydralazine nor minoxidil is a first-line drug for the treatment of hypertension. Hydralazine is recommended for hypertensive emergencies (parenteral use) and is safe for the treatment of preeclampsia in pregnant women.

❗ Tech Alert!

The following drugs have look-alike/sound-alike issues:
hydRALAZINE, hydrOXYzine, and hydroCHLOROthiazide;
Loniten and Lipitor

Adverse Reactions

The adverse drug reactions for hydralazine and minoxidil include orthostatic hypotension, headache, gastrointestinal upset, sodium and fluid retention, palpitations, and arrhythmia. Hydralazine can cause a lupus-like syndrome, and minoxidil causes facial hair growth. The discovery that minoxidil increases hair growth resulted in the drug being formulated for topical use for the treatment of baldness.

Direct Renin Inhibitors

Aliskiren is the first of a new class of drugs called direct renin inhibitors. It acts to block the conversion of angiotensinogen to angiotensin I, the first step in RAAS cascade (Fig. 18.3). Renin inhibitors block the formation of both angiotensin I and angiotensin II (vasoconstrictor), and aldosterone release by interrupting the RAAS at the beginning. Aliskiren may be used as monotherapy or in combination with other antihypertensive agents.

α₂-Agonists

Generic Name	US Brand Name / Canadian Brand(s)	Dosage Forms and Strengths
clonidine[a]	Catapres, Catapres-TTS, Duraclon, Kapvay, Nexiclon XR Generics	**Injection, epidural solution (Duraclon)**[b]: 0.1 mg/mL, 0.5 mg/mL, **Patch, transdermal**[b]: 0.1 mg/24 h (Catapres TTS-1), 0.2 mg/24 h (Catapres TTS-2) 0.3 mg/24 h (Catapres TTS-3) **Tablets:** 0.025 mg[c], 0.1 mg, 0.2 mg, 0.3 mg,[c] **Tablet, extended release**[b]: 0.1 mg (Kapvay), 0.17 (Nexiclon)
guanfacine[a]	Intuniv Generics	**Tablets:** 1 mg, 2 mg, **Tablets, extended release (Intuniv):** 1 mg, 2 mg, 3 mg, 4 mg,
methyldopa[a]	Generics Generics	**Tablets:** 125 mg[c], 250 mg, 500 mg,[c]

[a]Generic available.
[b]Available in the United States only.
[c]Available in Canada only.

Vasodilators

Generic Name	US Brand Name / Canadian Brand(s)	Dosage Forms and Strengths
hydralazine[a]	Generics	**Injection, solution:** 20 mg/mL (1 mL),
	Generics	**Tablets:** 10 mg, 25 mg, 50 mg, 100 mg,[b]
hydralazine + hydrochlorothiazide[a]	Generics	**Capsule:** hydralazine 25 mg + hydrochlorothiazide 25 mg,
	Not available	hydralazine 50 mg + hydrochlorothiazide 50 mg,
minoxidil[a]	Generics	**Tablets:** 2.5 mg, 10 mg,
	Not available	

[a]Generic available.
[b]Available in the United States only.

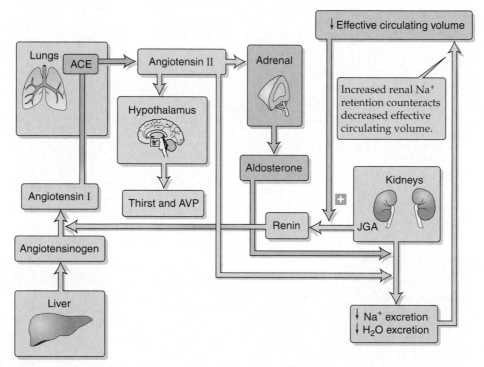

• **Fig. 18.3** The renin–aldosterone–angiotensin system. (From Boron WF, Boulpaep EL: *Medical physiology*, ed 3, Philadelphia, 2017, Elsevier.)

Adverse Reactions and Precautions

The most common side effect of aliskiren is diarrhea (2.3%). The drug may also cause dizziness, headache, and hyperkalemia; may aggravate gout; and, in rare cases, may cause acute renal failure.

Concurrent use of ACE inhibitors and ARBs with aliskiren is contraindicated, especially in patients with diabetes. The US Food and Drug Administration requires a boxed warning in the package labeling regarding the risk for fetal toxicity when aliskiren is taken during pregnancy.

Renin Inhibitors

Generic Name	US Brand Name / Canadian Brand(s)	Dosage Forms and Strengths
aliskiren[a]	Tekturna	**Tablets:** 150 mg, 300 mg,
	Rasilez	

[a]Generic available.

Summary of Drugs Used in the Treatment and Management of Hypertension

	Drug Name	Usual Dose and Dosing Schedule	Warning Label(s)
Diuretics			
Thiazides			
	chlorothiazide	500–1000 mg 1–2 times a day	TAKE WITH FOOD.
	chlorthalidone	12.5–50 mg once daily	MAY BE ADVISABLE TO EAT BANANAS OR DRINK ORANGE JUICE.
	hydrochlorothiazide (HCTZ)[a]	12.5–50 mg once daily	AVOID PROLONGED EXPOSURE TO SUNLIGHT. SOME OTC DRUGS CAN AGGRAVATE YOUR CONDITION.
	indapamide	1.25–2.5 mg once daily	
	metolazone	2.5–10 mg once daily	
Loop			
	bumetanide	0.5–2 mg once daily (typically 1 mg/day for hypertension)	MAY BE ADVISABLE TO EAT BANANAS OR DRINK ORANGE JUICE.
	furosemide[a]	20–80 mg daily in 1–2 divided doses	MAY CAUSE DIZZINESS OR LIGHT-HEADEDNESS. AVOID PROLONGED EXPOSURE TO SUNLIGHT. SOME OTC DRUGS CAN AGGRAVATE YOUR CONDITION.
	torsemide	5–10 mg once daily	
Aldosterone Receptor Antagonists			
	spironolactone[a]	25–100 mg daily in single or divided doses	TAKE WITH FOOD. MAY CAUSE DIZZINESS OR LIGHT-HEADEDNESS. AVOID SALT SUBSTITUTES. AVOID GRAPEFRUIT JUICE.
	eplerenone	50 mg 1–2 times daily	
Aldosterone Receptor Antagonist Combination			
	spironolactone + hydrochlorothiazide	1–4 tablets daily in 1–2 divided doses (25–100 mg spironolactone + 25–100 mg HCTZ once daily)	AVOID SALT SUBSTITUTES AND POTASSIUM-RICH DIETS. MAY CAUSE DIZZINESS OR LIGHT-HEADEDNESS. AVOID PROLONGED EXPOSURE TO SUNLIGHT.
Potassium-Sparing Diuretics			
	amiloride	5–20 mg once daily	
	triamterene	50–100 mg daily	
Potassium-Sparing Combination			
	triamterene + hydrochlorothiazide[a]	37.5–75 mg triamterene + 25–50 mg HCTZ once daily	AVOID SALT SUBSTITUTES. MAY CAUSE DIZZINESS OR LIGHT-HEADEDNESS. AVOID PROLONGED EXPOSURE TO SUNLIGHT.
β-Blockers			
	acebutolol	200–600 mg twice daily	DO NOT DISCONTINUE WITHOUT MEDICAL SUPERVISION.
	atenolol[a]	25–100 mg daily	MAY CAUSE DIZZINESS OR LIGHT-HEADEDNESS.
	betaxolol	10–20 mg once daily	TAKE WITH FOOD—immediate-release metoprolol.
	bisoprolol	2.5–10 mg once daily	SWALLOW WHOLE; DO NOT CRUSH OR CHEW— sustained release.
	metoprolol[a] metoprolol extended release[a]	50–100 mg 1–2 times a day 25–100 mg once daily	
	nadolol	40–320 mg once daily (typically 40–80 mg daily)	
	nebivolol[a]	5–40 mg once daily	

Summary of Drugs Used in the Treatment and Management of Hypertension—cont'd

	Drug Name	Usual Dose and Dosing Schedule	Warning Label(s)
	propranolol[a] propranolol long acting	40–120 mg twice daily (maximum up to 640 mg daily) 80–180 mg once daily	
	timolol	20–60 mg daily in 2 divided doses	

Combined α- and β-Blockers

	Drug Name	Usual Dose and Dosing Schedule	Warning Label(s)
	carvedilol[a] carvedilol CR[a]	6.25–25 mg twice daily 20–80 mg once daily	TAKE WITH FOOD. DO NOT DISCONTINUE WITHOUT MEDICAL SUPERVISION. MAY CAUSE DIZZINESS OR LIGHT-HEADEDNESS.
	labetalol	200–400 mg twice daily (up to 2400 mg/day)	

β-Blockers + Diuretic Combination

Drug Name	Usual Dose and Dosing Schedule	Warning Label(s)
atenolol + chlorthalidone	50–100 mg atenolol + 25 mg chlorthalidone once daily	Same warnings for thiazides plus β-blockers.
bisoprolol + hydrochlorothiazide	2.5–20 mg bisoprolol + 6.25–12.5 mg HCTZ once daily	
metoprolol + hydrochlorothiazide	100–200 mg metoprolol + 25–50 mg HCTZ once daily	
pindolol + hydrochlorothiazide	1–2 tablets once daily	

Angiotensin-Converting Enzyme Inhibitors

	Drug Name	Usual Dose and Dosing Schedule	Warning Label(s)
	benazepril[a]	10–40 mg once a day or 2 divided doses	DO NOT DISCONTINUE WITHOUT MEDICAL SUPERVISION. MAY CAUSE DIZZINESS OR LIGHT-HEADEDNESS. AVOID SALT SUBSTITUTES. DO NOT TAKE THIS DRUG IF YOU BECOME PREGNANT. MAY CAUSE A DRY COUGH; IF IT PERSISTS, REPORT IT TO YOUR DOCTOR. TAKE ON AN EMPTY STOMACH—captopril, moexipril. TAKE WITH FOOD—perindopril.
	captopril	25–50 mg 2–3 times a day	
	enalapril[a]	5–40 mg daily in single or divided doses	
	fosinopril	10–40 mg once a day or 2 divided doses (up to 80 mg daily if needed)	
	lisinopril[a]	10–40 mg once a day	
	moexipril	7.5–30 mg once a day or 2 divided doses	
	perindopril	4–8 mg once a day or 2 divided doses (up to 16 mg daily if needed)	
	quinapril	10–80 mg once a day or 2 divided doses	

Continued

Summary of Drugs Used in the Treatment and Management of Hypertension—cont'd

	Drug Name	Usual Dose and Dosing Schedule	Warning Label(s)
	ramipril[a]	2.5–20 mg once a day or 2 divided doses	
	trandolapril	1–4 mg once or twice a day	

Angiotensin-Converting Enzyme Inhibitor + Diuretic Combination

	Drug Name	Usual Dose and Dosing Schedule	Warning Label(s)
	benazepril + hydrochlorothiazide	10–40 mg benazepril + 12.5–50 mg HCTZ once daily	Same warnings for thiazides plus ACE inhibitors.
	captopril + hydrochlorothiazide	25–50 mg captopril + 15–50 mg HCTZ 2–3 times a day	
	enalapril + hydrochlorothiazide	10–20 mg enalapril + 12.5–50 mg HCTZ once daily	
	fosinopril + hydrochlorothiazide	10–20 mg fosinopril + 12.5 mg HCTZ once daily	
	lisinopril + hydrochlorothiazide	10–80 mg lisinopril + 12.5–50 mg HCTZ once daily	
	moexipril + hydrochlorothiazide	7.5–30 mg moexipril + 12.5–50 mg HCTZ once daily	
	quinapril + hydrochlorothiazide	10–40 mg quinapril + 12.5–25 mg HCTZ once daily	
	ramipril + hydrochlorothiazide	Maximum dose 10 mg ramipril + 50 mg HCTZ daily	

Angiotensin II Antagonists

	Drug Name	Usual Dose and Dosing Schedule	Warning Label(s)
	azilsartan	40–80 mg once daily	DO NOT DISCONTINUE WITHOUT MEDICAL SUPERVISION.
	candesartan	16–32 mg once daily or 2 divided doses	MAY CAUSE DIZZINESS OR LIGHT-HEADEDNESS.
	eprosartan	400–800 mg once daily or 2 divided doses	DO NOT TAKE THIS DRUG IF YOU BECOME PREGNANT.
	irbesartan	150–300 mg once daily	AVOID SALT SUBSTITUTES.
	losartan	50–100 mg once daily or 2 divided doses	
	olmesartan	20–40 mg once daily	
	telmisartan	20–80 mg once daily	
	valsartan	80–320 mg once daily	

Summary of Drugs Used in the Treatment and Management of Hypertension—cont'd

Drug Name	Usual Dose and Dosing Schedule	Warning Label(s)
Angiotensin II Receptor Antagonist + Diuretic Combination		
azilsartan + chlorthalidone	40–80 mg azilsartan + chlorthalidone 12.5–25 mg once daily	Same warnings as for ARBs and thiazide diuretics.
candesartan + hydrochlorothiazide	8–32 mg candesartan + 12.5–50 mg HCTZ once daily or 2 divided doses	
eprosartan + hydrochlorothiazide	600 mg eprosartan + 12.5 mg HCTZ once daily	
irbesartan + hydrochlorothiazide	150–300 mg irbesartan + 12.5–25 mg HCTZ once daily	
losartan + hydrochlorothiazide	50–100 mg losartan + 12.5–25 mg HCTZ once daily	
olmesartan + hydrochlorothiazide	20–40 mg olmesartan + 12.5–25 mg HCTZ once daily	
telmisartan + hydrochlorothiazide	80–160 mg telmisartan + 12.5–25 mg HCTZ once daily	
valsartan + hydrochlorothiazide	160–320 mg valsartan + 12.5–25 mg HCTZ once daily	
Calcium Channel Blockers		
amlodipine	2.5–10 mg once daily	SHAKE WELL—suspension. MAY CAUSE DIZZINESS. USE CAUTION WHEN DRIVING OR PERFORMING TASKS REQUIRING ALERTNESS. SWALLOW WHOLE; DO NOT CRUSH OR CHEW—sustained release. AVOID GRAPEFRUIT JUICE. TAKE ON AN EMPTY STOMACH—nisoldipine.
diltiazem extended release	240–360 mg once daily	
diltiazem long acting	120–540 mg once a day	
felodipine	2.5–10 mg once a day	
isradipine	2.5–10 mg twice a day	
levamlodipine	1.25–2.5 mg once daily (maximum dose 5 mg daily)	
nicardipine sustained release	30–60 mg twice a day	
nicardipine IV	5–15 mg/h IV	
nifedipine long acting	30–60 mg once daily	
nisoldipine	17–34 mg once daily	
verapamil immediate release	80 mg 3 times a day	
verapamil long acting	180–240 mg 1–2 times a day	
verapamil extended release	120–480 mg once daily	
Calcium Channel Blockers + Angiotensin-Converting Enzyme Inhibitor Combination		
amlodipine + benazepril	2.5–10 mg amlodipine + 10–40 mg benazepril once daily	Same warnings as calcium channel blockers plus ACE inhibitors.
amlodipine + perindopril	2.5–10 mg amlodipine + 3.5–14 mg perindopril once daily	
verapamil + trandolapril	1–4 mg trandolapril + 120–480 mg verapamil daily in 1 or 2 divided doses	

Continued

Summary of Drugs Used in the Treatment and Management of Hypertension—cont'd

Drug Name	Usual Dose and Dosing Schedule	Warning Label(s)
Combination Calcium Channel Blocker and Angiotensin II Receptor Blockers		
amlodipine + olmesartan	5–10 mg amlodipine + 20–40 mg olmesartan once daily	Same warnings as calcium channel blockers plus ARBs plus thiazides
amlodipine + olmesartan + hydrochlorothiazide	10 mg amlodipine + 40 mg olmesartan + 12.5 mg hydrochlorothiazide once daily	
amlodipine + telmisartan	2.5–10 mg amlodipine + 20–80 mg telmisartan once daily	
amlodipine + valsartan + hydrochlorothiazide	Dose once daily; maximum dose 10 mg amlodipine + 320 mg valsartan + 25 mg hydrochlorothiazide	
Combination Calcium Channel Blocker + Anticholesterol		
amlodipine + atorvastatin	5–10 mg amlodipine + 10–80 mg atorvastatin	AVOID PREGNANCY.
Centrally Acting α2-Agonist and Other Central-Acting Drugs		
clonidine	0.1–0.3 mg twice a day	ROTATE SITE OF APPLICATION—patch. DO NOT DISCONTINUE WITHOUT MEDICAL SUPERVISION. MAY CAUSE DIZZINESS OR LIGHT-HEADEDNESS.
clonidine patch	0.1–0.3 mg once a week	
methyldopa	250–1000 mg 2–3 daily	
guanfacine	1–2 mg once daily at bedtime	
α1-Antagonists		
doxazosin	1–16 mg once a day	DO NOT DISCONTINUE WITHOUT MEDICAL SUPERVISION. MAY CAUSE DIZZINESS OR LIGHT-HEADEDNESS.
prazosin	1–20 mg 2–3 times a day (maximum 40 mg/day)	
terazosin	1–5 mg 1–2 times a day (maximum 20 mg/day)	
Direct Vasodilators		
hydralazine	10–50 mg 4 times a day 20–40 mg IM or IV bolus as needed	DO NOT DISCONTINUE WITHOUT MEDICAL SUPERVISION. TAKE WITH FOOD. MAY CAUSE DIZZINESS OR LIGHT-HEADEDNESS. FOR HYPERTENSIVE EMERGENCIES.
minoxidil	4–40 mg daily in 1–2 doses	
enalaprilat	1.25–5 mg over 5 minutes every 6 hours IV	
Renin Inhibitors		
aliskiren	150–300 mg once daily	MAY CAUSE DIZZINESS. AVOID SALT SUBSTITUTES. AVOID PROLONGED EXPOSURE TO SUNLIGHT— Tekturna HCT. MAY CAUSE PERSISTENT COUGH. MAY UPSET STOMACH.
aliskiren + HCTZ	1 tablet once daily; begin with 150 mg aliskiren/12.5 mg HCTZ and increase to 300 mg aliskiren/25 mg HCTZ as needed	

ACE, Angiotensin-converting enzyme; *HCTZ*, hydrochlorothiazide; *IM*, intramuscular; *OTC*, over the counter.

TECHNICIAN'S CORNER

1. Patients with hypertension are often advised to "cut your salt intake in half" as part of their treatment. What is the rationale for this advice? What is the daily healthy limit?
2. Sites for blood pressure control are the kidneys, heart, blood vessels, CNS, and sympathetic nerves. Provide two examples of drugs that work at each of the sites of action.

Key Points

- Blood pressure is a ratio of the pressure when the heart's ventricles are contracting (systole) and the pressure measured when the heart is at rest (diastole).
- Average normal blood pressure is less than 120 mm Hg (systolic)/less than 80 mm Hg (diastolic).
- Sites for blood pressure control are the kidneys, heart, blood vessels, CNS, and sympathetic nerves.
- The CNS senses changes in blood pressure and signals sympathetic nerves to release neurotransmitters that control heart rate and blood flow through the arteries.
- Risk factors for high blood pressure are age (older than 55 years in men and 65 years in women), diabetes mellitus, family history of heart disease, metabolic syndrome, obesity, tobacco usage, decreased physical activity, increased total low-density lipoprotein or low high-density lipoprotein, diet high in salt and saturated fats, and excessive alcohol consumption.
- Reduction of blood pressure to normal levels is beneficial for persons with elevated blood pressure with and without preexisting disease.
- Isolated systolic hypertension is a condition whereby SBP is elevated and DBP is within the normal range.
- White coat hypertension is an abnormally high blood pressure when the measurement is taken by a health care professional.
- Hypertension is sometimes called the "silent killer" because it can cause damage to the body without any obvious symptoms. Hypertension can weaken arteries and cause aneurysms in the brain, aorta, or abdomen; blindness; kidney disease; and ischemic heart disease.
- Adoption of a healthy lifestyle can reduce blood pressure in patients with elevated blood pressure.
- Lifestyle modifications to reduce blood pressure include weight loss, a diet low in salt and cholesterol, increased physical activity, and decreased alcohol and tobacco consumption.
- The diuretics are classified as thiazide, loop, and potassium sparing.
- The thiazide diuretics promote water, sodium, potassium, and chloride ion elimination; decrease blood volume; and lower peripheral resistance.
- The loop diuretics block the sodium–potassium cotransporter in the ascending loop of Henle and are the most potent diuretics.

- The diuretics should be taken in the morning to avoid the need to urinate in the middle of the night.
- The effect of the loop diuretics and thiazides is reduced if they are taken concurrently with nonsteroidal antiinflammatory drugs.
- The potassium-sparing diuretics inhibit sodium reabsorption while avoiding potassium loss. They are less effective than the loop and thiazide diuretics.
- Patients taking potassium-sparing diuretics should be advised to avoid salt substitutes because they contain potassium chloride.
- Spironolactone and eplerenone are aldosterone receptor antagonists. Spironolactone is sometimes classified as a potassium-sparing diuretic.
- The ACE inhibitors decrease blood pressure by blocking the conversion of angiotensin I to angiotensin II, a potent vasoconstrictor.
- Dry cough is a common side effect of the ACE inhibitors.
- The ACE inhibitors are contraindicated in pregnancy because they can interfere with fetal development of the kidneys.
- The ARBs are competitive antagonists at the angiotensin II receptor site.
- The β-adrenergic blockers (β-blockers) lower blood pressure by decreasing heart rate and peripheral resistance.
- The α_1-blockers lower blood pressure by producing vascular relaxation, which reduces peripheral resistance.
- The calcium channel blockers are effective at lowering blood pressure because of their ability to relax blood vessels. They also decrease heart rate and force of contractions, lowering the cardiac output.
- Methyldopa is a prodrug that mimics the autoinhibitory effects of norepinephrine.
- Clonidine inhibits norepinephrine release from the CNS and peripheral sites.
- Hydralazine and minoxidil decrease peripheral resistance and reduce blood pressure by relaxing vascular smooth muscle.
- Hydralazine is recommended for hypertensive emergencies (parenteral use) and is safe for use in pregnant women.
- The direct renin inhibitors (e.g., aliskiren) prevent the formation of both angiotensin I and angiotensin II. They have a lower risk for dry cough and angioedema than ACE inhibitors.

Review Questions

1. _____ is the most often diagnosed medical condition in the United States.
   a. Myocardial infarction
   b. Hypertension
   c. Diabetes
   d. Cancer

2. Lifestyle modification is not an important strategy for the prevention and management of hypertension.
   a. true
   b. false

3. The _____ play(s) a major role in regulating blood pressure and is(are) the site of action for diuretics.
   a. liver
   b. brain
   c. heart
   d. kidneys

4. There are several classifications of diuretics. Which of the following is *not* a class of diuretics?
   a. thiazide
   b. loop
   c. sodium sparing
   d. potassium sparing

5. Diuretics should be taken in the _____ to avoid the need to urinate in the middle of the night (nocturia).
   a. evening
   b. morning
   c. afternoon
   d. night

6. Spironolactone blocks the effect of _____.
   a. aldosterone
   b. antidiuretic hormone
   c. epinephrine
   d. norepinephrine

7. A common ending for ACE inhibitors is
   a. -pine
   b. -statin
   c. -pril
   d. -olol

8. Doxazosin and terazosin are examples of what class of drugs?
   a. ACE inhibitors
   b. β-Blocker
   c. α1-Blocker
   d. Calcium channel blocker

9. Calcium channel blockers are effective at lowering blood pressure because of their ability to constrict blood vessels.
   a. true
   b. false

10. _____ is recommended for hypertensive emergencies (parenteral use) and is safe for use in pregnant women.
   a. Hydralazine
   b. Hydroxyzine
   c. HydroDiuril
   d. Hydrocodone

Bibliography

Al-Makki A, DiPette D, Whelton PK, et al. Clinical statements and guidelines. Hypertension pharmacological treatment in adults: a World Health Organization guideline executive summary. *Hypertension.* 2022;79:293–301.

Campbell N.R.C., Paccot Burnens M., Whelton P.K., et al: 2021 World Health Organization guideline on pharmacological treatment of hypertension: policy implications for the region of the Americas, *Lancet Regional Health Am* 9:100219, 2022.

Centers for Disease Control and Prevention. (2022). Making Healthy Living Easier, Obesity Fact Sheet. Division of Nutrition, Physical Activity, and Obesity. Retrieved October 28, 2022, from https://www.cdc.gov/obesity/about-obesity/index.html.

Health Canada. (2022). Drug Product Database, 2022. Retrieved October 18, 2022, from https://health-products.canada.ca/dpd-bdpp/index-eng.jsp.

Institute for Safe Medication Practices. (2016). FDA and ISMP Lists of Look-Alike Drug Names with Recommended Tall Man Letters. Retrieved October 18, 2022, from https://www.ismp.org/recommendations/tall-man-letters-list.

Institute for Safe Medication Practices. (2019). List of Confused Drugs. Retrieved October 18, 2022, from https://www.ismp.org/tools/confuseddrugnames.pdf.

Iqbal AM, Jamal SF. *Essential hypertension. StatPearls [Internet].* Treasure Island (FL): StatPearls Publishing; 2022.available from. https://www.ncbi.nlm.nih.gov/books/NBK539859/.

James PA, Oparil S, Carter BL, et al. 2014 evidence-based guideline for the management of high blood pressure in adults report from the panel members appointed to the eighth Joint National Committee (JNC 8). *JAMA.* 2014;311(5):507–520.

Kalant H, Grant D, Mitchell J. *Principles of medical pharmacology.* ed 7. Toronto: Elsevier Canada, A Division of Reed Elsevier Canada; 2007:157–169 449–464.

Klabunde R.E. (2022). Cardiovascular Pharmacology Concepts. Calcium Channel Blockers (CCBs). Retrieved October 27, 2022, from https://www.cvpharmacology.com/vasodilator/CCB.

Leung AA, Nerenberg K, Daskalopoulou SS, et al. Hypertension Canada's 2016 Canadian hypertension education program guidelines for blood pressure measurement, diagnosis, assessment of risk, prevention, and treatment of hypertension. *Can J Cardiol.* 2016;32:569–588.

Nerenberg KA, Zarnke KB, Leung AA, et al. Hypertension Canada's 2018 guidelines for diagnosis, risk assessment, prevention, and treatment of hypertension in adults and children. *Can J Cardiol.* 2018;34(5):506–525.

Ojha U, Ruddaraju S, Sabapathy N, et al. Current and emerging classes of pharmacological agents for the management of hypertension. *Am J Cardiovasc Drugs.* 2022;22(3):271–285.

Page C, Curtis M, Sutter M, et al. *Integrated pharmacology.* Philadelphia: Mosby; 2005:395–408.

Rabi DM, McBrien KA, Sapir-Pichhadze R, et al. Hypertension Canada's 2020 comprehensive guidelines for the prevention, diagnosis, risk assessment, and treatment of hypertension in adults and children. *Can J Cardiol.* 2020;36:596–624.

U.S. Food and Drug Administration. (nd). Drugs@FDA: FDA Approved Drug Products. Retrieved October 18, 2022, from http://www.accessdata.fda.gov/scripts/cder/daf/.

19

Treatment of Heart Disease and Stroke

LEARNING OBJECTIVES

1. Learn the terminology associated with heart failure, myocardial infarction, and stroke.
2. List the risk factors for heart failure, myocardial infarction, and stroke.
3. List the symptoms of heart failure, myocardial infarction, and stroke.
4. List and categorize medications used to treat heart failure, myocardial infarction, stroke, and hyperlipidemia.
5. Describe mechanism of action for each class of drugs used to treat heart failure, myocardial infarction, stroke, and hyperlipidemia.
6. Identify warning labels and precautionary messages associated with medications used to treat heart failure, myocardial infarction, stroke, and hyperlipidemia.

KEY TERMS

Anticoagulant Drug that prolongs coagulation time and is used to prevent clot formation.

Antiplatelet drug Drug that prevents accumulation of platelets, thereby blocking an important step in the clot formation process.

Antithrombotic Drug that inhibits clot formation by reducing the coagulation action of the blood protein thrombin.

Atherosclerosis Buildup of lipids and plaque inside artery walls, impeding the flow of blood and oxygen.

Atherothrombosis Formation of a blood clot in an artery.

Automaticity Spontaneous depolarization (contraction) of heart cells.

Cholesterol Naturally occurring, waxy substance produced by the liver and found in foods; it maintains cell membranes and is needed for vitamin D production. Excess cholesterol can cause atherosclerosis.

Ejection fraction Percentage of blood ejected from the left ventricle with each heartbeat.

Heart failure Clinical syndrome in which the heart is unable to pump blood at a rate necessary to meet the body's metabolic needs.

High-density lipoprotein "Good cholesterol"; lipoproteins that transport cholesterol, triglycerides, and other lipids from blood to body tissues.

Hyperlipidemia Excess lipids or fatty substances in the blood.

Ischemia Reduction of blood supplied to tissues that is typically caused by blood vessel obstruction due to atherosclerosis, stenosis, or plaque.

Low-density lipoprotein Compound consisting of a lipid and a protein that carries most of the total cholesterol in the blood and deposits the excess along the inside of arterial walls; also known as "bad cholesterol."

Myocardial infarction Sudden loss of blood supply in the heart; also known as a heart attack.

Natriuretic peptides Hormones that play a role in cardiac homeostasis.

Partial thromboplastin time Test given to determine effectiveness of heparin in reducing antithrombotic activity.

Plaque Fatty cholesterol deposits.

Platelets Structures found in the blood that are involved in the coagulation process.

Prothrombin time Test given to determine the effectiveness of warfarin in reducing clotting time.

Thrombolytic Drug used to dissolve blood clots.

Tissue plasminogen activator Naturally occurring thrombolytic substance.

Transient ischemic attack Stroke that typically lasts for a few minutes; also known as a ministroke.

Triglycerides Storage form of energy found in fat tissue muscle; metabolize to very-low-density lipoproteins.

Overview

Heart disease is the number one cause of death in the United States and the second leading cause of death in Canada. Coronary heart disease (CHD) is the leading cause of heart attack and is a risk factor for stroke and heart failure.

Heart Failure

Heart failure (HF) is a clinical syndrome in which the heart is unable to pump blood at a rate necessary to meet the body's metabolic needs. HF affects nearly 6.2 million people in the United States and is responsible for more than 1 million hospital visits and nearly 300,000 deaths annually. The syndrome affects 1.5% to 1.9% of the adult population in the United States and Canada. The percentage of the population living with HF increases with age and is projected to rise to 8.5% in individuals 65 to 70 years of age by 2030. The prevalence of HF is higher in men, but after age 75 years, the prevalence is higher in women. HF disproportionately affects Black patients. Recent studies have revealed social determinants of health, including racism, as the root cause for the disparity.

Disease, lifestyle, and drugs can contribute to the onset or aggravation of HF. Kidney dysfunction, diabetes, metabolic syndrome, ischemic heart disease, hypertension, hypothyroidism, hyperthyroidism, bradyarrhythmia, tachyarrhythmia, pulmonary embolism, HIV/AIDS, and myocardial infarction can contribute to HF. Obesity, cocaine abuse, excessive salt, alcohol consumption, and lack of physical activity can worsen HF. Nonsteroidal antiinflammatory drugs (NSAIDs), for example, worsen edema and interfere with the effect of drugs used to treat HF (e.g., angiotensin-converting enzyme [ACE] inhibitors). Many other medications associated with causing edema can likewise contribute to the development or exacerbation of HF.

Heart Attack

More than 805,000 Americans have a heart attack annually. Nearly 1000 individuals experience sudden cardiac arrest daily. Approximately 1 in 20 people die from heart attacks. A heart attack (*myocardial infarction*) produces symptoms that are similar to those of angina. More than 40,000 Canadians will have a heart attack annually. Prompt treatment is essential to persons experiencing the symptoms listed in Table 19.1. If symptoms persist beyond 15 minutes, emergency assistance (dialing 911) should be sought.

TABLE 19.1	Characteristics of Myocardial Infarction Versus Angina	
Characteristics	Myocardial Infarction	Angina
Timing	Sudden onset Lasts longer than 30 min May occur at rest	Often occurs after exercise Lasts 1–5 min Rest may relieve symptoms
Location	Mid-chest radiating to jaw, neck, arms, and epigastric area	Mid-chest radiating to jaw, neck, arms, and epigastric area
Quality	Severe squeezing or heaviness in chest area	Heaviness, chest tightness, indigestion

Stroke

Strokes are the third leading cause of death in Canada and the fifth highest cause of death in the United States. Strokes occur when brain cells are deprived of oxygen or are damaged by sudden bleeding into the brain. Approximately 795,000 Americans have a stroke annually. An ischemic stroke is the most common type and accounts for 87% of all strokes. Approximately 50,000 Americans will have a *transient ischemic attack* (TIA). Persons who have had one stroke and recover are more likely to have another. All strokes produce similar symptoms. Symptoms (Table 19.2) appear suddenly.

Ischemic strokes are caused by oxygen deprivation. Anoxia (absence of oxygen) occurs when arteries are obstructed, causing brain infarcts. *Thrombotic* strokes are caused by an enlarged thrombus or blood clot. *Embolic* strokes are caused by an embolus (traveling clot) or *plaque* that has been dislodged. Blood clots (thrombi, emboli) are the most common cause of strokes.

Hemorrhagic strokes are caused by bleeding in the brain. The bleeding may be the result of an aneurysm, a weakened spot of the artery wall that has stretched or burst, filling the area with blood and causing damage. TIAs are also known as ministrokes. They typically last only a few minutes and symptoms usually resolve within 1 hour.

Pathophysiology of Heart Failure, Heart Attack, and Stroke

HF may affect the left side of the heart, the right side of the heart, or both sides. In left-sided systolic HF, the left ventricle is unable to effectively pump sufficient blood to the rest of the body. This is referred to as HF with reduced ejection fraction (HFrEF). The *ejection fraction* is the percentage of blood ejected from the left ventricle with each heartbeat. In left-sided diastolic HF, the ejection fraction is preserved (HFpEF) when the left ventricle is stiff and unable to fill sufficiently. This too reduces the amount of oxygen-rich blood and nutrients pumped to the rest of the body. In HFrEF, the ejection fraction is 40% or less, and in HFpEF, the ejection fraction is 50% or greater.

The right side of the heart pumps blood to the lungs to pick up oxygen. Right-sided HF reduces the capacity of the heart chambers to fill and pump blood to the lungs. Individuals with right-sided HF may have swelling in the legs and ankles. Fluid accumulation can result in weight gain, shortness of breath, and feelings of fatigue.

Compensatory mechanisms are "switched on" when heart function fails (Fig. 19.1). The renin–aldosterone–angiotensin system (RAAS) is activated in an attempt to satisfy the metabolic

TABLE 19.2	Symptoms of Stroke
Limbs	Numbness or weakness of arms or legs Difficulty walking Loss of balance or coordination
Ears, eyes, nose, and throat	Facial numbness or weakness Impaired speech Impaired vision
Cognitive	Confusion Difficulty understanding speech
Other	Dizziness Severe headache

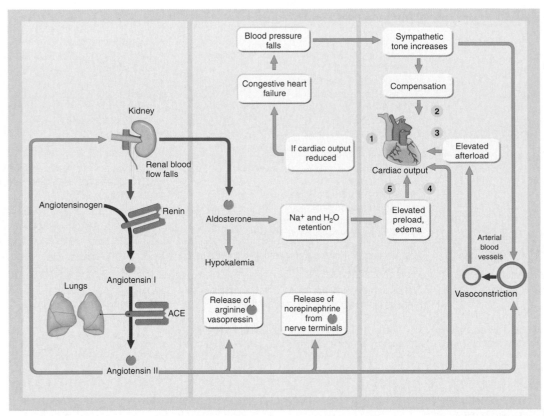

• **Fig. 19.1** Compensatory mechanisms in congestive heart failure. *ACE,* Angiotensin-converting enzyme. (From Page C, Curtis M, Sutter M, et al. *Integrated pharmacology,* ed 3, Philadelphia, 2005, Mosby.)

needs of the body. RAAS activation increases blood volume and cardiac output by increasing sodium and fluid retention. The sympathetic nervous system is activated to increase heart rate, heart contractility, and blood vessel relaxation to increase cardiac output. Unfortunately, although compensatory mechanisms are initially helpful, heart function progressively worsens over time.

Natriuretic peptides are hormones that also play a role in cardiac physiology. Atrial natriuretic peptide (ANP) and brain natriuretic peptide (BNP) are both found in cardiac tissue and are released in response to excessive stretching of heart muscle cells. Atrial stretching causes ANP release. Fluid accumulation and filling pressure in the left ventricle stimulates BNP release. Elevated BNP levels may be used to confirm a diagnosis of HF.

Stages of Heart Failure

There are four stages of HF. HF may also be described by functional class. The American College of Cardiology/American Heart Association (ACC/AHA) descriptions and New York Heart Association (NYHA) functional classifications are compared in Table 19.3.

Stroke and myocardial infarction occur when the blood supply to the brain (stroke) or heart (myocardial infarction) is interrupted. Cells become damaged from *ischemia* (reduction of blood supplied to tissues) or die when they are deprived of oxygen and nutrients. Chronic inflammation of the arteries that supply the heart and brain can also lead to stroke and myocardial infarction. The risk for chronic vascular inflammation increases with age. Vascular inflammation is a cause of atherosclerosis. *Atherosclerosis*

(a buildup of lipids and plaque inside of artery walls) can block blood flow through arteries. *Atherothrombosis* (the formation of a blood clot in the artery) can clog arteries and is triggered by atherosclerosis.

Risk Factors for Cardiovascular Disease

Risk factors for stroke and heart attack are categorized as modifiable and nonmodifiable. Nonmodifiable risk factors are age, gender, and family history. In addition, chronic diseases such as hypertension, ischemic heart disease, and diabetes place patients at increased risk for stroke.

Nonmodifiable Risk Factors

Age
Age is a significant risk factor for stroke and myocardial infarction. Although stroke can occur at any age, the risk increases exponentially with each increasing decade. Approximately 66% of strokes occur in persons older than 65 years. Strokes that occur in persons older than 65 years are more likely to be fatal.

Gender
Gender is an important risk factor for stroke. Men are 1.25 times more likely to have a stroke than are women, yet strokes in men are less likely to be fatal. This is probably because men are often younger than women when they have a stroke. As with stroke, men have a greater risk for heart attack than do women; however, older women are more likely to die within 3 weeks of a heart attack than are men.

TABLE 19.3 Classification[a] and Management of Heart Failure

ACC/AHA stage A	NYHA class I	• No symptoms • High risk for developing heart failure because of: • Hypertension • Coronary artery disease • Diabetes mellitus • History of cardiotoxic drug therapy • Alcohol abuse • History of rheumatic fever • Family history of cardiomyopathy	• Lifestyle modification • Diuretics if patient has fluid retention • ACE inhibitors • β-blockers • Treatment of underlying disease (e.g., diabetes, hypertension) • Antihyperlipidemics • Antiarrhythmics
ACC/AHA stage B	NYHA class II	• Structural heart disease but no prior symptoms of heart failure • Prior myocardial infarction • Left ventricular hypertrophy • Asymptomatic valvular disease • Left ventricular dilation or hypocontractility	• All of stage A treatment options, plus • Structural repairs (e.g., heart valve replacement) if needed
ACC/AHA stage C	NYHA class II and III	Current or prior symptoms of heart failure associated with structural heart disease	Treatment of symptoms as per stage A and B recommendations plus digoxin
ACC/AHA stage D	NYHA class IV	Advanced structural heart disease plus heart failure symptoms at rest despite medical therapy	Treatment of symptoms as per stage A and B recommendations plus digoxin

[a]American College of Cardiology/American Heart Association guidelines for evaluation and management and NYHA functional classes.
ACC/AHA, American College of Cardiology/American Heart Association; *ACE*, angiotensin-converting enzyme; *NYHA*, New York Heart Association.

Modifiable Risk Factors

Modifiable risk factors for stroke and myocardial infarction are smoking, alcohol consumption, and diet. Smoking promotes atherosclerosis, increases clotting factors in the blood (fibrinogen), stimulates vasoconstriction, and weakens the endothelial wall. These factors contribute to the risk for ischemic stroke and hemorrhagic stroke. Excessive alcohol consumption and binge drinking lead to an increase in blood pressure and can reduce *platelets*, which increase the risk for hemorrhagic stroke. After heavy drinking, a rebound effect occurs that increases platelets and thickens the blood significantly, increasing the risk of ischemic stroke. A diet high in *cholesterol* may increase the risk for atherosclerosis, and a diet high in salt can aggravate hypertension.

Hypertension

Hypertension increases the risk for stroke four to six times above that of persons without hypertension, and 90% of persons who have had a stroke have hypertension.

Atrial Fibrillation

Atrial fibrillation (see Chapter 20), a rapid and irregular beating of the atrium chamber of the heart, can increase the risk for clots. If the clots are dislodged, they can block an artery, leading to stroke or myocardial infarction. Malformations of the heart valves (e.g., mitral valve stenosis) can also lead to clot formation, increasing the risk of stroke or myocardial infarction.

High Cholesterol

High cholesterol levels are a risk factor for stroke and myocardial infarction. Cholesterol may be in the form of *high-density lipoproteins* (HDLs) and *low-density lipoproteins* (LDLs). LDLs can build up within artery walls and harden. This hardened material is called plaque, and it can impede blood supply to the heart and brain. Plaque can become dislodged, interrupting blood

supply and causing stroke or myocardial infarction. Diabetes also increases the development of atherosclerosis and therefore is a risk factor for stroke and myocardial infarction.

Infection and Inflammation

Infection is a risk factor for stroke and myocardial infarction. The immune system response to bacterial and viral infections is to release cytokines, leukotrienes, macrophages, and other infection-fighting substances that increase inflammation. Inflammation can increase the risk for ischemic and embolic stroke.

Drugs Used to Treat Heart Disease

Most of the treatments used in HF focus on treating symptoms, underlying causes, and factors that worsen HF. Many of the same drugs administered in the treatment of hypertension are also used in the treatment of HF. They include diuretics, aldosterone antagonists, β-blockers, ACE inhibitors, and angiotensin II receptor blockers (ARBs). These drugs are covered in detail in Chapter 18. An angiotensin receptor-neprilysin inhibitor (ARNI) or sodium-glucose cotransporter-2 (SGLT2) inhibitor may also be prescribed. SGLT2 inhibitors are covered in detail in Chapter 26.

Cardioglycosides

The cardioglycosides are the oldest class of drugs used in the treatment of HF. Digitalis is a cardioglycoside derived from the foxglove plant. Digoxin is the only commercially available cardioglycoside in the United States and Canada. Despite its historical use, studies by the Digitalis Investigation Group trial show that although digoxin reduces hospitalization and improves exercise tolerance in symptomatic patients with HFrEF, it fails to increase survival in patients with HF. In fact, digoxin may increase mortality in women.

> **Tech Note!**
>
> Lifestyle modification is recommended for people with HF to reduce symptoms and complications (see Box 19.1).

Mechanism of Action

Cardioglycosides such as digoxin have a *positive inotropic effect* on the heart; they increase the force of myocardial contractions. The greater force of contractions increases the cardiac output and reduces heart size. As end-diastolic pressures decrease, pulmonary and systemic venous pressures are reduced.

The positive inotropic effect is produced by the inhibition of the Na^+/K^+ ATPase pump. Digoxin-induced inhibition of the Na^+/Ca^{2+} exchanger leads to increased intracellular calcium, an electrolyte involved in the contraction of cardiac smooth muscle.

Digoxin increases cardiac output and decreases compensatory sympathetic activity, which slows heart rate. Heart rate is also slowed by stimulation of parasympathetic nervous system activity (increased vagal tone). Digoxin decreases intracellular potassium. Potassium depletion can increase automaticity and can cause arrhythmias. *Automaticity* is the spontaneous depolarization (contraction) of heart cells. Digoxin produces significant effects on the heart's conduction system. It decreases conduction velocity through the atrioventricular (AV) node, prolonging the time between contractions (refractory period). The number of depolarizations is reduced, too. There is moderate to low quality evidence to support digoxin use in patients with HFrEF in sinus rhythm who continue to have moderate to severe symptoms. A further description of digoxin's effect on the conduction system is described in Chapter 20.

Pharmacokinetics

Digoxin is marketed in several dosage forms, including tablets, oral solution, and parenteral solution. Oral absorption is good (60% to 85%), and the bioavailability of orally administered digoxin is between 70% and 85%. The bioavailability of digoxin differs among commercial manufacturers, so attempts should be made to consistently dispense the same manufacturer's product each time. Food can decrease absorption.

The peak effect of digoxin occurs 1.5 to 5 hours after administration, and the half-life of digoxin is approximately 36 hours. Between 30% and 50% is eliminated unchanged by the kidneys, and clearance is reduced in HF.

Adverse Reactions

Adverse drug reactions produced by digoxin include diarrhea, constipation, nausea, vomiting, fatigue, weakness, visual disturbances (altered color perception, hazy vision), photophobia, impotence, and gynecomastia. Signs of digitalis toxicity are arrhythmia, dizziness, headache, convulsions, delusions, and coma.

Precautions

Digitalis has a narrow therapeutic index, and the dosage range between the therapeutic dose and lethal dose is narrow; therefore patients should watch for signs of digitalis toxicity. According to current ACC/AHA recommendations, digoxin is not recommended for the treatment of HFrEF in men or women who also have sinoatrial or AV block.

> **Tech Note!**
>
> DigiFab (digoxin immune Fab) is an antidote for digoxin toxicity.

Diuretics

The diuretics are administered to treat volume overload. They also lower blood pressure and reduce pulmonary edema and swelling in the ankles, legs, and feet (peripheral edema). When diuretics are administered, potassium levels should be monitored because loop and thiazide diuretics can cause hypokalemia (see Chapter 18). Hypokalemia can increase the effects of digoxin, leading to toxicity. The drug summary table provides doses used for the treatment of HF.

Cardioglycosides

	Generic Name	US Brand Name(s) / Canadian Brand(s)	Dosage Forms and Strengths
	digoxin[a]	Lanoxin, Lanoxin Pediatric Toloxin	**Elixir/solution, oral**: 0.05 mg/mL **Solution for injection**: 0.1 mg/mL[b], 0.25 mg/mL **Tablets (Lanoxin)**: 0.0625 mg, 0.125 mg, 0.25 mg

Digoxin Antidote

	Generic Name	US Brand Name(s) / Canadian Brand(s)	Dosage Forms and Strengths
	digoxin immune Fab	Not available DigiFab	**Injection**: 40 mg (Digifab) lyophilized powder for reconstitution

[a]Generic available.
[b]Available in the United States only.

Aldosterone Antagonists

Aldosterone is a hormone that promotes Na$^+$ retention and water accumulation. Spironolactone and eplerenone are aldosterone antagonists. They are administered with other drugs to decrease Na$^+$ and water levels. Both drugs can increase K$^+$ levels in the body (hyperkalemia). Excess potassium may produce arrhythmias, so potassium levels should be monitored. Spironolactone is recommended to treat moderate to severe HF when the ability to pump blood out of the left ventricle is compromised. Eplerenone is specifically marketed for reducing cardiovascular risk in patients after myocardial infarction.

Beta Blockers

The β-blockers reduce heart rate, lower peripheral arterial resistance, lower blood pressure, and decrease the workload of the heart. They also reduce left ventricular hypertrophy. Studies show that β-blockers can lower the risk of mortality associated with HFrEF. β-Blockers block excess sympathetic stimulation induced by HF resulting from compensatory mechanisms. The β-blockers drug table in this chapter shows doses used for the treatment of HF. Adverse reactions requiring management are fluid retention, worsening HF, bradycardia, and heart block. Patients may also experience fatigue and hypotension.

Angiotensin-Converting Enzyme Inhibitors and Angiotensin II Receptor Blockers

The ACE inhibitors are one of the few classes of drugs used in the treatment of HFrEF that have been shown to reduce mortality. They are recommended for patients who have HFrEF with an acute myocardial infarction and post–myocardial infarction. They reduce left ventricular hypertrophy, improve diastolic filling, increase cardiac output, and reduce peripheral vascular resistance. Sympathetic tone, aldosterone-mediated sodium level, and blood volume expansion are reduced because angiotensin II levels are decreased. The ARBs are also administered for the treatment of HF. The ARBs improve exercise tolerance and diastolic filling in patients with HF. In this chapter, dosages for ACE inhibitors and ARBs used for the treatment of HF are shown.

Vasodilators

Isosorbide dinitrate and hydralazine are used in combination for the treatment of HF for their vasodilating effects. This reduces peripheral resistance along with cardiac preload and afterload. Moreover, hydralazine has been shown to indirectly increase the force of myocardial contractions (positive inotropic effect). Current Canadian guidelines report only moderate to low quality evidence to support the use of hydralazine + isosorbide dinitrate in patients with HFrEF unable to tolerate ACE inhibitors, ARBs, or ARNIs because of hyperkalemia renal dysfunction.

Angiotensin Receptor-Neprilysin Inhibitor

The Angiotensin Receptor-Neprilysin Inhibitor (ARNI) sacubitril/valsartan (Entresto) is recommended as a first-line treatment of HFrEF. Sacubitril is a prodrug that slows the degradation of natriuretic peptides and bradykinin. Diuresis, natriuresis, myocardial relaxation, and antiremodeling are enhanced. Valsartan, an ARB, inhibits angiotensin II and aldosterone. Hypotension and hyperkalemia are side effects of sacubitril/valsartan. ARBs are described in detail in Chapter 18.

If-Channel Blocker

Ivabradine (Corlanor, Lancora) is an If-channel blocker. It is a sinus node inhibitor. The most common adverse reactions are bradycardia, hypertension, and atrial fibrillation. Although food delays absorption, bioavailability is increased so ivabradine should be taken with food. Bioavailability of oral doses is reduced by approximately 40% because of the first pass effect in the liver and gut.

Guanylate Cyclase Stimulator

Vericiguat is indicated for the treatment of adults who have chronic symptomatic HFrEF. It is a guanylate cyclase (sGC) stimulator. Guanylate cyclase is an enzyme that is involved in the nitric oxide signaling pathway. When nitric oxide binds to sGC, the enzyme catalyzes the synthesis of cGMP, a nucleotide that is involved in the regulation of vascular tone, cardiac contractility, and cardiac remodeling. Vericiguat is the only drug in its class. The drug has a boxed warning that it should not be prescribed to pregnant women because it may cause fetal harm. Common side effects are hypotension and anemia.

Miscellaneous Agents for Treatment of Heart Failure

Generic Name	US Brand Name(s) Canadian Brand(s)	Dosage Forms and Strengths
ivabradine[a]	Corlanor	**Solution, oral**[b]: 1 mg/mL **Tablet**: 5 mg, 7.5 mg
	Lancora	
sacubitril/valsartan	Entresto	**Tablet**: 24 mg sacubitril + 26 mg valsartan, 49 mg sacubitril + 51 mg valsartan, 97 mg sacubitril + 103 mg valsartan
	Entresto	
vericiguat	Verquvo	**Tablet**: 2.5 mg, 5 mg, 10 mg
	Not available	

[a]Generic available in the United States only
[b]Available in the United States only

SGLT2 Inhibitors

SGLT2 inhibitors (e.g., canagliflozin) are antidiabetic agents that are recommended for the treatment of HF*r*EF in patients with or without diabetes. SGLT2 inhibitors used by patients who have HF*r*EF are dapagliflozin, empagliflozin, and canagliflozin. The mechanism of action and side effects of SGLT2 inhibitors are described in Chapter 26.

Drugs That Control Hemostasis

Clotting is a normal process without which one would bleed to death if an injury occurred (Fig. 19.2). Clots that form in arteries may dislodge and obstruct the supply of blood and oxygen to the brain or heart. Drugs that control hemostasis (the process of stopping the flow of blood) are administered to patients at risk for heart attack or stroke to prevent blood clots from forming in an artery. Drugs that control the rate of clot formation and clot dissolution are classified as ***antithrombotics***. Antithrombotic drugs include (1) agents that inhibit platelets; (2) ***anticoagulants***, which lessen coagulation; and (3) fibrinolytic agents. Fibrinolytic drugs dissolve existing clots.

Antiplatelet Drugs

Antiplatelet drugs produce their effect by interfering with steps in the clot formation process (Fig. 19.3). When an injury occurs, platelets cluster at the site and start to stick to the damaged cell wall (adhesion). The platelets are activated by natural substances in the blood such as thromboxane A2 (TXA_2), thrombin, and collagen. After platelets are activated, a cascade of events occurs that attracts more platelets to the region (aggregation) and causes fibrin to combine with the platelets. This strengthens the clot.

Although aspirin is a nonprescription drug, it is effective for the management of post–myocardial infarction and stroke. In addition to its antiplatelet activity, aspirin blocks the enzyme cyclo-oxygenase (see Chapter 10), reducing plaque formation. Aspirin inhibits prostaglandin synthesis, which decreases TXA_2.

Eptifibatide and tirofiban are glycoprotein IIb/IIIa inhibitors that block the final pathway of platelet aggregation. Abciximab is an anti–glycoprotein IIb/IIIa receptor antibody that also inhibits platelet aggregation. They are administered parenterally to reduce clot formation. Ticlopidine interferes with platelet adhesion and aggregation. Ticlopidine also decreases the thickness or viscosity of blood by reducing the concentration of fibrinogen. Clopidogrel's mechanism of action is similar to ticlopidine. Dipyridamole inhibits platelet aggregation and is a coronary vasodilator.

Pharmacokinetics

Oral absorption of aspirin, clopidogrel, and ticlopidine is good. The bioavailability of ticlopidine is enhanced by administering the drug with food. The peak effect of clopidogrel and ticlopidine is delayed and may take up to 4 days to be reached. The bioavailability of clopidogrel and aspirin is unaffected by food; however, food may decrease the bioavailability of dipyridamole.

A continuous infusion of abciximab must be given to maintain therapeutic blood levels. The effect on platelets lasts longer when abciximab is administered rather than tirofiban. Tirofiban has an elimination half-life of 2 hours.

Adverse Reactions and Precautions

Bleeding is a common side effect of antiplatelet drugs. Black, tarry stools; blood in vomit, urine, or stools; nosebleeds; and red or purple spots on the skin may indicate bleeding. Many drugs can enhance the effects of antiplatelet drugs and increase the potential for bleeding or hemorrhage. Nonprescription drugs such as NSAIDs (e.g., ibuprofen), vitamin supplements (fish oil), and herbs (feverfew, garlic, ginger) can increase the risk for bleeding.

Other side effects associated with antiplatelet drugs are skin rash or itching, stomach pain, and pain at the injection site (abciximab). Less commonly, patients may experience difficulty breathing, dizziness, weakness, joint pain, and bone marrow toxicity.

> ### ❶ *Tech Alert!*
> The following drugs have look-alike/sound-alike issues:
> Plavix and Paxil

Anticoagulants

Parenterally Administered Anticoagulants

Heparin is an anticoagulant that is derived from pig intestines or cow lungs. The extraction process results in a mixture of fragments of varied molecular weights. Low-molecular-weight heparins (LMWHs) are produced by separating the heparin fragments.

Heparin and LMWH are administered parenterally to prevent the formation of blood clots. Their uses include:

- Treatment of deep venous thrombosis and arterial thromboembolism
- Early treatment and prevention of myocardial infarction
- Prevention of pulmonary embolism
- Prevention of clotting medical devices (e.g., indwelling catheters, stents, or prosthetic valves)
- Prevention of acute ischemic stroke

Mechanism of Action and Pharmacokinetics

Heparin and LMWH increase the activity of antithrombin III. This inhibits clotting factors of the common pathway, Xa and IIa (thrombin), and prevents clot formation (Fig. 19.4). Fondaparinux and tinzaparin also inhibit Xa activity.

To test the effectiveness of heparin and to determine whether dosage adjustments are necessary, an activated ***partial thromboplastin time*** (aPTT) test is performed. This test measures antithrombic activity. The aPTT is a test of the intrinsic anticoagulation pathway. It tests the time it takes for the blood to clot. If heparin is effective in reducing antithrombotic activity, the clotting time will be prolonged. The test is not performed when LMWH is administered because increases in the aPTT may occur even when antithrombotic activity has not increased. Anti-Xa activity is monitored when tinzaparin or fondaparinux is administered.

Heparin and LMWH are administered by intravenous or subcutaneous injection. Oral absorption is poor. LMWH differs from heparin in a variety of ways. LMWH can be dosed less frequently than heparin, yet they are equally effective. Heparin is dosed two or three times a day, and LMWH is dosed once daily. LMWH has higher bioavailability, an increased half-life, fewer side effects (lower risk of thrombocytopenia and osteoporosis), and less protein binding. Higher doses of heparin must be administered because of protein binding.

Adverse Reactions

The most common adverse reaction is bleeding. Heparin and LMWH can cause osteoporosis.

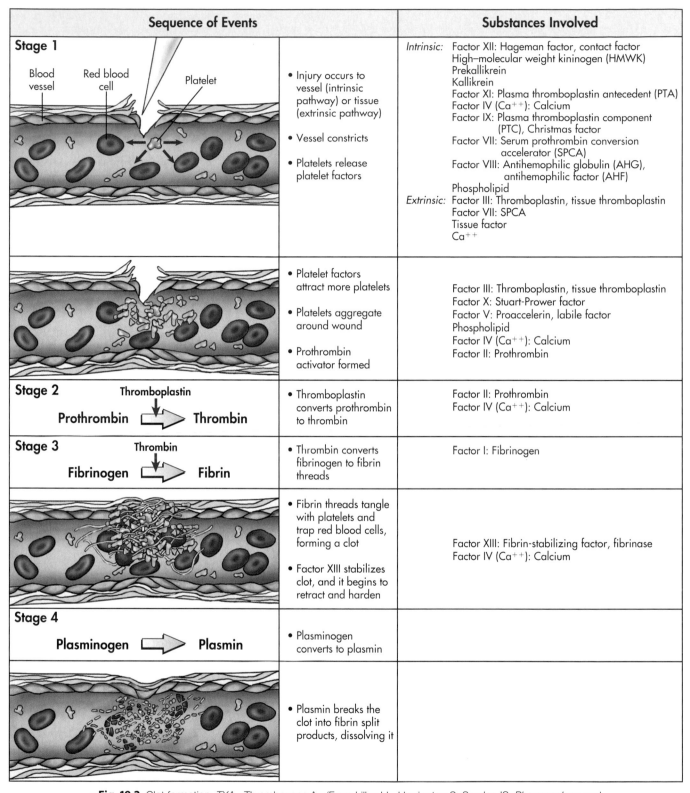

Sequence of Events		Substances Involved
Stage 1 Blood vessel Red blood cell Platelet	• Injury occurs to vessel (intrinsic pathway) or tissue (extrinsic pathway) • Vessel constricts • Platelets release platelet factors	*Intrinsic:* Factor XII: Hageman factor, contact factor High–molecular weight kininogen (HMWK) Prekallikrein Kallikrein Factor XI: Plasma thromboplastin antecedent (PTA) Factor IV (Ca⁺⁺): Calcium Factor IX: Plasma thromboplastin component (PTC), Christmas factor Factor VII: Serum prothrombin conversion accelerator (SPCA) Factor VIII: Antihemophilic globulin (AHG), antihemophilic factor (AHF) Phospholipid *Extrinsic:* Factor III: Thromboplastin, tissue thromboplastin Factor VII: SPCA Tissue factor Ca⁺⁺
	• Platelet factors attract more platelets • Platelets aggregate around wound • Prothrombin activator formed	Factor III: Thromboplastin, tissue thromboplastin Factor X: Stuart-Prower factor Factor V: Proaccelerin, labile factor Phospholipid Factor IV (Ca⁺⁺): Calcium Factor II: Prothrombin
Stage 2 Thromboplastin Prothrombin ⟹ Thrombin	• Thromboplastin converts prothrombin to thrombin	Factor II: Prothrombin Factor IV (Ca⁺⁺): Calcium
Stage 3 Thrombin Fibrinogen ⟹ Fibrin	• Thrombin converts fibrinogen to fibrin threads	Factor I: Fibrinogen
	• Fibrin threads tangle with platelets and trap red blood cells, forming a clot • Factor XIII stabilizes clot, and it begins to retract and harden	Factor XIII: Fibrin-stabilizing factor, fibrinase Factor IV (Ca⁺⁺): Calcium
Stage 4 Plasminogen ⟹ Plasmin	• Plasminogen converts to plasmin	
	• Plasmin breaks the clot into fibrin split products, dissolving it	

• **Fig. 19.2** Clot formation. *TXA₂*, Thromboxane A₂. (From Lilley LL, Harrington S, Snyder JS. *Pharmacology and the nursing process*, ed 5, St Louis, 2007, Mosby.)

⬤ *Tech Note!*

Low-molecular-weight heparins are not substitutable in accordance with product substitution laws. They must be dispensed as written because they differ in manufacturing process, molecular weight, dosage, units, and antithrombotic activity.

Orally Administered Anticoagulants

Warfarin and dabigatran are orally administered anticoagulants. Warfarin is used to prevent pulmonary embolism, thrombotic and embolic stroke, acute myocardial infarction, and atrial fibrillation. Dabigatran is indicated to reduce the risk of stroke and systemic embolism in patients with nonvalvular atrial fibrillation. It is also

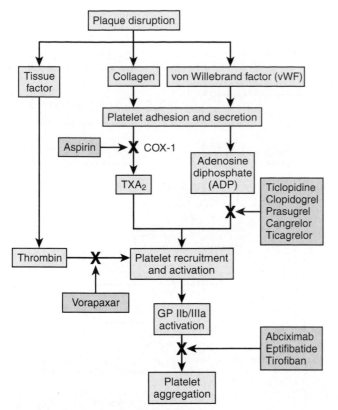

• **Fig. 19.3** Action for antiplatelet drugs. *ADP,* Adenosine diphosphate; *vWF,* von Willebrand factor. (Modified from Lilley LL, Harrington S, Snyder JS. *Pharmacology and the nursing process,* ed 5, St Louis, 2007, Mosby.)

approved in Canada and Europe to prevent clots in patients who have undergone hip and knee replacement surgeries.

Mechanism of Action and Pharmacokinetics

Dabigatran is an oral direct thrombin inhibitor. Warfarin interferes with the formation of vitamin K–Dependent clotting factors. ***Prothrombin time*** (PT) is a test to determine how well warfarin is working to prevent clotting and to determine whether dosage adjustments are necessary. This test is also called an international normalized ratio test. The effectiveness of warfarin may be decreased by consumption of foods rich in vitamin K and nutritional supplements with vitamin K. Foods and beverages rich in vitamin K are chickpeas, kale, turnip greens, broccoli, beef and pork liver, parsley, spinach, and green tea.

Warfarin has good oral absorption and bioavailability. The maximum effects of warfarin are not achieved until 4 to 5 days after initiating therapy because warfarin does not block the activity of existing coagulation factors. Stores of existing clotting factors must be depleted before the maximum effect of warfarin on clotting is achieved. Warfarin is highly protein bound, so it interacts with many other drugs. Pharmacy technicians should alert a pharmacist whenever a drug interaction is reported.

> ● *Tech Note!*
>
> Warfarin is the active ingredient in some rodent poisons.

Adverse Reactions

The most common adverse reaction is bleeding. Signs of bleeding are bruising, swollen joints, bleeding gums, red spots on the skin or in the eye, nosebleeds, coughing up blood, and heavy menstrual

Antiplatelet Drugs

Generic Name	US Brand Name(s)	Dosage Forms and Strengths
	Canadian Brand(s)	
aspirin[a] (Numerous—see Chapter 10)	Bayer, Bayer Low Dose, Ecotrin, Ecotrin Low Strength, St. Joseph Low Dose	**Tablets:** 81 mg, 325 mg, 500 mg **Tablets, chewable:** 81 mg **Tablets, delayed release:** 81 mg, 325 mg
	Bayer Aspirin, Bayer Aspirin Low Dose	
clopidogrel[a]	Plavix	**Tablets:** 75 mg, 300 mg
	Plavix	
dipyridamole[a]	Persantine	**Injection:** 5 mg/mL **Tablets**[b]**:** 25 mg, 50 mg, 75 mg
	Persantine	
ticlopidine[a]	Generics	**Tablets:** 250 mg
	Not available	
vorapaxar	Zontivity	**Tablet:** 2.08 mg
	Zontivity (Approved only)	
dipyridamole + aspirin[a]	Generics	**Capsule, extended release:** 200 mg dipyridamole + 25 mg aspirin
	Generics	

[a]Generic available.
[b]Available in the United States only.

Glycoprotein IIb/IIIa Inhibitors

Generic Name	US Brand Name(s) Canadian Brand(s)	Dosage Forms and Strengths
abciximab	ReoPro	Solution for injection: 2 mg/mL
	Not available	
eptifibatide[a,b]	Generics	Solution for injection: 0.75 mg/mL, 2 mg/mL
	Not available	
tirofiban	Aggrastat	Solution for injection[b]: 0.25 mg/mL
	Aggrastat	Solution for IV infusion[c]: 12.5 mg/250 mL

[a]Generic available.
[b]Available in the United States only.
[c]Available in Canada only.

bleeding. In addition to bleeding, dabigatran may cause dyspepsia, gastroesophageal reflux disease, and peptic ulcers.

❶ Tech Alert!

Warfarin can cause fetal abnormalities, so pharmacy technicians should apply the warning label "AVOID PREGNANCY" to prescription vials.

Precautions

Pharmacy technicians should remind patients taking anticoagulants to seek the advice of a pharmacist before taking prescription and nonprescription drugs. Many drugs interact with anticoagulants, causing serious bleeding or hemorrhaging. Anticoagulants should not be combined with antiplatelet drugs, aspirin, NSAIDs, vitamin supplements, and herbs (e.g., feverfew, fish oil supplements, garlic, ginger, ginkgo biloba).

Treating Overdose

Overdose of warfarin or heparin can result in hemorrhage and death. Overdose may be treated by giving a blood transfusion. In some cases, warfarin overdose can be reversed by the administration of vitamin K. Heparin overdose may be treated by the administration of protamine sulfate.

● Tech Note!

Warfarin tablets are color coded to reduce medication errors.

● Tech Note!

Idarucizumab (Praxbind) reverses the effects of dabigatran.

❶ Tech Alert!

Argatroban injection must be diluted.

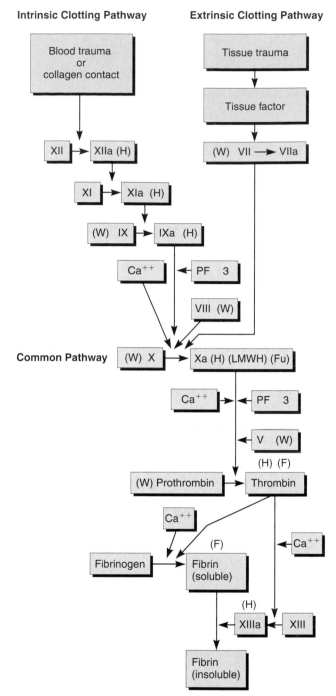

• **Fig. 19.4** Clotting pathways. *LMWHs,* Low-molecular-weight heparins; *PF 3,* platelet factor 3. (From Clayton BD, Willihnganz MJ. *Basic pharmacology for nurses,* ed 17, St Louis, 2017, Elsevier.)

Thrombolytics

Just as the body has a mechanism to form clots at the site of injury to prevent hemorrhage, the body also has a system to stop excessive clot formation, thereby avoiding obstruction to blood flow in blood vessels. **Thrombolytics,** also called fibrinolytics, are drugs that can dissolve blood clots. The drugs are administered in the early stage of stroke to open blood vessels in the brain. They are also used in the treatment of acute myocardial infarction.

Anticoagulant Drugs

Generic Name	US Brand Name(s) Canadian Brand(s)	Dosage Forms and Strengths
warfarin[a]	Jantoven Generics	**Tablets:** 1 mg, 2 mg, 2.5 mg, 3 mg, 4 mg, 5 mg, 6 mg, 7.5 mg, 10 mg
dalteparin	Fragmin Fragmin	**Injection, prefilled syringe:** 2500 units/0.2 mL, 3500 units/0.28 mL, 5000 units/0.2 mL, 7500 units/0.3 mL, 10,000 units/0.4 mL[c], 12,500 units/0.5 mL, 15,000 units/0.6 mL, 18,000 units/0.72 mL
enoxaparin[a]	Lovenox, Lovenox Preservative Free Inclunox, Inclunox HP, Lovenox, Lovenox HP	**Solution, for injection:** 300 mg/3 mL (100 mg/mL) **Injection, prefilled syringe:** 30 mg/0.3 mL, 40 mg/0.4 mL, 60 mg/0.6 mL, 80 mg/0.8 mL, 100 mg/1 mL, 120 mg/0.8 mL, 150 mg/mL
heparin sodium[a]	Generics Heparin Leo	**Solution, for irrigation (Heparin Leo):** 100 units/mL **Solution, for injection:** 1000 units/mL, 5000 units/mL, 10,000 units/mL, 20,000 units/mL[b]
tinzaparin	Not available Innohep	**Solution, for injection:** 10,000 units/mL, 20,000 units/mL
fondaparinux[a]	Arixtra Arixtra	**Solution, for injection:** 2.5 mg/0.5 mL, 5 mg/0.4 mL[b], 7.5 mg/0.6 mL, 10 mg/0.8 mL[b]
argatroban[a]	Argatroban Argatroban	**Solution, for injection:** 100 mg/mL
dabigatran	Pradaxa Pradaxa	**Capsule:** 75 mg, 110 mg, 150 mg **Pellets:** 20 mg/packet, 30 mg/packet, 40 mg/packet, 50 mg/packet, 110 mg/packet, 150 mg/packet

[a]Generic available.
[b]Available in the United States only.
[c]Available in Canada only.

Mechanism of Action

Thrombolytic agents currently in use in the United States and Canada are alteplase and tenecteplase. Reteplase is marketed in the United States only. All activate the fibrinolytic system, the body's normal system for preventing excess clotting. Alteplase is a ***tissue plasminogen activator*** produced by recombinant DNA technology. Tissue plasminogen activator is a naturally occurring thrombolytic substance. Thrombolytic agents dissolve blood clots that have formed in blood vessels. They increase the activity of plasmin, an enzyme that digests fibrin and other clotting factors. Without fibrin, the structure of the thrombin clot is weakened, and the clot dissolves.

Pharmacokinetics

Thrombolytic medications work rapidly. They can reopen an obstructed blood vessel within 90 minutes of administration. Alteplase and tenecteplase differ in specificity and half-life. The half-life for alteplase is 30 to 45 minutes; it is 20 to 24 minutes for tenecteplase. All thrombolytic agents lose shelf life rapidly after reconstitution. They must be stored in the refrigerator and used within 24 hours.

> ● **Tech Note!**
>
> Thrombolytic agents are very expensive. A single dose can cost more than $4500.

Adverse Reactions

Thrombolytic drugs must be administered within the first 1 to 3 hours after a stroke occurs. Thereafter, the risk of hemorrhage exceeds the benefit of administering clot-dissolving drugs. The risk of intracranial hemorrhage, leading to irreversible damage or death, increases exponentially over time. Thrombolytic agents can cause bruising and bleeding in the gastrointestinal tract, genitourinary tract, and mouth (gums) in addition to bleeding in the brain. Other adverse reactions are nausea, vomiting, hypotension, transient arrhythmia, allergic reaction, and fever.

Thrombolytic Agents

Generic Name	US Brand Name(s)	Dosage Forms and Strengths
	Canadian Brand(s)	
alteplase (t-PA)	Activase, Cathflo Activase	**Injection, powder for reconstitution (Activase):** 50 mg vial, 100 mg vial; 2 mg vial (Cathflo Activase)
	Activase, Cathflo Activase	
reteplase (r-PA)	Retavase	**Injection, powder for reconstitution:** 18.8 mg/vial
	Not available	
tenecteplase	TNKase	**Injection, powder for reconstitution:** 50 mg vial
	TNKase	

> **⓵ Tech Alert!**
>
> The following drugs have look-alike/sound-alike issues:
> Activase and Cathflo Activase;
> Activase and TNKase

Drugs That Treat Hyperlipidemia

Atherosclerosis and atherothrombosis are important risk factors for stroke and myocardial infarction. Drugs that control the buildup of lipids and plaque and drugs that reduce the formation of blood clots are administered to prevent stroke, myocardial infarction, and acute coronary syndrome. *Hyperlipidemia* is a disorder associated with dysfunctional fat metabolism. Although fats are necessary to form steroid hormones, bile, prostaglandins, and cell membranes, excessive buildup in the blood (hyperlipidemia) is a significant risk factor for stroke and myocardial infarction. A principal focus for prevention of cardiovascular disease is treatment of hyperlipidemia. The emphasis is on reducing LDLs and raising HDL levels.

LDL is known as "bad cholesterol" because elevated LDL cholesterol levels promote plaque buildup in arteries, atherothrombosis, and vasoconstriction. All increase the risk of cardiovascular disease and stroke. HDL controls excessive levels of LDL by transporting cholesterol from cells in the artery wall back to the liver for removal. Atherosclerosis is a chronic inflammatory disorder, and HF is also linked to inflammation. HDL has protective antiinflammatory properties and acts as an antioxidant to diminish LDL oxidation, thereby reducing inflammation and oxidative stress. HDL also has antithrombotic, vasodilatory, and antiinfectious properties, all of which protect against cardiovascular disease.

Recent evidence has shown that increasing HDL ("good cholesterol") in addition to reducing LDL cholesterol can lower the risk for cardiovascular disease, even in persons who have normal HDL levels before starting HDL drug therapy. Lipid-lowering drugs interfere with steps in the lipid metabolism pathway (Fig. 19.5). They may affect cholesterol synthesis or elimination in bile or act on LDL metabolism. Although the mechanisms of action may vary, all lipid-lowering drugs reduce LDL and *triglyceride* levels.

Hydroxymethylglutaryl Coenzyme A Reductase Inhibitors

Hydroxymethylglutaryl (HMG) coenzyme A (CoA) reductase inhibitors are also called "statins." Atorvastatin, lovastatin, pravastatin, rosuvastatin, and simvastatin are all HMG CoA reductase inhibitors. HMG CoA reductase is an enzyme that is involved in the final step of cholesterol synthesis.

> **● Tech Note!**
>
> All hydroxymethylglutaryl CoA inhibitors have the common ending "-statin."

Mechanism of Action and Pharmacokinetics

Statins increase LDL clearance. They are more effective than other lipid-lowering drugs at lowering LDL (up to 60%). They minimally elevate HDL (up to 16%) above predrug levels. Simvastatin and lovastatin are prodrugs and must undergo metabolic changes before they are pharmacologically active.

Adverse Reactions

Common side effects include diarrhea, gas, headache, joint pain, nausea, vomiting, stomach upset or pain, and tiredness. Serious, life-threatening muscle disorders caused by statins are myositis (inflammation of muscle) and rhabdomyolysis (breakdown of muscle fibers and release of contents into the circulation). Statins can also elevate liver enzymes, resulting in liver dysfunction.

> **⓵ Tech Alert!**
>
> The following drugs have look-alike/sound-alike issues:
> Lipitor and Loniten

Fibric Acid Derivatives

Fibric acid derivatives, or fibrates, are regarded as broad-spectrum lipid-lowering drugs. Fibrates increase the clearance of very-low-density lipoprotein (VLDL). Fibrates are less effective than statins at reducing LDL (≈10%) and in elevating HDL (up to 10% above pretherapy levels).

Mechanism of Action

Fibrates appear to activate the protein peroxisome proliferator-activated receptor-α (PPAR-α). PPAR-α activates the enzyme lipoprotein lipase. Activating these enzymes decreases VLDL cholesterol (which is converted into LDL cholesterol) and triglycerides. Fibrates also increase HDL cholesterol.

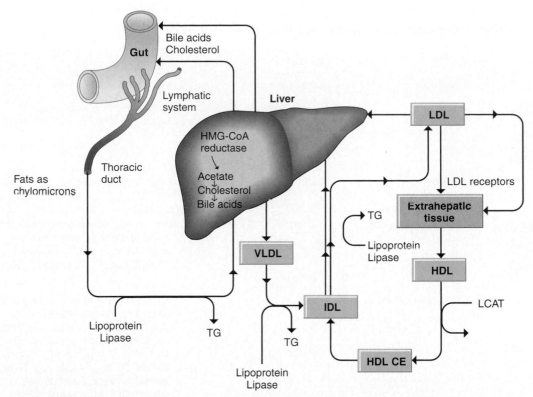

• **Fig. 19.5** Lipid metabolism pathways. *HDL*, high-density lipoprotein; *LDL*, low-density lipoprotein; *VLDL*, very-low-density lipoprotein; *IDL*, intermediate-density lipoprotein; *LCAT*, lecithin–cholesterol acyltransferase; *TG*, tri-glyceride. (From Lilley LL, Harrington S, Snyder JS. *Pharmacology and the nursing process*, ed 5, St Louis, 2007, Mosby.)

Statins (Hydroxymethylglutaryl CoA Inhibitors)

	Generic Name	US Brand Name(s) Canadian Brand(s)	Dosage Forms and Strengths
	atorvastatin[a]	Lipitor Lipitor	**Tablets:** 10 mg, 20 mg, 40 mg, 80 mg
	fluvastatin[a]	Lescol XL Generics	**Capsules (Lescol):** 20 mg, 40 mg **Tablets, extended release (Lescol XL):** 80 mg
	lovastatin[a]	Altoprev Generics	**Tablets:** 20 mg, 40 mg **Tablets, extended release (Altoprev):** 20 mg, 40 mg, 60 mg
	pravastatin[a]	Generics Generics	**Tablets:** 10 mg, 20 mg, 40 mg, 80 mg[b]
	rosuvastatin[a]	Crestor, Ezallor Sprinkle Crestor	**Sprinkles:** 5 mg, 10 mg, 20 mg, 40 mg **Tablets:** 5 mg, 10 mg, 20 mg, 40 mg

Continued

Statins (Hydroxymethylglutaryl CoA Inhibitors)—cont'd

	Generic Name	US Brand Name(s) / Canadian Brand(s)	Dosage Forms and Strengths
	simvastatin[a]	FloLipid, Zocor / Zocor	**Solution, oral:** 20 mg/5 mL, 40 mg/5 mL **Tablets:** 5 mg, 10 mg, 20 mg, 40 mg, 80 mg
	pitavastatin	Livalo, Zypitamag / Not available	**Tablets:** 1 mg, 2 mg, 4 mg
	ezetimibe + simvastatin[a]	Vytorin / Not available	**Tablets:** 10 mg ezetimibe + 10 mg simvastatin, 10 mg ezetimibe + 20 mg simvastatin, 10 mg ezetimibe + 40 mg simvastatin, 10 mg ezetimibe + 80 mg simvastatin,
	atorvastatin + amlodipine[a]	Caduet / Caduet	**Tablets:** atorvastatin 10 mg + amlodipine 2.5 mg,[b] atorvastatin 10 mg + amlodipine 5 mg, atorvastatin 10 mg + amlodipine 10 mg, atorvastatin 20 mg + amlodipine 2.5 mg,[b] atorvastatin 20 mg + amlodipine 5 mg, atorvastatin 20 mg + amlodipine 10 mg, atorvastatin 40 mg + amlodipine 2.5 mg,[b] atorvastatin 40 mg + amlodipine 5 mg, atorvastatin 40 mg + amlodipine 10 mg, atorvastatin 80 mg + amlodipine 5 mg, atorvastatin 80 mg + amlodipine 10 mg,
	atorvastatin + ezetimibe[b]	Lypqozet / Not available	**Tablets:** atorvastatin 10 mg + ezetimibe 10 mg, atorvastatin 20 mg + ezetimibe 10 mg, atorvastatin 40 mg + ezetimibe 10 mg, atorvastatin 80 mg + ezetimibe 10 mg,

[a]Generic available.
[b]Available in the United States only.

Miscellaneous Cholesterol-Lowering Agents

	Generic Name	US Brand Name(s) / Canadian Brand(s)	Dosage Forms and Strengths
	ezetimibe[a]	Zetia / Ezetrol	**Tablets:** 10 mg

[a]Generic available.

Precautions

If administered together, statins and fibrates produce a drug interaction that may increase the likelihood of development of myopathies.

Bile Acid Sequestrants

Bile acid sequestrants promote intestinal clearance of cholesterol. They are administered to reduce LDL levels. They are not absorbed and therefore are the drugs of choice for use in pregnancy.

Mechanism of Action

Bile acid sequestrants bind to cholesterol-containing bile acids in the intestine. The bound complex is insoluble and is excreted in the feces. Cholesterol depletion increases LDL receptor activity, which increases removal of LDLs from the blood.

Fibric Acid Derivatives

Generic Name	US Brand Name(s) Canadian Brand(s)	Dosage Forms and Strengths
gemfibrozil[a]	Lopid	**Tablets:** 600 mg
	Generic	
fenofibric acid[a]	Generics	**Capsule, extended release:** 45 mg, 135 mg
	Not available	
fenofibrate[a]	Antara, Fenoglide, Lipofen, Tricor, Triglide	**Capsules (Lipofen):** 50 mg, 150 mg
	Lipidil EZ, Lipidil Supra	**Capsules, micronized:** 30 mg[b], 43 mg[b], 90 mg[b], 130 mg[b] (Antara); 67 mg, 134 mg[b], 200 mg **Tablets:** 160 mg (Triglide); 40 mg, 120 mg (Fenoglide); 48 mg, 145 mg (Lipidil EZ, Tricor) **Tablets, micronized:** 100 mg, 160 mg (Lipidil Supra)

[a]Generic available.
[b]Available in United States only.

Bile Acid Sequestrants

Generic Name	US Brand Name(s) Canadian Brand(s)	Dosage Forms and Strengths
cholestyramine[a]	Prevalite	**Powder, for reconstitution (regular and sugar free):** 4 g/packet or scoop
	Olestyr	
colesevelam[a]	Welchol	**Tablets:** 625 mg **Powder, for suspension:** 3.75 g/packet
	Lodalis	
colestipol[a,b]	Colestid	**Granules, for reconstitution[b]:** 5 g/packet or scoop **Tablets:** 1 g
	Colestid	

[a]Generic available.
[b]Available in the United States only.

Adverse Effects and Precautions

Bile acid sequestrants produce bloating and gas. They must be administered at least 1 hour before or 4 hours after other medications to avoid decreasing the absorption of the other drugs. Bile acid sequestrants can lower body levels of fat-soluble vitamins such as vitamins A, D, E, and K. Unfortunately, the resins can increase triglyceride levels.

Nicotinic Acid Derivatives

Niacin is vitamin B_3. It is the most effective lipid-lowering agent for increasing HDL (up to 35%).

Mechanism of Action

The mechanism of niacin's antilipemic action is unknown. It is thought that effects may be linked to decreased VLDL synthesis and clearance in the liver, decreased VLDL triglyceride transport, and actions on free fatty acid release, lipoprotein lipase activity, and triglyceride synthesis. The elevation of HDL by nicotinic acid is possibly associated with an increase in serum levels of

Nicotinic Acid

Generic Name	US Brand Name(s) Canadian Brand(s)	Dosage Forms and Strengths
niacin[a]	Niacor, Slo-Niacin	**Tablets:** 500 mg (Niacor)
	Slo-Niacin (OTC)	**Tablets, time released:** 500 mg, 750 mg, 1000 mg

[a]Generic available.
OTC, Over the counter.

apolipoprotein A-I and lipoprotein A-I and a decrease in serum levels of apolipoprotein B.

Adverse Effects

The most common side effect of niacin is skin flushing, dizziness, and itchiness. Individuals may also experience nausea and vomiting. The consumption of high-dose niacin may cause liver damage.

Usual Dose and Dosing Schedule for Drugs Used in the Treatment of Cardiovascular Diseases

	Drug Name	Usual Dose and Dosing Schedule	Warning Labels
Cardioglycosides			
	digoxin	0.0625–0.25 mg once daily	TAKE AS DIRECTED; DO NOT SKIP OR EXCEED DOSAGE. IF YOU MISS A DOSE, TAKE IT AS SOON AS YOU REMEMBER UNLESS THE NEXT DOSE IS SCHEDULED TO BE TAKEN IN LESS THAN 12 HOURS.
Digoxin Antidote			
	DigiFab	Varies according to the amount of digoxin to be neutralized	
I*f*-Channel Blocker			
	ivabradine	2.5–7.5 mg 2 times a day	AVOID PREGNANCY.
Guanylate Cyclase Stimulator			
	vericiguat	2.5–10 mg daily	AVOID PREGNANCY.
Thiazides			
	chlorothiazide	500–1000 mg 1–2 times a day	See Chapter 18.
	chlorthalidone	50–100 mg/day (maximum 200 mg/day)	
	hydrochlorothiazide (HCTZ)	25–100 mg 1–2 times/day	
	indapamide	2.5–5 mg/day	
	metolazone	5–20 mg once daily (maximum 20 mg/day)	
Loop			
	bumetanide	0.5–2 mg typically as a single dose (maximum 10 mg/day)	See Chapter 18.
	furosemide	20–80 mg PO 1–2 times per day (maximum 600 mg/day PO) 20–40 mg IM or slow IV, over 1–2 minutes; may repeat same dosage 2 h later	
	torsemide	10–20 mg PO or IV daily (maximum 200 mg/day)	
Aldosterone Receptor Antagonists			
	eplerenone	25–50 mg once daily	
	spironolactone	25–50 mg once daily	
β-Blockers			
	bisoprolol	1.25–10 mg once daily	See Chapter 18.
	metoprolol extended release	Begin 12.5 mg/day; increase up to 200 mg/day	

Usual Dose and Dosing Schedule for Drugs Used in the Treatment of Cardiovascular Diseases—cont'd

	Drug Name	Usual Dose and Dosing Schedule	Warning Labels
Combined α- and β-Blockers			
	carvedilol	**Immediate release:** Begin 3.125 mg twice daily; increase to 25–50 mg twice daily **Controlled release:** Begin 10 mg/day; increase up to 80 mg/day	See Chapter 18.
Angiotensin-Converting Enzyme Inhibitors			
	benazepril	2–20 mg once daily	See Chapter 18.
	captopril	6.25–50 mg 3 times a day	
	enalapril	2.5–20 mg twice daily	
	fosinopril	5–40 mg once daily	
	lisinopril	2.5–40 mg once daily	
	perindopril	2–8 mg once daily	
	quinapril	5–20 mg twice daily	
	ramipril	1.25–10 mg/day in 2 divided doses	
	trandolapril	1–4 mg once daily	
Angiotensin II Antagonists			
	candesartan	Begin 4 mg once daily; increase to 32 mg/day	See Chapter 18.
	losartan	25–150 mg once daily	
	valsartan	40–160 mg twice daily	
	valsartan + sacubitril (Entresto)	1 tablet twice a day	

Continued

Usual Dose and Dosing Schedule for Drugs Used in the Treatment of Cardiovascular Diseases —cont'd

Drug Name	Usual Dose and Dosing Schedule	Warning Labels
Vasodilators (Hydralazine + Isosorbide in Combination)		
hydralazine + isosorbide (BiDil)	1–2 tablets 3 times a day	
hydralazine	Initiate at 10–25 mg 3 times a day; maintenance 200 mg/day in 2–4 divided doses (maximum, 300 mg/day) for systolic heart failure	
Antiplatelet Drugs		
abciximab	0.25 mg/kg bolus followed by 0.125 mcg/kg/min infusion for up to 12 h	REPORT SIGNS OF BLEEDING—all. DO NOT SHAKE—abciximab, eptifibatide, tirofiban. REFRIGERATE AT 2°C–8°C; DO NOT FREEZE—abciximab, eptifibatide, tirofiban. AVOID PREGNANCY—aspirin. PROTECT FROM LIGHT—tirofiban. STORE AT ROOM TEMPERATURE—tirofiban. TAKE ON AN EMPTY STOMACH—dipyridamole. TAKE WITH FOOD—aspirin, ticlopidine. SWALLOW WHOLE; DO NOT CRUSH OR CHEW—aspirin + dipyridamole.
aspirin	81–325 mg once daily	
eptifibatide	180 mcg/kg IV bolus (maximum, 22.6 mg); 2 mcg/kg/min continuous IV infusion (maximum, 15 mg/h)	
tirofiban	25 mcg/kg/min IV for 5 min followed by 0.15 mcg/kg/min IV	
clopidogrel	75 mg once daily	
dipyridamole	75–100 mg 4 times/day	
ticlopidine	250 mg twice daily	
aspirin + dipyridamole	Take 1 capsule twice daily	
Anticoagulants		
dalteparin	120 international units/kg/day SC every 12 h with aspirin (non-Q-wave myocardial infarction)	REPORT SIGNS OF BLEEDING—all. AVOID OTC WITHOUT MEDICAL SUPERVISION—vitamins, herbals, analgesics (aspirin and NSAIDs)—warfarin, dabigatran. AVOID PREGNANCY—warfarin. SWALLOW WHOLE; DO NOT CRUSH OR CHEW—dabigatran. PROTECT FROM MOISTURE—dabigatran. STORE IN MANUFACTURER'S ORIGINAL PACKAGING—dabigatran.
enoxaparin	30 mg IV bolus followed by 1 mg/kg SC every 12 h for up to 7 days	
heparin Na⁺	60 international units/kg IV bolus with initial dose of thrombolytic therapy; then 12 international units/kg/h IV	
tinzaparin	175 units/kg (or 0.00875 mL/kg) SC once daily	
dabigatran	75–150 mg orally twice daily	
warfarin	Individualized	
Thrombolytics		
alteplase (t-PA)	Based on weight; not to exceed 100 mg total dose	REFRIGERATE RECONSTITUTED SOLUTION (2°C–8°C)—all. DO NOT SHAKE—all. STABLE FOR 8 HOURS AFTER RECONSTITUTION—tenecteplase.
tenecteplase	Based on weight; not to exceed 50 mg/dose	
reteplase (r-PA)	10 units IV bolus over 2 min followed by another 10-unit bolus	

Usual Dose and Dosing Schedule for Drugs Used in the Treatment of Cardiovascular Diseases—cont'd

	Drug Name	Usual Dose and Dosing Schedule	Warning Labels
HMG CoA Reductase Inhibitors (Statins)			
	atorvastatin	10–80 mg once daily	AVOID GRAPEFRUIT JUICE—atorvastatin, lovastatin, simvastatin. AVOID PREGNANCY—all. SWALLOW WHOLE; DO NOT CHEW—extended release.
	lovastatin	10–80 mg once daily	
	fluvastatin	20–80 mg once daily	
	pravastatin	40–80 mg once daily	
	rosuvastatin	5–40 mg once daily	
	simvastatin	5–40 mg once daily	
	pitavastatin	1–4 mg once daily	
Fibric Acid Derivatives			
	fenofibrate	1 capsule/tablet daily; dose varies according to manufacturer's product, e.g., 40–120 mg once a day (Fenoglide®), 50–150 mg daily (Lipofen®), 54–160 mg daily (Tricor®, Triglide)	TAKE ON AN EMPTY STOMACH—gemfibrozil.
	fenofibric acid	45–135 mg once daily	
	gemfibrozil	600 mg twice daily	
Bile Acid Sequestrants			
	cholestyramine	4–24 g daily in 1–2 divided doses	TAKE 1 HOUR BEFORE OR 4 HOURS AFTER OTHER DRUGS.
	colestipol	5–30 g in 1–2 divided doses	RECONSTITUTE WITH 2–6 OZ OF LIQUID; SHAKE WELL—all.
	colesevelam	3.75 g daily in 1–2 doses	SWALLOW WHOLE, TAKE WITH HALF GLASS WATER AND FOOD.
Miscellaneous			
	ezetimibe	10 mg once daily	

Continued

Usual Dose and Dosing Schedule for Drugs Used in the Treatment of Cardiovascular Diseases—cont'd

	Drug Name	Usual Dose and Dosing Schedule	Warning Labels
	niacin (vitamin B₃)	**Immediate release:** 1–2 g 2–3 times/day (Niacor) **Extended release:** 1–2 g once daily	TAKE WITH FOOD—niacin.
	ezetimibe + atorvastatin	1 tablet daily	SWALLOW WHOLE; DO NOT CRUSH OR CHEW. AVOID PREGNANCY. AVOID GRAPEFRUIT JUICE.
	ezetimibe + simvastatin	1 tablet once daily in the evening	AVOID GRAPEFRUIT JUICE. TAKE WITH FOOD. AVOID PREGNANCY.

NSAIDs, Nonsteroidal antiinflammatory drugs; *PO,* oral; *IM,* intramuscular; *IV,* intravenous; *SC,* subcutaneous.

TECHNICIAN'S CORNER

1. Research and make a list of over-the-counter medications that should be avoided by patients taking digoxin and warfarin.
2. Patients with cardiovascular disease are always advised to make lifestyle modifications as part of their treatment. Why is that process so important and so difficult to do?

Key Points

- Heart failure is a clinical syndrome in which the heart is unable to pump blood at a rate necessary to meet the body's metabolic needs.
- Heart failure may affect the left side of the heart, the right side of the heart, or both sides.
- Compensatory mechanisms are "switched on" when the heart function fails. Compensatory mechanisms attempt to satisfy the metabolic needs of the body.
- There are four stages of heart failure: stage A, high risk for developing heart failure; stage B, structural changes without symptoms; stage C, symptomatic; and stage D, advanced structural heart disease plus heart failure symptoms.
- Diuretics are administered for heart failure to reduce edema. Diuretics that produce hypokalemia can increase the effects of digoxin, leading to toxicity.
- Drugs used in the treatment of heart failure include the cardioglycosides, diuretics, aldosterone antagonists, β-blockers, angiotensin-converting enzyme (ACE) inhibitors, angiotensin receptor blockers (ARBs), angiotensin receptor-neprilysin inhibitor, sodium-glucose cotransporter-2 inhibitor, and vasodilators.
- Digoxin has a positive inotropic effect on the heart; the result is an increase in the force of myocardial contractions.
- Spironolactone and eplerenone are aldosterone antagonists that can increase potassium levels. Potassium levels should be monitored because hyperkalemia can produce arrhythmias.

- ACE inhibitors and ARBs may reduce mortality. They reduce left ventricular hypertrophy, improve diastolic filling, increase cardiac output, and reduce peripheral vascular resistance.
- Isosorbide dinitrate and hydralazine are used in combination for the treatment of heart failure to decrease mortality and effectively reduce cardiac congestion.
- Strokes occur when brain cells are deprived of oxygen or are damaged by sudden bleeding into the brain.
- Transient ischemic attacks are also known as ministrokes and last only a few minutes.
- Chronic inflammation of arteries that supply the heart and brain can also lead to stroke and myocardial infarction because vascular inflammation is a cause of atherosclerosis.
- Atherosclerosis (a buildup of lipids and plaque inside of artery walls) can block blood flow through arteries.
- Atherothrombosis (the formation of a blood clot in the artery) is triggered by atherosclerosis and can also cause clogged arteries.
- The risk for heart failure, stroke, and myocardial infarction is increased by nonmodifiable risk factors, modifiable risk factors, and chronic disease.
- Nonmodifiable risk factors are age, gender, and family history of stroke and myocardial infarction.
- Modifiable risk factors are smoking, heavy alcohol consumption, and diet high in cholesterol.
- Drugs administered to prevent stroke and myocardial infarction control the buildup of lipids and plaque and reduce the formation of blood clots.

- Drugs that control hemostasis (the process of stopping the flow of blood) prevent the formation of clots that can obstruct the supply of blood to the brain and heart.
- Antithrombotic drugs include (1) agents that inhibit platelets; (2) anticoagulants, which lessen coagulation; and (3) fibrinolytic agents. Fibrinolytic drugs dissolve existing clots.
- Antiplatelet drugs interfere with early steps in the clot formation process.
- Aspirin is a nonprescription drug that has antiplatelet activity.
- Dabigatran is an oral direct thrombin inhibitor indicated to reduce the risk of stroke and systemic embolism in patients with nonvalvular atrial fibrillation.
- Abciximab, eptifibatide, and tirofiban are parenteral antiplatelet drugs. They block the final pathway for platelet aggregation.
- Ticlopidine, clopidogrel, and dipyridamole are orally administered antiplatelet drugs.
- Bleeding is a common side effect of all antiplatelet drugs. Other side effects associated with antiplatelet drugs are skin rash or itching, stomach pain, and pain at the injection site (abciximab).
- Nonprescription drugs, vitamin supplements, and herbs can enhance the effects of antiplatelet drugs. These drugs include nonsteroidal antiinflammatory drugs (e.g., ibuprofen), feverfew, fish oil supplements, garlic, and ginger.

- Heparin and low-molecular-weight heparin are anticoagulants that are administered to prevent the formation of blood clots.
- The activated partial thromboplastin time test is performed to measure the effectiveness of heparin and to determine whether dosage adjustments are necessary.
- Warfarin interferes with the formation of vitamin K–dependent clotting factors. Prothrombin time is a test to determine how well warfarin is working to reduce clotting.
- Warfarin can cause fetal abnormalities, so pharmacy technicians should apply the warning label "AVOID PREGNANCY" to prescription vials.
- Warfarin overdose is reversed by the administration of vitamin K. Heparin overdose is treated with protamine sulfate.
- Thrombolytics, also called fibrinolytics, are drugs that can dissolve blood clots and must be administered within the first few hours of a stroke.
- Statins are hydroxymethylglutaryl coenzyme A reductase inhibitors and block the final step of cholesterol synthesis and promote low-density lipoprotein elimination.
- Bile acid sequestrants promote intestinal clearance of cholesterol.
- Niacin is vitamin B_3. It is effective for increasing high-density lipoproteins.

Review Questions

1. Drugs that control the rate of clot formation and clot dissolution are classified as _____ and can prevent stroke and myocardial infarction.
   a. antihyperlipidemics
   b. antifibrinolytics
   c. antithrombotics
   d. antihemorrhagics
2. The _____ are the oldest class of drugs used in the treatment of heart failure.
   a. aminoglycosides
   b. cardioglycosides
   c. diuretics
   d. antibiotics
3. Digitalis is a cardioglycoside derived from the foxglove plant.
   a. true
   b. false
4. Statin drugs primarily lower what kind of cholesterol?
   a. LDL
   b. bile
   c. HDL
   d. all of the above
5. _____ is a parenteral antiplatelet drug.
   a. Ticlopidine
   b. Dipyridamole
   c. Abciximab
   d. Simvastatin
6. Thiazide diuretics can cause _____.
   a. hyperkalemia
   b. hypernatremia
   c. hypokalemia
   d. hypocalcemia

7. The mechanism of action for β-blockers used in the treatent of heart failure is to block excess _____ stimulation induced by heart failure.
   a. sympathetic
   b. parasympathetic
8. Spironolactone may be used in the treatment of moderate to severe heart failure to _____.
   a. reduce water and K+ accumulation
   b. reduce water and Ca++ accumulation
   c. reduce water and Na+ accumulation
   d. reduce water and Cl− accumulation
9. Thrombolytics must be administered within the first _____ hours after a stroke occurs.
   a. 1 to 3
   b. 2 to 4
   c. 3 to 5
   d. 4 to 6
10. Isosorbide dinitrate and hydralazine are used in combination for the treatment of heart failure for their _____ effects.
    a. vasodilating
    b. vasoconstricting
    c. sympathetic
    d. parasympathetic

Bibliography

Abramson BL, Al-Omran M, Anand SS, et al. Canadian Cardiovascular Society 2022 Guidelines for peripheral arterial disease. *Can J Cardiol.* 2022;38(5):560–587.

American Heart Association. (2022). AHA releases Heart and Stroke Statistics – 2022 Update. Retrieved November 14, 2022, from https://www.sca-aware.org/sca-news/aha-releases-heart-and-stroke-statistics-2022-update.

Aronow W. Epidemiology, pathophysiology, prognosis, and treatment of systolic and diastolic heart failure. *Cardiol Rev.* 2006;14:108–124.

Centers for Disease Control and Prevention. (2021). Coronary Artery Disease. Retrieved November 14, 2022, from https://www.cdc.gov/heartdisease/coronary_ad.htm.

Chapman J. Therapeutic elevation of HDL-cholesterol to prevent atherosclerosis and coronary heart disease. *Pharmacol Ther.* 2006;111:893–908.

D'Andrea E, Hey SP, Ramirez CL, Kesselheim AS. Assessment of the role of niacin in managing cardiovascular disease outcomes: a systematic review and meta-analysis. *JAMA Netw Open.* 2019;2(4):e192224.

Health Canada. (2022). Drug Product Database. Retrieved November 14, 2022, from https://health-products.canada.ca/dpd-bdpp/index-eng.jsp.

Hoffman R, Benz E, Shattil S, et al: *Hematology: Basic principles and practice*, ed 4, 2005. figure 130-1, Chapter 130.

Howlett JG, Chan M, Ezekowitz JA, et al. The Canadian Cardiovascular Society heart failure companion: bridging guidelines to your practice. *Can J Cardiol.* 2016;32:296e310.

Institute for Safe Medication Practices. (2016). FDA and ISMP Lists of Look-Alike Drug Names with Recommended Tall Man Letters. Retrieved November 14, 2022, from https://www.ismp.org/recommendations/tall-man-letters-list.

Institute for Safe Medication Practices. (2019). List of Confused Drugs. Retrieved November 14, 2022, from https://www.ismp.org/tools/confuseddrugnames.pdf.

Kalant H, Grant D, Mitchell J. *Principles of medical pharmacology.* ed 7. Toronto: Elsevier Canada, A Division of Reed Elsevier Canada; 2007:22–27 451, 453–454, 472–482, 503–504.

May H, Muhlestein J, Carlquist J, et al. Relation of serum total cholesterol, C-reactive protein levels, and statin therapy to survival in heart failure. *Am J Cardiol.* 2006;98:653–658.

McDonald M, Virani S, Chan M, et al. CCS/CHFS Heart Failure Guidelines Update: defining a new pharmacologic standard of care for heart failure with reduced ejection fraction. *Can J Cardiol.* 2021;37(4):531–546.

National Heart, Lung, and Blood Institute. *Heart attack.* Bethesda, MD: National Institutes of Health, US Department of Health and Human Services; 2022. Retrieved November 14, 2022, from. http://www.nhlbi.nih.gov/health/dci/Diseases/HeartAttack/HeartAttack_All.html.

National Heart, Lung, and Blood Institute. *High blood cholesterol.* Bethesda, MD: National Institutes of Health, US Department of Health and Human Services; 2022.Retrieved November 14, 2022, from. https://www.nhlbi.nih.gov/health/blood-cholesterol.

National Heart, Lung, and Blood Institute. *What is heart failure? Diseases and conditions index.* Bethesda, MD: National Institutes of Health, US Department of Health and Human Services; 2022. Retrieved November 14, 2022, from. https://www.nhlbi.nih.gov/health/heart-failure.

Page C, Curtis M, Sutter M, et al. *Integrated pharmacology.* Philadelphia: Mosby; 2005:386–391 393–395.

Pearson GJ, Thanassoulis G, Anderson TJ, et al. Canadian Cardiovascular Society Guidelines for the management of dyslipidemia for the prevention of cardiovascular disease in adults 2021. *Can J Cardiol.* 2021;37(8):1129–1150.

Roger VL. Epidemiology of heart failure: a contemporary perspective. *Circ Res.* 2021;128:1421–1434.

Secondary Prevention of Stroke Module, in Lindsay MP, Mountain A, Gubitz G, et al (eds), on behalf of the Canadian Stroke Best Practices and Quality Advisory Committee in collaboration with the Canadian Stroke Consortium and the Canadian Partnership for Stroke Recovery: *Canadian stroke best practice recommendations,* ed 7, Toronto, 2020, Heart and Stroke Foundation.

U.S. Food and Drug Administration. (nd). Drugs@FDA: FDA Approved Drug Products. Retrieved November 14, 2022, from https://www.accessdata.fda.gov/scripts/cder/daf/index.cfm.

20

Treatment of Arrhythmia

LEARNING OBJECTIVES

1. Learn the terminology associated with arrhythmias.
2. List risk factors for arrhythmias.
3. Describe the types of arrhythmias.
4. List and categorize medications used to treat arrhythmias.
5. Describe mechanism of action for each class of drugs used to treat arrhythmias.
6. Identify significant drug look-alike and sound-alike issues.
7. Identify warning labels and precautionary messages associated with medications used to treat arrhythmias.

KEY TERMS

Atrial fibrillation Rapid and uncoordinated contractions. The heart may beat between 300 and 400 beats/min.

Atrial flutter Irregular heartbeat in which contractions in atrium exceed the number of contractions in the ventricle. The heart rate is between 160 and 350 beats/min.

Automaticity Spontaneous contraction of heart muscle cells.

Depolarization Process during which the heart muscle conducts an electrical impulse, causing a contraction.

Ectopic Occurring in an abnormal location.

Electrical cardioversion Process of applying an electrical shock to the heart with a defibrillator to convert the heart to a normal rhythm.

Refractory period Time between contractions that it takes for repolarization to occur.

Repolarization Period when the heart is recharging and preparing for another contraction.

Supraventricular tachycardia Heart rate up to 200 beats/min that originates in an area above the ventricles.

Ventricular fibrillation Life-threatening arrhythmia during which the heart beats up to 600 beats/min.

Ventricular tachycardia Ventricles beat faster than 200 beats/min.

Overview

The heart normally beats at a rate between 60 and 100 beats/min or approximately 100,000 beats/day. With each beat or contraction, blood is pumped throughout the body, supplying oxygen and nutrients to cells and organs, including the heart. An arrhythmia is defined as an irregular heart rhythm or a heart rate that is too rapid or too slow. Arrhythmias can produce heart rates that exceed 600 beats/min. An arrhythmia can impair the heart's ability to distribute blood. Symptoms of arrhythmia are listed in Box 20.1.

Atrial fibrillation (Afib) is the most common arrhythmia, and although not usually life-threatening, individuals with Afib are at up to five times greater risk for stroke. One in three persons who have had a stroke have Afib. Afib can lead to stroke because the condition causes uncoordinated contractions that interfere with pumping blood out of the heart. If the blood pools, it may form a clot. Should the clot dislodge, it may travel to the brain and block one of the arteries, which causes the stroke.

Afib affects approximately 1% to 3% of the population, and it is estimated that it will affect nearly 12.1 million Americans by 2030. Nearly 350,000 Canadians are affected. Risk factors for Afib are similar to risk factors for coronary heart disease (CHD) and are similarly categorized as nonmodifiable risk factors, modifiable risk factors, and disease risk factors (Table 20.1). Afib affects women more than men primarily because age is a risk factor and women typically live longer. A description of these risk factors is found in chapters on hypertension, heart failure, myocardial infarction, and stroke (see Chapters 18 and 19).

Ventricular fibrillation is the leading cause of sudden cardiac death, killing nearly 600,000 people in the United States and Europe each year. The root causes are insufficient blood flow to the heart muscle, as occurs from damage to the heart muscle resulting from a heart attack.

How Arrhythmias Are Formed

Heart contractions occur when cardiac cells "fire." This is known as *depolarization*. During depolarization, positively charged ions enter heart cells through specialized ion exchange channels. Sodium entry initiates depolarization of the atria and ventricles,

BOX 20.1 Symptoms of Arrhythmia

- Palpitations or fluttering in the chest
- Rapid, irregular heart rate
- Sweating or nausea
- Chest pain
- Shortness of breath
- Light-headedness or dizziness
- Fainting

TABLE 20.1 Risk Factors for Atrial Fibrillation

Nonmodifiable	Increasing age, gender
Modifiable	Obesity, smoking, excessive alcohol consumption, stimulant use
Disease	Hypertension, heart failure, ischemic heart disease, enlarged chambers on the left side of the heart, diabetes, hyperthyroidism, chronic kidney disease, obstructive sleep apnea

and calcium entry results in depolarization of the sinoatrial (SA) and atrioventricular (AV) nodes. When the heart cells have fired, another contraction cannot occur until repolarization occurs. **Repolarization** is the process of returning the cells to their resting state. The time it takes for repolarization to occur is called the **refractory period**.

Arrhythmias occur when the cardiac ion exchange channels function improperly. This can result in excessive firing, extra currents during the refractory period, and establishment of sinus rhythm by nonpacemaker cells. These conditions may occur after a heart attack because fibrous scar tissue may develop in the healing process. Conduction is poor across fibrous tissue. Inflammation and oxidative stress (see Chapter 19) can also cause arrhythmias. In addition, having an arrhythmia may stimulate the formation of other arrhythmias.

Types of Arrhythmias

Atrial Flutter

Atrial flutter refers to an irregular heartbeat in which contractions in the atrium exceed the number of contractions in the ventricle. The heart rate may be between 160 and 350 beats/min. It usually occurs in the right atrium and is treated by inserting a catheter into the atrium (catheter ablation) rather than by drug therapy.

Atrial Fibrillation

Atrial fibrillation is defined as rapid and uncoordinated contractions of the atria. The heart may beat between 300 and 400 beats/min. There are three forms of Afib. They are temporary/recurrent (paroxysmal), persistent (>7 days), and permanent (>1 year).

Supraventricular Tachycardia

Supraventricular tachycardia (SVT) occurs in areas of the heart that lay above the ventricles. SVT may occur intermittently (paroxysmal) or frequently. The heartbeat may increase up to 200 beats/min and last several seconds to a few hours.

Ventricular Tachycardia

Ventricular tachycardia causes the ventricles to beat faster than 200 beats/min. It may occur when the spread of electrical impulses between heart chambers is "short-circuited" across scar tissue caused by a heart attack.

Ventricular Fibrillation

Ventricular fibrillation may cause the ventricles to beat faster than 600 beats/min. Ventricular fibrillation is life-threatening because the ventricles are unable to fill with blood, and blood is not effectively pumped throughout the body. Ventricular fibrillation is typically reversed only after electrical cardioversion. **Electrical cardioversion** is the process of applying an electrical shock to the heart with a defibrillator to return the heart to a normal rhythm.

Multiple mechanisms are involved in ventricular fibrillation, such as self-generated reentry of unstable wavelets and rapid, intermittent excitation alternating of the heart muscle with conduction block.

Treatment of Arrhythmia

Afib is treated with antiarrhythmic drugs to manage irregular heart rhythms and rate. Drugs that reduce clot formation, such as antiplatelet drugs (e.g., aspirin, clopidogrel) or anticoagulants (e.g., warfarin, dabigatran), may also be administered. All antiarrhythmic agents are proarrhythmic (can cause other arrhythmias).

Mechanism of Action

Antiarrhythmic drugs are categorized into four classes (classes I, II, III, and IV) according to their mechanisms of action and structural similarities. Class I antiarrhythmics are further subdivided into classes IA, IB, and IC. Antiarrhythmic drugs are listed in Table 20.2.

Class I Antiarrhythmic Drugs

Quinidine is the prototype class IA antiarrhythmic agent and has been widely used since the 1920s. It is the active ingredient in cinchona bark. Class I agents act on sodium channels and slow the

TABLE 20.2 Antiarrhythmic Drugs

Class	Category	Generic Name
Class IA	Na$^+$ channel blocker	quinidine sulfate, quinidine gluconate, procainamide, disopyramide
Class IB	Na$^+$ channel blocker	lidocaine, mexiletine, tocainide
Class IC	Na$^+$ channel blocker	flecainide, propafenone
Class II	β-blocker	propranolol, esmolol, acebutolol
Class III	K$^+$ channel blocker	amiodarone, dofetilide, dronedarone, ranolazine, sotalol, tilide, vernakalant
Class IV	Ca^{2+} channel blocker	verapamil

rate of depolarization. They also reduce **automaticity** (spontaneous contraction of heart muscle cells), delay conduction, and prolong the time between contractions (refractory period). Class IA agents have a moderate effect on depolarization and intermediate effects on the sodium channel. Class IB agents have a minimal effect on depolarization, and their effect on the sodium channel is rapid. The effect of class IC antiarrhythmic drugs on sodium channels is very slow, and they produce marked effects on depolarization. They are 80% to 90% effective at suppressing arrhythmias. All class I antiarrhythmic agents may be administered orally except lidocaine.

> **❶ Tech Alert!**
>
> The following drugs have look-alike/sound-alike issues:
>
> quiNIDine and quiNINE

Adverse Reactions and Precautions

Common side effects of antiarrhythmic agents are bradycardia, hypotension, and dizziness. Most antiarrhythmic agents cause nausea and vomiting, diarrhea, or constipation. Class I antiarrhythmic agents can produce local anesthesia and itchy, flaky rashes. Quinidine and procainamide can also produce a lupus-like syndrome, causing arthritis and chest pain. Tinnitus (ringing in the ears) is a sign of quinidine toxicity.

Class IA Antiarrhythmic Drugs

Generic Name	US Brand Name(s)	Dosage Forms and Strengths
	Canadian Brand(s)	
disopyramide[a]	Norpace, Norpace CR	**Capsules:** 100 mg, 150 mg[b]
	Rythmodan	**Capsules, extended release (Norpace CR)[b]:** 100 mg, 150 mg
procainamide[a]	Generics	**Solution, injection:** 100 mg/mL
	Generics	
quinidine gluconate[a]	Generics	**Tablets, extended release:** 324 mg
	Not available	
quinidine sulfate[a]	Generics	**Tablet[b]:** 200 mg, 300 mg
	Not available	

[a]Available in Canada only.
[b]Generic available.
[c]Available in the United States only.

Class IB Antiarrhythmic Drugs

Generic Name	US Brand Name(s)	Dosage Forms and Strengths
	Canadian Brand(s)	
lidocaine[a]	Generics	**Solution, injection[b]:** 20 mg/mL (2%)
	Xylocard	
mexiletine[a]	Generic	**Capsules:** 100 mg[b], 150 mg[c], 200 mg, 250 mg[c]
	Generic	

[a]Generic available.
[b]Available in Canada only.
[c]Available in the United States only.

Class IC Antiarrhythmic Drugs

Generic Name	US Brand Name(s)	Dosage Forms and Strengths
	Canadian Brand(s)	
flecainide[a]	Tambocor	**Tablets:** 50 mg, 100 mg, 150 mg[b]
	Generic only	
propafenone[a]	Rythmol SR	**Capsules, extended release (Rythmol SR)[b]:** 225 mg, 325 mg, 425 mg
	Rythmol	**Tablets:** 150 mg, 225 mg[b], 300 mg

[a]Generic available.
[b]Strength available in the United States only.

Class II Antiarrhythmic Drugs

Class II antiarrhythmic agents are β-adrenergic antagonists. The β-blockers antagonize the stimulation of the AV and SA nodes. They increase the refractory period, decrease automaticity, and slow conduction velocity. β-Blockers are indicated for primary management of ventricular arrhythmias. They are effective in suppressing **ectopic** (occurring in an abnormal location) beats and arrhythmias. The β-blockers that are recommended for long-term atrial fibrillation rate control in the Canadian Cardiovascular Society guidelines (2020) are bisoprolol, carvedilol, and metoprolol.

Adverse Reactions and Precautions

Adverse reactions for class II antiarrhythmic drugs (β-blockers) are described in detail in Chapter 18. They should be used with caution in patients with asthma, diabetes, and heart failure because they can cause bronchospasm, mask the signs of hypoglycemia, and may increase or decrease blood sugar levels.

> **❶ Tech Alert!**
>
> The following drugs have look-alike/sound-alike issues:
>
> Brevibloc and Brevital

Class III Antiarrhythmic Drugs

Amiodarone, dofetilide, dronedarone, ibutilide, ranolazine, sotalol, and vernakalant are class III antiarrhythmic agents. Class III antiarrhythmic drugs prolong depolarization and the refractory period by their action on ion channels. Ibutilide promotes the influx of sodium through slow inward sodium channels. All other class III drugs block potassium channels. Dronedarone is a multichannel ion

Class II Antiarrhythmic Drugs

Generic Name	US Brand Name(s) / Canadian Brand(s)	Dosage Forms and Strengths
acebutolol[a]	Generics Generics	**Capsules**[c]: 100 mg, 200 mg, 400 mg **Tablet**[b]: 100 mg, 200 mg, 400 mg
bisoprolol[a]	Generics Generics	**Tablet:** 5 mg, 10 mg
carvedilol[a]	Coreg, Coreg CR Generics	**Capsule, extended release**[c]: 10 mg, 20 mg, 40 mg, 80 mg **Tablet:** 3.125 mg, 6.25 mg, 12.5 mg, 25 mg
esmolol[a]	Brevibloc, Brevibloc Double Strength Brevibloc	**Solution, injection:** 10 mg/mL (Brevibloc), 20 mg/mL (Brevibloc Double Strength)[c]
propranolol[a]	Inderal LA, InnoPran XL Generics	**Capsules, extended release (Inderal LA, InnoPran XL):** 60 mg, 80 mg, 120 mg, 160 mg **Solution, injection:** 1 mg/mL **Solution, oral**[c]: 20 mg/5 mL, 40 mg/5 mL **Tablets:** 10 mg, 20 mg, 40 mg, 60 mg[c], 80 mg

[a]Generic available.
[b]Available in Canada only.
[c]Available in United States only.

blocker that also inhibits sodium and calcium ion channels. Ranolazine and vernakalant primarily act on the atria. Amiodarone can suppress both supraventricular and ventricular arrhythmias, notably by increasing reentry time. Dofetilide, ibutilide, ranolazine, sotalol, and vernakalant are indicated for the treatment of Afib. Dronedarone is indicated only for the treatment of Afib. Sotalol is also indicated for ventricular tachycardia and atrial flutter.

Adverse Reactions and Precautions

Side effects of amiodarone are photosensitivity, skin discoloration, stomach upset, visual disturbances (sun sensitivity, blurred vision, dry eyes), and corneal deposits. Serious side effects of amiodarone include thyroid disease and fatal hepatotoxicity (amiodarone). Vernakalant produces hypotension, nausea, paresthesia, and taste disturbances (dysgeusia). It is contraindicated in patients who have class III or IV heart failure, acute coronary syndrome, and several other severe heart conditions. Dofetilide is contraindicated in renal failure (creatine clearance <20 mL/min). Ibutilide should be avoided in women who are pregnant or breastfeeding.

❶ Tech Alert!

The following drugs have look-alike/sound-alike issues:

amiodarone and amantadine

Class IV Antiarrhythmic Drugs

Class IV antiarrhythmic agents are calcium channel blockers. Only nondihydropyridine calcium channel blockers (verapamil

Class III Antiarrhythmic Drugs

Generic Name	US Brand Name(s) / Canadian Brand(s)	Dosage Forms and Strengths
amiodarone[a]	Nexterone, Pacerone Generic only	**Solution, injection (Nexterone):** 1.5 mg/mL[b], 1.8 mg/mL[b], 50 mg/mL[c] **Tablets:** 100 mg, 200 mg, 400 mg[b]
dofetilide[a]	Tikosyn Not available	**Capsules:** 0.125 mg, 0.25 mg, 0.5 mg
dronedarone	Multaq Multaq	**Tablets:** 400 mg
ibutilide[ab]	Corvert Corvert	**Solution, injection:** 0.1 mg/mL
ranolazine[a]	Aspruzyo, Ranexa Corzyna	**Granules**[b]: 500 mg, 1000 mg **Tablets, extended release:** 500 mg, 1000 mg[b]
sotalol[a] sotalol AF[a]	Betapace, Betapace AF, Sorine, Sotylize Generics	**Tablets:** 80 mg, 120 mg[b], 160 mg, 240 mg[b], 320 mg[b] **Tablets (AF)**[b]: 40 mg, 60 mg, 80 mg, 100 mg, 120 mg, 160 mg **Solution, injection**[b]: 150 mg/10 mL (15 mg/mL) **Solution, oral (Sotylize)**[b]: 5 mg/mL
vernakalant	Not available Brinavess	**Solution, intravenous:** 20 mg/mL

[a]Generic available.
[b]Available in the United States only.
[c]Available in Canada only.
[ab]Generic available in the United States only.

and diltiazem) are indicated for the treatment of supraventricular arrhythmias, Afib, and atrial flutter. Calcium channel blockers produce headache, flushing, and peripheral edema. Additional adverse reactions and precautions are described in Chapters 17 and 18.

Miscellaneous

Digoxin, a drug used to treat heart failure, is also approved for the treatment of Afib. It reduces arrhythmias by slowing the conduction velocity and prolonging the refractory period in the Purkinje fibers and AV node. In the atria and ventricles, digoxin shortens the refractory period. Digoxin also reduces electrical discharges from the SA node. It may be administered intravenously or orally. Digoxin has a narrow therapeutic index, so it is important to avoid excessive doses. The adverse effects of digoxin are described in Chapter 19.

Drug Used to Prevent Arrhythmias

Arrhythmia management is currently focused on prevention. Prevention is important because Afib is a risk factor for stroke (see Chapter 19). Hypertension doubles the risk for Afib; therefore hypertension should be treated to reduce the risk. Angiotensin-converting enzyme (ACE) inhibitors and angiotensin II receptor blockers (ARBs) type 1 can significantly reduce the risk for first-time Afib in patients with hypertension or heart failure and post–myocardial infarction. The use of ACE inhibitors and ARBs to treat hypertension is discussed in Chapter 18.

TECHNICIAN'S CORNER

1. What is the difference between a palpitation and an arrhythmia?
2. Make a list of antiarrhythmic drugs that are administered parenterally. Make a list of orally administered antiarrhythmic drugs.

Class IV Antiarrhythmic Drugs

Generic Name	US Brand Name(s)	Dosage Forms and Strengths
	Canadian Brand(s)	
diltiazem	Generics	**Solution, injection[b]:** 5 mg/mL
	Generics	
verapamil[a]	Generics	**Solution, injection[b]:** 2.5 mg/mL
	Generics	

[a]Generic available.
[b]See Chapter 18 for additional dosage forms and strengths.

Summary of Drugs Used in the Treatment of Arrhythmia*

Generic Name	Usual Dose and Dosing Schedule	Warning Labels
Antiarrhythmic Drugs		
Class IA		
disopyramide[a]	**Ventricular arrhythmia:** Start with 200–300 mg immediate release; then 400–800 mg/day in divided doses (every 6 h for immediate release or every 12 h for controlled release)	MAY CAUSE DIZZINESS OR DROWSINESS. SWALLOW WHOLE; DO NOT CRUSH OR CHEW—extended release.
procainamide[a]	**Advanced cardiac life support—ventricular arrhythmia:** 20–50 mg/min IV until the arrhythmia is suppressed, or additional conditions met; maintenance infusion rate is 1–4 mg/min OR 100 mg IV every 5 minutes until arrhythmia is controlled or additional conditions are met **Ventricular arrhythmia, life-threatening:** Initial, direct IV injection 100 mg every 5 min to max dose 1 g OR IV loading infusion 20 mg/mL at 1 mL/min for 25–30 min to max dose 1 g; maintenance IV infusion, 2–6 mg/min	TAKE ON AN EMPTY STOMACH—procainamide. AVOID GRAPEFRUIT JUICE—quinidine sulfate. REFRIGERATE; DO NOT FREEZE—Diluted quinidine gluconate solution may be stored for up to 48 h at 4°C (39 °F) or 24 h at room temperature.
quinidine gluconate[a]	**Atrial flutter/atrial fibrillation:** 324–648 mg PO every 8–12 h **Ventricular arrhythmia, life-threatening:** 0.25 mg/kg/min IV infusion until sinus rhythm restored; max total dose 10 mg/kg	
quinidine sulfate[a]	**Atrial flutter/atrial fibrillation/ventricular arrhythmia:** 200–400 mg every 6–8 h (immediate release); 300 mg every 8–12 h (extended release)	

Continued

Summary of Drugs Used in the Treatment of Arrhythmia*—cont'd

	Generic Name	Usual Dose and Dosing Schedule	Warning Labels
Class IB			
	lidocaine[a]	50–100 mg IV infused 25–50 mg/min; may repeat dose in 10 min if necessary **Continuous infusion:** 1–2 mg/min until basic cardiac rhythm is stabilized	MAY CAUSE DIZZINESS OR DROWSINESS. TAKE WITH FOOD—mexiletine.
	mexiletine[a]	**Ventricular arrhythmia:** 200–300 mg every 8 h	
Class IC			
	flecainide[a] (max daily dose of 400 mg)	**Atrial flutter, atrial fibrillation, paroxysmal supraventricular tachycardia:** 50–300 mg/day dosed every 12 h **Ventricular arrhythmia:** 100–400 mg/day dosed every 12 h	DO NOT SKIP OR EXCEED DOSE.
	propafenone[a]	**Atrial flutter, atrial fibrillation, paroxysmal supraventricular tachycardia, ventricular arrhythmia:** 150–300 mg every 8 h (immediate release) **Atrial flutter, atrial fibrillation:** 225–425 mg every 12 h (extended release)	WEAR SUNGLASSES— propafenone. AVOID GRAPEFRUIT JUICE. SWALLOW WHOLE; DO NOT CRUSH OR CHEW—extended release.
Class II			
	acebutolol[a]	**Ventricular arrhythmia:** 400–1200 mg/day in 2–3 divided doses	MAY CAUSE DIZZINESS OR DROWSINESS. CONCENTRATE; MUST BE DILUTED—esmolol. ORAL CONCENTRATE; MUST BE DILUTED—propranolol. SWALLOW WHOLE; DO NOT CRUSH OR CHEW—extended release. DO NOT SKIP DOSES.
	esmolol[a]	**Ventricular/supraventricular tachycardia:** 500 mcg/kg IV loading dose over 1 min **May repeat:** 50–200 mcg/kg/min IV every 4 min based on ventricular response	
	propranolol[a]	**Cardiac dysrhythmia:** 10–30 mg 3–4 times daily (immediate-release tab) **Cardiac dysrhythmia:** 1–3 mg IV (don't exceed 1 mg/min), may repeat after 2 min; additional doses may be given after 4 h	
Class III			
	amiodarone[a]	**Atrial fibrillation prevention (heart surgery):** optimal dosage has not been established; off-label use **Supraventricular arrhythmia:** 400–600 mg/day orally in divided doses for 2–4 weeks, then 100–200 mg orally daily (sinus rhythm maintenance in atrial fibrillation) **Ventricular arrhythmia, life-threatening:** various IV, oral treatment and prophylaxis: initial, 800–1600 mg daily in divided doses for 1–3 weeks, then decrease to 600–800 mg orally daily for 1 month; maintenance, 400–600 mg daily in 1–2 doses	AVOID PROLONGED EXPOSURE TO SUNLIGHT—amiodarone. MAY CAUSE DIZZINESS OR DROWSINESS. AVOID GRAPEFRUIT JUICE— amiodarone, dofetilide, dronedarone, ranolazine. SHOULD NOT BE ADMINISTERED DURING PREGNANCY— ibutilide. TAKE ON AN EMPTY STOMACH— sotalol. AVOID SALT SUBSTITUTES— sotalol. PROTECT FROM MOISTURE— dofetilide. SWALLOW WHOLE; DO NOT CRUSH OR CHEW—extended release. DILUTE BEFORE USE— vernakalant.
	ibutilide	**Atrial arrhythmia:** varies, up to 1 mg/IV infused over at least 10 min; repeat as needed	
	dofetilide	**Atrial fibrillation/atrial flutter:** individualized, up to 1000 mcg/day PO; initiation of dofetilide in a hospitalized setting for a minimum of 3 days	
	dronedarone	**Atrial fibrillation:** 400 mg 2 times a day with meals	
	ranolazine	**Atrial fibrillation/cardioversion:** 750–1000 mg twice a day or 1500 mg as a single dose (off-label dosage for adjunct therapy with amiodarone or dronedarone)	
	sotalol[a]	**Atrial fibrillation, ventricular arrhythmia:** 80–160 mg 2 times a day; Betapace is usually taken twice a day, and Betapace AF is taken once or twice a day	
	vernakalant	**Atrial fibrillation:** 3 mg/kg dosed according to body weight	

Summary of Drugs Used in the Treatment of Arrhythmia*—cont'd

Generic Name	Usual Dose and Dosing Schedule	Warning Labels
Class IV		
verapamil[a]	**Paroxysmal supraventricular tachycardia:** 240–480 mg/day PO in 3–4 divided doses (immediate release) 2.5–5 mg IV over 2–4 min; may repeat 5–10 mg every 15–30 min up to 20 mg IV **Atrial fibrillation/flutter or paroxysmal supraventricular tachycardia:** 240–320 mg daily by mouth in 3–4 divided doses (immediate-release tabs); maximum 480 mg/day **Atrial fibrillation/atrial flutter, paroxysmal supraventricular tachycardia:** 0.075–0.15 mg/kg (5–10 mg) IV over 2–3 min; may give additional 10 mg after 30 min if necessary	TAKE WITH FOOD.
Angiotensin-Converting Enzyme Inhibitors—See Chapter 18		
Angiotensin II Receptor Antagonists Type 1—See Chapter 18		
Miscellaneous		
digoxin[a]	**Atrial fibrillation (rapid digitalization): Loading dose:** 10–15 mcg/kg PO or IV given in 3 divided doses every 6–8 h **Maintenance:** 125–500 mcg PO or IV once a day	TAKE ON AN EMPTY STOMACH. AVOID HIGH-FIBER DIET. ASK PHARMACIST BEFORE TAKING OTC MEDICINES.

[a]Generic available.
*Dosing can vary significantly based on patient-specific factors and the arrhythmia being treated.
IV, Intravenously; *PO,* orally or "by mouth"; *OTC,* over the counter.

Key Points

- An arrhythmia is defined as an irregular heart rhythm or a heart rate that is too rapid or too slow.
- An arrhythmia can impair the heart's ability to distribute blood.
- Atrial fibrillation is the most common arrhythmia; it can increase the risk for stroke.
- Nonmodifiable risk factors for arrhythmia are age and gender.
- Modifiable risk factors for arrhythmia are obesity, smoking, excessive alcohol consumption, and stimulant use.
- Disease-specific risk factors for arrhythmia are hypertension, heart failure, coronary heart disease, previous stroke, infection, diabetes, thyroid disease, and obstructive sleep apnea.
- Ventricular fibrillation is the leading cause of sudden cardiac death.
- Excessive firing, extra currents during the refractory period, and establishment of sinus rhythm by nonpacemaker cells can lead to arrhythmias.
- Antiarrhythmic drugs are categorized into four classes (classes I, II, III, and IV) according to their mechanisms of action and structural similarities.
- Class I antiarrhythmic drugs produce a sodium channel blockade.

- Class I antiarrhythmic drugs reduce automaticity (spontaneous contraction of heart muscle cells), delay conduction, and prolong the time between contractions (refractory period).
- Class II antiarrhythmic drugs are β-adrenergic blockers.
- The β-blockers antagonize stimulation at the AV and SA nodes. They increase the refractory period, decrease automaticity, and slow conduction velocity.
- Class III antiarrhythmic drugs produce potassium channel blockade.
- Class III antiarrhythmic drugs prolong depolarization and the refractory period.
- Class IV antiarrhythmic drugs produce calcium channel blockade.
- Digoxin is approved for the treatment of atrial fibrillation. It reduces arrhythmias by slowing the conduction velocity and prolonging the refractory period in the Purkinje fibers and AV node.
- In the atria and ventricles, digoxin shortens the refractory period. Digoxin also reduces electrical discharges from the SA node.
- The ACE inhibitors and ARBs can significantly reduce the risk for first-time atrial fibrillation in patients with hypertension or heart failure and post–myocardial infarction.

Review Questions

1. Only nondihydropyridine calcium channel blockers (ND-CCBs) are indicated for the treatment of Afib. Select the pair of ND-CCBs.
   a. nifedipine and nicardipine
   b. nisoldipine and isradipine
   c. amlodipine and felodipine
   d. verapamil and diltiazem

2. _____fibrillation is the most common arrhythmia.
   a. Atrial
   b. Ventricular
   c. Aortic
   d. Pulmonary

3. All of the following antiarrhythmic drugs are marketed as a parenteral dosage form EXCEPT _____.
   a. digoxin
   b. ranolazine
   c. esmolol
   d. amiodarone

4. Select the drug that is NOT indicated for the management of atrial arrhythmias.
   a. ranolazine
   b. propranolol
   c. nitroglycerin
   d. sotalol

5. All antiarrhythmic agents are proarrhythmic (can cause other arrhythmias). They also can cause all of the following symptoms except _____.
   a. bradycardia
   b. hypotension
   c. hypertension
   d. dizziness

6. Digoxin has a narrow therapeutic index, so it is important to avoid excessive doses.
   a. true
   b. false

7. Arrhythmia management is currently focused on _____.
   a. cure
   b. prevention
   c. medication
   d. all of the above

8. Select the drug that is classified as an ion channel blocker.
   a. propranolol
   b. verapamil
   c. ranolazine
   d. lidocaine

9. Dofetilide is placed in which class of drugs for arrhythmias?
   a. class I
   b. class II
   c. class III
   d. class IV

10. Select the Brand, generic pair that is INCORRECT.
    a. Cordarone, amiodarone
    b. Corvert, ibutilde
    c. Rhythmol, propranolol
    d. Ranexa, ranolazine

Bibliography

Canadian Cardiovascular Society. The 2020 Canadian Cardiovascular Society/Canadian Heart Rhythm Society Comprehensive Guidelines for the Management of Atrial Fibrillation. *Can J Cardiol.* 2020;361847e1948.

Centers for Disease Control and Prevention. (2022). Heart disease: atrial fibrillation. Retrieved November 4, 2022, from https://www.cdc.gov/heartdisease/atrial_fibrillation.htm.

Correa A, Rochlani Y, Aronow WS. Current pharmacotherapeutic strategies for cardiac arrhythmias in heart failure. *Expert Opin Pharmacother.* 2020;21(3):339–352.

Fragakis N, Vassilikos VP. New antiarrhythmic drugs for atrial fibrillation. *Continuing Cardiol Educ.* 2016;2(3).

Health Canada. (2022). Drug Product Database. Retrieved November 1, 2022, from https://health-products.canada.ca/dpd-bdpp/index-eng.jsp.

Hindricks G, Potpara T, Dagres N, et al. 2020 ESC Guidelines for the diagnosis and management of atrial fibrillation developed in collaboration with the European Association for Cardio-Thoracic Surgery (EACTS). *Eur Heart J.* 2021;42:373–498.

Institute for Safe Medication Practices. (2016). FDA and ISMP Lists of Look-Alike Drug Names with Recommended Tall Man Letters. Retrieved November 1, 2022, from https://www.ismp.org/recommendations/tall-man-letters-list.

Institute for Safe Medication Practices. (2019). List of Confused Drugs. Retrieved November 1, 2022, from https://www.ismp.org/tools/confuseddrugnames.pdf.

Kalant H, Grant D, Mitchell J. *Principles of medical pharmacology.* ed 7. Toronto: Elsevier Canada, A Division of Reed Elsevier Canada; 2007:366–376.

Lance L, Lacy C, Armstrong L, et al. *Drug information handbook for the allied health professional.* ed 12. Hudson, OH: APhA Lexi-Comp; 2005.

Nash M, Mourad A, Clayton R, et al. Evidence for multiple mechanism in human ventricular fibrillation. *Circulation.* 2006;114:536–542.

Page C, Curtis M, Sutter M, et al. *Integrated pharmacology.* Philadelphia: Mosby; 2005:432–446.

U.S. Food and Drug Administration. (nd). Drugs@FDA: FDA Approved Drug Products. Retrieved November 1, 2022, from http://www.accessdata.fda.gov/scripts/cder/daf/.

Zipes DP, et al. ACC/AHA/ESC practice guidelines. *J Am Coll Cardiol.* 2006;48:e268–e270.

UNIT VI

Drugs Affecting the Gastrointestinal System

The organs of the digestive system work together to perform the vital function of preparing food for absorption and for use by the millions of body cells. Digested food must be modified in its chemical composition and physical state so that nutrients can be absorbed and used by the body's cells. Structures of the digestive system are the mouth (lips, cheeks, tongue, and palate), esophagus, stomach, intestines, appendix, liver, gallbladder, and pancreas. To protect the stomach from self-erosion (autodigestion) by digestive juices, epithelial cells in the stomach produce and secrete a bicarbonate-rich solution that coats the stomach mucosa. Bicarbonate is alkaline, a base, and neutralizes the hydrochloric acid secreted by the parietal cells, producing water in the process. Bicarbonate secretions that neutralize the acid from the stomach are also produced in the intestines and pancreas. The end products such as glucose and amino acids are absorbed and enter cells for use as an energy source or for other metabolic functions.

In Unit VI, the pharmacotherapy for gastroesophageal reflux disease (GERD), peptic ulcer disease (PUD), irritable bowel syndrome (IBS), ulcerative colitis, Crohn's disease, constipation, and diarrhea is described. A brief description of each disorder is provided, followed by a description of the drugs indicated for treatment that includes mechanisms of action, adverse reactions, strength(s), dosage forms, OTC or prescription status, and drug schedules. Laxatives and stool softeners used for the treatment of constipation and antidiarrheals used for the treatment of diarrhea are also presented.

21

Treatment of Gastroesophageal Reflux Disease, Laryngopharyngeal Reflux, and Peptic Ulcer Disease

LEARNING OBJECTIVES

1. Learn the terminology associated with gastroesophageal reflux disease (GERD), laryngopharyngeal reflux (LPR), and peptic ulcer disease (PUD).
2. List the symptoms of GERD, LPR, and PUD.
3. List risk factors for GERD and PUD.
4. List and categorize medications used to treat GERD, LPR, and PUD.
5. Describe mechanism of action for drugs used to treat GERD, LPR, and PUD.
6. Identify significant drug look-alike and sound-alike issues.
7. List common endings for drug classes used for the treatment of GERD, LPR, and PUD.
8. Identify warning labels and precautionary messages associated with medications used to treat GERD and PUD.

KEY TERMS

Duodenal ulcer Ulcer located in the upper portion of the small intestine or duodenum.

Gastric ulcer Ulcer located in the stomach.

Gastroesophageal reflux A condition whereby the stomach contents occasionally flow up into the esophagus, producing heartburn.

Gastroesophageal reflux disease Motility disorder associated with impaired peristalsis that results in persistent backflow of gastric contents into the esophagus.

Hiatal hernia Condition in which the lower esophageal sphincter shifts above the diaphragm.

Laryngopharyngeal reflux Reflux of gastric contents into the larynx and pharynx.

Lower esophageal sphincter A ring of muscle separating the esophagus and the stomach that permits food and liquids to pass into the stomach and prevents stomach contents from returning to the esophagus.

Peptic ulcer disease Term used to describe ulcers located in the duodenum or stomach.

Peristalsis Forceful wave of contractions in the esophagus that moves food and liquids from the mouth to the stomach.

Reflux Backflow of gastric contents into esophagus or laryngopharyngeal region.

Ulcer Open wound or sore.

Upper esophageal sphincter A ring of muscle separating the pharynx and esophagus.

Overview

Gastroesophageal reflux disease (GERD), *peptic ulcer disease* (PUD), and *laryngopharyngeal reflux* (LPR) are diseases that affect millions of Americans and Canadians. Direct and indirect health care costs (e.g., missed days of work) are estimated to be greater than $10 billion annually.

Gastroesophageal Reflux Disease

Gastroesophageal reflux (GER) is a condition whereby the stomach contents flow up into the esophagus, producing symptoms described as heartburn. Persistent GER, more than twice a week, is a sign of GERD. GERD is estimated to affect up to 20% of the global population.

GER and GERD may initially produce minor discomfort, such as heartburn and chronic cough. Excessive or chronic exposure to gastric acid, pepsin, and bile may produce inflammation, ulceration, or hemorrhage and changes to the epithelial cells that can lead to esophageal or stomach cancer. Persons of any age can develop GERD. Infants may have GERD because their digestive system is immature; however, many will outgrow GERD by their first birthday. Obesity, smoking, and pregnancy are additional risk factors.

What Causes Reflux?

GERD is a motility disorder associated with impaired peristalsis. *Peristalsis* is a forceful wave of contractions in the esophagus that moves food and other orally ingested contents from the mouth to the stomach. The ***lower esophageal sphincter*** (LES) is a muscle located at the junction between the esophagus and upper stomach that relaxes to permit food and liquids to pass from the esophagus into the stomach and then contracts to prevent stomach contents from returning to the esophagus. GER occurs when there is a buildup of pressure in the stomach causing the LES to open and leak stomach contents back up into the esophagus.

Normally the LES lies below the diaphragm, which helps to keep the stomach contents from flowing back into the esophagus. Delayed gastric emptying or transient relaxation of the LES, especially after eating, may also cause reflux.

Hiatal hernia is a significant risk factor for GERD in persons older than 50 years. When a hiatal hernia occurs, the diaphragm muscle is unable to hold the LES in normal position, and the sphincter shifts above the diaphragm. Larger hiatal hernias are linked to more severe esophagitis (Fig. 21.1).

Factors Contributing to Gastroesophageal Reflux Disease

Many factors can aggravate GERD; these include foods, lifestyle, prescription and over-the-counter (OTC) medicines, and even body position. Foods that can aggravate GERD are listed in Table 21.1. Lifestyle factors that aggravate GERD include alcohol consumption and cigarette smoking. GERD symptoms are made worse when the body is in a prone position (lying down).

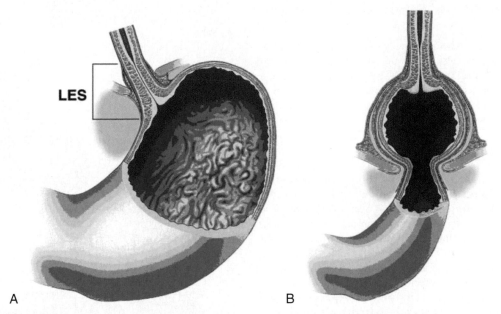

LES

A   B

• **Fig. 21.1** Gastroesophageal junction. (**A**) Location of the lower esophageal sphincter *(LES)*. (**B**) Hiatal hernia. (Courtesy Dr. J.T. Laitman, Mount Sinai School of Medicine, Center for Anatomy and Functional Morphology, New York.)

TABLE 21.1	Natural Alternatives for Gastroesophageal Reflux Disease	
Safe Foods	**Food to Avoid**	**Natural Alternative**
Fruits—apples, bananas	Fruits—tomatoes, citrus fruits and juice (e.g., lemon)	Magnesium oxide—increases lower esophageal sphincter tone
Vegetables—broccoli, carrots, cabbage, peas, green beans, baked potato	Juice—orange juice, cranberry juice, grapefruit juice, fried vegetables (e.g., French fries), raw onion, garlic, mint	Almonds—chew on a few almonds after each meal
Meat products—skinless chicken breast, extra lean ground beef, London broil, egg whites and substitutes, nonfatty fish	Fried and fatty meat products—ground beef, chicken nuggets, buffalo wings, marbled sirloin	Fennel tea or chamomile tea—soothing effect, sip slowly
Dairy—fat-free cream cheese, goat cheese, low-fat soy cheese, fat-free sour cream	Dairy products—regular cottage cheese, sour cream, ice cream, milk shake	Ginger (any form)—reduces acid in stomach
Grains—brown or white rice, multigrain or white bread, cereal (e.g., bran, oatmeal), cornbread, graham crackers, pretzels, rice cakes	Grains—spaghetti (pasta) with tomato sauce, macaroni and cheese	Organic apple cider—shake well; pulp contains enzymes to reduce acid
Salad—low-fat salad dressing	Salad—creamy and oil and vinegar salad dressings	Chewing gum—produces saliva, which dilutes stomach acid
Sweets, fat-free (e.g., fat-free cookies, jellybeans, red licorice, baked potato chips)	Sweets, high fat (e.g., butter cookies, chocolate, doughnuts, corn chips, brownies)	
Beverage—mineral water	Beverages—wine, liquor, caffeinated beverages (e.g., coffee, tea, cola)	

Raising the head of the bed 6 to 8 inches can reduce symptoms. Pregnancy and obesity can also aggravate GERD. Many prescription and OTC medicines can worsen GERD (Box 21.1). These drugs impair peristalsis, delay gastric emptying, decrease esophageal sphincter tone, decrease the protective mucosal lining, and/or increase gastric acid levels.

Laryngopharyngeal Reflux

LPR is closely related to GERD and can occur simultaneously. When gastric contents reflux into the larynx and pharynx, located in the head and neck region, inflammation occurs that may cause hoarseness, voice fatigue, laryngitis, sore throat, chronic cough, bad breath, sinusitis, wheezing, aggravation of asthma, and even middle ear infections.

As in GERD, LPR occurs when the normal reflux barriers fail. Anatomic barriers that protect against LPR are the gastroesophageal junction (includes the LES) and the ***upper esophageal sphincter*** (UES). The UES separates the pharynx and esophagus. It relaxes to permit the passage of food and liquids during swallowing, prevent air from entering the esophagus during breathing, and prevent gastric secretions from entering the pharynx via the esophagus. If the UES is damaged by exposure to stomach contents, it can become less sensitive and lose its ability to function properly. This increases the likelihood of reflux and more damage (Fig. 21.2). Laryngeal mucosal resistance protects the larynx from damage caused by reflux.

Peptic Ulcer Disease

An ***ulcer*** is an open wound or sore. Ulcers can occur anywhere on the body. In the gastrointestinal (GI) tract, ***gastric ulcers*** form in the stomach (Fig. 21.3), ***duodenal ulcers*** form in the upper region of the small intestines, and peptic ulcers form in the stomach or duodenum.

Risk Factors for Peptic Ulcer Disease

Helicobacter pylori infection is the primary cause of PUD. Almost two-thirds of the global population have the infection. More than 90% of people who have duodenal ulcers and 80% of people who have gastric ulcers are infected with *H. pylori*. *H. pylori* infection is also a risk factor for the development of stomach cancer. Worldwide, most people infected with *H. pylori* develop the infection in childhood. Infections are transmitted person to person by the gastric-oral route. Once the bacteria are ingested, they release

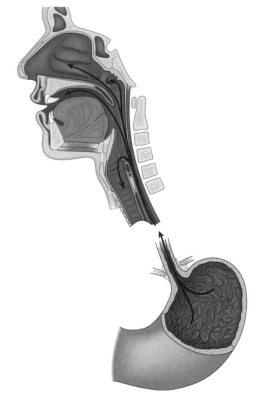

• **Fig. 21.2** Laryngopharyngeal reflux—direction of backflow into head and neck regions. (Courtesy Dr. J.T. Laitman, Mount Sinai School of Medicine, Center for Anatomy and Functional Morphology, New York.)

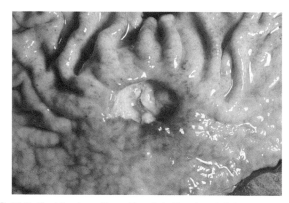

• **FIG. 21.3** Gastric ulcer. (From Rosai J: *Rosai and Ackerman's surgical pathology*, ed 9, Philadelphia, 2004, Mosby.)

buffers that enable the bacteria to survive in the acidic contents of the stomach. The bacteria also release virulence factors that are responsible for inflammation and tissue damage. Fortunately, most people who are infected with *H. pylori* will not develop chronic gastritis or PUD. Researchers are working to develop a vaccine that can be administered in childhood to prevent *H. pylori* infection. Persons with a family history of ulcers or living with close relatives who have PUD, those older than 50 years, and people who use medicines such as salicylates (e.g., aspirin), nonsteroidal antiinflammatory drugs (NSAIDs) (e.g., naproxen), and corticosteroids (e.g., prednisone) are at increased risk for PUD.

TABLE 21.2	**Symptoms of Gastroesophageal Reflux Disease, Laryngopharyngeal Reflux, and Peptic Ulcer Disease**	
Disease	Unique Symptoms	Common Symptoms
Gastroesophageal reflux disease	Difficulty swallowing Dry cough Bad breath Bloated stomach Rumbling noise in stomach Belching or burping Respiratory problems Hoarseness	Heartburn Stomachache Hunger pains Nausea or vomiting Chest pain
Laryngopharyngeal reflux	Hoarseness Voice fatigue or breaks Sore throat Excessive phlegm or saliva Chronic cough Bad breath Middle ear infection Wheezing Chronic sinusitis	
Peptic ulcer disease	Burning pain in the gut beginning 2–3 h after a meal Weight loss Loss of appetite	

When a person exhibits symptoms of PUD, several simple tests can be performed to see whether the person has an *H. pylori* infection. A sample of blood may be drawn to look for antibodies and other evidence of past or current infection, or a breath test may be done to check for evidence of urease, an enzyme released by *H. pylori*. An endoscopy may be performed to look for ulcers inside the stomach and small intestine using an endoscope, a thin flexible tube with a small video camera and light attached to one end that is passed down the esophagus into the stomach.

Symptoms of Gastroesophageal Reflux Disease, Laryngopharyngeal Reflux, and Peptic Ulcer Disease

Some of the symptoms of GERD, LPR, and PUD are common to all three conditions, whereas others are disease specific. Symptoms associated with GERD, LPR, and PUD are categorized in Table 21.2.

Lifestyle Modification

Lifestyle changes to reduce the risk for GERD and PUD or their symptoms include eating small, frequent meals; avoiding foods that aggravate GERD and PUD; limiting alcohol consumption; and stopping smoking. Cigarette smoking interferes with the healing of an ulcer by constricting blood vessels in the ulcerated area. Alcohol is a gastric irritant. See Box 21.2 for lifestyle modifications recommended for people with GERD and PUD.

• BOX 21.2	**Lifestyle Modifications Recommended for People With Gastroesophageal Reflux Disease or Peptic Ulcer Disease**

- Avoid lying down after eating (wait at least 3 hours).
- Elevate the head of the bed 6 to 8 inches.
- Eat small meals.
- Lose weight if you are overweight.
- Quit smoking if you smoke.
- Do not drink alcohol.
- Limit use of aspirin and nonsteroidal antiinflammatory drugs.

Drugs Used in the Treatment of Gastroesophageal Reflux Disease, Laryngopharyngeal Reflux, and Peptic Ulcer Disease

The treatment of GERD, LPR, and PUD is aimed at reducing GI irritants (e.g., volume of gastric acid and digestive enzymes such as pepsin) and increasing protective factors (e.g., mucus secretion by epithelial cells). Drugs used in the treatment of PUD, GERD, and LPR are classified according to their pharmacologic effects: (1) acid-suppressing drugs (e.g., histamine 2 [H2] receptor antagonists, proton pump inhibitors [PPIs]); (2) mucosal protectants (e.g., prostaglandins, sucralfate, alginates); (3) prokinetic drugs (e.g., metoclopramide); (4) acid-neutralizing drugs (e.g., antacids); and (5) drugs that eliminate *H. pylori* (e.g., antiinfective drugs).

> **● Tech Note!**
>
> It is a myth that stress and spicy foods can cause ulcers; however, some foods can aggravate existing GERD (see Table 21.1).

> **● Tech Note!**
>
> A common ending for H2 blockers is -*tidine*.

Histamine 2 Receptor Antagonist Drugs

There are four H2 receptor antagonists marketed in the United States and Canada—cimetidine, famotidine, nizatidine, and ranitidine. All H2 receptor antagonists are available in prescription and nonprescription strengths.

Mechanism of Action and Pharmacokinetics

Histamine stimulates acid secretion by gastric parietal cells. H2 receptor antagonists competitively and reversibly bind to H2 receptors, blocking histamine-mediated acid secretion. The secretion of pepsin, a digestive enzyme, occurs when the volume of acid in the stomach is high, such as when food is present in the stomach. Pepsin secretion decreases as gastric acid levels decrease. Chronic exposure to pepsin can cause inflammation and peptic ulcers.

The effect of H2 receptor antagonists on nocturnal (nighttime) acid secretion is significantly greater than on acid secretion after meals. The duration of effect on nocturnal secretion ranges from

8 hours (cimetidine) to 13 hours (ranitidine). The duration of effect on secretion after meals is reduced to 3 to 5 hours. The most potent H2 receptor antagonist is ranitidine. It is approximately 10 times more effective than cimetidine.

Adverse Reactions

H2 receptor antagonists can produce dizziness or drowsiness, constipation or diarrhea, bloating, headache, and confusion when taken at therapeutic doses. Older adults are more susceptible to these adverse effects. Less common adverse effects include skin rash, agitation, depression, hepatitis, and decreased libido. High-dose cimetidine may produce breast swelling or tenderness in males (gynecomastia).

Precautions

Cimetidine inhibits several metabolic enzymes and is responsible for increasing the elimination of more than 25 different drugs. The pharmacist should be alerted to all drug interactions that are flagged by prescription-filling software.

❶ Tech Alert!

The following drugs have look-alike/sound-alike issues:
raNITIdine, riMANTAdine;
Zantac, Xanax, and ZyrTEC

Proton Pump Inhibitor Drugs

There are six PPIs currently marketed in the United States and Canada—dexlansoprazole, esomeprazole, lansoprazole, omeprazole, pantoprazole, and rabeprazole. Esomeprazole is an S isomer (mirror image) of omeprazole. PPIs are effective in treating GERD, LPR, and PUD because they decrease gastric acid levels. They are more potent than H2 receptor antagonists. Esomeprazole, lansoprazole, and omeprazole are available OTC. All other PPIs are only commercially available in prescription strengths. OTC PPIs are marketed for the treatment of heartburn.

● Tech Note!

PPIs have the common ending -prazole.

Mechanism of Action and Pharmacokinetics

PPIs decrease gastric acids by interfering with the final step in gastric acid production. PPIs interfere with hydrogen and potassium ion exchange via the H^+/K^+-ATPase proton pump located on parietal cells in the stomach. Maximum effects are not achieved until there is sufficient drug in the parietal cells to inhibit the proton pumps.

PPIs can be destroyed in gastric acids. Zegerid is a formulation combining an antacid with omeprazole to reduce the destruction of omeprazole by gastric acids. PPIs are delayed-release formulations.

Histamine 2 Receptor Antagonists (H2 Blockers)

	Generic Name	US Brand Name(s) / Canadian Brand Name(s)	Dosage Forms and Strengths
	cimetidine[a]	Tagamet HB[b]	**Tablet:** 200 mg[b] **Solution, oral:** 300 mg/5 mL
		Tagamet Prevent[b]	
	famotidine[a]	Pepcid AC, Zantac 360 Maximum Strength	**Tablet:** 10 mg[b], 20 mg[b], 40 mg **Tablet, chewable:** 20 mg[b,c] **Injection, solution:** 10 mg/mL **Powder for oral suspension:** 40 mg/5 mL[c]
		Pepcid AC[b]	
	nizatidine[a]	Axid AR[b]	**Capsule:** 150 mg, 300 mg **Tablet:** 75 mg[b]
		Generics	
	ranitidine[a]	Zantac, Zantac-75[b], Zantac-150[b], Zantac-300	**Capsule**[c]**:** 150 mg, 300 mg **Tablet:** 75 mg[b], 150 mg, 300 mg **Injection, solution**[c]**:** 25 mg/mL **Oral solution/syrup**[c]**:** 15 mg/mL
		Zantac Maximum Strength Nonprescription	

H2 Receptor Antagonist Combinations

	famotidine + calcium carbonate + magnesium hydroxide	Pepcid Complete[b]	10 mg famotidine + 800 mg calcium carbonate + 165 mg magnesium hydroxide
		Pepcid Complete[b]	

[a]Generic available.
[b]Available over the counter in Canada and the United States.
[c]Available in the United States only.

They must not be crushed or chewed. Delayed-release tablets disintegrate in less than 1 minute.

Adverse Reactions

All the PPIs have a similar side effect profile. More common side effects are abdominal pain, headache, diarrhea or constipation, flatulence (gas), and nausea. Less common side effects are jaundice, skin rash, unusual tiredness or fatigue, agitation, vitamin B_{12} deficiency, dark yellow or brown urine, and vomiting.

> **🛈 Tech Alert!**
>
> The following drugs have look-alike/sound-alike issues:
> PriLOSEC and PROzac;
> Losec and Lasix;
> Protonix and protamine;
> RABEprazole and ARIPiprazole;
> Aciphex and Aricept

Proton Pump Inhibitors

	Generic Name	US Brand Name(s) / Canadian Brand Name(s)	Dosage Forms and Strengths
	dexlansoprazole[a]	Dexilant	**Capsules, delayed release:** 30 mg, 60 mg
		Generics	
	esomeprazole	Nexium, Nexium 24 HR[b]	**Capsules, delayed release:** 20 mg[b], 40 mg
		Nexium, Nexium 24 HR[b]	**Powder for oral suspension[c]:** 2.5 mg, 5 mg, 10 mg, 20 mg, 40 mg/packet **Powder for injection[c]:** 40 mg/vial **Tablet, delayed release[b]:** 20 mg
	lansoprazole[a]	Prevacid, Prevacid 24 HR[b]	**Capsules, delayed release (Prevacid, Prevacid 24 HR):** 15 mg[b], 30 mg
		Generics	**Tablets, disintegrating (Prevacid FasTab):** 15 mg, 30 mg
	omeprazole[a]	Prilosec, Prilosec OTC[b]	**Capsules, delayed release:** 10 mg[b], 20 mg[b,c], 40 mg[c] **Granules for suspension[c]:** 2.5 mg, 10 mg
		Losec, Losec MUPS	**Tablets, disintegrating[b,c]:** 20 mg **Tablets, delayed release:** 10 mg[b], 20 mg[b,c]
	pantoprazole sodium[a] pantoprazole magnesium	Protonix	**Granules, for oral suspension:** 40 mg[c] **Powder, for injection:** 40 mg base per vial
		Pantoloc, Tecta	**Tablet, delayed release, as sodium salt (Protonix, Pantoloc):** 20 mg, 40 mg **Tablet, enteric coated, as magnesium salt (Tecta):** 40 mg
	rabeprazole[a]	Aciphex	**Tablet, delayed release:** 10 mg[d], 20 mg
		Pariet	

PPI Combination Products

	Generic Name	US Brand Name(s) / Canadian Brand Name(s)	Dosage Forms and Strengths
	esomeprazole + naproxen[a]	Vimovo	**Tablet:** 20 mg esomeprazole + 375 mg naproxen, 20 mg esomeprazole + 500 mg naproxen[c]
		Vimovo	
	lansoprazole + amoxicillin + clarithromycin	Generic only	**Combo pack:** 30 mg lansoprazole capsule + 500 mg amoxicillin capsule + 500 mg clarithromycin tablet
		Generic	
	omeprazole + sodium bicarbonate	Zegerid, Zegerid OTC[b]	**Capsule:** 20 mg omeprazole + 1100 mg sodium bicarbonate[b], 40 mg omeprazole + 1100 mg sodium bicarbonate
		Not available	**Powder, for oral suspension:** 20 mg omeprazole + 1680 mg sodium bicarbonate[b] 40 mg omeprazole + 1680 mg sodium bicarbonate

[a]Generic available.
[b]Available over the counter.
[c]Available in the United States only.
[d]Available in Canada only.
OTC, over the counter.

Mucosal Protectants

Misoprostol and sucralfate are mucosal protectants. The drugs protect the epithelial cells that line the stomach and small intestine from damage by gastric acids, pepsin, and *H. pylori*. The drug is approved for the prevention of NSAID-induced peptic ulcers. Sucralfate is approved for the treatment and maintenance therapy of duodenal ulcers.

Mechanism of Action

Misoprostol is a synthetic prostaglandin E (PGE). It stimulates the production of protective mucus and bicarbonate in the stomach. It also increases the regeneration of gastric epithelial cells and enhances blood flow to the stomach.

Sucralfate binds to the ulcerated area and forms a protective barrier, much like a bandage protects a sore. It also promotes the regeneration of stomach epithelial cells. It is a weak inhibitor of *H. pylori*.

Adverse Reactions and Precautions

Misoprostol may produce abdominal cramps, diarrhea, menstrual irregularities, headache, and dizziness. It is contraindicated in pregnancy because it stimulates uterine contractions. Sucralfate may produce constipation, gas, dry mouth, and headache.

Sucralfate can block the absorption of several drugs, including H2 receptor antagonists, PPIs, and some antibiotics. To avoid drug interactions, the drugs should not be taken at the same time as sucralfate.

> **● Tech Note!**
>
> Misoprostol is labeled with a boxed warning that the drug may stimulate uterine contractions.

> **❶ Tech Alert!**
>
> The following drugs have look-alike/sound-alike issues:
> miSOPROStol and miFEPRIStone

Prokinetic Drugs

Prokinetic drugs are used for the treatment of GERD and LPR. They increase peristalsis (the wavelike movement throughout the GI tract), speed up gastric emptying, and improve LES tone.

Mucosal Protectant Drugs

Generic Name	US Brand Name(s) / Canadian Brand Name(s)	Dosage Forms and Strengths
misoprostol[a]	Cytotec	**Tablet:** 0.1 mg, 0.2 mg
	Generics	
sucralfate[a]	Carafate	**Suspension, oral:** 1 g/5 mL[b], 1 g/10 mL[c]
	Sulcrate, Sulcrate Suspension Plus	**Tablet:** 1 g

[a]Generic available.
[b]Available in Canada only.
[c]Available in the United States only.

Metoclopramide is currently the only prokinetic drug approved by the US Food and Drug Administration (FDA). Domperidone is approved in Canada for the symptomatic management of motility disorders associated with chronic gastritis and diabetic gastroparesis.

Mechanism of Action

Metoclopramide increases peristalsis by stimulating the release of acetylcholine in the periphery and increasing cholinergic activity. Domperidone blocks peripheral dopamine receptors to increase peristalsis. Both drugs enhance gastroduodenal coordination. Metoclopramide and domperidone block dopamine receptors centrally, which also decreases nausea.

Adverse Reactions

Common adverse effects associated with metoclopramide and domperidone include diarrhea, abdominal pain, constipation, restlessness, dizziness, and headache. Metoclopramide may cause drowsiness. Less common effects are leg cramps, skin rash, irregular heartbeat, and breast enlargement in men and women.

Antacids and Alginates

Antacids are one of the oldest drugs used for the treatment of GERD and PUD. Antacid use has declined since more potent drugs, requiring fewer daily doses, have been developed. Antacids can be obtained without prescription. Alginates are OTC agents that prevent reflux into the esophagus by creating a physical barrier protectant above the stomach contents. Alginates also inhibit pepsin and bile. Alginates are often found in antacid preparations.

Mechanism of Action

Antacids neutralize gastric acids and decrease pepsin secretion. The acid-neutralizing capacity (ANC) is a standard used to evaluate the potency of antacids. The ANC is a measure of the ability of an antacid to do the following: (1) neutralize approximately

Prokinetic Drugs

Generic Name	US Brand Name(s) / Canadian Brand Name(s)	Dosage Forms and Strengths
metoclopramide[a]	Gimoti, Reglan	**Nasal spray:** 15 mg/spray (Gimoti)
	Generics	**Tablet, oral disintegrating tablet:** 5 mg[b]
		Tablet: 5 mg, 10 mg[b]
		Solution, for injection: 5 mg/mL
		Solution, oral: 1 mg/mL
domperidone[a]	Not available	**Tablet:** 10 mg
	Generics	

[a]Generic available.
[b]Available in the United States only.

1 to 2 ounces hydrochloric acid (i.e., the volume of acid normally present between meals), and (2) raise the pH of the stomach to 3.5 within 10 minutes. Alginates are polysaccharide polymers. When alginates come in contact with acids, they form a gel-like barrier that prevents reflux of gastric contents.

Adverse Reactions

The side effects of antacids are related to their active ingredient and are dose related. Magnesium-containing antacids cause diarrhea; aluminum-containing antacids cause constipation and, in high doses, deplete phosphate levels in blood (hypophosphatemia). Calcium-containing antacids cause constipation and, in high doses, produce hypercalcemia and kidney stones. Sodium bicarbonate (baking soda) has been associated with rebound hyperacidity, metabolic alkalosis, edema, and hypertension.

Antimicrobials

Antimicrobial drugs are prescribed for the treatment of PUD to eradicate *H. pylori* infection. Clarithromycin, metronidazole, amoxicillin, and tetracycline are effective for eradicating *H. pylori*. They are prescribed in combination with drugs that decrease gastric acids and protect the gastric mucosa. Antimicrobial drugs will be described in detail in Chapter 29.

TECHNICIAN'S CORNER

1. Describe the function of the lower esophageal sphincter and how it is affected by gastroesophageal reflux disease.
2. Describe how alcohol consumption and cigarette smoking increase the risk for peptic ulcer disease and can aggravate existing disease. How do they interfere with healing of an ulcer?

Examples of Selected Antacids

Generic Name	US Brand Name(s) / Canadian Brand Name(s)
aluminum hydroxide[a]	Alternagel, Amphojel
	Not available
aluminum hydroxide + magnesium hydroxide[a]	Mag-Al, Mylanta Ultimate, Gaviscon Extra Strength
	Gelusil, Rolaids Extra Strength
aluminum hydroxide + magnesium hydroxide + simethicone	Mylanta Maximum Strength, Mylanta Regular Strength, Gelusil Antacid & Anti-Gas tablets for heartburn relief
	Diovol Plus
calcium carbonate[a]	Caltrate, Pepto Bismol Children's Chewable, Rolaids Extra Strength, TUMS, TUMS EX, TUMS Ultra, TUMS Chewy Bites Extra Strength
	Caltrate, TUMS, TUMS Ultra, TUMS Extra Strength
calcium carbonate + magnesium hydroxide[a]	Rolaids Chewable, Rolaids Extra Strength Chewable, Rolaids Ultra Strength, Mylanta Supreme Suspension, Mylanta Ultra Chewable
	Not available
calcium carbonate + simethicone	Titralac Plus, Tums Plus
	Rolaids Extra Strength Plus Gas
sodium alginate + calcium carbonate + aluminum hydroxide	Gaviscon
	Gaviscon, Gaviscon Max Relief, Gaviscon Extra Strength Liquid
alginic acid + magnesium carbonate	Gaviscon Extra Strength Chewable
	Gaviscon Extra Strength Chewable Foamtabs, Gaviscon Max Relief Chewable tabs
alginic acid + calcium carbonate	Not available
	Gaviscon Advanced Strength Chewable Mini Foamtabs
calcium carbonate + magnesium hydroxide + simethicone	Mylanta Coat & Cool, Mylanta Tonight, Rolaids Advanced
anhydrous citric acid + potassium bicarbonate + sodium bicarbonate	Alka Seltzer Gold

[a]Generic available.

Summary of Drugs Used for Treatment of Gastroesophageal Reflux Disease, Laryngopharyngeal Reflux, and Peptic Ulcer Disease

	Generic Name	US Brand Name	Usual Adult Oral Dosage and Dosing Schedule	Warning Labels
H2 Receptor Antagonists				
	cimetidine	Tagamet	**PUD:** 800 mg daily at bedtime or 400 mg twice daily or 300 mg 4 times daily for 8–12 weeks; Maintenance: 400 mg daily at bedtime **GERD:** 800 mg twice daily or 400 mg 4 times daily for 12 weeks	AVOID ANTACIDS WITHIN 2 HOURS OF DOSE (CIMETIDINE, NIZATIDINE). AVOID ALCOHOL—all. SHAKE SUSPENSION WELL. DISCARD FAMOTIDINE ORAL SUSPENSION 30 DAYS AFTER MIXING. STORE INJECTION IN THE REFRIGERATOR— famotidine, ranitidine. STORE INJECTION AT ROOM TEMPERATURE—cimetidine.
	famotidine	Pepcid	**PUD:** 40 mg once daily at bedtime or 20 mg twice daily for 4–8 weeks **GERD:** 20–40 mg twice daily for 6–12 weeks	
	nizatidine	Axid	**PUD:** 150 mg every 12 h or 300 mg at bedtime for up to 8 weeks **GERD:** 150 mg every 12 h for up to 12 weeks **Indigestion/heartburn:** 75 mg 30–60 min before food/beverage up to 150 mg/day	
	ranitidine	Zantac	**PUD:** 150 mg twice daily or 300 mg once daily at bedtime for 4–6 weeks **GERD:** 150 mg twice daily for 4–8 weeks **Indigestion/heartburn:** 75–150 mg orally 30–60 min before eating or drinking; max 300 mg/day	
Proton Pump Inhibitors				
	dexlansoprazole	Dexilant	**GERD:** 30 mg once or twice daily	SWALLOW WHOLE; DO NOT CRUSH OR CHEW (CAPSULES CAN BE SPRINKLED ONTO FOOD BUT DO NOT CRUSH THE CONTENTS INTO THE FOOD). DELAYED RELEASE—TAKE 30 MINUTES BEFORE A MEAL— lansoprazole. TAKE 60 MINUTES BEFORE A MEAL—esomeprazole. GRANULES FOR ORAL SUSPENSION MUST BE MIXED WITH 1–2 TABLESPOONFULS OF LIQUID. ALLOW MIXTURE TO STAND FOR 2–3 MINUTES, THEN IMMEDIATELY DRINK ENTIRE MIXTURE. DISSOLVE DISINTEGRATING TABLETS ON TONGUE.
	esomeprazole	Nexium	**PUD:** 40 mg daily in 1–2 divided doses as part of *H. pylori* triple drug therapy regimen **GERD:** 20–40 mg once daily for up to 4–8 weeks **Indigestion/heartburn:** 20 mg once daily for 14 days	
	lansoprazole	Prevacid	**PUD:** 15 mg once daily in the morning for up to 4 weeks or 30 mg twice daily as part of *H. pylori* triple and quadruple drug therapy regimens **GERD:** 15–30 mg once daily in the morning for up to 8 weeks **Indigestion/heartburn:** 15 mg orally once a day for 14 days	
	omeprazole	Prilosec	**PUD:** 40 mg once daily for 4–8 weeks or 20 mg twice daily as part of *H. pylori* triple drug therapy regimen **GERD:** 20 mg once daily for 4–8 weeks **Indigestion/heartburn:** 20 mg once daily for 14 days	
	pantoprazole	Protonix	**PUD:** 40 mg once daily after the morning meal for 4–8 weeks **GERD:** 40 mg once daily for up to 8 weeks	
	rabeprazole	Aciphex	**PUD:** 20 mg once daily after the morning meal for 3–6 weeks or 20–40 mg twice daily as part of the *H. pylori* triple drug therapy regimen **GERD:** 20 mg once daily for 4 weeks; repeat course of treatment if necessary	

Summary of Drugs Used for Treatment of Gastroesophageal Reflux Disease, Laryngopharyngeal Reflux, and Peptic Ulcer Disease —cont'd

	Generic Name	US Brand Name	Usual Adult Oral Dosage and Dosing Schedule	Warning Labels
Prokinetic Drugs				
	metoclopramide	Reglan	**GERD:** 10–15 mg up to 4 times a day	MAY CAUSE DROWSINESS. AVOID ALCOHOL. TAKE 15–30 MINUTES BEFORE MEALS.
	domperidone	Generics	10 mg 3–4 times a day	
Mucosal Protectants				
	misoprostol	Cytotec	**NSAID-induced PUD prevention:** 100–200 mcg 4 times a day for 4–8 weeks	AVOID PREGNANCY.
	sucralfate	Carafate	**Duodenal ulcer:** 1 g 4 times a day for 4–8 weeks	TAKE ON AN EMPTY STOMACH. SHAKE SUSPENSION WELL.
Antimicrobial Combinations for _H. pylori_ Eradication				
	lansoprazole + amoxicillin + clarithromycin	Generic	**_H. pylori_-associated ulcer:** 2 amoxicillin caps + 1 lansoprazole cap + 1 clarithromycin tablet twice daily for 10–14 days	SWALLOW WHOLE; DO NOT CRUSH OR CHEW. MAY DECREASE EFFECTIVENESS OF ORAL CONTRACEPTIVES. AVOID ALCOHOL—Talicia. TAKE WITH FOOD—Talicia.
	amoxicillin + omeprazole + rifabutin*	Talicia	**_H. pylori_-associated ulcer:** Take 4 capsules every 8 h for 14 days	

GERD, Gastroesophageal reflux disease; _NSAID_, nonsteroidal antiinflammatory drug; _PUD_, peptic ulcer disease.
*Rifabutin is a rifamycin antibacterial drug.

Key Points

- GERD, PUD, and LPR are diseases that affect millions of Americans and Canadians.
- GERD causes a chronic backflow (*reflux*) of acidic stomach contents and digestive enzymes up into the esophagus.
- Excessive or chronic exposure to gastric acids can lead to inflammation, ulceration, and changes to the epithelial cells that can cause stomach cancer.
- GERD may increase the risk for development of chronic disease, such as asthma.
- Hiatal hernia is a significant risk factor for GERD in persons older than 50 years.
- Fried food, mint, tomato-based foods, and citrus fruits are some foods that can aggravate GERD.
- Consumption of caffeinated beverages and alcohol and cigarette smoking are lifestyle factors that make GERD symptoms worse.
- Prescription and over-the-counter medicines can aggravate GERD.
- LPR occurs when gastric contents reflux into the larynx and pharynx.
- LPR causes hoarseness, voice fatigue, laryngitis, sore throat, chronic cough, bad breath, sinusitis, wheezing, aggravation of asthma, and even middle ear infections.
- Almost two-thirds of the world's population are infected with *H. pylori*, the primary cause of PUD.
- Medicines that can cause the development of ulcers are salicylates (e.g., aspirin), nonsteroidal antiinflammatory drugs (e.g., naproxen), and corticosteroids (e.g., prednisone).
- The treatment of GERD, LPR, and PUD is aimed at reducing GI irritants (e.g., gastric acid, digestive enzymes such as pepsin) and increasing protective factors (e.g., mucus secretion by epithelial cells).
- Acid-neutralizing drugs (antacids), acid-suppressing drugs (PPIs and H2 receptor antagonists), and mucosal protectants (e.g., misoprostol, sucralfate, alginates) are used to treat GERD, LPR, and PUD.
- Treatment of PUD also involves eliminating *H. pylori* infection with antimicrobial agents.
- Prokinetic drugs (e.g., metoclopramide) increase GI motility.
- The four H2 receptor antagonists marketed in the United States and Canada are cimetidine, famotidine, nizatidine, and ranitidine.
- H2 receptor antagonists competitively and reversibly bind to H2 receptors, blocking histamine-mediated acid secretion.
- The six PPIs currently marketed in the United States and Canada are dexlansoprazole, esomeprazole, lansoprazole, omeprazole, pantoprazole, and rabeprazole.
- PPIs decrease gastric acids by interfering with the final step in gastric acid production.
- PPIs are delayed-release formulations and must not be crushed or chewed.
- Misoprostol is synthetic prostaglandin E. It stimulates the production of protective mucus and bicarbonate in the stomach.
- Misoprostol is not indicated for NSAID-induced PUD prevention during pregnancy.
- Sucralfate binds to the ulcerated area and forms a protective barrier, much like a bandage protects a sore.

- Prokinetic drugs (e.g., metoclopramide, domperidone) increase peristalsis, speed gastric emptying, and improve LES tone.
- Antacids neutralize gastric acids and decrease pepsin secretion.
- Alginates create a mucosal barrier to prevent gastric reflux and inhibit pepsin and bile to further limit mucosal damage.

- Antimicrobial drugs are prescribed for the treatment of PUD to eradicate *H. pylori* infection. Clarithromycin, metronidazole, amoxicillin, and tetracycline are effective for eradicating *H. pylori*.

Review Questions

1. Which sphincter in the digestive system is affected by GERD?
   a. cardiac sphincter
   b. pyloric sphincter
   c. lower esophageal sphincter
   d. laryngeal sphincter
2. What bacteria contribute to peptic ulcer disease?
   a. *streptococcus*
   b. *helicobacter pylori*
   c. *staphylococcus*
   d. *helicobacter spirella*
3. Name two H2 receptor antagonist drugs.
   a. prilosec and cimetidine
   b. prevacid and ranitidine
   c. famotidine and diphenhydramine
   d. ranitidine and famotidine
4. Proton pump inhibitors are effective in treating GERD, LPR, and PUD because they _____.
   a. decrease gastric acid
   b. block histamine
   c. decrease respiratory mucus
   d. do none of the above
5. Name two proton pump inhibitor drugs.
   a. omeprazole and ketoconazole
   b. esomeprazole and lansoprazole
   c. pantoprazole and miconazole
   d. omeprazole and nizatidine

6. _____ is currently the only prokinetic drug approved by the FDA in the United States.
   a. Pantoprazole
   b. Misoprostol
   c. Metoclopramide
   d. Sucralfate
7. _____-containing antacids cause diarrhea; _____-containing antacids cause constipation.
   a. Calcium; aluminum
   b. Magnesium; sodium
   c. Calcium; magnesium
   d. Magnesium; calcium
8. Antacids are one of the oldest drugs used for the treatment of GERD and PUD. Is this statement true or false?
   a. true
   b. false
9. What is the brand name for esomeprazole?
   a. Aciphex
   b. Protonix
   c. Pepcid
   d. Nexium
10. Which drug binds to the ulcerated area and forms a protective barrier, much like a bandage protects a sore?
   a. sucralfate
   b. misoprostol
   c. axid
   d. nexium

Bibliography

Archer M., PharmD, Clinical Pharmacist, Oderda G., PharmD, M.P.H., Professor: University of Utah College of Pharmacy, Copyright © 2012 by University of Utah College of Pharmacy, Salt Lake City, Utah. All rights reserved. Drug Class review: Histamine H2 Receptor Antagonists March 2012.

Cleveland Clinic. (2021). *H. pylori* Infection. Retrieved December 29, 2022, from https://my.clevelandclinic.org/health/diseases/21463-h-pylori-infection.

Health Canada. (2022). Drug Product Database. Retrieved December 29, 2022, from https://health-products.canada.ca/dpd-bdpp/index-eng.jsp.

Institute for Safe Medication Practices. (2016). FDA and ISMP Lists of Look-Alike Drug Names with Recommended Tall Man Letters. Retrieved December 29, 2022, from https://www.ismp.org/recommendations/tall-man-letters-list.

Institute for Safe Medication Practices. (2019). List of Confused Drugs. Retrieved December 29, 2022, from https://www.ismp.org/tools/confuseddrugnames.pdf.

Kalant H, Grant D, Mitchell J. *Principles of medical pharmacology*. ed 7. Toronto: Elsevier Canada; 2007:557–571.

Kikuchi S, Imai H, Tani Y, et al. Proton pump inhibitors for chronic obstructive pulmonary disease. *Cochrane Database Syst Rev.* 2020;8(8):CD013113.

Krause AJ, Walsh EH, Weissbrod PA, et al. An update on current treatment strategies for laryngopharyngeal reflux symptoms. *Ann N Y Acad Sci.* 2020;1510:5–17.

Lipan M, Reidenberg J, Laitman J. *Anatomy of reflux: a growing health problem affecting structures of the head and neck, the anatomical record. Part B: new anatomy.* New York: Wiley-Liss; 2006:261–270.

National Institute of Diabetes and Digestive and Kidney Diseases. (2020). Acid Reflux (GER & GERD) in Adults. Retrieved December 28, 2022, from https://www.niddk.nih.gov/health-information/digestive-diseases/acid-reflux-ger-gerd-adults/all-content.

Pilotto A, Franceschi M, Leandro G, et al. Clinical features of reflux esophagitis in older people: a study of 840 consecutive patients. *J Am Geriatr Soc.* 2006;54:1537–1542.

Talley NJ, Zand Irani M. Optimal management of severe symptomatic gastroesophageal reflux disease. *J Intern Med.* 2021;289:162–178.

U.S. Food and Drug Administration. (nd). Drugs@FDA: FDA Approved Drug Products. Retrieved December 29, 2022, from https://www.accessdata.fda.gov/scripts/cder/daf/index.cfm.

22

Treatment of Irritable Bowel Syndrome, Ulcerative Colitis, and Crohn's Disease

LEARNING OBJECTIVES

1. Learn the terminology associated with irritable bowel syndrome (IBS), ulcerative colitis, and Crohn's disease.
2. List the symptoms of and risk factors for IBS, ulcerative colitis, and Crohn's disease.
3. List and categorize medications used to treat IBS, ulcerative colitis, and Crohn's disease.
4. Describe the mechanisms of action for drugs used to treat IBS, ulcerative colitis, and Crohn's disease.
5. Identify significant drug look-alike and sound-alike issues.
6. List common endings for drug classes used for the treatment of IBS, ulcerative colitis, and Crohn's disease.
7. Identify warning labels and precautionary messages associated with medications used to treat IBS, ulcerative colitis, and Crohn's disease.

KEY TERMS

Antidiarrheals Drugs that prevent or relieve diarrhea.
Constipation Abnormally delayed or infrequent passage of dry, hardened feces.
Crohn's disease Disease that produces inflammation and damage anywhere along the gastrointestinal tract.
Diarrhea Abnormally frequent passage of loose and watery stools.
Gastroenteritis Inflammation of the lining membrane of the stomach and the intestines.
Inflammatory bowel disease Chronic disorder of the gastrointestinal tract characterized by inflammation of the intestine, resulting in abdominal cramping and persistent diarrhea.

Irritable bowel syndrome Condition that causes abdominal distress and erratic movement of the contents of the large bowel, resulting in diarrhea and/or constipation.
Laxative Medicine that induces evacuation of the bowel.
Ulcerative colitis Disease that produces inflammation, ulcers, and damage to the colon.

Overview

Irritable bowel syndrome (IBS) and *inflammatory bowel disease* (IBD) are conditions of the gastrointestinal (GI) tract. The similar names sometimes cause confusion, but the root causes are not the same. The two major types of IBD are *ulcerative colitis* and *Crohn's disease*. Both conditions are linked to inflammation of the GI tract, unlike IBS. Diagnostic tests that are performed to diagnose ulcerative colitis and Crohn's disease include the testing of stool samples, taking x-rays, and performing a colonoscopy. A colonoscopy is performed by inserting a thin tube with a small light and camera at the end (i.e., an endoscope) into the anus, enabling the physician to examine the colon for inflammation and damage (Fig. 22.1).

Irritable Bowel Syndrome

An estimated 10% to 15% of people in North America have IBS. IBS affects quality of life and productivity for millions of people. Symptoms commonly occur before the age of 35 years. IBS is more common in women. IBS causes abdominal pain, bloating, and other discomfort. Movement of waste through the colon (large bowel) may occur too slowly, resulting in *constipation*, or it occurs too rapidly, causing *diarrhea*. Drugs selected to treat IBS with constipation (IBS-C) differ from treatment of IBS that mostly presents with diarrhea. Lubiprostone, linaclotide, plecanatide, and tenapanor are used to treat IBS-C.

What Causes Irritable Bowel Syndrome?

There is no one specific cause for IBS. Persons with IBS have an overly sensitive colon. Food allergies, stress, antibiotic use, chronic alcohol use, bile acid malabsorption, and infection are possible causes. Some infections may produce stomach and intestinal inflammation (*gastroenteritis*). Postinfectious IBS may follow an acute bout of gastroenteritis. IBS may also be associated with abnormally low levels of the neurotransmitter serotonin. Up to 95% of the body's serotonin (5-HT) is found in the stomach epithelium. The remaining 5% is found in neurons in the brain (see Chapter 6).

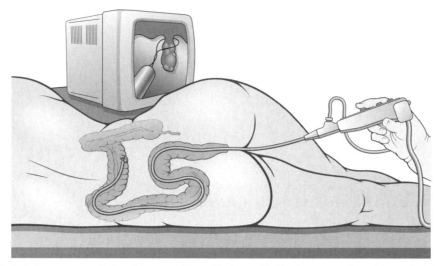

• **Fig. 22.1** Colonoscopy and sigmoidoscopy. (From Chabner DE: *The language of medicine*, ed 10, St Louis, 2014, Elsevier.)

Low levels of serotonin can cause GI motility problems and increase the sensitivity of pain receptors in the GI tract.

Drugs Used for the Treatment of Irritable Bowel Syndrome

Drugs used to treat IBS include serotonin receptor antagonists, ion channel activator/exchangers, opioid receptor agonists, guanylate cyclase-C agonists, sodium-hydrogen exchanger 3 (NHE3) inhibitors, laxatives, fiber supplements, antidiarrheal drugs, and anticholinergic agents.

Serotonin Receptor Antagonist

New medications have been developed that selectively target the serotonin receptors. The neurotransmitter serotonin controls GI motility. There are several types of serotonin receptors. Stimulation of 5-HT$_3$ receptors can cause diarrhea, whereas stimulation of 5-HT$_4$ receptors produces constipation. Not all drugs that act on 5-HT$_3$ receptors are used to treat IBS. Dolasetron, granisetron, ondansetron, and palonosetron are indicated for nausea and vomiting.

Mechanism of Action

Alosetron is a 5-HT$_3$ receptor antagonist. The drug decreases gastric motility and regulates transit through the colon, gastric secretions, and visceral pain.

> ● **Tech Note!**
>
> Alosetron is available only from health care providers who participate in a special prescribing program.

Adverse Reactions

The most common side effects of alosetron therapy are constipation, anxiety, difficulty sleeping or drowsiness, dry mouth, frequent urination, gas, headache, nausea, and restlessness. Alosetron's side effects limit its use. Alosetron may cause severe GI obstruction or impaction, leading to toxic megacolon—a life-threatening condition.

Precautions

Alosetron is approved only for women with severe IBS when other therapies have failed. The US Food and Drug Administration (FDA) requires physicians to obtain special training before prescribing the drug because it can significantly decrease blood flow to the colon, potentially causing ischemic colitis, toxic megacolon, and death.

Serotonin Receptor Antagonist

Generic Name	US Brand Name	Dosage Forms and Strengths
	Canadian Brand Name	
alosetron[a]	Lotronex	**Tablet:** 0.5 mg, 1 mg
	Not available	

[a]Generic available.

Ion Channel Activator and Ion Channel Exchanger

Lubiprostone and tenapanor are approved by the FDA for the treatment of IBS in women when constipation is the predominant symptom (IBS-C). The drugs treat constipation by their action on ion channels.

Mechanism of Action

Lubiprostone activates type 2 chloride channels in the gut, which increases secretions. The increased intestinal fluid volume softens the stool, increases motility in the intestine, and promotes spontaneous bowel movements. Tenapanor is an NHE3 inhibitor. It increases water in the intestine, which softens stools.

Adverse Reactions

The most common side effect of lubiprostone and tenapanor is nausea. Other GI side effects include abdominal pain and diarrhea.

Ion Channel Activator and Ion Channel Exchanger

Generic Name	US Brand Name / Canadian Brand Name	Dosage Forms and Strengths
lubiprostone	Amitiza / Not available	**Capsule:** 8 mcg, 24 mcg
tenapanor	Ibsrela / Ibsrela	**Tablet:** 50 mg

Non-GI side effects are dizziness and hypotension. Lubiprostone may also cause temporary shortness of breath.

Guanylate Cyclase-C Agonists

Linaclotide is indicated for the treatment of IBS when constipation is the predominant symptom (IBS-C). It is a guanylate cyclase-C agonist that acts on the receptors in the intestines to stimulate secretions that increase intestinal fluids and increase GI motility. Taking the drug with a fatty meal increases its effects on softening stool. The most common side effects are diarrhea, abdominal pain, gas, and bloating.

Guanylate Cyclase-C Agonist

Generic Name	US Brand Name / Canadian Brand Name	Dosage Forms and Strengths
linaclotide	Linzess / Constella	**Capsule:** 72 mcg, 145 mcg, 290 mcg

Opioid Receptor Agonist

Eluxadoline is indicated for IBS when the primary symptom is diarrhea (IBS-D). It is an opioid receptor agonist and is a controlled substance in the United States. Eluxadoline binds to μ-receptors and produces side effects similar to opioids, including constipation and dependence. Additional GI side effects are nausea and abdominal pain. Use may produce more serious side effects, including pancreatitis, severe constipation, or serious allergic reactions.

Opioid Receptor Agonist

Generic Name	US Brand Name / Canadian Brand Name	Dosage Forms and Strengths
eluxadoline	Viberzi / Viberzi	**Tablet:** 75 mg, 100 mg

> ● *Tech Note!*
> Eluxadoline is a C-IV controlled substance in the United States.

Bulk-Forming Laxatives and Fiber Supplements

Bulk-forming laxative and fiber supplements are administered to relieve constipation and diarrhea. Polycarbophil is a bulk-forming laxative that is approved by the FDA for the treatment of IBS. It can be obtained without a prescription.

Mechanism of Action

Bulk-forming *laxatives* swell in the presence of liquid. Polycarbophil can absorb 60 to 100 times its weight in water to form a gel. Bacteria that normally live in the colon digest the cellulose and polysaccharide fibers. As the bacteria colony grows, colonic bulk increases. The increased bulk causes the bowel to feel full and stimulates peristalsis and transit of contents through the bowel. It also promotes fluid accumulation in the colon.

Adverse Reactions

Bulk-forming laxatives can cause bloating, gas, abdominal cramps, nausea, diarrhea, or constipation.

Bulk-Forming Laxatives

Generic Name	US Brand Names / Canadian Brand Names	Dosage Forms and Strengths
polycarbophil[a,b]	Equalactin, FiberCon, Fiber-Lax / Mitrolan	**Tablet:** 500 mg, 625 mg

[a]Generic available.
[b]Available over the counter.

Opioid Antidiarrheal Drugs

Difenoxin, diphenoxylate, and loperamide are opioid *antidiarrheal drugs* that are administered to control watery and frequent stools. Difenoxin and loperamide are more potent than diphenoxylate. Difenoxin and diphenoxylate are Schedule C-V controlled substances in the United States. Loperamide is available without a prescription.

Mechanism of Action

Opioid antidiarrheal agents bind to receptors on the smooth muscle cells of the GI tract. They induce spasms that interfere with effective peristalsis. They decrease propulsive contractions by inhibiting the release of acetylcholine. Difenoxin is an active metabolite of diphenoxylate.

Adverse Reactions

Sedation and dizziness are the most common side effects of opioid antidiarrheal drugs. They may also produce constipation. Diphenoxylate and its metabolite difenoxin are controlled substances because they can produce tolerance and dependence.

Antidiarrheal Drugs

Generic Name	US Brand Names / Canadian Brand Names	Dosage Forms and Strengths	US Controlled Substance Schedule
difenoxin + atropine	Motofen / Not available	**Tablet:** 1 mg difenoxin + 0.025 mg atropine	C-IV
diphenoxylate + atropine[a]	Lomotil / Lomotil	**Solution, oral**[b]: 2.5 mg diphenoxylate + 0.025 mg atropine/5 mL **Tablet:** 2.5 mg diphenoxylate + 0.025 mg atropine	C-V (Schedule I narcotic in Canada)
loperamide[a,c]	Imodium-AD / Diarrhea Relief, Imodium Calming Liquid, Imodium Quick Dissolve, Imodium Liqui-gels	**Capsule:** 1 mg, 2 mg **Tablet, orally dissolving:** 2 mg **Tablet:** 2 mg **Solution, oral:** 1 mg/5 mL **Suspension, oral:** 1 mg/7.5 mL	OTC, not scheduled
loperamide + simethicone[c]	Imodium Multi-Symptom Relief / Imodium Complete	**Tablet:** 2 mg loperamide + 125 mg simethicone	OTC, not scheduled

[a]Generic available.
[b]Available in the United States only.
[c]Available over the counter (OTC).

⊘ Tech Alert!

The following drugs have look-alike/sound-alike issues:
difenoxin + atropine and diphenoxylate + atropine

Anticholinergic Drugs

Atropine and dicyclomine are anticholinergic drugs that are approved for the treatment of IBS. They are used for the treatment of IBS when diarrhea is the primary symptom. Anticholinergic drugs block the action of acetylcholine. Atropine and dicyclomine decrease GI muscular tone and motility by producing a nonspecific, direct spasmolytic action on GI smooth muscle. They treat a variety of GI conditions including urinary incontinence and overactive bladder.

Adverse Reactions

Anticholinergic agents may produce constipation, difficulty sleeping, dry mouth, change in taste, headache, photophobia (increased sensitivity of the eyes to light), nausea, sexual difficulty

Anticholinergic Drugs

Generic Name	US Brand Name / Canadian Brand Name	Dosage Forms and Strengths
dicyclomine[a]	Bentyl / Generics	**Capsule:** 10 mg **Solution, for injection**[b]: 10 mg/mL **Tablet:** 10 mg[c], 20 mg **Syrup**[b]: 10 mg/5 mL

[a]Generic available.
[b]Available in the United States only.
[c]Available in Canada only.

(e.g., impotence), fast or slow heartbeat, urinary retention, dizziness, or drowsiness. At higher doses, hallucinations may occur.

Inflammatory Bowel Disease (IBD)

IBD is thought to be an autoimmune disorder whereby the body reacts negatively to its own intestinal tract. It is not known what triggers the onset of the disease. Genetics, dysregulated immune responses, mucosal barrier dysfunction, disturbances in the gastrointestinal flora, and environmental and lifestyle factors are believed to play a role in the development of IBD. Chronic inflammation in the GI tract can lead to ulceration. High levels of tumor necrosis factor (TNF) and other substances that are released to fight infection are present in individuals who have IBD. The four inflammatory diseases of the bowel are ulcerative colitis, Crohn's disease, ulcerative proctitis, and pouchitis. Ulcerative colitis and Crohn's disease are the most common and are discussed in this chapter.

Ulcerative Colitis

Ulcerative colitis is an IBD that affects the colon. *Ulcers* (sores) form in the lining of the colon and rectum. Ulcerative colitis can occur at any age but most commonly begins between the ages of 15 and 30 years and affects men and women equally. Inflammation is limited to the bowel in ulcerative colitis.

Crohn's Disease

Crohn's disease is another IBD. It causes chronic inflammation anywhere along the entire length of the GI tube, from the mouth to the anus, although it typically affects the ileum (the lower part of the small intestine). The inflammation is formed deep within the intestinal wall, causing abdominal pain. Crohn's disease can involve any segment of the GI tract and may also cause inflammation in the eyes, mouth, and some joints.

TABLE 22.1	Symptoms of Irritable Bowel Syndrome, Ulcerative Colitis, and Crohn's Disease		
	Irritable Bowel Syndrome	**Ulcerative Colitis**	**Crohn's Disease**
Similar symptoms	Abdominal pain Diarrhea (mucus, pus) Cramping	Abdominal pain Diarrhea (bloody) Cramping	Abdominal pain Diarrhea Cramping
Disease-specific symptoms	Erratic bowel movements (diarrhea alternating with constipation) Abdominal pain relieved by having a bowel movement Bloating Constipation	Rectal bleeding Anemia Weight loss, loss of appetite Fatigue Loss of vitamins and minerals Skin lesions Joint pain (arthritis) Decreased growth in children Fever	Rectal bleeding Anemia Weight loss, loss of appetite Loss of vitamins and minerals Skin lesions Joint pain (arthritis) Decreased growth in children Fever

• BOX 22.1 Lifestyle Modifications to Reduce Symptoms of Irritable Bowel Syndrome, Ulcerative Colitis, and Crohn's Disease

- Eat small meals.
- Drink at least six to eight glasses of water daily.
- Avoid alcohol.
- Avoid caffeinated beverages (e.g., coffee, tea, cola drinks).
- Limit carbonated beverages.
- Avoid foods that worsen symptoms*.
- Engage in stress-reduction activities.

*Following a diet for celiac disease may reduce symptoms of irritable bowel syndrome. Avoid wheat, rye, barley, dairy, and chocolate.

Symptoms of Irritable Bowel Syndrome, Ulcerative Colitis, and Crohn's Disease

Many of the symptoms of IBS, ulcerative colitis, and Crohn's disease are similar; however, some symptoms are disease specific. Table 22.1 compares symptoms common to IBS, ulcerative colitis, and Crohn's disease.

Lifestyle Modification

Lifestyle changes can reduce symptoms of IBS, ulcerative colitis, and Crohn's disease. Foods and beverages that aggravate diarrhea, bloating, and gas should be avoided. Stress management may also reduce the frequency of symptoms. A list of lifestyle modifications is given in Box 22.1.

● Tech Note!

Drinking carbonated beverages and chewing gum can cause gas and bloating.

Drugs Used for the Treatment of Ulcerative Colitis and Crohn's Disease

Medicines administered for the management of ulcerative colitis are used to induce remission, reduce symptoms, and improve quality of life. Pharmacotherapy includes aminosalicylates, corticosteroids and immunomodulator biologic agents.

Aminosalicylates

Aminosalicylates are administered to patients with ulcerative colitis to reduce inflammation. The four aminosalicylate antiinflammatory agents available in the United States and Canada are sulfasalazine, olsalazine, mesalamine (mesalazine in Canada), and balsalazide.

● Tech Note!

A common ending for aminosalicylates is -salazine.

Mechanism of Action and Pharmacokinetics

Sulfasalazine, olsalazine, and mesalamine (mesalazine in Canada) are all formulations that contain 5-aminosalicylic acid (5-ASA). Sulfasalazine (sulfapyridine + 5-ASA) and olsalazine (two 5-ASA molecules) are also prodrugs. Balsalazide is a prodrug of mesalamine.

Several mechanisms of action for the antiinflammatory action of aminosalicylates have been proposed. They interfere with the metabolism of arachidonic acid and are thought to induce regulatory T cells in the colon. The release of proinflammatory substances by the body (e.g., leukotrienes, prostaglandins, cytokines) is inhibited, and cytokine production is decreased. Bacteria in the colon metabolize the drugs and release 5-ASA, the active metabolite of aminosalicylates. The effectiveness of sulfasalazine and olsalazine is reduced by factors that decrease the bacteria in the colon (e.g., antibiotics) and decrease the gut pH. Delayed-release formulations of 5-ASA are coated with a pH-dependent resin that releases the active drug in a less acidic environment. The optimal activity of 5-ASA depends on a rise in the pH to greater than 7 in the distal ileum. Pentasa is a time-release formulation.

❶ Tech Alert!

The following drugs have look-alike/sound-alike issues:
sulfaSALAzine and sulfADIAZINE;
Colazal and Clozaril

Adverse Reactions

The most common adverse effects of sulfasalazine, olsalazine, mesalamine (mesalazine), and balsalazide are nausea, vomiting, heartburn, headache, and watery diarrhea. Sulfasalazine may also cause sunburn, impaired folic acid absorption, crystalluria, and damage to white blood cells (cytopenia).

Aminosalicylates

Generic Name	US Brand Names / Canadian Brand Names	Dosage Forms and Strengths
balsalazide[a]	Colazal, Giazo	Capsule (Colazal): 750 mg
	Not available	Tablet (Giazo): 1.1 g
mesalamine[a] (known as mesalazine in Canada; 5-aminosalicylic acid [5-ASA])	Apriso, Canasa, Delzicol, Lialda, Pentasa, Rowasa, sfRowasa	Capsule, biphasic, extended release (Apriso): 0.375 g[b]
		Capsule, extended release: 250 mg[b], 400 mg, 500 mg[b]
	Mezavant, Mezera, Octasa, Pentasa, Salofalk	Suppository: 500 mg[c], 1 g[b]
		Suspension, rectal (Pentasa): 1 g/100 mL[c], 4 g/100 mL[c]
		Suspension, rectal (Salofalk, Rowasa): 2 g/60 mL[c]; 4 g/60 mL
		Tablet, delayed release (Octasa): 800 mg
		Tablet, delayed and extended release (Lialda, Mezavant): 1.2 g
		Tablet, enteric coated (Salofalk): 500 mg[c]
		Tablet, extended release (Pentasa): 500 mg[c], 1 g[c]
olsalazine	Dipentum	Capsule: 250 mg
	Dipentum	
sulfasalazine[a]	Azulfidine, Azulfidine EN Tabs	Tablet: 500 mg
	Salazopyrin, Salazopyrin EN Tabs	Tablet, enteric coated: 500 mg

[a]Generic available.
[b]Available in the United States only.
[c]Available in Canada only.

Corticosteroids

Corticosteroids (e.g., prednisone) are commonly prescribed to suppress inflammation, reduce flare-ups, and treat pain associated with ulcerative colitis and Crohn's disease. They decrease the synthesis of proinflammatory substances such as prostaglandins (see Chapter 10), leukotrienes, cytokines, arachidonic acid, and macrophages that are released as part of the inflammatory response. Corticosteroids have immunosuppressive actions that may inhibit the abnormal immune system activity associated with Crohn's disease and ulcerative colitis. Corticosteroids prescribed to treat ulcerative colitis and Crohn's disease may be administered by mouth or rectally in the form of an enema or suppository.

Corticosteroids

Generic Name	US Brand Names / Canadian Brand Names	Dosage Forms and Strengths
budesonide[a]	Entocort EC, Ortikos, Uceris	Capsule (Entocort): 3 mg
		Capsule, delayed release (Ortikos): 6 mg, 9 mg
	Entocort, Entocort Enema	Rectal foam (Uceris): 2 mg/metered dose
		Rectal suspension: 2.3 mg/115 mL
		Tablet, delayed and extended release (Cortiment, Uceris): 9 mg
hydrocortisone[a]	Colocort, Cortenema, Cortifoam	Foam, rectal (Colocort, Cortifoam): 10%
	Cortenema, Cortifoam, Cortiment	Suspension, rectal (Cortenema): 100 mg/60 mL
		Suppository (Cortiment): 10 mg, 40 mg
hydrocortisone + pramoxine	Proctofoam	Rectal foam: 1% hydrocortisone + 1% pramoxine
	Proctofoam	

[a]Generic available.

Adverse Reactions

Oral administration produces systemic effects (described in Chapter 15). Up to 40% of patients treated for Crohn's disease develop corticosteroid dependence. Adverse effects caused by rectal administration may be local (e.g., burning, itching) or systemic (e.g., nausea, constipation or diarrhea, appetite changes, headache). Only rectal and "gut-specific" formulations are presented in this chapter.

> **● Tech Note!**
>
> The contents of Entocort® delayed-release budesonide capsules may be sprinkled on food; however, patients should swallow the contents without chewing.

> **● Tech Note!**
>
> Given the similarity of symptoms and the similar mechanism of disease progression of Crohn's disease and ulcerative colitis, many agents used for the treatment of these diseases are the same.

> **❶ Tech Alert!**
>
> The following drugs have look-alike/sound-alike issues:
> azaTHIOprine and AzaCITIDine

Immunosuppressants

Azathioprine, 6-mercaptopurine, and methotrexate are classified as antimetabolites. They are used for the treatment of Crohn's disease to induce remission, but product package labeling does not list IBD as an indication. Azathioprine suppresses the T cell–mediated immune system response. Methotrexate decreases cytokine and immunoglobulin production and cyclooxygenase-2 activity. Decreasing these proinflammatory substances reduces both inflammation and immune system activity (see Chapter 13).

Immunomodulators

Adalimumab, certolizumab, golimumab, infliximab, and natalizumab are immunomodulators that have been approved for the treatment of moderate to severe Crohn's disease or ulcerative colitis. They are administered to induce remission of active disease and then continued as maintenance therapy in patients who have had unsuccessful results with other therapies.

> **● Tech Note!**
>
> A common ending for immunomodulators is *-mab*.

Mechanism of Action

Most immunomodulator biologic agents used for the treatment of Crohn's disease are genetically engineered TNF-α inhibitors. Infliximab blocks the inflammatory process by preventing cell lysis (destruction) and the release of substances that cause inflammation. A detailed description of the mechanism of action for TNF-α inhibitors is given in Chapter 13. Natalizumab is an α_4-integrin inhibitor. It reduces T cell–mediated intestinal inflammation. Additional immunomodulators are discussed in Chapter 32.

Adverse Reactions

Common adverse reactions to infliximab are nausea, stomach pain, headache, redness, and itching at the site of infusion. It may also increase susceptibility to opportunistic infections, reactivate dormant infections (e.g., tuberculosis), or worsen existing infection.

> **● Tech Note!**
>
> Infliximab package labeling contains a boxed warning that the drug may cause serious infections and malignancies.

> **● Tech Note!**
>
> Patients taking natalizumab (Tysabri) must be enrolled in an FDA Risk Evaluation and Mitigation Strategy (REMS) program.

Antiinfective Drugs

Patients who have Crohn's disease may develop fistulas. A fistula forms when an ulcer tunnels from the site of origin to surrounding tissues. Fistulas may be located in the bladder, vagina, or skin surrounding the anus and rectum. Antiinfective agents may be prescribed to treat infections that develop in the fistula. Fistulas may be treated with ampicillin, sulfonamides, cephalosporins, tetracycline, or metronidazole; these drugs are described in Chapter 29.

Immunomodulators

Biosimilar Name	US Brand Names		Dosage Forms and Strengths
	Canadian Brand Names		
adalimumab adalimumab- ADAZ adalimumab-AFZB adalimumab-ATTO adalimumab-ADBM adalimumab- AQVH adalimumab- BWWD adalimumab- FKJP	Abrilada, Amjevita, Cyltezo, Hadlima, Hulio, Humira, Hyrimoz, Yusimry		**Solution, for injection:** 10 mg/0.2 mL (Abrilada), 20 mg/0.4 mL[a] (Hulio, Hyrimoz), 40 mg/0.8 mL (Abrilada, Amjevita, Cyltezo, Hadlima, Hulio, Humira, Hyrimoz, Idacio, Simlandi, Yuflyma, Yusimry), 50 mg/mL[b] (Amgevita)
	Amgevita, Hadlima, Hulio, Humira, Hyrlmoz, Idacio, Simlandi, Yuflyma		
certolizumab	Cimzia		**Powder, for injection:** 200 mg/vial **Solution, for injection:** 200 mg/mL
	Cimzia		
golimumab	Simponi, Simponi Aria		**Solution, for injection:** 50 mg/0.5 mL, 100 mg/mL **Solution, intravenous (Simponi Aria, Simponi IV):** 50 mg/4 mL (12.5 mg/mL)
	Simponi, Simponi IV		
infliximab, infliximab-AXXQ, infliximab-DYYB, infliximab-QBTX infliximab-ADBA	Avsola, Inflectra, Ixifi, Remicade, Renflexis		**Powder, for injection:** 100 mg/vial, 120 mg/mL (Remsima SC)[b]
	Avsola, Inflectra, Renflexis, Remsima SC, Remicade		
natalizumab	Tysabri		**Solution for injection:** 300 mg/15 mL (20 mg/mL)
	Tysabri		

[a]Available in the United States only.
[b]Available in Canada only.

> ## TECHNICIAN'S CORNER
>
> 1. Why might bulk-forming laxatives be useful for treating irritable bowel syndrome with diarrhea or constipation?
> 2. Which lifestyle modifications might lessen the symptoms of irritable bowel syndrome?

Summary of Drugs Used for the Treatment of Irritable Bowel Disease, Ulcerative Colitis, and Crohn's Disease

Generic Name	US Brand Name	Usual Adult Oral Dose and Dosing Schedule	Warning Labels
Serotonin Receptor Antagonist			
alosetron	Lotronex	**IBS:** 0.5–1 mg twice daily	MAY CAUSE DIZZINESS OR DROWSINESS; AVOID DRIVING. AVOID ALCOHOL. TAKE WITH A FULL GLASS OF WATER.
Ion Channel Activator and Ion Channel Exchanger			
lubiprostone	Amitiza	**IBS:** 8–24 mcg twice daily	TAKE WITH A FULL GLASS OF WATER. TAKE WITH FOOD.
tenapanor	Ibsrela	**IBS:** 50 mg twice daily	TAKE IMMEDIATELY BEFORE BREAKFAST AND BEFORE DINNER.
Opioid Receptor Agonist			
eluxadoline	Viberzi	**IBS:** 100 mg twice daily	TAKE WITH FOOD.
Guanylate Cyclase-C Agonist			
linaclotide	Linzess	**IBS:** 290 mcg once daily	TAKE ON AN EMPTY STOMACH.
Bulk-Forming Laxatives			
polycarbophil	Equalactin	**IBS:** 2 tablets 1–4 times daily	TAKE WITH A FULL GLASS OF WATER.
Antidiarrheal Drugs			
difenoxin + atropine[a]	Motofen	**Acute diarrhea:** 2 tablets immediately; then 1 tablet after each loose stool every 3–4 h (maximum 8 tabs/day)	MAY CAUSE DIZZINESS OR DROWSINESS; AVOID DRIVING. AVOID ALCOHOL. DRINK LOTS OF FLUIDS.
diphenoxylate + atropine[a]	Lomotil	**Acute diarrhea:** 2 tablets immediately; then 1–2 tablet 4 times daily	
loperamide[a]	Imodium	**Acute diarrhea:** 2 tablets immediately; then 1 tablet after each loose stool (maximum 16 mg/day)	
Anticholinergic Agents			
dicyclomine	Bentyl	**IBS:** 20–40 mg orally 4 times daily, 10–20 mg IM 4 times a day; maximum 1–2 days	MAY CAUSE DIZZINESS OR DROWSINESS; AVOID DRIVING. AVOID ALCOHOL. DRINK LOTS OF FLUIDS. TAKE ON AN EMPTY STOMACH. AVOID ANTACIDS WITHIN 1–2 HOURS OF DOSE.
Aminosalicylate Drugs			
balsalazide	Colazal, Giazo	**Ulcerative colitis (UC):** 3 caps (2250 mg) 3 times daily for 8–12 weeks (Colazal); men, 3.3 g orally twice daily for up to 8 weeks (Giazo)	SWALLOW WHOLE; DO NOT CRUSH OR CHEW. CAPSULE CONTENTS MAY BE SPRINKLED ON APPLESAUCE.
mesalamine (5-ASA)	Canasa	**UC:** Insert 1 suppository rectally twice daily	REMOVE FOIL AND INSERT—suppository. MAY DISCOLOR CLOTHING OR SKIN—orange-yellow, suppository. SHAKE WELL—rectal suspension. SWALLOW WHOLE; DO NOT CRUSH OR CHEW—delayed release. TAKE WITH FOOD—delayed release. DO NOT SUBSTITUTE ASACOL HD WITH DELZICOL—not interchangeable.
	Rowasa	**UC:** 4 g enema nightly	
	Delzicol	**UC:** 1 tablet 3 times daily	
	Lialda	**UC:** 2–4 tablets once daily for up to 8 weeks	
	Pentasa, Salofalk	**UC:** 1 g 4 times daily	
olsalazine	Dipentum	**UC:** 1 g daily in 2 divided doses	SWALLOW WHOLE; DO NOT CRUSH OR CHEW. TAKE WITH FOOD.
sulfasalazine	Azulfidine	**UC:** 1 g 3 or 4 times daily	SWALLOW WHOLE; DO NOT CRUSH OR CHEW—enteric-coated tablets. AVOID PROLONGED EXPOSURE TO SUNLIGHT. DRINK LOTS OF FLUIDS.

Summary of Drugs Used for the Treatment of Irritable Bowel Disease, Ulcerative Colitis, and Crohn's Disease—cont'd

Generic Name	US Brand Name	Usual Adult Oral Dose and Dosing Schedule	Warning Labels
Corticosteroids			
budesonide	Entocort Enema, Uceris	**UC:** Insert 1 metered dose rectally twice daily (Uceris) **UC:** Add 1 tablet to enema solution and insert rectally nightly for 4 weeks (Entocort Enema)	SHAKE WELL.
	Ortikos, Entocort EC	**CD:** Take 1 capsule in the morning (delayed-release capsule)	SWALLOW WHOLE; DO NOT CRUSH OR CHEW— delayed release. AVOID GRAPEFRUIT JUICE. KEEP IN FOIL POUCH UNTIL READY FOR USE.
hydrocortisone	Cortema	**UC:** 100 mg rectal enema nightly for 21 days	SHAKE WELL.
	Anucort	**UC:** 1 suppository rectally 2–3 times daily for 2 weeks	REMOVE FOIL AND INSERT.
	Cortifoam	**UC:** 1 applicatorful 1–2 times daily for 2–3 weeks; then every other day	SHAKE WELL.
Immunomodulators			
adalimumab	Humira	**Crohn's and UC:** 160 mg followed by 80 mg in 2 weeks; then 40 mg maintenance dose every other week starting on day 29 of therapy	REPORT SIGNS OF INFECTION. DO NOT MISS DOSES.
certolizumab	Cimzia	**Crohn's:** 400 mg subcutaneously followed by 400 mg at weeks 2 and 4; then every 4 weeks thereafter if necessary	
golimumab	Simponi	**UC:** 200 mg subcutaneously followed by 100 mg at week 2 and every 4 weeks thereafter	
infliximab	Remicade	**Crohn's or UC:** 5 mg/kg IV at weeks 0, 2, and 6; then every 8 weeks	
natalizumab	Tysabri	**Crohn's:** 300 mg IV infusion given over 1 h every 4 weeks; reevaluate every 3 months	

IBS, Inflammatory bowel syndrome; *IM,* intramuscular; *IV,* intravenous; *UC,* ulcerative colitis.

Key Points

- Inflammatory bowel disease (IBD), ulcerative colitis, and Crohn's disease are conditions that are linked to inflammation of the GI tract.
- Abdominal pain, diarrhea, and cramping are common symptoms of IBS, ulcerative colitis, and Crohn's disease.
- Persons with IBS may have diarrhea or constipation.
- In ulcerative colitis and Crohn's disease, the body's immune system recognizes the bacteria that normally inhabit the GI tract as harmful invaders.
- Ulcerative colitis produces inflammation in the upper layers of the lining of the small intestine and colon.
- Crohn's disease may produce inflammation and can occur anywhere along the entire length of the GI tube, from the mouth to the anus, although typically it affects the ileum (the lower part of the small intestine). Inflammation occurs deep in the intestinal wall.

- Lifestyle modification such as stress management, eating small meals, and avoiding alcohol and caffeinated and carbonated beverages can reduce symptoms of IBS, ulcerative colitis, and Crohn's disease.
- Drugs used to treat IBS include serotonin receptor antagonists, ion channel activators/exchangers, opioid receptor agonists, guanylate cyclase-C agonists, sodium-hydrogen exchanger 3 (NHE3) inhibitors, laxatives, fiber supplements, antidiarrheal drugs, and anticholinergic agents.
- Alosetron is a 5-HT$_3$ receptor antagonist used in women to control diarrhea caused by severe IBS when other types of treatment have failed.
- Alosetron prescriptions cannot be refilled without a follow-up examination by the physician.
- Bulk-forming laxatives and fiber supplements are given to relieve constipation and diarrhea.

- Antidiarrheal drugs control watery, frequent stools.
- Diphenoxylate and difenoxin, which are controlled substances in the United States, may cause tolerance and dependence.
- Loperamide is not habit forming and is sold over the counter.
- Atropine and dicyclomine decrease diarrhea by reducing GI muscular tone and motility.
- The aminosalicylates sulfasalazine, olsalazine, balsalazide, and mesalamine (mesalazine) are administered to patients with ulcerative colitis and Crohn's disease to reduce inflammation.
- All commercially available aminosalicylates are formulated as delayed-release products.

- Glucocorticosteroids are prescribed commonly to suppress inflammation, reduce flare-ups, and treat pain associated with ulcerative colitis and Crohn's disease.
- Glucocorticosteroids have immunosuppressive actions that may inhibit the abnormal immune system activity associated with Crohn's disease and ulcerative colitis.
- Infliximab is an immunomodulator approved for the treatment of Crohn's disease; it is administered to induce remission.
- Infliximab is a TNF-α inhibitor that is genetically engineered to block the inflammatory process.
- Patients who have Crohn's disease may develop fistulas. Antiinfective agents may be prescribed to treat fistula infections.

Review Questions

1. Which disease(s) is/are linked to inflammation of the entire GI tract?
   a. irritable bowel syndrome
   b. ulcerative colitis
   c. Crohn's disease
   d. all of the above
2. How must adalimumab (Humira) be stored?
   a. at room temperature
   b. in the refrigerator
   c. kept frozen in the freezer
   d. either refrigerated or stored at room temperature
3. Which of the following drugs is marketed as a powder that must be reconstituted before administration?
   a. Cimzia
   b. Cortenema
   c. Sulfasalazine suspension
   d. Dicyclomine syrup
4. Name three common symptoms of irritable bowel syndrome, ulcerative colitis, and Crohn's disease.
   a. bloating, constipation, cramping
   b. abdominal pain, diarrhea, cramping
   c. rectal bleeding, bloating, diarrhea
   d. cramping, abdominal pain, bloating
5. Which of the following drugs is used to treat IBS in which constipation is the primary symptom?
   a. Amitiza
   b. Lotronex
   c. Lovenox
   d. Alosetron
6. _____ are administered to treat the symptoms of irritable bowel syndrome.
   a. Bulk-forming laxatives
   b. Fiber supplements
   c. Bile acid sequestrants
   d. a and b

7. An immunomodulator that has been approved for the treatment of Crohn's disease is _____.
   a. Golimumab
   b. Methotrexate
   c. Lomotil
   d. Budesonide
8. Patients who have Crohn's disease may develop _____, which form when an ulcer tunnels from the site of origin to surrounding tissues.
   a. ulcers
   b. fistulas
   c. diverticula
   d. none of the above
9. Select the corticosteroid that is formulated for rectal use.
   a. Enterocort EC
   b. Medrol
   c. prednisone
   d. Cortenema
10. These warning labels should be applied to prescription vials for which class of drugs used for IBS: "May cause dizziness or drowsiness, avoid driving, avoid alcohol, drink lots of fluids, take on an empty stomach."
   a. anticholinergics
   b. bulk-forming laxatives
   c. serotonin antagonists
   d. corticosteroids

Bibliography

Black CJ, Ford AC. Best management of irritable bowel syndrome. *Frontline Gastroenterol.* 2020;12:303–315.

Bressler B, Marshall J, Bernstein CN, et al. Clinical practice guidelines for the medical management of nonhospitalized ulcerative colitis: the Toronto consensus. *Gastroenterology.* 2015;148(5):1035–1958.

Cai Z, Wang S, Li J. Treatment of inflammatory bowel disease: a comprehensive review. *Front Med.* 2021;8:765474.

Chang J, Talley N. Current and emerging therapies in irritable bowel syndrome: from pathophysiology to treatment. *Trends Pharmacol Sci.* 2010;31:326–328.

Crohn's & Colitis Foundation. (2017). Immunomodulators Fact Sheet. Retrieved August 12, 2017, from http://www.crohnscolitisfoundation.org.

Ford AC, Moayyedi P, Chey WD, et al. ACG Task Force on Management of Irritable Bowel Syndrome: American College of Gastroenterology Monograph on Management of Irritable Bowel Syndrome. *Am J Gastroenterol.* 2018;113(Suppl 2):1–18.

Health Canada. (2022). Drug Product Database, 2022. Retrieved October 22, 2022, from https://health-products.canada.ca/dpd-bdpp/index-eng.jsp.

Institute for Safe Medication Practices. (2016). FDA and ISMP Lists of Look-Alike Drug Names with Recommended Tall Man Letters. Retrieved October 18, 2022, from https://www.ismp.org/recommendations/tall-man-letters-list.

Institute for Safe Medication Practices. (2019). List of Confused Drugs. Retrieved October 22, 2022, from https://www.ismp.org/tools/confuseddrugnames.pdf.

Kalant H, Grant D, Mitchell J. *Pharmacotherapy of intestinal motility disorders and inflammatory bowel disease principles of medical pharmacology.* ed 7. Toronto: Elsevier Canada; 2007:572–583.

Love BL. Pharmacotherapy for moderate to severe inflammatory bowel disease: evolving strategies. *Am J Manag Care.* 2016;22(3):s39–s50.

National Institute of Diabetes and Digestive and Kidney Diseases. (2017). Treatment of Crohn's Disease. Retrieved October 22, 2022, from https://www.niddk.nih.gov/health-information/digestive-diseases/crohns-disease/treatment.

National Institute of Diabetes and Digestive and Kidney Diseases. (2020). Treatment for Ulcerative Colitis. Retrieved October 22, 2022, from https://www.niddk.nih.gov/health-information/digestive-diseases/ulcerative-colitis/treatment.

Terdiman JP, Gruss CB, Heidelbaugh JJ, et al. American Gastroenterological Association Institute guideline on the use of thiopurines, methotrexate, and anti–TNF-a biologic drugs for the induction and maintenance of remission in inflammatory Crohn's disease. *Gastroenterology.* 2013;145:1459–1463.

U.S. Food and Drug Administration. (nd). Drugs@FDA: FDA Approved Drug Products. Retrieved October 22, 2022, from http://www.accessdata.fda.gov/scripts/cder/daf/.

Xia H. Post-infectious irritable bowel syndrome. *World J Gastroenterol.* 2009;15(29):3591–3596.

Drugs Affecting the Respiratory System

Respiration involves the exchange of oxygen (O_2) and carbon dioxide (CO_2) in the cells in the body. A properly functioning respiratory system ensures that the tissues of the body receive an adequate oxygen supply and carbon dioxide is promptly removed. In addition, the respiratory system effectively filters, warms, and humidifies the air we breathe. Respiratory organs also influence sound reproduction, including speech used in communicating oral language. Specialized epithelia in the respiratory tract make the sense of smell (olfaction) possible. The respiratory system also plays an important role in the regulation, or homeostasis, of pH (acid-base balance) in the body. Functionally, the respiratory system includes the lungs and accessory structures such as the oral cavity, rib cage, and respiratory muscles, including the diaphragm. Diseases of the respiratory tract, such as asthma, chronic obstructive pulmonary disease (COPD), and cystic fibrosis, affect the upper and lower respiratory tract. They impair breathing and gas exchange.

In Unit VII, the pharmacotherapy for asthma, COPD, and allergies is presented. A brief description of each disorder is provided, followed by a description of the drugs indicated for treatment that includes mechanisms of action, adverse reactions, strength(s), dosage forms, and OTC or prescription status.

23

Treatment of Asthma and Chronic Obstructive Pulmonary Disease

LEARNING OBJECTIVES

1. Learn the terminology associated with asthma and chronic obstructive pulmonary disease (COPD).
2. List risk factors for asthma and COPD.
3. List the symptoms of asthma and COPD.
4. List and categorize medications used in the treatment of asthma and COPD.
5. Describe the mechanism of action of drugs used to treat asthma and COPD.
6. Identify significant drug look-alike and sound-alike issues.
7. List common endings for drug classes used for the treatment of asthma and COPD.
8. Identify warning labels and precautionary messages associated with medications used to treat asthma and COPD.

KEY TERMS

Allergic asthma Asthma symptoms induced by a hypersensitivity reaction upon exposure to environmental allergens.

Asthma A chronic disease that affects the airways, producing irritation, inflammation, and difficulty breathing.

Bronchodilator A drug that relaxes tightened airway muscles and improves airflow through the airways.

Chronic obstructive pulmonary disease A progressive disease of the airways that produces a gradual loss of pulmonary function.

Forced expiratory volume The maximum volume of air that can be breathed out in 1 second; also called forced vital capacity.

Metered-dose inhaler A device used for delivering a dose of inhaled medication. A solution or powder is delivered as a mist and inhaled.

Nebulizer A device that converts a liquid drug into a mist that is inhaled.

Peak flow meter A handheld device used to measure the volume of air exhaled and how rapidly the air is moved out.

Spacer A device attached to the end of a metered-dose inhaler that facilitates drug delivery into the lungs (rather than to the back of the throat).

Spirometry A test that measures the volume of air that is expired (blown out of the lungs) after taking a deep breath and how rapidly the volume of air is expired.

Asthma

Overview

Asthma is a chronic disease that affects the airways, producing irritation, inflammation, and difficulty breathing. More than 21 million adults and 4.2 million children in the United States have been diagnosed with asthma, according to the US Centers for Disease Control and Prevention. Approximately 2.8 million Canadians 12 years of age and older have asthma, according to Statistics Canada. Females are more likely than males to report that they have asthma.

The burden of disease attributed to asthma is great because it is responsible for missed days at school and work and increased health care costs because of emergency department visits, hospitalization, and outpatient doctor visits. Asthma is the reason for more than 5 million physician office visits annually.

Asthma is classified according to the level of treatment necessary to control symptoms or keep symptoms from worsening, according to Global Initiative for Asthma (GINA) guidelines (2022) (Box 23.1).

It is not known exactly why some people develop asthma and others do not; however, there are factors that can increase the risk for asthma. A prime example is a positive family history of asthma or exposure to tobacco smoke. Research suggests that during pregnancy, secondhand smoke exposure may be just as damaging to the unborn baby as to the mother. Chronic exposure to other sources of air pollution and exposure to some allergens and infections early in life may also be risk factors.

Pathophysiology

Symptoms of asthma are linked to a progression of physiologic changes in the airways. Initially, the airways (bronchial tube and

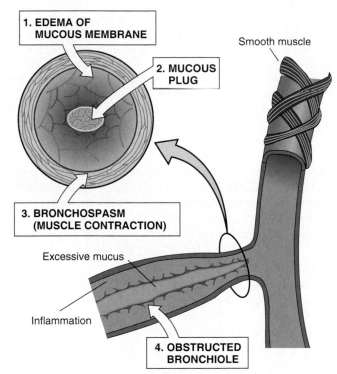

1. EDEMA OF MUCOUS MEMBRANE

2. MUCOUS PLUG

Smooth muscle

3. BRONCHOSPASM (MUSCLE CONTRACTION)

Excessive mucus

Inflammation

4. OBSTRUCTED BRONCHIOLE

• **Fig. 23.1** Airway changes during an asthma episode. (From VanMeter KC, Hubert RJ: *Gould's pathophysiology for the heart professions*, ed 5, St Louis, 2014, Elsevier.)

bronchioles) become irritated. This causes airway constriction, which makes the passage of air more difficult. Airways also become inflamed and swollen, further restricting the flow of air through the bronchial passages. Mucus production is increased above normal levels, which can obstruct breathing passages (Fig. 23.1).

Symptoms

Airway constriction, inflammation, and mucus produce characteristic asthma symptoms (Box 23.2) such as coughing, wheezing, shortness of breath (SOB), and chest tightness. Symptoms may be mild or severe (i.e., life-threatening) and vary for each individual. During an asthma episode (often called an asthma attack), breathing may be noisy and labored. A whistling or creaking sound may be heard with inspiration and expiration. Patients describe chest tightness that feels as though something or someone were "squeezing or sitting on their chest" and the feeling that they cannot get enough air into their lungs. Actually, SOB is associated with reduced expiration rather than decreased inspiration. Breathing may become faster and shallower. Nocturnal asthma is a condition characterized by decreased FEV_1 (***forced expiratory volume in 1 second***). The maximal volume of air that can be breathed out in 1 second is reduced. Increased airway inflammation is present, along with exaggerated bronchial constriction (hyperresponsiveness). Coughing at night may disrupt sleep. In one study of patients with asthma, as many as 74% reported nocturnal asthma symptoms at least once weekly. In nocturnal asthma, lung function and antiinflammatory hormones (e.g., cortisol) decrease and the release of proinflammatory mediators (e.g., leukotrienes, cytokines) increases in the middle of the night, according to the patient's circadian rhythm (biologic clock).

Asthma Triggers

Asthma triggers are things that can precipitate an asthma episode in individuals with asthma (Box 23.3). An asthma episode is also called an asthma attack. Examples of triggers are allergens such as animal dander, pollen, air pollution, cleaning fluid, mold, tobacco smoke, and even cold air. Exposure to cockroach droppings and air pollution is linked to the rise of asthma in inner-city youth. Other triggers are upper respiratory infection and strenuous exercise. The risk for exercise-induced asthma can be minimized by taking prescribed medicines before exercise.

Managing Asthma Symptoms

Asthma symptoms can be managed with a combination of medication, lifestyle modification, and home monitoring using a peak flow meter to measure volume of expired air flow. Medications that are administered for the treatment and management of asthma are divided into two classes. They treat the two main components of asthma: airway inflammation and acute bronchoconstriction (constriction of the airways). Rescue medicines treat the acute symptoms. They include short-acting β_2-adrenergic agonists such as albuterol (salbutamol in Canada) and short-acting anticholinergic agents (e.g., ipratropium bromide). Maintenance therapy is used to prevent asthma episodes. Maintenance medications include long-acting β_2-adrenergic agonists (e.g., salmeterol), inhaled corticosteroids (e.g., budesonide), leukotriene modifiers (e.g., montelukast), mast cell stabilizers (e.g., cromolyn sodium), long-acting anticholinergic drugs (e.g., tiotropium bromide), and xanthine derivatives (e.g., aminophylline). The key to preventing asthma attacks, hospitalizations, and death from asthma is reducing and preventing further inflammation. Sublingual immunotherapy has been administered with an aim to desensitize an individual to specific asthma triggers. The therapy involves exposing the individual to increasing doses of an allergen(s). Studies have shown mixed results regarding the effectiveness of sublingual immunotherapy.

A *peak flow meter* is a handheld device used to measure the volume of air exhaled and how fast the air is exhaled. Regular measurements can enable a person with asthma to spot trends that signal an impending attack. A peak flow meter permits patients to manage their asthma symptom control. Low peak flow numbers signal that asthma is not controlled. *Spirometry* is a test that is performed to measure the volume of air that is expired (blown out of the lungs) after taking a deep breath and how rapidly the volume of air is expired.

Drugs Used for the Treatment of Acute Symptoms: Relievers

Rescue medicines, also known as relievers, provide rapid and short-term relief of asthma symptoms. Current Global Initiative for Asthma (GINA) guidelines recommend as needed low-dose inhaled corticosteroid as the preferred symptom reliever; however, administration of a short-acting β_2-adrenergic agonist may alternatively be used. Albuterol (also known as salbutamol) is a short-acting β_2-adrenergic agonist (SABA) that relieves bronchospasm and opens airways. It is a *bronchodilator*. Other β_2-adrenergic agonists prescribed for the treatment of asthma include levalbuterol and terbutaline. β_2-Adrenergic agonists are commonly administered by oral inhalation using a *metered-dose inhaler* (MDI) or *nebulizer*. Ipratropium bromide is a short-acting anticholinergic that is administered by the inhalation route. Ipratropium bromide may be administered singularly or in combination with a short-acting β_2-adrenergic agonist for the relief of acute symptoms.

Mechanism of Action

Bronchial airways are composed of smooth muscle that is innervated by β_2, α_1, α_2, and muscarinic (M1 and M3) receptors. Short-acting β_2-adrenergic agonists relax bronchial smooth muscle, causing airways to dilate and thereby reversing bronchospasms. Levalbuterol is an isomer of albuterol and is a moderately selective β_2-adrenergic receptor agonist.

> **● *Tech Note!***
>
> To determine whether the contents of some metered-dose inhalers are low, patients should check the counter mechanism on the inhaler. The counter shows the number of doses that are left.

Pharmacokinetics

Short-acting β_2-adrenergic agonists have a rapid onset and short duration of action. The onset of action for albuterol is within 15 minutes, and the peak effect occurs within 30 minutes to 2 hours. The duration of action of albuterol is 2 to 6 hours compared with its isomer, levalbuterol, which has a duration of action of approximately 3 to 6 hours.

The bioavailability of ipratropium bromide is low, which accounts for the low incidence of adverse reactions.

Adverse Reactions

Drugs such as albuterol can produce nervousness, difficulty sleeping, dry mouth, mild headache, and throat irritation (inhalants only). β-Receptors are also located on heart and skeletal muscle, so the use of β_2-adrenergic agonists can increase the heart rate and lead to arrhythmias, hypertension, palpitations, tachycardia, and tremors. β_2-Adrenergic stimulation may also produce hyperglycemia, hypokalemia, and increased insulin secretion. Ipratropium bromide can cause difficulty urinating and blurred vision.

> **● *Tech Note!***
>
> Excessive use of reliever medication is a sign that the asthma is not well controlled.

Precautions

Store the canister at room temperature because exposure to excessive heat can cause the canister to explode. Excessive cold can reduce the effectiveness of albuterol. Keep the albuterol nebulizer solution in its foil package until time of use to protect it from light.

Maintenance Therapy to Prevent Asthma Flare-ups

Drugs that are intended for long-term use and taken daily to prevent asthma symptoms are called controllers. The five classes of drugs used for asthma prophylaxis are long-acting β_2-adrenergic agonists, inhaled corticosteroids, leukotriene modifiers, mast cell stabilizers, and xanthine derivatives.

Long-Acting β_2-Adrenergic Agonists

The US Food and Drug Administration (FDA) and Health Canada updated the indications for the use of long-acting β-agonists (LABAs) for the treatment of asthma because of safety concerns. To ensure the safe use of these products, the following guidelines are recommended:

- LABAs are contraindicated without the use of an inhaled corticosteroid. Single-ingredient LABAs should not be used alone.
- LABA use should be limited to the shortest duration of time required to achieve control of asthma symptoms and then discontinued.
- Long-term use of LABAs should be restricted to patients whose asthma cannot be adequately controlled with controller medications.
- Combination inhaled corticosteroid and a LABA are recommended for pediatric and adolescent patients when the addition of a LABA is required.

Short-Acting β₂-Adrenergic Agonists

Generic Name	US Brand Names / Canadian Brand Names	Dosage Forms and Strengths
albuterol[a] (salbutamol)	AccuNeb, Proair HFA, Proair Digihaler, Proair Respiclick, Proventil HFA, Ventolin HFA Airomir, Ventolin, Ventolin Diskus, Ventolin HFA	**Inhaler, metered dose (Proventil, Proair, Ventolin):** 90 mcg/actuation, 100 mcg/actuation (Airomir) **Solution, for inhalation:** 0.021%[b], 0.42%[b], 0.05%[c], 0.083%[b], 0.1%[c], 0.2%[c], 0.5%[c] **Powder, for inhalation (Proair Respiclick, Ventolin Diskus):** 90 mcg/dose, 200 mcg/dose **Solution, for IV use:** 1 mg/mL[c] **Solution, for respirator:** 5 mg/mL **Syrup:** 2 mg/5 mL[b] **Tablet, immediate release:** 2 mg, 4 mg
levalbuterol[a]	Xopenex, Xopenex HFA Not available	**Inhaler (Xopenex HFA):** 45 mcg/actuation **Inhalant solution (Xopenex):** 0.31 mg/3 mL (0.0103%), 0.63 mg/3 mL (0.021%), 1.25 mg/3 mL (0.042%), 1.25 mg/0.5 mL (0.25%)
terbutaline[a]	Brethine Bricanyl inhaler	**Inhaler (Canada only):** 0.5 mg/actuation[c] **Tablet:** 2.5 mg[b], 5 mg[b] **Solution, for injection:** 1 mg/mL[b]

Combination SABA + Short-Acting Anticholinergic/Antimuscarinic

albuterol + ipratropium bromide[a] (salbutamol + ipratropium bromide in Canada)	Combivent Respimat Combivent Respimat	**Inhaler, metered dose:** albuterol 100 mcg + ipratropium bromide 20 mcg/actuation **Inhalant solution:** salbutamol 2.5 mg + ipratropium bromide 0.5 mg/2.5 mL unit dose vial[c]; albuterol 3 mcg + ipratropium bromide 0.5 mg/3 mL unit dose vial[b]

[a]Generic available.
[b]Available in the United States only.
[c]Available in Canada only.

Long-Acting β₂-Adrenergic Agonists

Generic Name	US Brand Names / Canadian Brand Names	Dosage Forms and Strengths
arformoterol	Brovana Not available	**Solution, for inhalation:** 15 mcg/2 mL
formoterol	Foradil, Perforomist Foradil, Oxeze Turbuhaler	**Powder, for inhalation:** 6 mcg (Oxeze), 12 mcg/actuation (Foradil, Oxeze) **Solution, for inhalation (Perforomist):** 20 mcg/2 mL
olodaterol	Striverdi Respimat Not available	**Inhaler:** 2.5 mcg/actuation
salmeterol	Serevent Diskus Serevent Diskus	**Inhalation, powder:** 50 mcg/actuation

❶ Tech Alert!

The following drugs have look-alike/sound-alike issues:
Foradil and Toradol;
salmeterol and salbutamol

● Tech Note!

The FDA reports that long-acting β₂-adrenergic agonists, such as salmeterol (Serevent Diskus), may increase the risk for severe asthma exacerbations and asthma-related death; therefore a warning label advising patients not to exceed the prescribed dose is typically applied to dispensed prescriptions.

Glucocorticosteroids

Glucocorticosteroids are antiinflammatory drugs. They reduce the inflammatory response in airway cells, decreasing the mucus and swelling that make breathing difficult (see Fig. 23.1).

Mechanism of Action and Pharmacokinetics

Glucocorticoids decrease the synthesis of proinflammatory substances (e.g., prostaglandins, leukotrienes, cytokines, arachidonic acid, and macrophages) that are released as part of the inflammatory response. Further details about the mechanism of action and pharmacokinetics of glucocorticosteroids are discussed in detail in Chapter 13. The primary route of administration for corticosteroids used for the treatment of asthma is inhalation; however, they may be administered orally for more severe symptoms. Inhaled corticosteroids include beclomethasone, budesonide, ciclesonide, fluticasone, and mometasone.

Adverse Reactions

Adverse reactions to inhaled corticosteroids are primarily local and include coughing, hoarseness, throat irritation, dry mouth, flushing, loss of taste, or unpleasant taste. Some patients may develop an infection in the mouth or throat called thrush; however, the risk can be minimized by gargling or rinsing the mouth after administering each dose of medicine. Systemic effects are dose-dependent and more likely to occur at higher doses. Flovent HFA is contraindicated in children younger than 4 years of age, and budesonide, beclomethasone, and triamcinolone inhalers are contraindicated in children younger than 6 years of age. Symbicort and Advair HFA are contraindicated in children younger than 12 years.

> **❶ Tech Alert!**
>
> Arnuity Ellipta (fluticasone furoate) and Flovent Diskus (fluticasone propionate) are not substitutable.

Inhaled Corticosteroids

Generic Name	US Brand Names / Canadian Brand Names	Dosage Forms and Strengths
beclomethasone	Qvar Redihaler	**Inhaler:** 40 mcg/actuation[b], 50 mcg/actuation[c], 80 mcg/actuation[b], and 100 mcg/actuation[c]
	Qvar	
budesonide[a]	Pulmicort Flexhaler, Pulmicort Respules	**Inhalant powder (Pulmicort Flexhaler)**[b]: 80 mcg, 160 mcg/actuation
	Pulmicort Nebuamp, Pulmicort Turbuhaler	**Inhaler, metered dose (Pulmicort Turbuhaler):** 100 mcg, 200 mcg, 400 mcg/actuation
		Inhalant suspension (Pulmicort Nebuamp, Pulmicort Respules): 0.125 mg/mL[c], 0.25 mg/mL[c], 0.5 mg/mL[c], 0.25 mg/2 mL[b], 0.5 mg/2 mL[b], 1 mg/2 mL[b]
ciclesonide	Alvesco	**Inhalation aerosol:** 80 mcg/actuation[b], 100 mcg/actuation[c], 160 mcg/actuation[b], and 200 mcg/actuation[c]
	Alvesco	
fluticasone[a, c]	Armonair Respiclick, Arnuity Ellipta, Flovent Diskus, Flovent HFA	**Inhaler, metered dose (Flovent HFA):** 44 mcg/actuation[b], 50 mcg/actuation[c], 110 mcg/actuation[b], 125 mcg/actuation[c], 220 mcg/actuation[b], 250 mcg/actuation[c]
	Aermony Respiclick, Arnuity Ellipta, Flovent Diskus, Flovent HFA	**Powder, for inhalation (Flovent Diskus):** 50 mcg[b], 100 mcg, 250 mcg, 500 mcg/actuation[c]
		Powder, for inhalation (Aeromony Respiclick, Armonair Respiclick): 55 mcg, 113 mcg, 232 mcg/actuation
		Powder, for inhalation (Arnuity Ellipta): 50 mcg[b], 100 mcg, 200 mcg/actuation
mometasone	Asmanex HFA, Asmanex Twisthaler	**Inhaler, metered dose (Asmanex HFA):** 50 mcg, 100 mcg, 200 mcg/actuation
	Asmanex Twisthaler	**Powder, for inhalation (Asmanex Twisthaler):** 100 mcg[b], 110 mcg[c], 200 mcg[b], 220 mcg[c], 400 mcg[b]/actuation

Long-Acting β₂-Adrenergic Agonist + Corticosteroid

Generic Name	US/Canadian Brand Names	Dosage Forms and Strengths
formoterol + mometasone	Dulera	**Inhalation powder:** 5 mcg formoterol + 50 mcg mometasone, 5 mcg formoterol + 100 mcg mometasone, 5 mcg formoterol + 200 mcg mometasone/actuation
	Zenhale	
formoterol + budesonide	Breyna, Symbicort	**Inhaler, metered dose:** 4.5 mcg formoterol + 80 mcg budesonide/actuation[b]; 4.5 mcg formoterol + 160 mcg budesonide/actuation[b]; 6 mcg formoterol + 100 mcg budesonide/actuation[b]; 6 mcg formoterol + 200 mcg budesonide/actuation[b]
	Symbicort	

Inhaled Corticosteroids—cont'd

Generic Name	US Brand Names / Canadian Brand Names	Dosage Forms and Strengths
indacaterol + mometasone	Not available	**Powder for inhalation:** 150 mcg indacaterol + 80 mcg mometasone, 150 mcg indacaterol + 160 mcg mometasone, 150 mcg indacaterol + 320 mcg mometasone
	Atectura Breezhaler	
salmeterol + fluticasone[a]	Advair Diskus, Advair HFA, Airduo Digihaler, Airduo Respiclick	**Inhalant, powder (Advair Diskus, Wixela Inhub):** 50 mcg salmeterol + 100 mcg fluticasone, 50 mcg salmeterol + 250 mcg fluticasone, 50 mcg salmeterol + 500 mcg fluticasone
	Advair, Advair Diskus, Wixela Inhub	**Inhalant, powder (Airduo Respiclick, Airduo Digihaler):** 14 mcg salmeterol + 55 mcg fluticasone, 14 mcg salmeterol + 113 mcg fluticasone, 14 mcg salmeterol + 232 mcg fluticasone
		Inhaler, metered dose (Advair, Advair HFA): 21 mcg salmeterol + 45 mcg fluticasone[a], 21 mcg salmeterol + 115 mcg fluticasone[a], 21 mcg salmeterol + 230 mcg fluticasone[a], 25 mcg salmeterol + 125 mcg fluticasone[c], 25 mcg salmeterol + 250 mcg fluticasone[c]
vilanterol + fluticasone	Breo Ellipta	**Powder for inhalation:** 25 mcg vilanterol + 100 mcg fluticasone, 25 mcg vilanterol + 200 mcg fluticasone
	Breo Ellipta	

[a]Generic available.
[b]Available in the United States only.
[c]Available in Canada only.

Leukotriene Modifiers

Leukotrienes are proinflammatory substances that are released as part of the inflammatory response. Leukotriene modifiers are administered to patients with mild asthma to reduce inflammation.

> **● Tech Note!**
>
> A common ending for leukotriene modifiers is -lukast.

Mechanism of Action

Zileuton inhibits the action of the enzyme responsible for converting arachidonic acid to leukotriene A4. This is the first step in the leukotriene pathway.

Montelukast and zafirlukast interfere with the binding of leukotrienes on airway smooth muscle, reducing allergen-induced airway inflammation, airway relaxation, and edema.

Pharmacokinetics

Montelukast is readily absorbed when administered orally. The maximum concentration of oral tablets is reached within 3 to 4 hours. Chewable tablets work faster, reaching a maximum concentration within approximately 2.5 hours. Food does not decrease the bioavailability of montelukast, unlike zafirlukast, which must be taken on an empty stomach. Montelukast, zafirlukast, and zileuton are metabolized in the liver by cytochrome P-450 (CYP450) isozymes and can interfere with the metabolism of other drugs using the same metabolic pathway.

> **❶ Tech Alert!**
>
> The following drugs have look-alike/sound-alike issues:
> Singulair and SINEquan

Adverse Reactions

Montelukast and zafirlukast may produce a cough, hoarseness or sore throat, headache, indigestion, heartburn or stomach upset, and runny nose. Montelukast may also produce difficulty sleeping, dizziness, drowsiness, muscle aches or cramps, and unusual dreams. Zileuton extended-release tablets may produce abdominal pain in addition to the adverse reactions listed for montelukast and zafirlukast.

Precautions

The packet of montelukast granules should not be opened until ready for use. Once opened, packet contents (with or without mixing with food) must be administered within 15 minutes. Zileuton may cause abnormal liver function and jaundice, so liver function tests should be conducted every 2 to 3 months.

Mast Cell Stabilizers

Mast cells are released as part of the immune system's response to allergens. Mast cell degranulation leads to the release of histamine and mediators of inflammation (e.g., leukotrienes, eosinophils, basophils, cytokines, and prostaglandins). Cromolyn sodium is an example of a mast cell stabilizer. Cromolyn is administered for prophylaxis and does not control acute symptoms.

Mechanism of Action

Cromolyn sodium reduces the release of inflammatory substances responsible for producing the symptoms of asthma by making mast cells less reactive to antigens. It inhibits the degranulation of mast cells and prevents the release of histamine and the slow-reacting substance of anaphylaxis. Cromolyn sodium improves exercise tolerance and reaction to cold air and environmental pollutants by reducing hyperactivity of the bronchi.

Leukotriene Modifiers

Generic Name	US Brand Names / Canadian Brand Names	Dosage Forms and Strengths
montelukast[a]	Singulair Singulair	**Oral granules:** 4 mg/pack **Tablet:** 10 mg **Tablet, chewable:** 4 mg, 5 mg
zafirlukast[a]	Accolate Not available	**Tablet:** 10 mg, 20 mg
zileuton[a]	Zyflo, Zyflo CR Not available	**Tablet (Zyflo):** 600 mg **Tablet, controlled release (Zyflo CR):** 600 mg

[a]Generic available.

Pharmacokinetics

Cromolyn sodium is not used to treat acute symptoms. Several weeks of therapy are required before maximum response to the drug is achieved. Cromolyn produces a local effect on cell membranes. Only 1% of the drug is absorbed systemically.

Adverse Reactions

Cromolyn sodium may be administered using an MDI or nebulizer. Systemic absorption of cromolyn sodium is minimal, so side effects are generally localized. The most common adverse reactions are a bad taste in the mouth, irritated dry throat, and coughing or wheezing.

Mast Cell Stabilizers

Generic Name	US Brand Names / Canadian Brand Names	Dosage Forms and Strengths
cromolyn sodium[a]	Generics Generics	**Solution, for inhalation:** 1%

[a]Generic available.

Xanthine Derivatives

Theophylline is a xanthine drug. Xanthines are one of the oldest classes of drugs used for the treatment of asthma. Theophylline occurs naturally in tea and is chemically similar to caffeine.

> **❗ Tech Alert!**
>
> A common ending for xanthine derivatives is -phylline.

> **• BOX 23.4 Modifiers of Serum Blood Levels of Theophylline**
>
> **Drugs and Foods That Increase Levels**
> - Oral contraceptives
> - Erythromycin
> - Calcium channel blockers
> - Cimetidine
> - Caffeine
> - Chocolate
>
> **Drugs That Decrease Levels**
> - Phenobarbital
> - Phenytoin
> - Carbamazepine

Mechanism of Action

Xanthines have bronchodilator and antiinflammatory properties. The exact mechanism of action of xanthines is unknown; however, the drugs are known to inhibit the release of inflammatory substances and act on bronchial smooth muscle to reduce bronchospasms.

Pharmacokinetics

The half-life ($t_{1/2}$) of theophylline varies with the patient's age, liver function, smoking status, and use of concurrent drugs. Smoking decreases the drug's half-life by nearly 50%. In children ages 1 to 9 years, the half-life can be as much as 50% shorter than that in adults. Liver disease and pulmonary edema can prolong half-life up to 24 hours. Theophylline is extensively metabolized by the CYP450 enzyme system and is involved in numerous drug interactions (Box 23.4). The bioavailability of theophylline varies by manufacturer. It is recommended that patients receive the same manufacturer's product each time that their prescriptions are refilled.

Adverse Reactions

Xanthine derivatives (e.g., theophylline) may produce insomnia, dizziness, headache, irritability, decreased appetite, stomach cramps, and urinary retention.

Xanthine Derivatives

| Generic Name | US Brand Names | | Dosage Forms and Strengths |
	Canadian Brand Names		
theophylline[a]	Elixophyllin, Theo-24		**Capsule, extended release (Theo-24):** 400 mg
	Theo ER		**Elixir (Elixophyllin, Theolair):** 80 mg/15 mL
			Tablet, extended release (Theo ER): 300 mg, 400 mg, 450 mg, 600 mg

[a]Generic available.

Monoclonal Antibodies

Benralizumab, dupilumab, mepolizumab, omalizumab, reslizumab, and tezepelumab are monoclonal antibodies (anti-IgE) that are indicated for the treatment of moderate to severe *allergic asthma*. They decrease the body's response to asthma triggers. Asthma triggers and environmental allergens can cause a hypersensitivity reaction that produces overexpression of immunoglobulin E (IgE) antibodies that cause asthma symptoms. Monoclonal antibodies are indicated as add-on therapy for patients whose asthma is not controlled with inhaled corticosteroids and β_2-adrenergic agonists.

> **Tech Note!**
>
> A common ending for monoclonal antibody drugs is *-mab*.

Mechanism of Action and Pharmacokinetics

The action of monoclonal antibodies used for the treatment of asthma is specifically directed toward interleukin-5. They prevent early- and late-stage allergic responses as well as the release of inflammatory mediators (e.g., cytokines) because of their inhibitory action on interleukin-5.

Benralizumab, dupilumab, mepolizumab, omalizumab, and tezepelumab are administered by subcutaneous injection, and reslizumab is given by intravenous infusion once monthly. Maximum effects are achieved after 3 days to 2 weeks of administration depending on the agent administered.

Adverse Reactions

The most common adverse reactions are mild redness, itching, swelling, or bruising at the injection site; headache; and nausea. More serious adverse effects that may be a prelude to anaphylaxis are difficulty breathing, hives, and skin rash.

Precautions

Package labeling states that patients should be instructed to use aseptic technique and watch for signs and symptoms of anaphylaxis.

Monoclonal Antibodies

| Generic Name | US Brand Names | Dosage Forms and Strengths |
	Canadian Brand Names	
benralizumab	Fasenra	**Solution, for subcutaneous injection:** 30 mg/mL
	Fasenra, Fasenra Pen	
dupilumab	Dupixent	**Solution, for injection:** 150 mg/mL, 200 mg/1.14 mL
	Dupixent	
mepolizumab	Nucala	**Solution, for subcutaneous injection:** 100 mg/mL
	Nucala	**Powder, for injection:** 100 mg
omalizumab	Xolair	**Solution, for injection:** 75 mg/0.5 mL, 150 mg/mL
	Xolair	**Powder, for injection:** 75 mg, 150 mg
reslizumab	Cinqair	**Solution, for IV infusion:** 10 mg/mL
	Cinqair	
tezepelumab	Tezspire	**Solution, for subcutaneous injection:** 110 mg/mL
	Tezspire	

Chronic Obstructive Pulmonary Disease

Overview

Chronic obstructive pulmonary disease is a progressive disease of the airways that produces a gradual loss of pulmonary function. Emphysema, chronic bronchitis, and chronic obstructive bronchitis are all classified under the heading of COPD. The lungs and airways of patients with COPD are chronically inflamed and air sacs are destroyed. Inflammatory cells (e.g., CD8+ T lymphocytes and interleukin-6) infiltrate the airways.

Risk Factors

Age, disease, and various lifestyle and environmental factors contribute to the risk for developing COPD. COPD is more typical in individuals older than 40 years. Cigarette smoking (or exposure to secondhand smoke) is the leading cause of COPD; 75% of people with COPD are current or former smokers. Occupational irritants to the lungs such as asbestos, industrial chemicals, dust, and air pollution may all contribute to or worsen existing COPD. A history of chronic asthma is also a risk factor. Viral infections can aggravate COPD—in particular, respiratory syncytial virus and adenovirus.

Symptoms

Airflow obstruction produces SOB. Persons with COPD may also exhibit a chronic persistent cough and wheezing. Airways become clogged with mucus, making breathing more difficult.

Treatment

The aim of COPD management is to (1) relieve symptoms and airway obstruction, (2) increase oxygen, and (3) treat any precipitating factors and/or comorbidities. Pharmacologic treatment of COPD involves the administration of bronchodilators, glucocorticosteroids, and—when infections are present—antibiotics. Nonpharmacologic treatments include oxygen therapy and mechanical ventilation.

Pharmacologic Treatment

Current recommendations support the administration of bronchodilators and long-acting muscarinic antagonist (LAMA)/LABA combinations as first-line maintenance therapy (Table 23.1). The use of glucocorticosteroids to reduce inflammation and open airways was described earlier (see "***Maintenance Therapy to Prevent Asthma Flareups***"). Usual doses administered for the treatment of COPD are listed in the drug table at the end of this chapter. Additional drugs specifically indicated for the treatment of COPD are the anticholinergics (e.g., tiotropium).

Mechanism of Action

Aclidinium, glycopyrrolate (glycopyrronium in Canada), ipratropium, revefenacin, and umeclidinium are antimuscarinic anticholinergic drugs. Anticholinergics bind to muscarinic receptors and block the effects of acetylcholine (released by the vagus nerve), resulting in the relaxation of bronchial smooth muscle. Antagonism of cholinergic receptors relaxes bronchial smooth muscle, producing bronchodilation. Recall that parasympathetic nervous system stimulation produces increased mucus and bronchoconstriction, so antagonism decreases mucus and bronchoconstriction. Review the Unit II opener.

Aclidinium and tiotropium are dosed once daily and are indicated for the treatment of COPD. Ipratropium bromide prescribed for short-term relief of symptoms must be given three or four times daily.

Adverse Reactions

A stuffy or runny nose, upper respiratory tract infections (e.g., colds), and a cough are common side effecs of anticholinergic drugs. They may also produce urinary retention, blurred vision, constipation, hoarseness, dizziness, or headaches. Cardiac arrhythmias and asthma-related hospitalization and death have also been reported.

Phosphodiesterase 4 Inhibitor

Roflumilast is a phosphodiesterase-4 inhibitor. The exact mechanism for improving COPD symptoms is unknown; however, it is related to increasing cyclic AMP in lung cells.

TABLE 23.1 Chronic Obstructive Pulmonary Disease (COPD) Pharmacotherapy				
COPD Grade			**Recommended Pharmacotherapy**	
GOLD 1 Mild FEV$_1$ > 80% predicted	0 or 1 moderate exacerbations not leading to hospitalization	Category A Bronchodilator	Category B Long-acting β2-agonist (LABA) or Long-acting antimuscarinic (LAMA) or LAMA + LABA (if symptoms persist)	
GOLD 2 Moderate 50% < FEV$_1$ < 80% predicted				
GOLD 3 Severe 30% < FEV$_1$ < 50% predicted	2 or more exacerbations or 1 or more leading to hospitalization	Category E LAMA If further exacerbations ADD LAMA + LABA or LABA + inhaled corticosteroid (ICS) If persistent symptoms or further exacerbations LAMA + LABA + ICS If further exacerbations and/or lung function (FEV$_1$ < 50%) ADD roflumilast		
GOLD 4 Very severe FEV$_1$ < 30%				

Adapted from Global Initiative for Chronic Obstructive Pulmonary Disease 2023.

Anticholinergic Drugs

Generic Name	US Brand Names Canadian Brand Names	Dosage Forms and Strengths
aclidinium bromide	Tudorza Pressair Tudorza Genuair	**Powder, for inhalation**: 400 mcg/inhalation
glycopyrrolate (United States) glycopyrronium (Canada)	Lonhala Magnair Seebri Breezhaler	**Powder, for inhalation (Seebri)**: 50 mcg/inhalation **Solution, for inhalation (Lonhala Magnair)**: 25 mcg/mL
ipratropium bromide	Atrovent HFA Atrovent HFA	**Inhaler, metered dose**: 20 mcg/spray[b], 21 mcg/spray[a] **Solution, for inhalation**: 125 mcg/mL[b], 200 mcg/mL[a], 250 mcg/mL[b]
tiotropium bromide	Spiriva, Spiriva Respimat Spiriva, Spiriva Respimat	**Inhaler**: 1.25 mcg/inhalation[a], 2.5 mcg/inhalation **Powder, for inhalation**: 18 mcg/inhalation[a]
revefenacin	Yupelri Not available	**Solution, for inhalation**: 175 mcg/3 mL/vial
umeclidinium	Incruse Ellipta Incruse Ellipta	**Powder for inhalation**: 62.5 mcg/inhalation

Anticholinergic + Long-Acting β₂-Adrenergic Agonists Combinations

aclidinium + formoterol	Duaklir Pressair Duaklir Genuair	**Inhaler**: 400 mcg aclidinium + 12 mcg formoterol/ actuation
glycopyrrolate + formoterol	Bevespi Aerosphere Not available	**Inhaler**: 9 mcg glycopyrrolate + 4.8 mcg formoterol/ inhalation
glycopyrronium + indacaterol	Not available Ultibro Breezehaler	**Powder, for inhalation**: 50 mcg glycopyrronium + 110 mcg indacaterol
tiotropium + olodaterol	Stiolto Respimat Inspiolto Respimat, Spiolto Respimat	**Inhaler**: 2.5 mcg tiotropium + 2.5 mcg olodaterol/ actuation **Inhalation solution**: 2.5 mcg tiotropium + 2.5 mcg olodaterol
umeclidinium bromide + vilanterol	Anoro Ellipta Anoro Ellipta	**Powder for inhalation**: 62.5 mcg umeclidinium + 25 mcg vilanterol

Anticholinergic + corticosteroid + LABA

glycopyrronium + budesonide + formoterol	Not available Breztri Aerosphere	**Inhaler, metered dose**: 8.2 mcg glycopyrronium + 182 mcg budesonide + 5.8 mcg formoterol
umeclidinium + fluticasone + vilanterol	Trelegy Ellipta Trelegy Ellipta	**Powder, for inhalation**: 62.5 mcg umeclidinium + 100 mcg fluticasone + 25 mcg vilanterol, 62.5 mcg umeclidinium + 200 mcg fluticasone + 25 mcg vilanterol

[a]Available in the United States only.
[b]Available in Canada only.

Phosphodiesterase-4 Inhibitor

Generic Name	US Brand Names Canadian Brand Names	Dosage Forms and Strengths
roflumilast	Daliresp Daxas	**Tablet**: 250 mcg[a], 500 mcg

[a]Available in United States only.

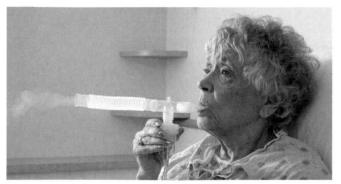

• **Fig. 23.2** Nebulizer. (From Hopper T: *Mosby's pharmacy technician*, ed 2, St Louis, 2007, WB Saunders.)

Drug-Delivery Devices for Use With Asthma and Chronic Obstructive Pulmonary Disease Medicines

Delivery of the prescribed dose of medication using an MDI is fast but may be challenging for some individuals and is inappropriate for small children. It is not uncommon for a substantial amount of the drug to be delivered to the back of the throat rather than into the lungs when an MDI is used. A dry powder inhaler (DPI) is similar to an MDI, but the medication is in powder form rather than in liquid form. A puff of the powder is inhaled rather than a mist of liquid. A nebulizer is a device that converts a liquid dose of medicine into an aerosolized mist that can be inhaled by normal breathing when used with a mask (Fig. 23.2). A mouthpiece may also be attached to the end of the nebulizer and the mist inhaled using slow deep breaths.

A *spacer* is a device that is attached to the end of the MDI (Fig. 23.3). The drug is sprayed into the device's chamber and then

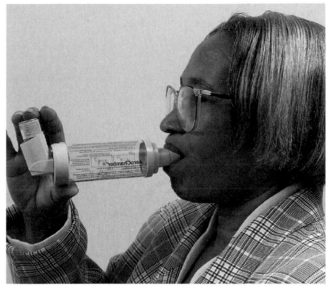

• **Fig. 23.3** Spacer. (From Potter PA, et al: *Fundamentals of nursing*, ed 9, St Louis, 2017, Elsevier.)

slowly inhaled into the lungs. Some devices produce a whistling sound to alert the patient when inhalation is too rapid or is not controlled.

TECHNICIAN'S CORNER

1. Can lung damage be reversed when a smoker stops smoking?
2. What are some lifestyle modifications that can be implemented to manage asthma?

Summary of Drugs Used for the Treatment of Asthma and Chronic Obstructive Pulmonary Disease

	Generic Name	US Brand Name	Usual Adult Oral Dose and Dosing Schedule[a]	Warning Labels
Short-Acting β$_2$-Adrenergic Agonists				
	albuterol (salbutamol)	Ventolin HFA	**Asthma Inhaler**: 1–2 puffs q 4–6 h as needed **Inhalant solution**: 2.5 mg q 6–8 h prn delivered over 5–15 min, *or* **AccuNeb**: 0.63–1.25 mg tid or qid; deliver over 5–15 min as needed **Solution or tablet, immediate release**: 2–4 mg q 6–8 h (max 32 mg/day) **Tablet, extended release**: 4–8 mg q 12 h (max 32 mg/day)	SHAKE WELL— inhaler.
	levalbuterol	Xopenex	**Asthma Inhalant solution**: 0.63–1.25 mg q 6–8 h **Inhaler**: 2 puffs q 4–6 h	DO NOT EXCEED RECOMMENDED DOSE.
	terbutaline	Generics	**Asthma and COPD Injection**: 0.25 mg SC; repeat in 15–30 min if needed **Tablet**: 2.5–5 mg 3 times a day **Asthma Inhaler**: 2 puffs q 4 h	

Summary of Drugs Used for the Treatment of Asthma and Chronic Obstructive Pulmonary Disease—cont'd

	Generic Name	US Brand Name	Usual Adult Oral Dose and Dosing Schedule[a]	Warning Labels
Long-Acting β₂-Adrenergic Agonists				
	formoterol	Foradil	**Asthma and COPD:** Inhale contents of 1 capsule q 12 h	DO NOT SWALLOW CAPSULES (FOR INHALATION DEVICE USE ONLY).
	salmeterol	Serevent Diskus	**Asthma and COPD:** 1 inhalation q 12 h	
β₂-Adrenergic Agonists + Anticholinergics				
	albuterol + ipratropium bromide	Combivent, DuoNeb	**COPD:** Inhale 1 puff 4 times daily (Combivent) or 3 mL qid (DuoNeb)	SHAKE WELL—inhaler.
	fenoterol hydrobromide + ipratropium bromide	DuoVent	**COPD:** Inhale 4 mL q 4–6 h	
Anticholinergics				
	aclidinium bromide	Tudorza	**COPD:** Inhale 1 puff twice daily	DISCARD 45 DAYS AFTER OPENING POUCH.
	glycopyrrolate (United States) glycopyrronium (Canada)	Lonhala Magnair (Seebri Breezhaler)	**COPD:** Inhale the contents of 1 vial twice daily (Lonhala Magnair) Inhale the contents of 1 capsule once daily (Seebri Breezhaler)	DO NOT SKIP DOSES.
	ipratropium bromide	Atrovent HFA	**COPD:** Inhale 2 sprays 3–4 times a day (MDI) or inhale 1 vial of nebulizer solution (500 mcg) q 6–8 h	SHAKE WELL. MAY CAUSE DIZZINESS OR BLURRED VISION; USE CAUTION WHEN DRIVING. DO NOT SWALLOW CAPSULES (FOR INHALATION DEVICE USE).
	tiotropium	Spiriva	**COPD:** Inhale contents of 1 capsule once daily	
	revefenacin	Yupelri	**COPD:** Inhale 175 mcg dose in nebulizer once daily	DO NOT SKIP DOSES.
	umeclidinium	Incruse Ellipta	**COPD:** Inhale powder once daily	DISCARD 6 WEEKS AFTER OPENING OR WHEN COUNTER IS AT ZERO.
Anticholinergic/Antimuscarinic + Long-Acting β₂-Adrenergic Agonists Combinations				
	aclidinium + formoterol	Duaklir Pressair	**COPD:** Inhale 1 puff twice daily	DO NOT SKIP DOSES—all. MAY CAUSE DIZZINESS OR BLURRED VISION; USE CAUTION WHEN DRIVING—all. RINSE MOUTH AFTER USE—Breztri Aerosphere, Trelegy Ellipta. DISCARD OPEN POUCHES 3 WEEKS AFTER OPENING (28 actuations/pouch) OR 3 MONTHS AFTER OPENING (120 actuations/pouch)— Breztri Aerosphere.
	glycopyrrolate + formoterol	Bevespi Aerosphere	**COPD:** Inhale 2 puffs twice daily	
	glycopyrronium + indacaterol	(Ultibro Breezehaler)	**COPD:** Inhale the contents of 1 capsule once daily	
	tiotropium + olodaterol	Stiolto Respimat (Spiolto Respimat)	**COPD:** Inhale 2 puffs once daily	
	umeclidinium bromide+ vilanterol	Anoro Ellipta	**COPD:** Inhale 1 puff once daily	
	formoterol + budesonide + glycopyrronium	(Breztri Aerosphere)	**COPD:** Inhale 2 puffs twice daily	
	vilanterol + fluticasone + umeclidinium	Trelegy Ellipta	**Asthma and COPD:** Inhale 1 puff once daily	

Continued

Summary of Drugs Used for the Treatment of Asthma and Chronic Obstructive Pulmonary Disease—cont'd

	Generic Name	US Brand Name	Usual Adult Oral Dose and Dosing Schedule[a]	Warning Labels
Inhaled Corticosteroids				
	beclomethasone	QVar	**Asthma:** 1–4 puffs twice daily (max 320 mcg/day)	SHAKE WELL—inhaler.
	budesonide	Pulmicort	**Asthma:** 1–2 puffs twice daily	
	ciclesonide	Alvesco	**Asthma:** 1–2 puffs once daily (800 mcg dose may be given as 400 mcg twice daily)	
	fluticasone	Flovent HFA	**Asthma:** 2 sprays up to twice daily (maximum dose varies for Armonair Respiclick, Flovent HFA, and Flovent Diskus)	
	mometasone	Asmanex	**Asthma:** 1–2 sprays once or twice daily (max 440 mcg/day)	
β2-Adrenergic Agonists + Inhaled Corticosteroids				
	formoterol + budesonide	Symbicort	**Asthma:** 2 puffs twice daily	SHAKE WELL—metered-dose inhalers.
	formoterol + mometasone	Dulera (Zenhale)	**Asthma:** 2 puffs twice daily	
	indacaterol + mometasone	Atectura Breezhaler	**Asthma:** Inhale contents of 1 capsule once daily	
	salmeterol + fluticasone	Advair HFA Advair Diskus	**Asthma and COPD:** 1 puff q 12 h (maximum fluticasone 500 mcg/salmeterol 50 mcg) (maximum dose varies for Advair Diskus, Advair HFA, and Airduo Respiclick)	
	vilanterol + fluticasone	Breo Ellipta	**Asthma:** Inhale 1 puff (100/25 mcg or 200/25 mcg) once daily **COPD:** Inhale 1 puff (100/25 mcg) once daily	DO NOT SKIP DOSES. DISCARD 6 WEEKS AFTER OPENING.
Leukotriene Modifiers				
	montelukast	Singulair	**Asthma:** 10 mg once daily in the evening	TAKE WITH A LARGE GLASS OF WATER—chewable tablets. DISCARD UNUSED PORTION OF GRANULES WITHIN 15 MINUTES.
	zafirlukast	Accolate	**Asthma:** 20 mg (1–2 tablets) twice daily	TAKE ON AN EMPTY STOMACH (1–2 HOURS AFTER EATING).
	zileuton	Zyflo	**Asthma:** 600 mg 4 times a day (immediate-release tabs) 1200 mg bid (extended-release tabs)	TAKE WITH FOOD (within 1 hour after morning and evening meals). SWALLOW WHOLE; DO NOT CRUSH OR CHEW.
Mast Cell Stabilizers				
	cromolyn sodium	Generics	**Asthma Inhaler:** 2 sprays 4 times a day **Nebulizer:** 20 mg (2 mL) 4 times a day	SHAKE WELL—inhaler.
Xanthine Derivatives				
	theophylline	Theo-24	**Asthma and COPD:** 300–800 mg/day (extended released) in divided doses q 12–24 h (Theo-24)	TAKE 30–60 MINUTES BEFORE MEALS WITH A FULL GLASS OF WATER.

Continued

Summary of Drugs Used for the Treatment of Asthma and Chronic Obstructive Pulmonary Disease—cont'd

	Generic Name	US Brand Name	Usual Adult Oral Dose and Dosing Schedule[a]	Warning Labels
Monoclonal Antibody				
	benralizumab	Fasenra	30 mg SC once every 4 weeks for 3 doses then q 8 weeks	REFRIGERATE AT 36°F–46°F (2°C–8°C) IN THE ORIGINAL CARTON TO PROTECT FROM LIGHT—benralizumab, dupilumab, mepolizumab, omalizumab, tezepelumab. DISCARD RECONSTITUTED SOLUTION AFTER 24 HOURS—omalizumab. DO NOT SHAKE. DISCARD IF SOLUTION IS DISCOLORED—reslizumab.
	dupilumab	Dupixent	Initial dose 400 or 600 mg SC followed by 200 or 300 mg every 2 weeks	
	mepolizumab	Nucala	**Severe asthma:** 100 mg SC once every 4 weeks	
	omalizumab	Xolair	**Asthma:** 150–375 mg SC q 2 or 4 weeks (based on baseline immunoglobulin E levels)	
	reslizumab	Cinqair	3 mg/kg IV once every 4 weeks	
	tezepelumab	Tezspire	210 mg SC administered once every 4 weeks	
Phosphodiesterase-4 Inhibitors				
	roflumilast	Daliresp	250 mcg once daily for 4 weeks then increase to 500 mcg once daily	MAY CAUSE DIZZINESS.

SC, subcutaneous; *IV,* intravenous.
[a]Adult dose for asthma and COPD unless specified.

Key Points

- Asthma is a chronic disease that affects the airways, producing irritation, inflammation, coughing, wheezing, shortness of breath, and chest tightness.
- Asthma is classified according to the level of treatment necessary to control symptoms or keep symptoms from worsening.
- Family history of asthma, smoking, exposure to secondhand smoke, chronic exposure to air pollution, exposure to some allergens, and infections early in life are risk factors for developing asthma.
- Symptoms of asthma are caused by airway irritation that results in bronchial constriction and impedes the passage of air. Airways also become inflamed, which produces swelling and restricts the flow of air. Mucus production is increased, which further obstructs breathing passages.
- Asthma "triggers" can precipitate an asthma attack. Examples are animal dander, cockroach droppings, environmental pollutants, cleaning fluids, mold, tobacco smoke, air pollution, upper respiratory infection, vigorous exercise, and even cold air.
- Asthma symptoms can be managed with a combination of medication, lifestyle modification, and home monitoring of breathing using a peak flow meter and medication.
- COPD is a progressive disease of the airways that produces gradual loss of pulmonary function, shortness of breath, chronic persistent cough, wheezing, and increased sputum production.
- Cigarette smoking or exposure to secondhand smoke, occupational irritants, industrial chemicals or dust, and age can increase the risk of developing COPD.
- Air pollution and viral infections may contribute to and worsen existing COPD.
- A peak flow meter permits self-management of asthma, similar to the way in which the monitoring of blood glucose levels enables self-management of diabetes.
- Low peak flow numbers signal that asthma is not controlled.
- Pharmacologic treatment of COPD involves the administration of bronchodilators, glucocorticosteroids, and antibiotics when infection is present.
- Nonpharmacologic treatments include oxygen therapy and mechanical ventilation.
- Drugs used for the treatment and management of asthma are divided into two classes. Drugs for the treatment of acute symptoms are classified as rescue or reliever medicines. Drugs administered to prevent asthma episodes are classified as maintenance therapies.
- Short-acting β_2-adrenergic agonists provide short-term relief of acute symptoms. Reliever medicines currently prescribed for the treatment of asthma include albuterol, levalbuterol, and terbutaline.
- Short-acting inhaled anticholinergic drugs (e.g., ipratropium bromide) are administered for the relief of acute symptoms. Long-acting inhaled cholinergic drugs (e.g., aclidinium,

tiotropium, umeclidinium) are used as COPD maintenance therapies.

- Short-acting β_2-adrenergic agonists can produce nervousness, difficulty sleeping, dry mouth, mild headache, and throat irritation (by inhalants).
- Glucocorticosteroids decrease inflammation and mucus in the airways.
- Inhaled corticosteroids include fluticasone (Flovent), budesonide (Pulmicort), mometasone (Asmanex), and beclomethasone (Qvar).
- Adverse reactions to inhaled corticosteroids are primarily local and include coughing, hoarseness, throat irritation, dry mouth, thrush, loss of taste, and/or unpleasant taste.
- Risks for thrush can be minimized by gargling or rinsing the mouth after administering the prescribed dose of glucocorticosteroid.
- Leukotriene modifiers are administered to patients with mild asthma to reduce inflammation.
- Leukotriene modifiers inhibit the release of proinflammatory leukotrienes, substances that are released as part of the inflammatory response.
- A packet of montelukast granules should not be opened until ready for use. Once opened, packet contents (with or without mixing with food) must be administered within 15 minutes.

- Cromolyn sodium is an example of a mast cell stabilizer; it makes mast cells less reactive to antigens and reduces the release of inflammatory substances responsible for producing the symptoms of asthma.
- Xanthines have bronchodilator and antiinflammatory properties.
- Smoking cigarettes decreases the half-life of theophylline by almost 50%.
- It is recommended that patients receive the same manufacturer's product each time their prescriptions for theophylline are refilled.
- Benralizumab, dupilumab, mepolizumab, omalizumab, reslizumab, and tezepelumab are monoclonal antibodies that are used for the treatment of moderate to severe allergic asthma as add-on therapy for patients whose asthma is not controlled with inhaled corticosteroids and β_2-adrenergic agonists.
- A nebulizer is a device that converts a liquid dose of medicine into an aerosolized mist.
- A spacer is a device attached to the end of the metered-dose inhaler that is used to control the delivery of an inhaled medicine.

Review Questions

1. A drug that relaxes tightened airway muscles and improves airflow through the airways is known as a _____.
   a. bronchodilator
   b. bronchoconstrictor
2. You receive a prescription for Advair Diskus 1 to 2 puffs every 4 to 6 hours. You consult with the pharmacist because _____.
   a. Advair is not marketed as a "Diskus"
   b. Advair is dosed once daily
   c. Advair is dosed twice a day
   d. Advair has been discontinued and is no longer marketed
3. All of the following are asthma triggers EXCEPT_____.
   a. family history
   b. exposure to cigarette smoke
   c. vigorous exercise
   d. exposure to environmental pollutants
4. A peak flow meter is a device _____.
   a. that is attached to the end of the metered-dose inhaler
   b. that aids in self-management of asthma
   c. that is used to administer asthma medication
   d. that is used to diagnose and treat COPD
5. Which of the following drugs used for the treatment of allergic asthma is administered by injection?
   a. Xolair
   b. Theolair
   c. Singulair
   d. Advair
6. Persons with _____ may also exhibit a chronic persistent cough, wheezing, and increased mucus production.
   a. a smoking habit
   b. COPD

   c. bronchitis
   d. none of the above
7. Nonpharmacologic treatments for COPD include which of the following?
   a. oxygen therapy
   b. mechanical ventilation
   c. inhalers
   d. a and b
8. All of the following drugs are marketed as an inhalant solution EXCEPT:
   a. albuterol
   b. ipratropium
   c. levalbuterol
   d. tiotropium
9. Dupixent is administered by the _____ route.
   a. oral
   b. subcutaneous injection
   c. transdermal
   d. intravenous
10. A(n) _____ is a device that converts a liquid dose of medicine into an aerosolized mist that can be inhaled by normal breathing when used with a mask.
   a. aerosolizer
   b. nebulizer
   c. spacer
   d. inhaler

Bibliography

Bollmeier SG, Hartmann AP. Management of chronic obstructive pulmonary disease: a review focusing on exacerbations. *Am J Health Syst Pharm*. 2020;77:4.

Centers for Disease Control and Prevention. (2022). National Center for Health Statistics—Asthma, 2022. Retrieved January 3, 2023, from https://www.cdc.gov/nchs/fastats/asthma.htm.

Centers for Disease Control and Prevention National Asthma Control Program. (2021). America Breathing Easier. Retrieved January 3, 2023, from https://www.cdc.gov/asthma/pdfs/breathing_easier_brochure.pdf.

Edris A, De Feyter S, Maes T, et al. Monoclonal antibodies in type 2 asthma: a systematic review and network meta-analysis. *Respir Res*. 2019;20:179.

Fortescue R, Kew KM, Leung Shiu Tsun M. Sublingual immunotherapy for asthma. *Cochrane Database Syst Rev*. 2020;9CD011293.

Global Initiative of COPD. (2023). Pocket Guide to COPD Diagnosis, Management and Prevention. Retrieved January 6, 2023, from https://goldcopd.org/2023-gold-report-2/.

Global Initiative for Asthma. (2022). Pocket Guide for Asthma Management and Treatment. Retrieved January 6, 2023, from https://ginasthma.org.

Health Canada. (2022). Drug Product Database. Retrieved January 3, 2023, from https://health-products.canada.ca/dpd-bdpp/index-eng.jsp.

Institute for Safe Medication Practices. (2016). FDA and ISMP Lists of Look-Alike Drug Names with Recommended Tall Man Letters. Retrieved December 29, 2023, from https://www.ismp.org/recommendations/tall-man-letters-list.

Institute for Safe Medication Practices. (2019). List of Confused Drugs. Retrieved December 29, 2023, from https://www.ismp.org/tools/confuseddrugnames.pdf.

National Heart Lung and Blood Institute. (2020). 2020 Focused Updates to the Asthma Management Guidelines: A Report from the National Asthma Education and Prevention Program Coordinating Committee Expert Panel Working Group. Retrieved January 3, 2023, from https://www.nhlbi.nih.gov/resources/2020-focused-updates-asthma-management-guidelines.

National Heart, Lung, and Blood Institute. (2022). A Quick Guide on COPD. NIH Publication No. 22-HL-8081, March 2022. Retrieved January 3, 2023, from https://www.nhlbi.nih.gov/resources/quick-guide-copd.

Page C, Curtis M, Sutter M, et al. *Integrated pharmacology*. Philadelphia: Mosby; 2005:415–423.

Papi A, Contoli M, Gaetano C, et al. Models of infection and exacerbations in COPD. *Curr Opin Pharmacol*. 2007;7:259–265.

Roman-Rodriguez M, Kaplan A. GOLD 2021 strategy report: implications for asthma-COPD overlap. *Int J Chron Obstruct Pulmon Dis*. 2021;16:1709–1715.

Shigemitsu H, Afshar K. Nocturnal asthma. *Curr Opin Pulm Med*. 2007;13:49–55.

Statistics Canada. (2022). Asthma, by age group, 2014. Retrieved January 3, 2023, from https://www150.statcan.gc.ca/t1/tbl1/en/tv.action?pid=1310009608.

U.S. Food and Drug Administration. (nd). Drugs@FDA: FDA Approved Drug Products. Retrieved January 3, 2023, from https://www.accessdata.fda.gov/scripts/cder/daf/index.cfm.

24

Treatment of Allergies

LEARNING OBJECTIVES

1. Learn the terminology associated with allergies.
2. Describe the causes and list the symptoms of allergic reactions.
3. List and categorize medications used for the treatment of allergies.
4. Describe the mechanism of action for drugs used to treat allergies.
5. Identify significant drug look-alike and sound-alike issues.
6. Identify warning labels and precautionary messages associated with medications used for the treatment of allergies.

KEY TERMS

Allergen Substance that produces an allergic reaction.
Allergic conjunctivitis Condition characterized by red, watering, itchy, or burning eyes.
Allergic rhinitis Seasonal condition characterized by inflammation and swelling of the nasal passageways (rhinitis) accompanied by runny nose (rhinorrhea).
Allergy Hypersensitivity reaction by the immune system on exposure to an allergen.
Anaphylaxis Life-threatening allergic reaction.
Angioedema Allergic skin disease characterized by patches of circumscribed swelling involving the skin and its subcutaneous layers, the mucous membranes, and sometimes the viscera.

Histamine An organic nitrogen compound involved in local immune responses, as well as regulating physiologic function in the gut and acting as a neurotransmitter.
Immunoglobulin E An antibody associated with allergies.
Leukotriene A proinflammatory mediator released as part of the allergic response. Leukotrienes also trigger contractions in the smooth muscles of airways.
Mast cells Granule-containing cells found in connective tissue. Histamine-containing granules are released during allergic reactions.
Urticaria Hives.
Wheal Raised blister-like area on the skin.

Overview

An *allergy* is a hypersensitivity reaction caused by exposure to an allergen. An *allergen* is any substance that produces an allergic reaction. Allergic conditions affect between 40 and 50 million people in the United States and are a public health issue because they affect the quality of life, productivity, and performance of sensitive individuals. Recent studies have shown a connection between climate change, urban heat islands in urban metropolitan areas, and allergies. As heat rises, air pollution and allergic sensitivity increase.

> ● *Tech Note!*
>
> Symptoms of an allergy and a cold are similar; however, cold symptoms rarely last longer than 1 to 2 weeks.

What Triggers an Allergic Response?

The immune system functions to defend the body against invading germs and other substances that it believes are harmful. When a person with allergies first comes into contact with an allergen,

the immune system treats the allergen as an invader and produces antibodies to the substance. The allergic reaction sequence is a cascade of events that begins with the ingestion or inhalation of an allergen. Exposure to the allergen triggers an immune system reaction and the production of specialized antibodies (immunoglobulin E [IgE]). Antibodies attach to *mast cells* containing *histamine*, which when released produces allergic reaction symptoms such as itching, runny nose, hives, and wheezing.

The production of allergen-specific *immunoglobulin E* antibodies develops within the first few years of life. Exposure to high levels of multiple endotoxins early in life, such as when children live with multiple pets, may reduce the risks for development of asthma and allergies. The degree of IgE antibody response varies, and allergens from some sources (e.g., dust mites, cat) are more potent than others.

Allergic Conditions

Allergic conditions affect adults and children. Seasonal allergic rhinitis (SAR), or hay fever, affects more than 7% of adults and children. SAR occurs on exposure to seasonal pollens. According to the US Centers for Disease Control and Prevention (CDC) National Center for Health Statistics, more than 7 million

Dermal
- Redness
- Swelling
- Urticaria
- Wheal

Respiratory
- Itchy eyes, nose, and throat
- Runny nose
- Stuffy nose
- Sneezing
- Coughing and postnasal drip
- Watery eyes
- Conjunctivitis
- Allergic shiners
- Allergic salute

respiratory allergies, 4.8 million food allergies, and 9 million skin allergies are reported in children younger than 18 years annually.

Allergic reactions may be localized to a specific area of contact, as with contact dermatitis, or may be more generalized. Persons with chronic airborne allergies may develop allergic shiners (dark circles under the eyes caused by increased blood flow near the sinuses) and an allergic salute (a crease across the bridge of the nose caused by persistent upward rubbing of the nose). Common allergy symptoms are listed in Box 24.1. *Urticaria* (also known as hives) is a condition characterized by itching and *angioedema* (swelling). Redness, swelling, and *wheals* (blister-like vesicles) appear on the skin. Urticaria may be caused by an insect bite, drug or food allergy, or injection of allergen extracts (allergy shots). The condition usually subsides within a few days but, if severe, may need to be managed by the administration of antihistamines and glucocorticosteroids. Acute pharyngeal or laryngeal angioedema must be managed by the administration of drugs that rapidly reduce swelling in the throat and restore breathing (e.g., short-acting β_2-adrenergic agonists).

Allergic Rhinitis

Allergic rhinitis is a condition characterized by nasal itching (rhinitis), runny nose (rhinorrhea), nasal congestion (stuffiness), and sneezing. Allergic rhinitis is typically self-limiting and will resolve without treatment with antiinfective agents. Symptoms are caused by inflammation and swelling of the nasal passageways and may occur throughout the year or seasonally. With SAR, allergy symptoms appear seasonally upon reexposure to allergens after a period of absence. The recurrence of allergic symptoms seasonally is believed to be caused by the presence of memory $CD4^+$ T cells. Memory $CD4^+$ T cells are allergen specific (e.g., tree, grass, weed pollen).

Allergic Conjunctivitis

Allergic conjunctivitis produces red, watering, itchy, or burning eyes. Sufferers may also have ocular puffiness and a stringy discharge from the eyes. Symptoms occur on exposure to an allergen. Seasonal allergic conjunctivitis may worsen during allergy and hay fever season. Overuse of decongestants to treat red eyes may result in *conjunctivitis medicamentosa*, or rebound eye redness

and congestion. More information about conjunctivitis is found in Chapter 15.

Occupational Allergens

Pharmacy technicians are at risk for developing latex allergy. Allergic reactions occur when latex-sensitive individuals breathe in or come into physical contact with latex proteins. Latex proteins in disposable gloves may form a complex with the lubricant powder used in some gloves. When the pharmacy technician changes gloves, the protein–powder particle complex may become airborne and then inhaled.

Latex allergy may produce mild reactions such as skin redness, rash, hives, or itching. Respiratory symptoms such as runny nose, sneezing, itchy eyes, and scratchy throat may occur. More severe reactions involve asthma (difficult breathing, coughing spells, and wheezing) and, rarely, *anaphylaxis*, which is life-threatening.

The National Institute for Occupational Safety and Health recommends taking the following steps to protect oneself from latex exposure and allergy in the workplace.
1. Avoid contact with latex gloves and products. Select nonlatex gloves when possible to provide barrier protection when handling infectious materials.
2. If you choose latex gloves, use powder-free gloves with reduced protein content.
3. Use appropriate work practices to reduce the chance of reactions to latex.
4. Do not use oil-based hand creams or lotions when wearing latex gloves because they can cause glove deterioration.
5. After removing latex gloves, wash hands with a mild soap and dry thoroughly.
6. Practice good housekeeping by frequently cleaning areas and equipment contaminated with latex-containing dust.
7. Avoid areas where you might inhale the powder from latex gloves worn by other workers.
8. Tell your employer and health care providers (e.g., physician, nurse, dentist) that you have a latex allergy.

Pharmacy technicians may encounter additional products containing latex in the workplace. Box 24.2 provides examples of products that may contain latex.

Pharmaceuticals Used in the Management of Allergies and Allergic Conditions

The pharmacologic treatment of allergies is aimed at reducing swelling and inflammation, suppressing the release of cells that mediate immune system and inflammatory responses, and blocking receptor sites of the mediators. Drugs used to treat allergic symptoms include antihistamines, corticosteroids (applied topically or inhaled depending on symptoms), mast cell stabilizers, immunotherapy (desensitization), and *leukotriene* receptor antagonists. Biologic therapies may be used to treat atopic disorders.

> ● *Tech Note!*
>
> Health Canada, the US Food and Drug Administration (FDA) Nonprescription Drug Advisory Committee, and the FDA Pediatric Advisory Committee recommend that cold and cough products be avoided in children younger than 6 years of age.

- Disposable gloves
- Intravenous tubing
- Intravenous bag ports
- Syringes
- Catheters
- Injection ports
- Rubber tops of multidose vials

Antihistamines

Antihistamines reduce allergic reactions. Some antihistamines also decrease nausea and vomiting (e.g., meclizine, cyclizine) or are used for the treatment of schizophrenia (phenothiazines). There are several classes of antihistamines: ethylenediamines, ethanolamines, alkylamines, piperazines, phenothiazines, phthalazinones, and piperidines. Most are available without prescription.

Mechanism of Action and Pharmacokinetics

Administration of antihistamines prevents histamine binding to H1 receptor sites. Azelastine, ketotifen, and olopatadine have a dual action. They also inhibit histamine release from mast cells and mediators of allergic reactions. Antihistamines compete with free histamine for binding at receptor sites. All H1 receptor antagonists have good oral absorption and reach maximum serum levels within 1 to 2 hours. The half-life ($t^{1/2}$) of the antihistamines varies, ranging from as short as 4 to 6 hours (e.g., diphenhydramine) to 24 hours (fexofenadine). Hydroxyzine is metabolized to the active metabolite cetirizine (Zyrtec). Fexofenadine and loratadine are formulated as disintegrating tablets for rapid dissolution and onset of action.

Adverse Reactions

Antihistamines that cross the blood-brain barrier decrease alertness and/or produce sedation. Sedation, dizziness, decreased alertness, dry mouth, blurred vision, lack of coordination, and urinary retention are the most common adverse reactions of antihistamines. Antihistamines that are classified as ethanolamines (e.g., diphenhydramine) and phenothiazines (e.g., promethazine) produce the most sedation and have the greatest anticholinergic effects. Ethylenediamines (e.g., pyrilamine) and piperazines (e.g., cetirizine) produce fewer sedative effects, and newer agents produce the least sedation. Piperidines (e.g., loratadine, fexofenadine) are relatively nonsedating.

> **Tech Note!**
>
> Because of its sedating effects, diphenhydramine is also administered for the treatment of insomnia.

Precautions

Antihistamines should be used cautiously in men with prostate disease, persons with asthma, and women who are breastfeeding. Antihistamine use in children younger than 2 years is not recommended. These drugs can decrease urination, thicken bronchial secretions, and decrease milk production.

> **Tech Alert!**
>
> The following drugs have look-alike/sound-alike issues:
> diphenhydramine and dimenhydrinate;
> Allegra and Viagra;
> ZyrTEC, Zantac, Zocor, and ZyPREXA;
> Claritin, and Clarinex

Over-the-Counter Antihistamines

Generic Name	US Brand Name(s) / Canadian Brand Name(s)	Dosage Forms and Strengths
cetirizine[a]	Zyrtec Allergy, Zyrtec Hives	**Capsule:** 5 mg[b], 10 mg
	Reactine, Reactine Allergy, Reactine Fast Melt	**Syrup:** 1 mg/mL **Tablet, chewable:** 5 mg, 10 mg **Tablet:** 5 mg, 10 mg, 20 mg[c] (Rx) **Tablet, ODT:** 10 mg
chlorpheniramine[a]	Generics	**Tablet:** 4 mg[c]
	Generics	**Tablet, extended release:** 12 mg[b]
diphenhydramine[a] (Selected products)	Benadryl Allergy, Benadryl Children's Allergy, Benadryl Itch Stopping Extra Strength	**Capsule:** 25 mg, 50 mg **Capsule, liquid filled:** 25 mg **Cream (Benadryl):** 1%, 2% **Elixir:** 12.5 mg/5 mL
	Benadryl, Benadryl Allergy Liquigel, Extra Strength Benedryl Allergy Nighttime, Benylin Night for Children	**Gel:** 2% **Liquid:** 6.25 mg/5 mL, 12.5 mg/5 mL **Solution, for injection:** 50 mg/mL **Spray:** 2% **Tablet:** 12.5 mg[c], 25 mg, 50 mg

Over-the-Counter Antihistamines—cont'd

	Generic Name	US Brand Name(s) / Canadian Brand Name(s)	Dosage Forms and Strengths
	fexofenadine[a]	Allegra Allergy, Allegra Hives, Children's Allegra Allergy / Allegra 12 Hour, Allegra 24 H	**Suspension**[b]: 30 mg/5 mL **Tablet**: 60 mg, 120 mg[c], 180 mg[b] **Tablet, oral disintegrating**: 30 mg
	levocetirizine[a]	Xyzal Allergy 24HR / Not available	**Solution, oral**: 2.5 mg/5 mL **Tablet**: 5 mg
	loratadine[a]	Alavert, Claritin, Children's Claritin, Claritin Hives Relief, Claritin RediTab, Claritin Liqui-gel / Claritin, Claritin Kids, Claritin Rapid Dissolve	**Capsule, liquid filled**: 10 mg **Suspension**: 1 mg/mL **Syrup**: 1 mg/mL **Tablet**: 10 mg **Tablet, chewable**: 5 mg **Tablet, oral disintegrating**: 5 mg, 10 mg

[a]Generic available.
[b]Available in the United States only.
[c]Available in Canada only.

Prescription Antihistamines

Generic Name	US Brand Name(s) / Canadian Brand Name(s)	Dosage Forms and Strengths
azelastine[a]	Astelin, Astepro / Not available	**Nasal spray solution**: 125 mcg (Astelin), 187.6 mcg (Astepro)/actuation **Ophthalmic solution**: 0.05%
bilastine	Not available / Blexten	**Tablet**: 20 mg
cetirizine	Quzyttir, Zerviate / Not available	**Solution, ophthalmic**: 0.24% **Solution, intravenous**: 10 mg/mL
clemastine[a]	Generic / Not available	**Tablet**: 2.68 mg
desloratadine[a] (prescription in United States and OTC in Canada)	Clarinex / Aerius, Aerius Kids (OTC)	**Liquid**: 0.5 mg/mL **Tablet**: 5 mg
dexchlorpheniramine[a]	Generics / Not available	**Syrup**: 2 mg/5 mL
ketotifen[a] (prescription in Canada and OTC in the United States)	Alaway (OTC), Zaditor (OTC) / Zaditen, Zaditor	**Solution, ophthalmic (Zaditor)**: 0.025% **Tablet (Zaditen)**: 1 mg
olopatadine[a] (prescription ophthamics in Canada and OTC in the United States)	Once Daily Relief, Pataday Twice Daily Relief, Patanase, Patanol, Pazeo / Pataday, Patanol, Pazeo	**Solution, ophthalmic**: 0.1% (Patanol), 0.2% (Pataday), 0.7% (Pazeo) **Spray, nasal (Patanase)**: 665 mcg/spray

Antihistamine + Glucocorticoid Combination

Generic Name	US / Canadian Brand Name(s)	Dosage Forms and Strengths
azelastine + fluticasone[a]	Dymista / Dymista	**Nasal spray solution**: 137 mcg azelastine + 50 mcg fluticasone/actuation
olopatadine + mometasone	Ryaltris / Not available	0.665 mg olopatadine + 0.025 mg mometasone/spray

[a]Generic available.
[b]Available in the United States only.
OTC, Over the counter.

Glucocorticosteroids

Glucocorticoids are antiinflammatory drugs. They are administered intranasally to control symptoms of allergic rhinitis. When administered intranasally, they inhibit the onset of the inflammatory response by reducing the permeability of the nasal mucosa cells to T-lymphocytes and eosinophils, thereby decreasing the release of mediators of the inflammatory response (e.g., cytokines). They also reduce the number of inflammatory cells. The result is reduction of mucus and swelling that makes breathing difficult. Additional mechanisms of action and pharmacokinetics of glucocorticosteroids are discussed in detail in Chapters 13 and 23. Fluticasone (Flonase®), budesonide (Rhinocort®), triamcinolone (Nasacort AQ®), mometasone (Nasonex®), and beclomethasone (Beconase AQ®) are examples of glucocorticoids that are marketed for use in the nose.

❶ Tech Alert!

The following drugs have look-alike/sound-alike issues:
Flonase and Flovent

Adverse Reactions

Side effects of glucocorticoids, when applied intranasally, are primarily local and include nasal irritation, throat irritation, and nosebleeds. Some patients may develop a *Candida* infection in their nose that may present as burning or stinging in the nostril(s).

Mast Cell Stabilizers

Cromolyn sodium, nedocromil, and lodoxamide are classified as mast cell stabilizers. The drugs make cells less reactive to allergens, decreasing the release of inflammatory substances.

Corticosteroids Used for Allergic Rhinitis or Allergic Conjunctivitis

Generic Name	US Brand Name(s) / Canadian Brand Name(s)	Dosage Forms and Strengths	Prescription Status
beclomethasone[a]	Beconase AQ, QNASL / Generics	**Pump nasal spray:** 40 mcg[b], 42 mcg[b], 50 mcg[c], 80 mcg/actuation[b]	Prescription only
budesonide[a]	Rhinocort, Rhinocort Allergy (OTC) / Rhinocort Aqua	**Pump nasal spray (suspension):** 32 mcg/actuation[b], 64 mcg/actuation[c], 100 mcg/actuation[c]	Prescription and OTC in the United States
ciclesonide[a]	Omnaris, Zetonna / Omnaris	**Nasal spray:** 37 mcg/actuation (Zetonna), 50 mcg/actuation (Omnaris)	Prescription
	Generics / Not available	**Pump nasal spray:** 25 mcg/actuation	Prescription only
fluticasone[a]	Flonase Allergy Relief (OTC), Flonase Sensimist (OTC), Xhance / Avamys, Flonase Allergy Relief (OTC)	**Pump nasal spray, as furoate (Avamys, Flonase Sensimist):** 27.5 mcg/actuation **Pump nasal spray, as propionate:** 50 mcg/actuation (Flonase Allergy Relief), 93 mcg/actuation (Xhance)	Prescription and OTC
loteprednol[a]	Alrex, Eysuvis, Lotemax, Lotemax SM / Alrex, Lotemax	**Gel, ophthalmic:** 0.35% (Lotemax SM), 0.5% (Lotemax) **Ointment, ophthalmic:** 0.5% **Suspension, ophthalmic:** 0.2% (Alrex), 0.25% (Eysuvis), 0.5% (Lotemax), 1% (Inveltys)	Prescription only
mometasone[a]	Nasonex 24HR (OTC) / Nasonex	**Pump nasal spray:** 50 mcg/actuation	Prescription and OTC in Canada
triamcinolone[a]	Nasacort Allergy 24H (OTC) / Nasacort Allergy 24H (OTC), Nasacort AQ	**Pump nasal spray:** 55 mcg/actuation	Prescription and OTC

[a]Generic available.
[b]Available in the United States only.
[c]Available in Canada only.
OTC, Over the counter.

Mast Cell Stabilizers

Generic Name	US Brand Name(s) / Canadian Brand Name(s)	Dosage Forms and Strengths*	Prescription Status
cromolyn sodium[a]	Nasalcrom (OTC) / Nalcrom (prescription)	Capsule (Nalcrom): 100 mg / Nasal spray (Nasalcrom): 5.2 mcg/actuation / Ophthalmic solution: 2%[b], 4%[c]	Prescription and OTC
lodoxamide	Alomide / Alomide	Solution, ophthalmic: 0.1%	
nedocromil	Alocril / Not available	Ophthalmic solution: 2%,	Prescription only

*Cromolyn is also marketed as an oral inhalant solution for use in nebulizers for the treatment of asthma.
[a]Generic available.
[b]Available in Canada only.
[c]Available in the United States only.
OTC, Over the counter.

Cromolyn is approved for intranasal and ophthalmic use, but nedocromil and lodoxamide are manufactured for ophthalmic use only. Mast cell stabilizers are not used to treat acute symptoms. Therapy should begin before coming into contact with allergens and continue for the duration of allergen exposure. For more details about the mechanisms of action, pharmacokinetics, and adverse reactions for mast cell stabilizers, read Chapter 23. Adverse effects include; bad taste in the mouth; cough; dry throat; difficulty breathing; headache; nosebleeds; runny nose; sneezing; and stinging, burning, or irritation inside the nose. Cromolyn eye drops and nasal spray do not require a prescription. Nedocromil and lodoxamide are prescription drugs.

Leukotriene Receptor Antagonists

The leukotriene receptor antagonist montelukast is used to control allergic rhinitis symptoms. Montelukast is a selective antagonist of the cysteinyl leukotriene D_4 receptor found in the human airway. Montelukast may produce cough, hoarseness, sore throat, headache, indigestion, heartburn, stomach upset, or runny nose. Montelukast may also produce difficulty sleeping, dizziness, drowsiness, muscle aches or cramps, or unusual dreams.

Immunotherapy and Biologic Agents

Allergy shots represent a form of immunotherapy. They may be administered to persons with perennial (symptoms all year round) or seasonal allergies. The rationale for immunotherapy is to reduce the level of IgE antibodies in the blood while at the same time stimulating the production of IgG, a protective antibody. Allergy shots are administered by subcutaneous injection as a series of shots; each injection has an increased concentration of the allergen that produces sensitivity. Allergy shots may reduce allergy symptoms over a longer period than all other treatments. Biologic therapies may be used to treat atopic disorders and chronic idiopathic urticaria that is resistant to treatment with antihistamines. Biologic agents will be described in Chapter 32.

TECHNICIAN'S CORNER

1. Some products used to treat allergic reactions are available over the counter, and others are prescription only. Make lists of both the OTC and prescription drugs used to treat allergic reactions.
2. Recent studies reveal socioeconomic and racial disparities related to food allergies and their management. Why do you think inequities might exist?

Leukotriene Receptor Antagonist for Allergic Rhinitis

Generic Name	US Brand Name(s) / Canadian Brand Name(s)	Dosage Forms and Strengths	Prescription Status
montelukast[a]	Singulair / Singulair	Oral granules: 4 mg / Tablet: 10 mg / Tablet, chewable: 4 mg, 5 mg	Prescription only

[a]Generic Available.

Summary of Drugs Used in the Treatment of Allergic Conditions

	Generic Name	US Brand Name(s)	Usual Adult Oral Dose and Dosing Schedule	Warning Labels
Antihistamine				
	azelastine	Astelin	**Allergic conjunctivitis:** 1 drop in affected eye(s) twice daily **Allergic rhinitis:** 1–2 sprays each nostril twice daily	PRIME INHALER BEFORE USE. MAY CAUSE SEDATION; DO NOT DRIVE OR OPERATE MACHINERY.
	chlorpheniramine	Generics	**Allergic rhinitis, immediate release**: 4 mg every 4–6 h up to 24 mg/day **Extended release**: 8 mg–12 mg 2–3 times a day	MAY CAUSE DIZZINESS OR DROWSINESS; ALCOHOL MAY INCREASE THIS EFFECT—chlorpheniramine, diphenhydramine, clemastine, cetirizine, desloratadine, loratadine, levocetirizine.
	diphenhydramine	Benadryl	**Allergic rhinitis, pruritus, and urticaria:** 25–50 mg 3–4 times a day	
	clemastine	Generics	**Allergic rhinitis and urticaria**: 1.34–2.68 mg 1–3 times daily **Pruritus and angioedema:** 2.68 mg 1–3 times daily	SWALLOW WHOLE; DO NOT CRUSH OR CHEW—extended release.
	cetirizine	Zyrtec	**Allergic rhinitis and urticaria:** 5–10 mg once daily	PROTECT FROM MOISTURE; LEAVE IN FOIL PACKET UNTIL READY FOR USE—disintegrating tablets.
	desloratadine	Clarinex	**Allergic rhinitis, pruritus, and urticaria:** 5 mg once daily	DISSOLVE REDITAB UNDER THE TONGUE—disintegrating tablets.
	fexofenadine	Allegra	**Allergic rhinitis and urticaria:** 60 mg bid or 180 mg once daily	WAIT 10 MINUTES BEFORE APPLYING ANY OTHER EYE DROPS OR CONTACT LENSES.
	ketotifen	Alaway, Zaditor	**Allergic conjunctivitis:** Instill 1 drop twice daily, every 8–12 h in each affected eye	MAY CAUSE DIZZINESS OR DROWSINESS—ketotifen.
	levocetirizine	Xyzal	**Allergic rhinitis and urticaria:** 5 mg once daily in the evening	AVOID ORANGE, GRAPEFRUIT, AND APPLE JUICE—fexofenadine.
	loratadine	Alavert, Claritin	**Allergic rhinitis and urticaria:** 10 mg once daily	
	olopatadine	Pataday Once Daily Relief	**Allergic conjunctivitis:** Instill 1 drop in affected eye(s) once a day	
Glucocorticoids				
	beclomethasone	Beconase AQ	**Allergic rhinitis:** 1–2 sprays each nostril twice daily	SHAKE WELL. RINSE AND DRY TIP AFTER EACH USE—all nasal inhalers.
	budesonide	Rhinocort	**Allergic rhinitis:** 1–2 sprays each nostril once daily	
	flunisolide	Generic	**Allergic rhinitis:** 2 sprays each nostril 2–3 times daily	
	fluticasone propionate	Flonase	**Allergic rhinitis:** 1 spray each nostril twice daily or 2 sprays in each nostril once daily	
	fluticasone furoate	Flonase Allergy Relief, Avamys	**Allergic rhinitis:** 1–2 sprays each nostril once daily	
	mometasone	Nasonex	**Allergic rhinitis:** 2 sprays each nostril once daily	
	triamcinolone	Nasacort Allergy 24 h	**Allergic rhinitis:** 1–2 sprays each nostril once daily	

Summary of Drugs Used in the Treatment of Allergic Conditions—cont'd

	Generic Name	US Brand Name(s)	Usual Adult Oral Dose and Dosing Schedule	Warning Labels
Mast Cell Stabilizer				
	cromolyn sodium	Generics	**Allergic rhinitis:** 1 spray each nostril tid or qid (up to 6 times daily) **Allergic conjunctivitis:** 1–2 drops in affected eye(s) 4–6 times a day **Food allergy:** 200 mg 4 times a day	RINSE AND DRY TIP AFTER EACH USE—nasal sprays. REMOVE SOFT CONTACT LENSES DURING TREATMENT. TAKE 15–20 MINUTES BEFORE MEALS—capsules.
	lodoxamide	Alomide	**Conjunctivitis:** Instill 1–2 drops in affected eyes 4 times a day	
	nedocromil	Alocril	**Allergic conjunctivitis:** Instill 1–2 drops in each eye twice a day	
Leukotriene Receptor Antagonist				
	montelukast	Singulair	**Allergic rhinitis:** 10 mg PO once daily **Adults, chewable tablets:** Chew 1 tablet (4 or 5 mg) once daily **Children and infants, 6 months to 2 years:** 4 mg PO once daily **Children, 2–5 years, oral granules:** Dissolve and consume 1 packet once daily	TAKE WITH A LARGE GLASS OF WATER— chewable tablet. DISCARD UNUSED PORTION OF SOLUTION WITHIN 15 MINUTES.
Antihistamine + Decongestant				
	naphazoline + pheniramine[a]	Visine-A[b], Naphcon-A[b], Opcon-A[b]	**Allergic conjunctivitis:** 1–2 drops in affected eye(s) up to qid	OVERUSE CAN LEAD TO CONJUNCTIVITIS MEDICAMENTOSA.

[a]Generic Available
[b]OTC

Key Points

- An allergy is a hypersensitivity reaction by the immune system upon exposure to an allergen.
- Allergic conditions affect the quality of life, productivity, and performance of sensitive individuals.
- When a person with allergies is first exposed to an allergen, the immune system treats the allergen as an invader and produces antibodies to the substance.
- Allergic rhinitis is a condition characterized by nasal itching (rhinitis), runny nose (rhinorrhea), nasal congestion (stuffiness), and sneezing. Allergic conjunctivitis produces itchy and watering eyes.
- Urticaria (also known as hives) is a condition characterized by itching and angioedema (swelling).
- Pharmacy technicians are at risk for developing a latex allergy. Allergic reactions occur when latex-sensitive individuals breathe in or come into physical contact with latex proteins.
- Latex allergies may produce mild reactions such as skin redness, rash, hives, or itching. Respiratory symptoms such as runny nose, sneezing, itchy eyes, and scratchy throat may occur.
- Pharmacologic treatment of allergies is aimed at reducing swelling and inflammation and suppressing the release of cells that mediate immune system and inflammatory responses, as well as blocking receptor sites of the mediators.
- Drugs used to treat allergic symptoms include antihistamines, inhaled corticosteroids, mast cell stabilizers, leukotriene modifiers, immunotherapy, and biologic therapies.

- Sedation, dizziness, decreased alertness, dry mouth, blurred vision, lack of coordination, and urinary retention are the most common adverse reactions of antihistamines.
- Antihistamines should be used cautiously in men with prostate disease, persons with asthma, and women who are breastfeeding. They are not recommended for use in children younger than 2 years.
- Glucocorticosteroids are administered intranasally to control symptoms of allergic rhinitis.
- Glucocorticosteroids for intranasal use include fluticasone (Flonase), budesonide (Rhinocort), triamcinolone (Nasacort), flunisolide, mometasone (Nasonex), and beclomethasone (Beconase AQ).
- Adverse reactions to corticosteroids administered intranasally are primarily local and include nasal irritation, throat irritation, and nosebleeds.
- Cromolyn sodium is a mast cell stabilizer available for intranasal and ophthalmic use. Nedocromil and lodoxamide are manufactured for ophthalmic use only.
- Therapy with cromolyn sodium should be initiated 1 week before exposure to allergens and continued for the duration of allergen exposure.
- Montelukast is a leukotriene receptor antagonist used to treat allergic rhinitis.
- Allergy shots are a form of immunotherapy that are administered as a series of subcutaneous injections; they may reduce allergy symptoms over a longer period than all other treatments.

Review Questions

1. Which of the following is a life-threatening allergic reaction?
   a. urticaria
   b. pruritus
   c. anaphylaxis
   d. wheal

2. All of the following drugs are nasal sprays for the treatment of allergic rhinitis EXCEPT_____.
   a. Astelin
   b. Rhinocort
   c. Pataday
   d. Beconase AQ

3. A condition characterized by nasal itching, runny nose, nasal congestion (stuffiness), and sneezing is called _____.
   a. Urticaria
   b. Allergic rhinitis
   c. Wheals
   d. Angioedema

4. Select the drug which may be purchased only by prescription.
   a. Dymista
   b. Claritin Children
   c. Allerga 24 HR
   d. Benadryl Allergy

5. All of the following drugs used to treat allergic conjunctivitis require a prescription EXCEPT_____.
   a. Alomide
   b. Alocril
   c. Alrex
   d. Alaway

6. Glucocorticosteroids are administered orally to control symptoms of rhinitis.
   a. Yrue
   b. False

7. Cromolyn sodium is a (an) _____ available for intranasal use.
   a. Mast cell stabilizer
   b. Glucocorticoid
   c. Antihistamine
   d. Leukotriene

8. Diphenhydramine has a side effect of _____.
   a. Insomnia
   b. Sedation
   c. Burning
   d. None of the above

9. Loratadine is the generic name for Clarinex (Aerius).
   a. true
   b. false

10. Cetirizine is available in which of the following dosage forms?
    a. tablet
    b. chewable tablet
    c. syrup
    d. all of the above

Bibliography

American College of Allergy, Asthma & Immunology: Treatment of seasonal allergic rhinitis: an evidence-based focused guideline update. *Ann Allergy Asthma Immunol.* 2017;119(6):489–511. 2017.

Centers for Disease Control and Prevention. (2021). Occupational latex allergies (NIOSH Alert No. 97–135), 2016 (update 2021). Retrieved January 8, 2023, from http://www.cdc.gov/niosh/docs/97-135.

Centers for Disease Control and Prevention (2022). Allergies and hay fever. National Center for Health Statistics. Retrieved January 8, 2023, from https://www.cdc.gov/nchs/fastats/allergies.htm.

Choi A, Jung YW, Choi H. The extrinsic factors important to the homeostasis of allergen-specific memory CD4 T cells. *Front Immunol.* 2022;13:1080855.

Fernandez J. (2022). Overview of Allergic and Atopic Disorders. Merck Manual Professional Version. Retrieved January 10, 2023, from https://www.merckmanuals.com/en-ca/professional/immunology-allergic-disorders/allergic,-autoimmune,-and-other-hypersensitivity-disorders/overview-of-allergic-and-atopic-disorders.

Health Canada. (2022). Drug Product Database. Retrieved January 8, 2023, from https://health-products.canada.ca/dpd-bdpp/index-eng.jsp.

Institute for Safe Medication Practices. (2016). FDA and ISMP Lists of Look-Alike Drug Names with Recommended Tall Man Letters. Retrieved January 8, 2023, from https://www.ismp.org/recommendations/tall-man-letters-list.

Institute for Safe Medication Practices. (2019). List of Confused Drugs. Retrieved January 8, 2023, from https://www.ismp.org/tools/confuseddrugnames.pdf.

Kaiser H, Naclerio R, Given J, et al. Fluticasone furoate nasal spray: a single treatment option for the symptoms of seasonal allergic rhinitis. *J Allergy Clin Immunol.* 2007;119:1430–1437.

Kalant H, Grant D, Mitchell J. *Principles of medical pharmacology.* ed 7. Toronto: Elsevier Canada; 2007:22–27 397–400, 451, 453–454.

National Institute of Allergy and Infectious Disease. (2003). Airborne Allergens: Something in the Air (NIH Publ. No. 03-7045). Retrieved January 8, 2023, from http://www.allergywatch.org/basic/airborne_allergens.pdf.

Page C, Curtis M, Sutter M, et al. *Integrated pharmacology.* Philadelphia: Mosby; 2005:330–336 428–430.

U.S. Food and Drug Administration. (nd). Drugs@FDA: FDA Approved Drug Products. Retrieved January 8, 2023, from https://www.accessdata.fda.gov/scripts/cder/daf/index.cfm.

Woodfolk J. T-cell responses to allergens, molecular mechanisms in allergy and clinical immunology. *J Allergy Clin Immunol.* 2007;119:280–294.

UNIT VIII

Drugs Affecting the Endocrine System

The endocrine system and nervous system both function to maintain the stability of the internal environment. In the endocrine system, regulatory function is performed by chemical messengers called hormones that diffuse into the blood to be carried to almost every point in the body. Their effects appear more slowly and last longer than the effects produced by neurotransmitters released by the nervous system. Endocrine glands are known as ductless glands because they secrete hormones directly into the blood.

Hormones are classified by their target site, their chemical composition (steroid or nonsteroid), whether they are hydrophilic or hydrophobic, and the mechanism by which they signal hormonal action. The effects of a particular hormone may be limited to specific tissues in the body (e.g., thyroid-releasing hormone) or the hormone may produce effects throughout the body (e.g., thyroid hormone). Endocrine regulation of body processes first begins during early development in the womb and continues throughout life, although the secretion of some hormones declines late in life (such as reproductive hormones). Through the secretion of hormones and autonomic nervous system regulation, almost every process in the human organism is kept in balance.

In Unit VIII, the pharmacotherapy for diseases of the endocrine system is described. Specific diseases covered in Unit VIII include hypothyroidism, hyperthyroidism, and diabetes. A brief description of each disorder is provided, followed by a description of the drugs indicated for treatment, mechanisms of action, adverse reactions, strength(s) and dosage forms.

25

Treatment of Thyroid Disorders

LEARNING OBJECTIVES

1. Learn the terminology associated with thyroid disorders.
2. Describe the pathophysiology of hyperthyroidism and hypothyroidism.
3. List symptoms of hyperthyroidism and hypothyroidism.
4. List and categorize medications used to treat hyperthyroidism and hypothyroidism.
5. Describe mechanism of action for each class of drugs used to treat hyperthyroidism and hypothyroidism.
6. Identify significant drug look-alike and sound-alike issues.
7. Identify warning labels and precautionary messages associated with medications used to treat hyperthyroidism and hypothyroidism.

KEY TERMS

Graves disease An autoimmune disorder that causes hyperthyroidism.
Hashimoto disease An autoimmune disorder that causes hypothyroidism.
Hyperthyroidism A condition in which there is an excessive production of thyroid hormones.
Hypothyroidism A condition in which there is insufficient production of thyroid hormones.
Thyroid-releasing factor A hormone released by the hypothalamus that stimulates the pituitary gland to release thyroid-stimulating hormone.

Thyroid-stimulating hormone A hormone released by the pituitary gland that stimulates the thyroid gland to produce and release thyroid hormones.
Tetraiodothyronine The most abundant thyroid hormone. It contains four atoms of iodine and is also known as thyroxine.
Triiodothyronine A hormone secreted by the thyroid gland containing three atoms of iodine.

Overview

The thyroid gland secretes hormones that have an effect on almost all cells in the body. The thyroid hormones *tetraiodothyronine* (T_4) and *triiodothyronine* (T_3) regulate growth and metabolism. The physiologic actions of thyroid hormone are listed in Box 25.1. Calcitonin, another hormone secreted by the thyroid gland, helps maintain calcium homeostasis.

Thyroid disorders result in overactivity or underactivity of the thyroid gland, causing hypersecretion or hyposecretion of thyroid hormones, respectively. More than 200 million persons worldwide have a thyroid disorder. Thyroid disease affects more than 20 million Americans and 3 million Canadians. Up to 50% of cases are undiagnosed. Thyroid disease is more common in women than in men. Having an autoimmune disease such as type 1 diabetes or rheumatoid arthritis is a risk factor for Graves disease (hyperthyroidism) and Hashimoto disease (hypothyroidism). Recent studies have identified an association between autoimmune thyroid diseases and vitamin D deficiency. Vitamin D decreases the secretion of proinflammatory cytokines that inhibit autoimmune responses. Additional studies have shown an association between depression and thyroid disease. The mechanism is unknown; however, a few studies found that both conditions affect mediators of immune response.

Thyroid Hormone Control

Thyroid levels are tightly controlled by a negative feedback loop. When the need for thyroid hormones increases, the hypothalamus secretes *thyroid-releasing factor* (TRF), a hormone that signals the pituitary gland to release *thyroid-stimulating hormone* (TSH). The target site of TSH is the thyroid gland, which produces and secretes T_4 and T_3. Once desired levels are achieved, TSH release is turned off (Fig. 25.1).

Synthesis of Thyroid Hormones

The thyroid gland is one of the few glands that produces and stores its hormones. Thyroid hormones (T_4, T_3) are synthesized by a coupling process in which atoms of iodine are bound to the thyroid protein thyroglobulin. T_3 is formed by three atoms of iodine bound to thyroglobulin. T_4 is formed by four atoms of iodine bound to thyroglobulin. In the body, T_4 (tetraiodothyronine) is converted to T_3.

Diagnosis of Thyroid Disorders

The TSH test measures the level of TSH in the blood. A low TSH level signals hyperthyroidism. This is to be expected because TSH release is turned off when the body recognizes that T_4 levels are

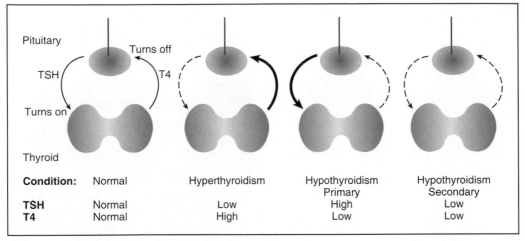

• **Fig. 25.1** Comparison of **thyroid-stimulating hormone** *(TSH)* and **tetraiodothyronine** *(T₄)* levels for normal function, hyperthyroidism, and hypothyroidism. (Courtesy American Thyroid Association, https://www.thyroid.org/thyroid-function-tests/.)

• BOX 25.1   Physiologic Actions of Thyroid Hormones

- Growth of skeletal tissues
- Fetal growth and development (cognitive and physical)
- Growth and development of the central nervous system
- Regulation of protein, lipid, and carbohydrate metabolism
- Regulation of hepatic metabolic enzymes
- Regulation of body temperature
- Cardiac function (heart rate and contractility)
- Circulatory volume
- Respiratory functions
- Peripheral vasodilation
- Bone turnover

---

high; the body therefore attempts to stop its further production and release. A high TSH level is a signal for hypothyroidism. A tetraiodothyronine test measures free T_4 (FT_4) and the FT_4 index (FT_4I). FT_4 and FT_4I tests measure circulating thyroid hormone. In hyperthyroidism, FT_4 levels are elevated, and TSH levels are depressed. The reverse is true in the case of hypothyroidism. The presence of thyroid-stimulating antibodies can be measured by a thyroid antibody test. When thyroid antibodies are present, autoimmune thyroid disease is diagnosed. A radioactive iodine uptake (RAIU) test may also be conducted to test for thyroid disease. Iodine is selectively taken up by the thyroid gland in the process of synthesizing T_4 and T_3 (Fig. 25.2); thus when a low dose of radioactive iodine (^{131}I) is administered, the amount of radioactivity in the thyroid gland can be measured. The RAIU is high when a person has hyperthyroidism and low when a person has hypothyroidism.

Types of Thyroid Disorders

Hyperthyroidism

Hyperthyroidism is a condition in which the thyroid gland secretes excessive amounts of thyroid hormones. It affects 1 in 100 Americans. Hyperthyroidism is most common in women between the ages of 20 and 40 years. *Graves disease* is an autoimmune disease and a primary cause of thyroid hyperactivity. In Graves disease, thyroid-stimulating antibodies mimic TSH and cause the thyroid gland to release its hormones (see Fig. 25.1). Graves disease is the

Thyroxine (T₄)

Triiodothyronine (T₃)

Dimethyl-isopropyl-thyronine (DIMIT)

• **Fig. 25.2** Structural formula of thyroid hormones. (From Kalant H, Grant DM, Mitchell J: *Principles of medical pharmacology,* ed 7, Philadelphia, 2007, WB Saunders.)

primary cause of hyperthyroidism. When it is left untreated, the severe hyperthyroidism that results may lead to cardiovascular disease and death. Additional causes of hyperthyroidism are (1) thyroid nodules (lumps on the thyroid gland that secrete thyroid hormone), and (2) inflammation of the thyroid gland (e.g., subacute thyroiditis, postpartum thyroiditis, lymphatic thyroiditis). Cigarette smoking increases the risk for developing thyroid-related eye disease. Smokers with Graves disease are five times more likely than nonsmokers to develop thyroid-associated ophthalmopathy.

● *Tech Note!*

Potassium iodide can protect the thyroid gland against exposure to radioactive iodine.

- Rapid heart rate and palpitations
- Muscle weakness
- Muscle wasting
- Tremor
- Weight loss
- Shortness of breath
- Nervousness or irritability
- Restlessness
- Sleeplessness
- Enlarged thyroid (goiter)
- Amenorrhea
- Diarrhea
- Breast enlargement
- Bulging eyes
- Rapid speech
- Sweating
- Heat intolerance, warm skin, facial flushing

Symptoms of Hyperthyroidism

Given that thyroid hormones have an effect on numerous cells throughout the body, it is not surprising that symptoms of thyroid disease are widespread. These are listed in Box 25.2.

Treatment of Hyperthyroidism

Treatment of hyperthyroidism involves the administration of either antithyroid drugs or radioactive iodine; it can also be treated with surgery.

Radioactive Iodine

Low-dose radioactive iodine is used for diagnosis, and higher-dose radioactive iodine is administered for the treatment of hyperthyroidism. It is selectively taken up by the thyroid gland, where it causes glandular destruction while minimizing damage to other tissues. The rate of cure is 61% to 86% depending on the dose administered. Pretreatment with an antithyroid drug is recommended for approximately 2 weeks to block the synthesis of thyroid hormone before the administration of ^{131}I. The full effects of ^{131}I therapy are achieved after 2 to 3 months in most people, but sometimes a second or third course of therapy is required. β-Blockers (see Chapter 18) may be administered concurrently with ^{131}I until tachycardia and tremors, symptoms of hyperthyroidism, subside. Radioactive iodine that is not retained by the thyroid is eliminated in the urine within 2 or 3 days.

> ● *Tech Note!*
>
> Radioactive iodine ^{131}I is made in nuclear pharmacies and is regulated by the Nuclear Regulatory Commission (NRC).

Adverse Reactions. Treatment with ^{131}I produces few adverse effects. The most common side effect is temporary inflammation of the salivary glands. Most patients also develop an underactive thyroid gland after treatment, requiring lifelong therapy for hypothyroidism.

Precautions. Radioactive iodine therapy is contraindicated in pregnant women because the drug can cross the placenta and cause thyroid damage in the developing fetus. Nursing mothers should also avoid breastfeeding until radioactive iodine can no longer be detected in the breast milk. Nonpregnant women and men treated with radioactive iodine should avoid close physical contact with pregnant women and young children for a few days after the dose is administered.

Radioactive Iodine (^{131}I)

Generic Name	US Brand Names	Dosage Forms and Strengths
	Canadian Brand Names	
radioactive iodine (^{131}I)[a]	No commercial preparations	Individualized
	No commercial preparations	

[a]Generic available.

Thioamides (Thionamides)

Propylthiouracil (PTU) and methimazole are antithyroid drugs. They are used for the primary treatment of hyperthyroidism or to reduce excess thyroid hormone levels in patients awaiting treatment with radioactive iodine or thyroid surgery.

> ● *Tech Alert!*
>
> The following drugs have look-alike/sound-alike issues:
>
> methimazole and metolazone;
> propylthiouracil and Purinethol

Mechanism of Action and Pharmacokinetics. PTU and methimazole block the synthesis of T_4 and T_3 by blocking the enzyme that catalyzes the coupling of iodinated tyrosine (MIT and DIT). PTU is also capable of blocking the conversion of T_4 to T_3. The maximal benefit of PTU therapy is not achieved until all the thyroid hormone that is stored in the thyroid gland's follicles is depleted. This can take 2 to 4 months of therapy.

> ● *Tech Alert!*
>
> The abbreviation PTU (propylthiouracil) has been misread as 6-MP (6-mercaptopurine).

Adverse Reactions. Methimazole and PTU may cause nausea or vomiting, muscle aches and pains, and/or minor rash or itching. Side effects requiring medical attention include fever accompanied by sore throat and hoarseness, goiter, severe redness or itching, hepatitis, arthritis, unusual bleeding, bruising, and red spots. Methimazole and PTU may also produce a dangerous decrease in the number of white blood cells (agranulocytosis), which increases the risk for serious infections. Dosages higher than 40 mg/day of methimazole may increase the risk for agranulocytosis.

Like radioactive thyroid therapy, treatment with antithyroid drugs typically induces hypothyroidism. Hypothyroidism may appear as soon as 6 months after the onset of therapy or as long as 25 years after disease remission and discontinuation of drug therapy.

• BOX 25.3 Symptoms of Hypothyroidism

- Slowed heart rate, slowed pulse
- Extreme fatigue
- Weight gain
- Dry skin and dry coarse hair
- Poor memory, slowed mental processes
- Constipation
- Deep coarse voice, slow speech, thick tongue
- Enlarged heart
- Enlarged thyroid (goiter)
- Cold intolerance
- Depression

• BOX 25.4 Medications That Interact With Thyroid Hormones

- Ferrous products (iron supplements)
- Calcium supplements and dairy products
- Proton pump inhibitors (e.g., omeprazole)
- Raloxifene
- Cholestyramine
- Colestipol
- Oral contraceptives
- Phenytoin
- Carbamazepine

Thioamides

Generic Name	US Brand Names / Canadian Brand Names	Dosage Forms and Strengths
methimazole[a]	Generics	Tablet: 5 mg, 10 mg
	Tapazole	
propylthiouracil[a]	Generics	Tablet: 50 mg
	Halycil	

[a]Generic available.

Hypothyroidism

Hypothyroidism is a condition in which the thyroid gland secretes deficient amounts of thyroid hormones. The following conditions are known to cause hypothyroidism: (1) treatment for hyperthyroidism with radioactive iodine and antithyroid drugs; (2) treatment with medications for non–thyroid-related conditions (e.g., lithium, amiodarone); (3) thyroidectomy (removal of all or a portion of the thyroid gland); (4) pituitary gland damage that affects TSH secretion; (5) congenital conditions (birth defects); and (6) thyroiditis. *Hashimoto disease* is an autoimmune disorder in which the body produces antibodies to its own thyroid cells. The antibodies and white blood cells attack and damage the thyroid. Hashimoto disease is the most common cause of non–iodine-deficiency hypothyroidism. The incidence of hypothyroidism increases with age. By age 60 years, up to 17% of women and 9% of men will have an underactive thyroid.

Symptoms

The effects of insufficient thyroid hormones can be felt throughout the body. Symptoms of hypothyroidism are listed in Box 25.3.

■ Tech Note!

Levothyroxine is the replacement for naturally occurring thyroxine.

Treatment of Hypothyroidism

Thyroid replacement therapy is the principal treatment for hypothyroidism. Replacement can be achieved by the administration of desiccated (dried, powdered) whole-gland animal thyroid or synthetic T_4 and synthetic T_3. The most widely prescribed treatment for hypothyroidism is synthetic T_4, which is converted in the body to T_3.

Mechanism of Action

Thyroid hormones derived from animal gland and synthetic T_4 and T_3 bind to the same receptor sites and produce the same actions as thyroid hormones made by the body. Synthetic T_4, known as levothyroxine (L-thyroxine), is generally the only thyroid hormone prescribed for the treatment of hypothyroidism. Additional administration of liothyronine is typically unnecessary because levothyroxine is converted to liothyronine in the body, just as naturally occurring T_4 is metabolized to T_3.

❶ Tech Alert!

The following drugs have look-alike/sound-alike issues:
levothyroxine and liothyronine

Pharmacokinetics

Liothyronine (T_3) and levothyroxine are dissimilar in their onset and duration of action. They also differ in potency and dosing frequency. Liothyronine has a rapid onset of action. Within 4 hours of an orally administered dose, 95% is absorbed from the gastrointestinal tract. The drug has a relatively long half-life of 2.5 days. In contrast, absorption of levothyroxine varies between 48% and 80% and is greatest when taken on an empty stomach. Levothyroxine is highly protein bound; thus the drug availability is affected by factors that affect plasma protein levels. When plasma proteins are increased, levothyroxine is decreased. Although bioavailability varies between different manufacturers' formulations of levothyroxine, switching between generic products does not have a significant impact on the level of TSH present in patients.

Numerous medications interact with thyroid hormones (Box 25.4). Ferrous products, calcium supplements, cholesterol-lowering agents (e.g., colestipol, cholestyramine), and didanosine interfere with the absorption of thyroid hormones. Food delays absorption. Antiseizure medicines such as phenytoin and carbamazepine accelerate the rate of metabolism of thyroid hormones. Soy isoflavones, oral contraceptives, and raloxifene reduce the clinical response to administered thyroid hormone by altering TSH, thyroglobulin, T_4, and T_3 levels. Thyroid hormones may increase the response to warfarin and decrease the response to oral antidiabetic agents. Close monitoring of the international normalized ratio and blood glucose levels is recommended.

Adverse Reactions. Given that thyroid replacement therapy is achieved by administering naturally occurring or synthetic thyroid hormone, adverse effects produced are the same as symptoms of hypothyroidism (subtherapeutic doses) or symptoms of hyperthyroidism (taking too much thyroid hormone).

Precautions. Diabetic patients may require an adjustment in their dose of diabetes medicine once thyroid replacement therapy is initiated. Thyroid hormones can affect blood sugar levels.

Congenital Hypothyroidism

Congenital hypothyroidism is a condition that occurs when the neonatal thyroid gland fails to develop or function properly. It may also occur if a woman has an iodine deficiency during pregnancy. If untreated, the condition causes severely stunted growth or dwarfism and intellectual disability. In the United States and Canada, all newborns are routinely tested for congenital hypothyroidism. Newborns diagnosed with the condition are treated with thyroid hormones.

> **Tech Note!**
>
> The various strengths of levothyroxine are color-coded to help avoid dispensing errors.

TECHNICIAN'S CORNER

1. What is an autoimmune disease, and what are the effects of an autoimmune disease such as Graves disease?
2. What types of food provide iodine?

Thyroid Replacements

Generic Name	US Brand Names / Canadian Brand Names	Dosage Forms and Strengths
levothyroxine[a] (T$_4$)	Ermeza, Euthyrox, Levoxyl, Levo-T, Synthroid, Thyquidity, Tirosint, Tirosint-sol Unithroid Eltroxin, Synthroid	**Capsule (Tirosint):** 13 mcg, 25 mcg, 37.5 mcg, 44 mcg, 50 mcg, 75 mcg, 88 mcg, 100 mcg, 112 mcg, 125 mcg, 137 mcg, 150 mcg, 175 mcg, 200 mcg **Powder, for injection:** 100 mcg/vial[b], 200 mcg/vial[b], 500 mcg/vial **Solution, for injection:** 20 mcg/mL[b], 40 mcg/mL, 100 mcg/mL **Solution, oral:** 13 mcg/mL, 25 mcg/ml, 37.5 mcg/mL, 44 mcg/mL, 50 mcg/mL, 62.5 mcg/mL, 75 mcg/mL, 88 mcg/mL, 100 mcg/mL, 125 mcg/mL, 137 mcg/mL, 150 mcg/mL, 175 mcg/mL, 100 mcg/5 mL (Thyquidity), 150 mcg/5 mL (Ermeza) **Tablet:** 25 mcg, 50 mcg, 75 mcg, 88 mcg, 100 mcg, 112 mcg, 125 mcg, 137 mcg, 150 mcg, 175 mcg, 200 mcg, 300 mcg
liothyronine[a] (T$_3$)	Cytomel, Triostat Cytomel	**Solution, injection (Triostat)[b]:** 10 mcg/mL **Tablet (Cytomel):** 5 mcg, 25 mcg, 50 mcg[b]
desiccated thyroid[a]	Not available Generics	**Tablet:** 30 mg, 60 mg, 125 mg

[a]Generic available.
[b]Available in the United States only.

Summary of Drugs Used in the Treatment of Thyroid Disorders

Generic Name	Brand Name	Usual Dose and Dosing Schedule	Warning Labels
Hyperthyroidism			
methimazole	Tapazole	Begin: 15–60 mg in 3 divided doses/day Maintenance: 5–15 mg daily	AVOID PREGNANCY.
propylthiouracil	Generics	Begin: 50–150 mg 3 times daily Maintenance: 50 mg 2–3 times a day	
radioactive iodine,[131]I	Manufactured in pharmacy	6–15 µCi as a single dose	
Hypothyroidism			
levothyroxine	Synthroid, Eltroxin	25–150 mcg once daily	AVOID ANTACIDS, DAIRY, CALCIUM, AND IRON PILLS WITHIN 4 HOURS OF DOSE. TAKE ON AN EMPTY STOMACH. TAKE WITH A FULL GLASS OF WATER. DO NOT SKIP DOSES.
liothyronine	Cytomel	25–75 mcg once daily	
desiccated thyroid	Generics	Initial: 30–300 mg daily Maintenance: 30–125 mg once daily	

Key Points

- Thyroid disorders result in either overactivity or underactivity of the thyroid gland.
- Hyperthyroidism is a condition in which the thyroid gland secretes excessive amounts of thyroid hormones.
- Graves disease is an autoimmune disease that causes hyperthyroidism.
- Hypothyroidism is a condition in which the thyroid gland secretes deficient amounts of thyroid hormones.
- Hashimoto disease is an autoimmune disorder that causes hypothyroidism.
- Hyperthyroidism and hypothyroidism are more prevalent in women than in men.
- The incidence of hypothyroidism increases with age.
- Patients with an autoimmune disease (e.g., type 1 diabetes) are at increased risk for developing thyroid disease.
- Cigarette smoking increases the risk for developing thyroid-related eye disease.
- The thyroid gland secretes hormones that affect almost all cells in the body. Thyroid hormones regulate growth and metabolism.
- The thyroid gland is one of the few glands that produces and stores its hormones.
- Treatment of hyperthyroidism involves the use of antithyroid drugs or high-dose radioactive iodine (^{131}I); it may also be treated with surgery.
- Radioactive iodine is selectively taken up by the thyroid gland, where it causes glandular destruction without producing damage to other tissues.
- Most patients treated with ^{131}I develop an underactive thyroid gland after treatment, requiring lifelong therapy for hypothyroidism.
- Radioactive iodine therapy is contraindicated in pregnant women because it can cause thyroid damage in the developing fetus.
- Radioactive iodine ^{131}I is made in nuclear pharmacies and is regulated by the Nuclear Regulatory Commission.
- Propylthiouracil and methimazole block the synthesis of T_4 and T_3. Propylthiouracil blocks the process that converts T_4 to T_3.
- Thyroid replacement therapy is the principal treatment for hypothyroidism. Synthetic T_4, known as levothyroxine (L-thyroxine), is the most commonly prescribed drug for the treatment of hypothyroidism.
- Levothyroxine is converted to liothyronine in the body, just as naturally occurring T_4 is metabolized to T_3.
- Ferrous products, calcium supplements, and food can decrease the absorption of thyroid hormones.
- The various strengths of levothyroxine are color-coded to help avoid dispensing errors.

Review Questions

1. Tetraiodothyronine is the most abundant thyroid hormone. It contains _____ atom(s) of iodine and is also known as thyroxine.
   a. three
   b. four
   c. two
   d. one

2. Hyperthyroidism and hypothyroidism are more prevalent in women than in men.
   a. true
   b. false

3. _____ is an autoimmune disease that is the primary cause of thyroid hyperactivity.
   a. Hashimoto disease
   b. TSH disease
   c. Graves disease
   d. All of the above

4. Treatment of hyperthyroidism involves the administration of _____.
   a. antithyroid drugs
   b. radioactive iodine
   c. surgery
   d. all of the above

5. Select the drug that is used to treat hypothyroidism.
   a. Propylthiouracil
   b. Tapazole
   c. Synthroid

   d. ^{131}I

6. Select the drug that is used to treat hyperthyroidism.
   a. Cytomel
   b. Synthroid
   c. Eltroxin
   d. Tapazole

7. A brand name for levothyroxine is _____.
   a. Cytomel
   b. Thyrolar
   c. Proloid
   d. Synthroid

8. Select the warning label that might be placed on a prescription filled for Synthroid.
   a. Take with food.
   b. Avoid antacids, dairy, and iron pills.
   c. May cause drowsiness.
   d. Avoid prolonged exposure to sunlight.

9. Hashimoto disease is an autoimmune disorder that causes _____.
   a. hypothyroidism
   b. hyperthyroidism

10. Diabetes is not a risk factor for thyroid disease.
    a. true
    b. false

Bibliography

Alexander EK, Pearce EN, Brent GA, et al. 2017 guidelines of the American Thyroid Association for the diagnosis and management of thyroid disease during pregnancy and the postpartum. *Thyroid.* 2017;27(3).

Brito JP, Deng Y, Ross JS, et al. Association between generic-to-generic levothyroxine switching and thyrotropin levels among US adults. *JAMA Intern Med.* 2022;182(4):418–425.

Burch H.B., Wartofsky L. (2021a). Graves' Disease. Retrieved October 21, 2022, from https://www.niddk.nih.gov/health-information/endocrine-diseases/graves-disease.

Burch H.B., Wartofsky L. (2021b). Hashimoto's Disease. Retrieved October 21, 2022, from https://www.niddk.nih.gov/health-information/endocrine-diseases/hashimotos-disease.

Cawood T, Moriarty P, O'Farrelly C, et al. Smoking and thyroid-associated ophthalmopathy: a novel explanation of the biological link. *J Clin Endocrinol Metab.* 2007;92:59–64.

Das D, Banerjee A, Jena AB, et al. Essentiality, relevance, and efficacy of adjuvant/combinational therapy in the management of thyroid dysfunctions. *Biomed Pharmacother.* 2022;146:112613.

Genovese BM, Noureldine SI, Gleeson EM, et al. What is the best definitive treatment for Graves' disease? A systematic review of the existing literature. *Ann Surg Oncol.* 2013;20:660–667.

Health Canada. (2022). Drug Product Database. Retrieved October 18, 2022, from https://health-products.canada.ca/dpd-bdpp/index-eng.jsp.

Institute for Safe Medication Practices. (2016). FDA and ISMP Lists of Look-Alike Drug Names with Recommended Tall Man Letters. Retrieved October 18, 2022, from https://www.ismp.org/recommendations/tall-man-letters-list.

Institute for Safe Medication Practices. (2019). List of Confused Drugs. Retrieved October 18, 2022, from https://www.ismp.org/tools/confuseddrugnames.pdf.

Kalant H, Grant D, Mitchell J. *Principles of medical pharmacology.* ed 7. Toronto: Elsevier Canada; 2007:613–619.

Kotkowska Z, Strzelecki D. Depression and autoimmune hypothyroidism—their relationship and the effects of treating psychiatric and thyroid disorders on changes in clinical and biochemical parameters including BDNF and other cytokines—a systematic review. *Pharmaceuticals.* 2022;15(4):391.

Okosieme OE, Lazarus JH. Current trends in antithyroid drug treatment of Graves' disease. *Expert Opin Pharmacother.* 2016;17(15):2005–2017.

Page C, Curtis M, Sutter M, et al. *Integrated pharmacology.* Philadelphia: Mosby; 2005:288–291.

Raffa R, Rawls S, Beyzarov E. , *Netter's illustrated pharmacology.* 136–142. Philadelphia: Saunders Elsevier; 2005:10–11.

Ross DS, Burch HB, Cooper DS, et al. American Thyroid Association guidelines for diagnosis and management of hyperthyroidism and other causes of thyrotoxicosis. *Thyroid.* 2016;26(10):2016.

Schellack N, Schellack G. A review of drugs acting on the thyroid gland. *S African Pharmaceut J.* 2013;80(2):12–17.

Sengupta J, Das H, Chellaiyan DVG, et al. An observational study of incidence of metabolic syndrome among patients with controlled Grave's disease. *Clin Epidemiol Global Health.* 2022;15.

U.S. Food and Drug Administration. (nd). Drugs@FDA: FDA Approved Drug Products. Retrieved October 20, 2022, from http://www.accessdata.fda.gov/scripts/cder/daf/.

Wang S, Baker Jr J. Targeting B cells in Graves' disease. *Endocrinology.* 2006;147:4559–4560.

Zhao R, Zhang W, Ma C, et al. Immunomodulatory function of vitamin D and its role in autoimmune thyroid disease. *Front Immunol.* 2021;12:574967.

26

Treatment of Diabetes Mellitus

LEARNING OBJECTIVES

1. Learn the terminology associated with diabetes mellitus.
2. Identify risk factors for diabetes mellitus.
3. Describe the causes of diabetes mellitus.
4. List the symptoms of diabetes mellitus.
5. List and categorize medications used to treat diabetes mellitus.
6. Describe mechanism of action for each class of drugs used to treat diabetes mellitus.
7. Identify significant drug look-alike and sound-alike issues.
8. List common endings for drug classes used in the treatment of diabetes mellitus.
9. Identify warning labels and precautionary messages associated with medications used to treat diabetes mellitus.

KEY TERMS

Diabetes mellitus Chronic condition in which the body is unable to use glucose (sugar) as energy properly.

Diabetic neuropathy Damage to peripheral nerves by diabetes that causes numbness in the lower limbs.

Fasting blood glucose Blood glucose level that is taken after a person has not eaten for 8 to 12 hours (usually overnight).

Gestational diabetes Diabetes that may be caused by the hormones of pregnancy or a shortage of insulin.

Hemoglobin A1c Blood test that measures a person's average blood glucose level over a period of 2 to 3 months.

Hyperglycemia Elevated blood glucose levels.

Hypoglycemia Low blood glucose levels.

Insulin resistance Condition in which the body does not respond to insulin; contributes to the development of type 2 diabetes.

Postprandial After a meal.

Prediabetes Condition of impaired fasting glucose and impaired glucose tolerance in which the body consistently has elevated glucose levels.

Type 1 diabetes An autoimmune disease that leads to high blood glucose levels. Pancreatic β-cells are destroyed, and insufficient amounts of insulin are produced.

Type 2 diabetes A condition that results in high blood glucose levels. People with type 2 diabetes have insulin resistance.

Overview

Diabetes mellitus is a disorder of metabolism that involves glucose use. It is a chronic condition in which the body cannot properly use glucose as energy. Glucose is the body's primary energy source. Under normal conditions, as glucose levels in the blood rise, hormones are released that move the glucose out of the bloodstream and into cells, where it is needed for growth and energy. In those with diabetes, glucose accumulates in the blood. Much like a person with sticky hands walking through a room, glucose in the bloodstream leaves a sticky residue over all the body's organs and cells and causes damage.

Diabetes affects approximately 422 million people globally. In the United States, more than 34 million adults have the disease, according to the National Institutes of Health, and 7 million are unaware that they have the disease. In Canada, nearly 6 million people are living with diabetes. Approximately 88 million adults in the United States and 5.7 million Canadians have prediabetes. Diabetes mellitus is one of the leading causes of disability in the United States. It is the leading cause of non-war-related amputations.

The global cost for treating diabetes is $825 billion annually! In the United States, one of every eight federal health care dollars is spent treating people with diabetes. National Institute of Diabetes and Digestive and Kidney Diseases (NIDDK) National Statistics has estimated the direct cost of diabetes in the United States is $105 billion. The costs in Canada were estimated to be $30 billion.

Hormone Regulation of Blood Glucose Level

The control of glucose levels occurs by a second-messenger reaction. Insulin, a hormone that is essential for the regulation of carbohydrates, fat, and protein metabolism, is secreted by the β-cells in the islets of Langerhans when the blood glucose level rises. Insulin binds to receptors on the cell membrane. This stimulates the docking of intracellular glucose transporters that carry glucose out of the bloodstream and into cells where it is needed. Insulin,

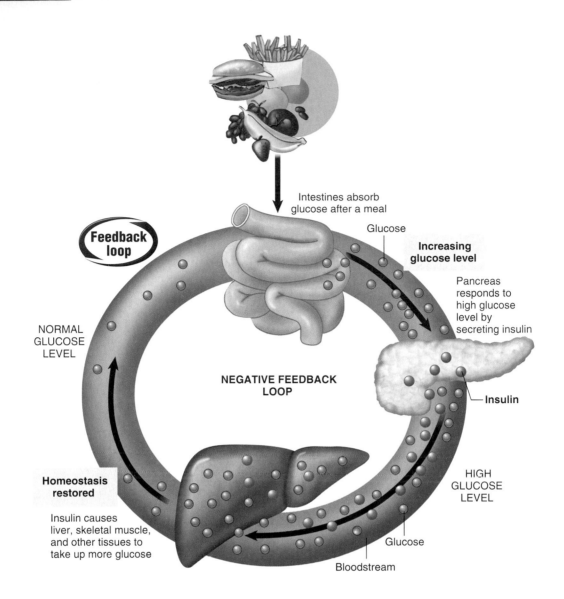

• **Fig. 26.1** Role of insulin. (From Patton KT, Thibodeau GA. *The human body in health and disease,* ed 7, St Louis, 2018, Elsevier.)

along with glucagon, is released by the pancreas in response to the rise and fall of blood glucose, amino acid, and gut-derived hormone levels (Fig. 26.1).

Excess glucose that is not needed for energy immediately is stored in the liver as glycogen, a reservoir for future energy needs (Fig. 26.2). When glucose levels drop, glucagon is secreted by α-cells in the islets of Langerhans. Glucagon stimulates the release of the stored energy. The physiologic effects of insulin are listed in Box 26.1.

Types of Diabetes Mellitus

Prediabetes, type 1 diabetes, type 2 diabetes, and gestational diabetes all produce elevated blood glucose levels *(hyperglycemia)*. Symptoms of *hyperglycemia* are listed in Box 26.2. A hemoglobin A1c test (Hb_{A1c}) is performed to diagnose prediabetes and diabetes. The Hb_{A1c} test measures the average blood glucose level over a 3-month period. An Hb_{A1c} result above 6.4% over 2 to 3 measurements is a sign of diabetes.

Prediabetes

Prediabetes causes impaired fasting glucose (IFG) and impaired glucose tolerance (IGT). Prediabetes is a risk factor for developing diabetes and also increases the risk of cardiovascular disease (CVD). An Hb_{A1c} level between 5.7% and 6.4% is a sign of prediabetes. A fasting blood glucose test and an oral glucose tolerance test (OGTT) may also be conducted. When blood glucose levels range between 100 and 125 mg/dL (6.1 to 6.9 mmol/L) after an overnight fast, glucose levels are said to be impaired. After a 2-hour OGTT, blood glucose levels are considered high when they range from 140 to 199 mg/dL (7.8 to 11.0 mmol/L) in individuals with IGT.

Type 1 Diabetes

Type 1 diabetes is an autoimmune disease. The immune system attacks and destroys the insulin-producing β-cells in the pancreas. Only 5% to 10% of all persons with diabetes have type 1 diabetes. People who have type 1 diabetes must inject insulin daily because their body no longer produces enough of the hormone insulin. The onset of type 1 diabetes is typically in childhood; hence the

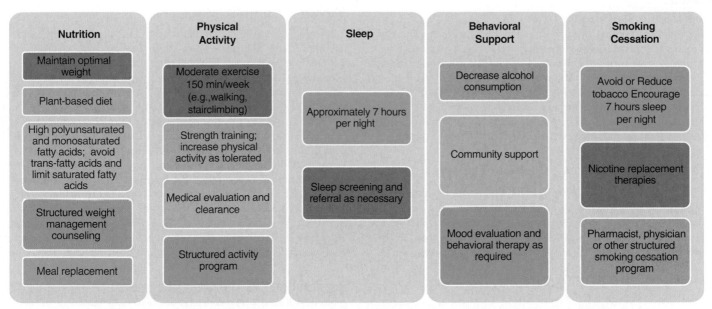

• **Fig. 26.2** Algorithm for management of diabetes (or equivalent). (From Garber AJ, Abrahamson MJ, Barzilay JI, et al. Consensus statement by the American Association of Clinical Endocrinologists and American College of Endocrinology on the comprehensive type 2 diabetes management algorithm—2017 executive summary, *Endocr Pract* 23(2):207–238, 2017.)

• BOX 26.1 Physiologic Effects of Insulin

Carbohydrate Metabolism
- Increased glycogen synthesis (liver)
- Decreased gluconeogenesis (liver)
- Increased glucose transport (muscle and fat cells)

Lipid Metabolism
- Sets the level of triglyceride production from free fatty acids
- Decreased lipolysis

Protein Metabolism
- Increased amino acid synthesis
- Increased amino acid transport (precursors for protein synthesis)

TABLE 26.1 Risk Factors for Diabetes Mellitus

Type of Risk Factor	Description
Nonmodifiable	Age (≥40 years), family history of diabetes
Modifiable	Overweight and obesity Physical inactivity Smoking
Disease	Hypertension, angina, myocardial infarction, stroke, metabolic syndrome, insulin resistance, hyperlipidemia, schizophrenia, polycystic ovary syndrome

---

• BOX 26.2 Symptoms of Hyperglycemia

Hyperglycemia
- Blurred vision
- Breath that smells fruity
- Decreased consciousness
- Dry mouth
- Elevated blood glucose level
- Extreme hunger
- Extreme thirst
- Frequent urination
- Shortness of breath
- Upset stomach and vomiting
- Weakness

---

condition was formerly called juvenile-onset diabetes mellitus. However, it can occur at any age.

Type 2 Diabetes

Type 2 diabetes is most common, accounting for 90% to 95% of all cases of diabetes. In type 2 diabetes, the pancreas initially produces sufficient amounts of insulin, but the body is unable to use the insulin effectively. This condition is called ***insulin resistance***. Insulin production eventually decreases; however, this may not occur for several years. Risk factors of type 2 diabetes are obesity, lack of physical activity, family history of diabetes, prior gestational diabetes, and increasing age (Table 26.1). Approximately 80% of persons diagnosed with type 2 diabetes are overweight. Type 2 diabetes was formerly called non-insulin-dependent diabetes (NIDDM) or adult-onset diabetes; however, these terms have been replaced because people with type 2 diabetes may sometimes be required to manage their condition with insulin and childhood obesity has caused children to become the fastest growing population with diabetes.

In Canada, the prevalence of type 2 diabetes is greater in Canadians of South Asian descent and First Nations and Métis peoples. In the United States, Black, Latino, and First Nations peoples have the highest prevalence. It is believed that internalized racism, chronic stress, and consumption of a "diabetes" diet that is high in fat and carbohydrates may contribute to the higher level of diabetes in these groups.

Gestational Diabetes

Gestational diabetes occurs in approximately 3% to 8% of all pregnant women. It typically occurs late in pregnancy and may be caused by the hormones of pregnancy or by a shortage of insulin. Pregnant women are routinely tested for gestational diabetes. An elevated blood glucose level is an early sign of gestational diabetes. Symptoms often disappear after delivery; however, women who have had gestational diabetes have a 20% to 50% increased risk for the development of type 2 diabetes within 5 to 10 years.

Insulin Resistance as a Cause of Diabetes

Insulin resistance is a condition in which the body does not respond to insulin. It is a precursor to type 2 diabetes. Insulin resistance is a syndrome that increases the risk for CVD, hypertension, dyslipidemia, elevated triglyceride and low-density lipoprotein (LDL) levels, decreased high-density lipoprotein (HDL) levels, microalbuminuria, and diabetes. It may also increase risk for obesity, a risk factor for type 2 diabetes, because insulin signals the body to increase food intake.

Symptoms and Diagnosis of Diabetes Mellitus

Symptoms

Symptoms of diabetes mellitus are listed in Box 26.3.

Diagnostic Tests

The **hemoglobin A1c** test is the principal method used to diagnose diabetes. It is the only test that provides information about blood glucose levels over a 2- to 3-month period. Additional tests are blood glucose levels measured after fasting or after the consumption of a dose of glucose (OGTT).

- **Fasting blood glucose** test: Blood glucose level 126 mg/dL or higher (≥7 mmol/L) or more after an 8-hour fast.
- OGTT: Blood glucose level 200 mg/dL or higher (≥11 mmol/L) 2 hours after drinking a beverage containing 75 g of glucose dissolved in water.
- Random blood glucose: Blood glucose level 200 mg/dL or higher (≥11 mmol/L), along with the presence of diabetes symptoms.

• BOX 26.3 Symptoms of Diabetes Mellitus

Type 1
- Blurred vision
- Constant hunger (polyphagia)
- Diabetic ketoacidosis
- Extreme fatigue
- Frequent urination (polyuria)
- Hyperglycemia
- Increased thirst (polydipsia)
- Weight loss

Type 2
- Blurred vision
- Fatigue
- Frequent urination
- Hunger
- Hyperglycemia
- Increased thirst
- Slow healing of wounds or sores
- Weight loss

Diabetes Complications

Untreated or poorly controlled diabetes mellitus produces damage throughout the body (Box 26.4). It may cause microvascular and macrovascular damage. Microvascular damage weakens blood vessels in the eye, and retinopathy can lead to blurred vision and blindness. Nephropathy (kidney damage) and **diabetic neuropathy** also occur. Diabetic neuropathy causes numbness in the lower limbs. Patients with diabetes must frequently inspect their feet because if they develop a foot injury, they might not feel it. Diabetes causes poor wound healing, so foot infections sometimes become serious enough to require limb amputation. Macrovascular changes can lead to hypertension, angina, and myocardial infarction. Diabetes can also cause hyperlipidemia. Individuals with untreated or poorly controlled type 1 diabetes may develop ketoacidosis, a condition in which the body breaks down fats to obtain its energy needs. Ketones are a byproduct of lipid metabolism, and their accumulation can lead to coma and death.

● Tech Note!

Alcohol, aspirin, and decongestants can alter blood glucose levels. A list of drugs that increase and decrease blood glucose levels is provided in Box 26.2.

● Tech Note!

It is recommended that alcohol consumption be limited in a patient with diabetes to no more than one or two drinks per day (maximum, 14 drinks/week for men and 9 drinks/week for women).

Management of Diabetes

Nonpharmacologic Management

Diabetes mellitus is sometimes classified as a disease of lifestyle because lifestyle factors can increase the risk for type 2 diabetes. All types of diabetes can be improved by weight loss, engaging in physical activity, consuming foods with a low glycemic index, quitting smoking, reducing alcohol consumption, and other lifestyle changes. Physical activity lowers the risk of type 2 diabetes

---

• BOX 26.4 Diabetes Complications

- Amputation
- Angina
- Blindness
- Blurred vision
- Heart attack
- Hyperlipidemia
- Hypertension
- Increased birth defects
- Infections
- Ketoacidosis
- Nephropathy
- Peripheral neuropathy
- Pregnancy complications
- Retinopathy
- Stroke

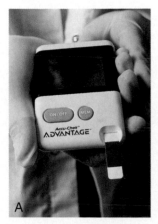
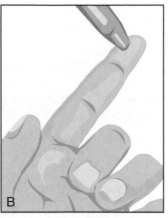
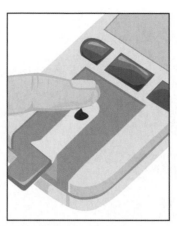
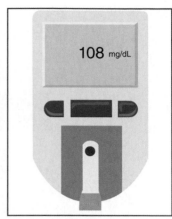

• **Fig. 26.3** (**A**) Blood glucose monitor. (**B**) Blood glucose testing using a blood glucose meter. ([**A**], From Bonewit-West K. *Clinical procedures for medical assistants*, ed 7, St Louis, 2008, Saunders. [**B**], From MedlinePlus: *Diabetes*. http://www.nlm.nih.gov/medlineplus/diabetes.html. 2017.)

by up to 30%. For those with diabetes, increased physical activity decreases risks of mortality from the disease. A minimum of 150 minutes of exercise weekly is recommended to maintain glycemic control, of which at least 90 minutes should be vigorous aerobic exercise. Loss of 5% to 7% of body weight through diet and increased physical activity can lower the risks of diabetes (Fig. 26.2).

Blood Glucose Monitoring

Blood glucose monitoring is an essential component of diabetes management (Fig. 26.3A). Measurement of blood glucose levels may be recommended 1 to 4 times daily, depending on the type of diabetes (type 1, type 2, or gestational) and the antihyperglycemic drug regimen that the patient is prescribed. Testing frequency is greatest for individuals using insulin. Blood glucose monitoring enables individuals with diabetes to take control of their disease by adjusting their level of diet, exercise, and insulin (see Fig. 26.3B).

Keeping the blood glucose level within a normal range has been shown to minimize the risk of diabetic complications. According to the Diabetes Control and Complications Trial, a 10-year study sponsored by the NIDDK and the United Kingdom Prospective Diabetes Study, intensive control of blood glucose and blood pressure reduces complications in types 1 and 2 diabetes.

> ● *Tech Note!*
>
> Pharmacy technicians knowledgeable about the various blood glucose monitors can help patients select the monitor that best suits their needs.

Pharmacologic Management

Type 1 diabetes is primarily managed with insulin. Type 2 diabetes may be managed with oral antidiabetic agents, insulin, and insulin analogs (Fig. 26.4). Pramlintide (Symlin) is a synthetic analog of the hormone amylin that is also used for the treatment of type 1 diabetes. Type 2 diabetes may be treated with oral agents (metformin, sulfonylureas, thiazolidinediones, sodium-glucose cotransporter-2 [SGLT2] inhibitors, glucagon-like peptide 1 [GLP-1] receptor agonists, dipeptidyl peptidase 4 [DPP-4] inhibitors) and injectable agents (insulin, insulin analogs, or GLP-1 receptor

agonists). Oral antidiabetic agents are indicated only as an adjunct to diet and exercise in the treatment of type 2 diabetes mellitus.

Insulin

Insulin is administered for the management of all types of diabetes. It helps the body metabolize carbohydrates, fats, and proteins from the diet. It may be the sole drug administered, as in type 1 diabetes, or may be added to oral therapy or replace oral therapy in type 2 diabetes. Insulin was originally manufactured from animal sources (pig and cow); however, genetically engineered insulin using recombinant DNA technology (see Chapter 1) to match human insulin has replaced animal source insulin. Pork and bovine insulins are no longer marketed in the United States but are still available in Canada and other parts of the world.

> ● *Tech Note!*
>
> Remember when mixing insulin that if one is cloudy, it gets drawn up second. Lantus or Levemir should not be mixed in a syringe with another form of insulin.

> ● *Tech Note!*
>
> Rapid-acting insulin (aspart, glulisine, lispro), regular insulin, and long-acting insulin (detemir, glargine) are clear solutions that should be discarded if they appear cloudy.

Mechanism of Action and Pharmacokinetics

Insulin facilitates the transport of glucose that is in the bloodstream into the body's cells where the glucose provides energy (Fig. 26.5). Insulin is administered parenterally. Solutions such as regular insulin may be administered intravenously; all other insulins are injected subcutaneously. Insulin is formulated in rapid-acting, short-acting, intermediate-acting, and long-acting forms. The onset of action for rapid-acting insulin (aspart, glulisine, lispro insulin) begins within 15 minutes, whereas the onset of action for long-acting insulin (detemir, glargine insulin) is 90 minutes (Table 26.2). Rapid-acting insulin is injected 5 to 15 minutes before eating, or even after a meal for some individuals. Long-acting basal insulin, administered at bedtime, has the advantage of lowering

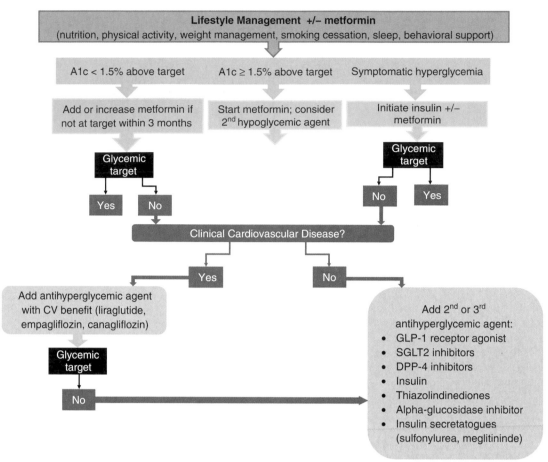

Lifestyle Management +/– metformin
(nutrition, physical activity, weight management, smoking cessation, sleep, behavioral support)

A1c < 1.5% above target | A1c ≥ 1.5% above target | Symptomatic hyperglycemia

Add or increase metformin if not at target within 3 months | Start metformin; consider 2nd hypoglycemic agent | Initiate insulin +/– metformin

Glycemic target
Yes No

Glycemic target
No Yes

Clinical Cardiovascular Disease?
Yes No

Add antihyperglycemic agent with CV benefit (liraglutide, empagliflozin, canagliflozin)

Glycemic target
No

Add 2nd or 3rd antihyperglycemic agent:
- GLP-1 receptor agonist
- SGLT2 inhibitors
- DPP-4 inhibitors
- Insulin
- Thiazolindinediones
- Alpha-glucosidase inhibitor
- Insulin secretatogues (sulfonylurea, meglitininde)

• **Fig. 26.4** Algorithm for glycemic control. (From Garber AJ, Abrahamson MJ, Barzilay JI, et al. Consensus statement by the American Association of Clinical Endocrinologists and American College of Endocrinology on the comprehensive type 2 diabetes management algorithm—2017 executive summary, *Endocr Pract* 23(2): 207–238, 2017.)

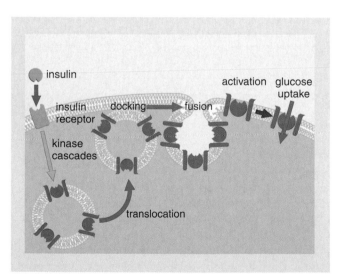

insulin

insulin receptor

kinase cascades

docking fusion

activation glucose uptake

translocation

• **Fig. 26.5** Insulin mechanism of action. (From Page C, Curtis M, Sutter M, et al. *Integrated pharmacology*, ed 3, Philadelphia, 2006, Mosby.)

the risk for nighttime *hypoglycemia* (low blood sugar) when compared with neutral protamine Hagedorn (NPH) insulin, which is also used for basal insulin needs. Basal bolus insulin administration is recommended by the Canadian Diabetes Association

Clinical Guidelines for people with type 1 diabetes. Intermediate- or long-acting basal insulin is typically administered once or twice daily, and rapid-acting prandial insulin is injected at mealtime.

Dosage delivery systems used for the administration of insulin are the insulin pump, vial and syringe, inhaler, and insulin pen (Fig. 26.6).

> **Tech Note!**
>
> Individuals with diabetes must eat scheduled meals. Basal bolus insulin administration mimics normal fluctuations of insulin levels throughout the day in response to preprandial and *postprandial* glucose levels.

> **Tech Note!**
>
> Insulin is the most effective agent for glycemic control and reduces the Hb$_{A1c}$ level by more than 2%.

Adverse Reactions

Insulin replacement therapy produces symptoms similar to the effects produced by the naturally secreted hormone at its target site. In addition to hypoglycemia, insulin therapy may cause

TABLE 26.2 Onset, Peak, and Duration of Action of Insulin

Insulin	Onset of Action	Peak Action	Duration of Action
Ultra-Rapid Acting (Prandial)			
insulin lispro	10–15 min	1–1.5 h	6–8 h
insulin aspart	10–15 min	1–2 h	3–5 h
insulin glulisine	10–15 min	1–1.5 h	5–6 h
Short Acting (Prandial)			
insulin regular	15 min (IV)	—	30–60 min (IV)
	30 min (SC)	2–3 h	8–12 h (SC)
Intermediate Acting (Basal)			
Neutral protamine Hagedorn (NPH), recombinant	1–3 h	5–8 h	Up to 18 h
Long Acting (Basal)			
insulin glargine - Lantus	1.5 h	—	Up to 24 h
- Basaglar	—	12 h	Up to 24 h
- Toujeo	6 h	12–16	Up to 24 h (blood glucose-lowering effect increases over time, up to 5 days)
insulin detemir	1.5 h	6–8 h	Up to 24 h

IV, intravenous; *SC,* subcutaneous.

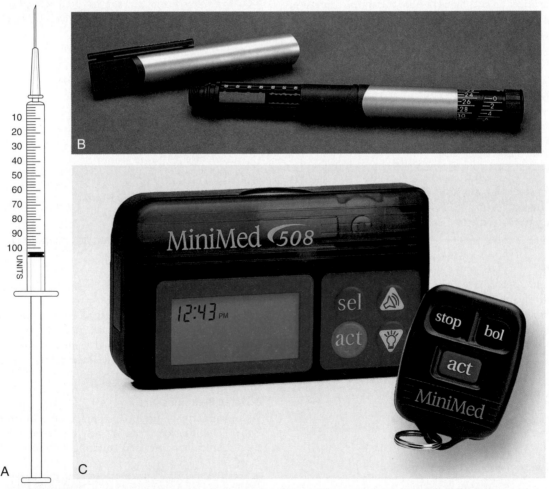

• **Fig. 26.6** Dosage delivery systems for the administration of insulin. (**A**) Standard insulin syringe. (**B**) Insulin pen. (**C**) Insulin pump. ([**A** and **B**], From Fulcher EM, Fulcher RM, Soto CD. *Pharmacology principles and applications*, ed 3, St Louis, 2012, Elsevier. [**C**], Courtesy of MiniMed, Sylmar, California. In Fulcher EM, Fulcher RM, Soto CD: *Pharmacology principles and applications*, ed 3, St Louis, 2012, Saunders.)

Hypoglycemia

- Anxiety, nervousness, irritability
- Blurred vision
- Cold sensations
- Confusion
- Difficulty concentrating
- Fatigue, uncontrolled yawning
- Headache
- Hunger
- Loss of consciousness
- Low blood glucose level
- Muscle weakness
- Nausea
- Numbness of the mouth
- Pale skin
- Palpitations, rapid heartbeat
- Shallow breathing
- Sweating
- Tingling in the fingers
- Tremors

TABLE 26.3 **Recommended Storage for Opened Vials and Cartridges of Insulin**

Type of Insulin	Storage
insulin aspart and insulin glulisine	Vials: Room temperature or refrigerated; discard after 28 days Cartridges: Store at room temperature; discard after 28 days
insulin detemir	Vials: Room temperature or refrigerated; discard after 42 days Cartridges: Store at room temperature; discard after 42 days
insulin glargine	Vials and cartridges: Refrigerated; discard after 28 days (5 and 10 mL)
insulin lispro	Vial, cartridges, and pens: Room temperature or refrigerated; once opened, discard after 28 days Insulin pump: Discard after 7 days
NPH insulin	Vial: Room temperature or refrigerated; discard after 42 days Cartridges: Room temperature or refrigerated; once opened, store at room temperature and discard after 14 days

NPH, Neutral protamine Hagedorn.

weight gain, pain, or irritation at the injection site and lipohypertrophy or lipoatrophy. Signs of lipohypertrophy are fat accumulation around the injection site. Signs of lipoatrophy are depressions around the site of injection caused by fat loss. Patients should be advised to rotate the site of injection to minimize these adverse reactions. Symptoms of hypoglycemia are listed in Box 26.5.

● Tech Note!

Insulin must be protected from extremes of heat and cold. Refrigerate unopened vials; do not freeze. Opened vials of insulin may be stored at room temperature, but this will shorten the expiry date for most insulin. Check the manufacturer's insert (Table 26.3).

● Tech Note!

Many drugs may produce hyperglycemia or hypoglycemia (Box 26.6).

Sulfonylureas

Sulfonylureas are sometimes categorized as oral hypoglycemic agents. They are effective only for the treatment of type 2 diabetes. They are very effective in producing glycemic control and can reduce the Hb$_{A1c}$ level by 1% to 2%.

---

❶ Tech Alert!

The following drugs have look-alike/sound-alike issues:
glyBURIDE, glipiZIDE, and gliclazide;
Microzide and Maxzide

Mechanism of Action and Pharmacokinetics

Sulfonylureas primarily stimulate insulin release from pancreatic β-cells. Sulfonylureas also decrease the breakdown of glycogen to glucose (glycogenolysis). Glycogen is the storage form of glucose.

Drugs Associated With Hyperglycemia

- Atypical antipsychotics
- β-Blockers
- Diuretics, thiazides (>25 mg hydrochlorothiazide)
- Glucocorticoids
- Growth hormone
- Nicotinic acid
- Pentamidine
- Phenytoin
- Protease inhibitors
- Sympathomimetics

Drugs Associated With Hypoglycemia

- Acetylsalicylic acid (ASA; salicylates)
- Alcohol
- Angiotensin-converting enzyme inhibitors; angiotensin II receptor blockers
- β-Blockers

Sulfonylureas differ in pharmacokinetics, pharmacodynamics, and incidence of hypoglycemic reactions. Glyburide and gliclazide have the highest risk for hypoglycemia, and glimepiride has the lowest risk. Glyburide has active metabolites that can accumulate in patients with kidney disease.

Adverse Reactions

Sulfonylureas can produce hypoglycemia, a serious side effect. Other common side effects are weight gain, abdominal pain, diarrhea, dyspepsia, nausea and vomiting, headache, and dizziness.

● Tech Note!

Conventional and micronized dosage forms of glyburide are not substitutable.

Insulin

Generic Name	US Brand Name(s) Canadian Brand Name(s)	Dosage Forms and Strengths
insulin aspart	Fiasp, Fiasp Fiasp Penfill, Novolog FlexPen, Novolog Penfill Fiasp, Kirsty, Novomix 30, Novorapid, Trurapi	**Suspension, for injection (vial, pen, cartridge):** 100 units/mL
insulin degludec	Tresiba Tresiba	**Solution:** 100 units/mL, 200 units/mL
insulin detemir	Levemir, Levemir FlexTouch Levemir Penfill, Levemir FlexTouch	**Solution, for injection (vial, pen, cartridge):** 100 units/mL
insulin glargine	Basaglar, Lantus, Lantus SoloStar, Rezvoglar, Semglee, Toujeo Basaglar, Lantus, Lantus SoloStar, Semglee, Toujeo Doublestar, Toujeo Solostar	**Solution, for injection (vial, pen, cartridge):** 100 units/mL, 300 units/mL (Toujeo)
insulin glulisine	Apidra, Apidra SoloStar Apidra, Apidra SoloStar, Apidra cartridge	**Injection, solution (vial, pen, cartridge):** 100 units/mL
insulin lispro	Admelog, Admelog Solostar, Humalog, Humalog Pen, Humalog Tempo Pen, Humalog KwikPen, LyumJev Admelog, Admelog Solostar, Humalog, Humalog cartridge, Humalog KwikPen	**Solution, for intravenous or subcutaneous injection (Admelog):** 100 units/mL **Solution, for injection (vial, pen, cartridge):** 100 units/mL, 200 units/mL
insulin, recombinant human	Afrezza Not available	**Powder, for inhalation:** 4 units/inhalation, 8 units/ inhalation, 12 units/inhalation
insulin regular recombinant human	Humulin R, Humulin R KwikPen, Myxredlin, Novolin R Entuzity KwikPen, Humulin R, Humulin R cartridge, Humulin R KwikPen	**Injection, solution (vial, pen, cartridge):** 100 units/mL, 500 units/mL (Entuzity)
insulin isophane recombinant human	Humulin N, Humulin N KwikPen, Novolin N Humulin N, Humulin N KwikPen, Humulin N cartridge, Novolin GE NPH, Novolin GE NPH pen, Novolin GE Toronto[a]	**Suspension, for injection (vial, pen, cartridge):** 100 units/mL
insulin isophane pork	Not available Hypurin NPH	**Suspension:** 100 units/mL
insulin regular pork	Not available Hypurin R	**Solution:** 100 units/mL
Insulin Mixtures		
insulin regular + insulin isophane	Humulin 70/30, Novolin 70/30 Humulin 30/70, Humulin 30/70 cartridge Novolin GE Penfill 30/70 Novolin GE Penfill 40/60 Novolin GE Penfill 50/50	**Suspension, for injection (vial, pen, cartridge):** 30 units/mL insulin + 70 units/mL insulin isophane 50 units/mL insulin + 50 units/mL insulin isophane[a] 40 units/mL insulin + 60 units/mL insulin isophane[a]
lispro insulin + lispro protamine suspension	Humalog Mix 50/50, Humalog Pen 50/50, Humalog KwikPen 50/50, Humalog Mix 75/25, Humalog Mix Pen 75/25, Humalog Mix KwikPen 75/25 Humalog Mix 25 (Cartridge), Humalog Mix 25 KwikPen, Humalog Mix 50 (Cartridge), Humalog Mix 50 KwikPen	**Suspension, for injection (cartridge, pen):** 75 units lispro protamine suspension + 25 units lispro insulin 50 units lispro insulin + 50 units lispro protamine suspension
insulin aspart + insulin aspart protamine	Novolog Mix 50/50, Novolog Mix 70/30, Novolog Mix Flexpen 70/30, Novomix Penfill 70/30 Novomix-30 Penfill	**Suspension, for injection (vial, pen, cartridge):** 30 units insulin aspart + 70 units insulin aspart protamine, 50 units insulin aspart + 50 units insulin aspart protamine
insulin degludec + liraglutide	Xultophy 100/3.6 Xultophy	**Solution:** 100 units insulin degludec + 3.6 mcg liraglutide/mL
insulin glargine + lixisenatide	Soliqua 100/33 Soliqua	**Solution:** 100 units insulin glargine/mL + 33 mcg lixisenatide/mL

[a]Strength available in Canada only.

Sulfonylureas

	Generic Name	US Brand Name(s) / Canadian Brand Name(s)	Dosage Forms and Strengths
	glyburide[a]	Diabeta, Glynase / Generics	**Tablet (Diabeta):** 1.25 mg[b], 2.5 mg, 5 mg **Tablet, micronized (Glynase)[b]:** 1.5 mg, 3 mg, 6 mg
	gliclazide[a]	Not available / Diamicron MR	**Tablet, immediate release:** 80 mg **Tablet, extended release:** 30 mg, 60 mg
	glipizide[a]	Glucotrol XL / Not available	**Tablet, immediate release:** 5 mg, 10 mg **Tablet, extended release (Glucotrol XL):** 2.5 mg, 5 mg, 10 mg
	glimepiride[a]	Amaryl / Generic	**Tablet:** 1 mg, 2 mg, 4 mg

[a]Generic available.
[b]Available in the United States only.

Biguanides

Metformin is classified as a biguanide antidiabetic agent. Metformin acts to control fasting blood glucose. It is effective in producing glycemic control and reduces Hb_{A1c} levels by 1% to 2% without producing hypoglycemia. This makes metformin a first-line drug for the treatment of type 2 diabetes. Unlike most other antihyperglycemic agents, metformin does not cause weight gain, which is a benefit when treating obese patients with type 2 diabetes.

Mechanism of Action and Pharmacokinetics

Metformin improves glucose tolerance and insulin resistance by increasing peripheral glucose uptake into skeletal muscles and adipose tissue. It increases glucose transport across cell membranes. Metformin also lowers postprandial plasma glucose levels, decreases hepatic gluconeogenesis (new glucose) production, and decreases intestinal absorption of glucose.

Metformin may be administered in immediate-release (tablets and solution) and extended-release dosage forms. Peak blood levels are achieved in 2.5 hours for immediate-release tablets, 2.2 hours for oral solution, and 7 hours for extended-release tablets. Food decreases the absorption of immediate-release tablets but increases the absorption of metformin solution and extended-release tablets. Glumetza, Glucophage XR, and Fortamet are all extended-release dosage forms of metformin; however, they are not substitutable because different processes are used to make the drug into an extended-release formulation. Glumetza is designed to remain in the stomach and deliver metformin to the upper gastrointestinal tract, where absorption is enhanced.

Adverse Reactions

Gastrointestinal adverse reactions are common. They include gas, heartburn, metallic taste in the mouth, mild stomachache, nausea, and weight loss. Metformin may produce lactic acidosis, a rare but potentially fatal condition. Metformin may stimulate ovulation in infertile women who have polycystic ovary syndrome.

⚠ Tech Alert!

Metformin immediate-release and extended-release forms are available in some of the same strengths. Check strength carefully to avoid dispensing errors.

■ Tech Note!

Extended-release dosage forms of metformin are not substitutable.

Alpha-Glucosidase Inhibitors

The α-glucosidase inhibitors prolong the digestion of carbohydrates and delay their absorption in the small intestine. They reduce peak plasma glucose levels. α-Glucosidase inhibitors do not promote insulin secretion like many other antidiabetic agents, nor do they cause hypoglycemia. They produce a minimal effect on reducing Hb_{A1c} levels (<1%) and therefore are not used as monotherapy.

Mechanism of Action and Pharmacokinetics

Acarbose and miglitol inhibit α-glucosidases, enzymes that break down carbohydrates. They must be administered with the first bite of each meal. The drugs compete for binding sites with oligosaccharides and disaccharides in foods. It is important to eat a diet rich in complex carbohydrates while taking acarbose and miglitol.

Adverse Reactions

The α-glucosidase inhibitors most commonly produce gastrointestinal side effects. Adverse reactions include a bloated feeling, diarrhea, stomach or intestinal gas, or rumbling stomach and stomach pain or discomfort.

Biguanides

Generic Name	US Brand Name(s) / Canadian Brand Name(s)	Dosage Forms and Strengths
metformin[a]	Fortamet, Glumetza / Glucophage, Glumetza	Tablet, immediate release (Glucophage): 500 mg, 850 mg Tablet, extended release: (Glumetza): 500 mg, 1000 mg (Fortamet): 1000 mg

Combination Biguanide + Sulfonylureas

Generic Name	US Brand Name(s) / Canadian Brand Name(s)	Dosage Forms and Strengths
metformin + glyburide[a]	Generic / Not available	Tablet: 250 mg metformin + 1.25 mg glyburide 500 mg metformin + 2.5 mg glyburide 500 mg metformin + 5 mg glyburide
metformin + glipizide[a]	Generic / Not available	Tablet: 250 mg metformin + 2.5 mg glipizide 500 mg metformin + 2.5 mg glipizide 500 mg metformin + 5 mg glipizide

[a]Generic available.

α-Glucosidase Inhibitors

Generic Name	US Brand Name(s) / Canadian Brand Name(s)	Dosage Forms and Strengths
acarbose	Generics / Glucobay	Tablet: 25 mg[a], 50 mg, 100 mg
miglitol	Glyset / Not available	Tablet: 25 mg, 50 mg, 100 mg

[a]Strength available in the United States only.

Meglitinides

Meglitinides are oral antidiabetic agents used for the treatment of type 2 diabetes. Meglitinides, like the sulfonylureas, are effective only in individuals who have functioning pancreatic β-cells. Repaglinide is more effective in producing glycemic control than nateglinide. Repaglinide reduces Hb_{A1c} levels by 1% to 2%, whereas nateglinide reduces Hb_{A1c} levels by less than 1%.

Tech Note!
A common ending for meglitinides is -glinide.

Mechanism of Action and Pharmacokinetics

Repaglinide and nateglinide lower postprandial blood glucose levels by stimulating insulin secretion from pancreatic β-cells. Repaglinide is rapidly and completely absorbed from the intestinal tract. The onset of action is within 15 to 30 minutes. Peak effects of repaglinide and nateglinide are achieved in approximately 1 to 1.5 hours, and elimination is equally as rapid. The drugs must be taken only with meals to avoid hypoglycemia. Their short half-life accounts for the multiple daily dosing required. Both drugs are metabolized via the cytochrome P-450 (CYP450) system and are subject to many drug-drug interactions.

Adverse Reactions

Meglitinides may cause hypoglycemia; however, the risk is lower than with sulfonylureas if they are taken appropriately with meals. Other side effects are headache, nausea, and vomiting. Nateglinide and repaglinide should be used with caution in patients with liver dysfunction.

Meglitinides

Generic Name	US Brand Name(s) / Canadian Brand Name(s)	Dosage Forms and Strengths
nateglinide[a]	Generics / Not available	Tablet: 60 mg, 120 mg
repaglinide[a]	Generics / Gluconorm	Tablet: 0.5 mg, 1 mg, 2 mg

[a]Generic available.

Thiazolidinediones

Thiazolidinediones are insulin sensitizers; they are used for the treatment of type 2 diabetes. They treat insulin resistance. Two agents are currently marketed in the United States and Canada: pioglitazone and rosiglitazone. Both drugs reduce fasting plasma glucose (FPG) and Hb_{A1c} levels by approximately 1% to 2%.

Tech Note!
A common ending for thiazolidinediones is -glitazone.

Thiazolidinediones

	Generic Name	US Brand Name(s) / Canadian Brand Name(s)	Dosage Forms and Strengths
	pioglitazone[a]	Actos / Generics	**Tablet:** 15 mg, 30 mg, 45 mg
	rosiglitazone[a]	Avandia / Avandia	**Tablet:** 2 mg, 4 mg, 8 mg[b]
Thiazolidinediones + Biguanides	pioglitazone + metformin[a]	Actosplus Met / Not available	**Tablet:** pioglitazone 15 mg + metformin 500 mg / pioglitazone 15 mg + metformin 850 mg
Thiazolidinediones + Sulfonylureas	pioglitazone + glimepiride[a]	Duetact / Not available	**Tablet:** pioglitazone 30 mg + glimepiride 2 mg / pioglitazone 30 mg + glimepiride 4 mg

[a]Generic available.
[b]Available in Canada only.

⊘ Tech Alert!

The following drugs have look-alike/sound-alike issues:
Avandia and Avandamet; Coumadin and Prandin;
Actos and Actonel

Mechanism of Action and Pharmacokinetics

Thiazolidinediones increase tissue sensitivity to insulin. They do not increase insulin secretion, so they do not produce hypoglycemia when used as monotherapy. Insulin receptor sensitivity is greatest in adipose tissue, skeletal muscle, and the liver. Pioglitazone and rosiglitazone increase the uptake of glucose in the liver and muscles. Pioglitazone also lowers free fatty acid and triglyceride levels, plasma glucose, insulin, and Hb_{A1c}. Pioglitazone and rosiglitazone are both administered orally. The time to reach peak plasma concentration is 1 hour for rosiglitazone and 2 hours for pioglitazone. Food doubles the time needed to reach the maximum concentration for pioglitazone but has no effect on rosiglitazone. Food does not reduce the bioavailability of either drug.

Adverse Reactions

The most common adverse reactions of therapy with pioglitazone and rosiglitazone are headache, weight gain, diarrhea, nausea, and vomiting. Serious side effects linked to pioglitazone and rosiglitazone are heart failure, heart attack, and liver failure. Patients should be instructed to report signs of muscle pain, jaundice, blurred vision, and signs of hypoglycemia or hyperglycemia.

Dipeptidyl Peptidase 4 Inhibitors

Alogliptin, linagliptin, saxagliptin, and sitagliptin are oral antidiabetic agents known as dipeptidyl peptidase 4 inhibitors. They are indicated for the treatment of type 2 diabetes. They increase insulin release and decrease glucagon levels by potentiating the activity of peptide hormones released in response to eating a meal. They decrease FPG, postprandial glucose, and Hb_{A1c} levels. The decrease in Hb_{A1c} levels is 0.5% to 1%, less than that produced by sulfonylureas and biguanides.

▪ Tech Note!

A common ending for DPP-4 inhibitors is *-gliptin.*

Mechanism of Action and Pharmacokinetics

DPP-4 is the enzyme responsible for the degradation of circulating GLP-1 and glucose-dependent insulinotropic peptide. These peptide hormones are key agents in glucose homeostasis. The action of the hormones is prolonged by DPP-4 inhibitors. DPP-4 inhibitors also increase β-cell responsiveness to glucose in the islets of Langerhans.

Oral absorption and bioavailability of DPP-4 inhibitors are good, and peak effects are reached 1 to 4 hours after administration. Sitagliptin and saxagliptin are primarily eliminated in the urine, so dosage adjustments may be required for individuals with kidney disease.

Adverse Reactions

The most common adverse reactions are intestinal upset, gas, heartburn, stomach pain, decreased appetite, metallic taste, and

Dipeptidyl Peptidase 4 Inhibitor

Generic Name	US Brand Name(s) Canadian Brand Name(s)	Dosage Forms and Strengths
alogliptin	Nesina Nesina	**Tablet:** 6.25 mg, 12.5 mg, 25 mg
linagliptin	Tradjenta Trajenta	**Tablet:** 5 mg
saxagliptin[a,b]	Onglyza Onglyza	**Tablet:** 2.5 mg, 5 mg
sitagliptin[a,b]	Januvia Januvia	**Tablet:** 25 mg, 50 mg, 100 mg
Combination Dipeptidyl Peptidase 4 Inhibitors		
alogliptin + metformin	Kazano Kazano	**Tablet:** alogliptin 12.5 mg + metformin 500 mg, alogliptin 12.5 mg + metformin 850 mg[b], alogliptin 12.5 mg + metformin 1000 mg
alogliptin + pioglitazone	Oseni Not available	**Tablet:** alogliptin 12.5 mg + pioglitazone 30 mg alogliptin 25 mg + pioglitazone 15 mg, alogliptin 25 mg + pioglitazone 30 mg, alogliptin 25 mg + pioglitazone 45 mg
linagliptin + metformin[a,c]	Jentadueto, Jentadueto XR Jentadueto	**Tablet:** linagliptin 2.5 mg + metformin 500 mg, linagliptin 2.5 mg + metformin 850 mg, linagliptin 2.5 mg + metformin 1000 mg **Tablet, extended release (Jentadueto XR):** linagliptin 2.5 mg + metformin 1000 mg, linagliptin 5 mg + metformin 1000 mg
saxagliptin + metformin	Kombiglyze XR Komboglyze	**Tablet (Komboglyze):** saxagliptin 2.5 mg + metformin 500 mg, saxagliptin 2.5 mg + metformin 850 mg, saxagliptin 2.5 mg + metformin 1000 mg **Tablet, extended release (Kombiglyze XR):** saxagliptin 2.5 mg + metformin 1000 mg, saxagliptin 5 mg + metformin 500 mg, saxagliptin 5 mg + metformin 1000 mg
sitagliptin + metformin[a,b]	Janumet, Janumet XR Janumet, Janumet XR	**Tablet:** sitagliptin 50 mg + metformin 500 mg sitagliptin 50 mg + metformin 850 mg[b] sitagliptin 50 mg + metformin 1000 mg **Tablet, extended release:** sitagliptin 50 mg + metformin 500 mg sitagliptin 50 mg + metformin 1000 mg sitagliptin 100 mg + metformin 1000 mg

[a]Generic available
[b]Available in Canada only.
[c]Available in the United States only.

stuffy or runny nose. Pancreatitis is a rare but serious adverse reaction associated with the use of sitagliptin. The drugs may cause hypoglycemia when used in combination with sulfonylureas.

Sodium-Glucose Cotransporter-2 Inhibitors

Canagliflozin, dapagliflozin, empagliflozin, and ertugliflozin are SGLT2 inhibitors used to treat type 2 diabetes. They increase urinary elimination of glucose, thereby reducing plasma glucose. They may be prescribed as monotherapy or in combination with other antidiabetic agents for adults with type 2 diabetes that is not well controlled. They lower Hb_{A1c} by approximately 0.5% to 1%.

Mechanism of Action and Pharmacokinetics

Glucose in the bloodstream is filtered by the kidney and then reabsorbed to be used by the body's cells. Sodium-glucose cotransporter inhibitors work by blocking the transporter proteins that are responsible for reabsorbing glucose (SGLT1 and SGLT2). SGLT2 is responsible for reabsorbing 90% of the glucose that is filtered by the kidneys. The SGLT2 inhibitors differ in selectivity for SGLT receptors. Empagliflozin has the greatest selectivity, and canagliflozin has the lowest selectivity. The drugs work best in patients who have normal kidney function.

Adverse Effects

Canagliflozin, dapagliflozin, or empagliflozin may increase urinary tract and genital infections. They promote weight loss, which is a beneficial side effect for treating obese patients. They may increase the risk for hypoglycemia if prescribed in combination with sulfonylureas (e.g., gliclazide and glyburide). They may also increase potassium levels.

> **● *Tech Note!***
>
> "gliflozin" is a common ending for sodium-glucose cotransporter-2 (SGLT2) inhibitors.

Sodium-Glucose Cotransporter-2 Inhibitors

Generic Name	US Brand Name(s) Canadian Brand Name(s)	Dosage Forms and Strengths
bexagliflozin	Brenzavvy Not available	**Tablet:** 20 mg
canagliflozin	Invokana Invokana	**Tablet:** 100 mg, 300 mg
dapagliflozin	Farxiga Forxiga	**Tablet:** 5 mg, 10 mg
empagliflozin[a]	Jardiance Jardiance	**Tablet:** 10 mg, 25 mg
ertugliflozin	Steglatro Not available	**Tablet:** 5 mg, 15 mg

Combination SGLT2 Inhibitors

Generic Name	US Brand Name(s) Canadian Brand Name(s)	Dosage Forms and Strengths
canagliflozin + metformin	Invokamet, Invokamet XR Invokamet	**Tablet:** canagliflozin 50 mg + metformin 500 mg, canagliflozin 50 mg + metformin 1000 mg, canagliflozin 150 mg + metformin 500 mg, canagliflozin 150 mg + metformin 1000 mg **Tablet, extended release:** canagliflozin 50 mg + metformin 500 mg, canagliflozin 50 mg + metformin 1000 mg, canagliflozin 150 mg + metformin 500 mg, canagliflozin 150 mg + metformin 1000 mg
dapagliflozin + metformin	Xigduo XR Xigduo	**Tablet (Xigduo):** dapagliflozin 5 mg + metformin 850 mg, dapagliflozin 5 mg + metformin 1000 mg **Tablet, extended release (Xigduo XR):** dapagliflozin 2.5 mg + metformin 1000 mg, dapagliflozin 5 mg + metformin 500 mg, dapagliflozin 5 mg + metformin 1000 mg, dapagliflozin 10 mg + metformin 500 mg, dapagliflozin 10 mg + metformin 1000 mg
dapagliflozin + saxagliptin	Qtern Not available	**Tablet:** dapagliflozin 10 mg + saxagliptin 5 mg
empagliflozin + metformin	Synjardy, Synjardy XR Synjardy	**Tablet:** empagliflozin 5 mg + metformin 500 mg, empagliflozin 5 mg + metformin 850 mg[b] empagliflozin 5 mg + metformin 1000 mg empagliflozin 12.5 mg + metformin 500 mg, empagliflozin 12.5 mg + metformin 850 mg[b] empagliflozin 12.5 mg + metformin 1000 mg **Tablet, extended release:** empagliflozin 5 mg + metformin 1000 mg, empagliflozin 10 mg + metformin 1000 mg, empagliflozin 12.5 mg + metformin 1000 mg, empagliflozin 25 mg + metformin 1000 mg

Sodium-Glucose Cotransporter-2 Inhibitors—cont'd

Generic Name	US Brand Name(s) Canadian Brand Name(s)	Dosage Forms and Strengths
empagliflozin + linagliptin	Glyxambi Glyxambi	**Tablet:** empagliflozin 10 mg + linagliptin 5 mg empagliflozin 25 mg + linagliptin 5 mg
empagliflozin + linagliptin + metformin	Trijardy XR Not available	**Tablet, extended release:** 5 mg empagliflozin + 2.5 mg linagliptin + 1000 mg metformin 10 mg empagliflozin + 5 mg linagliptin + 1000 mg metformin 12.5 mg empagliflozin + 2.5 mg linagliptin + 1000 mg metformin 25 mg empagliflozin + 5 mg linagliptin + 1000 mg metformin
ertugliflozin + sitagliptin	Steglujan Not available	**Tablet:** 5 mg ertugliflozin + 100 mg sitagliptin 15 mg ertugliflozin + 100 mg sitagliptin
ertugliflozin + metformin	Segluromet Not available	**Tablet:** 2.5 mg ertugliflozin + 500 mg metformin 2.5 mg ertugliflozin + 1000 mg metformin 7.5 mg ertugliflozin + 500 mg metformin 7.5 mg ertugliflozin + 1000 mg metformin

aGeneric available.
bAvailable in Canada only.

Glucagon-Like Peptide Receptor Agonists (Incretin Mimetics)

Dulaglutide, exenatide, lixisenatide, liraglutide, semaglutide, and tirzepatide are parenterally administered agents. GLP-1 receptor agonist drugs are administered as adjuncts to diet and exercise and may be administered only for type 2 diabetes mellitus. Exenatide is approved as monotherapy or in combination with other antidiabetic agents. Liraglutide is not approved as monotherapy. When GLP-1 receptor agonist and insulin therapy are prescribed, the drugs should be administered as separate doses.

Mechanism of Action and Pharmacokinetics

Dulaglutide, exenatide, lixisenatide, semaglutide, tirzepatide, and liraglutide stimulate GLP-1 receptors in the pancreatic α- and β-cells, stimulating insulin secretion when glucose levels are elevated. The α-cell stimulation suppresses glucagon release. GLP-1 receptor agonists also delay gastric emptying, slowing the rise of blood glucose levels after eating and decreasing appetite. GLP-1 receptor agonists are administered subcutaneously. They are formulated to be administered daily (liraglutide, lixisenatide, exenatide [Byetta]) or once weekly (dulaglutide, semaglutide, tirzepatide,

Glucagon-Like Peptide Receptor Agonists

Generic Name	US Brand Name(s) Canadian Brand Name(s)	Dosage Forms and Strengths
dulaglutide	Trulicity Trulicity	**Solution, for subcutaneous injection:** 0.75 mg/0.5 mL, 1.5 mg/0.5 mL
exenatide	Byetta, Bydureon BCISE Not available	**Solution, for injection (Byetta):** 250 mcg/mL **Suspension, for subcutaneous injection (extended release):** 2 mg/0.85 mL
liraglutide	Saxenda, Victoza Saxenda, Victoza	**Solution, for injection:** 18 mg/3 mL (6 mg/mL)
lixisenatide	Adlyxin Adlyxine	**Solution:** 0.05 mg/mL, 0.1 mg/mL
semaglutide	Ozempic, Rybelsus, Wegovy Ozempic, Rybelsus	**Solution, for subcutaneous injection:** 0.25 mg/0.5 mL, 0.5 mg/0.5 mL, 1 mg/0.5 mL, 1.7 mg/0.75 mL, 2 mg/1.5 mL, 2.4 mg/0.75 mL **Tablet (Rybelsus):** 3 mg, 7 mg, 14 mg
tirzepatide	Mounjaro Not available	**Solution, for subcutaneous injection:** 2.5 mg/0.5 mL, 5 mg/0.5 mg/mL, 7.5 mg/0.5 mL, 10 mg/0.5 mL, 12.5 mg/0.5 mL, 15 mg/0.5 mL

exenatide [Bydureon]). GLP-1 receptor agonists reduce Hb$_{A1c}$ levels by 0.5% to 1.7% depending on the specific agent.

Adverse Effects

Nausea is the most common side effect with exenatide and liraglutide, affecting up to 50% of patients. Gastrointestinal side effects are most common in the first month of therapy. Nausea associated with both drugs may be minimized by increasing the dose gradually. Other side effects include hypoglycemia; heartburn; itching, burning, swelling, or rash at the injection site; diarrhea or constipation; reduced appetite; and weight loss. Pancreatitis and thyroid-C cell tumors are rare but serious side effects of GLP-1 receptor agonists.

Amylin Analog

Pramlintide (Symlin) is a synthetic analog of the hormone amylin. Amylin levels are absent in type 1 diabetes and decreased in type 2 diabetes. Pramlintide is used with mealtime insulin to control blood sugar levels in people who have type 1 or 2 diabetes mellitus.

> **● Tech Note!**
>
> Pramlintide may cause hypoglycemia. The risk is greater during the first 3 hours after pramlintide is injected.

Mechanism of Action and Pharmacokinetics

Like amylin, pramlintide slows gastric emptying, reduces postprandial glucagon secretion, and reduces appetite. It should be injected subcutaneously immediately before each meal. The maximum concentration of pramlintide is reached within 20 minutes of administration, and the therapeutic effects last approximately 3 hours.

Adverse Reactions

Adverse reactions associated with pramlintide include hypoglycemia, loss of appetite, stomach pain, indigestion, upset stomach, excessive tiredness, dizziness, coughing, sore throat, joint pain, and redness, swelling, bruising, or itching at the injection site. Nausea and vomiting are dose dependent and may be reduced by gradually titrating the dose. This side effect decreases over time. To avoid lipodystrophy, patients should be advised to rotate the site of injection.

> **● Tech Note!**
>
> Rotate the site of injection to minimize risk of developing an increase or a decrease in fatty tissue under the skin at the injection site.

> **● Tech Note!**
>
> Do not mix pramlintide with any other injection, including insulin.

■ Amylin Analog

Generic Name	US Brand Name(s) — Canadian Brand Name(s)	Dosage Forms and Strengths
pramlintide	Symlin Not available	**Solution, for injection (pen cartridge):** 1.5 mg/1.5 mL, 2.7 mg/2.7 mL

Miscellaneous Agents

Colesevelam (Welchol) is a cholesterol-lowering agent approved by the US Food and Drug Administration for the management of type 2 diabetes. The mechanism of action for reducing FPG and Hb$_{A1c}$ levels is unknown. Bromocriptine (Cycloset) is a dopamine agonist that improves glycemic control; the mechanism of its effect on postprandial glucose levels is unknown. Both drugs are approved as an adjunct to diet and exercise. The most common side effects of colesevelam are heartburn and upset stomach. Nausea, drowsiness, and headache are side effects of bromocriptine.

■ Dopamine Agonist

Generic Name	US Brand Name(s) — Canadian Brand Name(s)	Dosage Forms and Strengths
bromocriptine	Cycloset Not available	**Tablet:** 0.8 mg

Management of Hypoglycemia

Some medicines used to treat diabetes cause hypoglycemia, especially when individuals increase exercise, do not eat regularly, or take other medicines that can also decrease blood sugar. Individuals experiencing symptoms of hypoglycemia may raise their blood sugar by consuming 3 or 4 glucose tablets or a tube of glucose gel; 1 tablespoon of sugar, honey, or corn syrup; 4 ounces (one-half cup) of juice or regular soda (not diet) or 8 ounces of nonfat or 1% milk; or several hard candies, jellybeans, or gumdrops. Severe hypoglycemia is treated by administering the hormone glucagon. It is administered by intravenous or intramuscular injection. Glucagon kits are available by prescription. The kit contains one vial with 1 mg of glucagon powder and a vial of diluent.

Complementary and Alternative Medicines and Diabetes

Six dietary supplements have been of particular interest in recent years as adjunct therapy for people with diabetes. They are α-lipoic acid (ALA), chromium, coenzyme Q10, garlic, magnesium, and omega-3 fatty acids. None has been extensively studied using randomized, double-blind studies. Of the six dietary supplements, ALA, magnesium, and omega-3 fatty acids have shown the most evidence of possible usefulness.

Alpha-Lipoic Acid

ALA is an antioxidant. Antioxidants prevent cell damage caused by oxidative stress from substances called free radicals. Elevated blood glucose levels can cause oxidative stress. ALA might lower the blood sugar level too much, so blood glucose levels must be monitored closely when it is used.

Magnesium

Magnesium is a mineral found in green leafy vegetables, nuts, seeds, and some whole grains. Magnesium levels are depressed in people with diabetes. Low magnesium levels may worsen glucose control in type 2 diabetes by interrupting insulin secretion and increasing insulin resistance.

Omega-3 Fatty Acids

Omega-3 fatty acids are naturally found in fish, fish oil, canola and soybean oils, walnuts, and wheat germ. Studies have shown that supplementation with omega-3 fatty acids can reduce the incidence of CVD and slow the progression of atherosclerosis. Omega-3 fatty acids have been of interest because diabetes increases the risk for developing CVD.

Garlic

Evidence about the value of garlic is mixed. It is believed that garlic may be involved in some biologic activities associated with type 2 diabetes, but the mechanism is not known.

TECHNICIAN'S CORNER

1. If your family has a history of type 2 diabetes, which lifestyle precautions should you take to reduce your risk for developing the disease?
2. What are some basic changes in diet that are recommended?

Summary of Drugs Used in the Treatment of Diabetes

	Generic Name	Brand Name	Usual Dose and Dosing Schedule	Warning Labels
Insulin				
	insulin	Afrezza, Apidra, Basaglar, Detemir, Entuzity, Fiasp, Humulin, Humalog, Lantus, Levemir, Myxredlin, Novolin, Novolog, Novolin GE Toronto, Ryzodeg, Tresiba	Individualized	STORE IN THE REFRIGERATOR; DO NOT FREEZE—all except Afrezza. USE AFREZZA CARTRIDGES ONLY WITH THE AFREZZA INHALER. DISCARD 14–15 DAYS AFTER FIRST USE—Afrezza cartridge, Soliqua.
	insulin/noninsulin combination	Soliqua, Xultophy		
Sulfonylureas				
	gliclazide	Diamicron, Diamicron MR 30 and MR 60	**Immediate-release** tabs: 80–160 mg twice daily (max 320 mg/day) **Extended-release** tabs: 30–120 mg once daily (max 120 mg/day)	AVOID PROLONGED EXPOSURE TO SUNLIGHT— glipizide, glimepiride. LIMIT OR AVOID ALCOHOL—all. TAKE 30 MINUTES BEFORE BREAKFAST—glipizide, glyburide. SWALLOW WHOLE; DO NOT CRUSH OR CHEW (SUSTAINED RELEASE). TAKE WITH A MEAL—gliclazide, glimepiride.
	glipizide	Glucotrol	5–40 mg daily in divided doses	
		Glucotrol XL	5–20 mg once daily	
	glyburide	Diabeta, Micronase	1.25–20 mg/day given in single or 2 divided doses	
		Glynase	0.75–12 mg/day, given in single or 2 divided doses	
	glimepiride	Amaryl	1–4 mg once daily (max 8 mg/day)	
Biguanides				
	metformin	Glucophage	**Maintenance:** 500–1000 mg twice daily or 850 mg PO 3 times daily (max 2000 mg/day)	TAKE WITH MEALS. SWALLOW WHOLE; DO NOT CRUSH OR CHEW—sustained release.
		Glumetza	1000 mg once or twice daily	
		Fortamet	500–1000 mg once daily	

Continued

Summary of Drugs Used in the Treatment of Diabetes—cont'd

	Generic Name	Brand Name	Usual Dose and Dosing Schedule	Warning Labels
Combination Biguanide + Sulfonylureas				
	metformin + glyburide	Generic	1 tablet (500 mg/2.5 mg or 500 mg/5 mg) twice daily	TAKE WITH MEALS.
	metformin + glipizide	Generic	1 tablet (500 mg/2.5 mg or 500/5 mg) twice daily	TAKE WITH MEALS.
α-Glucosidase Inhibitors				
	acarbose	Generic	25–100 mg 3 times a day	TAKE WITH THE FIRST BITE OF A MEAL.
	miglitol	Glyset	25–100 mg 3 times a day	
Dipeptidyl Peptidase 4 Inhibitors				
	alogliptin	Nesina	25 mg once daily	TAKE AT THE SAME TIME EACH DAY, WITH OR WITHOUT FOOD.
	linagliptin	Tradjenta	5 mg once daily	
	saxagliptin	Onglyza	2.5–5 mg once daily	
	sitagliptin	Januvia	100 mg once daily	
Combination Dipeptidyl Peptidase 4 Inhibitors				
	alogliptin + metformin	Kazano	1 tablet twice daily	TAKE WITH FOOD—all. SWALLOW WHOLE; DO NOT CRUSH OR CHEW—extended-release tabs.
	linagliptin + metformin	Jentadueto, Jentadueto XR	1 tablet twice daily 1 tablet once daily (XR tab)	
	saxagliptin + metformin	Kombiglyze XR, Komboglyze	1 tablet twice daily 1 tablet once daily (XR tab)	
	sitagliptin + metformin	Janumet, Janumet XR	1 tablet twice daily 1 tablet once daily (XR tab)	
Meglitinides				
	nateglinide	Starlix	60–120 mg 3 times a day	TAKE IMMEDIATELY BEFORE MEALS (SKIP DOSE IF THE MEAL IS MISSED). TAKE WITH A FULL GLASS OF WATER.
	repaglinide	Generic	1–4 mg before each meal, up to 4 times a day	
Thiazolidinediones				
	pioglitazone	Actos	15–45 mg once daily	LIMIT OR AVOID ALCOHOL. TAKE WITH A FULL GLASS OF WATER.
	rosiglitazone	Avandia	4–8 mg daily in single or divided doses	
Combination Thiazolidinediones				
	alogliptin + pioglitazone	Oseni	1 tablet once daily	TAKE WITH MEALS—all. LIMIT OR AVOID ALCOHOL—all. AVOID PROLONGED EXPOSURE TO SUNLIGHT— Metaglip, Glucovance.
	metformin + pioglitazone	Actoplus Met	1 tablet once or twice daily (max 2250 mg metformin + 45 mg pioglitazone/day)	
	pioglitazone + glimepiride	Duetact	1 tablet daily with first meal of the day	

Summary of Drugs Used in the Treatment of Diabetes—cont'd

Generic Name	Brand Name	Usual Dose and Dosing Schedule	Warning Labels
Glucagon-Like Peptide Receptor Agonist			
dulaglutide	Trulicity	Inject 0.75 mg–1.5 mg subcutaneously once weekly	REFRIGERATE; DO NOT FREEZE. DISCARD PEN UNIT 30 DAYS AFTER OPENING—Victoza, Byetta.
liraglutide	Victoza	Inject 0.6 mg subcutaneously once daily for 1 week, then increase to 1.2–1.8 mg subcutaneously once daily	INJECT 60 MINUTES BEFORE MORNING AND EVENING MEAL—Byetta. USE IMMEDIATELY AFTER RECONSTITUTION—Bydureon.
exenatide	Byetta	Initiate with 5 mcg subcutaneously twice daily, may increase to 10 mcg after 1 month	DO NOT USE DILUENT IF CLOUDY—Bydureon. INJECT 1 HOUR BEFORE FIRST MEAL OF THE DAY—Adlyxin.
	Bydureon	Inject 2 mg subcutaneously once every 7 days	TAKE 30 MINUTES BEFORE FIRST MEAL OF THE DAY—Rybelsus.
lixisenatide	Adlyxin	Inject 10–20 mcg once daily 1 hour before first meal of the day	SWALLOW WHOLE, DO NOT CRUSH OR CHEW—Rybelsus.
semaglutide	Ozempic, Rybelsus	Inject 0.25–1 mg subcutaneously once weekly **Tablet:** Take 3 mg once daily for 30 days; increase dose every 30 days up to 14 mg once daily	
tirzepatide	Mounjaro	Inject 2.5 mg subcutaneously once weekly; may increase dose every 4 weeks up to a maximum 15 mg once weekly	ROTATE SITE OF INJECTION.
Sodium-Glucose Cotransporter-2 (SGLT2) Inhibitors			
bexagliflozin	Brenzavvy	20 mg once daily	SWALLOW WHOLE, DO NOT CRUSH OR CHEW.
canagliflozin	Invokana	100–300 mg once daily	TAKE 1 HOUR BEFORE FIRST MEAL OF THE DAY—Invokana.
dapagliflozin	Farxiga, Forxiga	5–10 mg once daily in the morning	AVOID ALCOHOL
empagliflozin	Jardiance	10–25 mg once daily in the morning	TAKE WITH FOOD—Invokamet, Invokamet XR, Xigduo, Xigduo XR, Synjardy, Synjardy XR, Segluromet.
ertugliflozin	Steglatro	5–15 mg once daily	SWALLOW WHOLE, DO NOT CRUSH OR CHEW—extended-release tabs.
canagliflozin + metformin	Invokamet, Invokamet XR	1 tablet twice daily 1 tablet once daily (XR)	
dapagliflozin + metformin	Xigduo, Xigduo XR	1 tablet twice daily 1 tablet once daily (XR)	
dapagliflozin + saxagliptin	Qtern	1 tablet once daily in the morning	
empagliflozin + linagliptin + metformin	Trijardy XR	Take once daily with first meal of the day; maximum dose 25 mg empagliflozin + 5 mg linagliptin + 2 g metformin	
empagliflozin + metformin	Synjardy, Synjardy XR	1 tablet twice daily 1 tablet once daily (XR)	
ertugliflozin + metformin	Segluromet	1 tablet twice daily (maximum 15 mg ertugliflozin + 2000 mg metformin daily)	
empagliflozin + linagliptin	Glyxambi	1 tablet once daily in the morning	
ertugliflozin + sitagliptin	Steglujan	1 tablet once daily in the morning (maximum 15 mg ertugliflozin + 100 mg sitagliptin daily)	

Continued

Summary of Drugs Used in the Treatment of Diabetes—cont'd

	Generic Name	Brand Name	Usual Dose and Dosing Schedule	Warning Labels
	ertugliflozin + metformin	Segluromet	1 tablet twice daily	
Amylin Analog				
	pramlintide	Symlin	Inject 15–60 mcg before meals (type 1 diabetes) Inject 60–120 mcg before meals (type 2 diabetes)	REFRIGERATE; DO NOT FREEZE.
Dopamine Agonist				
	bromocriptine	Cycloset	1.6–4.8 mg once daily within 2 h after waking in the morning	TAKE WITH FOOD.

Key Points

- Diabetes mellitus is a disorder in which glucose accumulates in the blood.
- Insulin is released by the β-cells in the islets of Langerhans of the pancreas in response to the rise of blood glucose, amino acid, and gut-derived hormone levels.
- When glucose levels drop, glucagon is secreted by α-cells in the islets of Langerhans.
- Prediabetes causes impaired fasting glucose and impaired glucose tolerance.
- Type 1 diabetes is an autoimmune disease. The immune system attacks and destroys the insulin-producing β-cells in the pancreas.
- In type 1 diabetes, the body can no longer produce sufficient amounts of the hormone insulin.
- Type 2 diabetes is most common, accounting for 90% to 95% of all cases of diabetes.
- In type 2 diabetes, the pancreas usually produces sufficient amounts of insulin early in the disease, but the body is unable to use the insulin effectively.
- Gestational diabetes may be caused by the hormones of pregnancy or a shortage of insulin.
- Insulin resistance is a condition in which the body does not respond to insulin. It is a precursor to type 2 diabetes.
- The hemoglobin A1c (Hb_{A1c}) test provides information about blood glucose levels over a 2- to 3-month period.
- Individuals with type 1 or 2 diabetes can reduce risks for complications by weight loss, engaging in physical activity, consuming foods with a low glycemic index, quitting smoking, and other lifestyle changes.
- Insulin and insulin analogs are administered for the management of all types of diabetes.
- Insulin is formulated in rapid-acting, short-acting, intermediate-acting, and long-acting forms.

- Rapid-acting insulins are typically injected 5 to 15 minutes before eating.
- Rapid-acting insulin (aspart, glulisine, lispro), regular insulin, and long-acting insulin (detemir, glargine) are clear solutions that should be discarded if they appear cloudy.
- Sulfonylureas are also known as oral hypoglycemic agents. They are effective only for the treatment of type 2 diabetes because they stimulate insulin release from pancreatic β-cells.
- Metformin improves glucose tolerance and insulin resistance, lowers postprandial plasma glucose levels, decreases hepatic gluconeogenesis, and decreases the intestinal absorption of glucose.
- α-Glucosidase inhibitors (acarbose, miglitol) prolong the digestion of carbohydrates, delay their absorption in the small intestine, and are administered with the first bite of each meal.
- Meglitinides (nateglinide and repaglinide) stimulate insulin secretion from pancreatic β-cells, similar to sulfonylureas.
- Pioglitazone and rosiglitazone are insulin sensitizers that are used in the treatment of type 2 diabetes.
- Sitagliptin, saxagliptin, alogliptin, and linagliptin are dipeptidyl peptidase 4 inhibitors. They decrease fasting plasma glucose, postprandial glucose, and Hb_{A1c} levels.
- Exenatide, dulaglutide, lixisenatide, semaglutide, tirzepatide, and liraglutide are glucagon-like peptide receptor agonists.
- Colesevelam is a cholesterol-lowering agent that, along with diet and exercise, is approved for the treatment of type 2 diabetes.
- Bromocriptine is a dopamine agonist that, along with diet and exercise, is approved for the treatment of type 2 diabetes.
- α-Lipoic acid, magnesium, omega-3 fatty acids, and garlic are nutritional supplements that show some evidence of effectiveness for the treatment of diabetes mellitus.

Review Questions

1. The condition of elevated blood glucose levels is termed _____.
   a. hypoglycemia
   b. hyperglycemia
2. An autoimmune disease in which β-cells are destroyed and insufficient amounts of insulin are produced is _____.
   a. type 1 diabetes
   b. type 2 diabetes
   c. gestational diabetes
   d. all of the above
3. In diabetes, _____ accumulates in the blood.
   a. calcium
   b. glucose
   c. magnesium
   d. insulin
4. A hormone that is essential for the regulation of carbohydrate, fat, and protein metabolism is _____.
   a. aldosterone
   b. serotonin
   c. dopamine
   d. insulin
5. Type 2 diabetes is most common, accounting for 90% to 95% of all cases of diabetes.
   a. true
   b. false
6. Which insulin product is administered by inhalation?
   a. Afrezza
   b. Humulin N
   c. Humalog
   d. Soliqua
7. All of the following are recommendations for lifestyle changes to reduce the risk for diabetes mellitus EXCEPT_____.
   a. exercise 150 minutes week
   b. stop smoking
   c. limit alcohol
   d. eat carbohydrates
8. Insulin is administered only for the management of type 1 diabetes.
   a. true
   b. false
9. Januvia and Onglyza are examples of _____.
   a. sulfonylureas
   b. dipeptidyl peptidase 4 inhibitors
   c. thiazolidinediones
   d. nutritional supplements
10. Which of the following antidiabetic agents is administered by subcutaneous injection?
    a. Jardiance
    b. Glumetza
    c. Trulicity
    d. Januvia

Bibliography

Bilandzic A, Rosella L. The cost of diabetes in Canada over 10 years: applying attributable health care costs to a diabetes incidence prediction model. *Health Promot Chronic Dis Prev Can*. 2017;37(2):49–53.

Doyle-Delgado K, Chamberlain JJ, Shubrook JH, et al. Pharmacologic approaches to glycemic treatment of type 2 diabetes: synopsis of the 2020 American Diabetes Association's standards of medical care in diabetes clinical guideline. *Ann Intern Med*. 2020;173:813–821.

ElSayed NA, Aleppo G, Aroda VR, et al. Standards of care in diabetes—2023. *Diabetes Care*. 2022;46:S1–S4.

Garber AJ, Abrahamson MJ, Barzilay JI, et al. Consensus statement by the American Association of Clinical Endocrinologists and American College of Endocrinology on the comprehensive type 2 diabetes management algorithm—2017 executive summary. *Endocr Pract*. 2017;23(2):207–238. https://doi.org/10.4158/EP161682.CS.

Health Canada. (2022). Drug Product Database. Retrieved January 24, 2023, from https://health-products.canada.ca/dpd-bdpp/index-eng.jsp.

Jin S, Bajaj HS, Brazeau A-S, et al. Remission of type 2 diabetes: user's guide: Diabetes Canada clinical practice guidelines expert working group. *Can J Diabetes*. 2022;46:762–774.

Jude EB, Malecki MT, Gomez Huelgas R, et al. Expert panel guidance and narrative review of treatment simplification of complex insulin regimens to improve outcomes in type 2 diabetes. *Diabetes Ther*. 2022;13:619–634.

Kalant H, Grant D, Mitchell J. *Principles of medical pharmacology*. ed 7. Toronto: Elsevier Canada; 2007:635–642.

Kalra S. Sodium glucose co-transporter-2 (SGLT2) inhibitors: a review of their basic and clinical pharmacology. *Diabetes Ther*. 2014;5:355–366.

Mancini GBJ, O'Meara E, Zieroth S, et al. Canadian Cardiovascular Society guideline for use of GLP-1 receptor agonists and SGLT2 inhibitors for cardiorenal risk reduction in adults. *Can J Cardiol*. 2022;38:1153–1167. 2022.

Morrato E, Hill J, Wyatt H, et al. Physical activity in U.S. adults with diabetes and at risk for developing diabetes, 2003. *Diabetes Care*. 2007;30:203–209.

National Center for Complementary and Integrative Health. (2022). Type 2 Diabetes and Dietary Supplements. Retrieved January 24, 2023, from https://nccih.nih.gov/health/providers/digest/diabetes.

National Institute of Diabetes and Digestive and Kidney Diseases. (nd). Diabetes. Retrieved January 24, 2023, from https://www.niddk.nih.gov/health-information/diabetes.

National Institute of Diabetes and Digestive and Kidney Diseases. (2020). National Diabetes Statistics Report, 2020. Retrieved January 24, 2023, from https://www.niddk.nih.gov/health-information/health-statistics.

Page C, Curtis M, Sutter M, eds. *Integrated pharmacology*. Mosby: Philadelphia; 2006:293–299.

U.S. Food and Drug Administration. (nd). Drugs@FDA: FDA Approved Drug Products. Retrieved January 24, 2023, from http://www.accessdata.fda.gov/scripts/cder/daf/.

Williams DM, Jones H, Stephens JW. Personalized type 2 diabetes management: an update on recent advances and recommendations. *Diabetes Metab Syndr Obes*. 2022;15:281–295.

Drugs Affecting the Reproductive System

The human reproductive system undergoes change throughout its lifecycle. During puberty the male and female reproductive hormones surge, producing changes necessary for reproduction. The hypothalamus produces the hormones that signal the gonads (the testes in males and the ovaries in females) to produce the hormones testosterone, estrogen, and progesterone. These hormones stimulate sperm production, menstruation, ovulation, and secondary sexual characteristics such as facial hair, pubic hair, breast enlargement, and vaginal and uterine growth. Reproductive hormones decline with the onset of menopause in women, signaling changes that produce the symptoms of menopause (e.g., "hot flashes"), the cessation of ovarian function, and the end of reproduction capacity.

In Unit IX, diseases of the reproductive system including amenorrhea, infertility, endometriosis, premenstrual syndrome, abnormal uterine bleeding, prostate disease, and erectile dysfunction are covered. This unit also provides information about contraception and emergency contraception. A description of the drug indication, mechanism of action, adverse reactions, strength(s), and dosage forms is provided. It is important for pharmacy technicians to know about prescription and OTC agents that affect the reproductive system.

27

Drugs That Affect the Reproductive System

LEARNING OBJECTIVES

1. Learn the terminology associated with the reproductive system.
2. Describe the pathophysiology of reproductive system disorders.
3. Describe the physiology of pregnancy and methods of pregnancy prevention.
4. List and categorize medications that affect the reproductive system.
5. Describe the mechanism of action for each class of drugs that affects the reproductive system.
6. Identify significant drug look-alike and sound-alike issues.
7. List common endings for drug classes that affect the reproductive system.
8. Identify warning labels and precautionary messages associated with medications that affect the reproductive system.
9. Identify over-the-counter contraceptive methods.

KEY TERMS

Abnormal uterine bleeding Irregular or excessive uterine bleeding that results from a structural problem or hormonal imbalance.
Amenorrhea Absence of normal menstruation.
Atrophic vaginitis Postmenopausal thinning and dryness of the vaginal epithelium related to decreased estrogen levels.
Dysmenorrhea Difficult or painful menstruation.
Endometriosis Presence of functioning endometrial tissue outside the uterus.
Hypogonadism Inadequate production of sex hormones.
Hysterectomy Surgical removal of the uterus.
Infertility Inability to achieve pregnancy during 1 year or more of unprotected intercourse.
Menopause Termination of menstrual cycles; an event usually marked by the passage of at least 1 full year without menstruation.

Menorrhagia Excessive menstrual bleeding.
Pelvic inflammatory disease Infection of the uterus, fallopian tubes, and adjacent pelvic structures that is not associated with pregnancy or surgery.
Polycystic ovary disease Condition characterized by ovaries twice the normal size that contain fluid-filled cysts.
Premenstrual dysphoric disorder A condition associated with menstruation that is characterized by symptoms such as depression, anxiety, hopelessness, sad feelings, and self-deprecation.
Premenstrual syndrome Condition involving a set of symptoms (headache, irritability, depression, fatigue, sleep changes, weight gain) that occur before the start of the menstrual cycle.
Supraovulation Simultaneous rupture of multiple mature follicles.
Toxic shock syndrome Rare disorder caused by certain *Staphylococcus aureus* strains that occurs in women using tampons.

Overview

More than 72.7 million US women and 19 million Canadian women are of reproductive age (15–44 years). To prevent unintended pregnancy, nearly 65% of all women of reproductive age in the United States and Canada are using some contraceptive method.

Contraception: Prevention of Pregnancy

A variety of methods exist to prevent pregnancy. They are mechanical or barrier methods, hormonal methods, intrauterine devices (IUDs), abstinence, and emergency contraception (EC).

Mechanical and Barrier Methods of Contraception

Condoms, diaphragm, cervical cap, vaginal sponge, and spermicide (e.g., foams, jellies, creams) are mechanical barrier methods for contraception. They act to kill sperm or block sperm from entering the uterus.

A condom is a device, usually made of latex or polyurethane, which is placed on a man's erect penis before sexual intercourse to block ejaculated semen from physically entering the body of the sexual partner. Female condoms are placed in the vagina. Condoms are used to prevent pregnancy and transmission of sexually transmitted infections (STIs) such as gonorrhea, syphilis, and HIV. Condoms used with a spermicide provide greater protection.

Diaphragms

The diaphragm is a dome-shaped cup made of latex or silicone. The spring-molded rim creates a seal against the wall of the vagina. The rim of the diaphragm is squeezed into an arc shape for insertion. A water-based lubricant (usually spermicide) may be applied to the rim of the diaphragm to aid insertion. One teaspoonful (5 mL) of spermicide is placed in the dome of the diaphragm before insertion or with an applicator after insertion. The diaphragm must be inserted some time before sexual intercourse and remain in the vagina for 6 to 8 hours after a male's last ejaculation. The diaphragm must be removed for cleaning with warm soapy water at least once every 24 hours. The Omniflex diaphragm should be refitted after a weight change of 4.5 kg (10 lb) or more or after any pregnancy. The Caya diaphragm is described as one size fits most. In the United States, diaphragms are available by prescription only. Caya may be purchased without a prescription in Canada. Diaphragms are nonprescription in many countries globally.

Adverse Reactions

Diaphragms are associated with an increased risk of urinary tract infection. *Toxic shock syndrome* (TSS) occurs at a rate of 2.4 cases per 100,000 women using diaphragms, almost exclusively when the device is left in place longer than 24 hours.

Types of Diaphragms

Generic Name	US Brand Name(s) — Canadian Brand Name(s)	OTC/Prescription
diaphragm	Caya, Omniflex (50–105 mm)	Prescription (Omniflex) OTC (Caya)
	Caya Contoured Diaphragm (one size)	

OTC, Over the counter.

Cervical Cap, Contraceptive Sponge, and Vaginal Contraceptive Film

The cervical cap is placed over the cervix opening and is the size of a thimble. It is used with spermicide and has a 9% to 16% failure rate in women who have not previously been pregnant and is even less effective in women who have given birth. The cervical cap is a reusable silicone cup placed over the cervix and held in place by a one-way suction valve. It is also used with spermicide. It comes in one size and does not need to be specifically fitted to each woman. It is available by prescription in the United States, although it is obtainable over the counter in Europe and Canada. The contraceptive sponge (Today Sponge) is used with spermicide and has a 9% to 28% failure rate. It provides protection immediately after insertion and should remain inserted for 6 hours after intercourse. The vaginal contraceptive film (VCF) is a thin film that is impregnated with the spermicide nonoxynol-9. It is placed over the cervix 15 minutes before intercourse. The failure rate for VCF is approximately 6%.

Cervical Contraceptive Devices

Generic Name	US Brand Name(s) — Canadian Brand Name(s)	OTC/Prescription
cervical cap	FemCap	Prescription (US) OTC (Canada)
	FemCap	
cervical sponge	Today Sponge	OTC
	Today Sponge	
contraceptive film	VCF	OTC
	VCF	

OTC, Over the counter; *VCF*, vaginal contraceptive film.

Intrauterine Device

An IUD is a contraceptive device that is placed in the uterus and is the most widely used long-acting reversible birth control method globally. The device has to be inserted or removed from the uterus by a physician or qualified medical practitioner. Depending on the type, a single IUD is approved for 5 to 10 years of use. The IUD is more than 99% effective. There are two broad categories: copper-releasing and hormone-releasing IUDs. Levonorgestrel, a progestin, is released from hormone-releasing IUDs. In addition to contraception, levonorgestrel reduces menstrual bleeding, making it useful for the treatment of *menorrhagia* (heavy periods).

Mechanism of Action. The presence of an object in the uterus prompts the release of leukocytes and prostaglandins by the endometrium. These substances are hostile to sperm and eggs; the presence of the copper prevents the sperm from reaching the egg and the egg from attaching to the uterus. Progestin-releasing IUDs prevent ovulation and thicken cervical mucus, thus preventing the sperm from reaching the egg. IUDs do not protect against STIs, and their use is contraindicated in women with *pelvic inflammatory disease* (PID) or who are pregnant.

Intrauterine Devices

Generic Name	US Brand Name(s) — Canadian Brand Name(s)	Strength
copper-releasing T-shaped	ParaGard T 380 A	Copper: 380 mm^2
	Flex-T 300, Flex-T 380, Liberte TT, Liberte UT, Mona Lisa 5 NT, Mona Lisa 5 mini, Mona Lisa 10	Copper: 300 mm^2 (Flex-T 300, Mona Lisa N), 380 mm^2 (Liberte TT, Liberte UT, Flex-t 380, Mona Lisa 5, Mona Lisa Mini, Mona Lisa 10)
levonorgestrel-releasing	Liletta, Kyleena, Mirena, Skyla	Levonorgestrel-releasing IUD: 13.5 mg (Skyla), 19.5 mg (Kyleena), 52 mg (Liletta, Mirena)
	Kyleena, Mirena	

Adverse Reaction. Insertion of an IUD may introduce bacteria into the uterus. The insertion carries a small transient risk of PID in the first 20 days after insertion. If pregnancy does occur, presence of the IUD increases the risk of miscarriage, particularly during the second trimester.

Hormonal Methods of Contraception

Oral contraceptives (OCs), hormone-impregnated vaginal inserts, hormone injections, skin patches, surgical implants, and some IUDs are hormone dosage delivery systems marketed for contraception.

Oral Contraceptives

OCs have been collectively called the pill. Numerous OC products are available containing estrogen and progestin combinations, as well as progestin-only pills (Table 27.1). The pill can be used to regulate menstruation and prevent pregnancy. If used correctly and consistently, the pill is an extremely effective contraceptive, with an unintended pregnancy rate estimated at between 0.1% and 3%. In real life, the pill is approximately 91% effective.

Mechanism of Action. Hormonal contraceptives prevent pregnancy by initiating negative feedback inhibition of follicle-stimulating hormone (FSH) and luteinizing hormone (LH) secretion. As a result, mature follicles do not develop, and LH does not reach the level required to initiate ovulation. Menses takes place during the week with non-drug-containing pills (28-day cycle) or when the pill is stopped (21-day cycle). When the progestin and estrogen levels fall, as they normally do near the end of the cycle, menstruation occurs.

Adverse Reactions. Common side effects are breast tenderness and changes in menstrual pattern. Smoking increases the risk

of adverse reactions, including increased risk of thromboembolic events and heart attacks. Loss of appetite and constipation can also occur. Women taking OCs should immediately report shortness of breath, sudden loss of vision, unresolved leg or foot swelling, weight gain (>5 lb [2.3 kg]), breast tenderness that does not go away, acute abdominal cramping, signs of vaginal infection, changes in mood, or pain, muscle soreness, heat, or redness in calves.

Other Hormone-Releasing Contraceptive Dosage Forms

Etonogestrel (Nexplanon) and medroxyprogesterone (Depo-Provera) are progestins. They prevent pregnancy by preventing ovulation, thickening cervical mucus to inhibit the passage of sperm, and maintaining the endometrium. Depo-Provera is administered by injection, once every 3 months. Etonogestrel (Nexplanon) is

TABLE 27.1	Oral Contraceptives
Estrogen-Progestin Combination	**Description**
Monophasic	Provides a fixed dose of estrogen and progestin throughout cycle of 21- or 28-day package
Biphasic	Amount of estrogen remains the same throughout cycle; less progestin in first half of cycle, increased progestin in second half of cycle
Triphasic	Amount of estrogen is the same or varies throughout cycle; progestin amount varies

Oral Contraceptives

Generic Name	US Brand Name(s) Canadian Brand Name(s)	Dosage Forms and Strengths
Estrogen and Progestin Combinations		
estetrol + drospirenone	Nextstellis	**Tablet:** estetrol 14.2 mg + drospirenone 3 mg
	Nextstellis	
ethinyl estradiol + desogestrel[a]	Bekyree, Cyclessa, Enskyce, Isibloom, Kalliga, Kariva, Kimidess, Pimtrea, Simliya, Velivet, Viorele, Volnea	**Tablet, monophasic:** 21 days ethinyl estradiol 0.03 mg + desogestrel 0.15 mg (Apri, Freya, Marvelon, Mirvala) **Tablet, biphasic (Kariva):** 21 days ethinyl estradiol 0.02 mg + desogestrel 0.15 mg; 5 days ethinyl estradiol 0.01 mg
	Apri, Freya, Linessa, Marvelon, Mirvala	**Tablet, triphasic (Cyclessa, Linessa, Velivet):** 7 days ethinyl estradiol 0.025 mg + desogestrel 0.125 mg; 7 days ethinyl estradiol 0.025 mg + desogestrel 0.15 mg; 7 days ethinyl estradiol 0.025 mg + desogestrel 0.1 mg
ethinyl estradiol + drospirenone[a]	Angeliq, Loryna, Lo-Zumandimine, Melamisa, Nikki, Syeda, Yaela, Yasmin, Yaz, Zumandimine	**Tablet, monophasic:** ethinyl estradiol 0.02 mg + drospirenone 3 mg ethinyl estradiol 0.03 mg + drospirenone 3 mg (Zamine, Zarah)
	Angeliq, Mya, Yasmin, Yaz, Zamine, Zarah	
ethinyl estradiol + drospirenone + levomefolate[a]	Beyaz, Safyral, Tydemy	**Tablet, monophasic:** 24 days ethinyl estradiol 0.02 mg + drospirenone 3 mg + levomefolate 0.451 mg; 4 days levomefolate 0.451 mg
	Yaz Plus	

Oral Contraceptives—cont'd

Generic Name	US Brand Name(s) Canadian Brand Name(s)	Dosage Forms and Strengths
ethinyl estradiol + ethynodiol[a]	Kelnor, Lo-Malmorede, Malmorede, Zovia 1+ 50 E Not available	**Tablet, monophasic**: ethinyl estradiol 0.035 mg + ethynodiol 1 mg (Kelnor, Lo-Malmorede) ethinyl estradiol 0.05 mg + ethynodiol 1 mg (Malmorede, Zovia 1 + 50)
ethinyl estradiol + levonorgestrel[a]	Afirmelle, Altavera, Ashlyna, Aviane, Ayuna, Balcoltra, Daysee, Dolishale, Enpresse, Falmina, Iclevia, Introvale, Jaimiess, Kurvelo, Lessina, Levonest, Levora, Lo-Seasonique, Lo-Simpesse, Marlissa, Myzilra, Portia, Quartette, Quasense, Seasonale, Seasonique, Setlakin, Simpesse, Trivora, Tyblume, Vienva Alesse, Alysena, Aviane, Indayo, Min-Ovral, Ovima, Portia, Seasonale, Seasonique, Triquilar	**Tablet, monophasic:** ethinyl estradiol 0.03 mg + levonorgestrel 0.15 mg (Altavera, Ayuna, Indayo, Kurvelo, Levora, Min-Ovral, Nordette, Ovima, Portia) ethinyl estradiol 0.02 mg + levonorgestrel 0.1 mg (Afirmelle, Alesse, Alysena, Aviane, Balcoltra, Esme, Lessina) **Tablet, triphasic:** 6 days ethinyl estradiol 0.03 mg + levonorgestrel 0.05 mg; 10 days ethinyl estradiol 0.03 mg + levonorgestrel 0.125 mg; 5 days ethinyl estradiol 0.04 mg + levonorgestrel 0.75 mg (Enpresse, Triquilar, Trivora) **Tablet, 84-day extended cycle (Introvale, Seasonale):** 84 days each—ethinyl estradiol 0.03 mg + levonorgestrel 0.15 mg **Tablet, 84-day biphasic cycle (Lo-Seasonique, Seasonique):** 7 days ethinyl estradiol 0.01 mg; 84 days ethinyl estradiol 0.02 mg + levonorgestrel 0.1 mg
ethinyl estradiol + norethindrone[a] (selected products)	Alyacen, Amabelz, Aranelle, Aurovela, Balziva, Blisovi, Briellyn, Dasetta, Finzala, Gemmily, Hailey, Junel 1/20, Kaitlib, Larin 1/20, Merzee, Nortrel 7/7/7, Nylia, Philith, Rhuzdah, Taytulla, Tri-Norinyl, Vyfemla, Wera Brevicon 0.5/35, Brevicon 1/35, Lolo, Minestrin 1/20, Select 1/35, Synphasic	**Capsule:** ethinyl estradiol 0.02 mg + norethindrone 1 mg (Gemmily, Merzee, Taytulla) **Tablet, chewable:** ethinyl estradiol 0.025 mg + norethindrone 0.8 mg (Kaitlib) **Tablet, monophasic:** ethinyl estradiol 0.035 mg + norethindrone 0.4 mg (Balziva, Briellyn) ethinyl estradiol 0.035 mg + norethindrone 0.5 mg (Brevicon 0.5/35) ethinyl estradiol 0.035 mg + norethindrone 1 mg (Brevicon 1/ 35) ethinyl estradiol 0.03 mg + norethindrone 1.5 mg (Aurovela 1.5/30) ethinyl estradiol 0.02 mg + norethindrone 1 mg (Aurovela 1/20, Minestrin 1/20) **Tablet, biphasic:** 12 days ethinyl estradiol 0.035 mg + norethindrone, 0.5 mg; 9 days ethinyl estradiol 0.035 mg + norethindrone 1 mg (Aranelle, Synphasic, Tri-Norinyl) 10 days ethinyl estradiol 0.035 mg + norethindrone, 0.5 mg; 11 days ethinyl estradiol 0.035 mg + norethindrone 1 mg (generic) **Tablet, triphasic (Nortrel 7/7/7):** 7 days each—ethinyl estradiol 0.035 mg + norethindrone, 0.5 mg; 7 days each—ethinyl estradiol 0.035 mg + norethindrone 0.75 mg, 7 days each—ethinyl estradiol 0.035 mg + norethindrone 1 mg
ethinyl estradiol + norgestimate[a]	Estarylla, Mili, Mono-Linyah, Ortho-Cyclen, Ortho Tri-Cyclen-28, Previfem, Sprintec, Tri-Estarylla, Tri-Lo Estarylla, Tri-Lo-Mili, Tri-Mili, Tri-Sprintec, Tri-Lo-Sprintec, Tri-Linyah, Tri-lo-Linayh Tri-Cira, Tri-Cira Lo, Tri-Jordyna	**Tablet, monophasic (Cyclen, Ortho-Cyclen, Sprintec):** ethinyl estradiol 0.035 mg + norgestimate 0.25 mg **Triphasic formulation:** 7 days each—ethinyl estradiol 0.035 mg + norgestimate 0.18 mg; 7 days each—ethinyl estradiol 0.035 mg + norgestimate 0.215 mg; 7 days each—ethinyl estradiol 0.035 mg + norgestimate 0.25 mg (Tri-Cira, Tri-Jordyna, Tri-Sprintec) 7 days each—ethinyl estradiol 0.025 mg + norgestimate 0.18 mg; 7 days each—ethinyl estradiol 0.025 mg + norgestimate 0.215 mg; 7 days each—ethinyl estradiol 0.025 mg + norgestimate 0.25 mg (Tri-Cira Lo, Tri-Lo-Sprintec)

Progestins

norethindrone[a] norethindrone acetate[a]	Camila, Emzahh, Errin, Heather, Incassia, Jencycla, Nor QD Jencycla, Maeve, Movisse, Norlutate	**Tablet:** 0.35 mg, 5 mg[b] (Norlutate)

[a]Generic available.
[b]Strength not used for contraception; used for amenorrhea, abnormal uterine bleeding, and endometriosis.

formulated as a microsized rod, the size of a matchstick, that is surgically implanted. The medroxyprogesterone injection is 94% effective and the birth control implant is 99% effective at preventing pregnancy. Once inserted, Nexplanon prevents pregnancy for up to 4 years. Onsura and Xulane are transdermal patches containing a combination of estrogen and progestin. A single patch is applied each week for 3 weeks, followed by 1 patch-free week. Each patch should be applied on the same day each week, and only one patch should be worn at a time. No more than 7 days should pass during the patch-free interval. An advantage over other methods of contraception is that it is a weekly dose, noninvasive, and easy to use. The contraceptive patch is 91% effective in preventing pregnancy. Disadvantages are that the patch can become partially or completely detached and can irritate the skin.

NuvaRing is a hormonal vaginal ring inserted for 3 weeks and then removed for 1 week. A new ring is inserted 7 days after the last one was removed and should be inserted the same time as the insertion of the previous ring. Advantages are that it is easy to use and is a once-monthly dosing. Although rare, it is possible for the ring to slip outside the vagina; if this occurs, it must be replaced within 3 hours. The contraceptive ring is 91% effective in preventing pregnancy.

Adverse Reactions. Depo-Provera and Nexplanon may cause irritation, redness, or pain at the site of administration. Patients may also experience dizziness, weight gain, leg cramps or joint pain, lower sex drive, hot flashes, increased body hair (reversible when drug is discontinued), and loss of bone mineral density (prolonged use). Rarely, the Nexplanon is rejected by the body. The most common side effects for the birth control patches (Evra, Xulane) and birth control ring (NuvaRing) are breast tenderness, weight gain, changes in appetite, and vaginal infection. Smoking increases the risk of thromboembolic events, stroke, and heart attacks.

Emergency Contraception

ECs reduce the risk of pregnancy after unprotected intercourse. Levonorgestrel (various brands) is approximately 75% to 85% effective when taken as soon as possible after unprotected intercourse. It is most effective if taken within the first 72 hours after

Miscellaneous Contraceptive Dosage Forms

Generic Name	US Brand Name(s) / Canadian Brand Name(s)	Dosage Forms and Strengths
ethinyl estradiol + etonogestrel[a]	Eluryng, Haloette NuvaRing	**Intravaginal ring:** ethinyl estradiol 15 mcg/24 h + etonogestrel 120 mcg/24 h
	Haloette, NuvaRing	
ethinyl estradiol + levonorgestrel	Twirla	**Patch, weekly:** cthinyl estradiol 30 mcg + levonorgestrel 120 mcg/24 h
	Not available	
ethinyl estradiol + norelgestromin	Onsura, Xulane	**Patch, weekly:** ethinyl estradiol 35 mcg/24 h + norelgestromin 200 mcg/24 h (Evra) ethinyl estradiol 35 mcg/24 h + norelgestromin 150 mcg/24 h (Onsura, Xulane)
	Evra	
ethinyl estradiol + segesterone acetate	Annovera	**Intravaginal ring:** ethinyl estradiol 13 mcg/24 h + segesterone acetate 150 mcg/24 h
	Not available	
etonogestrel	Nexplanon	**Implantable rod:** etonogestrel 68 mg
	Nexplanon	
medroxyprogesterone[a]	Depo-Provera, Depo-subQ Provera 104	**Injection:** 104 mg/0.65 mL (Depo-SubQ Provera 104) 150 mg/mL (Depo-Provera)
	Depo-Provera	

[a]Generic available.

Emergency Contraceptives

Generic Name	US Brand Name(s) / Canadian Brand Name(s)	Dosage Forms and Strengths	OTC/Prescription Status
levonorgestrel[a]	Athentia Next, Fallback Solo, Her Style, Opcicon One Step, Plan B One-Step	**Tablet:** 1.5 mg	OTC
	Backup Plan Onestep, Contingency One, Plan B		
ulipristal	Ella, Logilia	**Tablet:** 30 mg	Prescription
	Ella		

[a]Generic available.

unprotected sexual intercourse. Levonorgestrel 1.5 mg is taken as a single dose. Ulipristal (Ella) is effective if taken within 5 days of unprotected intercourse. Ulipristal is a selective progesterone receptor modulator that delays ovulation and prevents implantation of a fertilized egg. EC may be used at any time during the menstrual cycle. If conception has already occurred, EC will not terminate pregnancy. EC use is contraindicated in pregnancy or suspected pregnancy. The most common side effects are nausea, headache, and abdominal pain.

The emergency insertion of a copper IUD also is highly effective, reducing the risk of pregnancy by as much as 99%.

Other Methods of Contraception

Surgical methods such as tubal ligation and male vasectomy result in permanent sterility. Behavioral methods involve abstaining from sexual intercourse for a specified number of days before, during, and after ovulation. The rhythm method is a natural method based on calculating the fertile period by the use of a calendar, on which the supposed infertile days are marked. The ovulation method includes keeping a temperature chart to detect a minute change in temperature at the time of ovulation or determining the time of ovulation by observing changes in cervical mucus.

Pregnancy Termination

Oral contraceptives, intrauterine devices, barrier birth control methods, and other pregnancy prevention methods are not 100% effective. Unintended pregnancy may result. When an unplanned pregnancy occurs, the decision to continue the pregnancy or consider options to obtain a safe, legal medical or surgical abortion is a deeply personal decision that can be made by the woman in Canada. In the United States, however, some states have restricted women's choices by passing legislation to ban or limit abortion. In both Canada and the United States, a medical abortion can be induced by the administration of the progestin antagonist mifepristone. The combination of mifepristone and misoprostol is taken. It is indicated only in early pregnancy, fewer than 70 days (10 weeks) since the woman's last menstrual period however federal regulation may influence if or when the drugs may be administered. Oral absorption of mifepristone is 69%. The drug is 98% protein bound and elimination is slow (only 83% is eliminated 11 days after administration). In the United States, mifepristone may be obtained only at certified pharmacies, and the patient must sign a patient agreement form as part of the U.S. Food and Drug Administration's Risk Evaluation and Mitigation Strategy requirements. The most common adverse reactions are heavy vaginal bleeding and cramping or abdominal pain. Dizziness and headache are additional side effects.

Menopause and Atrophic Vaginitis

Menopause is the termination of the menstrual cycle and is usually marked by the passage of at least 1 full year without menstruation. Natural menopause will occur in 25% of women by age 47, 50% by age 50, 75% by age 52, and 95% by age 55 years. Menopause caused by surgical removal of the ovaries *(hysterectomy)* occurs in almost 30% of US women who are 50 years or older.

Symptoms of menopause may last from a few months to years and vary from hardly noticeable to severe. Symptoms include mood changes, hot flashes (flushes), chills, fatigue, insomnia, palpitation, vertigo, headache, myalgia, urinary disturbances (e.g., incontinence), atrophic vaginitis, and various disorders of the gastrointestinal system. The long-range effects of lower estrogen levels are osteoporosis and atherosclerosis.

Atrophic vaginitis is the postmenopausal thinning and dryness of the vaginal epithelium related to decreased estrogen levels. Symptoms include burning and pain during intercourse. Hormone replacement therapy (HRT) or application of topical estrogen restores the integrity of the vaginal epithelium and relieves symptoms.

Hormone Replacement Therapy

HRT is prescribed to treat symptoms of menopause, such as hot flashes, vaginal dryness, mood swings, sleep disorders, and decreased sexual desire. HRT contains one or more female hormones, commonly estrogen plus progestin. Estrogen-only therapy is usually reserved for women who have had their uterus removed. It typically involves the administration of oral or vaginal estrogens, with or without progestins. The medication may be taken in the form of a pill, patch, or vaginal cream. The dosage form may vary according to the symptoms to be treated. For example, a vaginal cream can ease vaginal dryness but does not relieve hot flashes. Treatment protocols vary according to whether the woman has a uterus or has had a hysterectomy.

The Women's Health Initiative (WHI) HRT study (2002) showed that HRT increased the risk of developing breast cancer, heart attacks, strokes, and blood clots. The estrogen-progestin study showed that there was a 26% increase in the incidence of breast cancer, and the estrogen-only therapy study in women who no longer had a uterus showed that stroke risk was increased.

> **❗ Tech Alert!**
>
> The following drugs have look-alike/sound-alike issues:
> FemHRT and Femara;
> Alora and Aldara;
> Premphase and Prempro

Pregnancy Termination

Generic Name	US Brand Name(s) / Canadian Brand Name(s)	Dosage Forms and Strengths
mifepristone[a]	Mifeprex	**Tablet:** 200 mg
	Not available	
Combination Mifepristone		
mifepristone + misoprostol	Not available	**Tablet:** mifepristone 200 mg + misoprostol 200 mcg
	Mifegymiso	

[a]Generic available.

Hormone Replacement Therapy

Generic Name	US Brand Name(s) Canadian Brand Name(s)	Dosage Forms and Strengths
Estrogen		
conjugated estrogens	Premarin Premarin	**Vaginal cream**: 0.625 mg/g **Powder, for injection**: 25 mg/vial **Tablet**: 0.3 mg, 0.45 mg[b], 0.625 mg, 0.9 mg[b], 1.25 mg
estradiol[a]	Alora, Climara, Depo-Estradiol, Delestrogen, Divigel, Elestrin, Estrace, Estrogel, Evamist, Femring, Imvexxy, Menostar, Minivelle, Vagifem, Vivelle, Vivelle Dot Climara, Divigel, Estrace, Estraderm, Estra Dot, Estring, Estrogel, Oesclim, Vagifem	**Gel, topical**: 0.1% (Divigel), 0.06% (Elestrin, Estrogel) **Solution, for injection, as cypionate (Depo-Estradiol)**: 5 mg/mL **Solution, for injection, as valerate (Delestrogen)**: 10 mg/mL, 20 mg/mL, 40 mg/mL **Spray, topical (Evamist)**: 1.53 mg/spray **Tablet**: 0.5 mg, 1 mg, 2 mg **Transdermal patch, biweekly (Alora, Estraderm, Estradot, Minivelle, Oesclim, Vivelle, Vivelle dot)**: 0.025 mg/24 h, 0.0375 mg/24 h, 0.05 mg/24 h, 0.075 mg/24 h, 0.1 mg/24 h **Transdermal patch, weekly (Climara, Menostar)**: 0.014 mg/24 h, 0.025 mg/24 h, 0.0375 mg/24 h, 0.05 mg/24 h, 0.06 mg/24 h, 0.075 mg/24 h, 0.1 mg/24 h **Vaginal cream (Estrace)[b]**: 0.01% **Vaginal ring**: 0.5 mg/24 h, 0.1 mg/24 h (Femring); 2 mg (Estring) **Vaginal insert (Imvexxy)**: 4 mcg, 10 mcg **Vaginal tablet (Vagifem)**: 10 mcg/tablet
estrogen (esterified)	Menest Not available	**Tablet**: 0.3 mg, 0.625 mg, 1.25 mg, 2.5 mg
estropipate	Ogen 5 Not available	**Tablet**: 6 mg
Estrogen and Progestin Combinations		
estradiol + levonorgestrel	Climara Pro Not available	**Transdermal patch, weekly**: 0.45 mg/24 h estradiol + 0.15 mg/24 h levonorgestrel
estradiol + norethindrone[a]	Activella, Combipatch Activelle, Activelle LD, Estalis	**Tablet**: 0.5 mg estradiol + 0.1 mg norethindrone (Activella LD); 1 mg estradiol + 0.5 mg norethindrone (Activella, Activelle) **Transdermal patch, biweekly**: 0.05 mg/24 h estradiol + 0.14 mg/h norethindrone (Combipatch 50/140, Estalis 50/140); 0.05 mg/h estradiol + 0.25 mg/h norethindrone (Combipatch 50/250, Estalis 50/250)
estradiol + norgestimate	Generic Not available	**Tablet**: estradiol 1 mg + norgestimate 0.09 mg
conjugated estrogens + medroxypro- gesterone	Prempro, Premphase 14/14, Prempro/Premphase Not available	**Tablet (Premphase 14/14)**: conjugated estrogens 0.625 mg + medroxyprogesterone 5 mg (Premphase) **Tablet (Prempro)**: conjugated estrogens 0.3 mg + medroxyprogesterone 1.5 mg; conjugated estrogens 0.45 mg + medroxyprogesterone 1.5 mg; conjugated estrogens 0.625 mg + medroxyprogesterone 2.5 mg; conjugated estrogens 0.625 mg + medroxyprogesterone 5 mg
ethinyl estradiol + norethindrone	FemHRT Not available	**Tablet**: 0.005 mg ethinyl estradiol + 1 mg norethindrone
Estrogen Agonist-Antagonist		
conjugated estrogen + bazedoxifene	Duavee Duavive[c]	**Tablet**: 0.45 mg conjugated estrogens + 20 mg bazedoxifene

[a]Generic available.
[b]Available in the United States only.
[c]Product currently dormant in Canada.

Adverse Reactions

HRT may increase the risk of heart disease, pulmonary embolism, and breast and endometrial cancers. Other adverse effects are nausea, vomiting, bloating, cramping, breast tenderness, return of menstruation or spotting, migraine headaches, and weight gain.

Selective Serotonin Reuptake Inhibitors

Paroxetine is a selective serotonin reuptake inhibitor (SSRI) used to treat some symptoms of menopause, in addition to depression. Brisdelle is a low-dose paroxetine formulation approved for the treatment of moderate to severe vasomotor symptoms ("hot flashes"). The mechanism of action for the drug's effect on vasomotor symptoms is unknown.

Menstrual Disorders

Premenstrual Syndrome

Premenstrual syndrome (PMS) is a condition that involves a collection of symptoms that regularly occur in women before menstruation. Symptoms include headache, mood changes, fatigue, weight gain, sleep changes, and other problems that are distressing enough to limit activity and affect personal relationships. Because the causes of PMS are still unclear, current treatments focus on relieving the symptoms. A more severe form of PMS is *premenstrual dysphoric disorder* (PMDD). It is characterized by more pronounced features of PMS and occurs during the last week of the luteal phase in most menstrual cycles during the year preceding diagnosis. These symptoms disappear a few days after the onset of the menses. Symptoms may be accompanied by suicidal thoughts. Women commonly report that their symptoms worsen with age but go away with the onset of menopause. PMDD is treated with antidepressants including SSRIs such as fluoxetine, paroxetine, and sertraline. SSRIs and other antidepressants are described in Chapter 6.

⊘ Tech Alert!

The following drugs have look-alike/sound-alike issues:
FLUoxetine and DULoxetine;
PROzac, PriLOSEC, Prograf, and Provera;
Sarafem and Serophene;
PARoxetine, FLUoxetine, and piroxicam;
Sertraline and cetirizine

Dysmenorrhea

Dysmenorrhea, or painful menstruation, is the term used to describe menstrual cramps. Up to 85% of all women will have painful periods sometime during their reproductive years. Severe lower abdominal cramping and back pain accompanied by headache, nausea, and vomiting will disrupt their education, work, athletic, or other activities. Primary dysmenorrhea is the most common type, occurring primarily in adolescents and young women. Symptoms, which can last from hours to days, vary in severity from cycle to cycle and are caused by an abnormally increased concentration of certain prostaglandins produced by the uterine lining. High concentrations of prostaglandin E2 and prostaglandin F2 cause painful spasms by decreasing blood flow and oxygen to the uterine muscle.

Primary dysmenorrhea generally can be treated effectively with over-the-counter (OTC) drugs such as nonsteroidal antiinflammatory drugs (NSAIDs) like ibuprofen (Advil, Motrin, Midol), naproxen (Aleve, Pamprin), and prescription drugs ketoprofen and meclofenamate. Antiinflammatory drugs are listed and described in Chapter 10.

Amenorrhea

Amenorrhea is the absence of normal menstruation. Primary amenorrhea is the failure of the menstrual cycles to begin, and it may be caused by various factors, such as hormone imbalances, genetic disorders, or structural deformities of the reproductive

Pharmaceutical Treatment of Amenorrhea

Generic Name	US Brand Name(s) / Canadian Brand Name(s)	Dosage Forms and Strengths
bromocriptine[a,b]	Parlodel	**Tablet**: 2.5 mg
	Generics	**Capsule**: 5 mg
oral contraceptives	See earlier, "Oral Contraceptives"	See earlier, "Oral Contraceptives"

[a]Generic available.
[b]Also available as Cycloset (used to treat diabetes).

Selective Serotonin Reuptake Inhibitors for Menopause Symptoms

Generic Name	US Brand Name(s) / Canadian Brand Name(s)	Dosage Forms and Strengths
paroxetine[a]	Brisdelle	**Capsule**: 7.5 mg[b]
	Not available	

[a]Generic available.
[b]Available in the United States only.

organs. Secondary amenorrhea occurs when a woman who has previously menstruated slows to three or fewer cycles per year. Amenorrhea may be a symptom of excessive weight loss, pregnancy, lactation, menopause, or disease of the reproductive system. Amenorrhea is treated with bromocriptine, a dopamine receptor agonist that restores normal ovulatory menstrual cycles. Bromocriptine's mechanism of action and adverse effects are described in detail in Chapter 8. OCs may also be prescribed to establish a normal menstrual cycle.

Abnormal Uterine Bleeding

Abnormal uterine bleeding (AUB), a condition that causes heavy menstrual bleeding, affects up to one-third of all reproductive-age women. AUB may occur in women who have fibroids, but the exact association is unknown. In severe cases, excessive uterine bleeding from any cause can result in life-threatening anemia. In addition to excessive bleeding, women may experience cramping for an abnormal period beyond the normal menstrual cycle.

Treatment with NSAIDs and hormonal manipulation using gonadotropin-releasing hormone (GnRH) receptor antagonist may be prescribed. If conservative treatment fails to stop the endometrial lining from hemorrhaging, hysterectomy may be selected as a curative option.

Reproductive Disorders

Infertility

Conception is a biologic process that results in pregnancy. Conception may be aided by pharmacotherapy for men and women who are infertile. *Infertility* is often defined as a failure to conceive after 1 year of regular unprotected intercourse. It is caused by a wide variety of biologic, environmental, and even lifestyle factors, such as smoking or alcohol abuse. Infertility affects men and women. *Polycystic ovary disease*, characterized by enlarged ovaries that contain fluid-filled cysts, and *hypogonadism*, a condition in which the sex glands produce little or no hormones, are examples of medical conditions that can cause infertility. In men, gonads are the testes; in women, they are the ovaries.

Infertility may be treated with fertility drugs, alone or in combination with other assisted reproductive procedures, such as artificial insemination. Pharmaceutical treatment of infertility may involve the administration of selective estrogen receptor modulators (SERMs; e.g., clomiphene), menotropins (Menopur), GnRH antagonists (e.g., Ganirelix), and recombinant human FSH (follitropin alfa). FSH and LH stimulate normal follicular growth, maturation, and subsequent ovulation.

Selective Estrogen Receptor Modulator

Clomiphene is a SERM that stimulates ovulation. It is taken for 5 days, starting on day 3 to 5 of the menstrual cycle. If treatment is successful, ovulation begins 6 to 12 days after a course of the drug.

Mechanism of Action and Pharmacokinetics

Clomiphene competes with estrogen for estrogen-receptor binding sites. It works by effectively tricking the pituitary gland into producing FSH and LH, necessary for ovulation.

Adverse Reactions. Clomiphene may cause visual disturbances, dizziness, and headache. It should not be used during pregnancy. The incidence of multiple births when clomiphene is administered is approximately 5% to 7% (mostly twins). This percentage is much lower than occurs after direct administration (injection) of FSH and LH which produces multiple follicles before inducing ovulation.

> **! Tech Alert!**
> The following drugs have look-alike/sound-alike issues:
> clomiphene and clomipramine

Pharmacotherapy for Infertility

Generic Name	US Brand Name(s) / Canadian Brand Name(s)	Dosage Forms and Strengths
clomiphene	Generic	**Tablet**: 50 mg
	Not available	

Gonadotropins

Menotropins, human chorionic gonadotropin (hCG), choriogonadotropin alfa, and follitropin are gonadotropins that are administered to promote ovulation. Menotropins are purified combination preparations of FSH and LH that are derived from the urine of postmenopausal women. Urofollitropin is purified human follitropin derived from urine. Follitropin alfa and follitropin beta are recombinant version of human FSH. Choriogonadotropin alfa (rhCG) is a synthetic recombinant formulation of hCG.

Gonadotropins stimulate *superovulation*, or simultaneous rupture of multiple mature follicles, which is an infertility treatment option that may be used if clomiphene proves ineffective or if multiple ova are considered to be useful for assisted reproductive procedures, such as in vitro fertilization.

Mechanism of Action and Pharmacokinetics

Gonadotropins promote follicular growth, maturation, and ovulation. Menotropins, hCG, rhCG, and follitropin are peptides that are quickly destroyed in the gastrointestinal tract; therefore they must be administered parenterally as an intramuscular injection or, for select products, as a subcutaneous injection. Urine-derived hCG is administered intramuscularly, and recombinant hCG is administered subcutaneously.

Adverse Reactions

Side effects of gonadotropin administration include headache, light-headedness, nausea, abdominal discomfort, flushing, and local inflammation at the injection site.

Gonadotropin-Releasing Hormone

GnRH analogs may be agonists or antagonists. GnRH antagonists are approved for the treatment of infertility. GnRH agonists are indicated for the treatment of hypogonadism, endometriosis, AUB, and various other conditions.

Gonadotropin-Releasing Hormone Antagonists

Cetrorelix and ganirelix are GnRH antagonists approved for treating infertility. They are administered to prevent premature LH surges in women undergoing controlled ovarian hyperstimulation. GnRH antagonists decrease the production and release of LH by

Gonadotropins

Generic Name	US Brand Name(s) / Canadian Brand Name(s)	Dosage Forms and Strengths
follitropin alfa/beta	Follistim AQ	**Solution, for injection:** 150 units/ 0.18 mL, 300 units/0.36 mL, 600 units/0.72 mL, 900 units/1.08 mL
	Not available	
follitropin alfa	Gonal-f, Gonal-f RFF Redi-ject	**Powder, for subcutaneous injection:** 37.5 units/vial, 75 units (5.5 mcg)/vial, 150 units/vial, 300 units/vial[a], 450 units/vial (Gonal-F) 5.5 mcg/vial
	Gonal-f, Gonal-f pen	**Solution, for injection:** 150 units/0.25 mL[b], 300 units/0.5 mL, 450 units/0.75 mL, 900 units/1.5 mL (Gonal-F pen, Gonal-RFF Redi-ject)
follitropin beta	Not available	**Solution, for injection:** 833 units/1 mL
	Puregon	
urofollitropin	Bravelle	**Powder, for subcutaneous injection:** 75 units/vial
	Not available	
choriogonadotropin	Ovidrel	**Solution, prefilled syringe, for injection:** 0.25 mg/0.5 mL, 0.25 mg/vial
	Ovidrel	
menotropins	Menopur	**Powder, for injection:** 75 units/vial
	Menopur	

[a]Available in Canada only.
[b]Available in the United States only.

Gonadotropin-Releasing Hormone Antagonists

Generic Name	US Brand Name(s) / Canadian Brand Name(s)	Dosage Forms and Strengths
cetrorelix[a]	Cetrotide	**Powder, for injection:** 0.25 mg/vial
	Cetrotide	
elagolix	Orilissa	**Tablet:** 150 mg, 200 mg
	Orilissa	
ganirelix[a]	Fyremadel	**Solution, for injection (prefilled syringe):** 250 mcg/0.5 mL
	Orgalutran	

GnRH combinations

relugolix + norethindrone + estradiol	Myfembree	**Tablet:** relugolix 40 mg + norethindrone 0.5 mg + estradiol 1 mg
	Not available	

[a]Generic available.

competitively binding GnRH receptor sites. Elagolix and relugolix are GnRH antagonists indicated for moderate to severe pain associated with endometriosis and abnormal uterine bleeding caused by fibroids. Adverse drug reactions produced by elagolix and relugolix are bone loss because of decreases in estrogen levels, altered bleeding pattern that may mask pregnancy, and suicidal ideation.

Gonadotropin-Releasing Hormone Agonists

GnHR agonist analogs are used to treat endometriosis, endometrial thinning, and abnormal uterine bleeding (Lupron Depot, Suprefact-intranasal, Zoladex), hypogonadism (Luveris, Pergoveris), precocious puberty (Synarel), prostate cancer (Eligard, Suprefact, Zoladex), and advanced breast cancer (Zoladex).

Mechanism of Action
GnRH agonists produce initial stimulation followed by inhibition of the body's release of naturally occurring gonadotropins (LH and FSH). Busrelin is a luteinizing hormone-releasing hormone analog. Antagonists competitively bind to GnRH receptor sites to block the action of GnRH. Continuous administration of agonist and antagonist suppresses ovulation and decreases testosterone levels.

Adverse Reactions
Side effects of GnRH analogs include pain, redness, or swelling around the injection or implant site. Additional adverse reactions include headache, breast swelling and tenderness, postmenopausal symptoms, vaginal spotting, breakthrough bleeding, decreased libido, impotence, and bone loss. Recombinant human LH may also produce abdominal bloating, diarrhea, and gas.

> **⊘ Tech Alert!**
>
> The following drugs have look-alike/sound-alike issues:
> Lupron Depot-3 Month and Lupron Depot-Ped

Gonadotropin-Releasing Hormone Agonists

Generic Name	US Brand Name(s) / Canadian Brand Name(s)	Dosage Forms and Strengths
buserelin	Not available	**Implant (Suprefact Depot):** 6.3 mg (2 month), 9.45 mg (3 months)
	Suprefact, Suprefact Depot	**Nasal solution:** 1 mg/mL **Solution, injection:** 1 mg/mL
goserelin	Zoladex	**Injection (Zoladex), 1-month implant:** 3.6 mg
	Zoledex, Zoladex LA	**Injection (Zoladex LA), 3-month implant:** 10.8 mg
leuprolide[a]	Camcevi, Eligard, Fensolvi, Lupron Depot, Lupron Depot-Ped	**Emulsion, for subcutaneous injection:** 42 mg (Fensolvi) **Powder, for injection**[a]**:** 3.75 mg/vial (Zeulide Depot); 7.5 mg/vial, 22.5 mg/vial (Eligard kit, Zeulide Depot); 30 mg/vial, 45 mg/vial (Eligard kit); 15 mg (Lupron Depot-Ped)
	Eligard, Lupron Depot, Zeulide Depot	**Suspension, for injection:** 7.5 mg (1 month), 22.5 mg (3 months), 30 mg (4 months)/syringe (Eligard, Lupron Depot); 45 mg (6 months)/syringe (Eligard); 3.75 mg, 11.25 mg/syringe (Lupron Depot)
lutropin alfa	Not available	**Powder, for injection:** 75 units/vial
	Luveris	
lutropin alfa + follitropin alfa	Not available	**Powder, for injection:** 75 units lutropin alfa + 150 units follitropin alfa
	Pergoveris	**Solution, for subcutaneous injection:** 150 units lutropin alfa + 300 units follitropin alfa/0.48 mL; 225 units lutropin alfa + 450 units follitropin alfa/0.72 mL; 450 units lutropin alfa + 900 units follitropin alfa/1.44 mL
nafarelin	Synarel	**Solution, nasal spray:** 0.2 mg/spray
	Synarel	
histrelin	Supprelin LA	**Implant:** 50 mg
	Not available	

[a]Generic available.

Endometriosis

Endometriosis is a benign but painful condition that is characterized by the presence of functioning endometrial tissue outside the uterus. The displaced endometrial tissue is usually attached to an ovary or to the pelvic or abdominal organs; it is occasionally found in other areas of the body. Endometriosis often causes infertility, dysmenorrhea, and severe pain. Symptoms reflect the fact that displaced endometrial tissue reacts to ovarian hormones in the same way as the normal endometrium—exhibiting a cycle of growth and sloughing off. The disorder affects approximately 10% of women; most are aged 30 to 45 years. Endometriosis is treated with GnRH antagonists and agonists. GnRH antagonists prescribed for endometriosis are elagolix and relugolix in combination with estradiol and norethindrone. GnRH agonists used to treat endometriosis are buserelin and nafarelin.

Danazol

Danazol is an androgenic steroid that is used to treat endometriosis and fibrocystic breast disease. It reduces breast pain, tenderness, and nodules.

Mechanism of Action. Danazol works by suppressing the pituitary output of FSH and LH, resulting in anovulation and associated amenorrhea. It interrupts the progression and pain of endometriosis by shrinking normal and ectopic endometrial tissue.

Miscellaneous Treatment of Endometriosis*

Generic Name	US Brand Name(s) / Canadian Brand Name(s)	Dosage Forms and Strengths
danazol[a]	Generics	**Capsule:** 50 mg, 100 mg, 200 mg
	Cyclomen	

[a]Generic available.

*GnRH antagonists used to treat endometriosis are elagolix and relugolix. GnRH agonists used to treat endometriosis are buserelin and nafarelin.

Adverse Reactions. Adverse reactions include masculinity effects, gastrointestinal distress, diarrhea, jaundice, and menstrual irregularities.

Androgen Deficiency in Men

The male hormone testosterone and its derivatives are collectively called androgens. They are secreted by the anterior pituitary gland and are responsible for masculinization (development of male secondary sexual characteristics). Small amounts are produced by the adrenal gland.

Androgens and Anabolic Steroids

Anabolic steroids are synthetic drugs that closely resemble the androgen testosterone. They promote the tissue-building process and, in normal dosages, can have a minimal effect on accessory sex organs and secondary sex characteristics. Androgen therapy is used as replacement therapy for testosterone deficiency such as hypogonadism, select cases of delayed puberty, and postpuberty testosterone deficiency.

> **❶ Tech Alert!**
>
> Testosterone patches are not substitutable.

Mechanism of Action and Pharmacokinetics

Androgens aid in the development and maintenance of secondary sexual characteristics, such as facial hair, deepening of voice, growth of body hair, fat distribution, and muscle development, in adolescent boys. Testosterone stimulates the growth of accessory sex organs (penis, testes, vas deferens, prostate). Androgens also promote tissue-building processes (anabolism) and tissue-depleting processes (catabolism).

Androgens are available in different dosage forms as patches, gels, tablets, capsules, injections, transdermal patches, and pellets. The mucoadhesive form produces twice the androgen activity of oral tablets, the transdermal patch is applied daily to the scrotum or other parts of the body, and the gel is applied to the shoulder, upper arm, and abdomen (it should not be applied to the genitals).

Adverse Reactions

Androgens may produce gynecomastia (breast enlargement), testicular atrophy, impotence, decreased testicular function, penis enlargement, nausea, jaundice, headache, anxiety, male pattern baldness, acne, and depression. Fluid electrolyte imbalances (e.g., sodium, chloride, potassium, calcium, phosphate, water retention) may also occur. Prolonged use of anabolic steroids can cause many of the same serious adverse effects as androgens, as well as testicular atrophy, blood-filled cysts in the liver or spleen, malignant and benign liver tumors, increased risk of atherosclerosis, and mental changes (e.g., rage). These adverse effects are why androgens (anabolic steroids) are regulated as controlled substances.

> **❶ Tech Alert!**
>
> The following drugs have look-alike/sound-alike issues:
> Testoderm (scrotal patch) and Testoderm TTS (transdermal patch)

> **❶ Tech Alert!**
>
> Testosterone and other anabolic steroids are Schedule C-III controlled substances in the United States and C3 controlled substances in Canada.

TECHNICIAN'S CORNER

1. Since the WHI study, many women have turned to herbal preparations to combat menopausal symptoms. How effective are these preparations in improving these symptoms?
2. Many athletes have been using anabolic steroids to gain an edge in their sport. What are some long-term effects of these steroids on the body and mind?

Androgen Agonists

Generic Name	US Brand Name(s) / Canadian Brand Name(s)	Dosage Forms and Strengths
methyltestosterone[a]	Android 25	**Capsule**: 10 mg **Tablet (Android)**: 25 mg
	Not available	
testosterone[a]	Androderm, Androgel, Aveed, Fortesta, Jatenzo, Kyzatrex, Natesto, Testim, Testopel, Tlando, Vogelxo	**Capsule, as undecanoate**: 40 mg (Jatenzo), 100 mg, 150 mg, 200 mg (Kyzatrex), 112.5 mg (Tlando) **Gel, topical (Androgel, Testim, Vogelxo)**: 1% **Implant (Testopel)**: 75 mg **Nasal spray (Natesto)**: 5.5 mg/actuation (4.5%) **Spray, transdermal gel**: 10 mg/actuation (Fortesta), 12.5 mg/actuation (Androgel) **Solution, injection**: 100 mg/mL[b], 200 mg/mL, 250 mg/mL (Aveed) **Oil, as enanthate injection (Delestryl)**: 200 mg/mL **Solution, as enanthate (Xyosted)**: 50 mg/0.5 mL, 75 mg/0.5 mL, 100 mg/0.5 mL **Transdermal Patch (Androderm)**: 2 mg/24 h[c], 2.5 mg/24 h[b], 4 mg/24 h[c], 5 mg/24 h[b]
	Androgel, Delatestryl, Nastesto, Testim	

[a]Generic available.
[b]Available in Canada only.
[c]Available in the United States only.

Summary of Drugs That Affect the Reproductive System

	Generic Name	Brand Name	Usual Dose and Dosing Schedule	Warning Labels
Selective Serotonin Reuptake Inhibitors				
	fluoxetine	Prozac	**PMDD:** 20 mg/day dosed continuously or intermittently (starting 14 days before menstruation through the onset of menses)	MAY CAUSE DIZZINESS. MAY IMPAIR ABILITY TO DRIVE. SWALLOW WHOLE; DO NOT CRUSH OR CHEW—delayed release.
	sertraline	Zoloft	**PMDD:** 50–150 mg/day dosed continuously or intermittently (starting 14 days before menstruation through the onset of menses)	
	paroxetine	Brisdelle	**Menopause vasomotor symptoms:** 7.5 mg daily at bedtime	
Dopamine Receptor Agonist				
	bromocriptine	Parlodel	**Female infertility, in vitro fertilization:** 1.25 mg/day on days 4–6 of follicular phase, then 2.5 mg/day until 3 days after onset of menstruation	TAKE WITH FOOD OR MILK. MAY CAUSE DROWSINESS. LIMIT ALCOHOL USE.
Oral Contraceptives				
Estrogen and Progestin Combinations				
	ethinyl estradiol + desogestrel	Numerous (see OC table in chapter)	Take 1 tablet daily at same time every day for 21 days; off 7 days (21-day cycle), or take 1 tablet daily at same time every day (28-day cycle)	MAY TAKE WITH FOOD. TAKE AT THE SAME TIME EACH DAY. AVOID PROLONGED EXPOSURE TO SUNLIGHT. USE EXACTLY AS PRESCRIBED. AVOID SMOKING.
	ethinyl estradiol + drospirenone	Numerous (see OC table in chapter)		
	ethinyl estradiol + etonogestrel	NuvaRing	Insert ring vaginally and leave in place for 3 weeks; remove for 1 week; insert new ring 7 days after last one was removed	
	ethinyl estradiol + levonorgestrel	Numerous (see OC table in chapter)	Take 1 tablet at same time every day for 21 days; off 7 days (21-day cycle), or take 1 tablet daily at same time every day (28-day cycle)	
	ethinyl estradiol + norethindrone	Numerous (see OC table in chapter)		
	ethinyl estradiol + norgestimate	Numerous (see OC table in chapter)		
Intrauterine Devices				
	copper-releasing	ParaGard	**Intrauterine device:** Insert IUD into uterine cavity; replace 10 years after insertion	CALL YOUR HEALTH CARE PROVIDER IF YOU CANNOT FEEL THE IUD THREADS OR HAVE PELVIC PAIN OR PAIN DURING SEXUAL INTERCOURSE.
	levonorgestrel	Kyleena, Mirena	**Intrauterine device:** Insert IUD into uterine cavity; replace 5 years after insertion	
Contraceptive Implant				
	etonogestrel	Nexplanon	Insert 1 rod under the skin in upper arm; replace 3 years after insertion	CALL YOUR DOCTOR IF YOU CANNOT FEEL THE IMPLANT.

Summary of Drugs That Affect the Reproductive System—cont'd

	Generic Name	Brand Name	Usual Dose and Dosing Schedule	Warning Labels
Emergency Contraceptives				
	levonorgestrel	Plan B One Step	Take 1 tablet within 72 h of unprotected sexual intercourse	TAKE WITH FOOD. AVOID SMOKING.
Pregnancy Termination				
	mifepristone	Mifeprex	200 mg on day 1 followed by 800 mcg buccal misoprostol 28–48 hours later	MAY CAUSE DIZZINESS OR HEADACHE; EXERCISE CAUTION IF DRIVING.
	mifepristone + misoprostol	Mifegymiso	Take 1 tablet of mifepristone on day 1 followed by 4 tablets of misoprostol 24–48 hours later	
Hormone Replacement Therapy				
Estrogen				
	estradiol	Numerous (see Estrogen table in chapter)	**Moderate to severe symptoms of menopause (vasomotor symptoms or atrophic vulva) vaginal cream:** Insert 2–4 g/day intravaginally for 2 weeks; then reduce to half the initial dose for 2 weeks, followed by maintenance dose of 1 g 2 or 3 times/week **Tablet, oral:** 1–2 mg orally once daily in a cyclical pattern (3 weeks on, 1 week off) **Topical emulsion:** Apply 3.84 g once daily in the morning **Topical gel:** 1.25 g/day applied at same time daily **Transdermal spray (Evamist):** Apply 1 spray once daily to forearm; increase to 2 or 3 sprays daily based on clinical response **Patch:** Apply once weekly (Climara, Menostar) or twice weekly (Vivelle-Dot) **Vaginal ring:** Insert ring intravaginally; leave in for 3 months **Vaginal tablet:** Insert 1 tablet daily for 2 weeks; maintenance, insert 1 tablet twice weekly	ROTATE SITE OF APPLICATION— transdermal patch. AVOID SMOKING. TAKE WITH FOOD—tablet. INSERT PRESCRIBED DOSE VAGINALLY AS DIRECTED—vaginal cream, vaginal tablet.
	estrogens (conjugated)	Premarin	**Moderate to severe symptoms of menopause (vasomotor symptoms or atrophic vulva) vaginal cream:** Insert 0.5–2 g/day intravaginally for 3 weeks, then 1 week off (cyclically) **Tablet:** 0.3 mg/day cyclically or daily	
	estrogen (esterified)	Menest	0.3–1.25 mg/day tablet cyclically	
	estropipate	Ogen 5	1 tablet daily; administer cyclically	
Estrogen and Progesterone Combinations				
	estradiol + levonorgestrel	Climara Pro	**Transdermal:** Apply 1 patch weekly	ROTATE SITE OF APPLICATION. AVOID PROLONGED EXPOSURE TO SUNLIGHT.
	estradiol + norethindrone	Activella, CombiPatch, Estalis	**Transdermal patch:** Apply new patch twice weekly during 28-day cycle	
	estrogens + medroxyprogesterone acetates (MPA)	Premphase, Premplus, Prempro	**Premphase:** 1 maroon tablet days 1–14 followed by 1 light blue tablet days 15–28 **Prempro:** 1 tablet daily	

Continued

Summary of Drugs That Affect the Reproductive System—cont'd

	Generic Name	Brand Name	Usual Dose and Dosing Schedule	Warning Labels
Selective Estrogen Receptor Modulator				
	clomiphene	Generic	**Female infertility:** 50 mg once daily for 5 days starting on the 5th day of cycle; may repeat cycle in 30 days increasing dose to 100 mg if ovulation has not occurred **Male hypogonadism:** 25 mg once daily or 25–50 mg every other day	TAKE EXACTLY AS DIRECTED; DO NOT SKIP DOSES.
Gonadotropins				
	choriogonadotropin (recombinant)	Ovidrel	**Infertility:** Inject 250 mcg subcutaneously 1 day after the last dose of the follicle stimulating agent (Ovidrel) **Hypogonadism (males):** Inject 500–4000 units 3 times a weekly for 3 weeks to 6 months depending on protocol	DISCARD ANY UNUSED RECONSTITUTED SOLUTION.
	follitropin alfa	Gonal-f	**Ovulation induction:** 75 IU/day SC; if no response in 5–7 days, may increase by 37.5 IU weekly until max 300 IU **Hypogonadism (men):** 150 IU SC 3 times/week following hCG pretreatment, 1000 units	USE IMMEDIATELY AFTER RECONSTITUTION.
	menotropins	Menopur	On day 2 of cycle inject 225–450 IU daily for up to 20 days based on ovarian response	REFRIGERATE DILUTED POWDER; DO NOT FREEZE. PROTECT FROM LIGHT.
	urofollitropin	Bravelle	**Ovulation induction:** 150 units once daily SC or IM for 5 days according to protocol	USE IMMEDIATELY AFTER RECONSTITUTION.
Gonadotropin-Releasing Hormone Antagonists				
	cetrorelix	Cetrotide	**Ovulation induction:** Inject 0.25 mg SC once daily beginning on morning of stimulation day 5 or 6 and continue until hCG administration according to protocols	REFRIGERATE; DO NOT FREEZE—0.25 mg. STORE AT ROOM TEMPERATURE—3 mg cetrorelix, ganirelix.
	ganirelix	Fyremadel, Orgalutran	Inject 250 mg SC once daily during mid to late follicular phase	PROTECT FROM LIGHT—ganirelix.
Gonadotropin-Releasing Hormone Agonists				
	buserelin	Suprefact	**Endometriosis:** 2 sprays in each nostril 3 times daily for 6–9 months	DISCARD 5 WEEKS AFTER FIRST OPENING.
	goserelin	Zoladex	**Endometriosis:** Inject 3.6 mg SC every 28 days	STORE AT ROOM TEMPERATURE UNTIL READY FOR USE. DO NOT FREEZE.
	histrelin	Suprellin LA	**Precocious puberty:** Insert 1 implant SC annually	REFRIGERATE; DO NOT FREEZE.
	leuprolide	Eligard, Lupron Depot	**Endometriosis:** 11.25 mg IM every 3 months for 1–2 doses; max course of treatment is 12 months **Precocious puberty:** Dose varies by weight; 7.5–15 mg IM monthly or 11.25–30 mg IM depot once every 3 months **Anemia caused by uterine fibroids (Lupron Depot):** 3.5 mg monthly or 11.25 mg, max 3 months	SHAKE IF SETTLING OCCURS—suspension. DISCARD ANY UNUSED PORTION. STORE AT ROOM TEMPERATURE—solution. ROTATE INJECTION SITE.

Summary of Drugs That Affect the Reproductive System—cont'd

Generic Name	Brand Name	Usual Dose and Dosing Schedule	Warning Labels
lutropin alfa	Luveris	**Stimulate follicle development**: 75 IU SC once daily	DISCARD ANY UNUSED PORTION OF VIAL.
nafarelin	Synarel	**Endometriosis**: 1 spray in one nostril in the morning and 1 spray in the other nostril in the evening **Precocious puberty**: 2 sprays in each nostril every morning and evening	DO NOT USE NASAL DECONGESTANTS FOR 30 MINUTES AFTER USING NAFARELIN SPRAY.
lutropin alfa + follitropin alfa	Pergoveris	**Varies**	STORE AT ROOM TEMPERATURE. PROTECT FROM LIGHT.
Androgen Agonists			
fluoxymesterone	Generics	**Hypogonadism**: 5–20 mg/day	TAKE AS DIRECTED—all. TAKE WITH FOOD—all. ROTATE SITE OF APPLICATION—patch, injection. APPLY TO THE UPPER GUM ABOVE THE INCISOR TOOTH—buccal tablet. APPLY TO ARM, ABDOMEN, BACK, OR THIGH—Androderm. APPLY TO SCROTUM—Testoderm.
methyltestosterone	Android	**Hypogonadism**: 10–50 mg/day	
testosterone	Androderm, Delatestryl, Testoderm	**Hypogonadism** **Pellet**: SC implantation, 150–450 mg every 3–6 months **Scrotal patch (Testoderm)**: 6 mg daily to scrotum **Transdermal patch (Androderm, Testoderm TTS)**: Apply daily to back, abdomen, thigh, or arm **Injection**: 50–400 mg every 2–4 weeks **Gel**: 5 g daily **Nasal gel**: 2 pump actuations 3 times a day (max 33 mg/day)	
Miscellaneous			
danazol	Generics	**Endometriosis**: 200–800 mg daily in 2 divided doses	PROTECT FROM LIGHT AND MOISTURE.

OC, oral contraceptive; *IUD*, intrauterine device; *IU*, international unit; *IM*, intramuscularly; *SC*, subcutaneously; *PMDD*, premenstrual dysphoric disorder.

Key Points

- Infertility may be caused by a wide variety of medical, environmental, and even lifestyle factors, such as smoking or alcohol abuse.
- Symptoms of premenstrual syndrome include headache, mood changes, fatigue, weight gain, and sleep changes.
- Amenorrhea may be a symptom of weight loss, pregnancy, lactation, menopause, or disease of the reproductive system.
- Abnormal uterine bleeding is irregular or excessive uterine bleeding.
- Sexually transmitted infections are caused by communicable pathogens such as viruses, bacteria, fungi, and protozoa.
- Menopause is the termination of menstrual cycles and is usually marked by the passage of at least 1 full year without menstruation.
- Endometriosis is a benign but painful condition that is characterized by the presence of functioning endometrial tissue outside the uterus.
- Condoms are used to prevent pregnancy and transmission of sexually transmitted infections such as gonorrhea, syphilis, and HIV.
- Hormonal contraceptives initiate negative feedback inhibition of follicle-stimulating hormone and luteinizing hormone secretion.
- The diaphragm must be inserted sometime before sexual intercourse and remain in the vagina for 6 to 8 hours after a male's last ejaculation.
- The presence of an intrauterine device in the uterus prompts the release of leukocytes and prostaglandins by the endometrium interfering with fertilization and implantation.
- If used correctly and consistently, the pill is an extremely effective contraceptive, with an unintended pregnancy rate estimated at between 0.1% and 3%.
- Emergency contraceptive pills must be taken within 3 days (Plan B) or 5 days (Ella) after unprotected intercourse.
- The Women's Health Initiative (WHI) hormone replacement therapy study (2002) showed that it increases the risk of developing breast cancer, heart attacks, strokes, and blood clots.
- Gonadotropin-releasing hormone analogs are used to treat prostate cancer, endometriosis, advanced breast cancer, and endometrial thinning.
- The male hormone testosterone and its derivatives are androgens and Schedule C-III substances in the United States and Controlled drug C3, CDSA Schedule IV in Canada to limit misuse.

Review Questions

1. Hormonal contraceptives are manufactured in all of the following dosage forms EXCEPT _____.
   a. tablet
   b. transdermal patch
   c. vaginal cream
   d. implant

2. Select the contraceptive that is marketed as an over-the-counter (OTC) product.
   a. Contraceptive sponge
   b. Diaphragm
   c. Intrauterine device (IUD)
   d. Transdermal patch

3. Testoderm is applied to _____.
   a. back
   b. thigh
   c. abdomen
   d. scrotum

4. Select the emergency contraceptive that must be dispensed by prescription.
   a. Plan B One Step
   b. Next Choice
   c. Fallback Solo
   d. Ella

5. Menopause is the termination of menstrual cycles that is usually marked by the passage of at least 2 full years without menstruation.
   a. true
   b. false

6. Oral contraceptives (the pill) are 100% effective in preventing pregnancy.
   a. true
   b. false

7. The WHI study on hormonal replacement therapy concluded that hormonal replacement therapy may increase the risk for _____.
   a. heart disease and breast cancer
   b. heart attack and blood clots
   c. strokes
   d. all of the above

8. Clomiphene is a drug used to treat _____.
   a. contraception
   b. infertility
   c. hypogonadism
   d. amenorrhea

9. Gonadotropin-releasing hormone agonist, Synarel is a(n) _____.
   a. transdermal patch
   b. nasal spray
   c. injection
   d. capsule

10. Testosterone and anabolic steroids are _____ controlled substances in the United States and _____ in Canada.
    a. schedule I, C1
    b. schedule II, C2
    c. schedule III, C3
    d. schedule IV, C4

Bibliography

Bell C. Comparison of Copper Intrauterine Devices Available in Canada. MedSask Medication Information Service. 2018. Retrieved January 27, 2023, from https://www.medSask.usask.ca.

Borgelt L. Emergency Contraception: Key Concepts for the Pharmacy Technician. 2016. Retrieved January 31, 2023, from http://www.powerpak.com/course/preamble/115023.

Canadian Contraception Consensus Chapter 5 Barrier Methods. *J Obstet Gynaecol Can.* 2015;37(11):S12–S24.

Health Canada: Drug Product Database. Retrieved January 27, 2023, from https://health-products.canada.ca/dpd-bdpp/index-eng.jsp.

Hutten-Czapski P, Goertzen J. The occasional intrauterine contraceptive device insertion. *Can J Rural Med.* 2008;13:31–35.

Institute for Safe Medication Practices. FDA and ISMP Lists of Look-Alike Drug Names with Recommended Tall Man Letters. Retrieved July 20, 2022, from https://www.ismp.org/recommendations/tall-man-letters-list.

Institute for Safe Medication Practices List of Confused Drugs. Retrieved July 20, 2022, from https://www.ismp.org/tools/confuseddrugnames.pdf.

Kallmann's syndrome. *Tabers medical dictionary.* ed 20. Philadelphia: FA Davis; 2005:1163.

Kumar P, Sharma A. Gonadotropin-releasing hormone analogs: understanding advantages and limitations. *J Hum Reprod Sci.* 2014;7(3):170–174.

National Heart, Lung and Blood Institute. Facts About Menopausal Hormone Therapy. NIH Publ. No. 05-5200; 2005. Retrieved January 31, 2023, from http://www.nhlbi.nih.gov/health/women/pht_facts.pdf.

Rayani S, McInnes K. (2017). Hormonal and IUD Contraceptive Agents Available in Canada. BC Drug and Poison Information Centre. Retrieved January 27, 2023, from www.dpic.org/article/professional/hormonal-and-iud-contraceptive-agents-available-canada

Roach S. *Pharmacology for health professionals.* Baltimore: Lippincott, Williams & Wilkins; 2005.

Rovelli RJ, Cieri-Hutcherson NE, Hutcherson TC. Systematic review of oral pharmacotherapeutic options for the management of uterine fibroids. *J Am Pharm Assoc.* 2022;62:674–682.

Shannon M, Wilson B, Stang C. *Health professionals drug guide,* 2005–2006. Upper Saddle River, NJ: Prentice-Hall; 2006.

Syed YY. Relugolix/estradiol/norethisterone (norethindrone) acetate: a review in symptomatic uterine fibroids. *Drugs.* 2022;82:1549–1556.

Thibodeau G, Patton K. *Anatomy and physiology.* ed 6. St Louis: Mosby; 2007.

U.S. Department of Health and Human Services Office on Women's Health: Birth Control Methods. 2017. Retrieved January 27, 2023, from. https://www.womenshealth.gov/a-z-topics/birth-control-methods.

U.S. Food and Drug Administration Drugs@FDA: FDA Approved Drug Products. Retrieved January 26, 2023, from http://www.accessdata.fda.gov/scripts/cder/daf/.

Whitaker L, Critchley H. Abnormal uterine bleeding. *Best Pract Res Clin Obstet Gynaecol.* 2016;34:54–65.

Workowski KA, Berman SM. Sexually transmitted diseases treatment guidelines. *MMWR Recomm Rep.* 2021;70(3):1–187.

28

Treatment of Prostate Disease and Erectile Dysfunction

LEARNING OBJECTIVES

1. Learn the terminology associated with prostate disease and erectile dysfunction.
2. List symptoms of prostate disease and erectile dysfunction.
3. List and categorize medications used for the treatment of prostate disease and erectile dysfunction.
4. Describe mechanism of action for drugs used for the treatment of prostate disease and erectile dysfunction.

5. List common endings for drug classes used in the treatment of prostate disease and erectile dysfunction.
6. Identify significant drug look-alike and sound-alike issues.
7. Identify warning labels and precautionary messages associated with medications used for the treatment of prostate disease and erectile dysfunction.

KEY TERMS

Benign prostatic hyperplasia Noncancerous, abnormal increase in the growth of the prostate gland.
Erectile dysfunction Persistent inability to achieve and/or maintain an erection sufficient for satisfactory sexual intercourse.
Incontinence Loss of bladder or bowel control.
Prostate gland Gland in the male reproductive system just below the bladder surrounding the urethra.
Prostate-specific antigen Protein produced by the prostate gland. Levels are elevated in men with conditions ranging from prostate infection to prostate cancer.

Prostate-specific antigen test Blood test to measure the percentage of prostate-specific antigen that is unbound. Free prostate-specific antigen is linked to benign prostate hyperplasia but not to cancer.
Prostatitis Inflammation of the prostate gland.
Urinary frequency Need to urinate more often than is normal.

Benign Prostatic Hyperplasia

The ***prostate gland*** is a part of the male reproductive system located just below the bladder surrounding the urethra. The gland produces semen, the fluid that contains sperm. ***Prostatitis*** is an inflamed or infected prostate gland. Symptoms may be burning on urination, fever, body ache, difficulty urinating, urge ***incontinence***, painful ejaculation, decreased libido, and groin, rectal, or low back pain. Although some of the symptoms are similar, prostatitis is usually an acute condition, unlike ***benign prostatic hyperplasia*** (BPH). BPH is a condition in which noncancerous cells in the prostate grow and increase the size of the prostate gland (Fig. 28.1). It is a condition associated with bladder obstruction and lower urinary tract symptoms (LUTS) because as the gland grows, it begins to obstruct the flow of urine through the urethra. The urethra is a small tube that carries urine and semen through the penis.

The risk for developing BPH increases with age. By age 60, more than 50% of men will have the condition; 90% or more men will develop BPH/LUTS by 80 years old, and nearly all men

will have an enlarged prostate. The prevalence of BPH globally is rising from an estimated 51 million cases in the year 2000 to 91 million cases in 2019. The increase has been greatest in low- and middle-income countries. The global burden of disease was estimated to be nearly $74 billion annually.

Diagnosis

Several tests are available to check the health of the prostate. A digital rectal examination involves the insertion of a gloved finger into the rectum and palpating the prostate to determine whether it is enlarged. A ***prostate-specific antigen (PSA) test*** may be performed to determine whether levels of the PSA protein are elevated. A higher than normal level is a sign of BPH, infection, inflammation, or prostate cancer. A free PSA test, the percentage of PSA that is not attached to another chemical, may be conducted to differentiate between BPH and cancer. Free PSA is linked to BPH but not to cancer. Urinalysis and a biopsy of prostate tissue may also be taken.

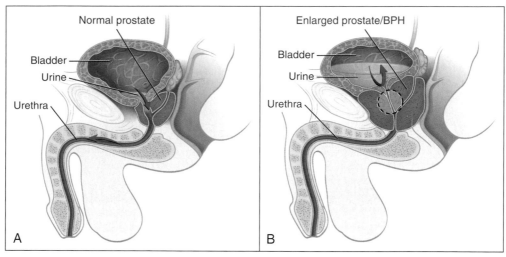

• **Fig. 28.1** (A) Normal prostate. (B) Enlarged prostate. *BPH*, Benign prostatic hyperplasia. (Courtesy National Institutes of Health, Bethesda, MD.)

• BOX 28.1 Symptoms of Benign Prostatic Hyperplasia

- Weak or slow stream of urine
- Delay in starting urination
- Urinary stream that starts and stops
- Frequent urination
- Urinary urgency
- Nighttime awakening to urinate
- Need to strain to urinate

Symptoms of Benign Prostatic Hyperplasia

The first symptom of an enlarged prostate gland is a weak or slow stream of urine (Box 28.1). There may also be a delayed start in the flow of urine or straining to urinate. As the disease progresses, the bladder becomes hypersensitive and the need to urinate becomes more frequent *(urinary frequency)*. Some men may develop urinary infection(s) from the condition. BPH may also produce bladder stones, sudden inability to urinate, or kidney damage.

Treatment of Benign Prostatic Hyperplasia

Pharmacotherapy for BPH is initiated when symptoms are uncomfortable enough to warrant treatment. Watchful waiting is recommended when patients are asymptomatic or when symptoms do not produce much discomfort. α-Blockers, 5α-reductase inhibitors, and combination drugs containing a 5-α reductase inhibitor and a phosphodiesterase-5 inhibitor may be administered to manage symptoms.

α₁-Adrenergic Antagonists

α_1-Adrenergic antagonists relax prostate and bladder smooth muscle, which reduces urethral resistance and improves the flow of urine. Some α-blockers are also prescribed for the treatment of hypertension (see Chapter 18).

❗ *Tech Alert!*

The following drugs have look-alike/sound-alike issues:
Cardura and Coumadin

Mechanism of Action and Pharmacokinetics

Alfuzosin, doxazosin, silodosin, tamsulosin, and terazosin bind to α_1-adrenergic receptor sites. Binding to α_1-adrenergic receptors blocks adrenergic-mediated vasoconstriction in the prostate.

Alfuzosin, doxazosin, and tamsulosin are available in extended-release dosage forms and are dosed once daily. The half-life ($t^{1/2}$) for all agents ranges between 10 and 22 hours. Absorption of tamsulosin is increased if the drug is taken with a high fat content meal, increasing the effects and side effects. Rapaflo (silodosin) should be taken with food. Urine flow rates are usually improved within the first 2 weeks of therapy.

Adverse Reactions

Adverse drug effects linked to the administration of α-adrenergic antagonists are postural hypotension, dizziness, reflex tachycardia, headache, stuffy nose, weakness, and fatigue.

5α-Reductase Inhibitors

High testosterone levels can stimulate growth of prostate tissue, whereas deprivation results in a reduction in glandular size. Finasteride and dutasteride are 5α-reductase inhibitors that reduce testosterone levels.

Mechanism of Action and Pharmacokinetics

Finasteride and dutasteride inhibit 5α-reductase, an enzyme that controls the production of dihydrotestosterone from testosterone. Drug effects accumulate over time, and it may take 6 to 12 months for full therapeutic effects to be achieved.

● *Tech Note!*

Finasteride 1 mg is prescribed for the treatment of male pattern baldness.

α₁-Adrenergic Antagonists

Generic Name	US Brand Name(s) / Canadian Brand Names(s)	Dosage Forms and Strengths
alfuzosin[a]	Uroxatral	Tablet, extended release: 10 mg
	Xatral	
doxazosin[a]	Cardura, Cardura XL	Tablet: 1 mg, 2 mg, 4 mg, 8 mg[b]
	Generics	Tablet, extended release (Cardura XL)[b]: 4 mg, 8 mg
silodosin[a]	Rapaflo	Capsule: 4 mg, 8 mg
	Generics	
tamsulosin[a]	Flomax	Capsule, controlled release[b]: 0.4 mg
	Flomax CR	Tablet, controlled release[c]: 0.4 mg
terazosin[a]	Generics	Capsule[b]: 1 mg, 2 mg, 5 mg, 10 mg
	Generics	Tablet[c]: 1 mg, 2 mg, 5 mg, 10 mg

[a]Generic available.
[b]Available in the United States only.
[c]Available in Canada only.

Adverse Reactions

Dutasteride and finasteride may decrease desire for sex, cause *erectile dysfunction* (ED), and/or reduce semen volume. Both drugs are harmful to the developing fetus; therefore pregnant women and women of childbearing age should be advised to avoid contact with broken or crushed tablets. The use of a barrier contraceptive, such as condoms, is also recommended.

> **● Tech Note!**
> A common ending for 5α-reductase inhibitors is -*steride*.

> **❶ Tech Alert!**
> Proscar and Provera have look-alike/sound-alike issues.

5α-Reductase Inhibitors

Generic Name	US Brand Name(s) / Canadian Brand Names(s)	Dosage Forms and Strengths
dutasteride[a]	Avodart	Capsule: 0.5 mg
	Avodart	
finasteride[a]	Proscar, Propecia	Tablet (Proscar): 5 mg
	Proscar, Propecia	Tablet (Propecia)[b]: 1 mg
Combination: 5α-Reductase Inhibitor and α-Blocker		
dutasteride + tamsulosin[a]	Jalyn	Capsule: 0.5 mg dutasteride + 0.4 mg tamsulosin
	Jalyn	
Combination: 5α-Reductase Inhibitor and Phosphodiesterase-5 Inhibitor		
finasteride + tadalafil	Entadfi	Capsule: 5 mg finasteride + 5 mg tadalafil
	Not available	

[a]Generic available.
[b]Propecia is used for hair loss.

Nonpharmacologic Treatment Options

When symptoms of BPH are severe, surgery is indicated. There are several surgical options. Some procedures are more invasive than others. The following are brief definitions of surgical procedures for BPH:

Prostatic stent: A stent (scaffolding) is inserted into the urethra to open a passage and improve urine flow.

Transurethral incision of the prostate (TUIP): One or two slits are made in the prostate to relieve the pressure and improve urine flow.

Transurethral microwave thermal therapy of the prostate (TUMT): Computer-regulated microwaves are sent through a catheter to heat portions of the prostate.

Transurethral needle ablation (TUNA): Delivers a low-level radio-frequency signal directly into the prostate and destroys the prostate tissue, improving the symptoms of BPH.

Transurethral resection of the prostate (TURP): Excess prostate tissue is trimmed away.

Transurethral vaporization of the prostate (TUVP): Excess prostate tissue is vaporized using an electrical current.

Erectile Dysfunction

An erection occurs when the arteries and sinusoids in the corpus cavernosum fill with blood (Fig. 28.2). Intracorporal blood pressure increases while at the same time venous outflow decreases, resulting in penile rigidity that enables effective intercourse. ED is defined as the total inability to achieve erection, an inconsistent ability to achieve erection, or difficulty maintaining erection long enough to sustain sexual intercourse. It is also known as impotence. Up to 52% of men globally have reported symptoms of ED, and it is anticipated that up to 322 million men will experience ED by 2025. ED increases with age; however, it is not an inevitable part of the aging process. By age 40 years, approximately 5% of men experience ED. By age 65, approximately 15% of men will have ED.

What Causes Erectile Dysfunction?

ED may have physiologic, psychological, neurologic, or endocrinologic causes. Physiologic causes include age-related changes and chronic disease (e.g., hypertension, hyperlipidemia, or multiple sclerosis). Neurologic and endocrinologic causes may be the result of

Summary of Drugs Used in the Treatment of Benign Prostatic Hyperplasia

	Generic Name	US Brand Name	Usual Adult Oral Dose and Dosing Schedule	Warning Labels
α₁-Adrenergic Antagonist				
	alfuzosin	Uroxatral	10 mg once daily	DO NOT DISCONTINUE WITHOUT MEDICAL SUPERVISION. MAY CAUSE DIZZINESS OR LIGHT-HEADEDNESS. AVOID DRIVING OR OPERATING HAZARDOUS MACHINERY. SWALLOW WHOLE; DO NOT CRUSH OR CHEW—Flomax, Cardura XL, Uroxatral. TAKE WITH MEAL—alfuzosin, silodosin.
	doxazosin	Cardura	1–8 mg once daily	
		Cardura XL	4–8 mg once daily	
	terazosin	Generics	1–10 mg at bedtime	
	silodosin	Rapaflo	8 mg daily	
	tamsulosin	Flomax	0.4–0.8 mg once daily	
5α-Reductase Inhibitors				
	dutasteride	Avodart	0.5 mg once daily	SWALLOW CAPSULES WHOLE; DO NOT CHEW—dutasteride. SWALLOW THE TABLETS WITH A DRINK OF WATER—finasteride. PREGNANT WOMEN SHOULD AVOID CONTACT WITH BROKEN OR CRUSHED TABLETS.
	finasteride	Proscar	5 mg once daily	
Combination: 5α-Reductase Inhibitor and α-Blocker				
	dutasteride + tamsulosin	Jalyn	1 capsule daily	MAY CAUSE DIZZINESS. SWALLOW CAPSULES WHOLE; DO NOT CHEW. PREGNANT WOMEN SHOULD AVOID CONTACT WITH BROKEN OR CRUSHED TABLETS.
Combination: 5α-Reductase Inhibitor and Phosphodiesterase-5 Inhibitor				
	finasteride + tadalafil	Entadfi	1 capsule daily	DO NOT TAKE WITH NITRATES. MAY CAUSE DIZZINESS.

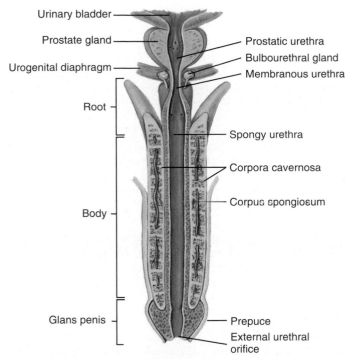

• Fig. 28.2 Structure of the penis. (From Page C, Hoffman B, Curtis M, et al. *Integrated pharmacology*, ed 3, Philadelphia, 2006, Mosby.)

Labels on figure:
Urinary bladder
Prostate gland
Urogenital diaphragm
Root
Body
Glans penis
Prostatic urethra
Bulbourethral gland
Membranous urethra
Spongy urethra
Corpora cavernosa
Corpus spongiosum
Prepuce
External urethral orifice

---

diabetes, a disease of the endocrine system that can cause vascular and nerve changes that affect erectile function. ED may also be caused by depression and lifestyle factors such as smoking, obesity, and alcoholism. Risk factors for erectile dysfunction are listed in Box 28.2.

Prescription and nonprescription drugs also can affect erectile function (Box 28.3). Therefore clinicians should take a patient medication history.

Drugs Used for the Treatment of Erectile Dysfunction

ED is managed by the administration of drugs that promote penile engorgement and slow the loss of erection. Neurotransmitters are involved in producing an erection (Box 28.4).

Nitric oxide (NO) is a mediator of smooth muscle relaxation that is released in response to sexual stimulation. It activates several intracellular enzymes such as phosphodiesterase type 5 (PDE5), an enzyme involved in the reversal of an erection. PDE5 inhibitors and prostaglandin E analogs are drugs used for the treatment of ED.

Phosphodiesterase Inhibitors

Sildenafil, tadalafil, avanafil, and vardenafil are prescribed for the treatment of ED. They are taken before intercourse to produce an erection. Sildenafil, avanafil, and tadalafil are taken 30 minutes before intercourse. Vardenafil is taken up to 60 minutes before sexual activity.

Mechanism of Action

Avanafil, sildenafil, tadalafil, and vardenafil relax smooth muscle and blood vessels that supply the corpus cavernosum and control penile engorgement (Fig. 28.3). At the cellular level, the drugs increase levels of NO in the corpus cavernosum, which blocks the opening of calcium voltage-gated channels and reduces calcium-mediated vascular contractions.

Pharmacokinetics

The oral absorption of sildenafil, vardenafil, and tadalafil is good, and maximum concentration (C_{max}) and onset of action of vardenafil are reached between 30 minutes and 2 hours after a dose of drug is administered. C_{max} for tadalafil and sildenafil is similar, averaging approximately 2 hours. The bioavailability of the drugs may be reduced by up to 50% when they are taken with a meal that is high in fat. Protein binding is approximately 96% for all PDE5s.

Adverse Reactions

Many of the adverse reactions associated with the use of phosphodiesterase inhibitors are a result of vasodilation. These side effects include dizziness, flushing, headache, and nasal congestion. Diarrhea and indigestion are gastrointestinal side effects. Sildenafil, avanafil, tadalafil, and vardenafil may also produce sudden hearing loss or visual effects that range from light sensitivity and difficulty distinguishing between green and blue to loss of

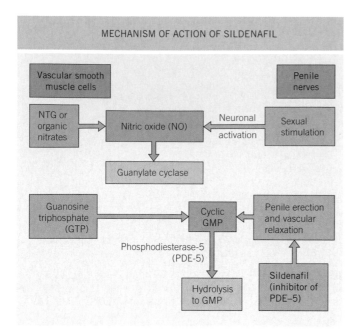

MECHANISM OF ACTION OF SILDENAFIL

• **Fig. 28.3** Mechanism of action for sildenafil. Sildenafil binds to receptors that block the degradation of cGMP and increase the effects of nitric oxide *(NO)* on the corpus cavernosum (relaxation and increased erectile response). *NTG,* Nitroglycerine; *GMP,* guanosine monophosphate. (From Page C, Hoffman B, Curtis M, et al. *Integrated pharmacology,* ed 3, Philadelphia, 2006, Mosby.)

vision. The incidence of visual disturbances is greater with sildenafil than with vardenafil and tadalafil.

Precautions

PDE5 inhibitors are involved in numerous drug interactions. A life-threatening drop in blood pressure has occurred in men who have taken nitrates such as nitroglycerin (for angina), so the use of nitrates, in all dosage forms, is contraindicated while taking PDE5 inhibitors. Concurrent administration of α-adrenergic agonists (e.g., alfuzosin, terazosin, doxazosin), used for the treatment of BPH, requires caution, and it is recommended that α-blockers should not be taken within 4 hours of PDE5 inhibitors. Patients taking PDE5 inhibitors should avoid antifungal agents *(-azoles),* cimetidine, grapefruit juice, macrolide antiinfective drugs (e.g., erythromycin, clarithromycin), and excessive alcohol consumption (more than five glasses of wine or five shots of whiskey). Drug interactions also occur with the coadministration of selective serotonin reuptake inhibitor and monoamine oxidase inhibitor (MAOI) antidepressants.

● *Tech Note!*

A common ending for phosphodiesterase inhibitors (PDE5) is *-afil.*

Prostaglandins

Alprostadil is naturally occurring prostaglandin E1 (PGE1) present in the seminal vesicles and cavernous tissues of males. It can also be found in the placenta of the fetus. PGE1 mediates the relaxation of penile smooth muscle.

Mechanism of Action and Pharmacokinetics

PGE1 mobilizes intracellular calcium in the corpus cavernosum, resulting in smooth muscle contraction; however, in the endothelium, PGE1 mediates the release of NO, which relaxes cavernous smooth muscle, causing an erection.

The oral absorption of alprostadil is poor; therefore the drug is formulated for intraurethral insertion and intracavernosal injection. The intracavernosal route of administration is more effective

Phosphodiesterase Inhibitors

	Generic Name	US Brand Name(s) / Canadian Brand Names(s)	Dosage Forms and Strengths
	avanafil	Stendra	**Tablet:** 50 mg, 100 mg, 200 mg
		Not available	
	sildenafil[a]	Viagra, Revatio[b]	**Solution, oral (Revatio)**[c]: 10 mg/mL
		Viagra, Revatio[b]	**Solution, IV (Revatio):** 0.8 mg/mL **Tablet (Viagra):** 25 mg, 50 mg, 100 mg **Tablet (Revatio):** 20 mg
	tadalafil[a]	Cialis, Adcirca[b]	**Tablet:** 2.5 mg, 5 mg, 10 mg, 20 mg
		Cialis, Adcirca[b]	
	vardenafil[a]	Generics	**Tablet:** 2.5 mg[c], 5 mg, 10 mg, 20 mg **Tablet, oral disintegrating:** 10 mg
		Levitra	

[a]Generic available.
[b]Indicated for pulmonary arterial hypertension (20 mg tablet only).
[c]Available in the United States only.

TABLE 28.1	Instructions for Administration of Intraurethral Pellets and Intracavernosal Injection
Administration of Intraurethral Pellets	**Administration of Intracavernosal Injection**
1. Gently and slowly stretch the penis upward to its full length. 2. Slowly insert the stem of the applicator into the urethra up to the collar; then gently and completely push down the button at the top of the applicator until it stops (and medicated pellet is released). 3. Hold the applicator in this position for 5 seconds; then remove applicator while keeping the penis upright. Roll the penis firmly between the hands for at least 10 seconds to ensure that the medication is adequately distributed along the walls of the urethra. 4. An erection should begin to form within 10 minutes of application.	1. Gently and slowly stretch the penis upward to its full length. 2. Insert the needle into the corpus cavernosum at 90 degrees until the metal portion of the needle is almost completely into the penis. Avoid visible veins, urethra, and corpus spongiosum. 3. Slowly inject the contents of the syringe over 5 to 10 seconds. 4. Withdraw syringe and apply pressure to injection site for 5 minutes or until bleeding stops.

than is the intraurethral route. Instructions for using alprostadil intraurethral inserts and alprostadil intracavernosal injection are provided in Table 28.1.

Adverse Reactions

Adverse reactions are specific to the route of administration. Hypotension, dizziness, bleeding, bruising, pain at the site of injection, and painful erection are associated with intracavernosal administration. Redness of the penis, warmth or burning sensation in the urethra, leg swelling, and itching in the penis, testicles, legs, and perineum are adverse effects associated with intraurethral

administration of alprostadil. Urethral bleeding or spotting may occur when the drug is administered improperly. Both dosage forms may produce prolonged erection (lasting >4 hours).

Nonpharmacologic Management of Erectile Dysfunction

ED may also be treated by attaching a mechanical vacuum device to the penis, which uses suction to produce engorgement. An alternative approach is to surgically implant a device with inflatable tubes that can cause the penis to become erect. Vascular surgery may be performed to reconstruct arteries that supply the penis and to block off veins that allow blood to leak from penile tissue.

Herbal Remedies for Benign Prostatic Hyperplasia and Erectile Dysfunction

The ripened fruit of saw palmetto contains fatty acids and plant sterols that inhibit 5α-reductase and cytosolic androgen binding, producing antiinflammatory and antiestrogenic effects. Saw palmetto may reduce urinary symptoms of BPH. Prostate cancer should be ruled out before taking saw palmetto. Yohimbe is an evergreen tree found in West Africa. Its bark contains an α_2-adrenergic blocker related to reserpine that may improve ED. Clinical trials have not been conducted, and evidence to support yohimbe's effectiveness is lacking. Adverse effects include increased blood pressure and heart rate, headache, insomnia, anxiety, nausea, and vomiting. Drug interactions may occur if yohimbe is taken concurrently with MAOIs, tricyclic antidepressants, and phenothiazines.

Prostaglandins

Generic Name	US Brand Name(s)		Dosage Forms and Strengths
	Canadian Brand Names(s)		
alprostadil[a]	Caverject, Caverject Impulse, Edex cartridge, Muse, Prostin VR[b]		**Powder, for injection (Caverject):** 10 mcg[c], 20 mcg, 40 mcg[c]/vial **Urethral insert (Muse):** 250 mcg, 500 mcg, 1000 mcg
	Caverject, Muse, Prostin VR[b]		**Injection, solution (Prostin VR):** 500 mcg/mL

[a]Generic available.
[b]Prostin VR is administered as a continuous infusion to neonates with congenital heart disease such as ductus arteriosus, pulmonary stenosis, or interruption of the aortic arch until corrective surgery can be performed.
[c]Available in the United States only.

TECHNICIAN'S CORNER

1. How are complementary and alternative medicines (e.g., herbs) used in managing BPH?
2. How might lifestyle changes reduce the risks of erectile dysfunction?

Summary of Drugs Used in the Treatment of Erectile Dysfunction

	Generic Name	US Brand Name	Usual Adult Oral Dose and Dosing Schedule	Warning Labels
Phosphodiesterase Inhibitors (PDE5)				
	avanafil	Stendra	50–200 mg 15 minutes before sexual activity	MAY CAUSE DIZZINESS. AVOID GRAPEFRUIT JUICE— avanafil, tadalafil, vardenafil. DISSOLVE ORAL DISINTEGRATING TABLETS UNDER TONGUE.
	sildenafil	Viagra	25–100 mg 30 min–4 h before sexual intercourse; not more than once daily	
	tadalafil	Cialis	10–20 mg before sexual intercourse; not more than once daily or 2.5–5 mg once daily	
	vardenafil	Levitra	5–20 mg up to 60 min before sexual intercourse; not more than once daily	
Prostaglandins				
	alprostadil	Muse	Insert 1 pellet 30–60 min before sexual intercourse; not more than once daily	REFRIGERATE (MAY BE STORED AT ROOM TEMPERATURE FOR 14 DAYS).
		Caverject	Inject individualized dose not more than once in 24 h or >3 times/week	ROTATE SITE OF INJECTION. MAY STORE AT ROOM TEMPERATURE FOR UP TO 3 MONTHS. AVOID DRUG EXPOSURE TO EXTREMES IN HEAT OR COLD.

Key Points

- The prostate gland is part of the male reproductive system.
- Prostatitis is an inflamed or infected prostate gland.
- Benign prostatic hyperplasia (BPH) is a condition in which noncancerous cells in the prostate grow and increase the size of the prostate gland.
- The risk for developing BPH increases with age; by 80 years old, nearly all men will have an enlarged prostate.
- Higher than normal ***prostate-specific antigen*** (PSA) levels are a sign of BPH, infection, inflammation, or prostate cancer.
- Two classes of drugs are administered to manage symptoms of BPH. They are α-blockers and 5α-reductase inhibitors.
- Alfuzosin, doxazosin, silodosin, terazosin, and tamsulosin are α_1-adrenergic blockers prescribed to treat BPH.
- Alfuzosin, doxazosin, and tamsulosin are available in extended-release dosage forms.
- Adverse drug effects linked to the administration of α-adrenergic antagonists are postural hypotension, dizziness, reflex tachycardia, headache, stuffy nose, weakness, and fatigue.
- Finasteride and dutasteride are 5α-reductase inhibitors that decrease testosterone levels. It may take 6 to 12 months to achieve maximum effects.
- Dutasteride and finasteride are harmful to the developing fetus. Pregnant women and women of childbearing age should be advised to avoid contact with broken or crushed tablets. The use of a barrier contraceptive is also recommended.

- Erectile dysfunction (ED) is defined as a total inability to achieve erection, an inconsistent ability to achieve erection, or difficulty maintaining erection long enough to sustain sexual intercourse.
- Drugs currently marketed for the treatment of ED are phosphodiesterase inhibitors (PDE5) and prostaglandin E analogs.
- Avanafil, sildenafil, tadalafil, and vardenafil are PDE5 inhibitors.
- PDE5 inhibitors relax smooth muscle and blood vessels that supply the corpus cavernosum and control penile engorgement by increasing levels of nitric oxide.
- Side effects of PDE5 inhibitors are dizziness, flushing, headache, nasal congestion, diarrhea, indigestion, and visual disturbances.
- The administration of nitrates, such as nitroglycerin, in all dosage forms, is contraindicated in patients taking PDE5 inhibitors.
- Patients taking PDE5 inhibitors should avoid consuming grapefruit juice with the drugs.
- Alprostadil is a naturally occurring prostaglandin E1 present in male seminal vesicles and cavernous tissues.
- Prostaglandin E1 mediates the relaxation of penile smooth muscle.
- Oral absorption of alprostadil is poor; therefore the drug is formulated for intraurethral insertion and intracavernosal injection.
- Both dosage forms may produce prolonged erection (lasting >4 hours).

Review Questions

1. Benign prostatic hyperplasia is a condition that is cancerous.
   a. true
   b. false
2. The first symptom(s) of an enlarged prostate gland is(are) _____.
   a. a weak or slow urine stream
   b. a delayed start in the flow of urine
   c. straining to urinate
   d. all of the above
3. Class(es) of drugs administered to manage the symptoms of benign prostatic hyperplasia are _____.
   a. α-blockers and β-blockers
   b. α-reductase inhibitors and β-blockers
   c. α-blockers and α-reductase inhibitors
   d. all of the above
4. Which warning label is NOT typically placed on prescription vials for avanafil, sildenafil, tadalafil, or vardenafil?
   a. Avoid grapefruit juice
   b. Avoid nitrates
   c. Report sudden hearing loss or vision disturbances
   d. Report signs of bleeding
5. The generic name for Flomax is _____.
   a. doxazosin
   b. tamsulosin
   c. alfuzosin
   d. terazosin
6. Which of the following is NOT an adverse effect of dutasteride and finasteride?
   a. Decreased desire for sex
   b. Erectile dysfunction
   c. Increased desire for sex
   d. Reduced semen
7. Select the agent that is NOT used for erectile dysfunction?
   a. sildenafil
   b. penadafil
   c. tadalafil
   d. vardenafil
8. Higher than normal levels of PSA may be a sign of _____.
   a. BPH
   b. infection and inflammation
   c. prostate cancer
   d. all of the above
9. Finasteride and dutasteride work by reducing testosterone levels.
   a. true
   b. false
10. _____ is(are) currently marketed for the treatment of erectile dysfunction.
   a. Phosphodiesterase inhibitors
   b. Prostaglandin E analogs
   c. Testosterone therapy
   d. All of the above

Bibliography

GBD. Benign Prostatic Hyperplasia Collaborators: The global, regional, and national burden of benign prostatic hyperplasia in 204 countries and territories from 2000 to 2019: a systematic analysis for the Global Burden of Disease Study 2019. *Lancet Healthy Longevity*. 2019;3(11):E754–E776, 2022.

Health Canada. Drug Product Database, 2023. Retrieved January 24, 2023, from https://www.canada.ca/en/health-canada/services/drugs-health-products/drug-products/drug-product-database.html.

Kapoor A. Benign prostatic hyperplasia (BPH) management in the primary care setting. *Can J Urol*. 2012;19(Suppl 1):10–17.

Knapp-Dlugosz C. *OTC advisor: popular herbal and dietary supplements*. Washington, DC: American Pharmacists Association; 2010.

Lakin M, Wood H. Erectile Dysfunction. *Cleveland Clinic Center for Continuing Education*. 2018. Retrieved January 24, 2023, from https://www.clevelandclinicmeded.com/medicalpubs/diseasemanagement/endocrinology/erectile-dysfunction/.

National Center for Complementary and Integrative Health Yohimbe. *U.S. Department of Health & Human Services, National Institutes of Health*. 2020. Retrieved January 24, 2023, from https://www.nccih.nih.gov/health/yohimbe.

National Center for Complementary and Integrative Health. Saw Palmetto. *U.S. Department of Health & Human Services, National Institutes of Health*. 2020. Retrieved January 24, 2023, from https://www.nccih.nih.gov/health/saw-palmetto.

National Kidney and Urologic Diseases Information Clearinghouse. Prostatitis: Inflammation of the Prostate. *National Institute of Diabetes and Digestive and Kidney Diseases*. 2014. Retrieved January 24, 2023, from https://www.niddk.nih.gov/health-information/urologic-diseases/prostate-problems/prostatitis-inflammation-prostate.

National Kidney and Urologic Diseases Information Clearinghouse. Prostate Enlargement: Benign Prostatic Hyperplasia. *The National Institute of Diabetes and Digestive and Kidney Diseases*. 2014. Retrieved January 24, 2023, from https://www.niddk.nih.gov/health-information/urologic-diseases/prostate-problems/prostate-enlargement-benign-prostatic-hyperplasia.

National Kidney and Urologic Diseases Information Clearinghouse. Erectile Dysfunction (NIH Publication No. 14–3923). *Bethesda: National Institute of Diabetes and Digestive and Kidney Diseases*. 2015. Retrieved January 24, 2023, from https://www.niddk.nih.gov/-/media/Files/Urologic-Diseases/Erectile_Dysfunction_Section_508.

Page C, Curtis M, Sutter M, et al. *Integrated pharmacology*. Philadelphia: Mosby; 2005:495–500.

Snoga J, Williams B, Courtney LA. Erectile dysfunction overview and treatment considerations in special populations. *US Pharmacist*. 2022;47(6):18–22.

U.S. Food and Drug Administration Drugs@FDA: FDA Approved Drug Products. Retrieved January 24, 2023, from https://www.accessdata.fda.gov/scripts/cder/daf/index.cfm.

Drugs Affecting the Immune System

The immune system, along with the nervous and endocrine systems, maintains the relative constancy of the body's internal environment. The immune system is made up of antibodies, proteins (immunoglobulins) on the surface of B cells, that mount an immune response and fight disease by recognizing and attacking antigens (foreign or abnormal substances). The immune system is continually patrolling the body for harmful or internal enemies. Our own cells have unique cell markers that identify our cells as self.

Cells that trigger immune responses are epithelial barrier cells, phagocytic cells (neutrophils, macrophages), natural killer (NK) cells, and cytokines, chemicals released from cells (e.g., interleukins, leukotrienes, and interferons) that are involved in innate immunity. Adaptive immunity involves mechanisms that recognize specific threatening agents and then adapt, or respond, by targeting their activity only against these agents. Lymphocytes (T cells and B cells) are the primary leukocytes (white blood cells) involved in adaptive immunity. The densest populations of lymphocytes occur in the bone marrow, thymus gland, lymph nodes, and spleen. Antibodies are proteins called immunoglobulins (Ig). There are five classes of antibodies, identified by letter names as immunoglobulins M, G, A, E, and D. The function of antibody molecules is to produce antibody-mediated immunity. They fight disease first by recognizing substances that are foreign or abnormal. Autoimmune disorders such as diabetes type 1 are a result of a hyperactive immune response. The body destroys β-cells in the pancreas that the body perceives as harmful invaders.

In Unit X, the treatment of bacterial infections, viral infections, and common types of cancers as well as vaccines, immunomodulators, and immunosuppressants are covered. A brief description of each disorder is provided, followed by a description of the drugs and antiviral agents indicated for treatment, mechanisms of action, adverse reactions, strength(s), and dosage forms.

29

Treatment of Bacterial Infections

LEARNING OBJECTIVES

1. Learn the terminology associated with treatments for infection.
2. Compare bacteriostatic with bactericidal.
3. Describe the morphology of bacterial cells.
4. Explain anti microbial resistance and list several reasons for its development.

5. List and categorize antiinfective agents.
6. Describe the mechanism of action for antiinfective agents.
7. List common beginnings and endings for antiinfective agents.
8. Identify significant drug look-alike and sound-alike issues.
9. Identify warning labels and precautionary messages associated with antiinfective agents.

KEY TERMS

Antibiotic A substance produced by or derived from a microorganism that is capable of destroying or inhibiting the growth of another microorganism (e.g., penicillin mold).
Antimicrobial A substance capable of destroying or inhibiting the growth of a microorganism.
Bactericidal Able to destroy bacteria.
Bacteriostatic Able to inhibit bacterial proliferation; host defense mechanisms destroy the bacteria.

Broad-spectrum antibiotic Antimicrobial that is capable of destroying a wide range of bacteria.
Antimicrobial resistance Ability of bacteria to overcome the bactericidal or bacteriostatic effects of an antiinfective agent. Resistance traits are encoded on bacterial genes and can be transferred to other bacteria.

Overview

Although chronic noninfectious disease is a leading cause of disability and death in high-income countries, infectious disease is still one of the leading causes of morbidity and mortality globally. In low- and middle-income countries, infectious diarrhea is a major cause of infant mortality. New infections of malaria and tuberculosis continue to grow. Poverty, malnutrition, lack of clean water, poor sanitation, and inadequate housing increase the risk for infectious disease and decrease the likelihood for adequate treatment.

Antimicrobial agents, also called antibiotic or antiinfective agents, play a key role in improving the survival of individuals with bacterial infections but do not treat viral infections. Technically, an *antibiotic* is a naturally occurring substance that is produced by or derived from a microorganism and is able to destroy or inhibit the growth of another microorganism. Bacteria that cause infection may be sensitive to the effects of one antiinfective agent but not another; therefore a culture and sensitivity test may also be performed. A small disk with antibiotic is placed in a culture from the infected patient and incubated in a petri dish. The larger the zone of inhibition (area of no bacterial growth) around the disk, the more effective the antibiotic will be in treating the bacterial infection. Effective treatment of bacterial infections is dependent on host factors, bacterial factors, and drug factors (Fig. 29.1). A drug factor that can influence how quickly a patient begins to "feel better"

after starting pharmacotherapy is whether the antiinfective agent is bactericidal or bacteriostatic. *Bactericidal* agents (e.g., penicillins) can destroy rapidly proliferating bacteria. Patients may begin to "feel better" within the first 24 hours. *Bacteriostatic* agents (e.g., tetracyclines) slow the growth of bacteria enough for the host's (our body's) defense mechanism to destroy the invading bacteria. It may take up to 3 days before patients start to "feel better."

Mechanisms of Antimicrobial Action

Antiinfective agents work by a variety of mechanisms of action, inhibiting (1) bacterial wall synthesis, (2) cell wall function, (3) protein synthesis, (4) bacterial deoxyribonucleic acid (DNA) or ribonucleic acid (RNA), and (5) folic acid. Fortunately, the anatomy of bacteria differs enough from humans that it is possible to destroy some bacteria without harming host cells.

Inhibition of Bacterial Cell Wall Synthesis

Many bacteria have a cell wall that is the target of some antibacterial agents. Because human cells lack cell walls, antibacterial agents that target the cell wall harm the bacteria without damaging the human host. Penicillins, cephalosporins, carbapenems, and monobactams are β-lactam antibiotics that inhibit cell wall synthesis (Fig. 29.2). The β-lactam ring is highlighted in pink (see Fig. 29.2). The β-lactam ring can be broken by some bacteria,

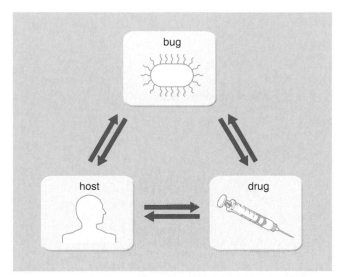

• **Fig. 29.1** Factors that influence successful antimicrobial therapy. (From Page C, Curtis M, Sutter M, et al. *Integrated pharmacology*, ed 3, Philadelphia, 2006, Mosby.)

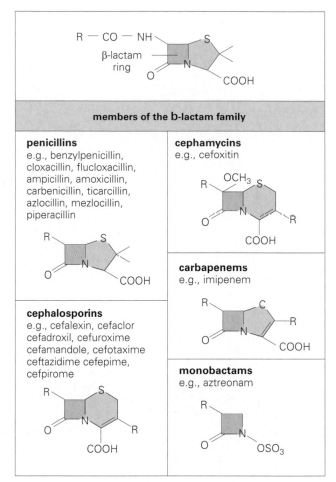

• **Fig. 29.2** Basic structure of β-lactam antibiotics. (From Page C, Curtis M, Sutter M, et al. *Integrated pharmacology*, ed 3, Philadelphia, 2006, Mosby.)

which inactivates the antibiotic's effects. Glycopeptides also target the bacterial cell wall. Vancomycin is the only glycopeptide antibiotic available in the United States and Canada.

Inhibition of Bacterial Cell Wall Function

Antibiotics that inhibit the function of the bacterial cell wall work by binding to bacterial membranes, where the antibiotic produces a detergent-like action that increases cell membrane permeability. This causes essential cell contents to leak out of the cell and destroys the bacteria. Polymyxin B is an example of an antibiotic that interferes with cell wall function.

Inhibition of Protein Synthesis

Aminoglycosides, macrolides, tetracyclines, amphenicols, and oxazolidinone are classes of antibacterial agents that inhibit the formation of the proteins that bacteria need to replicate. Specifically, they act to disrupt RNA function in the bacterial replication process (Fig. 29.3).

Inhibition of Bacterial Deoxyribonucleic Acid and Ribonucleic Acid Synthesis

Genetic code is stored in DNA. In the replication process, a strand of RNA forms along a strand of DNA. RNA regulates specific cell functions, such as editing strands of code. Without the ability to transfer the genetic code for the synthesis of bacteria cell constituents, bacteria are unable to replicate and spread. Fluoroquinolones and nitroimidazoles are classes of antibiotics capable of inhibiting DNA synthesis. Fluoroquinolones (e.g., ciprofloxacin) and nitroimidazoles (e.g., metronidazole) are predominantly bactericidal. Rifampin inhibits bacterial RNA synthesis.

Inhibition of Folic Acid

Folic acid is needed for the bacteria to synthesize DNA because unlike humans, bacteria cannot get folic acid from external sources. Bacteria synthesize folic acid from para-aminobenzoic acid (PABA). Antifolate agents and dihydrofolate reductase inhibitors block the bacterial synthesis of folic acid. Sulfonamides are antifolate drugs, and trimethoprim is a dihydrofolate reductase inhibitor (Fig. 29.4).

Antimicrobial Resistance

Microbes spread rapidly, mutate frequently, and adapt with relative ease to new environments and hosts. Unfortunately, microbes can learn how to withstand the effects of antibiotics. Superbugs are resistant to currently available antimicrobial agents. Multidrug resistance is a serious problem, and, although previously only a risk for hospitalized patients, multidrug-resistant tuberculosis, vancomycin-resistant enterococci, and methicillin-resistant *Staphylococcus aureus* are spreading outside of hospitals. **Antimicrobial resistance** is the ability of bacteria to overcome the bactericidal effects of an antibiotic. Bacteria may overcome the effects of antiinfective agents by secreting an enzyme (e.g., β-lactamase) that inactivates the β-lactam antibiotics like amoxicillin. There are three β-lactamase inhibitors: clavulanic acid (clavulanate), sulbactam, and tazobactam. Macrolide antibiotics are inactivated by bacterial production of enzymes (e.g., erythromycin ribosomal methylase). Bacteria can mutate to modify the site on the ribosome to which the antibiotic normally binds. This is a mechanism for resistance to macrolide antibiotics (e.g., erythromycin).

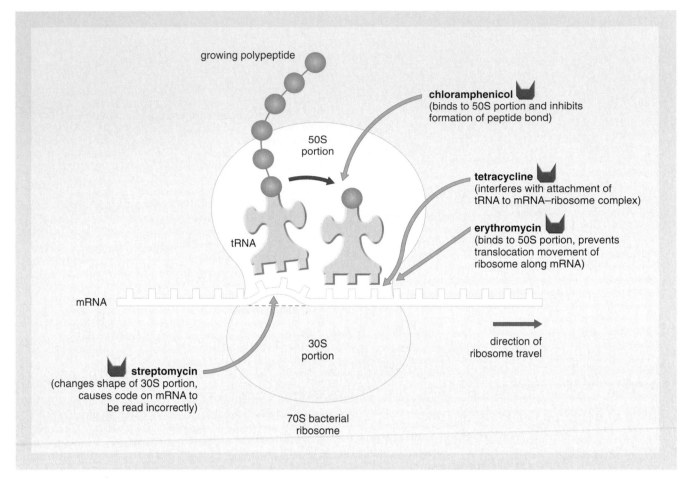

• **Fig. 29.3** Antibiotics that inhibit bacterial protein synthesis. (From Page C, Curtis M, Sutter M, et al. *Integrated pharmacology*, ed 3, Philadelphia, 2006, Mosby.)

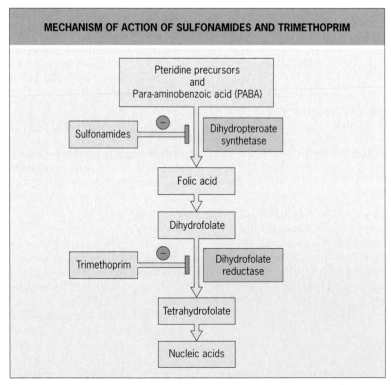

• **Fig. 29.4** The folate biosynthetic pathway. *DHFR*, Dihydrofolate reductase; *DHPS*, dihydropteroate synthase; *PABA*, para-aminobenzoic acid. (From Page C, Curtis M, Sutter M, et al. *Integrated pharmacology*, ed 3, Philadelphia, 2006, Mosby.)

Bacteria that are resistant to macrolides are capable of lowering the concentration of the antibiotic by transporting the antibiotic out of the cell. Bacteria previously sensitive to the effects of aminoglycosides can become resistant by adding an acetyl or phosphoryl group to the antibiotic, which inhibits the antibiotic's ability to reach the bacterial binding site. Bacteria that are resistant to tetracyclines have mutated to change the transport mechanism that causes the antibiotic to accumulate in the bacterial cell. Resistance traits can be transferred to other bacteria. Bacteria resistant to one penicillin antibiotic may also be resistant to most penicillins and other β-lactams, including cephalosporins.

Misuse of antimicrobial agents is a major cause for the development and spread of anti microbial resistance. Misuse includes the following: (1) inappropriate prescribing, (2) failure to complete the full course of therapy, (3) administration of antibacterial agents for viral infections (e.g., the common cold), (4) antibiotics in the food chain (agriculture, animal husbandry, fish farms), and (5) lack of guidelines for preventing the spread of infections in institutional care settings.

Classification of Antimicrobial Agents

Aminoglycosides

Aminoglycoside antiinfective agents are effective for treating serious infections of the bone, abdomen, heart, brain, urinary tract, reproductive system, skin, and kidneys caused by bacteria that are sensitive to their antimicrobial effects. Examples are peritonitis, septicemia, meningitis, pelvic inflammatory disease, and endocarditis. Aminoglycosides may also be administered to sterilize the bowel before bowel surgery. Ophthalmic dosage forms are also prescribed for the treatment of blepharitis and conjunctivitis (see Chapter 15).

Mechanism of Action and Pharmacokinetics

Aminoglycosides inhibit bacterial protein synthesis. They enter the bacterial cell via an oxygen-dependent transport system, which explains why they are effective against aerobic bacteria and not anaerobic bacteria. They bind to a site on the bacterial ribosome that causes the genetic code carried by messenger RNA (mRNA) to be read incorrectly.

Aminoglycosides are not absorbed systemically when administered by mouth. The only aminoglycoside that is administered orally (neomycin) is used to reduce the bacteria in the bowel before colorectal surgery. Other nonparenteral use is topical application for skin, eye, and ear infections. Aminoglycosides for topical use are commonly marketed in combination products that contain additional antiinfective agents, local anesthetic drugs, and/or antiinflammatory agents, such as Lanobiotic and Viaderm KC.

Adverse Reactions

Aminoglycosides may cause hearing loss (ototoxicity) and kidney damage (nephrotoxicity). These effects limit their use to the treatment of serious infections. There is little risk for this side effect when it is applied topically.

Cephalosporins

Cephalosporins have a β-lactam ring structure (see Fig. 29.2). Like penicillins, the different side chains added to the basic β-lactam ring structure can affect the antimicrobial spectrum of activity. They are classified as first-, second-, third-, and fourth-generation

cephalosporins. First-generation cephalosporins are most effective against staphylococcal infections and streptococcal infections of the skin and soft tissue caused by gram-positive aerobic (require oxygen) bacteria. Gram stain is a process used to identify types of bacteria. A crystal violet stain is applied to a sample taken from the site of the infection. When the stain is washed out, gram-positive bacteria retain a dark purple color. Gram-negative bacteria retain a pink color. Second-generation cephalosporins are effective for treating upper respiratory infections (URIs) such as *Haemophilus influenzae* caused by gram-positive and gram-negative bacteria. Third-generation cephalosporins are used to treat bacterial meningitis, gonorrhea, intraabdominal infections (e.g., peritonitis), and bone and joint infections caused by gram-negative anaerobic bacteria. The fourth-generation cephalosporin cefepime is administered to treat pneumonia (community-acquired and nosocomial) and urinary tract infections (UTIs).

Aminoglycosides

Generic Name	US Brand Name(s) / Canadian Brand Name(s)	Dosage Forms and Strengths
amikacin[a]	Generics / Generics	**Solution, for injection:** 50 mg/mL[b], 250 mg/mL
gentamicin[a]	Generics (except ophthalmic medications) / Generics	**Cream**[b]: 0.1% **Ointment**[b]: 0.1% **Solution, for injection:** 10 mg/mL, 40 mg/mL **Solution, in normal saline:** 0.8 mg/mL[b], 1 mg/mL, 1.2 mg/mL[b], 1.6 mg/mL, 2 mg/mL[b] **Ophthalmic ointment and solution:** see Chapter 15
neomycin[a]	Generics / Not available	**Tablet:** 500 mg
streptomycin[a]	Generics / Generics	**Powder, for injection:** 1 g/vial
tobramycin[a]	Bethkis, Kitabis Pak, Tobi, Tobi Podhaler / Tobi, Tobi Podhaler	**Capsule, for inhalation (Tobi Podhaler):** 28 mg **Powder, for injection:** 1.2 g/vial **Solution, for inhalation:** 300 mg/4 mL (Bethkis)[b], 300 mg/5 mL (Kitabis Pak, Tobi) **Solution, for injection:** 10 mg/mL, 40 mg/mL **Solution, for injection in normal saline (NS)**[b]: 1.2 mg/mL **Ophthalmic ointment and solution:** See Chapter 15

[a]Generic available.
[b]Available in the United States only.

Mechanism of Action

Cephalosporins inhibit the third and final stage of bacterial cell wall synthesis by binding to specific penicillin-binding proteins (PBPs) located inside the bacterial cell wall. Because PBPs vary among different bacterial species, cephalosporin spectrum of activity is dependent on the drug's ability to bind to a specified bacterial PBP.

Pharmacokinetics

Cephalosporins are formulated for oral, intramuscular, and intravenous use. Cefixime is the only third-generation cephalosporin that is administered orally. In contrast, all but two second-generation cephalosporins (cefotetan, cefoxitin) are available for oral use. First-generation cephalosporins do not penetrate the cerebrospinal fluid in adequate concentration to treat meningitis, whereas most third-generation agents reach a high-enough level. The fourth-generation agent has a greater ability to penetrate the bacterial cell wall of gram-negative bacteria than third-generation agents and is more resistant to destruction by β-lactamases.

Adverse Reactions

Adverse reactions produced by cephalosporins include diarrhea, headache, dizziness, nausea, vomiting, gas, abdominal pain, dry mouth, and heartburn.

Cephalosporins

Generic Name	US Brand Name(s) / Canadian Brand Name(s)	Dosage Forms and Strengths
First-Generation Cephalosporins		
cefazolin[a]	Generics / Generics	**Powder, for injection:** 0.5 g/vial, 1 g/vial, 2 g/vial[c], 10 g/vial, 100 g/bag[c]
cefadroxil[a]	Generics / Generics	**Capsule:** 500 mg **Powder, for oral suspension**[b]: 250 mg/5 mL, 500 mg/5 mL **Tablet**[b]: 1 g
cephalexin[a]	Generics / Generics	**Capsule:** 250 mg, 333 mg[b], 500 mg, 750 mg[b] **Powder, for oral suspension:** 125 mg/5 mL, 250 mg/5 mL **Tablet:** 250 mg, 500 mg
Second-Generation Cephalosporins		
cefaclor[a]	Generics / Not available	**Capsule:** 250 mg, 500 mg **Powder, for oral suspension:** 125 mg/5 mL, 187 mg/5 mL, 250 mg/5 mL, 375 mg/5 mL **Tablet, extended release:** 375 mg, 500 mg
cefotetan[a]	Cefotan / Not available	**Powder, for injection:** 1 g/vial, 2 g/vial, 10 g/vial
cefoxitin[a]	Generics / Generics	**Powder, for injection:** 1 g/vial, 2 g/vial, 10 g/vial
cefuroxime[a]	Zinacef / Ceftin	**Powder, for injection:** 750 mg/vial, 1.5 g/vial **Powder, for oral suspension**[c]: 125 mg/5 mL **Solution, for injection**[b]: 1.5 g/20 mL, 1.5 g/100 mL **Tablet:** 125 mg[b], 250 mg, 500 mg
Third-Generation Cephalosporins		
cefotaxime	Generics / Generics	**Powder, for injection:** 500 mg/vial[b], 1 g/vial, 2 g/vial, 10 g/vial[b]
ceftazidime[a]	Fortaz, Tazicef / Generic	**Powder, for injection:** 500 mg/vial[b], 1 g/vial, 2 g/vial, 6 g/vial

Cephalosporins—cont'd

Generic Name	US Brand Name(s) / Canadian Brand Name(s)	Dosage Forms and Strengths
ceftriaxone[a]	Generics Generics	**Powder, for injection:** 250 mg, 500 mg[b], 1 g, 2 g, 10 g **Solution, for injection**[c]: 20 mg/mL, 40 mg/mL
cefixime[a]	Suprax Suprax	**Capsule**[b]: 400 mg **Powder, for oral suspension:** 100 mg/5 mL, 200 mg/5 mL[b], 500 mg/5 mL[b], **Tablet:** 400 mg **Tablet, chewable**[b]: 100 mg, 150 mg, 200 mg
cefpodoxime[a]	Generics Not available	**Powder, for oral suspension:** 50 mg/5 mL, 100 mg/5 mL **Tablet:** 100 mg, 200 mg
Fourth-Generation Cephalosporin		
cefepime[a]	Maxipime Generics	**Powder, for injection:** 500 mg/vial[b], 1 g/vial, 2 g/vial

[a]Generic available.
[b]Available in the United States only.
[c]Available in Canada only.

Fluoroquinolones

Fluoroquinolones are indicated for the treatment of UTIs, sinusitis, sexually transmitted infections, bacterial conjunctivitis (see Chapter 15), infectious diarrhea, anthrax, and numerous other infections.

> **⊘ Tech Alert!**
>
> A common ending of fluoroquinolone is -floxacin.

> **⊘ Tech Alert!**
>
> The following drugs have look-alike/sound-alike issues:
> Noroxin and Neurontin

Mechanism of Action and Pharmacokinetics

Fluoroquinolones inhibit the enzyme DNA gyrase that is responsible for blocking one of the processes of DNA replication. This results in the inhibition of bacterial DNA synthesis.

Fluoroquinolones are formulated for oral, ophthalmic, and parenteral use. Oral absorption is good. The half-life ($t^{1/2}$) of the newer agents such as moxifloxacin is long, permitting once-daily dosing, whereas ciprofloxacin ($t^{1/2} \cong 4$ hours) is dosed every 12 hours.

Adverse Reactions and Precautions

Common adverse reactions are diarrhea, crystalluria, photosensitivity, dizziness, drowsiness, headache, nausea, and stomach upset. Cartilage deformities may occur in children and developing fetuses, so quinolones are contraindicated in children and pregnant women. Quinolones can also cause arrhythmias by prolongation of the QT interval, musculoskeletal pain, and, rarely, peripheral neuropathy.

Macrolides

Azithromycin, clarithromycin, and erythromycin are macrolide antibiotics that are primarily used for the treatment of URIs. Other important uses are the treatment of peptic ulcer disease (PUD), eye infections, and acne. Erythromycin, the prototype for the macrolides, is used for the prevention of neonatal eye infections and acne, in addition to treatment of URIs. Clarithromycin is one of the ingredients in multidrug treatment regimens for PUD caused by the bacterium *Helicobacter pylori* (see Chapter 21).

Mechanism of Action

Macrolides inhibit bacterial protein synthesis by binding to the 50 S ribosomal subunit and blocking the translocation movement along mRNA.

Pharmacokinetics

Macrolides are formulated for oral, parenteral, and ophthalmic use. Erythromycin base is formulated for immediate release and delayed release. Delayed-release tablets have a lower incidence of gastrointestinal (GI) side effects than do immediate-release tablets.

The expiration date of powder for the oral suspension of erythromycin, clarithromycin, and azithromycin is shortened once the drug is reconstituted. Refrigeration is recommended for oral suspensions of erythromycin; storage at room temperature is recommended for clarithromycin and azithromycin.

Adverse Reactions

GI upset is common with the use of macrolides. It occurs in up to 21% of those who take erythromycin. The incidence of GI upset is less with clarithromycin (10%) and azithromycin (5%). Erythromycin and clarithromycin can cause arrhythmias by prolongation of the QT interval. Other adverse reactions include headache and tinnitus. Macrolides may decrease the effectiveness of oral contraceptives.

Fluoroquinolones

Generic Name	US Brand Name(s) / Canadian Brand Name(s)	Dosage Forms and Strengths
ciprofloxacin[a]	Cetraxal, Ciloxan, Cipro, Cipro XR Ciloxan, Cipro, Cipro XL, Otixal	**Powder, for oral suspension (Cipro):** 250 mg/5 mL[b], 500 mg/5 mL **Tablet:** 250 mg, 500 mg, 750 mg **Tablet, extended release (Cipro XL, Cipro XR):** 500 mg, 1000 mg **Ophthalmic and otic solution (Ciloxan, Cetraxal, Otixal):** see Chapter 15 **Solution, for injection:** 2 mg/mL[c], 10 mg/mL[b]
gatifloxacin[a]	Zymar, Zymaxid Zymar	**Ophthalmic solution:** see Chapter 15
levofloxacin[a]	Generics Quinsair	**Ophthalmic solution:** see Chapter 15 **Solution, for injection:** 25 mg/mL[b] **Solution, for injection in 5% dextrose[c]:** 5 mg/mL **Solution, oral:** 25 mg/mL[b] **Solution, for inhalation (Quinsair)[c]:** 240 mg/2.4 mL **Tablet:** 250 mg, 500 mg, 750 mg
moxifloxacin[a]	Avelox, Moxeza, Vigamox Vigamox	**Ophthalmic solution (Moxeza, Vigamox):** see Chapter 15 **Tablet:** 400 mg **Solution, for IV:** 400 mg/250 mL
ofloxacin[a]	Generics (except ophthalmic) Ocuflox	**Ophthalmic and otic solution (Ocuflox):** see Chapter 15 **Tablet[b]:** 200 mg, 300 mg, 400 mg
norfloxacin[a]	Not available Generics	**Tablet:** 400 mg

[a]Generic available.
[b]Available in the United States only.
[c]Available in Canada only.

Macrolides and Related Antiinfective Agents

Generic Name	US Brand Name(s) / Canadian Brand Name(s)	Dosage Forms and Strengths
azithromycin[a]	Azasite, Zithromax Zithromax	**Ophthalmic solution (Azasite):** see Chapter 15 **Powder, for injection:** 500 mg/vial **Powder, for oral suspension (Zithromax):** 100 mg/5 mL, 200 mg/5 mL, 1 g (single dose) [b] **Tablet (Zithromax):** 250 mg, 500 mg[b], 600 mg
clarithromycin[a]	Biaxin XL Biaxin, Biaxin BID, Biaxin XL	**Powder, for suspension:** 125 mg/5 mL, 250 mg/5 mL **Tablet (Biaxin, Biaxin BID):** 250 mg, 500 mg **Tablet, extended release (Biaxin XL):** 250 mg[b], 500 mg
erythromycin base[a] (immediate release)	Ery-gel, Erytha-derm Generics	**Gel, topical (Ery-gel)[b]:** 2% **Ophthalmic ointment:** 0.5% **Tablet (generics)[b]:** 250 mg, 500 mg **Solution, topical[b]:** 2% **Swab[b]:** 2%
erythromycin base[a] (delayed release)	ERYC, Ery-Tab ERYC	**Capsule:** 250 mg[b], 333 mg[c] **Tablet, delayed release (Ery-Tab):** 250 mg, 333 mg, 500 mg
erythromycin stearate[a]	Erythrocin Generic	**Tablet:** 250 mg
erythromycin ethylsuccinate[a]	EES, EES 400, Eryped Not available	**Granules, for oral suspension:** 200 mg/5 mL, 400 mg/5 mL **Tablet:** 400 mg
erythromycin lactobionate[a]	Erythrocin Generic	**Powder, for injection:** 500 mg, 1 g[c]

[a]Generic available.
[b]Available in the United States only.
[c]Available in Canada only.

Oxazolidinones

Linezolid is a newer antimicrobial agent indicated for the treatment of gram-positive bacterial pneumonia and skin structure infections. Its use is limited because of adverse side effects and to limit the development of bacterial resistance.

Mechanism of Action and Pharmacokinetics

Linezolid inhibits bacterial protein synthesis. Its action on the bacterial ribosome blocks a key step in the translation process, which inhibits bacterial replication. The metabolism of linezolid is not well understood. Linezolid has no effect on cytochrome P-450 (CYP450) isoenzymes, so it has fewer drug interactions involving drug metabolism.

Adverse Reactions

The most common side effects of linezolid are skin rash, itching, change in taste, headache, mild diarrhea, dizziness, mild stomach upset, nausea, vomiting, and temporary tongue discoloration.

Oxazolidinones

Generic Name	US Brand Name(s) / Canadian Brand Name(s)	Dosage Forms and Strengths
linezolid[a]	Zyvox / Zyvoxam	**Powder, for suspension**: 100 mg/5 mL **Solution, for injection**: 2 mg/mL **Tablet**: 600 mg

[a]Generic available.

Penicillins and Carbapenems

Penicillin was one of the first antibiotics discovered. It is a naturally occurring substance originally produced by the mold *Penicillium chrysogenum* (also known as *Penicillium notatum*) and can grow on stale bread and fruit. Oral penicillins are used to treat many infections, including URIs, otitis media, skin infections, and strep throat, and to prevent recurrent rheumatic fever. Penicillins may be administered before dental and other medical procedures to prevent bacterial endocarditis in individuals with prosthetic heart valves. Parenteral penicillins are used for the treatment of numerous infections, including bone and joint infections, diabetic foot ulcers, infectious arthritis, sexually transmitted infections, meningitis, and septicemia.

> **⊘ Tech Alert!**
>
> A common ending of the penicillin family of drugs is *-cillin*.

> **⊘ Tech Alert!**
>
> Persons who are allergic to penicillin may also be allergic to cephalosporins.

> **⊘ Tech Alert!**
>
> The following drugs have look-alike/sound-alike issues:
> penicillin and penicillAMINE;
> Augmentin and Augmentin XR

Mechanism of Action

Penicillins are β-lactam antibiotics; they inhibit the synthesis of the cell wall of sensitive microbes. Side chains on this structure alter the antibacterial and pharmacologic properties of the basic penicillin molecule. The side chains can extend the antimicrobial spectrum. For example, amoxicillin and ticarcillin are effective against more types of bacteria than is penicillin. Antistaphylococcal penicillins are penicillinase resistant and are not inactivated by penicillinase (staphylococcal β-lactamase), a substance produced by the bacteria that destroys the antibiotic's β-lactam ring.

Carbapenems have a β-lactam ring fused with a penem ring. Carbapenems inhibit the third step in bacterial cell wall synthesis. Their spectrum of activity is broad, and they resist inactivation by microbial enzymes (e.g., β-lactamase).

Pharmacokinetics

Many penicillins lack stability in gastric acids, which is why most are administered intramuscularly or must be taken on an empty stomach. The exception is penicillin VK, which is relatively acid stable.

Procaine penicillin G and benzathine penicillin G are formulated to delay absorption and achieve prolonged blood levels. Levels of benzathine penicillin G can be detected in the blood up to 1 month after an intramuscular injection of the drug is given.

Penicillins that are formulated as powders for reconstitution have shortened expiration dates once mixed with water. Expiration dates range from 10 to 14 days, depending on the drug. Most suspensions should be refrigerated after they are reconstituted.

> **⊘ Tech Alert!**
>
> The quantity of clavulanic acid varies widely between products. It is important to read the stock bottle label carefully before making product substitutions.

Adverse Reactions

GI side effects such as diarrhea, loss of appetite, nausea, vomiting, sore mouth, stomach gas, and heartburn are the most common adverse reactions to penicillins. Other adverse effects include superinfection and hypersensitivity reactions. Penicillins may decrease the effectiveness of oral contraceptives.

Sulfonamides

Sulfonamides are the oldest antimicrobial agents. They were developed in the 1930s, but their use did not spread until the 1940s during World War II. Sulfonamides are commonly called sulfa drugs because the generic name of all agents begins with *sulf-*. Sulfonamides and trimethoprim are used in the treatment of various upper respiratory, urinary tract, and skin infections. They are also indicated for the treatment of AIDS-related pneumonia (caused by *Pneumocystis jirovecii*).

Penicillins

Generic Name	US Brand Name(s) / Canadian Brand Name(s)	Dosage Forms and Strengths
Penicillin		
penicillin G potassium[a]	Pfizerpen	**Powder, for injection:** 1 million units, 5 million units, 20 million units
	Not available for human use	
phenoxymethyl penicillin potassium[a] (penicillin VK)	Generics	**Powder, for oral suspension**[b]: 125 mg/5 mL, 250 mg/5 mL **Tablets:** 250 mg, 300 mg[c], 500 mg
	Not available	
benzathine penicillin G[a]	Bicillin L-A	**Suspension, for IM injection:** 600,000 units/mL
	Bicillin L-A	
benzylpenicillin (penicillin G sodium)	Generics	**Powder, for injection:** 1 million units/vial[c], 5 million units/vial, 10 million units/vial[c]
	Generics	
Aminopenicillins: Extended Spectrum		
amoxicillin[a]	Amoxil, Larotid	**Capsule:** 250 mg, 500 mg **Powder, for oral suspension:** 50 mg/mL[b], 125 mg/5 mL, 200 mg/5 mL[b], 250 mg/5 mL, 400 mg/5 mL[b] **Tablet**[b]: 500 mg, 875 mg **Tablet, chewable**[b]: 125 mg, 250 mg
	Generics	
ampicillin[a]	Generics	**Capsule:** 500 mg **Powder, for injection:** 125 mg[b], 250 mg, 500 mg, 1 g, 2 g, 10 g[b] **Powder, for oral suspension**[b]: 125 mg/5 mL, 250 mg/5 mL
	Generics	
Antistaphylococcal Penicillins: Penicillinase Resistant		
cloxacillin[a]	Not available	**Capsule:** 250 mg, 500 mg **Powder, for oral suspension:** 125 mg/5 mL **Powder, for injection:** 0.5 g, 1 g, 2 g, 10 g
	Generics	
dicloxacillin[a]	Generics	**Capsule:** 250 mg, 500 mg
	Not available	
nafcillin[a]	Nallpen	**Powder, for injection:** 1 g, 2 g, 10 g **Solution, for injection (Nallpen):** 20 mg/mL
	Not available	
oxacillin[a]	Bactocill	**Powder, for injection:** 1 g, 2 g, 10 g
	Not available	
Antipseudomonal Penicillins		
piperacillin[a]	Generic	**Powder, for injection:** 2 g, 3 g, 4 g, 40 g
	Not available	
Penicillin Combinations		
amoxicillin + clavulanic acid[a]	Augmentin, Augmentin ES, Augmentin XR	**Powder, for oral suspension:** amoxicillin 125 mg + clavulanic acid 31.25 mg/5 mL amoxicillin 200 mg + clavulanic acid 28.5 mg/5 mL amoxicillin 250 mg + clavulanic acid 62.5 mg/5 mL amoxicillin 400 mg + clavulanic acid 57 mg/5 mL amoxicillin 600 mg + clavulanic acid 42.9 mg/5 mL **Tablet:** amoxicillin 250 mg + clavulanic acid 125 mg amoxicillin 500 mg + clavulanic acid 125 mg amoxicillin 875 mg + clavulanic acid 125 mg **Tablet, chewable (Augmentin):** amoxicillin 200 mg + clavulanic acid 28.5 mg amoxicillin 400 mg + clavulanic acid 57 mg **Tablet, extended release**[b]: amoxicillin 1000 mg + clavulanic acid 62.5 mg
	Clavulin	

Penicillins—cont'd

Generic Name	US Brand Name(s) / Canadian Brand Name(s)	Dosage Forms and Strengths
ampicillin + sulbactam[a]	Unasyn	**Powder, for injection:** ampicillin 1 g + sulbactam 0.5 g
	Not available	ampicillin 2 g + sulbactam 1 g
		ampicillin 10 g + sulbactam 5 g
piperacillin + tazobactam	Zosyn	**Powder, for injection:** piperacillin 2 g + tazobactam 0.25 g/vial
	Tazocin	piperacillin 3 g + tazobactam 0.375 g/vial
		piperacillin 4 g + tazobactam 0.5 g/vial
		piperacillin 12 g + tazobactam 1.5 g/vial[c]
		pipcracillin 36 g + tazobactam 4.5 g/vial

[a]Generic available.
[b]Available in the United States only.
[c]Available in Canada only.

Carbapenems

Generic Name	US Brand Name(s) / Canadian Brand Name(s)	Dosage Forms and Strengths
ertapenem[a]	Invanz	**Powder, for injection:** 1 g/vial
	Invanz	
imipenem + cilastatin[a]	Primaxin	**Powder, for injection:** imipenem 250 mg + cilastatin 250 mg/vial[b], imipenem 500 mg + cilastatin 500 mg/vial
	Generics	
meropenem[a]	Merrem	**Powder, for injection:** 500 mg/vial, 1 g/vial
	Merrem	
meropenem + vaborbactam	Vabomere	**Powder, for injection:** meropenem 1 g + vaborbactam 1 g
	Not available	
imipenem + cilastatin + relebactam	Recarbrio	**Powder, intravenous:** imipenem + cilastatin + relebactam
	Not available	

[a]Generic available.
[b]Available in Canada only.

> **● Tech Note!**
>
> A common beginning for sulfonamides is *sulf-*.

> **❶ Tech Alert!**
>
> The following drugs have look-alike/sound-alike issues:
> sulfADIAZINE, sulfiSOXAZOLE, and sulfaSALAzine;
> sulfamethoxazole + trimethoprim single-strength and sulfamethoxazole + trimethoprim double-strength

Mechanism of Action and Pharmacokinetics

Sulfonamides and trimethoprim are antifolate drugs. They interfere with the microbial synthesis of folic acid at separate steps in the biosynthetic pathway that ultimately leads to bacterial DNA synthesis (see Fig. 29.4). Food may slightly decrease the absorption of sulfonamides; however, the drug may be taken with small amounts of food to reduce GI upset.

> **❶ Tech Alert!**
>
> The warning label "Take with Lots of Water" is put on prescription vials for sulfonamides. This reduces the risk of kidney damage caused by crystalluria.

Adverse Reactions

Common adverse reactions are nausea, vomiting, abdominal pain, headache, drowsiness, dizziness, diarrhea, and photosensitivity. Sulfonamides may promote the formation of crystals in the urine (crystalluria), especially if taken with acidic foods or beverages.

Tetracyclines

Tetracyclines are **broad-spectrum antibiotic** (antibacterial) agents. They may be bactericidal or bacteriostatic. They are used for the treatment of acne, sexually transmitted infections such as chlamydia, Lyme disease, and Rocky Mountain spotted fever.

> **● Tech Note!**
>
> A common ending for the tetracycline family of drugs is *-cycline*.

Mechanism of Action and Pharmacokinetics

Tetracyclines inhibit bacterial protein synthesis. Doxycycline and minocycline are more stable in the acidic stomach contents than tetracycline. They also have a longer duration of action. They are given once or twice daily compared with tetracycline, which is given four times daily. Tetracycline interacts with dairy products, calcium, aluminum, and ferrous supplements to form a chelated

Sulfonamides

	US Brand Name(s)	
Generic Name	Canadian Brand Name(s)	Dosage Forms and Strengths
Sulfonamides		
sulfadiazine[a]	Generics	**Tablet:** 500 mg
	Not available	
Combination Sulfonamides		
sulfamethoxazole + trimethoprim[a] (SMX-TMP; Cotrimox)	Bactrim, Bactrim DS, Septra, Septra DS, Sulfatrim Pediatric	**Solution, for injection:** sulfamethoxazole 80 mg/mL + trimethoprim 16 mg/mL
	Septra, Sulfatrim, Sulfatrim DS, Sulfatrim Pediatric	**Tablet:** sulfamethoxazole 100 mg + trimethoprim 20 mg[b] sulfamethoxazole 400 mg + trimethoprim 80 mg sulfamethoxazole 800 mg + trimethoprim 160 mg
		Suspension[c]: sulfamethoxazole 200 mg/5 mL + trimethoprim 40 mg/5 mL

[a]Generic available.
[b]Available in Canada only.
[c]Available in the United States only.

complex. The complex significantly reduces the absorption of tetracycline and should be avoided.

Adverse Reactions

The tetracyclines can cause nausea, vomiting, diarrhea, and photosensitivity. Serious but less common side effects include hepatotoxicity, pseudomembranous colitis, and kidney disease. Outdated tetracycline becomes toxic. Patients should be advised to discard old medicines. Tetracyclines may decrease the effectiveness of oral contraceptives.

Tetracyclines

	US Brand Name(s)	
Dosage Forms and Strengths	Canadian Brand Name(s)	Dosage Forms and Strengths
demeclocycline[a]	Generics	**Tablet:** 150 mg, 300 mg
	Not available	
doxycycline anhydrous	Oracea	**Capsule, immediate + delayed release (Oracea):** 40 mg
	Not available	
doxycycline calcium	Vibramycin	**Powder, for oral suspension:** 25 mg/5 mL, 50 mg/5 mL
	Not available	

Tetracyclines—cont'd

	Dosage Forms and Strengths	US Brand Name(s) / Canadian Brand Name(s)	Dosage Forms and Strengths
	doxycycline hyclate[a]	Acticlate, Doryx, Vibramycin Doxytab, Periostat	**Capsule:** 20 mg (Periostat)[b], 50 mg[c], 75 mg (Acticlate)[c], 100 mg **Powder, for injection**[c]: 100 mg/vial, 200 mg/vial **Suspension:** 25 mg/5 mL, 50 mg/5 mL **Tablet:** 50 mg[c], 75 mg[c], 100 mg, 150 mg[c] **Tablet, delayed release (Doryx)**[c]: 50 mg, 60 mg, 75 mg, 80 mg, 100 mg, 120 mg, 150 mg, 200 mg
	doxycycline monohydrate[a]	Monodox Apprilon	**Capsule:** 40 mg (Apprilon), 50 mg, 75 mg, 100 mg, 150 mg
	minocycline[a]	Amzeeq, Arestin, Dynacin, Minocin, Minolira, Solodyn, Ximino, Zilxi Arestin	**Capsule:** 50 mg, 75 mg[c], 100 mg **Capsule, extended release (Ximino):** 45 mg, 67.5 mg, 90 mg, 112.5 mg, 135 mg **Foam:** 1.5% (Zilxi), 4% Amzeeq **Powder, for injection**[c]: 100 mg/vial **Powder, periodontal sustained release (Arestin):** 1 mg **Tablet**[c]: 50 mg, 75 mg, 100 mg **Tablet, extended release (Minolira, Solodyn)**[c]: 55 mg, 65 mg, 80 mg, 115 mg (Solodyn) 105 mg, 135 mg (Minolira)
	tetracycline[a]	Achromycin V Generics	**Capsule:** 250 mg, 500 mg[c]
	tigecycline[a]	Tygacil Tygacil	**Powder, for injection:** 50 mg/vial

[a]Generic available.
[b]Available in Canada only.
[c]Available in the United States only.

Miscellaneous Antibacterial Agents

Isoniazid is used for the treatment of tuberculosis. It inhibits the synthesis of mycolic acid, an important constituent of the highly lipid cell wall of mycobacteria. Isoniazid may cause liver disease and nerve damage. Concurrent administration of vitamin B_6 is recommended to prevent neurotoxicity.

Metronidazole is an amebicide. It destroys the protozoa that cause giardiasis (traveler's diarrhea) and trichomoniasis (a sexually transmitted infection). It is the drug of choice for the treatment of *Clostridium difficile* enteritis, a condition that may cause pseudomembranous colitis. Topical preparations are used for the treatment of acne rosacea. It is formulated for oral, parenteral, vaginal, and topical use. Alcoholic beverages or medicines containing high levels of alcohol may produce nausea, vomiting, stomach pains, headache, and dizziness. The drug may also produce a metallic taste.

Mupirocin is a topically applied antimicrobial agent used to treat staphylococcal infections of the skin, such as impetigo.

Chloramphenicol is a broad-spectrum antimicrobial agent that inhibits protein synthesis. It is typically prescribed as a second-line therapy, when other less toxic drugs cannot be used (e.g., for drug allergy). It may be used for the treatment of bacterial meningitis, brain abscess, and Rocky Mountain spotted fever. It is contraindicated in neonates and children.

Clindamycin is an antimicrobial agent used topically for the treatment of acne and vaginosis. Systemic use of clindamycin is associated with the development of *C. difficile*, a bacterium that causes diarrhea and pseudomembranous colitis. Drinking plenty of fluids can lower the risk of the development of this condition.

Malaria is a parasitic infection caused by *Plasmodium falciparum*. The parasite infects humans bitten by an infected mosquito. Drugs prescribed to treat malaria are chloroquine, mefloquine, primaquine, tafenoquine, and artemether-lumefantrine. Tafenoquine is the newest antimalarial and the first new agent to be developed and marketed in more than 70 years. Tafenoquine is taken concurrently with chloroquine and is indicated to prevent relapse of malaria. The full course of therapy is taken as a single dose on day 1 or 2 of drug treatment with chloroquine. Primaquine is also administered to prevent relapsing malaria. Mefloquine (Malarone) is used to treat and prevent malaria. Its malaria treatment regimen differs from its malaria prevention regimen. When mefloquine is prescribed for the prevention of malaria, the drug must be taken for the entire period the individual is within the malaria area. Mefloquine (Malarone) and the combination drug artemether + lumefantrine (Coartem) can be taken by children. Malarone is marketed as a suspension and Coartem may be crushed and dissolved in water.

TECHNICIAN'S CORNER

1. With antimicrobial resistance developing against antibiotics, what steps should be taken by the pharmaceutical and food industries, patients, and health care providers to combat this problem?
2. Can the practice of universal precautions (e.g., handwashing) reduce the incidence of nosocomial infections?

Miscellaneous Antiinfective Agents

Generic Name	US Brand Name(s) / Canadian Brand Name(s)	Dosage Forms and Strengths
dalbavancin	Dalvance	**Powder, for infusion:** 500 mg/vial
	Not available	
oritavancin	Orbactiv	**Powder, for infusion:** 400 mg/vial
	Not available	
isoniazid[a]	Generics	**Solution, for injection:** 100 mg/mL[b]
	Generics	**Syrup, oral:** 50 mg/5 mL **Tablet:** 100 mg, 300 mg
metronidazole[a]	Flagyl, Metrocreme, Metrogel, Metrolotion, Noritate, Nuvessa, Vandazole	**Capsule (Flagyl):** 375 mg[b], 500 mg[c] **Cream:** 0.75% (Metrocreme), 1% (Noritate) **Cream, vaginal (Flagyl)[c]:** 10%
	Flagyl, Metrogel, Nidagel, Noritate	**Gel, topical (Metrogel):** 0.75%, 1% **Gel, vaginal:** 0.75% Metrogel, Nidagel, Vandazole), 1.3% (Nuvessa) **Lotion:** 0.75% (Metrolotion) **Tablet (Flagyl):** 250 mg, 500 mg[b] **Tablet, extended release:** 750 mg
mupirocin[a]	Centany	**Cream:** 2% **Ointment, topical:** 2%
	Bactroban, Bactroban Cream	
chloramphenicol[a]	Generics	**Powder, for injection:** 1 g/vial
	Chloromycetin	
clindamycin[a]	Cleocin, Cleocin T, Clinda-derm, Clindagel, Clindesse, Clindets, Evoclin	**Capsule:** 75 mg[b], 150 mg, 300 mg **Foam (Evoclin)[b]:** 1% **Swab (Clindets)[b]:** 1% **Solution, for injection:** 150 mg/mL
	Clinda-T, Dalacin C, Dalacin T 1%	**Solution, for infusion:** 6 mg/mL[b], 12 mg/mL, 18 mg/mL **Powder, for oral solution:** 75 mg/5 mL **Topical gel and lotion (Clinda-T, Cleocin T, Clindagel, Clindamax):** 1% **Topical solution (Cleocin T, Dalacin T):** 1% **Vaginal cream (Clindesse, Cleocin, Dalacin):** 2% **Vaginal suppositories (Cleocin)[b]:** 100 mg
telavancin	Vibativ	**Powder, for injection:** 250 mg[b], 750 mg
	Vibativ	
vancomycin	Firvanq Kit, Vancocin	**Capsule:** 125 mg, 250 mg **Powder, for oral solution (Firvanq Kit)[b]:** 25 mg/mL, 50 mg/mL
	Vancocin	**Powder, for injection:** 500 mg, 750 mg[b], 1 g, 5 g, 10 g/vial

Antimalarials

chloroquine[a]	Generics	**Tablet:** 250 mg, 500 mg
	Not available	

Miscellaneous Antiinfective Agents—cont'd

Generic Name	US Brand Name(s) / Canadian Brand Name(s)	Dosage Forms and Strengths
hydroxychloroquine[a]	Plaquenil	Tablet: 200 mg
	Plaquenil	
mefloquine[a]	Generics	Tablet: 250 mg
	Generics	
primaquine	Generic	Tablet: 15 mg
	Not available	
tafenoquine	Arakoda, Krintafel	Tablet: 100 mg (Arakoda), 150 mg (Krintafel)
	Not available	
artemether + lumefantrine	Coartem	Tablet: artemether 20 mg + lumefantrine 120 mg
	Not available	
atovaquone + proguanil[a]	Malarone, Malarone Pediatric	Tablet: 62.5 mg atovaquone + 25 mg proguanil, 250 mg atovaquone + 100 mg proguanil
	Malarone, Malarone Pediatric	Suspension: 750 mg/5 mL

[a]Generic available.
[b]Available in the United States only.
[c]Available in Canada only.

Summary of Drugs Used for the Treatment of Bacterial Infections

	Generic Name	Brand Name	Usual Dose and Dosing Schedule	Warning Labels
Cephalosporins				
	cefadroxil	Duricef	1 g orally/day given in 1 or 2 daily doses until course of therapy is finished	COMPLETE FULL COURSE OF THERAPY—all.
	cephalexin	Keflex	Varies (max, 4 g/day)	TAKE WITH FOOD—cefadroxil, delayed release. REFRIGERATE, SHAKE WELL, AND DISCARD AFTER 14 DAYS— cefadroxil, cephalexin, cefaclor oral suspensions.
	cefaclor	Generics	**Immediate release:** 250–500 mg orally every 8 h until course of therapy is finished **Extended release:** 375–500 mg every 12 h until course of therapy is finished (max, 1.5 g/day)	REFRIGERATE, SHAKE WELL, AND DISCARD AFTER 10 DAYS— cefuroxime suspension. REFRIGERATE OR STORE AT ROOM TEMPERATURE, SHAKE WELL, AND DISCARD AFTER 14 DAYS— cefixime oral suspension.
	cefuroxime	Ceftin	250–500 mg orally every 12 h until course of therapy is finished	
	cefixime	Suprax	400 mg orally once every 24 h until course of therapy is finished	

Continued

Summary of Drugs Used for the Treatment of Bacterial Infections—cont'd

	Generic Name	Brand Name	Usual Dose and Dosing Schedule	Warning Labels
Fluoroquinolones				
	ciprofloxacin	Cipro Cipro XR	**Immediate release:** 500–750 mg orally every 12 h until course of therapy is finished **Extended release:** 500–1000 mg once daily until course of therapy is finished	COMPLETE FULL COURSE OF THERAPY. TAKE WITH LOTS OF WATER. AVOID PROLONGED EXPOSURE TO SUNLIGHT. MAY CAUSE DIZZINESS OR DROWSINESS. AVOID ANTACIDS AND VITAMINS CONTAINING IRON AND ZINC. SHAKE WELL, AND DISCARD AFTER 14 DAYS—cipro suspension. SWALLOW WHOLE; DO NOT CRUSH OR CHEW—extended release. TAKE ON AN EMPTY STOMACH.
	levofloxacin	Levaquin	250–500 mg every 24 h (max, 750 mg/day) until course of therapy is finished	
	moxifloxacin	Avelox	400 mg orally or IV once daily until course of therapy is finished	
	norfloxacin	Noroxin	400 mg orally twice daily until course of therapy is finished	
Macrolides				
	azithromycin	Zithromax	500 mg day 1, followed by 250 mg once daily for 4 days	COMPLETE FULL COURSE OF THERAPY. SHAKE WELL—all suspensions. STORE AT ROOM TEMPERATURE AND DISCARD IN 14 DAYS—clarithromycin and azithromycin extended-release suspension. REFRIGERATE; DISCARD IN 10 DAYS—azithromycin suspension, immediate release. TAKE ON AN EMPTY STOMACH—azithromycin suspension. MAY DECREASE THE EFFECTIVENESS OF ORAL CONTRACEPTIVES. TAKE WITH FOOD—delayed release.
	clarithromycin	Biaxin, Biaxin XL	**Immediate release:** 250–500 mg every 12 h up to 1000 mg once daily until course of therapy is finished **Extended release:** 1000 mg once daily until course of therapy is finished	
	erythromycin base, delayed release	ERYC, PCE	250–500 mg every 6–8 h until course of therapy is finished	
	erythromycin ethylsuccinate	EES	400–800 mg every 6–8 h until course of therapy is finished (max, 4 g/day)	
Sulfonamides and Sulfonamide Combinations				
	sulfamethoxazole + trimethoprim	Septra, Bactrim	40–160 mg trimethoprim + 200–800 mg sulfamethoxazole every 12 h until course of therapy is finished	COMPLETE FULL COURSE OF THERAPY. TAKE WITH PLENTY OF WATER. AVOID PROLONGED SUNLIGHT. SHAKE WELL—suspension. STORE AT ROOM TEMPERATURE.
Penicillins				
	ampicillin	Generics	250–1000 mg orally every 6 h until course of therapy is finished	COMPLETE FULL COURSE OF THERAPY. TAKE ON AN EMPTY STOMACH—ampicillin, cloxacillin, dicloxacillin. REFRIGERATE, SHAKE WELL, AND DISCARD AFTER 14 DAYS—suspension ampicillin, dicloxacillin, penicillin VK. MAY DECREASE EFFECTIVENESS OF ORAL CONTRACEPTIVES. REFRIGERATE, SHAKE WELL, AND DISCARD AFTER 10 DAYS—suspension, amoxicillin + clavulanic acid.
	amoxicillin	Amoxil	Varies; 500–875 mg every 12 h or 250–500 mg PO every 8 h until course of therapy is finished	
	dicloxacillin	Generics	125–500 mg orally every 6 h until course of therapy is finished	
	penicillin VK	Generics	125–500 mg orally every 6 h until course of therapy is finished	
	amoxicillin + clavulanic acid	Augmentin	Varies; 250–500 mg every 8 h or 500–875 mg every 12 h until course of therapy is finished	
	penicillin G benzathine	Bicillin L-A	Varies	REFRIGERATE; DO NOT FREEZE.

Summary of Drugs Used for the Treatment of Bacterial Infections—cont'd

	Generic Name	Brand Name	Usual Dose and Dosing Schedule	Warning Labels
Tetracyclines				
	doxycycline	Vibramycin, Monodox	Varies; commonly 100 mg bid on day 1 followed by 100 mg daily or 100 mg bid until course of therapy is completed	COMPLETE FULL COURSE OF THERAPY. TAKE WITH LOTS OF WATER. AVOID PROLONGED SUNLIGHT. AVOID ANTACIDS AND VITAMINS CONTAINING IRON AND ZINC. MAY DECREASE EFFECTIVENESS OF ORAL CONTRACEPTIVES. SHAKE WELL—tetracycline suspension. TAKE ON AN EMPTY STOMACH—tetracycline.
	minocycline	Minocin	Varies (max, 350 mg on day 1, then 200 mg/day)	
	tetracycline	Generics	Varies (max, 4 g/day)	
Miscellaneous				
	metronidazole	Metrogel, Metrocreme, Noritate Flagyl	**Acne rosacea:** Apply a thin film once or twice daily **Bacterial vaginosis:** One applicatorful once daily at bedtime **Other infections:** Varies: 250–1000 mg 2–3 times daily until course of therapy is completed	COMPLETE FULL COURSE OF THERAPY. TAKE WITH A FULL GLASS OF WATER. AVOID ALCOHOL.
	isoniazid	Generics	**Tuberculosis prophylaxis:** 300 mg orally once daily or 900 mg/day twice weekly with pyridoxine (50 mg once daily or 100 mg twice weekly) for 9 months	COMPLETE FULL COURSE OF THERAPY. AVOID ANTACIDS. AVOID ALCOHOL.
	clindamycin	Cleocin	Varies: Take in 3–4 divided doses daily until course of therapy is completed	COMPLETE FULL COURSE OF THERAPY. TAKE WITH A FULL GLASS OF WATER. SHAKE WELL, STORE AT ROOM TEMPERATURE—suspension.
	mupirocin	Bactroban	Apply tid or bid for intranasal infections	COMPLETE FULL COURSE OF THERAPY.
	ertapenem	Invanz	Varies: 1 g IM or IV once daily for up to 14 days	
	imipenem + cilastatin + relebactam	Recarbrio	Reconstitute and administer by IV infusion over 30 min every 6 h	
	dalbavancin	Dalvance	Varies: administer by IV infusion	
	oritavancin	Orbactiv	Infuse 1200 mg as a single dose over 3 h	

Continued

Summary of Drugs Used for the Treatment of Bacterial Infections—cont'd

	Generic Name	Brand Name	Usual Dose and Dosing Schedule	Warning Labels
Antimalarial Agents				
	chloroquine	Generic	**Prevention:** 500 mg once weekly starting 2 weeks before traveling to the malaria area and continuing until 8 weeks after leaving the malaria area **Treatment:** 1000 mg on day 1 followed by 500 mg 6–8 h later and 500 mg on the second and third days of treatment	TAKE WITH FOOD OR MILK (to increase absorption)—tafenoquine, chloroquine, hydroxychloroquine. MAY CAUSE DIZZINESS. MAY CAUSE NAUSEA.
	hydroxychloroquine	Plaquenil	**Prevention:** 400 mg weekly; begin 2 weeks before travel to the malaria area and continue weekly doses until 4 weeks after leaving the malaria area **Treatment:** 800 mg followed by 400 mg every 6 h for 48 h after initial dose	
	primaquine		1 tablet daily for 14 days	
	mefloquine	generic	**Prevention:** Take 1 tablet daily; start 1–2 days before entering malaria area and continue for 7 days after leaving the malaria area **Treatment:** Take 4 tablets as a single dose × 3 days	
	tafenoquine	Akakoda Krintafel	Take 300 mg as a single dose on the first or second day of chloroquine (Krintafel) Take 200 mg (2 tablets) beginning 3 days before entering malaria area, 200 mg once weekly while in malaria area, and 200mg x 1 dose 7 days after leaving the malaria area. (Akakoda)	TAKE WITH FOOD. AVOID PREGNANCY. MAY CAUSE DIZZINESS OR HEADACHE. MAY CAUSE NAUSEA OR VOMITING.
	artemether + lumefantrine	Coartem	Take 1–4 tablets twice daily × 3 days (dose based on body weight)	MAY CRUSH AND MIX IN WATER.
	atovaquone + proguanil	Malarone	**Prevention:** Start 1–2 days before entering malaria area and continue for 7 days after leaving the malaria area Treatment: Take 4 tablets as a single dose × 3 days	

Key Points

- Chronic noninfectious disease is a leading cause of disability and death in high-income countries; however, infectious disease is still one of the leading causes of morbidity and mortality globally.
- Poverty, malnutrition, lack of clean water, poor sanitation, and inadequate housing increase the risk for infectious disease and decrease the likelihood for successful treatment.
- Microbes can learn how to resist the effects of antibiotics; superbugs are resistant to some currently available antimicrobial agents. Multidrug resistance is a serious problem.

- Antimicrobial resistance occurs because of the following: (1) inappropriate prescribing, (2) failure to complete the full course of therapy, (3) administration of antibacterial agents for viral infections (e.g., the common cold), (4) antibiotics in the food chain (agriculture, animal husbandry, fish farms), and (5) lack of guidelines for preventing the spread of infections in institutional care settings.
- Bactericidal agents can destroy rapidly proliferating, pathogenic bacteria.

- Bacteriostatic agents slow the growth of bacteria enough for the host's (our body's) defense mechanism to destroy the invading bacteria.
- β-Lactam antibiotics target the bacterial cell wall. Penicillins, cephalosporins, carbapenems, and monobactams are β-lactam antibiotics that inhibit cell wall synthesis.
- There are five classes of antiinfective agents that act to inhibit bacterial protein synthesis—aminoglycosides, macrolides, tetracyclines, amphenicols, and oxazolidinones.
- Fluoroquinolones (e.g., ciprofloxacin) and nitroimidazoles (e.g., metronidazole) inhibit bacterial DNA synthesis.
- Rifampin inhibits bacterial RNA synthesis.
- Sulfonamides are antifolate drugs; trimethoprim is a dihydrofolate reductase inhibitor that interferes with bacterial folic acid synthesis.
- Aminoglycosides are not absorbed systemically when administered by mouth but may be given orally to reduce the number of bacteria in the bowel before colorectal surgery.
- A common beginning for cephalosporin drugs is *ceph-* or *cef-*.
- Cephalosporins are classified as first-, second-, third-, and fourth-generation agents.
- A common ending of fluoroquinolones is *-floxacin*.

- Clarithromycin is a key component of treatment regimens for peptic ulcer disease caused by the bacterium *H. pylori*.
- Macrolides, penicillins, and tetracyclines may decrease the effectiveness of oral contraceptives.
- Penicillins may be administered before dental and other medical procedures to prevent bacterial endocarditis in individuals with prosthetic heart valves.
- Antistaphylococcal penicillins are penicillinase resistant.
- A common beginning for sulfonamides is *sulf-*.
- Tetracyclines are used for the treatment of acne, sexually transmitted infections such as chlamydia, Lyme disease, and Rocky Mountain spotted fever.
- Tetracyclines are contraindicated in pregnancy and small children because they can weaken fetal bone, retard bone growth, weaken tooth enamel, and stain teeth.
- Isoniazid is used for the treatment of tuberculosis. Vitamin B_6 should be taken with isoniazid to reduce neurotoxicity.
- Individuals taking metronidazole should avoid drinking alcoholic beverages or taking medicines containing alcohol.
- Mupirocin is a topically applied antimicrobial used to treat staphylococcal infections of the skin such as impetigo.

Review Questions

1. Antibiotics are used to treat_____.
   a. bacterial infections
   b. viral infections
   c. fungal infections
   d. none of the above
2. Misuse of antimicrobial agents is a major cause for the development and spread of anti microbial resistance.
   a. true
   b. false
3. Antibacterial agents may be classified as _____.
   a. bactericidal
   b. bacteriolytic
   c. bacteriostatic
   d. a and c
4. Each of the following antiinfective agents is marketed as a pediatric solution or suspension EXCEPT _____.
   a. amoxicillin
   b. trimethoprim + sulfamethoxazole
   c. vancomycin
   d. clindamycin
5. All of the following antiinfective agents must be refrigerated after reconstitution EXCEPT _____.
   a. Amoxil 250 mg/5 mL
   b. Keflex 250 mg/5 mL
   c. Augmentin 250 mg/5 mL
   d. Ceftin 250 mg/5 mL

6. Fluoroquinolones are formulated for oral, ophthalmic, and parenteral use.
   a. true
   b. false
7. All of the following antiinfective agents must be stored at room temperature EXCEPT: _____.
   a. Augmentin 250 mg/5 mL
   b. Septra 200 mg/40 mg/5 mL
   c. Biaxin 250 mg/5 mL
   d. Cleocin 75 mg/5 mL
8. Oral penicillins are used to treat many infections, including _____.
   a. upper respiratory infections
   b. otitis media, skin infections
   c. strep throat
   d. all of the above
9. Outdated tetracycline becomes toxic and should be discarded.
   a. true
   b. false
10. Isoniazid is used for the treatment of _____.
    a. upper respiratory infections
    b. AIDS
    c. tuberculosis
    d. peptic ulcers

Bibliography

Centers for Disease Control and Prevention. (2022). Treatment of Malaria: Guidelines for Clinicians (United States). Retrieved January 31, 2023, from https://www.cdc.gov/malaria/diagnosis_treatment/clinicians1.html.

Costello J, King E, Patel D. (2017). Core elements of antibiotic stewardship. Retrieved January 31, 2023, from http://www.powerpak.com/course/preamble/115367.

Government of Canada. (2021). Chapter 4 – Prevention-Chemoprophylaxis regimen: Canadian recommendations for the prevention and treatment of malaria. Retrieved January 31, 2023, from https://www.canada.ca/en/public-health/services/catmat/canadian-recommendations-prevention-treatment-malaria/chapter-4-prevention-chemoprophylaxis-regimen.html.

Health Canada. (2022). Drug Product Database. Retrieved January 29, 2023, from https://health-products.canada.ca/dpd-bdpp/index-eng.jsp.

Institute for Safe Medication Practices. (2016). FDA and ISMP Lists of Look-Alike Drug Names with Recommended Tall Man Letters. Retrieved October 18, 2022, from https://www.ismp.org/recommendations/tall-man-letters-list.

Institute for Safe Medication Practices. (2019). List of Confused Drugs. Retrieved October 18, 2022, from https://www.ismp.org/tools/confuseddrugnames.pdf.

Kalant H, Grant D, Mitchell J. *Principles of medical pharmacology*. ed 7. Toronto: Elsevier Canada; 2007:671–686 702–707, 713.

National Institute of Allergy and Infectious Diseases. (2006). Understanding Microbes in Sickness and in Health, 2006. (NIH Publication No. 06-4914). National Institutes of Health. Retrieved January 31, 2023, from https://www.niaid.nih.gov

Page C, Curtis M, Sutter M, et al. *Integrated pharmacology*. Philadelphia: Elsevier Mosby; 2005:111–134.

U.S. Food and Drug Administration. (nd). Drugs@FDA: FDA Approved Drug Products. Retrieved January 29, 2023, from http://www.accessdata.fda.gov/scripts/cder/daf/

30
Treatment of Viral Infections

LEARNING OBJECTIVES

1. Learn the terminology associated with the treatment of viral infections.
2. Describe the mechanism of virus entry into cells.
3. Describe antiviral resistance.
4. List and categorize antiviral agents.
5. Describe mechanism of action for antiviral agents.
6. List common endings for antiviral agents.
7. Identify significant drug look-alike and sound-alike issues.
8. Identify warning labels and precautionary messages associated with antiviral agents.

KEY TERMS

Acquired immunodeficiency syndrome (AIDS) The most severe form of human immunodeficiency virus (HIV) infection. HIV-infected patients are diagnosed with AIDS when their CD4 cell count falls below 200 cells/mm^3 or if they develop an AIDS-defining illness (an unusual illness in someone who is not HIV positive).

Antiretroviral Medication that interferes with the replication of a retrovirus (e.g., HIV).

Antiviral Medication that is able to inhibit viral replication.

Antiviral resistance Ability of a virus to overcome the suppressive action of antiviral agents.

CD4 T lymphocyte White blood cells that fight infection.

COVID-19 A contagious viral infection caused by SARS-CoV-2 coronavirus.

Cross-resistance Development of resistance to one drug in a particular class that results in resistance to other drugs in that class.

Highly active antiretroviral therapy (HAART) Combination of three or more antiretroviral medications taken in a regimen.

Human immunodeficiency virus (HIV) Virus that causes acquired immunodeficiency syndrome (AIDS).

Oncovirus A virus that is a causative agent in a cancer.

Virion Infectious particles of a virus.

Virustatic Able to suppress viral proliferation.

Virus Intracellular parasite that consists of a DNA and RNA core surrounded by a protein coat and sometimes an outer covering of lipoprotein.

Overview

A *virus* is an intracellular parasite that consists of a deoxyribonucleic acid (DNA) or ribonucleic acid (RNA) core surrounded by a protein coat and sometimes an outer covering of lipoprotein. The infectious particle (*virion*) does not have the cellular components necessary for reproduction, so they use the host's cellular machinery to replicate (Fig. 30.1). The virus attaches itself to susceptible host cells and then releases viral genetic material (RNA and DNA) into the host cell. The viral material takes control of the host cell machinery for replication. The host cell eventually dies because the virus keeps it from performing its normal functions. When it dies, the cell releases replicated viruses that proliferate and attack more and more host cells. The ability of viruses to transfer genetic material between cells is beneficial in the development of bioengineered drugs and vaccines (e.g., *Haemophilus influenzae* type B conjugate vaccine) (see Chapter 32).

Viruses may cause minor illnesses, such as the common cold and warts, or serious infections such as *human immunodeficiency virus* (HIV), smallpox, and hepatitis C infection. Some viral infections are linked to cancers. For example, human papillomavirus (HPV) is linked to cervical cancer. Epstein-Barr virus (EBV) is associated with nose and throat cancers, and hepatitis B and C viruses are associated with liver cancer. Viruses that can cause cancer are called *oncoviruses*.

An *antiviral* is a medication that can inhibit viral replication. Antiviral agents work best when the host (the individual with the infection) has a healthy immune system. This is because antivirals do not destroy viruses; they slow the rate of virus proliferation (*virustatic*). Macrophages, immunoglobulins, T cells, interleukins, interferons, and other cells released by the host in response to the virus's attack ultimately are responsible for recovery from the infection. Like bacterial infections, effective treatment of viral infections is dependent on host factors, virus factors, and antiviral agent factors. Fig. 30.1 shows factors that influence successful therapy.

The following factors influence the outcome of antiviral therapy: (1) stage of illness at the time therapy begins, (2) antiviral dose, (3) ability of the virus to penetrate the central nervous system, (4) ability of the virus to remain latent within its host, and (5) development of antiviral resistance. Herpes simplex virus types 1 and 2 (HSV-1, HSV-2) are viruses that demonstrate the

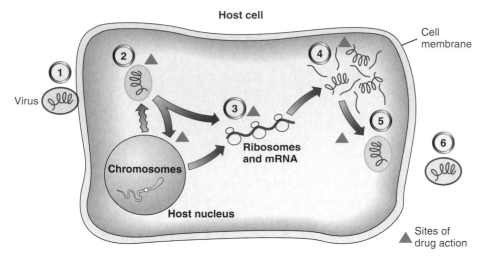

Host cell

Virus

Chromosomes

Host nucleus

Ribosomes and mRNA

Cell membrane

▲ Sites of drug action

1. Attachment to host cell
2. Uncoating of virus, and entry of viral nucleic acid into host cell nucleus
3. Control of DNA, RNA, and/or protein production
4. Production of viral subunits
5. Assembly of virions
6. Release of virions

• **Fig. 30.1** Virus invasion of a host cell, viral replication, and release of virions. (Adapted from Brody TM, Larner J, Minneman KP: *Human pharmacology: molecular to clinical*, ed 3, St Louis, 1998, Mosby.)

importance of timing related to the initiation of antiviral therapy. Antiviral therapy reduces the severity of the infection and symptoms only if it begins within the first 24 to 48 hours of exposure to the virus or the onset of symptoms. Other viral infections improved by early initiation of antiviral therapy are influenza and varicella zoster virus (VZV). HSV-1, HSV-2, and VZV are also examples of viruses that lay dormant in host cells and periodically awaken to cause recurrent disease.

Antiviral agents are typically effective against specific viral strains. For example, amantadine acts against influenza A but not influenza B. Oseltamivir (Tamiflu) is indicated for the treatment of influenza but is not effective for the treatment of HIV, HPV, or HSV. Antibiotics are not effective against viral infections.

Antiviral Resistance

The growth of viral colonies involves viral replication. In the process of replication, the virus may mutate. Mutations often result in adaptations that make it easier for the virus to exist in new environments and hosts. *Antiviral resistance* is the ability of a virus to overcome the suppressive action of antiviral agents. It may occur when an individual taking an antiviral drug skips doses or takes them irregularly. Vomiting may cause subtherapeutic levels of antiviral agents, resulting in insufficient levels to suppress viral replication yet sufficient residual exposure to permit antiviral resistance to develop. The virus may accidentally mutate into a form that is resistant to the antiviral drug(s) taken.

Because viruses continually mutate, it is difficult to develop a vaccine to prevent viral infections. For example, each year a new flu vaccine must be developed against the latest virulent strain of influenza. A triple cocktail of drugs is administered for the treatment of HIV and AIDS, known as *highly active antiretroviral therapy (HAART)*, to decrease mutations and improve antiretroviral therapy. There are several strains of HPV. Cervarix and Gardasil are effective against HPV types 16 and 18, which cause most cervical cancers. Gardasil is also effective against HPV types 6 and 11.

Mechanisms of Antiviral Action

Antivirals interfere with virus-specific steps in the replication cycle, specifically:
- virus attachment to the host cell receptors, cell penetration, and viral uncoating;
- virus regulatory proteins;
- virus cleavage;
- viral assembly; and
- release of virus.
- Antivirals inhibit:
- reverse transcriptase, transamidase, and other virion-associated enzymes;
- viral transcription; and
- viral messenger RNA (mRNA).

Treatment of Influenza

Two types of antiviral agents are used to prevent or treat influenza. They are adamantanes (amantadine and rimantadine) and neuraminidase inhibitors (oseltamivir, zanamivir, and peramivir).

> **❶ Tech Alert!**
>
> A common ending for antiviral agents that inhibit viral uncoating is -mantidine.

Adamantanes

Amantadine and rimantadine are classified as adamantane antivirals that are used for the prevention and treatment of influenza A.

> **❶ Tech Alert!**
>
> The following drugs have look-alike/sound-alike issues: amantadine and amiodarone

Mechanism of Action and Pharmacokinetics

Amantadine and rimantadine interfere with the uncoating of the influenza A virus, a necessary step in the viral replication process. More specifically, they inhibit the activity of the influenza virus M2 protein, which forms a channel in the virus membrane and enables replication after the virus enters the host cell. Amantadine is rapidly absorbed, and peak plasma levels are achieved within 2 to 4 hours of an oral dose. Peak plasma levels for rimantadine occur in approximately 6 hours. Rimantadine is approximately 40% protein bound. It is also highly metabolized in the liver and has active metabolites that account for the drug's long half-life of 13 to 65 hours.

Adverse Reactions and Precautions

Amantadine and rimantadine may produce anxiety, irritability, nervousness, drowsiness, confusion, and headache. They can also cause diarrhea or constipation, difficulty sleeping or nightmares, dry mouth, loss of appetite, nausea or vomiting, unusual tiredness, and, rarely, kidney damage. Antiviral resistance limits their effectiveness in treating influenza A and influenza B.

Neuraminidase Inhibitors

Oseltamivir, zanamivir, and peramivir are indicated for the treatment of influenza A and influenza B. Nearly 98% of H1N1 and H3N3 strains of influenza A are susceptible to the effects of oseltamivir and zanamivir; however, one strain of H1N1 influenza that is resistant to oseltamivir and zanamivir has been identified.

> **❶ Tech Alert!**
>
> Tamiflu and Theraflu have look-alike/sound-alike issues.

Mechanism of Action and Pharmacokinetics

The surfaces of influenza viruses are dotted with neuraminidase proteins. Neuraminidase inhibitors inhibit viral release by inhibiting the enzyme that breaks the bonds that hold the virus particle to the outside of the infected cell. They inhibit virus spread by blocking virus release from the host cell. Oseltamivir (Tamiflu) is formulated for oral use, zanamivir (Relenza) is a powder that is inhaled by mouth, and peramivir (Rapivab) is formulated for an intravenous infusion.

Adverse Reactions

Side effects common to the use of oseltamivir and zanamivir are nausea and vomiting, coughing, dizziness, and headache. Psychosis and other emotional changes have been reported with the use of neuraminidase inhibitors. Zanamivir is not recommended for patients with pulmonary disease because it has been reported to produce bronchospasm and deterioration of pulmonary function. Allergic reactions include oropharyngeal or facial edema. The most common side effect with Rapivab is diarrhea, although serious skin and hypersensitivity reactions may also occur.

Treatment of Hepatitis B and Hepatitis C

Hepatitis B and hepatitis C are viral infections that attack the liver. The viruses can spread when blood from an infected person enters the bloodstream of a noninfected person, as can occur with unsafe injection practices (e.g., sharing needles). Hepatitis B can also be transmitted in semen and other body fluids. Five percent of the global population is infected with hepatitis B, and 600,000 people die annually from liver damage and other complications of chronic infection. More than 170 million people worldwide are infected with hepatitis C. Interferons, nucleoside analogs, nucleotide analogs, and protease inhibitors (PIs) are used for the treatment of hepatitis B virus (HBV) and/or hepatitis C virus (HCV) infections. Nucleosides, nucleotides, and PIs are also used for the treatment of HIV infections and are described in the next section.

Interferons

Interferons are a family of naturally occurring proteins that are made and secreted by cells of the immune system. There are approximately 2000 interferon receptors on each normal and malignant cell. Interferons may also be produced by recombinant DNA technology. They are not technically antiviral agents. Instead, they protect uninfected cells by promoting resistance to virus infection.

Treatment of Influenza

Generic Name	U.S. Brand Name(s) / Canadian Brand Name(s)	Dosage Forms and Strengths
Adamantanes		
amantadine[a]	Gocovri[b], Osmolex ER[b] / Generics	**Capsule:** 100 mg **Capsule, extended release (Gocovri):** 68.5 mg, 137 mg **Oral solution:** 10 mg/mL **Tablet[c]:** 100 mg **Tablet, extended release:** 129 mg, 161 mg, 193 mg, 258 mg
rimantadine[a]	Flumadine / Not available	**Tablet:** 100 mg
Neuraminidase Inhibitors		
oseltamivir[a]	Tamiflu / Tamiflu	**Capsule:** 30 mg, 45 mg, 75 mg **Powder, for oral suspension:** 6 mg/mL, 12 mg/mL[c]
peramivir	Rapivab / Not available	**IV infusion:** 200 mg/20 mL
zanamivir	Relenza / Relenza	**Powder, for inhalation:** 5 mg/actuation

[a]Generic available.
[b]Gocovri and Osmolex ER are indicated for the treatment of Parkinson disease-related symptoms.
[c]Available in the United States only.

Interferon alfa-2b, interferon alfacon-1, peginterferon alfa-2a, and peginterferon alfa-2b are administered to treat viral infections. Peginterferon alfa-2b is indicated for the treatment of HCV. Interferon alfa-2b and peginterferon alfa-2a may be used for the treatment of HBV and HCV.

> ## ❶ *Tech Alert!*
> The following drugs have look-alike/sound-alike issues: peginterferon alfa-2a and peginterferon alfa-2b

Interferon Alfa and Interferon Alfa N3 Mechanism of Action and Pharmacokinetics

Interferons inhibit viral transcription by activating enzymes that cleave single-stranded viral RNA. Depending on the virus and cell type, they may also inhibit viral uncoating, inhibit the synthesis of mRNA, and interfere with the translation, assembly, and release of viral proteins.

Adverse Reactions and Precautions

The most common adverse reactions associated with interferons are flulike symptoms: fever, chills, headache, fatigue, muscle aches, and joint pain. They may also cause nausea, vomiting, diarrhea, dizziness, and depression. More serious adverse effects are neutropenia (a drop in the white blood cell count) and thrombocytopenia (a decrease in the platelet count).

Nucleoside and Nucleotide Analogs

Nucleoside and nucleotide analog antiviral agents used for the treatment of HBV are adefovir, lamivudine, entecavir, telbivudine, and tenofovir. Entecavir is effective against lamivudine-resistant HBV. Ribavirin is indicated for the treatment of hepatitis C when combined with peginterferon alfa. Ribavirin is also indicated for the treatment of respiratory syncytial virus.

Mechanism of Action

Nucleoside and nucleotide analogs inhibit at least one of the three steps of virus replication. Entecavir, lamivudine, ribavirin, and telbivudine are nucleoside analogs. They inhibit HBV reverse transcriptase. Telbivudine inhibits HBV DNA polymerase, resulting in DNA chain termination and inhibition of viral replication. Ribavirin is effective against RNA and DNA viruses. The mechanism of action is not completely understood, but it is believed that the drug increases the mutation rate of the virus, leading to a growing number of viruses unable to replicate. Adefovir and tenofovir are nucleotide analogs that inhibit HBV DNA polymerase, resulting in DNA chain termination and inhibition of viral replication. Sovaldi (sofosbuvir) is a nucleotide analog NS5B polymerase inhibitor that works by blocking a specific protein that the HCV needs to grow.

Adverse Effects and Precautions

The most common adverse effects of entecavir and lamivudine are headache, fatigue, dizziness, and nausea. Headache, abdominal pain, diarrhea, nausea, dyspepsia, flatulence, and asthenia are the most common side effects associated with adefovir. Adefovir, entecavir, and telbivudine have a boxed warning regarding worsening of hepatitis upon discontinuation. Tenofovir may increase the toxicity of adefovir.

> ## ❶ *Tech Alert!*
> The US Food and Drug Administration (FDA) requires a boxed warning for adefovir, entecavir, and tenofovir, informing prescribers of the following: (1) severe acute exacerbations of hepatitis B have been reported in patients who have discontinued anti-hepatitis B therapy; (2) fatal lactic acidosis; and (3) renal dysfunction (adefovir).

> ## ❶ *Tech Alert!*
> The FDA requires a boxed warning that entecavir is not recommended for patients coinfected with HIV and HBV unless also receiving HAART, to reduce the risk for the development of drug resistance.

Direct-Acting Antivirals

Direct-acting antivirals (DAAs) are approved by the FDA for the treatment of hepatitis C. Most of the DAAs are marketed as combination products or are taken in combination with ribavirin or interferons to improve effectiveness and/or reduce the development of antiviral resistance.

Mechanism of Actions

DAAs target specific nonstructural proteins of the HCV to disrupt viral replication and the infection. There are four classes of DAAs: (1) nonstructural proteins 3/4 A (NS3/4 A) PIs, (2) NS5B nucleoside polymerase inhibitors (NPIs), (3) NS5B nonnucleoside polymerase inhibitors (NNPIs), and (4) NS5A inhibitors.

NS3/4 A PIs include glecaprevir, grazoprevir, paritaprevir, and voxilaprevir. Sofosbuvir is an NS5B NPI. It is approved by the FDA for the treatment of HIV and HCV coinfection.

Elbasvir, ledipasvir, ombitasvir, pibrentasvir, and velpatasvir are NS5A inhibitors. NS5B NNPIs are in the clinical phase of development.

Epclusa oral pellets (sofosbuvir + velpatasvir) and Mavyret (glecaprevir + pibrentasvir) may be sprinkled on soft foods to improve palatability. The foods should be nonacidic and at room temperature or colder. Aluminum- and magnesium-containing antacids decrease the concentration of velpatasvir, so Vosevi and Epclusa should be taken 4 hours before or 4 hours after a dose of antacid.

Adverse Reactions

The most common side effects of DAA medications are headache, fatigue, and nausea. HBV reactivation has been reported upon initiation of therapy in patients coinfected with HCV and HBV, leading to the severe and sudden onset of hepatitis, hepatic failure, and death.

Treatment of Herpes Simplex, Herpes Zoster, and Cytomegalovirus

The virus that causes cold sores (HSV-1), the virus that causes genital warts (HSV-2), and the virus that causes chickenpox and shingles (varicella zoster) are treated with acyclovir, famciclovir, penciclovir, and valacyclovir. Acyclovir and valacyclovir are indicated for the treatment of cold sores, genital herpes, and shingles, whereas penciclovir is indicated only for the treatment of herpes labialis, commonly known as a cold sore. Trifluridine is used for

Treatment of Hepatitis B and Hepatitis C

Generic Name	US Brand Name(s) / Canadian Brand Name(s)	Dosage Forms and Strengths
Interferons		
interferon alfa-2b	Intron-A	**Powder, for injection:** 10 million international units (mIU)/vial, 18 mIU/vial, 25 mIU/vial
	Not available	
peginterferon alfa-2a	Pegasys	**Solution for injection, vial[b]:** 180 mcg/mL
	Pegasys	**Solution for injection, prefilled syringe:** 180 mcg/0.5 mL
peginterferon alfa-2b	PegIntron, Sylatron	**Powder for injection (Sylatron):** 296 mcg, 444 mcg, 888 mcg/vial
	Not available	**Solution, for injection (vial and pre-filled syringe):** 50 mcg/0.5 mL, 80 mcg/0.5 mL, 120 mcg/0.5 mL, 150 mcg/0.5 mL
Nucleoside/Nucleotide Analogs[d]		
adefovir[a]	Hepsera	**Tablet:** 10 mg
	Generic	
entecavir[a]	Baraclude	**Solution, oral:** 0.05 mg/mL[b]
	Baraclude	**Tablet:** 0.5 mg, 1 mg
lamivudine[a]	Epivir HBV	**Solution, oral:** 5 mg/mL[b], 10 mg/mL
	Generic	**Tablet:** 100 mg
ribavirin[a]	Generic	**Capsule:** 200 mg
	Ibavyr	**Tablet:** 200 mg, 400 mg[c]
tenofovir alafenamide	Vemlidy	**Tablet:** 25 mg
	Vemlidy	
tenofovir disoproxil[a]	Viread	**Tablet:** 150 mg[c], 200 mg[c], 250 mg[c], 300 mg
	Viread	
Direct-Acting Antivirals		
sofosbuvir	Sovaldi	**Tablet:** 400 mg
	Sovaldi	
Combination Direct-Acting Antivirals		
glecaprevir + pibrentasvir	Mavyret	**Tablet:** 100 mg glecaprevir + 40 mg pibrentasvir
	Maviret	
sofosbuvir + velpatasvir	Epclusa	**Pellets, oral[b]:** 150 mg sofosbuvir + 37.5 mg velpatasvir/packet, 200 mg sofosbuvir + 50 mg velpatasvir/packet
	Epclusa	**Tablet:** 200 mg sofosbuvir + 50 mg velpatasvir[b], 400 mg sofosbuvir + 100 mg velpatasvir
sofosbuvir + ledipasvir	Harvoni	**Pellets, oral[b]:** 150 mg sofosbuvir + 33.75 mg ledipasvir/packet, 400 mg + 45 mg/packet
	Harvoni	**Tablet:** 400 mg sofosbuvir + 90 mg ledipasvir
sofosbuvir + velpatasvir + voxilaprevir	Vosevi	**Tablet:** 400 mg sofosbuvir + 100 mg velpatasvir + 100 mg voxilaprevir
	Vosevi	
elbasvir + grazoprevir	Zepatier	**Tablet:** 50 mg elbasvir + 100 mg grazoprevir
	Not available	

[a]Generic available.
[b]Available in the United States only.
[c]Available in Canada only.
[d]Only brand names and strength of nucleoside/nucleotide analogs marketed for the treatment of hepatitis are shown in the table. Additional strengths or brand names may be marketed for the treatment of additional infections.

Prevention and Treatment of Respiratory Syncytial Virus: Inhibition of DNA and RNA Replication

Generic Name	US Brand Name(s)		Dosage Forms and Strengths
		Canadian Brand Name(s)	
palivizumab	Synagis		**Powder, for injection solution**[b]: 50 mg/vial, 100 mg/vial
	Synagis		**Solution, for injection**[c]: 50 mg/0.5 mL, 100 mg/mL
ribavirin[a]	Virazole		**Powder, for inhalation:** 6 g/vial
	Virazole		

[a]Generic available.
[b]Available in the United States only.
[c]Available in Canada only.

the treatment of keratoconjunctivitis of the eye caused by HSV-1 and HSV-2 (see Chapter 15). Cytomegalovirus (CMV) may be treated with cidofovir, ganciclovir, or foscarnet. Foscarnet is also indicated for the treatment of acyclovir-resistant HSV-1, HSV-2, and herpes labialis.

> **⊘ Tech Alert!**
>
> Common endings for antiviral agents used for the treatment of herpes virus infections are -cyclovir and -ciclovir.

> **⊘ Tech Alert!**
>
> The following drugs have look-alike/sound-alike issues:
> Zovirax and Zostrix

Mechanism of Action and Pharmacokinetics

Acyclovir inhibits viral DNA synthesis, which is an essential step in the process of viral replication because genetic code is stored in DNA. Acyclovir is approximately 10 times more potent against HSV-1 and HSV-2 than against VZV. Higher doses are required for the treatment of chickenpox and shingles. Acyclovir may be administered topically, orally, or parenterally. Gastrointestinal (GI) absorption is poor, and the bioavailability of orally administered acyclovir is much lower than parenterally administered acyclovir. Systemic effects from topical administration are limited.

Valacyclovir is an ester of acyclovir. It has greater oral absorption. It treats the same conditions as acyclovir but requires less frequent dosing. Cidofovir inhibits viral DNA polymerase, the enzyme responsible for the replication of new viral RNA and DNA.

Foscarnet inhibits the viral-specific DNA polymerases and reverse transcriptases. It also inhibits the replication of HSV, VZV, EBV, human herpesvirus 6, and CMV.

Ganciclovir is used for the treatment of CMV. It is similar in structure to acyclovir. Ganciclovir is a competitive inhibitor of viral DNA polymerases that results in the inhibition of viral DNA synthesis.

Famciclovir is metabolized to penciclovir. It has a similar spectrum of activity to acyclovir and is also indicated for the treatment of HSV-1, HSV-2 and acute herpes zoster infections. It has a longer duration of action than acyclovir.

Penciclovir is an active metabolite of famciclovir. It is administered topically.

Adverse Reactions

Adverse reactions that are common to acyclovir, famciclovir, ganciclovir, penciclovir, valacyclovir, and cidofovir are diarrhea, nausea, vomiting, headache, fatigue, dizziness, and confusion. Penciclovir and acyclovir topical cream or ointment may also cause local irritation. Cidofovir may produce neutropenia, hair loss, tinnitus, renal failure, and hearing loss. Foscarnet has a side effect profile similar to that of cidofovir but can also cause arrhythmias, heart failure, and peripheral neuropathy.

COVID-19 (SARS-CoV-2)

COVID-19, the disease caused by the deadly SARS-CoV-2 virus, has infected more than 670 million people globally and killed nearly 7 million people. In February 2023, the number of COVID-19 deaths surpassed 1 million in the United States and 50,000 in Canada. Infection prevention strategies include wearing an N-95 mask and getting vaccinated. **COVID-19** vaccines are described in Chapter 32. Masking and vaccination reduce the risk for COVID-19 acute infection and long COVID, a post-COVID syndrome that produces long-term physical and mental health effects.

Treatment options are limited for individuals who test positive for COVID-19.

Remdesivir (Veklury) is indicated only for severe SARS-CoV-2 infection in individuals who are at risk for hospitalization or death. An intravenous infusion of sotrovimab, a monoclonal antibody therapeutic, is a treatment option for mild to moderate infections. Paxlovid (nirmatrelvir + ritonavir) is an orally administered antiviral agent that is indicated for mild to moderate infection. Paxlovid must be administered within 5 days of symptom onset.

Access to Paxlovid is widely available in the United States. Its use is prioritized in Canada according to the patient's risk for severe infection and hospitalization. Paxlovid is recommended for individuals older than 60 years and those 18 to 59 years of age who are immunocompromised or have an additional medical condition (e.g., cancer, diabetes) or are living in a long-term care setting. Social determinants of health, such as poverty, racism, or homelessness, also increase the risk for severe infection and thus are also considered when determining eligibility to receive Paxlovid in Canada.

Mechanism of Action and Pharmacokinetics

Veklury solution must be diluted. Infusion bags of diluted VEKLURY solution can be stored up to 24 hours at room temperature (20°C to 25°C [68°F to 77°F]) prior to administration or 48 hours at refrigerated temperature (2°C to 8°C [36°F to 46°F]). A pregnancy exposure registry has been established to collect information about pregnancy outcomes when the antiviral agent is taken by pregnant individuals.

Treatment of Herpes Virus and Cytomegalovirus

Generic Name	US Brand Name(s) Canadian Brand Name(s)	Dosage Forms and Strengths
acyclovir[a]	Sitavig, Zovirax Zovirax	**Capsule**[b]: 200 mg **Cream:** 5% **Ointment:** 5% **Solution, for injection:** 25 mg/mL[c], 50 mg/mL **Suspension:** 200 mg/5 mL **Tablet:** 200 mg[c], 400 mg, 800 mg **Tablet, buccal (Sitavig):** 50 mg
acyclovir + hydrocortisone	Xerese Xerese	**Cream:** 5% acyclovir + 1% hydrocortisone
cidofovir[a]	Generics Generics	**Solution, for injection:** 75 mg/mL
famciclovir[a]	Generics Famvir	**Tablet:** 125 mg, 250 mg, 500 mg
foscarnet[a]	Foscavir Generics	**Solution, for injection:** 24 mg/mL
ganciclovir[a]	Ganzyk-RTU, Zirgan Cytovene	**Gel, ophthalmic (Zirgan)**[b]: 0.15% **Powder, for injection:** 500 mg/vial (50 mg/mL) **Solution, intravenous (Ganzyk-RTU):** 500 mg/250 mL (2 mg/mL)
penciclovir	Denavir Not available	**Cream:** 1%
trifluridine[a]	Viroptic Viroptic	**Ophthalmic solution:** 1%
valacyclovir[a]	Valtrex Valtrex	**Tablet:** 500 mg, 1 g
valganciclovir[a]	Valcyte Valcyte	**Powder, for oral solution:** 50 mg/mL **Tablet:** 450 mg

[a]Generic available.
[b]Available in the United States only.
[c]Available in Canada only.

Summary of Drugs Used for the Treatment of Influenza, Herpes, Hepatitis, Respiratory Syncytial Virus, and Cytomegalovirus Viral Infections

Generic Name	Brand Name	Usual Dose and Dosing Schedule	Warning Labels
Influenza A or B Treatment			
amantadine	Generics	**Influenza A treatment and prophylaxis:** 200 mg/day as 1 or 2 divided doses; begin within 24–48 h of onset of signs or symptoms and continue for 24–48 h after symptoms resolve or for prophylaxis at least 10 days	MAY CAUSE DIZZINESS OR DROWSINESS. COMPLETE FULL COURSE OF THERAPY.
rimantadine	Flumadine	**Influenza A treatment and prophylaxis:** 100 mg twice daily; begin within 24–48 h of onset of signs or symptoms, continue for 5–7 days	

Continued

Summary of Drugs Used for the Treatment of Influenza, Herpes, Hepatitis, Respiratory Syncytial Virus, and Cytomegalovirus Viral Infections—cont'd

Generic Name	Brand Name	Usual Dose and Dosing Schedule	Warning Labels
oseltamivir	Tamiflu	**Influenza A or B treatment and prophylaxis:** 75 mg twice daily within 48-72h of symptoms for 5 days for acute infection, once daily for 10 days—prophylaxis	REFRIGERATE; SHAKE WELL; DISCARD AFTER 10 DAYS—oseltamivir suspension. COMPLETE FULL COURSE OF THERAPY. INHALE USING DISKHALER DELIVERY DEVICE—zanamivir.
peramavir	Rapivab	**Influenza treatment:** 600 mg/100 mL IV infusion over 15–30 min	
zanamivir	Relenza	**Influenza A treatment:** 2 doses to start; then 2 oral inhalations twice daily for 5 days; begin within 48 h of onset of signs or symptoms. **Influenza A prophylaxis:** 2 oral inhalations daily for 10 or 28 days, as directed	

Hepatitis B

Generic Name	Brand Name	Usual Dose and Dosing Schedule	Warning Labels
adefovir[a]	Hepsera	10 mg once daily	TAKE WITH OR WITHOUT FOOD—adefovir, lamivudine, tenofovir. TAKE ON AN EMPTY STOMACH—entecavir. REFRIGERATE; DO NOT FREEZE—interferon alfa-2b, peginterferon alfa-2a.
entecavir	Baraclude	0.5–1 mg once daily	
interferon alfa-2b	Intron A	30–35 mIU weekly SC or IM for 16 weeks	
lamivudine	Epivir HBV	HIV-negative patients—100 mg once daily for up to 1 year	
peginterferon alfa-2a	Pegasys	180 mcg SC once weekly for 48 weeks	
tenofovir	Vemlidy	25 mg once daily	

Hepatitis C

Generic Name	Brand Name	Usual Dose and Dosing Schedule	Warning Labels
peginterferon alfa-2b	PEG-Intron	1.5 mcg/kg once weekly for 1 year	STORE IN ORIGINAL CONTAINER TO AVOID CONTACT WITH MOISTURE—Zepatier, Epclusa, Vosevi. TAKE WITH OR WITHOUT FOOD—Zepatier, Mavyret, Harvoni. DO NOT OPEN PELLET PACKETS UNTIL READY FOR USE—Harvoni, Solvadi, Epclusa. TAKE WITH FOOD—Vosevi. AVOID ANTACIDS—Vosevi, Epclusa.
ribavirin	Copegus	**Monoinfection:** 800–1200 mg daily according to body weight with 180 mcg of peginterferon alfa-2a for 24–48 weeks depending on the virus genotype **Coinfection with HIV:** 800 mg PO daily for 48 weeks with 180 mcg of peginterferon alfa-2a	
sofosbuvir	Sovaldi	400 mg once a day or 1 packet of pellets	
glecaprevir + pibrentasvir	Mavyret, Maviret	Take 3 tablets once daily	
sofosbuvir + velpatasvir	Epclusa	Take 1 tablet once daily	
sofosbuvir + ledipasvir	Harvoni	Take 1 tablet once daily	
sofosbuvir + velpatasvir + voxilaprevir	Vosevi	Take 1 tablet once daily	
elbasvir + grazoprevir	Zepatier	Take 1 tablet once daily	

Respiratory Syncytial Virus

Generic Name	Brand Name	Usual Dose and Dosing Schedule	Warning Labels
palivizumab	Synagis	**Prevention:** 15 mg/kg IM monthly	STORE AT ROOM TEMPERATURE PROTECT FROM LIGHT AND MOISTURE—virazole. DO NOT SHAKE—palivizumab.
ribavirin	Virazole	**Treatment:** 20 mg/mL administered as continuous aerosol administration for 12–18 h/day for 3–7 days	

Summary of Drugs Used for the Treatment of Influenza, Herpes, Hepatitis, Respiratory Syncytial Virus, and Cytomegalovirus Viral Infections—cont'd

Generic Name	Brand Name	Usual Dose and Dosing Schedule	Warning Labels
Herpes Simplex, Herpes Zoster Infections			
acyclovir	Zovirax	Varies according to type of infection (HSV-1, HSV-2, VZV) and acute versus recurrent infection **Dosage range:** **IV:** 5–10 mg/kg every 8 h for 5–10 days **Oral:** 200 mg 5 times/day or 400 mg tid for 5–10 days **Topical:** Apply every 3 h for 7 days	SHAKE WELL—acyclovir suspension. COMPLETE FULL COURSE OF THERAPY; BEGIN THERAPY WITHIN 72 HOURS OF ONSET OF SYMPTOMS. SWALLOW WHOLE; DO NOT CRUSH OR CHEW—ganciclovir. AVOID PREGNANCY—ganciclovir. TAKE WITH FOOD—ganciclovir.
famciclovir	Famvir	Varies according to type of infection (HSV-1, HSV-?, VZV) and acute versus recurrent infection **Dosage range:** 125–500 mg bid or tid for 5–10 days or 1000–1500 mg bid for 1 day	WASH YOUR HANDS WITH SOAP AND WATER AFTER USING—penciclovir. DO NOT SKIP DOSES—all. SHAKE WELL, STORE IN THE REFRIGERATOR, DISCARD AFTER 28 DAYS—valacyclovir suspension.
ganciclovir	Cytovene Ganzyk-RTU	Varies according to acute or recurrent CMV infection **Dosage range:** **IV:** 5 mg/kg IV every 12–24 h for 7–21 days **Oral:** 1000 mg tid or 500 mg 6 times daily **CMV prevention (posttransplant):** 5 mg/kg every 12 h for 7–14 days; then once daily 7 days per week, or 6 mg/kg for 5 days/week for 100–120 days	
penciclovir	Denavir	**Cold sores:** Apply every 2 h while awake for 4 days; start within 1 h of symptom onset	
valacyclovir	Valtrex	Varies according to type of infection (HSV-1, HSV-2, VZV) and acute versus recurrent infection **Dosage range:** 500 mg–2 g, 2–3 times a day for 5–10 days	
foscarnet	Foscavir	Varies according to type of infection (HSV-1, HSV-2, VZV, CMV) and acute versus recurrent infection **Dosage range:** 40–90 mg/kg IV every 8–12 h for 2–3 weeks	STORE AT ROOM TEMPERATURE; DISCARD DISCOLORED SOLUTION—foscarnet. REMOVE CONTACT LENSES BEFORE USE—trifluridine.
trifluridine	Viroptic	1 drop in affected eye(s) every 2 h while awake (max, 9 drops/day)	
Cytomegalovirus			
cidofovir	Vistide	**CMV retinitis:** 5 mg/kg IV once weekly for 2 weeks with probenecid **Prophylaxis:** 5 mg/kg IV once every other week	USE WITHIN 24 HOURS OF PREPARATION—cidofovir. STORE BETWEEN 2°C AND 8°C (36°C–46°F)—Cytogam. USE WITHIN 6 HOURS OPENING—Cytogam.[a]
cytomegalovirus immune globulin	Cytogam	100–150 mg/kg/dose	

[a]Generic available.

SC, subcutaneously; *IM*, intramuscularly; *PO*, orally; *IV*, intravenously; *RSV*, respiratory syncytial virus.

Adverse Reactions

Veklury is administered parenterally and may cause soreness or swelling at the injection site. It may also cause nausea and bleeding or bruising of the skin. Sotrovimab is administered by intravenous infusion. Diarrhea is the most common reaction; however, infusion-related anaphylaxis reactions have occurred. Paxlovid adverse reactions are altered taste, diarrhea, and muscle aches. Rebound infections may occur 2 to 8 days after treatment with Paxlovid in up to 9% of patients, according to the US Centers for Disease Control and Prevention.

Treatment of COVID-19

Generic Name	US Brand Name(s)	Dosage Forms and Strengths
	Canadian Brand Name(s)	
remdesivir[a]	Veklury	**Powder, for injection(?)[a]:** 100 mg/vial
		Solution, for injection: 5 mg/mL
	Veklury	
sotrovimab	Not available	**Solution, intravenous:** 500 mg/8 mL
	sotrovimab	
nirmatrelvir + ritonavir	Paxlovid	**Tablet:** 150 mg nirmatrelvir + 100 mg ritonavir
	Paxlovid	

[a]Available in the United States only.

Summary of Drugs Used to Treat COVID-19

Generic Name	Brand Name	Usual Dose and Dosing Schedule	Warning Labels
ritonavir	Veklury	**Hospitalized patients:** day 1, 200 mg; day 2, 100 mg once daily × 10 days **Outpatient:** × 3 days	
sotrovimab	sotrovimab	Infuse 500 mg over 1 h as a single dose	REFRIGERATE; DO NOT FREEZE. DO NOT SHAKE.
nirmatrelvir + ritonavir	Paxlovid	Take 2 tablets nirmatrelvir (300 mg) + 1 tablet ritonavir (100 mg) twice a day for 5 days	SWALLOW WHOLE; DO NOT CRUSH OR CHEW.

Human Immunodeficiency Virus and Acquired Immunodeficiency Syndrome

HIV/AIDS (*acquired immunodeficiency syndrome*) is a global public health issue. According to the Joint United Nations Programme on HIV/AIDS (UNAIDS), 39 million people were living with HIV in 2022. There were 1.3 million new HIV infections wordwide reported in 2022.

HIV/AIDS is worsened by poverty. Poverty creates the following conditions: (1) individuals knowingly engage in risky sexual behaviors such as the sex trade; (2) it increases malnutrition, which can weaken the immune system; (3) it decreases access to health care and HIV medicines, which can increase drug resistance; and (4) many HIV medicines should be taken with food, and access to regular meals may be limited.

HIV is the virus that causes AIDS. The virus attacks *CD4 T lymphocytes* and weakens the immune system. As the CD4 count declines below 200 cells/mm³ and the viral load increases, the risk for developing opportunistic infections such as tuberculosis, candidiasis, CMV, and other AIDS-defining conditions also increases. The viral load is the amount of materials from the virus that are released into the bloodstream when the HIV reproduces.

Human Immunodeficiency Virus Life Cycle

HIV, like other viruses, lacks the cellular machinery to reproduce itself. It incorporates its DNA into the DNA of the host cell; then, when the host cell tries to make new proteins, it accidentally makes new HIV as well. HIV treatments interfere with specific steps in the HIV life cycle and are briefly described here:

- Step 1. Binding: The HIV binds to CD4 surface receptors.
- Step 2. Fusion: The HIV is activated by proteins on the cell's surface, allowing the HIV envelope to fuse to the outside of the cell.
- Step 3. Uncoating: The virus is uncoated, permitting the contents of the viral capsid (viral RNA and enzymes) to be released into the infected host cell.
- Step 4. Reverse transcription: A viral enzyme called reverse transcriptase makes a DNA copy of the viral RNA.
- Step 5. Integration: Viral DNA is incorporated into the host cellular DNA.
- Step 6. Genome replication: The strands of viral DNA in the nucleus separate and mRNA provides instructions for making new virus (genome). This process is called transcription.
- Step 7. Protein synthesis: The HIV mRNA genome acts as a template for synthesizing viral proteins needed to make a new virus in a process called translation.
- Step 8. Protein cleavage and viral assembly: Protease is an enzyme that cuts the long chain of viral protein into smaller individual proteins. Some of the cleaved proteins become structural elements of new HIV and others become enzymes, such as reverse transcriptase. The new particles are assembled into new HIV.
- Step 9. Virus release: New virus buds off from the host cell.

Pharmacologic Treatment

UNAIDS 2020 treatment targets are: (1) 90% of people living with HIV know their HIV status, (2) 90% of people who know their HIV-positive status are accessing treatment, and (3) 90% of people on treatment have a suppressed viral load. Global HIV treatment and prevention programs have been credited with the 16% decline in new AIDS infections between 2010 and 2016 worldwide. *Antiretrovirals* are administered to reduce viral load, increase CD4 counts, delay the development of AIDS-related conditions and opportunistic infections, and improve survival. Antiretroviral agents fall into eight classes:

- Nucleoside/nucleotide reverse transcriptase inhibitors (NRTIs)
- Non-nucleoside reverse transcriptase inhibitors (NNRTIs)
- Protease inhibitors
- Fusion inhibitors
- Chemokine receptor antagonist type 5 (CCR5)
- HIV integrase strand inhibitors
- Attachment Inhibitors
- Postattachment Inhibitors

International treatment guidelines have been established for initiation of antiretroviral therapy based on CD4 counts and whether patients are symptomatic or asymptomatic. Antiretroviral therapy is a lifelong commitment and requires strict adherence to treatment regimens.

To reduce antiviral resistance, *HAART*—a regimen of three or more medications from two or more antiretroviral classes—is prescribed. Combination therapy improves effectiveness and decreases the risk of developing resistance but may increase adverse reactions. Antiretroviral agent resistance testing is recommended before the initiation of therapy with antiretroviral drugs and before changing therapy.

Nucleoside and Nucleotide Reverse Transcriptase Inhibitors

Many NRTIs are prodrugs that are activated by host cell enzymes. They competitively inhibit reverse transcriptase, the enzyme that makes a DNA copy of the viral RNA.

Abacavir

Abacavir (also called ABC) is an NRTI. It is an ingredient in the triple antiretroviral therapy that combines abacavir with zidovudine and lamivudine. It is also formulated with lamivudine as a dual combination therapy. It is linked to a fatal hypersensitivity reaction that necessitates discontinuation of the drug. Symptoms include fever and chills, muscle and joint pain, fatigue and feeling rundown, nausea and vomiting, skin rash, and shortness of breath.

Emtricitabine

Emtricitabine (commonly called FTC) is an NRTI similar to lamivudine. *Cross-resistance* occurs between lamivudine and emtricitabine. Cross-resistance refers to the development of resistance to one agent in a particular class that results in resistance to the other agents in that class. Emtricitabine is formulated as an oral capsule and an oral solution. Refrigeration is recommended for the oral solution; however, the solution is stable at room temperature for 3 months if refrigeration is not available.

Lamivudine

Lamivudine (commonly called 3TC) is an NRTI that is effective against HIV, including zidovudine-resistant strains of HIV. Lamivudine also inhibits replication of HBV. It is a good choice of therapy for those who have HIV and HBV coinfections. Lamivudine is an ingredient in HIV combination therapies. The drug has good oral absorption, and the relatively long intracellular half-life (12 hours) permits once-daily dosing.

Tenofovir

Tenofovir (or TDF, short for tenofovir disoproxil fumarate) is an NRTI. It is administered orally. Food increases bioavailability of the drug. It has a long intracellular half-life, up to 50 hours. Tenofovir-containing antiretrovirals are used for preexposure prevention (PrEP) of HIV infection. Tenofovir should not be administered concurrently with adefovir (used to treat hepatitis C) because it increases the risk of toxicity.

Zidovudine

Zidovudine (also known as AZT or azidothymidine) was the first available antiretroviral drug and was introduced in 1987. It is an NRTI and is formulated for oral and parenteral administration. The drug may be administered orally to pregnant women and intravenously during delivery, and as a suspension to neonates. It has been shown to decrease perinatal mother-to-child transmission of HIV from 25% to 8%.

Adverse Reactions

Common side effects associated with almost all NRTIs are headache, stomach upset, fatigue or insomnia, muscle ache, and diarrhea. Zidovudine may also cause nail discoloration. More severe, less common side effects are liver problems, muscle inflammation and weakness, diabetes, abnormal fat distribution (lipodystrophy syndrome),

Nucleoside Reverse Transcriptase Inhibitors Used for the Treatment of HIV and AIDS*

Generic Name	US Brand Name(s) Canadian Brand Name(s)	Dosage Forms and Strengths
abacavir[a] (ABC)	Ziagen	**Tablet:** 300 mg
	Ziagen	**Solution:** 20 mg/mL
emtricitabine[a] (FTC)	Emtriva	**Capsule:** 200 mg
	Not available	**Solution:** 10 mg/mL
lamivudine[a] (3TC)	Epivir	**Solution:** 10 mg/mL
	Epivir	**Tablet:** 150 mg, 300 mg

Continued

Nucleoside Reverse Transcriptase Inhibitors Used for the Treatment of HIV and AIDS*—cont'd

Generic Name	US Brand Name(s) Canadian Brand Name(s)	Dosage Forms and Strengths
tenofovir DF[a] (TDF)	Viread	**Powder, for oral suspension**[b]: 40 mg/scoopful **Tablet**: 150 mg[b], 200 mg[b], 250 mg[b], 300 mg
	Viread	
zidovudine[a] (AZT)	Retrovir	**Capsule**: 100 mg **Solution, injection**: 10 mg/mL **Syrup**: 10 mg/1 mL
	Retrovir	
Fixed-Dose Combinations		
abacavir + lamivudine[a]	Epzicom	**Tablet**: 600 mg abacavir + 300 mg lamivudine
	Kivexa	
emtricitabine + tenofovir DF[a]	Truvada	**Tablet**: 200 mg emtricitabine + 300 mg tenofovir DF 100 mg emtricitabine + 150 mg tenofovir[b] 133 mg emtricitabine + 200 mg tenofovir[b] 167 mg emtricitabine + 250 mg tenofovir[b]
	Truvada	
emtricitabine + tenofovir AF	Descovy	**Tablet**: 200 mg emtricitabine + 25 mg tenofovir AF 200 mg emtricitabine + 10 mg tenofovir AF[c] 120 mg emtricitabine + 15 mg tenofovir AF[b]
	Descovy	
lamivudine + zidovudine[a]	Combivir	**Tablet**: 150 mg lamivudine + 300 mg zidovudine
	Combivir	
efavirenz + emtricitabine + tenofovir[a]	Atripla	**Tablet**: 600 mg efavirenz + 200 mg emtricitabine + 300 mg tenofovir
	Generics	
abacavir + lamivudine + zidovudine[a]	Trizivir	**Tablet**: 300 mg abacavir + 150 mg lamivudine + 300 mg zidovudine
	Not available	
emtricitabine + rilpivirine + tenofovir DF	Complera	**Tablet**: 200 mg emtricitabine + 25 mg rilpivirine + 300 mg tenofovir
	Complera	
emtricitabine + rilpivirine + tenofovir AF	Odefsey	**Tablet**: 200 mg emtricitabine + 25 mg rilpivirine + 25 mg tenofovir
	Odefsey	
lamivudine + tenofovir + efavirenz	Symfi, Symfi Lo	**Tablet**: 300 mg lamivudine + 300 mg tenofovir + 600 mg efavirenz 300 mg lamivudine + 300 mg tenofovir + 400 mg efavirenz
	Not available	

[a]Generic available.
[b]Available in the United States only.
[c]Available in Canada only.
*Only brand names and strengths of NRTIs marketed for the treatment of HIV/AIDS are shown in the table. Additional strengths or brand names may be marketed for the treatment of additional infections.

high cholesterol, decreased bone density caused by osteonecrosis and osteopenia, skin rash, pancreatitis (inflammation of the pancreas), peripheral neuropathy, leukopenia (a drop in the white blood cell count), and increased bleeding in patients with hemophilia.

Non–Nucleoside Reverse Transcriptase Inhibitors

NNRTIs bind to viral transcriptase. They differ from NRTIs in three important ways:
1. NNRTIs are noncompetitive inhibitors of reverse transcriptase.
2. They do not need to be activated by host enzymes.
3. They are not effective against HIV-2.

Except for nevirapine, NNRTIs are used only in combination therapy with NRTIs and PIs because resistance develops rapidly. All NNRTIs are metabolized by cytochrome P-450 hepatic enzymes and reduce their own half-life as well as the half-life of other drugs coadministered with them that are metabolized by the same enzymes. Numerous drug interactions are seen when NNRTIs are administered concurrently with benzodiazepines, HMG-CoA inhibitors (-*statins*), and proton pump inhibitors (-*prazoles*).

Delavirdine

Delavirdine (also called DLV) has a short half-life and must be given in multiple daily doses. It is administered three times daily compared with nevirapine and efavirenz, which are dosed once daily. Cross-resistance, frequency of dosing, and the number of tablets per dose (four tablets) have limited the use of delavirdine.

Efavirenz

Efavirenz (or EFV) is an ingredient in several fixed-dose combination medicines used for the treatment of HIV-1 infection. It is also available as a single-ingredient product; however, monotherapy is not recommended because of the rapid development of resistance. The drug is administered by mouth, and because of its long half-life (40 to 55 hours) it may be given once daily.

Efavirenz is teratogenic. The drug should not be administered in the first trimester of pregnancy, and women taking the drug should be advised to avoid pregnancy.

Nevirapine

Nevirapine (or NVP) is the one NNRTI that may be administered as monotherapy for the prevention of mother-to-child transmission of HIV. It is administered as a single dose. Controversy exists about the use of single-dose nevirapine therapy because of the risk of developing drug resistance. Treatment of mothers with triple antiretroviral therapy reduces the risk for developing antiretroviral resistance.

Nevirapine is associated with fatal liver toxicity, and the FDA has required changes in the package labeling to warn of this adverse effect. Risk for the development of liver toxicity with the use of single doses of nevirapine to the mother and child for the prevention of perinatal HIV infection is minimal.

Adverse Reactions

Rash is a common side effect of all NNRTIs. Nevirapine is associated with fatal hepatotoxicity. The risk is greatest during the first 6 to 18 weeks of therapy and is more common in women than in men. Efavirenz may cause dizziness, drowsiness or insomnia, abnormal dreams, confusion, abnormal thinking, impaired concentration, amnesia, agitation, hallucinations, depersonalization, and euphoria.

Protease Inhibitors

PIs interfere with step 8 of the HIV life cycle. They block the cleavage of long-chain viral proteins into individual proteins that are assembled to make a new virus. PIs are administered as combination therapy; most are recommended to be given along with ritonavir.

> **⚠ Tech Alert!**
>
> A common ending for protease inhibitors is -navir.

Fosamprenavir

Fosamprenavir is indicated for the treatment of HIV-1 infection. Fosamprenavir is a prodrug that is metabolized to the active drug amprenavir. The effect of fosamprenavir is boosted with the coadministration of ritonavir.

Atazanavir

Atazanavir (or ATV) is another PI that is effective against HIV-1. Its effectiveness is increased when the drug is coadministered with ritonavir. Concurrent administration with the NNRTI efavirenz can decrease its bioavailability. Atazanavir may be given orally once daily. Administration with a light meal increases bioavailability compared with a heavy meal or fasting.

Darunavir

Darunavir (also called DRV) has advantages over other PIs because cross-resistance is low and it produces a greater reduction in viral

Non–Nucleoside Reverse Transcriptase Inhibitors Used for the Treatment of HIV and AIDS

Generic Name	US Brand Name(s) / Canadian Brand Name(s)	Dosage Forms and Strengths
doravirine (DOR)	Pifeltro / Pifeltro	**Tablet:** 100 mg
efavirenz (EFV)[a]	Sustiva / Sustiva	**Capsule:** 50 mg[b], 200 mg **Tablet**[b]: 600 mg
etravirine (ETV)	Intelence / Intelence	**Tablet:** 25 mg, 100 mg, 200 mg
nevirapine[a] (NVP)	Viramune, Viramune XR / Generics	**Suspension:** 10 mg/1 mL[c] **Tablet:** 200 mg **Tablet, extended release (Viramune XR)**[b]: 100 mg, 400 mg
rilpivirine (RIL)	Edurant / Edurant	**Tablet:** 25 mg

Combination Non-Nucleoside Reverse Transcriptase Inhibitors

doravirine + lamivudine + tenofovir DF	Delstrigo / Delstrigo	**Tablet:** 100 mg doravirine + 300 mg lamivudine + 300 mg tenofovir DF

[a]Generic available.
[b]Available in Canada only.
[c]Available in the United States only.

load after 24 weeks of treatment. Like other PIs, it must be administered along with ritonavir. Darunavir and atazanavir are also formulated as a combination product with cobicistat and other antiviral agents. Cobicistat (Tybost®) is a CYP3A inhibitor that decreases the metabolism of the drugs, thereby increasing systemic exposure to antiretroviral agents used for the treatment of HIV-1 infection.

Indinavir

Indinavir (or IDV) must be administered in three daily doses. Absorption is affected by food, so the drug is taken on an empty stomach. To avoid the formation of kidney stones, indinavir should be taken with at least 1.5 L of water daily. The effects of indinavir are boosted by the coadministration of ritonavir.

Nelfinavir

Nelfinavir (also called NFV) is a competitive inhibitor of HIV protease that is typically administered as part of a three-drug regimen that includes indinavir, efavirenz, and/or abacavir. Unlike indinavir and atazanavir, the absorption of nelfinavir is enhanced by a fatty meal. Nelfinavir should be taken with food. Nelfinavir oral powder is stable for 6 hours, once mixed with food or liquid, if refrigerated.

Ritonavir

Ritonavir (or RTV) is a competitive inhibitor of HIV protease. It differs from other PIs in that it is effective against HIV-1 and HIV-2 proteases. Ritonavir boosts the effects of other PIs by inhibiting their metabolism, and resistance appears to occur more slowly than with other PIs. Ritonavir inhibits the metabolic enzyme CYP3A4. It is formulated as a single entity and a fixed-dose combination with lopinavir (Kaletra). Lopinavir/ritonavir (LPV/r) is available in multiple formulations. The syrup formulation must be refrigerated, so the cold chain must be maintained until dispensing. It has good oral bioavailability, although adverse effects are common and occur in more than 85% of those taking the drug.

Tipranavir

Tipranavir is a sulfonamide that selectively binds to HIV-1 protease. It has a lower rate for the development of resistance than some other PIs. Like other PIs, tipranavir is not used for monotherapy but is administered with other antiretroviral drugs. It should be taken with food to increase absorption.

Adverse Reactions

PIs can elevate triglyceride, cholesterol (see Chapter 19), and blood glucose levels, and can produce insulin resistance (see Chapter 26). They also cause the redistribution of fat, causing its accumulation in the abdomen and loss in the face and limbs. All PIs produce nausea, vomiting, and diarrhea.

Fusion Inhibitors

Fusion inhibitors interfere with step 2 in the HIV life cycle. Fusion (the attachment of the HIV to the host cell membrane) is required for the virus capsid to release its contents (genetic material) into the host cell.

Enfuvirtide must be administered by subcutaneous injection in the thigh, arm, or abdomen. It is formulated as a powder that is reconstituted before administration. Once reconstituted, the solution is stable for only 24 hours if refrigerated. Enfuvirtide is intended to be administered in combination with other antiretroviral drugs.

Protease Inhibitors Used for the Treatment of HIV and AIDS

Generic Name	US Brand Name(s) / Canadian Brand Name(s)	Dosage Forms and Strengths
atazanavir (ATV)[a]	Reyataz / Reyataz	**Capsule:** 100 mg[b], 150 mg, 200 mg, 300 mg **Powder, oral**[b]: 50 mg/packet
darunavir (DRV)[a]	Prezista / Prezista	**Suspension:** 100 mg/mL **Tablet:** 75 mg, 150 mg, 300 mg[b], 400 mg[b], 600 mg, 800 mg
fosamprenavir (FPV)[a,b]	Lexiva / Telzir	**Suspension:** 50 mg/mL **Tablet:** 700 mg
nelfinavir (NFV)	Viracept / Not available	**Tablet:** 250 mg, 625 mg
ritonavir (RTV)[a]	Norvir / Norvir	**Powder, oral**[b]: 100 mg/packet **Solution, oral**[b]: 80 mg/mL **Tablet:** 100 mg
tipranavir	Aptivus / Aptivus	**Capsule:** 250 mg **Solution, oral**[b]: 100 mg/mL

Protease Inhibitor Combinations

atazanavir + cobicistat	Evotaz / Not available	**Tablet:** 300 mg atazanavir + 150 mg cobicistat
darunavir + cobicistat	Prezcobix / Prezcobix	**Tablet:** 800 mg darunavir + 150 mg cobicistat
lopinavir + ritonavir[a,b]	Kaletra / Kaletra	**Solution, oral:** 80 mg/mL lopinavir + 20 mg/mL ritonavir **Tablet:** 100 mg lopinavir + 25 mg ritonavir 200 mg lopinavir + 50 mg ritonavir
darunavir + cobicistat + emtricitabine + tenofovir	Symtuza / Symtuza	**Tablet:** 800 mg darunavir + 150 mg cobicistat + 200 mg emtricitabine + 10 mg tenofovir

[a]Generic available.
[b]Available in the United States only.

Adverse Reactions

Irritation, pain, redness, itchiness, and the formation of nodules and cysts at the site of injection are common adverse reactions. Allergic reactions also occur and produce rash, chills, fever, stiffness, hypotension, nausea, and vomiting.

Fusion Inhibitors Used for the Treatment of HIV and AIDS

Generic Name	US Brand Name(s) Canadian Brand Name(s)	Dosage Forms and Strengths
enfuvirtide (T-20)	Fuzeon Fuzeon	Powder, for solution: 90 mg/vial[a], 108 mg/vial[b]

[a]Available in the United States only.
[b]Available in Canada only.

Chemokine Receptor Type 5 Antagonist

Maraviroc is a human CCR5. It is the only agent in this class and is a novel drug for the treatment of HIV. It inhibits HIV entry into host cells.

Mechanism of Action

Maraviroc is a selective CCR5 antagonist of the G protein-coupled receptor found on the cell surface. It is associated with entry of HIV into human host cells. Maraviroc binding to the CCR5 receptor prevents CCR5-tropic HIV-1 entry into cells. It does not prevent cell entry mediated by CXCR4 receptor binding of dual or mixed receptor binding.

Adverse Effects

The most common side effects of maraviroc are colds, cough, fever, rash, and dizziness. Myocardial infarction, hepatotoxicity, and increased infections or cancers have also been reported.

CCR5 Antagonists Used for the Treatment of HIV and AIDS

Generic Name	US Brand Name(s) Canadian Brand Name(s)	Dosage Forms and Strengths
maraviroc	Selzentry Celsentri	Solution, oral[a]: 20 mg/mL Tablet: 25 mg[a], 75 mg[a], 150 mg, 300 mg

[a]Available in the United States only.

Human Immunodeficiency Virus Integrase Strand Inhibitors

Dolutegravir, elvitegravir, bictegravir, and raltegravir are HIV integrase strand inhibitors. HIV resistance to raltegravir can develop quickly, so it is indicated only in combination with other antiretroviral agents.

Mechanism of Action

HIV integrase strand inhibitors block the final step in the process of human host cell infection by HIV. The HIV-1 integrase viral enzyme binds to the double-stranded viral DNA and mediates its integration into the infected host cell's DNA to produce a functional provirus.

Adverse Effects

Raltegravir side effects include headache, dizziness, diarrhea, and GI upset. Rhabdomyolysis, depression, suicide ideation, thrombocytopenia, and increased cancers have also been reported.

> **! Tech Alert!**
>
> Isentress chewable tablets and suspension are not interchangeable. Do not substitute.

Attachment Inhibitors and Postattachment Inhibitors. Attachment inhibitors and postattachment inhibitors prevent HIV from entering cells. Fostemsavir is an attachment inhibitor that is administered orally. Ibalizumab is a monoclonal antibody. Ibalizumab is classified as a postattachment inhibitor. Fostemsavir and ibalizumab are used to treat multidrug-resistant HIV-1 infection. Fostemsavir and ibalizumab are taken concurrently with other antiretroviral medicines.

Mechanism of Action. Fostemsavir is a prodrug of temsavir. It is an attachment inhibitor. The antiretroviral agent binds to gp120 protein on the surface of HIV and entry into CD4 cell is blocked. Ibalizumab binds to CD4 T cell amino acid sites across from the gp120 protein site. The binding inhibits structural changes necessary for gp120 protein action to open access into cells. As a result, HIV is unable to enter the cells.

Adverse Reactions. Common adverse reactions to fostemsavir are headache, upset stomach, nausea, and fatigue. Common side effects of ibalizumab are diarrhea, nausea, rash, and dizziness.

Preexposure Prophylaxis. Individuals who are at risk for getting HIV can now take PrEP. PrEP is taken orally or by intramuscular injection once every 2 months. PrEP is up to 99% effective in reducing the risk for HIV from sex when taken as prescribed. PrEP is recommended for individuals (1) who have anal or vaginal sex without a condom with a sexual partner who has HIV, (2) who have had a sexually transmitted infection in the past 6 months, (3) who have injected drugs or shared needles/injection equipment with another individual who has HIV, and (4) whose HIV status is unknown. PrEP antiretroviral drugs include Truvada, Descovy, Apretude, and Vocabria. Should an individual be exposed to HIV, post-exposure (PEP) drugs may be taken. The CDC recommends the combination pill tenofovir + emtriciabine plus dolutegravir or raltegravir once or twice a day for 28 days.

TECHNICIAN'S CORNER

1. We have yet to find a cure for the common cold. Why is it difficult to find that cure?
2. HPV is spreading among teens. Why is it important to reduce the risk for HPV infection? Who should be vaccinated?

HIV Integrase Strand Inhibitors Used for the Treatment of HIV and AIDS

Generic Name	US Brand Name(s) Canadian Brand Name(s)	Dosage Forms and Strengths
cabotegravir (CAB)	Apretude, Vocabria Vocabria	**Suspension, intramuscular extended release (Apretude):** 200 mg/mL **Tablet (Vocabria):** 30 mg
dolutegravir (DTG)	Tivicay, Tivicay PD Tivicay	**Tablet:** 10 mg, 25 mg, 50 mg **Tablet, for suspension:** 5 mg
raltegravir (RAL)	Isentress, Isentress HD Isentress, Isentress HD	**Powder, oral**[a]**:** 100 mg/packet **Tablet, chewable:** 25 mg, 100 mg **Tablet:** 400 mg, 600 mg
Combination Integrase Strand Inhibitors		
cabotegravir + rilpivirine	Cabenuva Kit Cabenuva	**Suspension, for IM injection:** 200 mg/mL cabotegravir + 300 mg/mL rilpivirine
dolutegravir + lamivudine	Dovato Dovato	**Tablet:** 50 mg dolutegravir + 300 mg lamivudine
dolutegravir + rilpivirine	Juluca Juluca	**Tablet:** 50 mg dolutegravir + 25 mg rilpivirine
dolutegravir + abacavir + lamivudine	Triumeq, Triumeq PD Triumeq	**Tablet:** 50 mg dolutegravir + 600 mg abacavir + 300 mg lamivudine **Tablet, for suspension (Triumeq PD):** 5 mg dolutegravir + 60 mg abacavir + 30 mg lamivudine
elvitegravir + cobicistat (COBI) + emtricitabine + tenofovir DF	Stribild Stribild	**Tablet:** 150 mg elvitegravir + 150 mg cobicistat + 200 mg emtricitabine + 300 mg tenofovir DF
elvitegravir + cobicistat (COBI) + emtricitabine + tenofovir AF	Genvoya Genvoya	**Tablet:** 150 mg elvitegravir + 150 mg cobicistat + 200 mg emtricitabine + 10 mg tenofovir AF
bictegravir + emtricitabine + tenofovir AF	Biktarvy Biktarvy	**Tablet:** 30 mg bictegravir + 120 mg emtricitabine + 15 mg tenofovir AF[a], 50 mg bictegravir + 200 mg emtricitabine + 25 mg tenofovir AF

[a]Available in the United States only.

Attachment Inhibitors and Postattachment Inhibitors Used for the Treatment of HIV and AIDS

Generic Name	US Brand Name(s) Canadian Brand Name(s)	Dosage Forms and Strengths
Attachment Inhibitors		
fostemsavir	Rukobia Rukobia	**Tablet, extended release:** 600 mg
Postattachment Inhibitors		
ibalizumab-uiyk	Trogarzo Not available	**Solution, intravenous:** 150 mg/mL

Summary of Drugs Used for the Treatment of HIV and AIDS

Generic Name	Brand Name	Usual Dose and Dosing Schedule	Warning Labels
Nucleoside Reverse Transcriptase Inhibitors			
abacavir	Ziagen	300 mg bid or 600 mg once daily	TAKE EXACTLY AS DIRECTED; DO NOT SKIP DOSES—all.
emtricitabine	Emtriva	Varies according to body weight and dosage form **Capsule:** 200 mg once daily (>33 kg) **Oral solution:** 6 mg/kg up to 240 mg once daily	AVOID ALCOHOL—abacavir, lamivudine. PROTECT FROM MOISTURE—abacavir.
lamivudine	Epivir	300 mg once daily or 150 mg twice daily	REFRIGERATE; DO NOT FREEZE (SOLUTION)— emtricitabine.
tenofovir DF	Viread	300 mg once daily	REFRIGERATE DILUTED IV SOLUTION (STABLE FOR 24 HOURS AT ROOM TEMPERATURE)—
zidovudine	Retrovir	**Oral:** 300 mg PO twice daily or 200 mg PO 3 times a day **Intravenous:** 1 mg/kg IV given 5 or 6 times daily, around the clock	zIdovudine (IV). TAKE WITH FOOD—tenofovir DF. TAKE WITH LOTS OF WATER—zidovudine. DISCARD 48 HOURS AFTER MIXING—zidovudine (IV).
lamivudine + zidovudine	Combivir	1 tablet twice daily	AVOID ALCOHOL—Combivir. TAKE ON AN EMPTY STOMACH—Atripla, Symfi.
abacavir + lamivudine	Epzicom	1 tablet once daily	
emtricitabine + tenofovir	Truvada	1 tablet once daily	
efavirenz + emtricitabine + tenofovir	Atripla	1 tablet daily at bedtime	
efavirenz + lamivudine + tenofovir	Symfi	1 tablet daily	
abacavir + lamivudine + zidovudine	Trizivir	1 tablet twice daily	
emtricitabine + tenofovir AF	Descovy	1 tablet once daily	
emtricitabine + rilpivirine + tenofovir AF	Odefsey	1 tablet once daily	
Non–Nucleoside Reverse Transcriptase Inhibitors			
delavirdine	Rescriptor	400 mg 3 times a day	STORE IN ORIGINAL CONTAINER. PROTECT FROM MOISTURE—Pilfeltro, Delstrigo.
doravirine	Pilfeltro	100 mg tablet once daily	TAKE EXACTLY AS DIRECTED; DO NOT SKIP DOSES—all.
efavirenz	Sustiva	600 mg once daily	AVOID ANTACIDS WITHIN 1 HOUR OF DOSE—delavirdine.
etravirine	Intelence	200 mg twice a day	TAKE ON AN EMPTY STOMACH—efavirenz.
nevirapine	Viramune	200 mg once daily for the first 14 days, then 200 mg twice daily **Extended release:** 400 mg once daily	TAKE WITH FOOD—rilpivirine. MAY CAUSE DIZZINESS OR DROWSINESS; ALCOHOL INTENSIFIES THIS EFFECT—efavirenz.
rilpivirine	Edurant	25 mg once daily	AVOID PREGNANCY—efavirenz. SHAKE GENTLY (SUSPENSION)—nevirapine.
cabotegravir + rilpivirine	Cabenuva	Inject 3 mL IM every 3 months or 2 mL every 2 months	REFRIGERATE.

Continued

Summary of Drugs Used for the Treatment of HIV and AIDS—cont'd

Generic Name	Brand Name	Usual Dose and Dosing Schedule	Warning Labels
Protease Inhibitors			
atazanavir	Reyataz	400 mg once daily or 300 mg once daily (taken with ritonavir)	TAKE EXACTLY AS DIRECTED; DO NOT SKIP DOSES—all. AVOID ANTACIDS WITHIN 1 HOUR OF DOSE—atazanavir. SWALLOW WHOLE; DO NOT CRUSH OR CHEW—atazanavir, Kaletra. TAKE WITH FOOD—atazanavir, darunavir, fosamprenavir (pediatric suspension), nelfinavir, ritonavir, tipranavir, Kaletra. TAKE ON AN EMPTY STOMACH—indinavir. MAINTAIN ADEQUATE HYDRATION—indinavir. PROTECT FROM MOISTURE—indinavir. REFRIGERATE, DO NOT FREEZE—ritonavir, tipranavir, Kaletra. SHAKE WELL (SUSPENSION)—ritonavir. CAPSULE STABLE FOR 30 DAYS (ritonavir), 60 DAYS (tipranavir) AT ROOM TEMPERATURE. SOLUTION STABLE FOR 60 DAYS AT ROOM TEMPERATURE—Kaletra.
darunavir	Prezista	800 mg once daily or 600 mg twice daily (taken with ritonavir)	
fosamprenavir	Lexiva, Telzir	700 mg twice daily or 1400 mg once daily (taken with ritonavir) or 1400 mg twice daily	
nelfinavir	Viracept	1250 mg twice daily or 750 mg 3 times a day	
ritonavir	Norvir	600 mg twice daily (as sole PI) or 100–400 mg once daily when taken to boost the effect of other antiretrovirals	
tipranavir	Aptivus	500 mg twice daily (taken with ritonavir)	
lopinavir + ritonavir	Kaletra	3 capsules, 5 mL, or 2 tablets twice daily (400 mg lopinavir + 100 mg ritonavir) *or* 6 capsules, 10 mL, or 4 tablets once daily (800 mg lopinavir + 200 mg ritonavir)	
Fusion Inhibitor			
enfuvirtide	Fuzeon	90 mg subcutaneously twice daily	TAKE EXACTLY AS DIRECTED; DO NOT SKIP DOSES. REFRIGERATE DILUTED SOLUTION, DO NOT FREEZE; DISCARD AFTER 24 HOURS.
CCR5 Antagonist			
maraviroc	Selzentry, Celsentri	150–600 mg twice daily	TAKE EXACTLY AS DIRECTED; DO NOT SKIP DOSES. MAY CAUSE DIZZINESS OR DROWSINESS.

Summary of Drugs Used for the Treatment of HIV and AIDS—cont'd

Generic Name	Brand Name	Usual Dose and Dosing Schedule	Warning Labels
HIV Integrase Strand Inhibitor			
cabotegravir	Apretude Vocabria	**PrEP:** 30 mg Vocabria (1 tablet) once daily with 25 mg Endurant (1 tablet) for 28 days then start Apretude IM every 2 months	TAKE WITH FOOD—Vocabria. TAKE EXACTLY AS DIRECTED; DO NOT SKIP DOSES. SWALLOW WHOLE; DO NOT CRUSH OR CHEW—dolutegravir. TAKE SUSPENSION WITHIN 30 MINUTES AFTER MIXING—raltegravir. TAKE WITH FOOD—Juluca.
dolutegravir	Tivicay	50 mg once daily	
raltegravir	Isentress	400 mg twice daily	
dolutegravir + lamivudine	Dovato	1 tablet once daily	
dolutegravir + rilpivirine	Juluca	1 tablet once daily	
dolutegravir + abacavir + lamivudine	Triumeq	1 tablet once daily	TAKE EXACTLY AS DIRECTED; DO NOT SKIP DOSES. TAKE CALCIUM, IRON, OR ANTACIDS AT LEAST 2 HOURS BEFORE OR 6 HOURS AFTER DOSE—Genvoya, Stribild, Triumeq. TAKE WITH FOOD—Genvoya, Stribild.
elvitegravir + cobicistat (COBI) + emtricitabine + tenofovir DF	Stribild	1 tablet once daily	
elvitegravir + cobicistat (COBI) + emtricitabine + tenofovir AF	Genvoya	1 tablet once daily	
bictegravir + emtricitabine + tenofovir AF	Biktarvy	1 tablet once daily	STORE IN ORIGINAL CONTAINER.
Attachment Inhibitors			
fostemsavir	Rukobia	1 tablet twice daily	SWALLOW WHOLE, DO NOT CHEW.
Postattachment Inhibitors			
ibalizumab-uiyk	Trogarzo	2000 mg IV followed by a maintenance dose of 800 mg every 2 weeks	

IM, intramuscular; *IV*, intravenous; *PO*, orally.

Key Points

- A virus is an intracellular parasite that consists of a DNA or RNA core surrounded by a protein coat and sometimes an outer covering of lipoprotein.
- The infectious particles (virions) do not have the cellular components necessary for reproduction, so they use their host's cellular machinery to replicate.
- Viruses may cause minor illness, such as the common cold and warts, or serious infections, such as HIV infection, smallpox, and hepatitis C.
- Some viruses are linked to cancer; for example, human papillomavirus is associated with cervical cancer.
- An antiviral is a medication that is able to inhibit viral replication.
- Effective treatment of viral infections is dependent on host, virus, and antiviral agent factors.
- Some viruses can lay dormant in host cells and periodically awaken to cause recurrent disease.
- All antiviral agents work best when the host (the individual with the infection) has a healthy immune system.
- Antivirals are effective only against a specific virus.
- Antivirals inhibit virus-specific steps in the replication cycle.
- Antibiotics are not effective against viral infections.

- Viruses may become resistant to the suppressive action of antiviral agents.
- Amantadine and rimantadine inhibit viral uncoating of the influenza A virus, a necessary step in the virus replication process.
- Oseltamivir and zanamivir are indicated for the treatment of influenza A and influenza B. They are neuraminidase inhibitors. Neuraminidase inhibitors inhibit viral release.
- Interferons protect uninfected cells by promoting a resistance to virus infection.
- Interferon alfacon-1 and peginterferon alfa-2b are indicated for the treatment of hepatitis C virus.
- Interferon alfa-2b and peginterferon alfa-2a may be used for the treatment of hepatitis B and hepatitis C.
- Acyclovir, famciclovir, and valacyclovir are used for the treatment of HSV-1, the virus that causes cold sores; HSV-2, one of the viruses that cause genital warts; and VZV, the virus that causes chickenpox and shingles.
- Cidofovir, foscarnet, and ganciclovir are indicated for the treatment of cytomegalovirus infections.
- Penciclovir is a metabolite of famciclovir used for the treatment of cold sores.

- Trifluridine is used to treat herpes keratoconjunctivitis of the eye.
- Ribavirin is used to treat respiratory syncytial virus and hepatitis C when combined with interferon alfa.
- HIV is the virus that causes AIDS. The virus attacks CD4 T lymphocytes and weakens the immune system.
- The steps in the HIV life cycle are (1) binding, (2) fusion, (3) uncoating, (4) reverse transcription, (5) integration, (6) genome replication, (7) protein synthesis, (8) protein cleavage and assembly, and (9) virus release.
- Eight classes of antiretrovirals are used to treat HIV infections: (1) nucleoside/nucleotide reverse transcriptase inhibitors (NRTIs), (2) non-nucleoside reverse transcriptase inhibitors (NNRTIs), (3) protease inhibitors, (4) fusion inhibitors, (5) CCR5 antagonists, (6) HIV integrase strand inhibitors, (7) attachment inhibitors, and (8) postattachment inhibitors.
- Combination antiretrovirals are prescribed to reduce antiretroviral resistance.
- Many NRTIs are prodrugs.
- NRTIs competitively inhibit reverse transcriptase, the enzyme that makes a DNA copy of the viral RNA.
- NNRTIs are used only in combination therapy with NRTIs and protease inhibitors because resistance develops rapidly.
- Protease inhibitors (PIs) interfere with step 8 of the HIV life cycle. They block the cleavage of long-chain viral proteins into individual proteins that are assembled to make a new virus.
- Ritonavir is effective against HIV-1 and HIV-2 proteases.
- Enfuvirtide is a fusion inhibitor. It interferes with attachment of HIV to the host cell membrane (step 2 in the HIV life cycle).
- Maraviroc is a CCR5 antagonist that inhibits HIV entry into host cells.
- HIV integrase strand inhibitors block the final step in the process of human host cell infection by HIV.
- Cobicistat inhibits the metabolism of antivirals (e.g., darunavir and atazanavir), thereby increasing systemic exposure to the antiretroviral agents.

Review Questions

1. _____is the most severe form of HIV infection.
   a. CMV
   b. AIDS
   c. HPV
   d. HSV
2. The warning label TAKE WITH FOOD should be applied to the vial of all of the following prescriptions, EXCEPT_____.
   a. Genvoya
   b. Kaletra
   c. Norvir
   d. Atripla
3. An antiviral is a medication that is able to _____ viral replication.
   a. stimulate
   b. inhibit
   c. proliferate
   d. induce
4. All of the following antivirals are combination products used to treat hepatitis C except _____.
   a. Solvadi
   b. Epclusa
   c. Mavyret
   d. Harvoni
5. Which of the following antivirals is indicated for the treatment of cold sores?
   a. Acyclovir
   b. Ganciclovir
   c. Cidofovir
   d. Norvir
6. Human immunodeficiency virus (HIV) is the virus that causes acquired immunodeficiency syndrome (AIDS). The virus attacks _____ and weakens the immune system.
   a. CD4 monocytes
   b. CD4 T lymphocytes
   c. CD2 T lymphocytes
   d. None of the above

7. All of the following antiviral and antiretroviral liquids should be stored in the refrigerator, EXCEPT_____.
   a. Tamiflu suspension
   b. Valtrex suspension
   c. Kaletra suspension
   d. Rebetol solution
8. Lamivudine is an NRTI that is effective against _____.
   a. HIV
   b. HBV
   c. CMV
   d. a and b
9. All of the following antiretrovirals are marketed in liquid formulations for pediatric use, EXCEPT_____.
   a. tenofovir DF (Viread) and lamivudine (Epivir)
   b. lopinavir + ritonavir (Kaletra) and zidovudine (Retrovir)
   c. fosamprenavir (Lexiva, Telzir) and ritonavir (Norvir)
   d. dolutegravir + rilpivirine (Juluca) and nelfinavir (Viracept)
10. The warning label SWALLOW WHOLE; DO NOT CRUSH OR CHEW should be applied to the vial of all of the following prescriptions, EXCEPT_____.
    a. Viekira XR
    b. Rukobia
    c. Triumeq
    d. Kaletra

Bibliography

Beccari MV, Mogle BT, Sidman EF, et al. Ibalizumab, a novel monoclonal antibody for the management of multidrug-resistant HIV-1 infection. *Antimicrob Agents Chemother.* 2019;63(6):e00110–e00119.

Blair HA. Ibalizumab: a review in multidrug-resistant HIV-1 infection. *Drugs.* 2020;80(2):189–196.

Callaway E. COVID rebound is surprisingly common—even without Paxlovid. *Nature Epub.* August 11, 2022

Centers for Disease Control and Prevention. (2016). Antiviral Drug Resistance among Influenza Viruses, 2016. Retrieved February 14, 2023, from https://www.cdc.gov/flu/professionals/antivirals/antiviral-drug-resistance.htm.

Centers for Disease Control and Prevention. (2021). Vaccine (Shot) for Human Papillomavirus. Retrieved February 14, 2023, from https://www.cdc.gov/vaccines/parents/diseases/teen/hpv.html.

Chahine EB. Fostemsavir: the first oral attachment inhibitor for treatment of HIV-1 infection. *Am J Health Syst Pharm.* 2021;78(5):376–388.

Dorr P, Westby M, Dobbs S, et al. Maraviroc (UK-427,857), a potent, orally bioavailable, and selective small-molecule inhibitor of chemokine receptor CCR5 with broad-spectrum anti-human immunodeficiency virus type 1 activity. *Antimicrob Agents Chemother.* 2005;49:4721–4732.

Eggleton JS, Nagalli S. *Highly active antiretroviral therapy (HAART).* Treasure Island, FL: StatPearls Publishing; 2022.

Fiore AE, Fry A, Shay D, Centers for Disease Control and Prevention (CDC) : Antiviral agents for the treatment and chemoprophylaxis of influenza—recommendations of the Advisory Committee on Immunization Practices (ACIP). *MMWR Recomm Rep.* 2011;60:1–24.

Global AIDS update. (2023). Retrieved February 14, 2023, from http://www.unaids.org/.

Health Canada. (2023). Drug Product Database. Retrieved February 14, 2023, from https://health-products.canada.ca/dpd-bdpp/index-eng.jsp.

Institute for Safe Medication Practices. (2016). FDA and ISMP Lists of Look-Alike Drug Names with Recommended Tall Man Letters. Retrieved October 18, 2022, from https://www.ismp.org/recommendations/tall-man-letters-list.

Institute for Safe Medication Practices. (2019). List of Confused Drugs. Retrieved February 14, 2023, from https://www.ismp.org/tools/confuseddrugnames.pdf.

Kalant H, Grant D, Mitchell J. *Principles of medical pharmacology.* ed 7. Toronto: Elsevier Canada; 2007:739–759.

Kumar S, Jacobson IM. Antiviral therapy with nucleotide polymerase inhibitors for chronic hepatitis C. *J Hepatol.* 2014;61:S91–S97.

McColl DJ, Chen X. Strand transfer inhibitors of HIV-1 integrase: bringing in a new era of antiretroviral therapy. *Antiviral Res.* 2010;85:101–118.

Menendez-Arias L, Alvarez M, Pacheco B. Nucleoside/nucleotide analog inhibitors of hepatitis B virus polymerase: mechanism of action and resistance. *Curr Opin Virol.* 2014;8:1–9.

NIH. (2021). HIV treatment: The Basics. Retrieved February 14, 2023, from https://hivinfo.nih.gov/understanding-hiv/fact-sheets/print/19.

Page C, Curtis M, Sutter M, et al. *Integrated pharmacology.* Philadelphia: Elsevier Mosby; 2005:91–109.

Rathbun R.C., Liedtke M.D., Lockhart S.M.: Antiretroviral therapy for HIV infection, 2023. Retrieved February 14, 2023, from https://emedicine.medscape.com/article/1533218-overview.

University of Washington. (2023). Hepatitis C Online. Retrieved February 15, 2023, from https://www.hepatitisc.uw.edu/.

U.S. Food and Drug Administration. (nd). Drugs@FDA: FDA Approved Drug Products. Retrieved February 14, 2023, from http://www.accessdata.fda.gov/scripts/cder/daf/.

U.S. Food and Drug Administration. (2021). FDA Approves First Injectable Treatment for HIV Pre-Exposure Prevention. Retrieved February 14, 2023, from https://www.fda.gov/news-events/press-announcements/fda-approves-first-injectable-treatment-hiv-pre-exposure-prevention.

Wong GL-H, Wong VW-S, Chan HL-Y. Combination therapy of interferon and nucleotide/nucleoside analogues for chronic hepatitis B. *J Viral Hepat.* 2014;21:825–834.

World Health Organization *Implementation tool for pre-exposure prophylaxis (PrEP) of HIV infection, 2017. Module 6: Pharmacists.* Geneva: World Health Organization; 2017.

World Health Organization: Consolidated guidelines on the use of antiretroviral drugs for treating and preventing HIV infection: recommendations for a public health approach, 2016. Retrieved February 14, 2023, from http://www.who.int/hiv/pub/arv/arv-2016/en/.

31
Treatment of Cancers

LEARNING OBJECTIVES

1. Learn the terminology associated with cancer.
2. Identify risk factors for breast, colorectal, lung, prostate, skin, uterine, and ovarian cancer.
3. Identify causes for breast, colorectal, lung, prostate, skin, uterine, and ovarian cancer.
4. List, categorize, and describe the mechanism of action for medications used for the treatment of breast, colorectal, lung, prostate, skin, uterine, and ovarian cancer.
5. List common endings and/or beginnings of drug classes used for the treatment of breast, colorectal, lung, prostate, skin, uterine, and ovarian cancer.
6. Identify significant drug look-alike and sound-alike issues.
7. Identify warning labels and precautionary messages associated with medications used for the treatment of breast, colorectal, lung, prostate, skin, uterine, and ovarian cancer.

KEY TERMS

Benign Refers to a tumor that is not cancerous and does not spread to surrounding tissues or other parts of the body.

Cancer Term for diseases in which abnormal cells divide without control. Specific cancers are named according to the site at which the cancerous growth begins.

Chemotherapy Treatment with drugs that kill cancerous cells.

Complementary and alternative medicine Treatments that may include dietary supplements, herbal preparations, acupuncture, massage, magnet therapy, spiritual healing, and meditation.

Malignant Cancerous tumors that can invade and destroy nearby tissue and spread to other parts of the body.

Mammogram Screening examination to detect breast cancer in which a radiograph of the breast is taken.

Melanoma Form of skin cancer that arises in melanocytes, the cells that produce pigment.

Metastasis Spread of cancer from one part of the body to another.

Neoplasm An abnormal mass of tissue that results when cells divide more than they should or do not die when they should. Also called a tumor.

Oncovirus Virus that is a causative agent of a cancer.

Pap test Procedure to detect cervical cancer that involves removal and examination of a few cells from the cervix.

Polyp Growth that protrudes from a mucous membrane.

Prostate-specific antigen test Test that measures the level of free prostate-specific antigen, a protein produced by the prostate gland. Levels are elevated in men who have prostate cancer, infection or inflammation of the prostate gland, and benign prostatic hyperplasia.

Radiation therapy Use of high-energy radiation from X-rays, gamma rays, neutrons, and other sources to kill cancer cells and shrink tumors.

Stage Extent of a cancer within the body. Staging is based on the size of the tumor, whether lymph nodes contain cancer, and whether the disease has spread from the original site to other parts of the body.

Stem cell Undifferentiated cells that can develop into many different cell types.

Tumor marker Substance sometimes found in the blood, other body fluids, or tissues that may signal the presence of a certain type of cancer; for example, a high level of prostate-specific antigen is a signal for possible prostate cancer.

What Is Cancer?

Cancer is a disease that occurs when the normal cell renewal process fails. When old cells fail to die and new cells form more rapidly than needed, the cells may accumulate and form a mass called a *neoplasm* (also called a tumor). Tumors are caused by abnormal cell division. They may be benign or malignant. A *malignant* tumor is cancerous and can invade and destroy nearby tissue and spread via *metastasis* to other parts of the body, whereas a *benign* tumor is not cancerous and does not spread. Specific cancers are named according to the site

at which the cancerous growth began. This is the site of the primary tumor. For example, with melanoma, cancerous cells form in the skin; cancerous cells in blood-forming tissues lead to leukemia; in osteosarcoma, bone-forming cells become cancerous; and in lymphoma, cancerous cells form in the immune system.

Risk Factors for Cancer

There are many risk factors for cancer, including age, tobacco use, and exposure to ionizing radiation (Box 31.1).

• BOX 31.1 Risk Factors for Cancer

Increasing age
- Tobacco use
- Environmental pollutants
- Ionizing radiation
- Sunlight and tanning salons (UV light)
- Carcinogenic chemicals (e.g., benzene)
- Viruses (e.g., HPV, EBV)
- Bacteria (e.g., *Helicobacter pylori*)
- Hormone therapy (e.g., DES)
- Family history
- Alcohol use

Age

The risk for developing cancer increases with age. Cancers are more prevalent in persons over the age of 65 years.

Tobacco

Inhalation of cigarette, cigar, and pipe tobacco smoke may increase the risk for developing cancer of the lungs, larynx, mouth, esophagus, bladder, kidney, throat, stomach, pancreas, and cervix, as well as the risk for acute myeloid leukemia. Smokers and nonsmokers exposed to secondhand tobacco smoke are at increased risk. Chewing tobacco may increase the risk for oral cancer.

Ionizing Radiation and Sunlight

X-rays, nuclear fallout (from atomic weapons testing or leaks from nuclear power plants), and radon gas are examples of ionizing radiation. Exposure increases the risk for the development of leukemia, thyroid cancer, and breast cancer. Exposure to radon gas may increase the risk for developing lung cancer.

Exposure to sunlight is necessary for the skin to make the hormone vitamin D. Excessive exposure to the sun's ultraviolet (UV) radiation can increase the risk for skin cancer (**melanoma**). The ozone layer of the atmosphere provides protection from excessive exposure to UV radiation, prompting concerns over depletion of the earth's ozone layer. UVA levels are highest during midday, whereas UVB levels are found throughout the day. Exposure to UV light from sunlamps and tanning booths also increases cancer risk.

Hazardous Chemicals and Environmental Pollutants

Cancer-causing chemicals (carcinogens) are found in the workplace, home, and environment through pollution. Industrial solvents, cleaning fluids, pesticides, and used engine oil are examples of hazardous chemicals. Known workplace carcinogens include benzene, vinyl chloride, polychlorinated biphenyls (commonly called PCBs), asbestos, cadmium, and nickel. These carcinogens may get into the environment through improper disposal or chemical spills, or they are particulates that are released into the air in the process of incineration.

Bacterial and Viral Infection

Exposure to some viruses or bacteria may increase the risk of developing certain cancers. *Helicobacter pylori* is a bacterium known to cause peptic ulcer disease (PUD). PUD is associated with stomach cancer. An **oncovirus** is a virus known to cause cancer. Epstein-Barr virus (EBV), a common virus that remains dormant in most people, has been associated with lymphomas such as Burkitt lymphoma and immunoblastic lymphoma. The virus is also linked to nasopharyngeal carcinoma. Hepatitis B virus and hepatitis C virus are linked to liver cancer. Human papillomavirus (HPV) is a virus that causes genital warts and cancer of the cervix. Human immunodeficiency virus (HIV) and human herpesvirus 8 can cause Kaposi sarcoma. Human T-cell leukemia virus type 1 is a retrovirus that can cause leukemia and lymphoma.

Hormone Therapy

Hormone replacement therapy (HRT) and diethylstilbestrol (DES) have been linked to specific cancers. HRT, once the principal treatment for menopausal symptoms, is now limited because of the risk for the development of breast cancer, heart attack, stroke, and blood clots. DES is an estrogen-type drug that was taken by pregnant women between 1940 and 1971. Girls born to women who took DES have a higher risk for cancer of the cervix than girls born to women who did not take the drug. Women who took DES also have a higher incidence of breast cancer.

Family History

It is not known why one individual will develop cancer and another does not. Except for cancers of the breast, ovary, prostate, skin, and colon, most cancers do not run in families. For example, if a father develops stomach cancer, his children have no greater risk for stomach cancer than would a nonfamily member.

Alcohol

Chronic alcohol consumption (up to two drinks daily over a period of years) may increase the risk for cancer of the liver, mouth, throat, esophagus, larynx, and breast.

Diet, Physical Inactivity, and Obesity

A diet that is high in fat may increase the risk of cancers of the colon, uterus, and prostate. Cancers of the breast, colon, esophagus, kidney, and uterus are higher in individuals who have little physical activity and are overweight.

Types of Cancers

In this chapter, information is provided about the most common cancers in Canada and the United States. In 2022, the most common cancers in the United States were breast, prostate, lung, colorectal, and skin cancer. In Canada, breast, prostate, colorectal, skin, and thyroid cancer accounted for more than 55% of all cancers in 2015. Cancer of the breast and prostate were most common in Canada and the United States.

Breast Cancer

Breast cancer is the most common cancer in the United States and Canada. In 2022, there were an estimated 287,850 new cases of breast cancer in the United States. One percent of the cases were men. Approximately 3,771,794 women were living with breast cancer. The survival rate is approximately 90.6%. The death rate is 19.6 per 100,000. In Canada, 28,600 women were diagnosed with breast cancer in 2022. The median age at the time of diagnosis is 61 years. One or both breasts may be involved. The following are risk factors for breast cancer: (1) family history and inherited susceptibility (*BRCA1* and *BRCA2* genes), (2) nulliparity (no pregnancies), (3) early onset of menses (periods), (4) advanced age, (5) dense breast tissue, (6) history of HRT, and (7) excess alcohol intake.

Prostate Cancer

The incidence of prostate cancer increases as men grow older. The median age of diagnosis is 66 years old. Levels begin to slowly decline again after the age of 75. In 2022, there were an estimated 268,490 new cases diagnosed and 34,500 deaths in the United States. The 5-year survival rate is 96.8%. In 2014, an estimated 3,253,416 men were living with prostate cancer in the United States. In Canada, an estimated 24,600 new cases were diagnosed in 2022. It is estimated that one in eight males will be diagnosed with prostate cancer within their lifetime. Prostate disease, diagnosis, and treatment are described in Chapter 28.

Lung Cancer

Lung cancer is the second most common cancer in men and women. Only breast cancer and prostate cancer are more common. In the United States, the incidence of lung cancer was 52 cases per 100,000 in 2019, almost 237,000 men and women. In Canada, 30,000 Canadians were diagnosed in 2022. Lung cancer is the leading cause of cancer-related death. The 5-year survival rate is only 19%. There are two types of lung cancer: small cell lung cancer (SCLC) and non-small cell lung cancer (NSCLC). A history of smoking tobacco is the primary cause of SCLC. Other risk factors are increasing age, exposure to cancer-causing substances (e.g., secondhand smoke, asbestos, radon, atomic radiation), **radiation therapy** and medical imaging (e.g., x-ray to the breast or chest, computed tomography scans), air pollution, and family history.

Colorectal Cancer

Cancer of the colon and rectum affects millions of American and Canadian men and women. In the United States, there were an estimated 151,030 new cases of colorectal cancer in 2022. Approximately 1.36 million Americans were living with colorectal cancer in 2019 and 37.7 cases per 100,000 are diagnosed annually. In Canada, 24,300 new cases were diagnosed in 2022. Risk factors are obesity, physical inactivity, consumption of red and processed meat, and tobacco use. The first signs of colon cancer may be the appearance of a small **polyp** and blood in the stool. Early detection through the administration of screening examinations helps reduce the numbers of deaths from the disease. Colonoscopy and a fecal occult blood test (FOBT) are screening tests for colorectal cancer.

Skin Cancer

Skin cancer is one of the top five most common cancers. Skin cancer is divided into two categories: melanoma and nonmelanoma. The most treatable form is nonmelanoma. In 2019 there were an estimated 21.5 new cases of melanoma of the skin per 100,000 in the United States. In Canada in 2022, there were an estimated 9000 new cases diagnosed.

Nonmodifiable risk factors for developing skin cancer are having a fair complexion, personal and family history of skin cancer, or weakened immune system. Modifiable risk factors are excessive exposure to UV light from the sun or UV lights used in tanning salons, or a history of severe blistering sunburn(s). Protection from harmful UV light is the best way to prevent skin cancer. This can be achieved by wearing protective clothing when outdoors and using sunscreen.

Cancer of the Uterus and Ovaries

The cervix is located at the neck of the uterus, and the endometrium lines its inner surface (Fig. 31.1). More than 823,000 women are living with uterine cancer. Uterine cancers represent approximately 3.4% of all cancers. There were an estimated 27.8 new cases of endometrial cancer per 100,000 (65,950 total) in the United States in 2022. Endometrial cancer most commonly affects postmenopausal women.

Cancer of the cervix is linked to HPV and exposure to the drug DES while the fetus is still in the uterus. Approximately 7.8 per 100,000 women are diagnosed annually with cancer of the cervix, and it was estimated that 295,382 women were living with cervical cancer in 2019. Cancer of the uterus, obesity, diabetes, genetic predisposition, and never having been pregnant or birthed a child are all risk factors for cancer of the cervix. Disorders of the reproductive system may also cause excessive growth of the endometrium, prevent ovulation, and produce estrogen-secreting ovarian tumors.

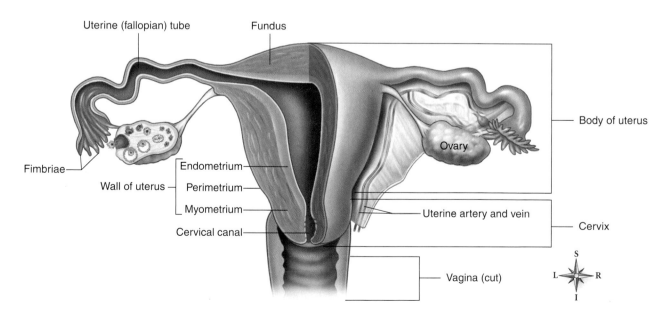

• **Fig. 31.1** Anatomy of the uterus. (From Patton KT, Thibodeau GA: *The human body in health and disease*, ed 7, St Louis, 2018, Elsevier.)

Cancer Screening Tests

Early diagnosis is critical to successful treatment. Screening tests are recommended for the early diagnosis of breast cancer, colorectal cancer, cancer of the cervix, and prostate cancer. A ***mammogram*** is a screening examination used to detect breast cancer. A radiograph is taken of the breast and inspected for evidence of tumors. Sonography is an alternative method for screening for breast cancers. If a lump is found, a biopsy is performed. A biopsy is a procedure whereby the cells or tissue is removed for examination by a pathologist. Regular self-examination of the breast is another important method of screening for breast cancer.

Tests to screen for colorectal cancer are the FOBT, colonoscopy, sigmoidoscopy, double-contrast barium enema, and digital rectal examination (see Chapter 28). The FOBT is a test that screens for blood in stool. Bleeding may indicate the presence of polyps or cancer. A colonoscopy and sigmoidoscopy involve the insertion of a lighted tube into the colon to inspect for abnormal growths. The procedure for X-ray screening is to administer a double-contrast barium enema to the patient to permit greater visualization of the bowel.

Another method of detection is to identify the presence of a ***tumor marker*** in the blood, other body fluids, or tissues that may signal the presence of a certain type of cancer. For example, a ***prostate-specific antigen*** (PSA) test is performed to screen for prostate cancer. PSA is a protein produced by the prostate gland. A high level of PSA is a signal for possible prostate cancer, although benign prostatic hypertrophy and prostate infection may also cause elevated PSA levels (see Chapter 28). A ***Pap test*** is a screening test for cancer of the cervix. The Pap test is a simple procedure in which cells from the cervix are removed and examined to detect cancer and changes that may lead to cancer.

Treatment of Cancer

Cancer may be treated with chemotherapy, biologic therapy, radiation therapy, and surgery. ***Chemotherapy*** is the use of drugs to kill or slow the growth of cancerous cells. Biologic therapy is the administration of immune system modulators to boost the body's natural defense against abnormal, invasive, and cancerous cells. Radiation therapy, the use of high-energy radiation from X-rays, gamma rays, neutrons, and other sources, can be used to kill cancer cells and shrink tumors. Radiation can be administered externally or as brachytherapy, a procedure in which radioactive material sealed in needles, seeds, wires, or catheters is placed directly into or near a tumor.

Some patients may try ***complementary and alternative medicine***, which may include dietary supplements, herbal preparations, acupuncture, massage, magnet therapy, spiritual healing, and meditation. ***Stem cell transplantation***, another form of treatment, is a procedure that replaces cells that were destroyed by cancer treatment with stem cells. *Stem cells* are undifferentiated cells that can develop into many different cell types. For example, blood cells develop from blood-forming stem cells. Stem cells act as the body's internal repair system by replenishing cells.

The following factors influence the selection of treatment options: (1) type of cancer, (2) ***stage*** of cancer, (3) individual tolerance for adverse effects of treatment, (4) patient's age, (5) histologic and nuclear grade of the primary tumor, and (6) capacity of the cancer to metastasize. Staging is a method used to describe how far the cancer has progressed within the body. It is based on the size of the tumor, whether lymph nodes contain the cancer, and whether the cancer has spread from the original site to other parts of the body.

This chapter focuses on chemotherapy and immunotherapy of the most common cancers. The therapeutic agents may be administered parenterally or by mouth. They work by various mechanisms to interrupt the cell replication cycle. Some agents are specific to cell cycle, that is, they interrupt a specific stage of the cell cycle (Table 31.1). Examples include mitotic inhibitors, microtubule inhibitors, and deoxyribonucleic acid (DNA) synthesis inhibitors. Other antineoplastic agents are nonspecific. The site of action of chemotherapeutic agents is shown in Fig. 31.2.

TABLE 31.1	Summary of the Cell Life Cycle
Phase of Cell Life Cycle	**Description**
Cell Growth	Interphase
Protein synthesis	Proteins are manufactured according to the cell's genetic code; functional proteins, the enzymes, direct the synthesis of other molecules in the cells, and thus the production of more and larger organelles and plasma membrane; sometimes called the first growth phase, or the G1 phase of interphase
Deoxyribonucleic acid (DNA) replication	Nucleotides, influenced by newly synthesized enzymes, arrange themselves along the open sides of an unzipped DNA molecule, thereby creating two identical daughter DNA molecules; they produce two identical sets of the cell's genetic code, which enables the cell later to split into two different cells, each with its own complete set of DNA; sometimes called the (DNA) synthesis stage or S phase of interphase
Protein synthesis	After DNA is replicated, the cell continues to grow by means of protein synthesis and the resulting synthesis of other molecules and various organelles; this second growth phase is called the G2 phase
Cell Reproduction	M phase
Mitosis or meiosis	The parent cell's replicated set of DNA is divided into two sets separated by an orderly process into distinct cell nuclei; mitosis is subdivided into at least four phases: prophase, metaphase, anaphase, and telophase
Cytokinesis	The plasma membrane of the parent cell pinches in and eventually separates the cytoplasm and two daughter nuclei into two genetically identical daughter cells

From Patton KT, Thibodeau GA: *Anatomy and physiology*, ed 9, St Louis, 2016, Elsevier.

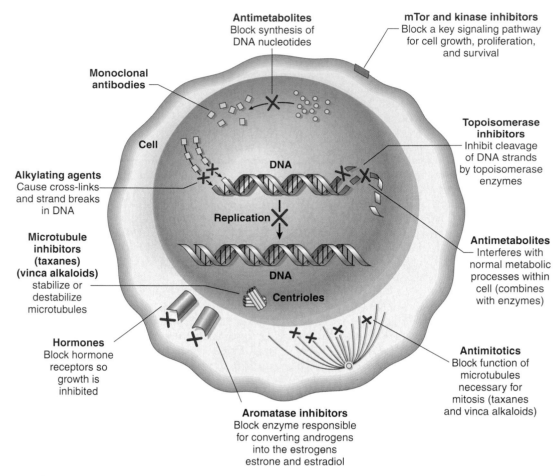

Fig. 31.2 Site of action of chemotherapeutic agents. (From Raffa RB, Rawls SM, Beyzarov EP: *Netter's illustrated pharmacology*, Philadelphia, 2005, WB Saunders.)

Pharmacotherapy for Breast Cancer

Pharmacotherapy for breast cancer includes the administration of selective estrogen receptor (ER) modulators (e.g., tamoxifen), ER downregulators (e.g., elacestrant, fulvestrant), aromatase inhibitors (e.g., anastrozole), and kinase inhibitors (e.g., palbociclib).

> **⚠ Tech Alert!**
>
> All parenteral chemotherapeutic agents should be prepared in a Class II biohazard safety cabinet or a vertical flow hood containing a high-efficiency particulate air (HEPA) filter with a vertical downward flow of air. The pharmacy technician is protected by a glass front and wears a fluid-proof gown, double gloves, mask, bonnet, shoe covers, and goggles. US Pharmacopeia (USP) guidelines for safety equipment and gear are described in USP General Chapter 800 Hazardous Drugs—Handling in Healthcare Settings.

Selective Estrogen Receptor Modulators

The hormones estrogen and progesterone can promote the growth of ER-positive and/or progesterone receptor (PR)-positive breast cancer. The administration of a selective ER modulator (antiestrogen) can reduce the risk of breast cancer recurrence for up to 5 years after treatment of the primary tumor. Treatment decisions are influenced by the woman's menopausal status, the affinity of the tumor for ERs and PRs, and the human epidermal growth

factor receptor 2 (HER2/neu) status (overexpression), in addition to the other factors listed earlier.

Tamoxifen and toremifene are indicated for the treatment of ER-positive breast cancer that is noninvasive or invasive (metastatic). Tamoxifen is approved for the treatment of metastatic breast cancer in premenopausal and postmenopausal women. It is also approved for the treatment of metastatic breast cancer in men. Toremifene is a derivative of tamoxifen that is indicated for the treatment of metastatic breast cancer in postmenopausal women. Raloxifene is indicated for the treatment of osteoporosis, not the treatment of breast cancer (see Chapter 14). It has a secondary indication to reduce the risk for invasive breast cancer in postmenopausal women with osteoporosis and/or for those at high risk of invasive breast cancer.

> **⚠ Tech Alert!**
>
> Tamoxifen should not be taken during pregnancy. The warning label "Avoid Pregnancy" should be applied to the prescription vial.

Mechanism of Action and Pharmacokinetics

Tamoxifen, toremifene, and raloxifene are selective estrogen receptor modulators (SERMs) that compete with estrogen for binding sites. When SERMS occupy the ERs in breast cells, they block the effects of estrogen (estrogen antagonist). SERMS can have estrogenic activities in other tissues. For example, raloxifene has agonist effects on bone cell turnover (remodeling), which can decrease postmenopausal bone loss. Tamoxifen has an active metabolite and long half-life and accumulates with continued administration. It may be given once or twice daily.

Adverse Reactions

Tamoxifen and toremifene commonly produce menopause-like symptoms such as hot flashes, sweating, vaginal bleeding, vaginal itchiness, discharge or dryness, nausea, and vomiting. They may also cause menstrual changes. Agonist effects on the endometrium double the risks for endometrial cancer. Other adverse effects are pelvic pain and ocular changes (e.g., cataracts). Tamoxifen and toremifene are contraindicated during pregnancy.

> **⊘ Tech Alert!**
>
> A dangerous drug-drug interaction that may cause hemorrhage can occur when tamoxifen is taken with the anticoagulant warfarin.

Selective Estrogen Receptor Modulators

Generic Name	US Brand Name(s)		Dosage Forms and Strengths
	Canadian Brand Name(s)		
tamoxifen[a]	Soltamox		**Solution (Soltamox)**[b]: 10 mg/5 mL
	Nolvadex-D		**Tablet:** 10 mg, 20 mg
toremifene	Fareston		**Tablet:** 60 mg
	Not available		

[a]Generic available.
[b]Available in the United States only.

Estrogen Receptor Antagonist

Fulvestrant is indicated for the treatment of ER-positive, HER2-negative metastatic breast cancer in postmenopausal women with disease progression after antiestrogen therapy.

Mechanism of Action and Pharmacokinetics

Fulvestrant is an ER antagonist that produces downregulation of ER protein. It is an analog of estradiol that acts as a competitive antagonist. When fulvestrant binds to ERs, it inhibits estrogen activity, causes changes in ER function, and triggers ER degradation. Unlike SERMS (e.g., tamoxifen), it does not have partial estrogenic activity. Fulvestrant is administered intramuscularly. Plasma concentrations are maintained at therapeutic levels for up to 1 month.

Adverse Reactions

Adverse effects caused by fulvestrant include pain at the injection site, generalized bone and back pain, hot flashes, headache, nausea and vomiting, diarrhea or constipation, and weakness. Fulvestrant is contraindicated during pregnancy.

Estrogen Receptor Downregulator

Generic Name	US Brand Name(s)	Dosage Forms and Strengths
	Canadian Brand Name(s)	
elacestrant	Orserdu	**Tablet:** 86 mg, 345 mg
	Not available	
fulvestrant	Faslodex	**Solution, for injection:** 50 mg/mL
	Faslodex	

Aromatase Inhibitors

Anastrozole, exemestane, and letrozole are aromatase inhibitors. They may be prescribed alone or in combination with tamoxifen. They are approved by the US Food and Drug Administration (FDA) for the first-line treatment of advanced or metastatic ER-positive breast cancer in postmenopausal women. They are also approved as an adjuvant for the treatment of early-stage breast cancer.

> **⊘ Tech Alert!**
>
> A common ending for aromatase inhibitors is -trozole.

Mechanism of Action and Pharmacokinetics

The adrenal gland is the primary source of estrogen after menopause. Aromatase is an enzyme responsible for converting androgens produced by the adrenal gland into the estrogens, estrone, and estradiol in the peripheral tissues. Aromatase inhibitors block this process. Anastrozole and letrozole are nonsteroidal aromatase inhibitors and are potent inhibitors of serum estradiol levels. Exemestane is a steroidal aromatase inhibitor. It is a more potent inhibitor of estrogen than the other aromatase inhibitors.

Adverse Reactions

Like tamoxifen, aromatase inhibitors produce menopause-like symptoms, nausea, and vomiting. Additional adverse effects include dizziness, cough, headache, hair loss, constipation, mood changes, and bone pain. Administration of steroid aromatase inhibitors requires adrenal HRT to replenish depleted glucocorticoids (cortisol) and mineralocorticoids (aldosterone). Symptoms of adrenal hormone insufficiency are fatigue, weight gain, and edema.

> **⊘ Tech Alert!**
>
> Femara and FemHRT have look-alike/sound-alike issues.

Kinase and mTOR Inhibitors

Abemaciclib (Verzenio), palbociclib (Ibrance), ribociclib (Kisqali), lapatinib (Tykerb), and neratinib (Nerlynx) are kinase inhibitors that are indicated for the treatment of hormone receptor (HR)-positive, HER2-negative advanced or metastatic breast cancer in postmenopausal women. Abemaciclib, palbociclib, and ribociclib

Aromatase Inhibitors

Generic Name	US Brand Name(s) Canadian Brand Name(s)	Dosage Forms and Strengths
anastrozole[a]	Arimidex	**Tablet:** 1 mg
	Arimidex	
exemestane[a]	Aromasin	**Tablet:** 25 mg
	Aromasin	
letrozole[a]	Femara	**Tablet:** 2.5 mg
	Femara	

[a]Generic available.

are used in combination with an aromatase inhibitor (e.g., anastrozole or letrozole) as initial therapy or with fulvestrant in women with advanced metastatic breast cancer. Lapatinib is approved for the treatment of breast cancer when taken with capecitabine. Neratinib is indicated as adjuvant therapy for early stage HER2-overexpressed breast cancer after treatment with the monoclonal antibody trastuzumab.

Everolimus (Afinitor) is an mTOR inhibitor that is used in combination with exemestane to treat postmenopausal women with advanced HR-positive, HER2-negative breast cancer who have already received other medicines for their cancer.

Mechanism of Action and Pharmacokinetics

Kinase inhibitors and mTOR inhibitors block a key signaling pathway for cell growth, proliferation, and survival.

Adverse Reactions

The most common adverse effects of abemaciclib, palbociclib, and ribociclib are diarrhea, anemia, increased infections, fatigue, hair loss, nausea, headache, stomatitis, and fever. Side effects of everolimus are stomatitis, infections, rash, fatigue, diarrhea, edema, abdominal pain, nausea, fever, asthenia, cough, headache, and decreased appetite.

Taxanes

Taxanes are cytotoxic drugs that are naturally derived from the Western yew tree (paclitaxel) and European yew tree (docetaxel). They are approved for the treatment of breast cancer.

❗ Tech Alert!

A common ending for taxanes is *-taxel*.

❗ Tech Alert!

The following drugs have look-alike/sound-alike issues:
PACLitaxel and PACLitaxel protein-bound particles;
Taxotere and Taxol;
Taxol and Paxil.

Kinase and mTOR Inhibitors

Generic Name	US Brand Name(s) Canadian Brand Name(s)	Dosage Forms and Strengths
abemaciclib	Verzenio	**Tablet:** 50 mg, 100 mg, 150 mg, 200 mg
	Not available	
alpelisib	Piqray, Vijoice	**Tablet:** 50 mg, 125 mg (Vijoice), 150 mg (Piqray), 200 mg
	Piqray	
everolimus	Afinitor, Afinitor Disperz	**Tablet, for suspension (Afinitor Disperz):** 2 mg, 3 mg, 5 mg **Tablet (Afinitor):** 2.5 mg, 5 mg, 7.5 mg, 10 mg
	Afinitor, Afinitor Disperz	
lapatinib	Tykerb	**Tablet:** 250 mg
	Tykerb	
neratinib	Nerlynx	**Tablet:** 40 mg
	Not available	
palbociclib	Ibrance	**Capsule:** 75 mg, 100 mg, 125 mg
	Ibrance	
ribociclib	Kisqali	**Tablet:** 200 mg
	Kisqali	
letrozole + ribociclib	Kisqali Femara Co-Pak	**Tablet:** 2.5 mg letrozole + 200 mg ribociclib
	Not available	

Mechanism of Action and Pharmacokinetics

Taxanes interfere with the process of mitosis. Mitosis is a key step in the process of cell division and is the stage at which DNA is organized and distributed.

Adverse Reactions

Common adverse reactions produced by taxanes are diarrhea, total body hair loss, nausea, muscle pain, joint and low back pain, flushing, and sweating. Taxanes also decrease white blood cell, red blood cell, and platelet counts. When white blood cell levels drop, individuals may get infections more easily. Docetaxel may also cause discoloration of fingernails and loosening of fingernails from the nail bed. Paclitaxel may cause mouth sores.

Microtubule Inhibitors

Ixabepilone and eribulin are microtubule inhibitors. Eribulin is isolated from the marine sponge. Both drugs are used to treat metastatic or locally advanced breast cancer.

Mechanism of Action and Pharmacokinetics

Like taxanes, eribulin and ixabepilone interfere with cell mitosis. Drug action leads to cell death.

Taxanes

Generic Name	US Brand Name(s) / Canadian Brand Name(s)	Dosage Forms and Strengths
docetaxel[a]	Taxotere	Solution, for injection: 10 mg/mL, 20 mg/mL, 40 mg/mL
	Taxotere	
paclitaxel[a]	Taxol	Solution, for injection: 6 mg/mL
	Generics	
paclitaxel albumin-bound particles	Abraxane	Powder, for suspension: 100 mg/vial
	Abraxane	

[a]Generic available.

Adverse Reactions

Nausea, vomiting, constipation, neutropenia, weight loss, anorexia, and diarrhea are the most common side effects of eribulin. Muscle, joint, and bone pain may also occur.

Microtubule Inhibitors

Generic Name	US Brand Name(s) / Canadian Brand Name(s)	Dosage Forms and Strengths
eribulin	Halaven	Solution, for injection: 0.5 mg/mL
	Halaven	
ixabepilone	Ixempra	Powder, for injection: 15 mg/vial, 45 mg/vial
	Not available	

Miscellaneous Chemotherapy Agents Used to Treat Breast Cancer

Talazoparib and olaparib are used for the treatment of germline *BRCA*-mutated (gBRCAm) HER2-negative locally advanced or metastatic breast cancer and ovarian cancer. Their antitumor activity is due to the inhibition of poly(ADP-ribose) polymerase (PARP). PARP is an enzyme that is involved in cell DNA repair. Inhibition of PARP damages tumor cells, increases cell death, and decreases the spread of cancer cells.

Miscellaneous Chemotherapy Agents

Generic Name	US Brand Name(s) / Canadian Brand Name(s)	Dosage Forms and Strengths
olaparib	Lynparza	Tablet: 100 mg, 150 mg
	Lynparza	
talazoparib	Talzenna	Capsule: 0.25 mg, 0.5 mg, 0.75 mg, 1 mg
	Not available	

Immunotherapy for Breast Cancer

Monoclonal Antibodies

Margetuximab, pertuzumab, and trastuzumab are monoclonal antibodies that are used in the treatment of HER2-positive breast cancer. HER2-positive tumors are characterized by increased invasiveness and cell proliferation to other sites (metastasis) and decreased cell death.

> **❶ Tech Alert!**
>
> A common ending for monoclonal antibody immunotherapeutic agents is *-mab*.

Mechanism of Action and Pharmacokinetics

Margetuximab-cmkb and trastuzumab are anti-HER2/neu antibodies that are effective when used as adjuvant therapy for HER2-overexpressing breast cancer. Pertuzumab is a monoclonal antibody that reduces tumor growth and invasion by blocking epidermal growth factor receptor (EGFR) and HER2 dimerization (a process that results in joining the two proteins). Hyaluronidase is an enzyme that is added to some formulations to increase the absorption and dispersion of pertuzumab and trastuzumab.

Adverse Reactions

Common side effects of margetuximab, pertuzumab, and trastuzumab are fatigue, nausea, diarrhea, skin rash, fever, chills, infection, joint and muscle pain, anemia, and headache. Pertuzumab and trastuzumab have been linked to an increased risk for heart failure.

Pharmacotherapy for Prostate Cancer

Gonadotropin-Releasing Hormone Agonists, Luteinizing Hormone-Releasing Hormone Agonists, and Luteinizing Hormone-Releasing Hormone Antagonists

Gonadotropin-releasing hormone (GnRH) is also known as luteinizing hormone-releasing hormone (LHRH). Goserelin is a GnRH agonist indicated for the treatment of prostate cancer in men and advanced breast cancer in premenopausal and perimenopausal women with ER-positive disease. The drug initially increases hormone levels and is followed by desensitization to the hormone's effects. When used for the treatment of prostate cancer, goserelin is given to patients with hormone-dependent advanced carcinoma of the prostate. It is used in combination with antiandrogens and radiation therapy for the management of locally advanced or bulky carcinoma of the prostate. When used for the treatment of breast cancer, GnRH agonists may be prescribed to treat premenopausal women, whereas SERMs and aromatase inhibitors are indicated for use only in postmenopausal women. GnRH and its analogs are described in depth in Chapter 27. LHRH antagonists decrease testosterone levels to treat prostate cancer.

Antiandrogens

Prostate cancer cell growth is mediated by androgens that connect to an androgen receptor. When antiandrogen drugs

Monoclonal Antibodies

Generic Name	US Brand Name(s) Canadian Brand Name(s)	Dosage Forms and Strengths
margetuximab-cmkb	Margenza Not available	**Solution, for intravenous use:** 25 mg/mL
pertuzumab	Perjeta Perjeta	**Solution, for infusion:** 420 mg/14 mL
trastuzumab	Herceptin Herceptin	**Powder, for injection:** 150 mg/vial, 440 mg/vial
trastuzumab-anns	Kanjinti Kanjinti	**Powder, for injection:** 150 mg/vial, 420 mg/vial
trastuzumab-dttb	Ontruzant Ontruzant	**Powder, for infusion:** 150 mg/vial, 420 mg/vial
trastuzumab-dkst	Ogivri Ogivri	**Powder, for injection:** 150 mg/vial[a], 420 mg/vial[b], 440 mg/vial[a]
trastuzumab-pkrb	Herzuma Herzuma	**Powder, for injection:** 150 mg/vial[a], 420 mg/vial
trastuzumab-qyyp	Trazimera Trazimera	**Powder, for injection:** 150 mg/vial[a], 420 mg/vial[b], 440 mg/vial[a]
ado-trastuzumab emtansine	Kadcyla Kadcyla	**Powder, for injection:** 100 mg/vial, 160 mg/vial
fam-trastuzumab deruxtecan-nxki	Enhertu Enhertu	**Powder, for injection:** 100 mg/vial
pertuzumab + trastuzumab	Not available Perjeta-Herceptin	**Kit**[a]: 420 mg/14 mL pertuzumab + 440 mg/vial trastuzumab
trastuzumab + hyaluronidase-oysk	Herceptin Hylecta Herceptin SC	**Solution, for subcutaneous injection:** 600 mg trastuzumab + 10,000 units hyaluronidase-oysk/5 mL
pertuzumab + trastuzumab + hyaluronidase-zzxf	Phesgo Phesgo	**Solution, for subcutaneous injection:** 80 mg pertuzumab + 40 mg trastuzumab + 2000 units hyaluronidase-zzxf/mL 60 mg pertuzumab + 60 mg trastuzumab + 2000 units hyaluronidase-zzxf/mL

[a]Available in Canada only.
[b]Available in the United States only.

GnRH Agonists, LHRH Agonists, and LHRH Antagonists

Generic Name	US Brand Name(s) Canadian Brand Name(s)	Dosage Forms and Strengths
degarelix	Firmagon Firmagon	**Powder, for subcutaneous injection:** 80 mg/vial, 120 mg/vial
goserelin	Zoladex Zoladex, Zoladex LA	**Implant (1 month):** 3.6 mg **Implant (3 months):** 10.8 mg
relugolix	Orgovyx Not available	**Tablet:** 120 mg

compete for the androgen receptor binding sites, binding interferes with steps in the androgen receptor signaling pathway. This inhibits tumor growth. Antiandrogens are used to treat metastatic and nonmetastatic prostate cancer. They are commonly prescribed as adjunct therapy with other prostate cancer treatments such as LHRH agonists or orchiectomy (surgical removal of the gonads). Antiandrogens may affect sexual interest or erection and may also cause nausea, diarrhea, fatigue, dizziness, and hot flashes.

> ● **Tech Note!**
>
> A common ending for antiandrogens is -*lutamide*.

Antiandrogens Used to Treat Prostate Cancer

Generic Name	US Brand Name(s) / Canadian Brand Name(s)	Dosage Forms and Strengths
apalutamide	Erleada	**Tablet:** 60 mg, 240 mg
	Erleada	
bicalutamide[a]	Casodex	**Tablet:** 50 mg
	Casodex	
darolutamide	Nubeqa	**Tablet:** 300 mg
	Nubeqa	
enzalutamide	Xtandi	**Capsule:** 40 mg **Tablet[b]:** 40 mg, 80 mg
	Xtandi	
flutamide[a]	Generic	**Capsule:** 125 mg **Tablet:** 250 mg
	Generic	
nilutamide	Nilandron	**Tablet:** 50 mg (Anandron), 150 mg (Nilandron)
	Anandron	

Miscellaneous Agents Used to Treat Prostate Cancer

Estramustine has antigonadotropic effects. It is approved for the treatment of hormone-refractory prostate cancer in Canada and the United States. Estramustine may inhibit DNA synthesis and cause dose-related DNA strand breaks. Abiraterone is a CYP17 inhibitor that is coadministered with methylprednisolone to treat metastatic prostate cancer.

Adverse Reactions

The most common side effects of estramustine are breast tenderness, gynecomastia, elevated liver function tests, nausea, myalgia, and edema. Abiraterone has similar side effects. It may produce hot flashes, joint or muscle pain, diarrhea, and fatigue.

Miscellaneous Drugs Used to Treat Cancer

Generic Name	US Brand Name(s) / Canadian Brand Name(s)	Dosage Forms and Strengths
abiraterone[a]	Yonsa, Zytiga	**Tablet:** 125 mg (Yonsa), 250 mg, 500 mg (Zytiga)
	Zytiga	
estramustine	Emcyt	**Capsule:** 140 mg
	Emcyt	

[a]Generic available.

Pharmacotherapy for Lung Cancer

Lung cancer may be treated with surgery, radiation, chemotherapy, immunotherapy, and targeted agents. Drugs used in the treatment of lung cancer are typically effective against one but not both forms of the disease. Only treatments for NSCLC are covered in this chapter because chemotherapy for SCLC has limited effect on overall survival. Pharmacotherapy includes platinum-based compounds (e.g., cisplatin or carboplatin) with paclitaxel, gemcitabine, docetaxel, vinorelbine, protein-bound paclitaxel, pemetrexed, or etoposide. Agents used for immunotherapy are monoclonal antibodies (e.g., bevacizumab, necitumumab). EGFR tyrosine kinase inhibitors (gefitinib, afatinib), anaplastic lymphoma kinase inhibitors (crizotinib and ceritinib), *BRAF* and *MEK* inhibitors (dabrafenib and trametinib), and programmed death receptor (PD-1) and programmed death ligand (PD-L1) blocking antibodies are targeted agents used to treat NSCLC.

Kinase Inhibitors

Afatinib (Gilotrif), ceritinib (Zykadia), crizotinib (Xalkiori), erlotinib (Tarceva), and gefitinib (Iressa) are kinase inhibitors that are used in the treatment of lung cancer. They block signaling pathways that are needed for tumor growth and spread to other parts of the body.

All of the kinase inhibitors may cause diarrhea, regardless of the type of cancer they are used to treat. Other adverse reactions common to the kinase inhibitors used for treating NSCLC are nausea, fatigue, and skin rashes. Additionally, Xalkori may produce vision disorders and upper respiratory infection; Tarceva can cause shortness of breath and cough. Additional details about the mechanism of action and adverse reactions of kinase inhibitors are described in this chapter under Breast Cancer.

Antimetabolites

Methotrexate (MTX) is the principal drug in this class. It is indicated for the treatment of lung cancer, breast cancer, bladder cancer, acute lymphocytic leukemia (ALL), cutaneous T-cell lymphoma, non-Hodgkin lymphoma, leukemia, and osteogenic sarcoma. It is also indicated for the treatment of rheumatoid arthritis (see Chapter 13). Pemetrexed, a related compound, is indicated for the treatment of lung cancer. The purine antimetabolites 6-mercaptopurine and 6-thioguanine are primarily indicated for the treatment of ALL. Pentostatin is a structural analog of the purine adenosine and is indicated for the treatment of hairy cell leukemia.

Kinase Inhibitors

Generic Name	US Brand Name(s) / Canadian Brand Name(s)	Dosage Forms and Strengths
afatinib	Gilotrif / Giotrif	**Tablet:** 20 mg, 30 mg, 40 mg
ceritinib	Zykadia / Zykadia	**Capsule:** 150 mg
crizotinib	Xalkori / Xalkori	**Capsule:** 200 mg, 250 mg
dacomitinib	Vizimpro / Not available	**Tablet:** 15 mg, 30 mg, 45 mg
entrectinib	Rozlytrek / Rozlytrek	**Capsule:** 100 mg, 200 mg
erlotinib[a]	Tarceva / Tarceva	**Tablet:** 25 mg, 100 mg, 150 mg
gefitinib[a,b]	Iressa / Iressa	**Tablet:** 250 mg
lorlatinib	Lorbrena / Lorbrena	**Tablet:** 25 mg, 100 mg
osimertinib	Tagrisso / Tagrisso	**Tablet:** 40 mg, 80 mg
pralsetinib	Gavreto / Gavreto	**Capsule:** 100 mg
selpercatinib	Retevmo / Retevmo	**Capsule:** 40 mg, 80 mg
tepotinib	Tepmetko / Tepmetko	**Tablet:** 225 mg
trametinib	Mekinist / Mekinist	**Tablet:** 0.5 mg, 2 mg[c] **Powder for solution:**[c] 4.7 mg/vial **Solution:**[c] 0.05 mg/mL

[a]Generic available.
[b]Available in Canada.
[c]Available in the United States only

Mechanism of Action and Pharmacokinetics

Antimetabolites are chemotherapeutic agents that work most effectively against rapidly dividing cancerous cells. They inhibit normal DNA synthesis by forming abnormal nucleic acid base pairs, resulting in abnormal DNA. MTX is structurally similar to the vitamin folic acid and inhibits folate metabolism, which is essential to the formation of the purines. Pentostatin, 6-mercaptopurine, and 6-thioguanine are purine analogs. Purine bases, along with pyrimidine bases, make up the DNA strand. MTX also causes the depletion of thymidine, a DNA nucleoside, so DNA synthesis ceases and cells die.

Adverse Reactions

MTX and pemetrexed commonly cause hair loss, photosensitivity, loss of appetite, and nausea. They also decrease the numbers of white and red blood cells and platelets. When white blood cell levels drop, individuals may get infections more easily. Similar adverse reactions are produced by 6-mercaptopurine and 6-thioguanine, with the exception of photosensitivity. Folic acid is commonly prescribed to patients being treated for rheumatoid arthritis with MTX. It has been shown to reduce gastrointestinal side effects and risks for megaloblastic anemia. Supplementation with folic acid is controversial in patients treated for cancer with MTX. Folic acid may reduce the effectiveness of MTX by interfering with its antifolate action.

> **⊘ Tech Alert!**
>
> The warning label "Avoid aspirin, APAP, and NSAIDs" should be applied to prescription vials for MTX because these drugs may decrease MTX clearance and cause toxicity. (APAP is acetaminophen; NSAIDs are nonsteroidal antiinflammatory drugs.)

> **⊘ Tech Alert!**
>
> The following drugs have look-alike/sound-alike issues:
> purinethol and propylthiouracil;
> pentostatin and Pentosan

Antimetabolites

Generic Name	US Brand Name(s) / Canadian Brand Name(s)	Dosage Forms and Strengths
methotrexate[a] (MTX)	Otrexup, Rasuvo, Trexall, Xatmep / Generics	**Powder, for injection (generics)**[b]: 1 g/vial **Solution, oral (Xatmep):** 2 mg/mL **Solution, for injection:** 10 mg/mL, 25 mg/mL **Tablet (Trexall):** 2.5 mg, 5 mg[b], 7.5 mg[b], 10 mg, 15 mg[b]
pemetrexed[a,c]	Alimta / Alimta	**Powder, for injection:** 100 mg/vial, 500 mg/vial
mercaptopurine[a]	Purinethol, Purixan / Purinethol	**Suspension, oral**[b]: 20 mg/mL **Tablet:** 50 mg
thioguanine	Thioguanine / Lanvis	**Tablet:** 40 mg
pentostatin[a]	Nipent / Not available	**Powder, for injection:** 10 mg/vial

Methotrexate marketed under the name of Otrexup and Rasuvo is prescribed for arthritis.
[a]Generic available.
[b]Available in the United States only.
[c]Available in Canada only.

Immunotherapy for Lung Cancer

Monoclonal Antibodies

Atezolizumab (Tecentriq), durvalumab (Imfinzi), ipilimumab (Yervoy), nivolumab (Opdivo), and pembrolizumab (Keytruda) are monoclonal antibodies that are used in immunotherapy for treating NSCLC. Keytruda and Opdivo are classified as PD-1 blocking antibodies. Tecentriq is a PD-L1 blocking antibody.

Mechanism of Action and Pharmacokinetics

The PD-1 and PD-L1 blocking antibody antitumor activity stems from their blockade of the signaling pathway that regulates late immune response and the spread of tumor-causing cells.

Adverse Reactions

The most common adverse reactions of Tecentriq, Opdiva, and Keytruda are fatigue, decreased appetite, dyspnea, cough, nausea, musculoskeletal pain, and constipation.

PD-1 and PD-L1 Blocking Antibodies

Generic Name	US Brand Name(s) Canadian Brand Name(s)	Dosage Forms and Strengths
atezolizumab	Tecentriq	Solution, for injection: 60 mg/mL
	Tecentriq	
nivolumab	Opdivo	Solution, for injection: 10 mg/mL
	Opdivo	
durvalumab	Imfinzi	Solution, for intravenous injection: 50 mg/mL
	Imfinzi	
ipilimumab	Yervoy	Solution, for injection: 5 mg/mL
	Yervoy	
necitumumab	Portrazza	Solution, for injection: 16 mg/mL
	Not available	
pembrolizumab	Keytruda	Powder, for injection: 50 mg/vial
	Keytruda	Solution, for infusion[a]: 25 mg/mL

[a]Available in Canada only.

Pharmacotherapy for Colorectal Cancer

Colorectal cancer is treated with surgery, radiation, chemotherapy, immunotherapy, and targeted agents. Chemotherapeutic agents include fluoropyrimidines, MTX, and platinum compounds. Bevacizumab (Avastin) is a monoclonal antibody that is used as immunotherapy. It is a biological response modifying agent.

Platinum Compounds

Carboplatin, cisplatin, and oxaliplatin are platinum compounds. Cisplatin is approved by the FDA for the treatment of testicular and ovarian cancers. Carboplatin is approved for the treatment of ovarian cancer, and oxaliplatin is approved for the treatment of colorectal cancer.

> **❶ Tech Alert!**
> Platinum compounds have the common ending -platin.

Mechanism of Action and Pharmacokinetics

The action of platinum compounds on purine bases (adenine and guanine) results in the formation of faulty cross-linkages and defective DNA.

Adverse Reactions

Side effects of platinum compounds are fatigue, loss of appetite, loss of hair, metallic taste, pain at the site of injection, increased infections, bleeding, bruising, and nausea. Cisplatin may also cause irreversible hearing loss and neurotoxicity. Sensory neurotoxicity produced by oxaliplatin is reversible.

> **❶ Tech Alert!**
> The following drugs have look-alike/sound-alike issues:
> CARBOplatin and CISplatin;
> Platinol and Patanol

Platinum Compounds

Generic Name	US Brand Name(s) Canadian Brand Name(s)	Dosage Forms and Strengths
carboplatin[a]	Generics	Solution, for infusion: 10 mg/mL
	Generics	
cisplatin[a]	Generics	Solution, for injection: 1 mg/mL
	Generics	
oxaliplatin[a]	Eloxatin	Solution, for infusion: 5 mg/mL
	Generics	

[a]Generic available.

Fluoropyrimidines

Capecitabine, cytarabine, gemcitabine, and 5-fluorouracil (5-FU) are fluoropyrimidines, also known as fluorinated pyrimidines. These drugs are indicated for the treatment of several cancers, including colorectal cancer (capecitabine, 5-FU), leukemia (cytarabine), gastric cancer (5-FU), basal cell carcinoma (5-FU), metastatic breast cancer (capecitabine, gemcitabine, 5-FU), lung cancer (gemcitabine), ovarian cancer (gemcitabine), and pancreatic cancer (gemcitabine, 5-FU).

Mechanism of Action and Pharmacokinetics

Capecitabine and 5-FU are prodrugs. Capecitabine is converted to 5-FU by an enzyme that is present in high levels in tumors. 5-FU must also be activated. Once activated, 5-FU inhibits the enzyme responsible for making thymidine (a DNA nucleoside), inhibits RNA formation, and causes mismatched DNA base pairs (Fig. 31.3).

Adverse Reactions

Adverse effects linked to capecitabine and 5-FU are stomach upset, loss of appetite, diarrhea or constipation, fatigue, muscle and bone pain, insomnia, headache, and dry, itchy skin. Additional adverse reactions include paresthesia (prickling or tingling sensation) in the hands and feet, jaundice, bone marrow suppression, fatal autoimmune anemias, increased opportunistic infections, and cardiotoxicity (capecitabine, 5-FU, and fludarabine).

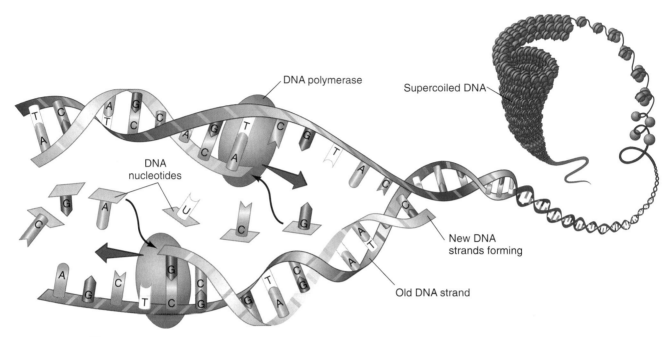

• **Fig. 31.3** Deoxyribonucleic acid replication. (From Patton KT, Thibodeau GA: *Anatomy and physiology*, ed 9, St Louis, 2016, Elsevier.)

Fluoropyrimidines Used in the Treatment of Colorectal Cancer

Generic Name	US Brand Name(s) / Canadian Brand Name(s)	Dosage Forms and Strengths
capecitabine	Xeloda	**Tablet:** 150 mg, 500 mg
	Xeloda	
fluorouracil (5-FU)[a]	Carac, Efudex, Tolak	**Cream:** 0.5% (Carac)[b], 4% (Tolak), 5% (Efudex)
	Generics	**Solution, intravenous:** 50 mg/mL (5%)
		Solution, topical[b]**:** 2%, 5%
cytarabine[a]	Generics	**Powder, for injection**[b]**:** 100 mg/vial, 500 mg/vial, 1 g/vial, 2 g/vial
	Generics	**Solution, for injection:** 20 mg/mL, 100 mg/mL
fludarabine[a]	Generics	**Powder, for injection**[b]**:** 50 mg/vial
	Fludara	**Solution, for injection:** 25 mg/mL
		Tablet: 10 mg[c]
gemcitabine[a]	Infugem	**Powder, for injection:** 200 mg, 1 g/vial, 2 g/vial[c]
	Generics	**Solution, for injection**[c]**:** 38 mg/mL, 40 mg/mL
		Solution, for IV infusion (Infugem)[b]**:** 1200 mg, 1300 mg, 1400 mg, 1500 mg, 1600 mg, 1700 mg, 1800 mg, 1900 mg, 2000 mg, 2200 mg in solutions equivalent to 10 mg/mL

[a]Generic available.
[b]Available in the United States only.
[c]Available in Canada only.

Topoisomerase Inhibitors

Irinotecan (Camptosar, Onivyde) is a topoisomerase inhibitor that is indicated for the treatment of colorectal cancer. The other drugs in this class are used to treat various other cancers. Etoposide (Vepesid) is indicated for the treatment of testicular cancer, SCLC, and NSCLC. Topotecan (Hycamtin) is indicated for the treatment of ovarian cancer, cervical cancer, and SCLC. Etoposide is a semisynthetic derivative of an extract from the mandrake plant. Irinotecan and topotecan are derived from *Camptotheca acuminata* (a Chinese tree).

> ### ❶ Tech Alert!
> Common endings for topoisomerase inhibitors are -*poside* and -*tecan*.

Mechanism of Action and Pharmacokinetics

Topoisomerases are enzymes that cleave DNA strands, a step needed for DNA replication and RNA transcription (Fig. 31.4). Topoisomerase II plays a role in mitosis. Oral absorption of the drugs is good, but penetration in the central nervous system is poor. Irinotecan is a prodrug that has an active metabolite that is 1000 times more potent in inhibiting topoisomerase.

Adverse Reactions

Etoposide may cause diarrhea, hair loss, nausea, skin rash, fatigue, irritation at the injection site, flulike symptoms, bleeding, or bruising. Irinotecan and topotecan produce similar side effects plus headache, gas, and weight loss. Rarely, individuals on high-dose etoposide therapy may develop acute nonlymphocytic leukemia.

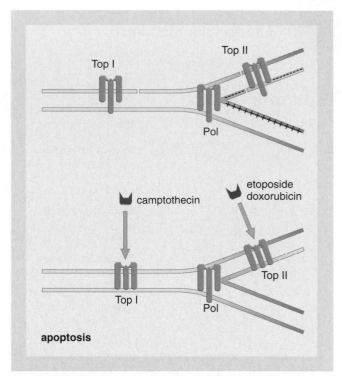

• **Fig. 31.4** Site of action of topoisomerase inhibitors. *Top I*, Topoisomerase I; *Top II*, topoisomerase II; *Pol*, DNA polymerase. (From Page C, Curtis M, Sutter M, et al: *Integrated pharmacology*, ed 3, Philadelphia, 2006, Mosby.)

Topoisomerase Inhibitors

Generic Name	US Brand Name(s) / Canadian Brand(s)	Dosage Forms and Strengths
etoposide[a]	Generics	**Capsule (Vepesid):** 50 mg
	Vepesid	**Solution, for injection:** 20 mg/mL
irinotecan[a]	Camptosar, Onivyde	**Solution, for injection:** 20 mg/mL
	Onivyde	**Suspension, for injection (Onivyde):** 4.3 mg/mL
topotecan[a]	Hycamtin	**Capsule**[b]: 0.25 mg, 1 mg
	Generics	**Powder, injection:** 4 mg/vial
		Solution, for injection: 1 mg/mL

[a]Generic available.
[b]Available in the United States only.

Kinase Inhibitors

Two kinase inhibitors are currently approved for the treatment of metastatic colorectal cancer. They are regorafenib and tucatinib. The mechanism of action and adverse reactions for kinase inhibitors used in the treatment of cancers are described earlier in this chapter.

Kinase Inhibitors

Generic Name	US Brand Name(s) / Canadian Brand Name(s)	Dosage Forms and Strengths
regorafenib	Stivarga	**Tablet:** 40 mg
	Stivarga	
tucatinib	Tukysa	**Tablet:** 50 mg, 150 mg
	Tukysa	

Immunotherapy for Colorectal Cancer

Monoclonal Antibodies

Numerous monoclonal antibodies and their biosimilars are used for the treatment of several cancers, including colorectal cancer with 5-FU, NSCLC in combination with carboplatin and paclitaxel, renal cancer, and glioblastoma. They include bevacizumab, ipilimumab, nivolumab, panitumumab, pembrolizumab, and ramucirumab. The mechanism of action of monoclonal antibody biological response modifiers is described in Chapter 13 and in this chapter in the sections on Breast Cancer. The mechanism of action for the monoclonal antibodies bevacizumab, panitumumab, pembrolizumab, and ramucirumab used for the treatment of colorectal cancer that has not been described previously is human vascular endothelial growth factor receptor 2 antagonists.

Monoclonal Antibodies

Generic Name	US Brand Name(s) / Canadian Brand Name(s)	Dosage Forms and Strengths
bevacizumab	Avastin	**Powder, for injection[a]:** 100 mg/vial, 400 mg/vial **Solution, for injection:** 100 mg/4 mL, 400 mg/16 mL (25 mg/mL)
	Avastin, Aybinto, Bambevi	
bevacizumab-awwb	Mvasi	**Solution, for injection:** 100 mg/4 mL, 400 mg/16 mL (25 mg/mL)
	Mvasi	
bevacizumab-adcd	Vegzelma	**Solution, for injection:** 100 mg/4 mL, 400 mg/16 mL (25 mg/mL)
	Vegzelma	
bevacizumab-bvzr	Zirabev	**Solution, for injection:** 100 mg/4 mL, 400 mg/16 mL (25 mg/mL)
	Zirabev	
bevacizumab-maly	Alymsys	**Solution, for injection:** 100 mg/4 mL, 400 mg/16 mL (25 mg/mL)
	Abevmy	
cetuximab	Erbitux	**Powder, for intravenous solution[a]:** 100 mg/vial **Solution for intravenous use[b]:** 2 mg/mL
	Erbitux	
panitumumab	Vectibix	**Solution, for infusion:** 100 mg/5 mL, 200 mg/10 mL[a], 400 mg/20 mL
	Vectibix	
ramucirumab	Cyramza	**Solution, for injection:** 100 mg/10 mL, 500 mg/50 mL (10 mg/mL)
	Cyramza	

[a]Available in the United States only.
[b]Available in Canada only.

Pharmacotherapy for Melanoma (Skin Cancer)

Melanoma is treated with chemotherapy, immunotherapy, and targeted agents (e.g., kinase inhibitors).

Kinase Inhibitors

Binimetinib, cobimetinib (Cotellic), dabrafenib (Tafinlar), encorafenib (Braftovi), trametinib (Mekinist), and vemurafenib (Zelboraf) are kinase inhibitors that are used in the treatment of melanoma. Dabrafenib and trametinib are also indicated for the treatment of NSCLC. They block signaling pathways that are needed for tumor growth and spread to other parts of the body. Melanoma may mutate and develop alternate signaling pathways. This type of resistance quickly develops when the drugs are used as monotherapy; therefore combination therapy is often used. Mutations may lead to secondary cancers.

Kinase inhibitors may cause diarrhea, regardless of which cancer they are used to treat. Other common adverse reactions are thickening skin, headache, and joint pain (dabrafenib); fatigue, fever, and skin rash (trametinib); and photosensitivity, hair loss, joint pain, and itchy skin (vemurafenib). Additional details about the mechanism of action and adverse reactions of kinase inhibitors are described in this chapter under Breast Cancer.

Kinase Inhibitors

Generic Name	US Brand Name(s) / Canadian Brand Name(s)	Dosage Forms and Strengths
binimetinib	Mektovi	**Tablet:** 15 mg
	Mektovi	
cobimetinib	Cotellic	**Tablet:** 20 mg
	Cotellic	
dabrafenib	Tafinlar	**Capsule:** 50 mg, 75 mg
	Tafinlar	
encorafenib	Braftovi	**Capsule:** 75 mg
	Braftovi	
trametinib	Mekinist	**Tablet:** 0.5 mg, 2 mg
	Mekinist	
vemurafenib	Zelboraf	**Tablet:** 240 mg
	Zelboraf	

Immunotherapy for Melanoma (Skin Cancer)

Monoclonal Antibodies

Nivolumab (Opdivo) and pembrolizumab (Keytruda) are PD-1 blocking antibodies that are indicated for metastatic melanoma and NSCLC. The mechanism of action for Keytruda and other PD-1 and PD-L1 blocking antibodies is described in this chapter in the section on Lung Cancer. Ipilimumab is a monoclonal antibody that blocks cytotoxic T-lymphocyte antigen 4 (CTLA-4) binding. Human CTLA-4 blocking antibodies are also called "check point" inhibitors. Nivolumab is marketed in combination with relatlimab, a lymphocyte-activation gene 3 (LAG-3) blocking antibody. The combination of the two monoclonal antibodies that act by different mechanisms increases T-cell activation more than individual administration.

Pharmacotherapy for Cancer of the Uterus and Ovaries

Progestins

Megestrol acetate and medroxyprogesterone acetate are progestins. Megestrol is approved for the treatment of inoperable, advanced metastatic cancer of the endometrium and breast, as well as for palliative treatment of advanced stage, hormone-responsive prostate cancer. Medroxyprogesterone acetate is indicated for the

PD-1, PD-L1, CTLA-4, and LAG-3 Blocking Antibodies

Generic Name	US Brand Name(s) / Canadian Brand Name(s)	Dosage Forms and Strengths
ipilimumab	Yervoy / Yervoy	**Solution, for injection:** 5 mg/mL
nivolumab + relatlimab-rmbw	Opdualag / Not available	**Solution, for intravenous injection:** 240 mg nivolumab + 80 mg relatlimab

adjunctive and/or palliative treatment of recurrent and/or metastatic cancer of the endometrium and hormone-dependent metastatic cancer of the breast.

❶ Tech Alert!

Megestrol suspension is prescribed to increase the appetite and combat the wasting syndrome in patients with AIDS and cancer.

Mechanism of Action

Megestrol binds to PRs where it stimulates cell maturation. It inhibits overgrowth of endometrial tissue in women who have endometrial cancer. It has androgenic properties that act on the pituitary, when taken with diethylstilbestrol, to suppress androgens in the testes, which is useful for treating prostate cancer. It is not fully known how megestrol works to suppress estrogen-dependent breast tumors; however, suppression of luteinizing hormone release from the pituitary and increased estrogen metabolism are believed to be involved.

Adverse Reactions

The most common adverse effects associated with megestrol use are hot flashes, breakthrough menstrual bleeding, and weight gain. Breast tenderness, hair loss, and hyperglycemia may also occur.

Progestins

Generic Name	US Brand Name(s) / Canadian Brand Name(s)	Dosage Forms and Strengths
medroxyprogesterone[a]	Provera / Provera	See Chapter 27
megestrol acetate[a]	Megace ES / Generics	**Suspension, oral (Megace ES):** 125 mg/mL **Tablet:** 20 mg[b], 40 mg, 160 mg[c]

[a]Generic available.
[b]Available in the United States only.
[c]Available in Canada only.

Immunotherapy for Endometrial Cancer of the Uterus

Immunotherapeutic agents have recently been approved for the treatment of endometrial, cervical, and ovarian cancers. They include pembrolizumab (Keytruda), dostarlimab-gxly (Jemperli), and the kinase inhibitor lenvatinib (Lenvima). Olaparib is used to treat ovarian and other cancers that have a *BRCA* mutation. It also is used to treat breast cancer, prostate cancer, and pancreatic cancer. Megestrol is used for the treatment of endometrial cancer.

Immunotherapy for Endometrial Cancer

Generic Name	US Brand Name(s) / Canadian Brand Name(s)	Dosage Forms and Strengths
dostarlimab-gxly	Jemperli / Jemperli	**Solution, for injection:** 50 mg/mL
lenvatinib	Lenvima / Lenvima	**Capsule:** 4 mg, 8 mg[a], 10 mg, 12 mg[a], 14 mg[a], 18 mg[a], 20 mg[a], 24 mg[a]
olaparib	Lynparza / Lynparza	See Breast Cancer

[a]Available in Canada only.

Summary of Antineoplastic Agents That Treat Various Other Cancers

Alkylating Agents

Alkylating agents are one of the oldest classes of antineoplastic agents. They are related to nitrogen mustard, a lethal gas that was used for chemical warfare in World War I. Cyclophosphamide (Procytox), busulfan (Busulfex, Myleran), ifosfamide (Ifex), melphalan (Alkeran, Evomela), mechlorethamine (Mustargen), and chlorambucil (Leukeran) are all alkylating agents. Only cyclophosphamide and melphalan are approved for the treatment of one of the top six cancers described in this chapter. Cyclophosphamide is indicated for breast cancer and ovarian cancer, as well as Hodgkin disease, non-Hodgkin lymphoma, ALL, multiple myeloma, chronic lymphocytic leukemia, mycosis fungoides, and retinoblastoma. Melphalan is indicated for ovarian cancer and multiple myeloma. The alkylating agents vary in their antitumor effects and toxicity, but their mechanism of action is the same. All alkylating agents damage DNA and impair DNA replication and the growth phase of the cell life cycle (see Table 31.1). Alkylating agents are toxic to cancer cells and noncancerous cells, and they can cause cell mutations that lead to other cancers. Resistance to the effects of cyclophosphamide and other alkylating agents can develop.

Cyclophosphamide commonly causes hair loss, appetite and weight loss, skin discoloration, mouth sores, and fatigue. The side effects of melphalan are fatigue, diarrhea, nausea, vomiting, and anemia.

Alkylating Agents

Generic Name	US Brand Name(s) / Canadian Brand Name(s)	Dosage Forms and Strengths
cyclophosphamide[a]	Cytoxan / Procytox	**Capsule**[c]: 25 mg, 50 mg **Powder, for solution (Cytoxan, Procytox):** 200 mg/vial[b], 500 mg/vial, 1000 mg/vial, 2000 mg/vial **Tablet**[b]: 25 mg, 50 mg
melphalan[a]	Evomela / Alkeran	**Powder, for infusion:** 50 mg/vial **Tablet:** 2 mg

[a]Generic available.
[b]Available in Canada only.
[c]Available in the United States only.

Anthracyclines

Doxorubicin (Caelyx, Doxil), epirubicin (Ellence), and idarubicin (Idamycin PFS) are anthracyclines. Mitoxantrone is a related compound and is classified as an anthracenedione. Doxorubicin is indicated for the treatment of numerous cancers such as ovarian cancer, bladder cancer, lung cancer, Hodgkin disease, leukemia, gastric cancer, soft tissue sarcoma, and thyroid cancer. Doxorubicin liposomal is approved for the treatment of ovarian cancer, Kaposi sarcoma, and multiple myeloma. Doxorubicin and epirubicin are indicated for the treatment of breast cancer, typically in combination with other antineoplastic agents. Idarubicin and mitoxantrone are approved for the treatment of acute myelogenous leukemia.

Anthracyclines damage cellular DNA and inhibit the DNA and RNA enzymes that promote protein synthesis (see Fig. 31.3). This impairs DNA replication and the growth phase of the cell life cycle (see Table 31.1). Anthracyclines also inhibit the activity of the enzyme topoisomerase (see the section Topoisomerase Inhibitors) as a secondary mechanism for cellular destruction. Doxorubicin is a prodrug that is metabolized to the active metabolite idarubicin.

① Tech Alert!

Doxorubicin and doxorubicin liposomal are not substitutable.

① Tech Alert!

The following drugs have look-alike/sound-alike issues:
DOXOrubicin and DOXOrubicin liposomal;
mitoXANtrone and mitoMYcin

Anthracyclines

Generic Name	US Brand Name(s) / Canadian Brand Name(s)	Dosage Forms and Strengths
doxorubicin[a]	Generics / Adriamycin PFS	**Powder, for injection:** 10 mg/vial, 20 mg/vial[b], 50 mg/vial, 150 mg/vial[c] **Solution, for injection:** 2 mg/mL
doxorubicin liposomal	Doxil / Caelyx	**Solution, for injection:** 2 mg/mL
epirubicin[a]	Ellence / Generics	**Solution, for injection (Ellence, Pharmorubicin PFS):** 2 mg/mL
mitoxantrone[a]	Generics / Generics	**Solution, for injection:** 2 mg/mL

[a]Generic available.
[b]Available in the United States only.
[c]Available in Canada only.

Vinca Alkaloids

Vinorelbine (Navelbine), vincristine (Marqibo Kit), and vinblastine are vinca alkaloids. They are naturally derived from the periwinkle plant. Vinorelbine is used for the treatment of NSCLC. Vinblastine is indicated for the treatment of breast cancer, Kaposi sarcoma, Hodgkin disease, non-Hodgkin lymphoma, and testicular cancer. Vincristine is indicated for the treatment of leukemia. The mechanism of action of vinca alkaloids is similar to that of taxanes. Both drugs act on microtubules to inhibit mitosis. Vinca alkaloids inhibit microtubule formation (taxanes inhibit microtubule degradation).

The side effects linked to vinca alkaloids are similar to those for taxanes and include hair loss, nausea and vomiting, constipation, joint and muscle pain, mouth sores, increased risk for infections, and pain at the injection site.

① Tech Alert!

A common beginning for vinca alkaloids is *vin-*.

① Tech Alert!

VinBLAStine and vinCRIStine have look-alike/sound-alike issues.

① Tech Alert!

Vincristine is usually stored in the refrigerator.

Miscellaneous Agents

Bleomycin, dactinomycin (Cosmegen), and mitomycin are antineoplastic agents approved for the treatment of various cancers.

Vinca Alkaloids

Generic Name	US Brand Name(s) / Canadian Brand Name(s)		Dosage Forms and Strengths
vinorelbine[a]	Generics	Generics	**Solution, for injection:** 10 mg/mL
vinblastine[a]	Generics	Generics	**Powder, for injection[b]:** 10 mg/vial **Solution, for injection:** 1 mg/mL
vincristine PFS[a]	Generics	Generics	**Solution, for injection:** 1 mg/mL

[a]Generic available.
[b]Available in the United States only.

Miscellaneous Antineoplastic Agents

Generic Name	US Brand Name(s) / Canadian Brand Name(s)		Dosage Forms and Strengths
bleomycin[a]	Generics	Generics	**Powder, for injection:** 15 units/vial, 30 units/vial[b]
dactinomycin[c] (actinomycin D)	Cosmegen	Cosmegen	**Powder, for injection:** 500 mcg/vial
mitomycin[a]	Jelmyto, Mitosol	Generics	**Powder, for injection:** 20 mg/vial, 40 mg/vial[b] **Solution, topical (Mitosol):** 0.2 mg/vial[b]
porfimer	Photofrin	Not available	**Powder, for injection:** 75 mg/vial

[a]Generic available.
[b]Available in the United States only.
[c]Generic available in the United States only.

Bleomycin is indicated for the treatment of cervical, penile, testicular, and vulvar cancers, in addition to Hodgkin disease and head and neck cancers. Dactinomycin is indicated for the treatment of testicular cancer, choriocarcinoma, and rhabdomyosarcoma. Mitomycin is approved for gastric and pancreatic cancer treatment. Mitomycin (as Mitosol) is also indicated as an adjunct to glaucoma surgery, where it is used to reduce scarring that might result in increased intraocular pressure. Hydroxyurea is indicated for the treatment of head and neck cancers, leukemia, and sickle cell anemia. Porfimer is used for the treatment of NSCLC.

The primary mechanism of action for bleomycin and mitomycin is to impair DNA replication by producing breaks in the DNA strands. Mitomycin also binds to DNA to form abnormal cross-links. Dactinomycin causes the DNA helix to uncoil and inhibits DNA, RNA, and protein synthesis. Porfimer produces its cytotoxic and antitumor effects only after exposure to light. Photodynamic therapy is administered 40 to 50 hours after administration to activate the drug.

Bleomycin, dactinomycin, and mitomycin may produce pain at the injection site, fatigue, nausea, vomiting, decreased appetite, hair loss, and darkened skin color. Mitomycin may discolor the urine and nails. Dactinomycin may cause bone marrow suppression and severe anemias, thereby increasing the risk for infection.

❗ Tech Alert!

The following drugs have look-alike/sound-alike issues:
DACTINomycin and DAPTOmycin

❗ Tech Alert!

Exercise precautions for handling, preparing, and administering cytotoxic drugs.

TECHNICIAN'S CORNER

1. There have been many reports of the destruction of the rain forests and the possibility of losing potential cures for cancer. What can we do to prevent this from happening?
2. What are some new innovations being used to deliver chemotherapeutic agents in doses that will not harm good cells?

Summary of Drugs Used for the Treatment of Breast, Prostate, Lung, Colorectal, Skin, Uterine, and Ovarian Cancer

Generic Name	US Brand Name(s)	Usual Dose and Dosing Schedule	Warning Labels
Hormones			
Selective Estrogen Receptor Modulators			
tamoxifen	Soltamox	**Breast cancer:** 20–40 mg PO twice a day in divided doses	SWALLOW WHOLE— tamoxifen. AVOID PREGNANCY. AVOID GRAPEFRUIT JUICE— toremifene.
toremifene	Fareston	**Breast cancer:** 60 mg PO once a day	

Continued

Summary of Drugs Used for the Treatment of Breast, Prostate, Lung, Colorectal, Skin, Uterine, and Ovarian Cancer—cont'd

Generic Name	US Brand Name(s)	Usual Dose and Dosing Schedule	Warning Labels
Estrogen Receptor Downregulator			
elacestrant	Orserdu	**Breast cancer:** 345 mg once daily	TAKE WITH FOOD.
fulvestrant	Faslodex	**Breast cancer:** 500 mg IM as two 5-mL injections, on days 1, 15, 29 and once monthly thereafter	AVOID PREGNANCY. REFRIGERATE; DO NOT FREEZE. STORE IN ORIGINAL CONTAINER. PROTECT FROM LIGHT.
Aromatase Inhibitors			
anastrozole	Arimidex	**Breast cancer:** 1 mg PO once daily	AVOID PREGNANCY. TAKE AT THE SAME TIME EACH DAY WITH A DRINK OF WATER.
exemestane	Aromasin	**Breast cancer:** 25 mg PO once daily; increase to 50 mg daily if taken with CYP3A4 inhibitor	TAKE WITH MEALS—exemestane. MAY CAUSE DIZZINESS OR DROWSINESS—
letrozole	Femara	**Breast cancer:** 2.5 mg PO once daily	letrozole.
GnRH Agonist and LHRH Antagonists			
degarelix	Firmagon	**Prostate cancer:** 240 mg given as 2 subcut injections followed by 80 mg every 28 days	RECONSTITUTE WITH STERILE WATER. DO NOT SHAKE.
goserelin	Zoladex	**Breast cancer:** 3.6 mg subcut into upper abdominal wall every 28 days **Prostate cancer (advanced):** 3.6 mg subcut implanted into upper abdominal wall every 28 days or 10.8 mg every 12 weeks	AVOID PREGNANCY. STORE AT ROOM TEMPERATURE.
relugolix	Orgovyx	**Prostate cancer:** 360 mg to start, then 120 mg once daily	SWALLOW WHOLE; DO NOT CRUSH OR CHEW.
Progestins			
megestrol acetate	Megace	**Breast cancer:** 40 mg PO 4 times daily **Endometrial cancer:** 40–320 mg PO daily in divided doses	SHAKE WELL—suspension.
Antiandrogens			
apalutamide	Erleada	**Prostate cancer:** 240 mg once daily	SWALLOW WHOLE; DO NOT CRUSH OR CHEW—apalutamide, darolutamide. MAY CAUSE DIZZINESS.
bicalutamide	Casodex	**Prostate cancer:** 50 mg once daily	
darolutamide	Nubeqa	**Prostate cancer:** 600 mg twice daily	
enzalutamide	Xtandi	**Prostate cancer:** 160 mg once daily	
flutamide[a]	Generic	**Prostate cancer:** 250 mg 3 times a day	
nilutamide	Nilandron	**Prostate cancer:** 300 mg once daily for 30 days, followed by 150 mg once daily	TAKE AS DIRECTED; DO NOT SKIP DOSES—all.

Summary of Drugs Used for the Treatment of Breast, Prostate, Lung, Colorectal, Skin, Uterine, and Ovarian Cancer—cont'd

Generic Name	US Brand Name(s)	Usual Dose and Dosing Schedule	Warning Labels
Kinase and mTOR Inhibitors			
abemaciclib	Verzenio	**Breast cancer:** Take 200 mg twice daily (monotherapy) or 150 mg twice daily with fulvestrant	SWALLOW WHOLE; DO NOT CRUSH OR CHEW—abemaciclib, crizotinib, dabrafenib, everolimus, gefitinib, palbociclib, ribociclib.
afatinib	Gilotrif	**Lung cancer (NSCLC):** Take 40 mg once daily	AVOID GRAPEFRUIT JUICE AND/OR POMEGRANATE JUICE—abemaciclib,
alpelisib	Piqray	**Breast cancer:** 300 mg once daily	lapatinib, neratinib, palbociclib, ribociclib, encorafenib, entrectinib.
ceritinib	Zykadia	**Lung cancer (NSCLC):** Take 450 mg once daily	TAKE ON AN EMPTY STOMACH—afatinib,
cobimetinib	Cotellic	**Melanoma:** Take 60 mg once daily for 21 of a 28-day cycle	ceritinib, dabrafenib, erlotinib, lapatinib, pralsetinib, trametinib.
crizotinib	Xalkori	**Lung cancer (NSCLC):** Take 250 mg twice daily	TAKE WITH FOOD— alpelisib, neratinib, palbociclib, tepotinib.
dabrafenib	Tafinlar	**Melanoma:** Take 150 mg twice daily	TAKE AS DIRECTED; DO NOT SKIP DOSES—all.
dacomitinib	Vizimpro	**Lung cancer (NSCLC):** 45 mg once daily	AVOID PREGNANCY—abemaciclib, afatinib,
encorafenib	Braftovi	**Melanoma:** 450 mg once daily in combination with binimetinib **Colorectal cancer:** 300 mg once daily in combination with cetuximab	ceritinib, crizotinib, dabrafenib, erlotinib, everolimus, lapatinib, neratinib, palbociclib, ribociclib, trametinib, vemurafenib.
entrectinib	Rozlytrek	**Lung cancer (NSCLC):** 600 mg once daily	AVOID PROLONGED EXPOSURE TO SUNLIGHT—erlotinib, vemurafenib.
erlotinib	Tarceva	**Lung cancer (NSCLC):** 150 mg once daily	DISSOLVE IN 4–8 OUNCES OF WATER; THEN DRINK SOLUTION—Afinitor Disperz,
everolimus	Afinitor, Afinitor Disperz	**Breast cancer:** Take 10 mg once daily	gefitinib.
gefitinib	Iressa	**Lung cancer (NSCLC):** Take 250 mg once daily	AVOID ANTACIDS—lapatinib, neratinib.
lapatinib	Tykerb	**Breast cancer:** Take 1250 mg once daily on days 1–21 plus capecitabine twice daily on days 1–14 in a repeating 21-day cycle	REFRIGERATE; DO NOT FREEZE—trametinib. MAY CAUSE DIZZINESS OR DROWSINESS; AVOID DRIVING OR OPERATING MACHINERY—entrectinib.
lenvatinib	Lenvima	**Endometrial Cancer:** 20 mg once daily in combination with pembrolizumab 200 mg administered as an intravenous infusion every 3 weeks.	
lorlatinib	Lorbrena	**Lung cancer (NSCLC):** 100mg once daily	
neratinib	Nerlynx	**Breast cancer:** Take 240 mg once daily	
olaparib	Lynparza	**Breast cancer or Ovarian cancer:** 300 mg taken orally twice daily	
osimertinib	Tagrisso	**Lung cancer (NSCLC):** 80 mg once daily	
palbociclib	Ibrance	**Breast cancer:** Take 125 mg once daily for 21 consecutive days; off 7 days then repeat	
pralsetinib	Gavreto	**Lung cancer (NSCLC):** 400 mg orally once daily	
regorafenib	Stivarga	**Colorectal cancer:** 160 mg orally, once daily for the first 21 days of each 28-day cycle	
ribociclib	Kisqali	**Breast cancer:** Take 600 mg once daily for 21 consecutive days; off 7 days then repeat	
selpercatinib	Retevmo	**Lung cancer (NSCLC):** Less than 50 kg: 120 mg orally twice daily. 50 kg or greater: 160 mg orally twice daily	
tepotinib	Tepmetko	**Lung cancer (NSCLC):** 450 mg orally once dailyer	
trametinib	Mekinist	**Melanoma:** Take 2 mg once daily	
tucatinib	Tukysa	**Breast Cancer or Colorectal cancer:** 300 mg taken orally twice daily	
vemurafenib	Zelboraf	**Melanoma:** Take 960 mg twice daily	
letrozole + ribociclib	Kisqali Femara Co-Pak	**Breast cancer:** Take 3 Kisqali tablets (600 mg) once daily for 21 consecutive days; off 7 days. Take 1 letrozole tablet (2.5 mg) daily for 28 days; repeat cycle	

Continued

Summary of Drugs Used for the Treatment of Breast, Prostate, Lung, Colorectal, Skin, Uterine, and Ovarian Cancer—cont'd

Generic Name	US Brand Name(s)	Usual Dose and Dosing Schedule	Warning Labels
Anthracyclines			
doxorubicin	Generics	**Breast cancer:** 50–60 mg/m² IV bolus on day 1 of every 21 days with other agents, this is one of several dosage regimens used in combination with other agents (e.g., cyclophosphamide and fluorouracil, paclitaxel, docetaxel) **Ovarian cancer and SCLC:** 40–50 mg/m² per dose IV once monthly in combination with various other antineoplastic agents	AVOID PREGNANCY. SHAKE WELL—powder, for injection. REFRIGERATE—doxorubicin, epirubicin. PROTECT FROM LIGHT—doxorubicin, epirubicin. MAY CAUSE DISCOLORATION OF URINE—doxorubicin. STORE AT ROOM TEMPERATURE—mitoxantrone. SHAKE VIGOROUSLY TO DISSOLVE—epirubicin powder, for injection.
epirubicin	Ellence	**Breast cancer:** 100 mg/m² IV on day 1 in combination with fluorouracil and cyclophosphamide (FEC regimen) every 21 days for 6 cycles or 60 mg/m² IV on days 1 and 8 in combination with oral cyclophosphamide and fluorouracil every 28 days for 6 cycles	
mitoxantrone	Generics	**Prostate cancer:** 12–14 mg/m² IV every 21 days in combination with prednisone or hydrocortisone	
Taxanes			
docetaxel	Taxotere	**Breast cancer (advanced, metastatic):** 60–100 mg/m² IV over 1 h once every 3 weeks	AVOID PREGNANCY. DO NOT SHAKE—docetaxel. REFRIGERATE; DO NOT FREEZE—docetaxel. RECONSTITUTED SOLUTION IS STABLE FOR A CERTAIN LENGTH OF TIME: docetaxel (4 h), paclitaxel (27 h), protein-bound paclitaxel (24 h). STORE AT ROOM TEMPERATURE—paclitaxel. PROTECT FROM LIGHT—docetaxel, paclitaxel. DO NOT MIX IN PVC BAGS OR USE PVC SETS—docetaxel, paclitaxel. AVOID ASPIRIN, APAP, AND NSAIDS.
paclitaxel	Taxol	**Breast cancer (metastatic):** 175 mg/m² IV over 3 h every 3 weeks	
paclitaxel protein-bound particles	Abraxane	**Breast cancer:** 260 mg/m² IV over 30 min once per week for 3 weeks, then 1 week off, every 28 days (dose depends on previously untreated or taxane-refractory)	
Fluoropyrimidines			
5-fluorouracil	Generics	**Breast cancer (palliative):** 12 mg/kg IV daily for 4 days, if tolerated then 6 mg/kg IV daily on days 6, 8, 10, 12 (max dose 800 mg/day). Maintenance: if tolerated, repeat cycle every 30 days. Regimens also for colorectal, gastric, and pancreatic cancer	ONCE THE PHARMACY BULK VIAL IS OPENED, ANY UNUSED PORTION SHOULD BE DISCARDED AFTER 1 HOUR. AVOID PREGNANCY. AVOID PROLONGED EXPOSURE TO SUNLIGHT. AVOID ASPIRIN, APAP, AND NSAIDS. STORE AT ROOM TEMPERATURE. PROTECT DRUG FROM LIGHT.
capecitabine	Xeloda	**Breast cancer:** 2500 mg/m²/day PO in 2 divided doses for 2 weeks, repeated every 3 weeks **Colorectal cancer:** 1250 mg/m² PO twice daily within 30 min for 2 weeks, repeated every 3 weeks for a total of 8 cycles	TAKE WITH FOOD—capecitabine. AVOID PREGNANCY. AVOID ASPIRIN, APAP, AND NSAIDS. STORE AT ROOM TEMPERATURE—gemcitabine.
gemcitabine	Gemzar	**Breast cancer (metastatic):** 1250 mg/m² IV over 30 min on days 1 and 8 of a 21-day cycle in combination with paclitaxel **Lung cancer (NSCLC):** 1000 mg/m² IV on days 1, 8, 15 of a 28-day cycle or 1250 mg/m² on days 1 and 8 of a 21-day cycle. Cisplatin (100 mg/m² IV) is given after the gemcitabine infusion on day 1 of either regimen. **Ovarian cancer:** 1000 mg/m² IV over 30 min on days 1 and 8 of a 21-day cycle in combination with carboplatin on day 1 after gemcitabine infusion	

Summary of Drugs Used for the Treatment of Breast, Prostate, Lung, Colorectal, Skin, Uterine, and Ovarian Cancer—cont'd

Generic Name	US Brand Name(s)	Usual Dose and Dosing Schedule	Warning Labels
Antimetabolites			
methotrexate	Generics	**Lung cancer (SCLC): PO:** 10 mg/m^2 PO twice weekly ×4 doses every 3 weeks in combination with lomustine and cyclophosphamide **IV:** 20 mg/m^2 IV as a single dose with cisplatin, doxorubicin, and cyclophosphamide, every 28 days or numerous other regimens. **Breast cancer:** 40–60 mg/m^2 IV given on day 1 of every 21–28 days along with cyclophosphamide and fluorouracil. Also regimens for bladder cancer, non-Hodgkin lymphoma, and acute lymphocytic leukemia	PROTECT FROM LIGHT—methotrexate. STORE AT ROOM TEMPERATURE. RECONSTITUTE POWDER IMMEDIATELY BEFORE USE AND DISCARD ANY UNUSED PORTION— methotrexate. TAKE WITH A FULL GLASS OF WATER. MAY MAKE SKIN MORE SENSITIVE TO SUNLIGHT. AVOID PREGNANCY. DO NOT DRINK ALCOHOLIC BEVERAGES— methotrexate. REFRIGERATE AND USE WITHIN 24 HOURS OF RECONSTITUTION; DISCARD ANY UNUSED PORTION—pemetrexed.
pemetrexed	Alimta	**Lung cancer (NSCLC):** 500 mg/m^2 over 10 min on day 1 of each 21-day cycle	
Vinca Alkaloids			
vinorelbine	Navelbine	**Breast cancer:** 30 mg/m^2 IV over 6–10 min weekly or on days 1 and 8 repeated every 21 days **Lung cancer (NSCLC):** 30 mg/m^2 IV over 6–10 min once weekly or 25–30 mg/m^2 once weekly with cisplatin	REFRIGERATE; DO NOT FREEZE—vinorelbine. PROTECT FROM LIGHT—vinorelbine. AVOID ASPIRIN, APAP, AND NSAIDS. SYRINGES MUST BE LABELED "FOR IV USE ONLY—FATAL IF GIVEN INTRATHECALLY."
vinblastine	Generics	**Breast cancer:** 4.5 mg/m^2 IV on day 1 of every 21 days in combination with doxorubicin and thiotepa	
Platinum Compounds			
carboplatin	Generics	**Ovarian cancer:** 300 mg/m^2 IV on day 1 in combination with cyclophosphamide, repeated every 4 weeks for 6 cycles or 360 mg/m^2 IV on day 1, repeated every 4 weeks. Other regimens also recommended	AVOID PREGNANCY. AVOID ASPIRIN, APAP, AND NSAIDS. STABLE FOR 28 DAYS ONCE VIAL IS PENETRATED—cisplatin. PROTECT FROM LIGHT. STORE AT ROOM TEMPERATURE. RECONSTITUTED SOLUTION IS STABLE FOR 24 HOURS IF REFRIGERATED.
cisplatin	Generics	**Lung cancer (NSCLC):** 75 mg/m^2 IV as a single dose after administration of paclitaxel or docetaxel every 3 weeks. Other regimens also recommended	
oxaliplatin	Eloxatin	**Colorectal cancer:** Day 1, oxaliplatin 85 mg/m^2 IV infusion with leucovorin IV infusion given over 2 h, followed by 5-FU IV bolus over 2–4 min; then 5-FU IV infusion over 22 h. Day 2, leucovorin 200 mg/m^2 IV over 2 h followed by 5-FU IV bolus over 2–4 min, then 5-FU IV continuous infusion over 22 h. The 2-day regimen is repeated every 2 weeks	
Topoisomerase Inhibitors			
etoposide	Vepesid	**Lung cancer (SCLC):** 35 mg/m^2/day IV for 4 days to 50 mg/m^2/day IV for 5 days in combination with other antineoplastic agents 100–200 mg/m^2 orally for 5 days	TAKE WITH A FULL GLASS OF WATER— etoposide capsule. SWALLOW WHOLE; DO NOT CRUSH OR CHEW—etoposide capsule. AVOID PREGNANCY. RECONSTITUTED SOLUTION IS STABLE FOR 24 HOURS AT ROOM TEMPERATURE. MAY CAUSE DIZZINESS OR DROWSINESS. AVOID ASPIRIN, APAP, AND NSAIDS.

Continued

Summary of Drugs Used for the Treatment of Breast, Prostate, Lung, Colorectal, Skin, Uterine, and Ovarian Cancer—cont'd

Generic Name	US Brand Name(s)	Usual Dose and Dosing Schedule	Warning Labels
irinotecan	Camptosar	**Colorectal cancer:** 125 mg/m² IV over 90 min, once weekly for 4 weeks, every 6 weeks or 350 mg/m² by IV infusion over 90 min, once every 3 weeks. Other regimens with irinotecan followed by leucovorin and 5-FU	SWALLOW WHOLE; DO NOT CRUSH OR CHEW—topotecan capsules. TAKE WITH A FULL GLASS OF WATER—topotecan capsules. PROTECT FROM LIGHT. AVOID ASPIRIN, APAP, AND NSAIDS. RECONSTITUTED SOLUTION IS STABLE FOR 24 HOURS AT ROOM TEMPERATURE—topotecan.
topotecan	Hycamtin	**Ovarian cancer:** 1.5 mg/m²/day IV on days 1–5 of a 21-day course **Cervical cancers:** 0.75 mg/m² IV on days 1–3 in combination with cisplatin IV day 1 only, every 3 weeks **Lung cancer (SCLC):** 1.5–2.3 mg/m²/day PO on days 1–5 of a 21-day course	

Microtubule Inhibitors

Generic Name	US Brand Name(s)	Usual Dose and Dosing Schedule	Warning Labels
eribulin	Halaven	**Breast cancer:** 1.4 mg/m² IV over 2–5 min on days 1 and 8, repeated every 21 days	AVOID PREGNANCY. AVOID ASPIRIN, APAP, AND NSAIDS. STORE AT ROOM TEMPERATURE.
estramustine	Emcyt	**Prostate cancer:** 14 mg/kg/day or 600 mg/m²/day PO in 3–4 divided doses	AVOID PREGNANCY. AVOID ASPIRIN, APAP, AND NSAIDS. TAKE ON AN EMPTY STOMACH. AVOID DAIRY PRODUCTS WITHIN 2–3 HOURS OF DOSE.
ixabepilone	Ixempra	**Breast cancer:** 40 mg/m² IV over 3 h, given every 3 weeks in regimens with and without capecitabine	AVOID PREGNANCY. MAY CAUSE DIZZINESS OR DROWSINESS. AVOID ASPIRIN, APAP, AND NSAIDS. RECONSTITUTED SOLUTION IS STABLE FOR 6 HOURS AT ROOM TEMPERATURE.

Immunotherapeutic Agents
Monoclonal Antibodies

Generic Name	US Brand Name(s)	Usual Dose and Dosing Schedule	Warning Labels
bevacizumab	Avastin Mvasi Vegzalma Zirabev Alymsys Abevmy	**Colorectal cancer:** 5 or 10 mg/kg IV every 14 days in combination with 5-FU. **Lung cancer (NSCLC):** 15 mg/kg IV every 3 weeks in combination with carboplatin and paclitaxel	REFRIGERATE; DO NOT FREEZE—bevacizumab, pertuzumab, trastuzumab, ado-trastuzumab. PROTECT FROM LIGHT—pertuzumab. DO NOT SHAKE—pertuzumab, ado-trastuzumab, fam-trastuzumab. AVOID PREGNANCY—bevacizumab, pertuzumab, trastuzumab.
cetuximab	Erbitux	**Colorectal cancer:** 400 mg/m² by infusion 1 week before radiation therapy followed by 250 mg/m² every week for the duration of radiation therapy	
margetuximab	Margenza	**Breast cancer:** Administer 15 mg/kg margetuximab IV infusion to start, then every 3 weeks	
pertuzumab	Perjeta	**Breast cancer:** Initiate with 840 mg IV infusion, then 420 mg every 3 weeks thereafter	
ramucirumab	Cyramza	**Colorectal cancer:** 8 mg/kg every 2 weeks with Folfiri **Lung cancer (NSCLC):** 10 mg/kg every 2 weeks with erlotinib	
trastuzumab	Herceptin Kanjinti Ontruzant Ogivri Herzuma Trazimera	**Breast cancer:** 4 mg/kg IV infusion on week 1; if tolerated, at week 2, decrease to 2 mg/kg infused IV once weekly. Several other regimens are recommended	
ado-trastuzumab	Kadcyla	**Breast cancer:** 3.6 mg/kg given by IV infusion	
fam-trastuzumab	Enhertu	**Breast cancer:** 5.4 mg/kg given by IV infusion	

Summary of Drugs Used for the Treatment of Breast, Prostate, Lung, Colorectal, Skin, Uterine, and Ovarian Cancer—cont'd

Generic Name	US Brand Name(s)	Usual Dose and Dosing Schedule	Warning Labels
pertuzumab + trastuzumab + hyaluronidase-zzxf	Phesgo	**Breast cancer:** First dose of 1200 mg pertuzumab, 600 mg trastuzumab, and 30,000 units hyaluronidase subcut followed by 600 mg pertuzumab, 600 mg trastuzumab, and 20,000 units hyaluronidase every 3 weeks	
PD-1- and PD-L1–Blocking Antibodies			
atezolizumab	Tecentriq	**Lung cancer:** 1200 mg IV infusion every 3 weeks	REFRIGERATE; DO NOT FREEZE— atezolizumab, nivolumab, pembrolizumab, Opdualag. DO NOT SHAKE—atezolizumab, nivolumab, pembrolizumab, Opdualag. AVOID PREGNANCY—atezolizumab, nivolumab, pembrolizumab. PROTECT FROM LIGHT—pembrolizumab.
dostarlimab-gxly	Jemperli	**Endometrial cancer:** 500 mg every 3 weeks by infusion for 4 weeks followed by 1000 mg for 6 weeks	
durvalumab	Imfinzi	**Lung cancer (NSCLC):** 10 mg/kg every 2 weeks or 1500 mg every 4 weeks administered by infusion	
nivolumab	Opdivo	**Melanoma and lung cancer:** 3 mg/kg IV infusion every 2 weeks	
pembrolizumab	Keytruda	**Melanoma and lung cancer:** Inject 200 mg every 3 weeks	
nivolumab + relatlimab-rmbw	Opdualag	**Melanoma:** 480 mg nivolumab and 160 mg relatlimab intravenously every 4 weeks	
CTLA-4 Blocking Antibody			
ipilimumab	Yervoy	**Melanoma:** 3 mg/kg IV every 3 weeks for 4 doses	REFRIGERATE; DO NOT FREEZE. AVOID PREGNANCY. PROTECT FROM LIGHT.
necitumumab	Portrazza	**Lung cancer (NSCLC):** 800 mg by IV infusion on days 1 and 8 of a 3-week cycle	
Miscellaneous Agents			
abiraterone	Zytiga	**Prostate cancer:** 1000 mg orally daily	TAKE ON AN EMPTY STOMACH—abiraterone. SWALLOW WHOLE; DO NOT CRUSH OR CHEW—abiraterone, olaparib, talazoparib.
olaparib	Lynparza	**Breast cancer, ovarian cancer, prostate cancer:** 300 mg twice daily	
porfimer	Photofrin	**Lung cancer (NSCLC):** 2 mg/kg IV administered over 3–5 min followed 40–50 h later by laser illumination at the site(s) of tumor involvement	AVOID PREGNANCY. PROTECT EYES FROM SUNLIGHT.
talazoparib	Talzenna	**Breast cancer:** 1 mg orally once daily	SWALLOW WHOLE; DO NOT CRUSH OR CHEW— talazoparib.

Key Points

- Cancer is a disease that occurs when new cells form more rapidly than needed; the cells accumulate and form a mass called a tumor.
- A malignant tumor is cancerous and can invade and destroy nearby tissue and spread to other parts of the body; a benign tumor is not cancerous and does not spread.
- Cancers are named according to the site at which the cancerous growth began. This is the site of the primary tumor.
- Age, smoking or chewing tobacco, ionizing radiation and sunlight, hazardous chemicals, environmental pollutants, bacterial and viral infection, hormone therapy, family history, alcohol consumption, and diet, obesity, and lack of physical activity are all risk factors for cancer.

- Advancing age (>61 years) and history of hormone replacement therapy increase the risk for breast cancer.
- Cancer of the cervix is linked to human papillomavirus and exposure to the drug diethylstilbestrol.
- Endometrial cancer most commonly affects postmenopausal women.
- Skin cancer is associated with excessive exposure to ultraviolet (UV) light from the sun or UV lights used in tanning salons. Wearing protective clothing or using a sunscreen when outdoors is recommended.
- There are two types of lung cancer: small cell lung cancer (SCLC) and non–small cell lung cancer (NSCLC).
- The incidence of prostate cancer increases as men grow older.

- Staging is a method used to describe how far the cancer has progressed within the body.
- Cancer may be treated with chemotherapy, immunotherapy, radiation therapy, and surgery.
- Chemotherapy is the use of drugs to kill or slow the growth of cancerous cells.
- Immunotherapy is the administration of immune system modulators, vaccines, or synthetically generated immune components to boost the body's natural defense against abnormal, invasive and cancerous cells.
- A common ending for monoclonal antibodies is -*mab*.
- Bevacizumab (Avastin) and trastuzumab (Herceptin) are monoclonal antibodies used for the treatment of metastatic breast cancer.
- Ipilimumab (Yervoy) is an immunotherapeutic antibody that works by blocking cytotoxic T-lymphocyte antigen 4. It is used to treat melanoma. Programmed death receptor (PD-1)– and programmed death ligand (PD-L1)–blocking antibodies (atezolizumab, nivolumab, and pembrolizumab) are used to treat melanoma or lung cancer.
- The hormones estrogen and progesterone can promote the growth of estrogen receptor (ER)-positive and/or progesterone receptor (PR)-positive breast cancer.
- Antiestrogens are used for the treatment of ER-positive breast cancer.
- Tamoxifen and toremifene are selective ER modulators indicated for the treatment of ER-positive breast cancer.
- The warning label "Avoid Pregnancy" should be applied to the prescription vial of most antineoplastic agents.
- Elacestrant and fulvestrant are ER downregulators approved for the treatment of breast cancer.
- Anastrozole, exemestane, and letrozole are aromatase inhibitors approved for the treatment of breast cancer.
- Goserelin is a gonadotropin-releasing hormone agonist indicated for the treatment of advanced breast cancer in premenopausal and perimenopausal women with ER-positive disease, and for prostate cancer in men.
- Megestrol acetate is a progestin approved for the treatment of breast cancer.
- Medroxyprogesterone acetate is approved for the treatment of inoperable metastatic endometrial cancer.

- Cyclophosphamide (Cytoxan) and melphalan (Alkeran) are alkylating agents that are used to treat ovarian cancer. Cyclophosphamide is also used to treat breast cancer.
- A common ending for taxanes is -*taxel*.
- Taxanes are cytotoxic drugs that are naturally derived from the Western yew (paclitaxel) and the European yew (docetaxel) trees.
- Vinorelbine, vincristine, and vinblastine are vinca alkaloids. They are naturally derived from the periwinkle plant. A common beginning for vinca alkaloids is *vin*-.
- A common ending for anthracyclines is -*rubicin*.
- Doxorubicin, epirubicin, and idarubicin are anthracyclines.
- Doxorubicin and epirubicin are indicated for the treatment of breast cancer. Doxorubicin liposomal is approved for the treatment of ovarian cancer.
- The anthracyclines may turn urine and nails red, whereas mitoxantrone causes them to turn blue-green.
- Etoposide, irinotecan, and topotecan are topoisomerase inhibitors.
- Topotecan is indicated for the treatment of ovarian cancer, cervical cancer, and SCLC. Irinotecan is indicated only for the treatment of colorectal cancer.
- Platinum compounds have the common ending -*platin*.
- Cisplatin is approved for the treatment of testicular and ovarian cancer; carboplatin is approved for the treatment of ovarian cancer; and oxaliplatin is approved for the treatment of colorectal cancer.
- Capecitabine, cytarabine, gemcitabine, and 5-fluorouracil (5-FU) are fluoropyrimidines, which are also known as fluorinated pyrimidines.
- Antimetabolites are chemotherapeutic agents that work by inhibiting normal DNA synthesis.
- Bleomycin, dactinomycin, and mitomycin are antineoplastic agents approved for the treatment of various cancers. They interfere with DNA, RNA, and protein synthesis.
- Porfimer is used for the treatment of lung cancer. It produces its cytotoxic and antitumor effects only after exposure to light.
- Kinase inhibitors are used for the treatment of breast cancer, lung cancer, and melanoma. Two common endings for kinase inhibitors are -*ciclib* and -*tinib*.

Review Questions

1. All of the following are agents used in the treatment of breast cancer, EXCEPT _____.
   a. palbociclib (Ibrance)
   b. letrozole (Femara)
   c. gefitinib (Iressa)
   d. ribociclib (Kisqali)
2. Cancerous tumors that can invade and destroy nearby tissue and spread to other parts of the body are termed _____.
   a. benign
   b. malignant
   c. invasive
   d. tumors
3. Cancers are more prevalent in persons older than 65 years.
   a. true
   b. false

4. Cancer of the cervix is linked to the _____.
   a. herpes simplex virus (HSV)
   b. human immunodeficiency virus (HIV)
   c. varicella zoster virus (VZV)
   d. human papillomavirus (HPV)
5. Select the chemotherapeutic agent that must be stored in the refrigerator.
   a. Trametinib (Mekinist)
   b. Vemurafenib (Zalboraf)
   c. Palbociclib (Ibrance)
   d. Lapatinib (Tykerb)
6. Cancer may be treated with _____.
   a. chemotherapy
   b. immunotherapy
   c. radiation therapy
   d. all of the above

7. The warning label AVOID GRAPEFRUIT JUICE should be applied to each of the following chemotherapeutic agents, EXCEPT _____.
   a. toremifene (Fareston)
   b. abemaciclib (Verzenio)
   c. crizotinib (Xalkori)
   d. ribociclib (Kisqali)
8. Kinase inhibitors are used for the treatment of all of the following cancers, EXCEPT_____.
   a. prostate cancer
   b. lung cancer
   c. breast cancer
   d. skin cancer (melanoma)

9. Which one of the following is not a vinca alkaloid?
   a. Vinorelbine
   b. Vincristine
   c. Vinblastine
   d. Venlafaxine
10. _____ does NOT require the warning TAKE ON AN EMPTY STOMACH.
   a. Erlotinib (Tarceva)
   b. Capecitabine (Xeloda)
   c. Estramustine (Emcyt)
   d. Dabrafenib (Tarfinlar)

Bibliography

Canadian Cancer Statistics Advisory, in collaboration with the Canadian Cancer Society, Statistics Canada and the Public Health Agency of Canada. *Canadian Cancer Statistics: a 2022 special report on cancer prevalence.* 2022. Retrieved March 14, 2023, from. cancer.ca/canadian-cancer-statistics-2022-en.

Gombos A, Awada A. Advances in chemical pharmacotherapy to manage advanced breast cancer. *Expert Opin Pharmacother.* 2017;18(1):95–103.

Health Canada. *Drug Product Database.* 2022. Retrieved October 18, 2022, from. https://health-products.canada.ca/dpd-bdpp/index-eng.jsp.

Huang L, Jiang S, Shi Y. Tyrosine kinase inhibitors for solid tumors in the past 20 years (2001–2020). *J Hematol Oncol.* 2020;13:143.

Institute for Safe Medication Practices. *FDA and ISMP Lists of Look-Alike Drug Names with Recommended Tall Man Letters.* 2016Retrieved October 18, 2022, from. https://www.ismp.org/recommendations/tall-man-letters-list.

Institute for Safe Medication Practices. *List of Confused Drugs.* 2019Retrieved October 18, 2022, from. https://www.ismp.org/tools/confuseddrugnames.pdf.

Iwai Y, Hamanishi J, Chamoto K, et al. Cancer immunotherapies targeting the PD-1 signaling pathway. *J Biomed Sci.* 2017;24(26).

Jeon M, You D, Bae SY, et al. Dimerization of EGFR and HER2 induces breast cancer cell motility through STAT1-dependent ACTA2 induction. *Oncotarget.* 2017;8(31):50570–50581.

Jinga DC, Ciuleanu T, Negru S, et al. Effectiveness and safety profile of ipilimumab therapy in previously treated patients with unresectable or metastatic melanoma—the Romanian Patient Access Program. *J BUON.* 2017;22(5):1287–1295.

Kalant H, Grant D, Mitchell J. *Principles of medical pharmacology.* ed 7. Toronto: Elsevier Canada; 2007:777–790.

National Institutes of Health National Cancer Institute. Surveillance Epidemiology and End Results Program: Cancer statistics. *Cancer Stat Facts..* 2017Retrieved March 14, 2023, from. https://seer.cancer.gov/statfacts/.

National Institutes of Health Drugs Approved for Breast Cancer. *National Cancer Institute.* 2023Retrieved March 14, 2023, from. https://www.cancer.gov/about-cancer/treatment/drugs/breast.

National Institutes of Health Drugs Approved for Colon and Rectal Cancer. *National Cancer Institute.* 2023Retrieved March 14, 2023, from. https://www.cancer.gov/about-cancer/treatment/drugs/colorectal.

National Institutes of Health Drugs Approved for Endometrial Cancer. *National Cancer Institute.* 2021Retrieved March 14, 2023, from. https://www.cancer.gov/about-cancer/treatment/drugs/endometrial.

National Institutes of Health Drugs Approved for Lung Cancer. *National Cancer Institute.* 2023Retrieved March 14, 2023, from. https://www.cancer.gov/about-cancer/treatment/drugs/lung.

National Institutes of Health Drugs Approved for Prostate Cancer. *National Cancer Institute..* 2022Retrieved March 14, 2023, from. https://www.cancer.gov/about-cancer/treatment/drugs/prostate.

National Institutes of Health Drugs Approved for Skin Cancer. *National Cancer Institute..* 2022Retrieved March 14, 2023, from. https://www.cancer.gov/about-cancer/treatment/drugs/skin.

Page C, Curtis M, Sutter M, et al. *Integrated pharmacology.* Philadelphia: Elsevier Mosby; 2005:163–185.

Thibodeau G, Patton K. *Anatomy and physiology.* ed 6. St. Louis: Mosby; 2007:121–133.

U.S. Food and Drug Administration. (nd). Drugs@FDA: FDA Approved Drug Products. Retrieved October 18, 2022, from http://www.accessdata.fda.gov/scripts/cder/daf/.

Ventriglia J, Paciolla I, Pisano C, et al. Immunotherapy in ovarian, endometrial and cervical cancer: state of the art and future perspectives. *Cancer Treat Rev.* 2017;59:109–116.

Wellbrock C, Arozarena I. The complexity of the ERK/MAP-kinase pathway and the treatment of melanoma skin cancer. *Front Cell Dev Biol.* 2016;4(33).

32

Vaccines and Immunomodulators

LEARNING OBJECTIVES

1. Learn the terminology associated with vaccines and immunomodulators.
2. Describe types of vaccines and how they work.
3. Discuss the importance of the cold chain and identify vaccines requiring cold storage.
4. Provide examples of the pharmacy technician's role in maintaining the cold chain.
5. List procedures that must be followed if the cold chain is broken.
6. List and categorize immunomodulators and immunosuppressants.
7. Describe the mechanism of action for immunomodulators and immunosuppressants.
8. List common endings for selected vaccines and immunomodulators and immunosuppressants.
9. Identify warning labels and precautionary messages associated with select vaccines and immunomodulators and immunosuppressants.

KEY TERMS

Antigen Substance, usually a protein fragment, that causes an immune response.

Cold chain Set of safe handling practices ensuring that vaccines and immunologic agents requiring refrigeration are maintained at the required temperature from the time of manufacture until the time of administration to patients.

Conjugate vaccine Vaccine that links antigens or toxoids to the polysaccharide or sugar molecules that certain bacteria use as a protective device to disguise themselves.

Immunomodulator Agent that modifies the immune response or the functioning of the immune system.

Immunosuppressant Agent that inhibits a rapid increase of the cells of the immune system; also known as an immunopharmacologic agent.

Immunization Deliberate artificial exposure to disease to produce acquired immunity.

Inactivated killed vaccine Killed vaccine; provides less immunity than a live vaccine but has fewer risks for vaccine-induced disease.

Interferons Antiviral proteins that enhance T-cell recognition of antigens (interferon-γ) and produce immune system suppression (interferon-α, interferon-β).

Live attenuated vaccine Nonvirulent, live, weakened version of the invader that does not cause disease in nonimmunocompromised individuals.

Subunit vaccine Contains an isolated part of the bacterium or its coating.

Toxoid vaccine Vaccine that stimulates the immune system to produce antibodies to a specific toxin that causes illness.

Vaccine Substance that prevents disease by taking advantage of your body's ability to make antibodies and prime killer cells to fight disease.

Overview

An *immunization* is defined as a deliberate artificial exposure to disease to produce acquired immunity. Vaccines are administered to immunize individuals against disease. They prevent disease by taking advantage of your body's ability to make antibodies and prime killer cells to destroy disease-causing microbes and viruses. Under normal circumstances, cells of your immune system can distinguish between the cells that are part of your body, harmless bacteria normally found in your body, and harmful invaders that need to be destroyed. The first time that your body is exposed to a harmful virus or bacterium, the immune system releases macrophages, cytotoxic T cells, and B cells. The macrophages digest most parts of the virus or bacterium but not the *antigens*. B cells secrete antibodies to the antigens and if the person is exposed to the virus or bacteria again, the antibodies will inactivate the antigen. Cytotoxic T cells designed to destroy the virus or bacteria are also released on exposure to antigens. A *vaccine* is an altered antigen injected into your body that does not cause disease but stimulates your immune system's production of antibodies and cytotoxic T cells, providing protection against the disease if you are exposed to it again.

Types of Vaccines

- *Live attenuated vaccines* are a living, but weakened, version of the invader virus and do not cause disease in healthy individuals. However, they can mutate to a virulent strain of the virus. Measles, mumps, and rubella, chicken pox, shingles, influenza nasal spray, and rotavirus vaccines are live attenuated vaccines.

- *Inactivated killed vaccines* are advantageous because they cannot mutate; however, they produce less immunity compared with live vaccines. Booster shots are usually required to ensure continued immunity. Flu, hepatitis A, polio, and rabies vaccines are inactivated killed vaccines.
- *Toxoid vaccines* stimulate the immune system to produce antibodies to the toxins that cause illness (e.g., tetanus and diphtheria).
- *Subunit vaccines* contain an isolated part of the bacterium or its coating. The vaccines may be genetically engineered by inserting a virus protein or gene coding into another virus that when it replicates produces the vaccine. Hepatitis B and human papillomavirus vaccines are subunit vaccines.
- *Conjugate vaccines* link pieces of the bacterium or virus coating to a carrier protein or carbohydrate that allows the immune system to recognize and attack these disguised pathogens. *Haemophilus influenzae* type b (Hib) is a conjugate vaccine.

Special Handling Conditions for Vaccines

Cold Chain

Vaccines and immunologic agents requiring refrigeration must be protected from extremes in temperature. Exposure to freezing temperatures or heat can destroy their integrity and make them unusable.

The *cold chain* (Fig. 32.1) refers to a set of safe handling practices that ensure vaccines and immunologic agents requiring refrigeration are maintained at the required temperature from the time of manufacture until the time of administration to patients. This means that they must be maintained at a constant temperature from 2°C to 8°C (36°F to 46°F) throughout the transport process and placed in appropriate storage units once they are delivered to their final destination. Trained personnel, proper transportation and equipment, and efficient management procedures are key to effective maintenance of the cold chain.

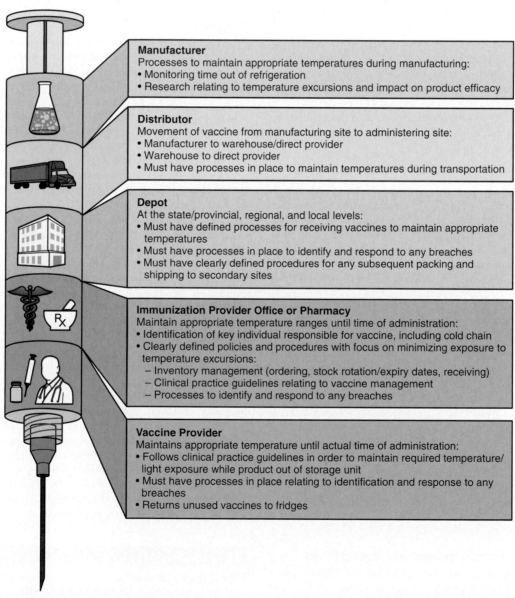

Manufacturer
Processes to maintain appropriate temperatures during manufacturing:
- Monitoring time out of refrigeration
- Research relating to temperature excursions and impact on product efficacy

Distributor
Movement of vaccine from manufacturing site to administering site:
- Manufacturer to warehouse/direct provider
- Warehouse to direct provider
- Must have processes in place to maintain temperatures during transportation

Depot
At the state/provincial, regional, and local levels:
- Must have defined processes for receiving vaccines to maintain appropriate temperatures
- Must have processes in place to identify and respond to any breaches
- Must have clearly defined procedures for any subsequent packing and shipping to secondary sites

Immunization Provider Office or Pharmacy
Maintain appropriate temperature ranges until time of administration:
- Identification of key individual responsible for vaccine, including cold chain
- Clearly defined policies and procedures with focus on minimizing exposure to temperature excursions:
  - Inventory management (ordering, stock rotation/expiry dates, receiving)
  - Clinical practice guidelines relating to vaccine management
  - Processes to identify and respond to any breaches

Vaccine Provider
Maintains appropriate temperature until actual time of administration:
- Follows clinical practice guidelines in order to maintain required temperature/light exposure while product out of storage unit
- Must have processes in place relating to identification and response to any breaches
- Returns unused vaccines to fridges

- **Fig. 32.1** The cold chain. (Adapted from Public Health Agency Canada Vaccine Storage Guidelines Task Group: National Vaccine Storage and Handling Guidelines for Immunization Providers – 2015, Ottawa, 2015, Canada.)

Why Cold Storage Is Important

Disruption of the cold chain is a public health threat. When the cold chain is disrupted, the effectiveness and shelf life of vaccines are reduced, and stability of the vaccine decreases exponentially with each increase in temperature. Once the integrity of the vaccine is compromised, it cannot be restored by returning the vaccine to the refrigerator. Loss of potency and effectiveness is cumulative, so each time the cold chain is breached, the vaccine's effectiveness is further reduced. Ultimately, patients are placed at risk when suboptimal vaccines are administered. In addition to vaccine failure, patients may experience increased reactions at the injection site. Disruption of the cold chain is also costly. Vaccines that expire or that have been stored improperly must be destroyed.

The severity of problems linked to disruption of the cold chain is dependent on whether the vaccine is chemical or biologic and whether the dosage form is an aqueous solution, suspension, or dry powder. Dry powders and chemicals are the least affected by breaches in the cold chain. Vaccines and other biologic solutions and suspensions are most sensitive to breaches in the cold chain. They are more sensitive to degradation.

Cold Chain Maintenance and Safety

The cold chain starts with storing the vaccines in a cold storage unit at the manufacturing plant. Maintenance of the cold chain involves appropriate selection and maintenance of refrigeration units and transport containers capable of storing drug products at required temperatures. Real-time tracking of shipments (including temperature monitoring) is used with technology that alerts providers if interventions are required to keep shipments safe until delivery.

Refrigeration Units

Once a vaccine is received, the pharmacy should place it in a refrigerator designated solely for vaccines. If a separate refrigerator is not feasible, vaccines should be kept separate from other refrigerated pharmaceutical agents. Pharmacies that handle a large volume of vaccines should purchase a walk-in refrigeration unit. If the refrigerator is overstocked, air circulation is insufficient to maintain constant temperatures. The refrigeration unit should be equipped with a continuous temperature-recording device and a minimum-maximum thermometer to monitor temperature fluctuations. An alarm that signals when the refrigeration unit is out of range should be installed in the refrigerator. Monitors and thermometers should be calibrated routinely. It is important to place the refrigerator in a location away from a heat source because this can affect the performance of the unit.

Protocols for Receiving, Stocking, and Storing Drugs

An important component of the cold chain is establishment and adherence to protocols for receiving, stocking, storing, and transporting drugs requiring refrigeration. The pharmacy team should develop these protocols in accordance with national guidelines. Protocols for receiving vaccines should include

accurate assessment of the condition of vaccines received by the pharmacy. Pharmacy personnel should be alert for warning signs that the cold chain has been broken during shipment. This might be as simple as noticing that freezer packs have thawed or that the dry ice placed in the transport container with a vaccine has evaporated. Unfortunately, exposure to heat or freezing that results in damage to the vaccine is not easy to detect because no changes in color or appearance occur. There are no visual indicators. Shaking the vaccine may reveal clumps in the vaccine that indicate freezing; however, often no clumps are visible, making this method unreliable.

A procedure should be established to ensure that stocked vaccines are rotated to avoid wastage caused by outdated supplies. Expiry dates should be checked and vaccines stocked so that those that expire soon are placed in front of vaccines that expire later. Vaccines should not be removed from the refrigerator until the time of dispensing unless the vaccine must be transported. This is especially important for pneumococcal or influenza vaccines that are purchased in multidose vials.

Transport

Pharmacy personnel in charge of transporting vaccines are responsible for making sure that vaccines arrive at their destination at the proper temperature. How long the vaccine will be out of the refrigerator must be considered when determining the type of transport container. In most cases, vaccines should be transported in an insulated container. Protocols should be followed regarding the number of ice packs needed. Vaccines should always be positioned to avoid direct contact with the ice packs. Heat and cold monitors should be placed in the transport container, if necessary.

Vaccines should be dispensed to patients with accurate advice for transport and storage. Extremes in heat and cold must be avoided; never place vaccines in the hot glove compartment of a car. If the travel time between the pharmacy and the patient's destination, where a refrigerator is located, is less than 20 minutes, dispense the vaccine in an insulated bag. If transport time is longer than 20 minutes, the vaccine should be transported with ice packs in an insulated container. See Fig. 32.2 for a diagram explaining the importance of the pharmacy technician in cold chain management.

Immunizations

Vaccines are administered to provide immunity to a wide variety of childhood diseases, as well as influenza, hepatitis, pneumonia, COVID-19, viral meningitis, rabies, and other conditions. Sufficient immunity may be achieved after a single immunization; however, many vaccines must be administered as a series or require a booster shot. Epidemiologists track flu infections from sentinel sites around the globe to determine which strains of the flu virus are most virulent. Vaccines are developed for the most infectious strains of the virus. Flu vaccines must be reformulated each year. See Fig. 32.3 for age-specific immunization schedules recommended by the Centers for Disease Control and Prevention (CDC).

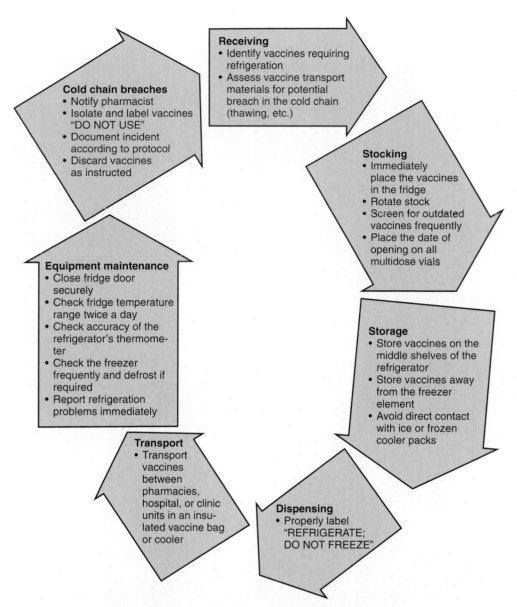

• **Fig. 32.2** Pharmacy technician's role in maintaining the cold chain.

COVID-19 Vaccine

In 2019, SARS-CoV-2 (which causes COVID-19), a previously unknown virus, was discovered. The deadly virus infected more than 676 million people globally and led to nearly 7 million deaths. As of 2023, more than 4.6 million Covid-19 infections and nearly 52 thousand deaths were reported in Canada. More than 100 million cases of COVID-19 were reported in the United States and more than 1.1 million people died of COVID-19. Untold numbers are living with debilitating long COVID symptoms. Long COVID is a syndrome that causes fatigue, shortness of breath, chest pain, trouble speaking, anxiety or depression, muscle aches, fever, loss of smell, loss of taste, and more. Measures to prevent COVID-19 infection are vaccination, wearing medical grade face masks (e.g., N-95 or KN-95), and handwashing. Four types of vaccines are approved for the prevention of COVID-19 infection. They are messenger RNA (mRNA) vaccines, viral vector-based vaccines, protein subunit vaccines, and plant-based vaccines.

Messenger RNA Vaccines

mRNA vaccines (Comiraty, Spikevax) provide instructions to the cells to make the SARS-CoV-2 spike protein to trigger an immune response. The instructions are then destroyed. Bivalent mRNA vaccines provide greater protection against COVID-19 because they target two strains of the virus.

Viral Vector-Based Vaccines

Viral vector-based vaccines (Vaxzevria, Jcovden) are a modified common cold adenovirus. The adenovirus is modified to produce the SARS-CoV-2 spike protein when injected in the body. This results in an immune response in which the body creates antibodies against the spike protein and the adenovirus is eliminated.

Protein Subunit Vaccines

Nuvaxovid is a protein subunit vaccine. It contains 5 mcg of SARS-CoV-2 spike protein (original strain) with 50 mcg of Matrix-M adjuvant to boost the effectiveness.

Plant-Based Vaccines

Covifenz is created from plant leaves in which SARS-CoV-2 genetic code has been inserted by a nonpathogenic bacterium.

Figure 1. Recommended Immunization Schedule for Children and Adolescents Aged 18 Years or Younger—United States, 2018.

(FOR THOSE WHO FALL BEHIND OR START LATE, SEE THE CATCH-UP SCHEDULE [FIGURE 2]).

These recommendations must be read with the footnotes that follow. For those who fall behind or start late, provide catch-up vaccination at the earliest opportunity as indicated by the green bars in Figure 1. To determine minimum intervals between doses, see the catch-up schedule (Figure 2). School entry and adolescent vaccine age groups are shaded in gray.

Vaccine	Birth	1 mo	2 mos	4 mos	6 mos	9 mos	12 mos	15 mos	18 mos	19–23 mos	2–3 yrs	4–6 yrs	7–10 yrs	11–12 yrs	13–15 yrs	16 yrs	17–18 yrs
Hepatitis B¹ (HepB)	1st dose	◄── 2nd dose ──►			◄──────── 3rd dose ────────►												
Rotavirus² (RV) RV1 (2-dose series); RV5 (3-dose series)			1st dose	2nd dose	See footnote 2												
Diphtheria, tetanus, & acellular pertussis³ (DTaP: <7 yrs)			1st dose	2nd dose	3rd dose		◄─── 4th dose ───►					5th dose					
Haemophilus influenzae type b⁴ (Hib)			1st dose	2nd dose	See footnote 4		◄─ 3rd or 4th dose, See footnote 4 ─►										
Pneumococcal conjugate⁵ (PCV13)			1st dose	2nd dose	3rd dose		◄─── 4th dose ───►										
Inactivated poliovirus⁶ (IPV: <18 yrs)			1st dose	2nd dose	◄──────── 3rd dose ────────►							4th dose					
Influenza⁷ (IIV)						Annual vaccination (IIV) 1 or 2 doses								Annual vaccination (IIV) 1 dose only			
Measles, mumps, rubella⁸ (MMR)							◄─ 1st dose ─►					2nd dose					
Varicella⁹ (VAR)							◄─ 1st dose ─►					2nd dose					
Hepatitis A¹⁰ (HepA)							◄─ 2-dose series, See footnote 10 ─►										
Meningococcal¹¹ (MenACWY-D ≥9 mos; MenACWY-CRM ≥2 mos)					See footnote 11									1st dose		2nd dose	
Tetanus, diphtheria, & acellular pertussis³ (Tdap: ≥7 yrs)														Tdap			
Human papillomavirus¹⁴ (HPV)													See footnote 14				
Meningococcal B¹²														See footnote 12			
Pneumococcal polysaccharide⁵ (PPSV23)												See footnote 5					

Range of recommended ages for all children | Range of recommended ages for catch-up immunization | Range of recommended ages for certain high-risk groups | Range of recommended ages for non-high-risk groups that may receive vaccine, subject to individual clinical decision making | No recommendation

For complete information go to https://www.cdc.gov/vaccines/schedules/downloads/child/0-18yrs-child-combined-schedule.pdf.

• **Fig. 32.3** Recommended immunization schedule for children and adolescents aged 18 years or younger, United States, 2023. (From US Department of Health and Human Services, Centers for Disease Control and Prevention (CDC), available at https://www.cdc.gov/vaccines/schedules/downloads/child/0-18yrs-child-combined-schedule.pdf.)

Selected Vaccines, Dosage Forms, and Strength

Generic Name	US Brand Name(s) / Canadian Brand Name(s)	Dosage Forms (Pediatric/Adult Use)	Storage
diphtheria and tetanus toxoids (Td)	TD Vax, Tenivac / TD Adsorbed	**Suspension, for injection** (children 6 weeks to 6 years)	Refrigerate 2°C–8°C (35°F–46°F)
diphtheria + tetanus toxoids + acellular pertussis (DTaP)	Adacel, Boostrix, Daptacel, Infanrix / Adacel, Boostrix	**Suspension, for Intramuscular injection:** Daptacel (children 6 weeks to 6 years); Infanrix (children 6 weeks to 7 years) **Suspension, for injection:** Adacel, Boostrix (booster for individuals 10 years and older)	Refrigerate 2°C–8°C (35°F–46°F)
diphtheria + tetanus toxoid + acellular pertussis + inactivated polio vaccine	Quadracel, Kinrix / Adacel-Polio, Boostrix-Polio	**Suspension, for Intramuscular injection:** Adacel-Polio, Boostrix-Polio, Quadracel (booster for individuals 4 years and older); Kinrix (children 4–6 years)	Refrigerate 2°C–8°C (35°F–46°F)
diphtheria toxoid + tetanus toxoid + acellular pertussis + *Haemophilus influenzae* B conjugate + poliovirus vaccine	Pentacel / Pediacel	**Suspension, for Intramuscular injection:** Pentacel (children 6 weeks to 4 years); Pediacel (2 months to 6 years)	Refrigerate 2°C–8°C (35°F–46°F)
diphtheria toxoid + tetanus toxoid + acellular pertussis + hepatitis B surface antigen + inactivated poliovirus vaccine	Pediarix / Infanrix-Hexa	**Suspension, for Intramuscular injection** (children 6 weeks to 6 years)	Refrigerate 2°C–8°C (35°F–46°F)
tetanus immune globulin	Not available / Hypertet	**Solution, for injection** Adults	Refrigerate 2°C–8°C (35°F–46°F)
Haemophilus influenzae b (Hib) conjugate vaccine (meningococcal protein)	PedvaxHIB / Not available	**Liquid, for intramuscular injection** (children 2–71 months)	Refrigerate 2°C–8°C (35°F–46°F)
Haemophilus influenzae b (Hib) conjugate vaccine (tetanus protein)	ActHIB, Hiberix / ActHIB, Hiberix	**Powder, for Intramuscular injection solution:** (children 2 months to 5 years)	Refrigerate 2°C–8°C (35°F–46°F)
inactivated polio vaccine	Ipol, Poliovax / Imovax Polio	**Suspension, for injection:** trivalent, inactivated (children 2 months to adult)	Refrigerate 2°C–8°C (35°F–46°F)
measles, mumps, and rubella (MMR) vaccine	M-M-R II, Priorix / M-M-R II, Priorix	**Powder, for injection solution:** (12 months and older)	Keep frozen until use; store at −50°C to +8°C—M-M-R II Refrigerate 2°C–8°C (35°F–46°F)—Priorix
measles, mumps, and rubella (MMR) vaccine + varicella zoster	ProQuad / Priorix-Tetra, ProQuad	**Powder, for injection solution:** Priorix-Tetra (children 9 months to 12 years); ProQuad (children 12 months to 12 years)	Refrigerate 2°C–8°C (35°F–46°F)—Priorix-Tetra Keep frozen until use; store at −0°C to +8°C—ProQuad
hepatitis A vaccine (inactivated)	Havrix, VAQTA / Avaxim, Havrix, Havrix Jr., VAQTA	**Suspension, for Intramuscular injection:** Avaxim (individuals 12 years and older); Havrix (19 years and older); Havrix Jr. (children 12 months to 18 years)	Refrigerate 2°C–8°C (35°F–46°F)
hepatitis B vaccine surface antigen, recombinant	Energix-B, Prehevbrio, Recombivax HB / Energix-B, Recombivax HB, Recombivax HB (Dialysis)	**Suspension, for Intramuscular injection:** Energix-B, Recombivax HB (all ages); Recombivax HB (Dialysis) (adults only); Prehevbrio (adults 18+ years)	Refrigerate 2°C–8°C (35°F–46°F)
hepatitis B immunoglobulin	Hepagam B, Nabi-B / Hepagam B, Hyperhep B, Hyperhep B S/D	**Solution, for injection** (newborn and older)	Refrigerate 2°C–8°C (35°F–46°F)

Continued

Selected Vaccines, Dosage Forms, and Strength—cont'd

Generic Name	US Brand Name(s) / Canadian Brand Name(s)	Dosage Forms (Pediatric/Adult Use)	Storage
hepatitis A vaccine + hepatitis B vaccine	Twinrix Twinrix, Twinrix Jr.	**Suspension, for Intramuscular injection:** (all ages)	Refrigerate 2°C–8°C (35°F–46°F)
influenza vaccine, adjuvanted (formulated annually for selected strains each flu season)	Audenz, Fluad, Fluad Quadrivalent Fluad, Fluad Pediatric	**Suspension, for IM injection:** (individuals 6 months and older)	Refrigerate 2°C–8°C (35°F–46°F)
influenza, trivalent type A and B and quadrivalent type A and type B	Afluria, Agriflu, FluLaval, FluMist, Fluarix, Fluvirin, Fluzone, Fluzone High Dose, Fluzone Intradermal Quadrivalent, Flucelvax, Flublok, Flubok Quadrivalent, Flurix Quadrivalent, Fluzone Quadrivalent Afluria Tetra, FluLaval Tetra, Flumist, Fluzone Quadrivalent, Fluzone High Dose Quadrivalent	**Solution, nasal:** Flumist (individuals 2–59 years), Fluzone High Dose (65 years and older) **Suspension, for intradermal injection:** Fluzone Intradermal (individuals 18–64 years)	
meningococcal (groups A/C/Y/W-135) oligosaccharide conjugate vaccine	Menveo Menveo	**Powder, for Intramuscular injection:** (individuals 2 months to 55 years)	Refrigerate 2°C–8°C (35°F–46°F)
meningococcal (groups A/C/Y/W-135) polysaccharide tetanus toxoid conjugate vaccine	Menomune Nimenrix	**Powder, for IM injection:** Nimenrix (individuals 12 months to 55 years); Menomune (older than 2 years)	Refrigerate 2°C–8°C (35°F–46°F)
meningococcal (groups A/C/Y/W-135) polysaccharide diphtheria toxoid conjugate vaccine	Menactra Menactra	**Solution, for Intramuscular injection:** (individuals 9 months to 55 years)	Refrigerate 2°C–8°C (35°F–46°F)
meningococcal group B conjugate vaccine	Bexsero, Trumenba Trumenba	**Suspension, for Intramuscular injectioin:** (individuals 10–25 years)	Refrigerate 2°C–8°C (35°F–46°F)
meningococcal group C conjugate vaccine	Not available Menjugate, NeisVac-C	**Suspension, for Intramuscular injection:** (children 2 months old to adult)	Refrigerate 2°C–8°C (35°F–46°F)
pneumococcal polysaccharide 13-polyvalent vaccine	Prevnar 13 Prevnar 13, Prevnar 20	**Suspension, for Intramuscular injection:** (individuals 6 weeks and older)	Refrigerate 2°C–8°C (35°F–46°F)
pneumococcal polysaccharide 15-polyvalent vaccine	Vaxneuvance Vaxneuvance	**Suspension, for IM injection:** (Children 7 months to 17 years; 18 years and older):	Refrigerate 2°C–8°C (36°F to 46°F). Protect from light.
pneumococcal polysaccharide 23-polyvalent vaccine	Pneumovax 23 Pneumovax 23	**Solution, for Intramuscular or subutaneously injection:** (individuals 2 years and older)	Refrigerate 2°C–8°C (35°F–46°F)
rabies vaccine	Imovax rabies, RabAvert Imovax rabies, RabAvert	**Powder, for Intramuscular injection:** Imovax rabies (adults); RabAvert (all ages)	Refrigerate 2°C–8°C (35°F–46°F)
rotavirus	RotaTeq, Rotarix RotaTeq, Rotarix	**Solution, oral:** RotaTeq (children 6–32 weeks old); Rotarix (children 6–24 weeks old)	Refrigerate 2°C–8°C (35°F–46°F)
varicella vaccine (live)	Varivax Varivax III, Varilrix,	**Powder, for Subcutaneous injection:** Varivax III, Varilrix (individuals 12 months and older)	Keep frozen until use; store at −50°C to +8°C—Varivax Ship frozen; then refrigerate at 2°C–8°C (35°F–46°F)—Varivax III

Selected Vaccines, Dosage Forms, and Strength—cont'd

Generic Name	US Brand Name(s) / Canadian Brand Name(s)	Dosage Forms (Pediatric/Adult Use)	Storage
zoster vaccine, live	Zostavax / Not available	**Powder, for Subcutaneous injection:** (individuals 50 years and older)	Keep frozen before reconstitution at −50°C to −15°C (−58°F to +5°F); protect from light
zoster, adjuvanted	Shingrix / Shingrix	**Powder, for Intramuscular injection plus adjuvant:** (Individuals 50 years and older [18 years and older if at increased risk for herpes zoster infection due to immunodeficiency or immunosuppression]).	Refrigerate at 2°C–8°C (35°F–46°F); protect from light
COVID-19 vaccine	Comirnaty, Spikevax / Comirnaty, Spikevax, Vaxzevria, Jcovden, Nuvaxovid, Covifenz	**Primary dose only**[a]: Comirnaty (6 months and older); Comirnaty, bivalent (BA.4/5) (5 years and older); Spikevax (6 months and older); Intramuscular injection Spikevax, bivalent (BA.1) (6 years and older); Spikevax, bivalent (BA.4/5) (18 years and older); Vaxzevria (18 years and older); Jcovden (18 years and older); Nuvaxovid (12 years and older); Covifenz (ages 18–64 years)	Keep frozen until use at −50°C to −15°C (−58°F to +5°F)
human papillomavirus	Gardasil, Gardasil 9, Cervarix / Gardiasil 9, Cervarix	**Suspension, for Intramuscular injection:** (individuals 9–26 years old)	Refrigerate 2°C–8°C (35°F–46°F)
mpox/smallpox	Jynneos / Imvamune	**Suspension, for Subcutaneous injection:** (adults 18 years and older)	Keep frozen until use at −25°C to −15°C (−13°F to +5°F)

[a]Approved ages for administration of COVID-19 vaccine booster doses vary.

A protein virus-like particle (VLP) is produced by the plants' natural metabolic processes. The body responds to the VLP like the COVID-19 spike protein and mounts an immune response.

Adverse Reactions

Common side effects of COVID-19 vaccines and boosters are redness, soreness, and swelling at the injection site. Systemic side effects are headache, muscle or joint aches, fever, fatigue, and nausea.

Mpox

Mpox, formerly called monkeypox, is a viral infection similar to smallpox. It produces lesions on the skin, genitals, mouth, and perianal area, along with fever and swollen lymph nodes. Individuals who have mpox are contagious until the scabs on the lesions fall off and the lesions have healed. The smallpox vaccine (Imvamune, Jynneos) is administered to prevent infection and to reduce risk for infection postexposure.

Imvamune and Jynneos are classified as a modified vaccinia Ankara (MVA) vaccine. The live virus vaccine is modified so that it cannot replicate. Once administered, the body creates antibodies to the virus. Maximum protection is achieved 14 days after vaccination. The vaccine is authorized for use in adults 18 years and older. The MVA vaccine is a live attenuated vaccine and must be stored frozen.

Adverse Reactions

Common side effects of Imvamune and Jynneos are pain, redness, swelling, and itching at the injection site. Systemic side effects are headache, muscle or joint aches, fever, fatigue, chills, and nausea.

Immunomodulators and Immunosuppressants

Drugs that primarily act on cells of the immune system are called immunomodulators. An *immunomodulator* is an agent that modifies the immune response or the functioning of the immune system. Vaccines, corticosteroids (e.g., prednisone), antimetabolites (e.g., mycophenolate mofetil), calcineurin inhibitors (e.g., cyclosporine and tacrolimus), mTOR kinase inhibitors (e.g., everolimus and sirolimus), monoclonal antibodies (e.g., basiliximab and belatacept), and interferons and immunoglobulins (e.g., antithymocyte globulin [ATG], intravenous immunoglobulin [IVIG], and Rh_o(D) immune globulin) are all categorized as immunopharmacologic agents. They are used for the treatment of inflammatory autoimmune diseases, such as multiple sclerosis (see Chapter 12), rheumatoid arthritis, systemic lupus erythematosus (see Chapter 13), and Crohn's disease (see Chapter 22), as well as to prevent organ transplant (liver, heart, or kidney) rejection and treat specific cancers (Chapter 31). Immunomodulators that suppress, or reduce, the strength of the body's immune system and inhibit the rapid increase and spread (proliferation) of cells of the immune system are called *immunosuppressants*. Their actions may be cell specific or nonspecific.

Calcineurin Inhibitors

Cyclosporine, pimecrolimus, and tacrolimus are classified as calcineurin inhibitors. Cyclosporine is produced by a fungus (*Tolypocladium inflatum*) and is used to improve survival rates for individuals with organ transplants. It suppresses cell destruction in graft-versus-host reactions. Cyclosporine ophthalmic solution is used to treat chronic dry eye syndrome.

Tacrolimus and pimecrolimus are immunosuppressants. Tacrolimus is derived from a fungus (*Streptomyces tsukubaensis*). Like cyclosporine, tacrolimus is prescribed to prevent transplant rejection. Tacrolimus ointment and pimecrolimus cream are used for the treatment of mild to moderate chronic atopic dermatitis (see Chapter 36).

Mechanism of Action and Pharmacokinetics

T cells are important to the immune response. Cyclosporine reduces cellular responsiveness to inflammatory stimuli by inhibiting T-lymphocyte cell activation and suppressing interferon gamma (IFN-γ). Cyclosporine is formulated as capsules, modified and nonmodified oral solutions, and solution for injection. Cyclosporine-modified solution has greater absorption than capsules. Cyclosporine inhibits cytochrome P-450 microsomal pathways, which are responsible for several drug-drug interactions.

Tacrolimus and pimecrolimus inhibit the first phase of T-cell activation and proliferation. Pimecrolimus inhibits T-cell activation by blocking transcription of early cytokines and inhibits **interferons** and interleukins that are mediators of the inflammatory response. The exact mechanism of action for pimecrolimus effects on atopic dermatitis is unknown. Tacrolimus is more potent than cyclosporine.

Adverse Reactions

Adverse reactions of cyclosporine include acne, bleeding or tender gums, overgrowth of gum tissue, diarrhea, hirsutism, headache, leg cramps, anorexia, nausea and vomiting, and tremors. More serious adverse reactions are nephrotoxicity, neurotoxicity, and seizures. Because cyclosporine is an immunosuppressant, it can increase risk for infections. Tacrolimus may increase the risk for bacterial, fungal, protozoal, and viral infections (e.g., thrush, urinary tract infection, and upper respiratory infections). It may also produce gastrointestinal adverse reactions such as diarrhea or constipation, loss of appetite, nausea, and vomiting. Other common side effects are headache and visual disturbances. The most common side effects of tacrolimus ointment and pimecrolimus cream are burning, itching, and skin infections.

> **❶ *Tech Alert!***
>
> Cyclosporine, oral liquid nonmodified (Sandimmune), is not substitutable for cyclosporine, oral liquid modified (Neoral, Gengraf).

mTOR Kinase Inhibitors

Everolimus and sirolimus are mTOR kinase inhibitors that are used to prevent organ rejection in kidney transplant patients. Temsirolimus is indicated for the treatment of metastatic cancer of the kidneys.

Mechanism of Action and Pharmacokinetics

Sirolimus is the active metabolite of the immunosuppressant temsirolimus. Sirolimus and everolimus interfere with the second phase of T-cell activation and proliferation. Sirolimus also decreases the levels of immunoglobulins IgM, IgG, and IgA. Everolimus inhibits activation and proliferation of B lymphocytes in addition to T cells. Eating fatty foods can reduce the absorption of tacrolimus and sirolimus.

Calcineurin Inhibitors

Generic Name	US Brand Name(s) / Canadian Brand Name(s)	Dosage Forms and Strengths
cyclosporine[a] (cyclosporin)	Cequa, Gengraf, Neoral, Restasis, Sandimmune, Verkazia	**Capsule (Sandimmune):** 25 mg, 50 mg, 100 mg
		Capsule, modified (Gengraf, Neoral): 10 mg[b], 25 mg, 50 mg[b], 100 mg
	Neoral, Restasis, Sandimmune	**Solution, for injection (Sandimmune):** 50 mg/mL
		Solution, oral (Sandimmune): 100 mg/mL
		Solution, modified, oral (Gengraf, Neoral): 100 mg/mL
		Ophthalmic: 0.05% (Restasis), 0.09% (Cequa), 0.1% (Verkazia)
pimecrolimus[a,c]	Elidel	**Cream:** 1%
	Elidel	
tacrolimus[a]	Astagraf XL, Envarsus XR, Prograf, Protopic	**Capsule (Prograf):** 0.5 mg, 1 mg, 5 mg
		Capsule, extended release (Advagraf, Astagraf XL): 0.5 mg, 1 mg, 3 mg[b], 5 mg
	Advagraf, Envarsus PA, Prograf, Protopic	**Intravenous solution (Prograf):** 5 mg/mL
		Ointment (Protopic): 0.03%, 0.1%
		Powder, for oral suspension (Prograf)[c]: 0.2 mg/packet, 1 mg/packet
		Tablet, extended release (Envarsus PA, Envarsus XR): 0.75 mg, 1 mg, 4 mg

[a]Generic available.
[b]Available in Canada only.
[c]Available in the United States only.

Adverse Reactions

Everolimus and sirolimus may increase the risk for bacterial, fungal, protozoal, and viral infections (e.g., thrush, urinary tract infection, or pneumonia) and produce gastrointestinal adverse reactions, such as diarrhea or constipation, nausea, and vomiting. Other side effects are mouth ulcers and stomatitis, insomnia, dizziness or drowsiness, hair loss or unusual hair growth, headache, mood changes, depression, confusion, and tremor. More serious adverse reactions include seizures, hepatitis, and hemolytic anemia.

---

❶ Tech Alert!

Sirolimus tablets and oral solution are not bioequivalent and thus are not substitutable.

---

mTOR Kinase Inhibitors

Generic Name	US Brand Name(s) / Canadian Brand Name(s)	Dosage Forms and Strengths
everolimus[a]	Afinitor, Afinitor Disperz, Zortress Afinitor, Afinitor Disperz	**Tablet:** 0.25 mg, 0.5 mg, 0.75 mg, 1 mg (Zortress)[b]; 2.5 mg, 5 mg, 7.5 mg[b], 10 mg (Afinitor) **Tablet, for suspension (Afinitor Disperz):** 2 mg, 3 mg, 5 mg
sirolimus[a]	Rapamune Rapamune	**Solution, oral:** 1 mg/mL **Tablet:** 0.5 mg[b], 1 mg, 2 mg[b]
temsirolimus[a]	Torisel Torisel	**Solution, for intravenous injection:** 25 mg/mL

[a]Generic available.
[b]Available in the United States only.

Antimetabolites

Azathioprine, mycophenolate mofetil, and mycophenolic acid are antimetabolites that are used in conjunction with corticosteroids and cyclosporine to decrease the rejection of transplanted organs.

Mechanism of Action and Pharmacokinetics

Mycophenolate mofetil is a prodrug that is metabolized to mycophenolic acid. Mycophenolic acid is an immunosuppressive agent that inhibits the enzyme required for the synthesis of purines. Purines are needed for T-cell and B-cell proliferation. Azathioprine interferes with purine metabolism, inhibiting the synthesis of cell building blocks DNA and RNA. Azathioprine is most commonly used for long-term immunosuppression rather than acute rejection episodes.

Adverse Reactions

Gastrointestinal side effects are common and include constipation, diarrhea or soft stools, gas, loss of appetite, nausea, vomiting, stomach pain, or indigestion. Mycophenolate mofetil, like other immunosuppressives, can increase the risk of bacterial and viral infections. Other serious adverse effects are leukopenia, infections, lymphoma, and other malignancies.

Antimetabolites

Generic Name	US Brand Name(s) / Canadian Brand Name(s)	Dosage Forms and Strengths
azathioprine[a]	Azasan, Imuran Imuran	**Powder, for injection**[b]: 100 mg/vial **Tablet:** 25 mg[b], 50 mg, 75 mg[b], 100 mg[b]
mycophenolate mofetil[a], mycophenolic acid[a,c]	CellCept CellCept, Myfortic	**Capsule:** 250 mg **Powder, for injection:** 500 mg/vial **Powder, for oral suspension:** 200 mg/mL **Tablet:** 500 mg **Tablet, delayed release (Myfortic):** 180 mg, 360 mg

[a]Generic available.
[b]Available in the United States only.
[c]Available in Canada only.

Monovclonal Antibodies

Monoclonal antibody immunomodulators are used for the treatment of COVID-19 (casirivimab + imdevimab, tocilizumab), numerous autoimmune and immune system disorders, such as multiple sclerosis (daclizumab and natalizumab), rheumatoid arthritis (adalimumab), and Crohn's disease (infliximab), and specific cancers. Basiliximab is used to reduce transplant rejections and prolong the life of transplanted organs. Sotrovimab and bebtelovimab are no longer authorized for emergency use in treating COVID-19 viral infection in the United States because of lack of effectiveness against currently circulating strains of the virus. Additional monoclonal antibody immunomodulators are described in Chapters 13, 14, 22, 31, and 36.

● Tech Note!

A common ending for monoclonal antibody immunomodulators is -mab.

Mechanism of Action

Monoclonal antibodies act on B cells, T cells, and surface proteins important to the immune system, specifically leukocyte surface antigens, including CD3, CD4 (T helper cells), and T-cell activation markers (IL-2, IL-6, CD20, and CD25).

Adverse Reactions

Monoclonal antibodies may increase susceptibility to opportunistic infections, reactivation of dormant infections (e.g., tuberculosis), or worsening of existing infection. Other common side effects are itching at the site of infusion, nausea, and stomach pain.

Monoclonal Antibody Immuno-modulators*

Generic Name	US Brand Name(s) / Canadian Brand Name(s)	Dosage Forms and Strengths
adalimumab	Humira	See Chapter 22
	Humira	
basiliximab	Simulect	**Powder, for injection:** 10 mg/vial[a], 20 mg/vial
	Simulect	
certolizumab	Cimzia	See Chapter 22
	Cimzia	
daclizumab	Zinbryta	**Solution, injection:** 150 mg/mL
	Not available	
golimumab	Simponi	See Chapter 22
	Simponi	
infliximab	Remicade	See Chapter 22
	Remicade	
natalizumab	Tysabri	See Chapter 22
	Tysabri	
rituximab	Rituxan	See Chapter 13
	Rituxan, Rituxan SC	
tocilizumab	Actemra	**Solution, for intravenous use:** 80 mg/4 mL. See also Chapter 13
	Actemra	
casirivimab + imdevimab	Regen-COV[b]	**Solution, for intravenous infusion:** 1332 mg/11.1 mL casirivimab + 1332 mg imdevimab/11.1 mL
	Generic	
cilgavimab + tixagevimab	Evusheld[b]	**Solution, for intravenous infusion:** 150 mg/1.5 mL cilgavimab + 150 mg/1.5 mL tixagevimab
	Evusheld	

[a]Strength available in the United States only.
[b]Currently not authorized for treatment of COVID-19 in the United States.
*See Chapter 31 for monoclonal antibody immunomodulators used to treat specific cancers.

Interferons

There are approximately 2000 interferon (IFN) receptors on each normal and malignant cell. These receptors recognize and bind interferons (proteins with antigenic properties). IFN-α2b is used to treat hepatitis B and C. It is also used to treat cancers such as multiple myeloma and chronic myelogenous leukemia. IFN-β1a and IFN-β1b are first-line therapies for the treatment of multiple sclerosis. They alter the actions of T cells, B cells, and other cytokines that produce immune response and inflammation. They reduce the development of the brain lesions that cause disability in

Interferons

Generic Name	US Brand Name(s) / Canadian Brand(s)	Dosage Forms and Strengths
interferon-α2b	Intron A	**Powder, for injection:** 10 million units/vial, 18 million units/vial, 25 million units/vial
	Not available	
interferon-β1a	Avonex, Rebif	**Injection, powder for reconstitution (Avonex): Solution, for injection (Avonex):** 30 mcg/0.5 mL **Solution, for injection (Rebif):** 22 mcg, 44 mcg, 66 mcg[a] (0.2, 0.5, and 1.5 mL prefilled syringe)
	Avonex, Rebif	
interferon-β1b	Betaseron, Extavia	**Injection, powder for reconstitution:** 0.3 mg/vial
	Betaseron	

[a]Available in Canada only.

people who have multiple sclerosis. Adverse reactions of IFN-β1a and IFN-β1b include flulike symptoms, headache, fatigue, weight loss, anorexia, and neutropenia.

Immunoglobulins

ATG, IVIG, and Rho(D) immune globulin are immunoglobulins. ATG is primarily administered to reduce the rejection associated with organ and bone marrow transplantation. Rho(D) immune globulin is administered to pregnant women who are Rh negative and have been exposed to blood that is Rh positive. This may occur through exposure to fetal blood, amniocentesis, ectopic pregnancy, abdominal trauma during pregnancy, or whole blood transfusions. When an Rh incompatibility exists between the pregnant woman and fetus, maternal antibodies are produced that act against the fetal red blood cells, causing erythroblastosis fetalis, a severe hemolytic disease of the fetus. Anti-D, administered within 72 hours of delivery, can prevent erythroblastosis fetalis in a subsequent pregnancy. Rho(D) is also used in the treatment of idiopathic thrombocytopenic purpura (ITP), a condition that causes excessive bruising or bleeding. IVIG is used for the treatment of a variety of infections and chronic lymphatic leukemia.

Mechanism of Action and Pharmacokinetics

ATG is prepared by immunizing horses or rabbits with human thymocytes. The resulting horse immunoglobulin (Atgam) or rabbit immunoglobulin (Thymoglobulin) that fights against human T cells is then collected and purified. ATG reduces the number of T-cell lymphocytes. T-cell depletion persists for several days after a single dose of ATG and takes approximately 2 months before T-cell levels return to normal. When Rho(D) immune globulin (anti-D) is administered to an Rho(D) mother, antibodies contained in Rho(D) immune globulin suppress the maternal immune system response, preventing maternal antibodies to fetal red blood cells. In the treatment of ITP, anti-D blocks platelet destruction and increases platelet count in patients with a spleen. Anti-D binding to $Rh_o(D)$ is thought to result in an anti-D–coated RBC complex. It may cause immunosuppression by stimulating cytokines. It is formulated for intramuscular and intravenous administration. IVIG is collected from human plasma. It is classified as a biologic response modifier.

Adverse Reactions

Side effects associated with ATG administration are fever, chills, leukopenia, and skin rash. Additional adverse reactions are headache, dizziness, tiredness, and diarrhea. Rh_o immune globulin side effects are headache, muscle aches and pains, pain and tenderness at the injection site, chills, fever, and allergic reactions. Dizziness, weight gain, and difficulty breathing are additional side effects.

hypertension, pyrexia, graft dysfunction, cough, nausea, vomiting, headache, hypokalemia, hyperkalemia, and leukopenia. Persons taking belatacept should not receive immunizations with live viruses. Fingolimod (Gilenya) is an immunosuppressant that is used to treat multiple sclerosis. Fingolimod is believed to reduce lymphocyte migration into the central nervous system. The most common side effects are headache, diarrhea, cough, influenza, sinusitis, back pain, abdominal pain, and pain in extremities. Glatiramer is an immunostimulant that is used for the treatment of multiple sclerosis. The most common side effects are local injection site reactions, itching, dyspnea, vasodilation, or hypersensitivity reactions; however, patients should be monitored for more serious postinjection reactions.

Immunoglobulins

Generic Name	US Brand Name(s) / Canadian Brand Name(s)	Dosage Forms and Strengths
antithymocyte globulin (lymphocyte immune globulin)	Thymoglobulin / Atgam, Thymoglobulin	**Powder, for injection (Thymoglobulin):** 25 mg/vial **Solution, for injection (Atgam):** 50 mg/mL
immune globulin, intravenous (IVIG)	Bivigam, Carimune, Flebogamma, Gammagard, Gammaplex, Gamunex-C, Panzyga, Octagam / Gammagard, Gammagard S/D, Gamastan S/D, Gamunex, IVIGnex, Octagam, Panzyga, Privigen	**Powder, for injection (Gammagard S/D, Gammunex):** 5 g/vial, 10 g/vial **Solution, for IM injection:** 10% (IVIGnex, Octagam, Panzyga, Privigen), 18% (Gamastan S/D)
immune globulin (human), subcutaneous	Hizentra, Vivaglobulin, Cuvitru / Hizentra, Cutaquig, Cuvitru	**Solution, for injection:** 20% (Cuvitru, Hizentra), 16% (Vivaglobulin), 16.5% (Cutaquig)
Rh_o immune globulin	Rhophylac, WinRho SDF / WinRho SDF	**Solution, for injection:** 600 units/vial, 1500 units/vial, 5000 units/vial

Miscellaneous Immunomodulators

Generic Name	US Brand Name(s) / Canadian Brand Name(s)	Dosage Forms and Strengths
belatacept	Nulojix / Not available	**Powder, for injection:** 250 mg/vial
fingolimod[a]	Gilenya, Tascenso ODT / Gilenya	**Capsule:** 0.25 mg, 0.5 mg **Tablet, disintegrating:** 0.25 mg, 0.5 mg
glatiramer[a]	Copaxone, Glatopa / Copaxone, Glatect	**Solution, for injection:** 20 mg/mL, 40 mg/mL

[a]Generic available.

Future of Vaccines

Scientists are researching innovative ways to deliver vaccines. Current delivery systems include nasal sprays (e.g., the flu vaccine). Future delivery forms may be plant based. Scientists are conducting research on "edible vaccines" made from genetically engineered foods such as potatoes and bananas. They have engineered a potato-based vaccine against hepatitis and are also modifying bananas to prevent norovirus. Covifenz is a plant-based vaccine to prevent COVID-19 infection. Other food-based vaccines are also being researched.

Miscellaneous Immunomodulators

Belatacept (Nulojix) is a selective, T-cell costimulation blocker that is used to prevent posttransplantation rejection in adults receiving a kidney transplant. Adverse effects include anemia, diarrhea, urinary tract infection, peripheral edema, constipation,

TECHNICIAN'S CORNER

1. If a patient receives a vaccine, can that patient still become ill with the disease related to the vaccine?
2. Why does the body reject transplanted organs and how can this risk be minimized?

Summary of Selected Immunomodulators

Generic Name	Brand Name	Use	Warning Labels
Calcineurin Inhibitors			
cyclosporine	Neoral, Sandimmune	Heart and kidney transplantation prophylaxis	AVOID PREGNANCY. DILUTE ORAL SOLUTION IN LIQUID. SWALLOW CAPSULES WHOLE; DO NOT CRUSH OR CHEW. AVOID GRAPEFRUIT JUICE. DO NOT REFRIGERATE. ORAL SOLUTION MUST BE USED WITHIN 2 MONTHS OF OPENING. DISCARD DISCOLORED OR CLOUDY SOLUTION FOR INJECTION.
pimecrolimus	Elidel	Atopic dermatitis, see Chapter 36.	See Chapter 36
tacrolimus	Prograf, Protoptic	Heart and kidney transplantation prophylaxis Atopic dermatitis, see Chapter 36.	AVOID GRAPEFRUIT JUICE. TAKE ON AN EMPTY STOMACH.
mTOR Kinase Inhibitors			
everolimus	Afinitor	Kidney transplantation prophylaxis	AVOID PREGNANCY. AVOID PROLONGED EXPOSURE TO SUNLIGHT; USE SUNSCREEN. AVOID ASPIRIN, ACETAMINOPHEN, AND NSAIDS. AVOID GRAPEFRUIT JUICE.
sirolimus	Rapamune	Kidney transplantation prophylaxis	AVOID PREGNANCY. AVOID GRAPEFRUIT JUICE. AVOID PROLONGED EXPOSURE TO SUNLIGHT; USE SUNSCREEN. DILUTE ORAL SOLUTION WITH WATER OR ORANGE JUICE. REFRIGERATE; DISCARD WITHIN 30 DAYS OF OPENING—oral solution.
Immunoglobulins			
antithymocyte globulin	Atgam	Bone marrow and kidney transplant prophylaxis	GENTLY ROTATE SOLUTION; DO NOT SHAKE. REFRIGERATE DILUTED SOLUTION.
intravenous immunoglobulin (IVIG)	Gammagard	Primary immunodeficiency	PROTECT FROM LIGHT. DO NOT FREEZE.
Rh_o immune globulin	WinRho	Rh isoimmunization prophylaxis	REFRIGERATE; DO NOT FREEZE. PROTECT FROM LIGHT.
Antimetabolites			
azathioprine	Imuran	Treatment of rheumatoid arthritis, see Chapter 13	See Chapter 13
mycophenolate mofetil	CellCept	Heart, kidney, and liver transplant prophylaxis	SHAKE WELL—suspension. SWALLOW WHOLE; DO NOT CRUSH OR CHEW. TAKE ON AN EMPTY STOMACH. STORE RECONSTITUTED SUSPENSION AT ROOM TEMPERATURE AND DISCARD IN 60 DAYS.

Summary of Selected Immunomodulators—cont'd

Generic Name	Brand Name	Use	Warning Labels
Monoclonal Antibody Immunomodulators			
adalimumab	Humira	Crohn's disease, rheumatoid arthritis, ulcerative colitis, see Chapter 22	REFRIGERATE (2°C to 8°C); DO NOT FREEZE—all.
basiliximab	Simulect	Prevent kidney transplant rejection	MIX GENTLY; DO NOT SHAKE—golimumab, infliximab, rituximab, tocilizumab.
certolizumab	Cimzia	Crohn's disease, rheumatoid arthritis, ulcerative colitis, see Chapter 22	PROTECT FROM LIGHT—Evusheld, Regen-COV.
daclizumab	Zinbryta	Multiple sclerosis, see Chapter 12	
golimumab	Simponi	Crohn's disease, rheumatoid arthritis, ulcerative colitis, see Chapter 22	
infliximab	Remicade	Crohn's disease, rheumatoid arthritis, ulcerative colitis, see Chapter 22	
natalizumab	Tysabri	Crohn's disease, rheumatoid arthritis, ulcerative colitis, see Chapter 22	
rituximab	Rituxan	Rheumatoid arthritis, see Chapter 13	
tocilizumab	Actemra	COVID-19, rheumatoid arthritis, see Chapter 13	
casirivimab + imdevimab	Regen-COV	COVID-19	
cilgavimab + tixagevimab	Evusheld	COVID-19	
Miscellaneous			
belatacept	Nujolix	Kidney transplantation prophylaxis	AVOID PROLONGED EXPOSURE TO SUNLIGHT. REFRIGERATE; DO NOT FREEZE. PROTECT DRUG FROM LIGHT.
fingolimod	Gilenya	Multiple sclerosis	AVOID PREGNANCY.
glatiramer	Copaxone	Multiple sclerosis	REFRIGERATE; DO NOT FREEZE. PROTECT DRUG FROM LIGHT.

Key Points

- An immunization is defined as a deliberate artificial exposure to disease to produce acquired immunity.
- Vaccines prevent disease by taking advantage of your body's ability to make antibodies and prime killer cells to combat disease-causing microbes and viruses.
- Live attenuated vaccines are a living, but weakened, nonvirulent version of the invader microbe or virus.
- Inactivated killed vaccines are advantageous because they cannot mutate; however, they produce less immunity than live vaccines.
- Toxoid vaccines stimulate the immune system to produce antibodies to the toxins that cause illness.
- Conjugate vaccines link antigens or toxoids to the polysaccharide or sugar molecules that certain bacteria use as a protective device to disguise themselves.
- The cold chain refers to a set of safe handling practices that ensure vaccines and immunologic agents requiring refrigeration are maintained at the required temperature from the time of manufacture until the time of administration to patients.

- When the cold chain is disrupted, the effectiveness and shelf life of vaccines are reduced.
- Loss of potency and effectiveness is cumulative. Each time the cold chain is breached, the vaccine's effectiveness is further reduced.
- Patients are placed at risk when suboptimal vaccines are administered.
- Vaccines and other biologic solutions and suspensions are most sensitive to breaches in the cold chain.
- Vaccines should be placed in a refrigerator designated solely for vaccines or, if a separate refrigerator is not feasible, vaccines should be separated from other refrigerated pharmaceutical agents.
- An important component of the cold chain is establishment and adherence to protocols for receiving, stocking, storing, and transporting drugs requiring refrigeration.
- Pharmacy personnel should be alert for warning signs that the cold chain has been broken during shipment. This might be as simple as noticing that freezer packs have thawed or that

dry ice placed in the transport container with a vaccine has evaporated.

- Vaccine stock should be rotated to avoid wastage because of outdated supplies. Expiration dates should be checked frequently.
- Vaccines should not be removed from the refrigerator until the time of dispensing or until the vaccine must be transported.
- In most cases, vaccines should be transported in an insulated container.
- Extremes in heat and cold must be avoided; vaccines should never be placed in the hot glove compartment of a car.
- Vaccines are administered to provide immunity to a wide variety of childhood diseases, influenza, hepatitis, pneumonia, viral meningitis, rabies, and other conditions.
- Immunosuppressants inhibit proliferation of cells of the immune system.
- Drugs that have their primary action on cells of the immune system are used to treat autoimmune diseases, such as multiple sclerosis, rheumatoid arthritis, systemic lupus erythematosus, and Crohn's disease, prevent tissue or organ rejection after transplantation surgery, and treat cancer.
- Corticosteroids, antimetabolites, calcineurin inhibitors, mTOR kinase inhibitors, immunoglobulins, and monoclonal antibodies are all immunopharmacologic agents.
- Cyclosporine is used to improve survival rates for individuals with organ transplants.

- Everolimus and sirolimus are mTOR kinase inhibitors that are used to prevent transplant rejection.
- Tacrolimus interferes with the first phase of T-cell activation, and sirolimus interferes with a key enzyme that regulates the second phase of T-cell activation and proliferation.
- T-cell depletion persists for several days after a single dose of antithymocyte globulin and takes approximately 2 months before T-cell levels return to normal.
- Mycophenolate mofetil is a prodrug. It inhibits T-cell and B-cell proliferation.
- Basiliximab, daclizumab, and muromonab are monoclonal antibody immunomodulators that are used to reduce transplant rejections and prolong the life of transplanted organs.
- Intravenous immunoglobulin is collected from human plasma. It is used for the treatment of a variety of infections and chronic lymphatic leukemia.
- $Rh_o(D)$ immune globulin is administered to pregnant women who are Rh negative and have been exposed to blood that is Rh positive.
- COVID-19 is prevented by vaccination, handwashing, and wearing medical-grade face masks.
- The four types of COVID-19 vaccines are mRNA, plant based, protein subunit, and viral vector.
- The mpox/smallpox vaccine is a live virus that must be stored frozen.

Review Questions

1. A living but weakened version of an invader that does not cause disease (nonvirulent) is called a _____.
   a. live attenuated vaccine
   b. dead attenuated vaccine
   c. live encapsulated vaccine
   d. live strengthened vaccine
2. All of the following immunosuppressants are used to prevent organ transplant rejection, EXCEPT: _____.
   a. cyclosporine
   b. mycophenolate mofetil
   c. tacrolimus
   d. pimecrolimus
3. Immunization is not always achieved by administering vaccines.
   a. true
   b. false
4. Examples of inactivated killed vaccine(s) are _____ vaccines.
   a. flu
   b. hepatitis A
   c. polio
   d. all of the above
5. These vaccines stimulate the immune system to produce antibodies to the toxins that cause illnesses such as tetanus and diphtheria.
   a. Conjugated vaccine
   b. Live attenuated vaccines
   c. Toxoid vaccines
   d. Inactivated killed vaccines

6. Which of the following statements is FALSE?
   a. Pharmacy technicians must protect against breaches in the cold chain by assessing integrity of refrigerated items received in the pharmacy.
   b. Pharmacy technicians must protect against breaches in the cold chain by placing vaccines directly on ice packs or cold packs during transport.
   c. Pharmacy technicians must protect against breaches in the cold chain by checking the refrigerator temperature up to twice daily.
   d. Pharmacy technicians must protect against breaches in the cold chain by selecting the appropriate transport containers/packaging for vaccines that must be stored between 2°C and 8°C.
7. Select the vaccine that is NOT used to prevent COVID-19 viral infection?
   a. Spikevax
   b. Jynneos
   c. Comirnaty
   d. Jcovden
8. Select the immunosuppressant that is available as a topical dosage form.
   a. CellCept
   b. Imuran
   c. Protoptic
   d. Rapimune

9. A common ending for monoclonal antibody immunomodulators is _____.
   a. *-tan*
   b. *-mab*
   c. *-ine*
   d. *-olol*

10. Rho(D) immune globulin is administered to pregnant women who are Rh _____ who have been exposed to blood that is Rh _____.
    a. negative, positive
    b. positive, negative
    c. both a and b
    d. Rho(D), negative

Bibliography

Ali ES, Mitra K, Akter S, et al. Recent advances and limitations of mTOR inhibitors in the treatment of cancer. *Cancer Cell Int*. 2022;22:284.

Collins B.H. (2021). Renal Transplantation Medication. Retrieved February 26, 2023, from https://emedicine.medscape.com/article/430128-medication#showall.

COVID-19 Treatment Guidelines Panel. (2023). Coronavirus Disease 2019 (COVID-19) Treatment Guidelines. National Institutes of Health. Retrieved February 26, 2023, from https://www.covid19treatmentguidelines.nih.gov/.

College of Physicians of Philadelphia. (nd). Different Types of Vaccines. Retrieved February 26, 2023, from https://www.historyofvaccines.org/content/articles/different-types-vaccines.

Government of Canada. (2022). Storage and handling of immunizing agents: Canadian Immunization Guide. Retrieved February 26, 2023, from https://www.canada.ca/en/public-health/services/publications/healthy-living/canadian-immunization-guide-part-1-key-immunization-information/page-9-storage-handling-immunizing-agents.html.

Health Canada. (2023). Drug Product Database. Retrieved February 26, 2023, from https://health-products.canada.ca/dpd-bdpp/index-eng.jsp.

Institute for Safe Medication Practices. (2016). FDA and ISMP Lists of Look-Alike Drug Names with Recommended Tall Man Letters. Retrieved February 26, 2023, from https://www.ismp.org/recommendations/tall-man-letters-list.

Institute for Safe Medication Practices. (2019). List of Confused Drugs. Retrieved February 26, 2023, from https://www.ismp.org/tools/confuseddrugnames.pdf.

Kalant H, Grant D, Mitchell J. *Principles of medical pharmacology*, ed 7, Toronto, Elsevier; 2007:546–552.

Kurup VM, Thomas J. Edible vaccines: promises and challenges. *Mol Biotechnol*. 2020;62(2):79–90.

Lloyd EC, Gandhi TN, Petty LA. Monoclonal antibodies for COVID-19. *JAMA*. 2021;325(10):1015.

Moscou K. (2015). Tech Talk CE: The Vaccine Cold-Chain. Retrieved February 26, 2023, from https://www.yumpu.com/en/document/view/40273160/vaccine-cold-chain-canadian-healthcare-network.

Murdoch J. Chill out: what pharmacists need to know about the room temperature stability of refrigerated pharmaceutical products. *Pharm Pract*. 2006;22:32–42.

Patil US, Jaydeokar AV, Bandawane DD. Immunomodulators: pharmacological review. *Int J Pharm Pharm Sci*. 2012;4(S1).

Seto J, Marra F. Keeping it cool: a pharmacist's guide. Executive summary, University of British Columbia, Continuing Pharmacy Professional Development, Home Study Program, 2005, Rogers, pp 1–7.

U.S. Food and Drug Administration. (nd). Drugs@FDA: FDA Approved Drug Products. Retrieved February 26, 2023, from http://www.accessdata.fda.gov/scripts/cder/daf/.

U.S. Food and Drug Administration. (2023). Licensed Biological Products with Supporting Documents. Retrieved February 26, 2023, from https://www.fda.gov/vaccines-blood-biologics/licensed-biological-products-supporting-documents#I.

Weir E, Hatch K. Preventing cold-chain failure: vaccine storage and handling. *JAMC*. 2004;171

Drugs Affecting the Integumentary System

The integumentary system or skin is classified as a cutaneous membrane. The primary layers are the epidermis, a superficial thin layer composed of squamous tissue; the dermis, a deep, thicker layer of connective cells; and the hypodermis, a layer of loose subcutaneous tissue, rich in fat and areolar tissue beneath the dermis. The skin forms a self-repairing and protective boundary between the internal environment of the body and the outside elements that could potentially damage vital, life-sustaining organs. The epidermis has the ability to create new cells and repair itself after injury or disease. The dermis is sometimes called the true skin because it protects against mechanical injury and compression. Additional functions of the skin are sensation detection, growth, synthesis of important chemicals and hormones (vitamin D), excretion, temperature regulation, and immunity.

In Unit XI, the various types of medications used to treat diseases of the integumentary system, such as fungal infections, pressure injuries, burns, atopic dermatitis, psoriasis, acne, lice, and scabies, are described. A brief description of each disorder is provided, followed by a description of the drugs indicated for treatment that includes mechanisms of action, adverse reactions, strength(s), and dosage forms. Pharmacy technicians need to be familiar with various types of skin products applied to treat skin conditions because customers may ask questions about OTC skin and hair products and lice treatments sold in the pharmacy.

33

Treatment of Fungal Infections

LEARNING OBJECTIVES

1. Learn the terminology associated with fungal infections.
2. Identify risk factors for fungal infections.
3. List and categorize medications used for the treatment of fungal infections.
4. Describe the mechanism of action for drugs used for the treatment of fungal infections.
5. List common endings for drug classes used for the treatment of specific fungal infections.
6. Identify significant drug look-alike and sound-alike issues, warning labels, and precautionary messages associated with medications used for the treatment of fungal infections.

KEY TERMS

Antifungal Drug used to treat a fungal infection.
Candida Genus of a type of fungus. It is also called yeast.
Fungus (*pl.,* fungi) Organism similar to plants but lacking chlorophyll and capable of producing mycotic (fungal) infections.
Mycosis General term for a fungal infection.

Onychomycosis Fungal infection involving the fingernails or toenails, also known as tinea unguium.
Ringworm Group of tinea infections involving the body or scalp that have a characteristic ring-like shape. Ringworm is spread person to person and animal to person.
Vulvovaginal candidiasis Yeast vaginitis.

What Are Fungi and Yeast?

Fungi are organisms similar to plants but lacking chlorophyll and capable of producing mycotic (fungal) infections. Thousands of different fungi exist. Mold, mildew, yeast, and mushrooms are all types of fungi. Many fungi are beneficial and do not cause disease. For example, some mushrooms and fungi are edible. The antibiotic penicillin is derived from a mold, and yeast causes bread to rise. Other fungi can cause severe illness. *Pneumocystis jirovecii* is a fungus that can cause pneumonia in individuals who have a decreased immune system response (are immunocompromised); *Aspergillus fumigatus* is a mold that also causes serious respiratory infection. Fungal infections are common and are estimated to affect 5.7 billion individuals globally and lead to the death of 1.6 million people annually.

Fungal Infections of the Skin and Nails

The general term used to describe a fungal infection is *mycosis*. Most fungal infections of the skin are caused by a group of fungi called dermatophytes. Dermatophyte infections are common and affect up to 20% to 25% of the global population. This is because fungi are ubiquitous (found everywhere). They are found in the air, soil, plants, and water. They are also found on surfaces in the home, office, schools, and gyms and even occur normally on our bodies. Fungi that are part of the normal body flora may become pathogenic (cause infection) only when the normal balance of

flora is upset. For example, women who take broad-spectrum antibiotics may get a yeast infection because the bacteria and fungi that keep the yeast that are normally present in the vagina from overgrowing are killed by the antibiotic. Dermatophytes thrive on dead keratin, a tough protein substance found in the top layer of skin, nails, and hair.

Fungal infections caused by the dermatophyte tinea are named for the site of the infection. For example, tinea manus is a fungal infection on the hands, while tinea corporis is an infection on the body, and tinea capitis is located on the head (hence cap). Tinea infections are also commonly called *ringworm*.

> ● *Tech Note!*
>
> Ringworm is caused by a fungus, not a worm as the name implies!

Athlete's Foot

Athlete's foot (tinea pedis) (Fig. 33.1) is a common fungal infection that affects athletes and nonathletes. Symptoms are peeling, flaking skin between the toes, redness, itchiness, burning or stinging, blisters, and thickening of skin on the soles of the feet and heels. It may be accompanied by a foul odor. If severe, it may cause cracking of the skin, oozing, and secondary bacterial infection.

Individuals who have abrasions on the feet, as caused by improperly fitted shoes that rub against the skin, are more

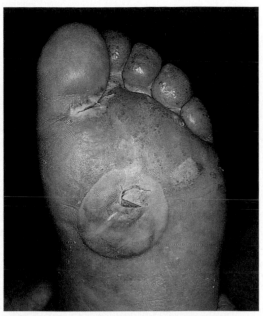

• **Fig. 33.1** Athlete's foot. (From Callen JP, Greer KE, Hood A, et al. *Color atlas of dermatology*, Philadelphia, 1993, WB Saunders.)

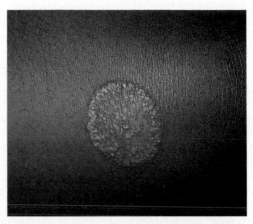

• **Fig. 33.2** Tinea corporis. (From Zitelli BJ, McIntire S, Nowalk AJ. *Zitelli and Davis' atlas of pediatric physical diagnosis*, ed 6, Philadelphia, 2012, Elsevier.)

• BOX 33.1 Prevention of Athlete's Foot

- Keep your feet clean and dry.
  - Dry between your toes after swimming or bathing.
  - Wear leather shoes or sandals that allow your feet to breathe.
  - When indoors, wear socks without shoes.
  - Wear cotton socks to absorb sweat. Change your socks twice a day. (White socks do not prevent athlete's foot, as some people believe.)
  - Use talcum or antifungal powder on your feet.
- Allow your shoes to air for at least 24 hours before you wear them again.
- Wear shower sandals in public pools and showers.

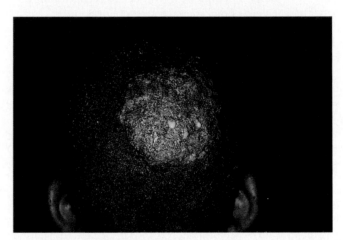

• **Fig. 33.3** Ringworm of the scalp. (From Callen JP, Greer KE, Paller LJ, et al. *Color atlas of dermatology*, ed 2, Philadelphia, 2000, Saunders.)

susceptible to athlete's foot. Tips for prevention of athlete's foot are listed in Box 33.1.

"Ringworm"

Ringworm infections are caused by tinea fungi. Ringworm may occur on the scalp, body, feet, fingernails, or toenails. Ringworm is contagious and is spread person to person by physical contact with infected surfaces or lesions. Ringworm can also spread between humans and animals. Cats and dogs may be carriers of the fungus.

Ringworm of the body is also known as tinea corporis. Patches and plaques appear pink to red, with raised scaly borders. They form in a distinctive circular pattern that gives the name of "ring" worm (Fig. 33.2).

Tinea capitis is also called ringworm of the scalp. It occurs more frequently in children than in adults and is spread by sharing contaminated hats, combs, clothing, bedding, and linens. It may also be spread from animal to person. The fungus can cause bald patches on the scalp (Fig. 33.3).

Tinea manus affects the hands, and tinea unguium affects the nails. A fungal infection of the nails is also called **onychomycosis**. Infected nails become discolored and thick and may crumble or fall off. Onychomycosis is hard to treat with topically applied **antifungals** because it is difficult for drugs to penetrate the nails and nail bed (Fig. 33.4).

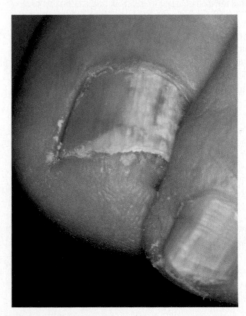

• **Fig. 33.4** Onychomycosis.

Candidiasis

Candida, also called "yeast," is a type of fungus that thrives in warm moist areas and can cause fungal infections in the vagina, groin, penis, skin folds, corners of the mouth, and nail beds. Invasive candidiasis is a serious infection that can affect the stomach, intestines, heart, and lungs. Premature neonates and individuals who have COVID-19 infection treated with corticosteroids are at increased risk for developing invasive candidiasis.

Vulvovaginal candidiasis is also known as yeast vaginitis. *Candida* is normally present in the gastrointestinal tract and vagina but causes infection only when conditions are favorable for the overgrowth of yeast. The risk for getting yeast vaginitis increases with age. Changes in hormone levels, such as occurs during pregnancy or when taking oral contraceptives or hormone replacement therapy, can also increase the risk of infection. When the body's ability to fight infection is suppressed because of infections such as human immunodeficiency virus (HIV) or if taking immunosuppressive drugs (e.g., corticosteroids, antineoplastic agents), fungal infections may flourish. Risk factors of vulvovaginal candidiasis are listed in Box 33.2. Signs and symptoms of vulvovaginal candidiasis are shown in Box 33.3.

Candida can also cause infections in the oral cavity and area surrounding the mouth. A *Candida* infection in the oral cavity is termed *thrush* (Fig. 33.5). Thrush is most common in infants. A thrush infection in adults is a sign that the immune system is compromised. Thrush is an opportunistic infection that occurs in individuals with diseases that affect the immune system (such as HIV), persons who take immunosuppressive medicines for cancer treatment or after stem cell and organ transplantation, and individuals taking broad-spectrum antiinfective agents.

● **BOX 33.2** **Risk Factors for Vulvovaginal Candidiasis**

- Age
- Decreased immune status
- Diabetes
- Drug therapy (e.g., hormone replacement therapy, oral contraceptives, antibiotics, immunosuppressives, corticosteroids)
- Douching
- Diet
- Menses
- Pregnancy
- Sexual activity
- Stress
- Tight-fitting clothing and synthetic underwear

● **BOX 33.3** **Signs of Vulvovaginal Candidiasis**

- Itching
- Cottage cheese-like vaginal discharge
- Burning
- Pain during intercourse

Treatment of Fungal and Yeast Infections

Some fungal infections can be treated with nonprescription antifungal agents. Ringworm, vulvovaginal candidiasis, jock itch, and athlete's foot are examples of fungal infections that are cured using over-the-counter (OTC) drugs. Onychomycosis and systemic fungal infections must be treated with prescription antifungal agents.

Antifungal agents are categorized by their mechanism of action. Classifications are *imidazoles* and *triazoles*, *-polyenes*, echinocandins, and drugs that interfere with the synthesis of fungal nucleic acids (RNA) needed for replication.

Imidazoles and Triazoles

Imidazoles and triazoles are formulated for the treatment of cutaneous (skin) fungal infections and systemic infections in patients who are immunocompromised. Tinidazole is indicated for amebiasis, trichomoniasis, and giardiasis.

Clotrimazole and miconazole are topical imidazoles that are available without prescription (OTC) in the United States and Canada. Butoconazole, ketoconazole, and tioconazole are OTC antifungal agents used to treat athlete's foot, vulvovaginal candidiasis, jock itch, ringworm, and oral candidiasis. The remaining imidazoles (econazole, oteseconazole, oxiconazole, sulconazole, sertaconazole) are restricted to prescription use in both countries. Fluconazole, itraconazole, posaconazole, terconazole, and voriconazole are triazoles. All require a prescription in the United States. Fluconazole is available without prescription in Canada.

Levoketoconazole (Recorlev) is an *-azole* that is not used to treat fungal infections. It inhibits cortisol synthesis and is used to reduce hypercortisolemia in patients with Cushing syndrome.

Mechanism of Action and Pharmacokinetics

The imidazoles and triazoles interfere with ergosterol, an essential component needed for the synthesis of the fungal cell membrane.

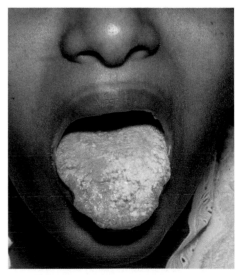

● **Fig. 33.5** Thrush.

This causes cellular contents to leak out, and the cell dies. Topical azoles are formulated for application to the skin (creams, gel, lotion), mucous membranes (vaginal creams, suppositories), and scalp (shampoo).

Adverse Effects

The most common adverse effects for topical imidazoles and triazoles are stinging or burning at the application site, redness, itchiness, or blistering. Nausea and vomiting, skin rash, liver toxicity, heart rhythm disturbances, and photophobia are adverse reactions linked to oral itraconazole and ketoconazole.

> **⚠ Tech Alert!**
>
> Fluconazole, itraconazole, ketoconazole, and posaconazole interact with numerous drugs (e.g., macrolide antibiotics, quinidine, protease inhibitors, statins, cimetidine, and calcium channel blockers).

> **⚠ Tech Alert!**
>
> Fungicure, Zeasorb, Lotrimin, Lamisil, and other antifungal products are marketed in formulations that contain clotrimazole, terbinafine, tolnaftate, or undecylenic acid. Read labels carefully to select the desired product.

Allylamine Antifungals

Butenafine, naftifine, and terbinafine are classified as allylamine antifungal agents. Lamisil (terbinafine) is effective for treating fungal infections involving the nails.

Mechanism of Action and Pharmacokinetics

Allylamine antifungal agents inhibit the synthesis of the cell membrane of susceptible fungi by blocking an enzyme needed for the synthesis of ergosterol. Butenafine and naftifine are available only for topical application. Terbinafine is formulated for topical and oral use. Terbinafine is fungicidal (kills fungi), whereas "azole" antifungal agents (e.g., clotrimazole and miconazole) are only

Imidazoles and Triazoles

Generic Name	US Brand Name(s) / Canadian Brand Name(s)	Dosage Forms and Strengths	Prescription/OTC Status
butoconazole[a]	Gynezole-1 / Not available	**Cream, vaginal:** 2%	OTC
clotrimazole[a]	Fungicure Intensive, Lotrimin AF, Mycelex, Trivagizole 3 / Canasten, Canesten Cream 1, Canesten Cream 3, Canesten Cream 6, Canesten Comfortab 1, Canesten Comfortab 3, Canasten Comfortab Combi-Pak-1, Canasten Comfortab Combi-Pak-3, Clotrimaderm Cream, Clotrimaderm Vaginal Cream Clotrimaderm Vaginal 3 Clotrimaderm Vaginal 6	**Cream, topical:** 1% **Solution, topical:** 1% **Cream, vaginal:** 1%, 2%, 10%[b] **Tablet, vaginal tab:** 200 mg, 500 mg **Vaginal tab + cream (Combipak):** 500-mg vaginal tab + 1% cream, 200-mg vaginal tab + 1% cream **Troche:** 10 mg	OTC, prescription
econazole[a]	Ecoza / Not available	**Cream:** 1% **Foam, topical (Ecoza):** 1%	Prescription
fluconazole[a]	Diflucan / Canesoral, Diflucan, Diflucan One, Monicure	**Capsule (Canesoral, Diflucan One, Monicure)[b]:** 150 mg **Powder, for oral suspension:** 10 mg/mL, 40 mg/mL[c] **Solution, for injection:** 2 mg/mL **Tablet:** 50 mg, 100 mg, 150 mg[c], 200 mg[c]	OTC, prescription (Canada), prescription (United States)
itraconazole[a]	Sporonox, Tolsura / Sporonox	**Capsule:** 65 mg (Tolsura), 100 mg **Solution, oral:** 10 mg/mL	Prescription
ketoconazole[a]	Extina, Nizoral A-D, Ketozole / Ketoderm, Nizoral Cream	**Cream (Ketoderm, Ketozole, Nizoral):** 2% **Foam, topical (Extina):** 2% **Shampoo:** 1% (Nizoral A-D)[c], 2% **Tablet:** 200 mg	OTC—cream and shampoo, prescription—other formulations
levoketoconazole	Recorlev / Not available	**Tablet:** 150 mg	Prescription

Continued

Imidazoles and Triazoles—cont'd

Generic Name	US Brand Name(s) / Canadian Brand Name(s)	Dosage Forms and Strengths	Prescription/OTC Status
miconazole[a]	Desenex AF, Micatin, Monistat 3, Monistat 7, Monistat 1 Day or Night Combination Pack, Monistat 3 combination pack, M-Zole 3 Combination Pack, Oravig, Ting, Zeasorb AF Micatin, Micoderm, Monistat 7, Monistat Derm, Monistat 1 Combination Pack, Monistat 3 Dual-Pak, Monistat 7 Dual-Pak, Monistat 1 Vaginal Ovule, Monistat 3 Vaginal Ovules, Monistat 3 Vaginal cream, Monicure Combo	**Cream (Micatin Derm, Monistat Derm)**: 2% **Ointment**: 2% **Buccal tablet (Oravig)**: 50 mg **Powder, topical (Micatin, Desenex AF, Zeasorb AF)**: 2% **Spray, solution**: 2% **Spray, powder (Desenex Jock Itch)**: 2% **Vaginal cream**: 2% (Monistat-7), 4% (Monistat-3) **Vaginal suppository**: 100 mg[c] (Monistat 7), 200 mg[c] (Monistat 3), 400 mg[b] (Monistat 3), 1200 mg (Monistat 1) **Vaginal suppository + cream**: 100 mg suppository + 2% cream (Monistat 7 Dual-Pak), 200 mg suppository + 2% cream (Monistat 3 combination pack, M-Zole 3 combination), 400 mg suppository + 2% cream (Monistat 3 Dual-Pak), 1200 mg suppository + 2% cream (Monistat 1 combination pack) **Vaginal cream 2% + topical cream 4%**: Monistat 3 combination pack	OTC (topical), prescription (oral)
miconazole + zinc oxide + petrolatum	Vusion Not available	**Ointment**: 0.25% miconazole + 15% zinc oxide + 81.35% petrolatum	Prescription
oteseconazole	Vivjoa Not available	**Capsule**: 150 mg	Prescription
oxiconazole	Oxistat Not available	**Cream**: 1% **Lotion**: 1%	Prescription
posaconazole	Noxafil Posanol	**Solution, IV**: 18 mg/mL **Suspension, oral**: 40 mg/mL **Tablet, delayed release**: 100 mg	Prescription
sertaconazole	Ertaczo Not available	**Cream**: 2%	Prescription
sulconazole	Exelderm Not available	**Cream**: 1% **Topical solution**: 1%	Prescription
terconazole[a]	Generic Generic	**Vaginal cream**: 0.8%[c], 0.4% **Vaginal suppository**[c]: 80 mg	Prescription
tinidazole	Tindamax Not available	**Tablet**: 250 mg, 500 mg	Prescription
tioconazole[a]	Vagistat-1 Not available	**Vaginal ointment**: 6.5%	OTC

Imidazoles and Triazoles—cont'd

Generic Name	US Brand Name(s) / Canadian Brand Name(s)	Dosage Forms and Strengths	Prescription/OTC Status
voriconazole[a]	Vfend / Vfend	**Powder, for injection**: 200 mg/vial **Powder, for oral suspension**: 40 mg/mL **Tablet**: 50 mg, 200 mg	Prescription
clotrimazole + fluconazole	Not available / Canesoral Combipak	**Vaginal cream + capsule**: 1% clotrimazole cream + 150 mg fluconazole	OTC
clotrimazole + betamethasone[a]	Lotrisone / Lotriderm	**Cream**: 1% clotrimazole cream + betamethasone 0.05% **Lotion**[c]: 1% clotrimazole cream + betamethasone 0.05%	Prescription

[a]Generic available.
[b]Available in Canada only.
[c]Available in the United States only.
OTC, Over the counter.

Allylamines

Generic Name	US Brand Name(s) / Canadian Brand Name(s)	Dosage Form and Strength	Prescription/OTC Status
butenafine[a]	Mentax, Lotrimin Ultra / Not available	**Cream**: 1%	Prescription (Mentax), OTC (Lotrimin Ultra)
naftifine[a]	Naftin / Not available	**Cream**: 1%, 2% **Gel**: 1%, 2%	Prescription
terbinafine[a]	Lamisil, Lamisil AT / Lamisil	**Cream**: 1% **Gel**[b]: 1% **Tablet**: 250 mg **Spray**: 1% **Topical solution**[b]: 1%	Prescription, OTC (all Lamisil topical formulations)[b]

[a]Generic available.
[b]Available in the United States only.
OTC, Over the counter.

fungistatic (slow the growth of fungi). When administered orally, therapeutic levels are reached within 3 to 18 weeks. Therapeutic levels persist in the skin for 2 to 3 weeks after terbinafine has been discontinued.

Adverse Effects

Orally administered terbinafine may produce nausea, vomiting, altered taste, headache, and tiredness. Topical application of terbinafine, butenafine, or naftifine may produce burning, stinging, redness, itchiness, and drying of the skin.

Polyene Class of Antifungals

Nystatin, natamycin, and amphotericin B are derived from the fungi-like bacteria *Streptomyces*. They belong to the class of antifungal agents called polyenes. Nystatin is used for the treatment of *Candida* infections on the skin and mucous membranes. Nystatin

suspension is commonly prescribed for the treatment of thrush. Amphotericin B is prescribed for systemic infections caused by various fungi, including candidiasis, histoplasmosis, and aspergillosis. Natamycin is used to treat fungal infections in the eye (e.g., blepharitis, conjunctivitis, keratitis). These infections are described in Chapter 15.

Mechanism of Action and Pharmacokinetics

Nystatin, natamycin, and amphotericin B inhibit the synthesis of the fungal cell membrane by binding irreversibly to ergosterol. Nystatin is available only for oral and topical use. Oral absorption of amphotericin B is low, so the drug is administered parenterally. Natamycin is formulated for ophthalmic use.

Adverse Effects

Systemic absorption of nystatin is low when administered topically and orally, so adverse effects are minimal. Oral administration may

Polyenes

Generic Name	US Brand Name(s) / Canadian Brand Name(s)	Dosage Form and Strength	Prescription/OTC Status
amphotericin B[a]	Abelcet, Ambisome Abelcet, Ambisome, Fungizone	**Powder, for injection (Ambisome, Fungizone):** 50 mg/vial **Suspension, for IV (Abelcet):** 5 mg/mL	Prescription
natamycin	Natacyn Not available	**Ophthalmic suspension:** 5%	Prescription
nystatin[a]	Nystop Nyaderm	**Cream:** 100,000 units/g **Tablet, oral[b]:** 500,000 units **Ointment[b]:** 100,000 units/g **Powder, topical (Nystop)[b]:** 100,000 units **Suspension, oral:** 100,000 units/mL **Vaginal cream:** 25,000 units/g	Prescription, OTC (topical cream)[c]
nystatin + triamcinolone acetonide[a]	Mykacet Not available	**Cream:** 100,000 units nystatin + 1% triamcinolone **Ointment:** 100,000 units nystatin + 1% triamcinolone	Prescription

[a]Generic available.
[b]Available in the United States only.
[c]Available in the Canada only.
OTC, Over the counter.

produce nausea or diarrhea. Amphotericin B may produce nausea, vomiting, kidney damage, fever, chills, headache, and thrombophlebitis when administered intravenously. Amphotericin B may also cause potassium loss (hypokalemia).

Thiocarbamates

Tolnaftate is the only antifungal belonging to the thiocarbamate class. It is approved for the treatment and prevention of athlete's foot. It is also indicated for the treatment of ringworm and jock itch. Tolnaftate is available without prescription.

Mechanism of Action and Pharmacokinetics

The mechanism of action for tolnaftate is similar to that of terbinafine and naftifine.

Adverse Effects

Adverse reactions are mild; they include irritation at the site of application, itching, or burning.

Echinocandins

Anidulafungin, caspofungin, and micafungin belong to a class of antifungal agents called echinocandins. They are effective for treating infections caused by *Candida* and *Aspergillus*.

❶ *Tech Alert!*

A common ending for echinocandin antifungals is *-fungin.*

Mechanism of Action and Pharmacokinetics

Echinocandins interfere with the synthesis of the fungal cell wall. They are not toxic to human cells because their target is a cell wall component that does not exist in human cells. Oral absorption is poor, so echinocandins are formulated for parenteral use.

Adverse Effects

Echinocandins have fewer adverse effects and drug interactions than other oral or parenterally administered antifungal

Thiocarbamates

Generic Name	US Brand Name(s) / Canadian Brand Name(s)	Dosage Forms and Strengths	Prescription/OTC status
tolnaftate[a]	Tinactin, Tinactin Jock Itch Odor Eaters, Tinactin, Tinactin Chill Deodorant Powder Spray, Pro Clerz Antifungal Liquid	**Cream:** 1% **Foam:** 1% **Spray:** 1% **Topical powder:** 1% **Topical solution:** 1%	OTC

[a]Generic available.
OTC, Over the counter.

Echinocandins

Generic Name	US Brand Name(s) Canadian Brand Name(s)	Dosage Forms and Strengths	Prescription/OTC status
anidulafungin	Eraxis	**Powder, for IV infusion:** 50 mg/vial, 100 mg/vial	Prescription
	Eraxis		
caspofungin[a]	Cancidas	**Powder, for IV infusion:** 50 mg/vial, 70 mg/vial	Prescription
	Cancidas		
micafungin[a]	Mycamine	**Powder, for IV infusion:** 50 mg/vial, 100 mg/vial	Prescription
	Mycamine		

[a]Generic available.

agents. They can cause elevated liver enzyme levels, diarrhea, and hypokalemia.

Miscellaneous Agents

The remaining antifungal agents work by various mechanisms of action. Ciclopirox and undecylenic acid are effective for treating athlete's foot and jock itch. Ciclopirox is a broad-spectrum antifungal agent and is also approved for the treatment of ringworm and mild onychomycosis. Griseofulvin is an orally administered drug used to treat onychomycosis. Povidone-iodine is used to treat thrush and is also used as an antiseptic wash (orally and topically).

Mechanism of Action and Pharmacokinetics

Ciclopirox, povidone-iodine, and undecylenic acid are topical antifungal agents. Ciclopirox interferes with DNA and RNA synthesis. Undecylenic acid and zinc undecylate are combined to produce a drug that decreases the spread of susceptible fungi. Formulations must contain at least 10% undecylenate to be effective. In addition, zinc undecylenate is an astringent and reduces irritation.

Griseofulvin interferes with fungal mitosis and disrupts the ability of the fungus to replicate. Griseofulvin formulations made with ultramicronized crystals (Gris-PEG) offer the best absorption. Absorption is also increased when the drug is taken with a fatty meal.

❶ Tech Alert!

Griseofulvin microsize and griseofulvin ultramicrosize have look-alike/sound-alike issues.

Adverse Effects

Topically applied antifungal agents may produce mild burning, stinging, itching, swelling, or other signs of skin irritation. Common adverse effects caused by the administration of griseofulvin are nausea, vomiting, headache, dizziness, gas, and heartburn.

TECHNICIAN'S CORNER

1. There are many reports of onychomycosis caused by artificial nails. What is causing these infections, and how can they be prevented?
2. Describe one potential dispensing error associated with antifungal agents. How would you prevent this error?

Miscellaneous Antifungal Agents

Generic Name	US Brand Name(s) Canadian Brand Name(s)	Dosage Forms and Strengths	Prescription/ OTC Status
ciclopirox[a]	Loprox, Penlac	**Cream:** 0.77%[b], 1%[c] **Lotion/suspension:** 0.77%[b], 1%[c] **Nail lacquer (Penlac):** 8% **Shampoo:** 1% (Loprox), 1.5% (Steiprox)	Prescription
	Loprox, Steiprox		
griseofulvin[a]	Fulvicin P/G, Fulvicin P/G 165, Fulvicin P/G 330, Fulvicin U/F, Gris-PEG	**Suspension, microsize:** 125 mg/5 mL **Tablet, microsize:** 250 mg, 500 mg **Tablet, ultramicrosize:** 125 mg, 165 mg, 250 mg, 330 mg	Prescription
	Not available		

Continued

Miscellaneous Antifungal Agents—cont'd

Generic Name	US Brand Name(s) / Canadian Brand Name(s)	Dosage Forms and Strengths	Prescription/ OTC Status
povidone-iodine[a]	Betadine First Aid	**Ointment**: 10% **Scrub, cleanser**: 7.5% **Solution**: 5%, 10% **Spray**: 5% **Sponge**: 10% **Swab sticks**: 10%	OTC
undecylenic acid[a]	Fungicure Liquid, Fungi Nail Antifungal, Nail Max Fungicure Liquid	**Solution, topical**: 25%	OTC

[a]Generic available.
[b]Available in the United States only.
[c]Available in Canada only.
OTC, Over the counter.

Summary of Drugs Used for the Treatment of Fungal and Yeast Infections

	Generic Name	US Brand Name(s)	Usual Dose and Dosing Schedule[a]	Warning Labels
Imidazoles and Triazoles				
	butoconazole	Gynezole-1	**Vaginal cream:** One applicatorful vaginally at bedtime for 3–7 days depending on product formulation	COMPLETE THE FULL COURSE OF THERAPY—all.
	clotrimazole	Canasten Mycelex	**Vaginal cream:** One applicatorful at bedtime for 3–14 days depending on product formulation **Vaginal tablet:** Insert once daily for 1–3 days depending on product formulation **Topical cream:** Apply twice daily	
	econazole	Ecoza	**Topical:** Apply twice daily	
	fluconazole	Diflucan	**Oral or IV:** 200 mg on day 1, then 100 mg daily for 2 weeks (esophageal or oropharyngeal candidiasis) *or* 150–200 mg as a single dose or 3 doses for 3 days each (vulvovaginal candidiasis)	SHAKE WELL (SUSPENSION)—fluconazole, posaconazole.
	itraconazole	Sporonox	**Oral:** 100–400 mg once daily **Topical:** Apply 1–2 times daily	TAKE WITH FOOD (CAPSULES). AVOID GRAPEFRUIT JUICE (CAPSULES)—itraconazole, voriconazole.

Summary of Drugs Used for the Treatment of Fungal and Yeast Infections—cont'd

Generic Name	US Brand Name(s)	Usual Dose and Dosing Schedule[a]	Warning Labels
ketoconazole	Nizoral	**Oral:** 200–400 mg once daily **Topical:** Apply daily for up to 6 weeks **For dandruff:** Use shampoo every 3–4 days for up to 8 weeks	TAKE WITH FOOD (TABLETS)—ketoconazole, posaconazole. AVOID ALCOHOL—ketoconazole, voriconazole.
miconazole	Monistat	**Vaginal:** One applicatorful or one suppository at bedtime for 1–14 days depending on product formulation **Topical:** Apply twice a day	
oxiconazole	Oxistat	**Topical:** Apply once or twice daily	
posaconazole	Noxafil	**Oral:** 200 mg 3 times a day	
sulconazole	Exelderm	**Topical:** Apply once or twice daily	
terconazole	Generic	**Vaginal:** One applicatorful or one suppository at bedtime for 3–7 days depending on product formulation	
tioconazole	Vagistat-1	**Vaginal:** One applicatorful as a single dose	
sertaconazole	Ertaczo	Apply a thin layer of 2% cream to cleansed, dry, infected area twice daily for 4 weeks	
voriconazole	Vfend	**Parenteral:** 6 mg/kg IV every 12 h	TAKE ON AN EMPTY STOMACH—voriconazole.
		Oral: 400 mg every 12 h loading dose on day 1, followed by 200 mg every 12 h	
Allylamines			
butenafine	Mentax	**Topical:** Apply once daily for 2–4 weeks	COMPLETE THE FULL COURSE OF THERAPY—all. TAKE WITH FOOD (TABLETS)—terbinafine.
naftifine	Naftin	**Topical:** Apply cream once daily and apply gel twice daily	
terbinafine	Lamisil	**Topical:** Apply cream twice daily and apply gel once daily for 1–4 weeks **Oral:** 250 mg once daily for 6–12 weeks	
Polyenes			
amphotericin B	Fungizone	**IV:** 0.25–1.5/kg/day (max 1.5 mg/day)	PROTECT FROM LIGHT (IV SOLUTION)—amphotericin B. REFRIGERATE—amphotericin B.
natamycin	Natacyn	**Ophthalmic:** See Chapter 15	SHAKE WELL—natamycin.

Continued

Summary of Drugs Used for the Treatment of Fungal and Yeast Infections—cont'd

	Generic Name	US Brand Name(s)	Usual Dose and Dosing Schedule[a]	Warning Labels
	nystatin	Generics	**Capsule:** 1 cap 3 times a day **Suspension:** 4–6 mL swished in mouth 4 times a day **Topical:** Apply twice daily **Vaginal:** One insert nightly for 14 days	COMPLETE THE FULL COURSE OF THERAPY—natamycin. SHAKE WELL (SUSPENSION)—natamycin.
Thiocarbamates				
	tolnaftate	Tinactin	**Topical:** Apply twice daily for 2–4 weeks	COMPLETE THE FULL COURSE OF THERAPY.
Echinocandins				
	anidulafungin	Eraxis	100-mg IV loading dose on day 1, followed by 50 mg IV daily for 7 days after symptoms resolve	REFRIGERATE; DO NOT FREEZE—anidulafungin, caspofungin. TO MIX, GENTLY SWIRL; DO NOT SHAKE—micafungin. MAY BE STORED AT ROOM TEMPERATURE FOR 24 HOURS—micafungin.
	caspofungin	Cancidas	70-mg IV infusion as a loading dose on day 1, followed by 50-mg IV infusion once daily for at least 14 days	
	micafungin	Mycamine	150 mg IV daily for 10–30 days	
Miscellaneous Agents				
	griseofulvin	Gris-PEG	375–750 mg daily or in 1 or 2 divided doses	COMPLETE THE FULL COURSE OF THERAPY—all. TAKE WITH FOOD—griseofulvin. SHAKE WELL (LOTION)—ciclopirox.
	ciclopirox	Loprox	**Topical:** Apply twice daily	

[a]Usual dose for candidiasis or tinea.

Key Points

- Some fungi are beneficial to humans, whereas others cause serious infections.
- The general term used to describe a fungal infection is *mycosis*.
- Fungal infections caused by the dermatophyte tinea are named for the site of the infection. For example, tinea manus is a fungal infection on the hands, while tinea corporis is an infection on the body, and tinea capitis is located on the head (cap).
- Athlete's foot (tinea pedis) is a common fungal infection that affects athletes and nonathletes.
- Tinea infections are also called *ringworm*. Ringworm has a characteristic ring-like shape and may affect the body, scalp, nails, or feet.
- Ringworm is contagious and is spread via person-to-person and animal-to-person contact.
- Women who take broad-spectrum antiinfective agents may get a yeast infection because the bacteria and fungi that keep the yeast normally present in the vagina from overgrowing are killed by the antibiotic.
- *Candida*, also called yeast, is a type of fungus that thrives in warm moist areas and causes fungal infections in the vagina, groin, and mouth.
- Vulvovaginal candidiasis is also known as yeast vaginitis.

- A *Candida* infection in the oral cavity is called thrush.
- Fungal infections such as vulvovaginal candidiasis, jock itch, and athlete's foot can be cured using over-the-counter drugs. Some of these drugs can also be used as prophylaxis.
- Topical antifungal agents are formulated for application to the skin (creams, gel, lotion), mucous membranes (vaginal creams, suppositories), and scalp (shampoo).
- Butenafine, naftifine, and terbinafine are classified as allylamine antifungal agents.
- Nystatin, natamycin, and amphotericin B are all derived from the fungi-like bacteria *Streptomyces* and belong to the class of antifungals called polyenes.
- Nystatin, natamycin, and amphotericin B inhibit the synthesis of the fungal cell membrane.
- Tolnaftate is the only antifungal belonging to the thiocarbamate class. It is approved for the treatment and prevention of athlete's foot.
- Anidulafungin, caspofungin, and micafungin belong to a class of antifungal agents called echinocandins.
- Echinocandins interfere with the synthesis of the fungal cell wall.

Review Questions

1. *Candida* is a type of _____. It is also called yeast.
   a. virus
   b. bacteria
   c. fungus
   d. protozoan
2. Select the antifungal that is not an OTC product applied or inserted vaginally to treat vaginal yeast infections.
   a. Gynezole-1
   b. Canesten Comfortab 1
   c. Diflucan
   d. Monistat-3
3. Ringworm is caused by a _____.
   a. worm
   b. fungus
   c. bacteria
   d. insect
4. Fungal infections of the _____ are called onychomycosis.
   a. hair
   b. skin
   c. scalp
   d. nails
5. Which of the following is the primary mechanism of action for antifungal agents?
   a. Destroying the cell membrane of the fungus
   b. Interfering with the synthesis of nucleic acids needed for replication
   c. Inhibiting the synthesis of the fungal cell wall
   d. All of the above
6. _____ is effective for treating fungal infections involving the nails.
   a. Terbinafine
   b. Tioconazole
   c. Nystatin
   d. Clotrimazole
7. Nystatin suspension is commonly prescribed for the treatment of thrush.
   a. true
   b. false
8. All of the following antifungal agents are marketed as OTC formulations EXCEPT _____.
   a. povidone
   b. clotrimazole
   c. miconazole
   d. itraconazole
9. Echinocandins are formulated for oral use.
   a. true
   b. false
10. Sporonox may be administered _____.
   a. topically
   b. orally
   c. parenterally
   d. a and b

Bibliography

Aaron DM. (2022). Candidiasis (Mucocutaneous). Moniliasis. Retrieved October 21, 2022, from https://www.merckmanuals.com/professional/dermatologic-disorders/fungal-skin-infections/candidiasis-mucocutaneous#top.

Aaron DM. (2022). Overview of Dermatophytoses. Retrieved October 21, 2022, from https://www.merckmanuals.com/professional/dermatologic-disorders/fungal-skin-infections/overview-of-dermatophytoses?qt=ringwormandalt=sh.

Burchacka E, Pięta P, Łupicka-Słowik A. Recent advances in fungal serine protease inhibitors. *Biomed Pharmacother*. 2022;146:112523.

Cappelletty D, Eiselstein-McKitrick K. The echinocandins. *Pharmacotherapy*. 2007;27:369–388.

Centers for Disease Control and Prevention. (2022). Types of Fungal Diseases. Retrieved October 21, 2022, from https://www.cdc.gov/fungal/diseases/index.html.

Health Canada. (2022). Drug Product Database. Retrieved October 21, 2022, from https://health-products.canada.ca/dpd-bdpp/index-eng.jsp.

Hornik CD, Bondi DS, Greene NM, et al. Review of fluconazole treatment and prophylaxis for invasive candidiasis in neonates. *J Pediatr Pharmacol Ther*. 2021;26(2):115–122.

Institute for Safe Medication Practices. (2016). FDA and ISMP Lists of Look-Alike Drug Names with Recommended Tall Man Letters. Retrieved October 18, 2022, from https://www.ismp.org/recommendations/tall-man-letters-list.

Institute for Safe Medication Practices. (2019). List of Confused Drugs. Retrieved October 18, 2022, from https://www.ismp.org/tools/confuseddrugnames.pdf.

Jaulim Z, Salmon N, Fuller C. Fungal skin infections: current approaches to management. *Prescriber*. 2015;26(19):31–35.

Kalant H, Grant D, Mitchell J. *Principles of medical pharmacology*, ed 7. Toronto: Elsevier Canada; 2007;688:691–695.

Lance L, Lacy C, Armstrong L, et al. *Drug information handbook for the allied health professional*, ed 12. Hudson, OH: APhA Lexi-Comp; 2005.

National Institute of Allergy and Infectious Diseases: Understanding Microbes in Sickness and in Health, Bethesda, 2006, US Department of Health and Human Services, National Institutes of Health. NIH Publication No. 06-4914.

Pray W. *Nonprescription product therapeutics*. Baltimore: Lippincott Williams and Wilkins; 1999:542–551.

U.S. Food and Drug Administration. (nd). Drugs@FDA: FDA Approved Drug Products. Retrieved October 21, 2022, from http://www.accessdata.fda.gov/scripts/cder/daf/.

34

Treatment of Pressure Injuries and Burns

LEARNING OBJECTIVES

1. Learn the terminology associated with pressure injuries and burns.
2. Describe the stages of pressure injuries and degrees of burns.
3. List and categorize medications used to treat pressure injuries and burns.
4. Describe the mechanism of action for each class of drugs used

to treat pressure injuries and burns.
5. Identify significant drug look-alike and sound-alike issues.
6. Identify warning labels and precautionary messages associated with medications used to treat pressure injuries and burns.

KEY TERMS

Blister Collection of fluid below or within the epidermis.
Debridement Surgical removal of foreign material and dead tissue from a wound to prevent infection and promote healing.
Eschar Blackened necrotic tissue of a pressure injury.
Escharotomy Removal of necrotic skin and underlying tissue.
First-degree burn Minor discomfort and reddening of the skin.
Full-thickness burn Third-degree burn where the epidermis and dermis are destroyed.
Partial-thickness burns First- and second-degree burns.
Pressure injury Pressure sore or "bedsore."

Rule of palms Rule for determining the extent of a burn surface area. A palm size of a burn victim is about 1% of total body surface area.
Rule of nines Formula for estimating the percentage of adult body surface covered by burns dividing the body into 11 areas, each representing 9% of the body surface area.
Second-degree burn A burn that involves deep epidermal layers and causes damage to the upper layers of dermis.
Third-degree burn A burn that is characterized by destruction of the epidermis and dermis.

Pressure Injuries

A *pressure injury* (formerly termed "decubitus ulcer") is commonly called a "bedsore" (Fig. 34.1). A common cause of pressure injuries is lying in a prone position for long periods. Pressure injuries typically occur in patients who are confined to a bed or chair. Patients with sensory or mobility deficits such as spinal cord injury, stroke, coma, multiple sclerosis, peripheral vascular disease, or diabetes; hospitalized older patients; nursing home residents; and malnourished patients are all at risk.

All pressure injuries have a course of injury similar to a burn and are classified in stages according to severity. Pressure injuries can range from a mild pink coloration of the skin, which disappears in a few hours after pressure is relieved on the area, to a deep wound extending to and sometimes through a bone into internal organs. Burns can cause a mild redness of the skin and/or blistering (*first-degree burn*) or produce a deep open wound with blackened tissue (*eschar*), such as with a *third-degree burn*.

Nonpharmacologic Management of Pressure Injuries and Burns

A pressure injury typically forms from continuous pressure to an area; however, it can also occur from friction caused by rubbing against

something, such as a bedsheet, cast, or brace, or prolonged exposure to cold. The most common places for pressure injuries to form are over bones close to the skin, such as the elbows, heels, hips, sacrum, ankles, shoulders, back, and back of the head. The weight of a body presses on the bone, and the bone presses on the tissue and skin that it covers. This tissue begins to decay from lack of blood circulation.

The Norton scale and Braden scale are simple assessment tools used to determine a patient's risk for developing a pressure injury. The Norton scale assesses patients on five risk factors (physical condition, mental state, level of activity, mobility, and continence). A rating scale of 1 to 4 is used. The Braden scale has six categories. They are sensory perception, moisture, activity, mobility, nutrition, and friction/shear. Patients with the lowest score are at the highest risk for pressure injuries on both scales.

The most important principle is to prevent initial skin damage, which promotes ulceration. In at-risk patients, aggressive nursing practices, such as frequent turning of immobile patients (changing position every 2 hours or more frequently if needed) and the application of skin protection to bony body parts can be effective. This 2-hour time frame is generally accepted as the maximum interval that the tissue can tolerate pressure without damage. Range-of-motion exercises and early ambulation are encouraged along with the use of low-pressure mattresses and special beds.

(A) Stage 1 Pressure Injury – Edema

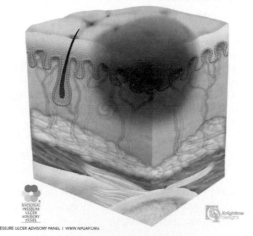

(B) Stage 2 Pressure Injury

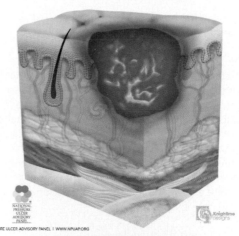

(C) Stage 3 Pressure Injury

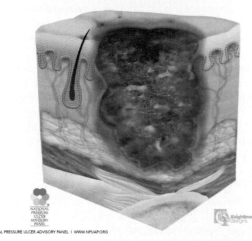

(D) Stage 4 Pressure Injury

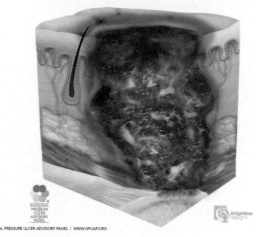

(E) Unstageable Pressure Injury - Slough and Eschar

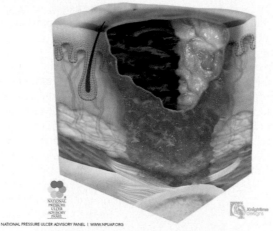

• **Fig. 34.1** Pressure injury. (A) Stage 1. (B) Stage 2. (C) Stage 3. (D) Stage 4. (E) Unstageable. (From National Pressure Ulcer Advisory Panel: Pressure injury staging illustrations, available at https://npiap.com/page/PressureInjuryStages.)

Wound Stages

Pressure injuries and burns are often categorized according to stages of severity.

Stage 1 Wounds

This stage is characterized by a surface reddening of the skin. The skin is unbroken, and the wound is superficial. The pressure injury quickly fades when pressure is relieved on that area. Changes in sensation, temperature, or firmness may precede visual changes. The key factors to consider in a stage 1 wound are the causes of the wound, how to alleviate the pressure on the area to prevent it from worsening, and improving the nutritional status of the individual. The presence of a stage 1 wound is an indication or early warning of a problem and a signal to take preventive action.

Stage 2 Wounds

This stage is characterized by broken skin. The wound can appear as a **blister**, abrasion, or shallow crater. A partial layer of the skin is injured, and the dermis is exposed. The goal of care is to cover, protect, and clean the area. Coverings are designed to insulate, absorb, and protect. Close attention to prevention, protection, nutrition, and hydration is also important. With quick attention, a stage 2 wound can heal rapidly. In general, pressure wounds developing beyond stage 2 are the result of lack of aggressive intervention when first noted at stage 1.

Stage 3 Wounds

In stage 3, the wound has extended through all layers of the skin. Fatty tissue may be exposed. It is the primary site for a serious infection to occur. The depth of tissue damage varies by the part of the body that is affected. The goal of treatment is to alleviate pressure, cover and protect the wound, and place an increased emphasis on nutrition and hydration. Medical care is necessary to promote healing and to treat and prevent infection. If left unattended, this type of wound will worsen rapidly. Infection is a grave concern.

Stage 4 Wounds

Stage 4 wounds extend through the skin and involve underlying muscle, tendons, and bone. The diameter of the wound is not as important as the depth. Stage 4 wounds are very serious and can produce life-threatening infections. Treatment involves protecting, cleaning, and alleviating pressure on the area. Nutrition and hydration are now critical because without adequate nutrition, this wound will not heal. Anyone with a stage 4 wound requires medical care by someone skilled in wound care. A skilled wound care physician, physical therapist, or nurse can sometimes successfully treat a smaller diameter wound without surgery. Surgical removal of the necrotic or decayed tissue (**escharotomy**) is often necessary for wounds of larger diameter.

Drug Therapy for Pressure Injuries

The treatment for a pressure injury involves keeping the area clean and removing necrotic (dead) tissue, which can form a breeding ground for infection. There are many procedures and products available for this purpose. Topical treatments aid the healing of partial-thickness sores (Box 34.1).

Recombinant Platelet-Derived Growth Factor

Becaplermin is a biologically engineered platelet-derived growth factor. It promotes wound repair by increasing the recruitment

---

> **• BOX 34.1   Topical Treatment of Pressure Injuries**
>
> - Occlusive hydrocolloid dressings
> - Polyurethane films
> - Absorbable gelatin sponges
> - Karaya gum patches
> - Antiseptic irrigations
> - Antibiotic ointments
> - Air-permeable occlusive clear dressings (allow aspiration of collected fluids)
> - Supportive adhesive-backed foam padding
> - Absorptive dextranomer beads

and proliferation of cells involved in wound healing and formation of granulation tissue. It is indicated for the treatment of diabetic neuropathic ulcers.

Collagenase

Collagenase is used to promote **debridement** (removal of foreign material and dead tissue from a wound) in dermal ulcers and severe burns. Collagenase is a water-soluble proteinase that specifically breaks down collagen into gelatin, allowing less-specific enzymes to act. Commercially available preparations of collagenase (e.g., Santyl) are derived from the bacterium *Clostridium histolyticum*. There is evidence that elastin and fibrin are also degraded by collagenase, but to a lesser degree. Additional indications for collagenase are treatment of moderate to severe cellulite in the buttocks (Qwo® subcutaneous injection) and Dupuytren contracture (Xiaflex®).

Antibacterial Drugs

Antibacterial drugs may be used if the pressure injury is not healing or if it continues to ooze after 2 weeks of proper cleansing and bandage changes. Most antibacterial preparations can be applied directly to the skin. Antiinfective agents given by mouth or injection are typically needed only for individuals who have developed sepsis or have infections in the skin or underlying bone. Antiinfective agents are also given when the injury requires surgical repair.

Burns

Typically we think of a burn as a thermal injury or lesion caused by contact of the skin with some hot object or fire. In addition, overexposure to ultraviolet (UV) light (sunburn) or contact with an electric current, corrosive chemical, or radioactive agents can cause injury or death to skin cells. The injuries that result can be classified as burns. The effects may be local or systemic, involving primary shock (which occurs immediately after injury and rarely is fatal) or secondary shock (which develops insidiously after severe burns and is often fatal). Worldwide, more than 8 million people are burned annually and 180,000 die from their injuries (World Health Organization). Burns result in 3000 deaths annually in the United States. More than 2 million people in the United States and 450,000 Canadians receive medical treatment for burns annually. More than 50,000 of these burn victims require hospitalization.

Estimating Burn Surface Area

Treatment and the prognosis for recovery of burns depends in large part on the total area involved and severity of the burn. The severity of a burn is determined by the depth and extent (percentage

Topical Drugs Used for the Treatment of Ulcerated Wounds

Generic Name	US Brand Name(s) / Canadian Brand Name(s)	Dosage Forms and Strengths
becaplermin	Regranex / Not available	**Gel:** 100 mcg/g (0.01%)
collagenase	Santyl / Santyl	**Ointment (Santyl):** 250 units/g
Topical Antibacterials		
bacitracin zinc[a]	Generics / Bacitin (OTC)	**Ointment:** 500 units/g
gentamicin[a]	Generics / Not available	**Cream:** 0.1% **Ointment:** 0.1%
mupirocin[a]	Centany / Generics	**Cream:** 2% **Ointment:** 2%
Combination Topical Antibacterials		
bacitracin + neomycin+ polymyxin[a]	Neosporin Original (OTC) / Not available	**Ointment:** 400 IU bacitracin + 3.5 mg neomycin+ 5000 units polymyxin
bacitracin + polymyxin[a]	Polysporin (OTC) / Band-Aid adhesive bandages plus antibiotic (OTC), Bioderm (OTC), Polyderm (OTC), Polysporin (OTC), Sterisporin (OTC)	**Ointment:** 500 g bacitracin + 10,000 units polymyxin/gram
bacitracin + gramacidin + polymyxin[a]	Not available / Triple antibiotic ointment (OTC)	**Ointment:** 500 IU bacitracin, 0.25 mg gramicidin + 10,000 units polymyxin
bacitracin + gramacidin + polymyxin + lidocaine[a]	Not available / Polysporin Complete (OTC)	**Ointment:** 500 IU bacitracin, 0.25 mg gramicidin + 10,000 units polymyxin + 50 mg/g lidocaine
bacitracin + neomycin + polymyxin B + pramoxine[a]	Triple antibiotic ointment pain relief (OTC) / Not available	**Cream:** 500 units bacitracin zinc + 3.5 mg neomycin +10,000 units polymyxin B + 10 mg pramoxine
Antiseptics		
povidone-iodine[a]	Betadine (OTC) / Generics	**Ointment:** 10% **Prep pads:** 10% **Scrub, cleanser:** 7.5%, 10% **Solution:** 10% **Spray:** 10% See Chapter 33 for additional dosage forms

[a]Generic available.
OTC, Over the counter.

of body surface area [BSA]) of the lesion. There are several ways to estimate the extent of BSA burned. *The **rule of palms** method* is based on the assumption that the palm size of a burn victim is about 1% of the total BSA. Estimating the number of palms that are burned approximates the percentage of BSA involved.

Another method is the ***rule of nines*** (Fig. 34.2). In this technique, the body is divided into 11 areas of 9%, with the area around the genitals, called the perineum, representing the additional 1% of BSA (see Fig. 34.2). The rule of nines works well with adults but does not reflect the differences of BSA in small children. Special tables called Lund-Browder charts, which take the large surface area of certain body areas (e.g., the head) in a growing child into account, are used by physicians to estimate burn percentages in children.

The depth of a burn injury depends on the tissue layers of the skin that are involved (Fig. 34.3). A first-degree or superficial burn (typical sunburn) causes minor discomfort and some reddening of the skin. Although the surface layers of the burned area may peel

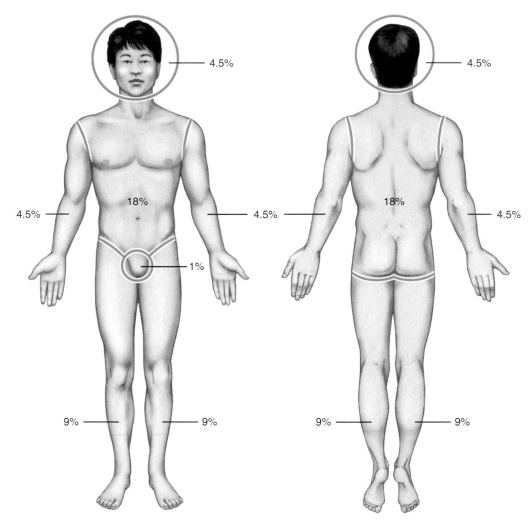

• **Fig. 34.2** Rule of nines. (From Patton KT, Thibodeau GA. *The human body in health and disease*, ed 6, St Louis, 2014, Elsevier.)

in 1 or 2 days, no blistering occurs, and the actual tissue destruction is minimal. It can be treated with medications to relieve pain and barrier protectants such as aloe vera gel or cream.

Second-degree burns are called ***partial-thickness burns***. Second-degree burns may involve the papillary or upper dermis or involve the deeper epidermal layers. Injury to the upper dermal layers can heal in 1 to 2 weeks. Injury from deep second-degree burns can damage sweat glands, hair follicles, and sebaceous glands, but tissue death is not complete. Blisters, severe pain, generalized swelling, and edema characterize this type of burn. Healing typically takes more than 2 weeks. Scarring is common. Over-the-counter pain medications and antibiotic cream may be applied to reduce pain and reduce risk of infection.

Third-degree or ***full-thickness burns*** are characterized by destruction of both the epidermis and dermis. Tissue death extends below the follicles and sweat glands. The burn may also involve underlying muscles, fasciae, or bone. A full-thickness burn is insensitive to pain immediately after injury because of destruction of the nerve endings. Scarring is a serious problem. Full-thickness burns are best managed in specialized burn centers.

Complications

Sloughing of skin, gangrene, scarring, erysipelas (skin infection caused by group A staphylococci), nephritis (kidney infection), pneumonia, immune system impairment, and intestinal disturbances are possible complications of burns. The risk for infection and dehydration is greatest when more than 25% of the body surface is burned.

Signs of infection are as follows:
- Change in color of the burned area or surrounding skin
- Purplish discoloration, particularly if swelling is also present
- Change in thickness of the burn
- Greenish discharge or pus
- Fever
- Signs of dehydration are as follows:
- Thirst
- Light-headedness or dizziness (when moving from lying or sitting to standing)
- Weakness
- Dry skin
- Urinating less often than usual

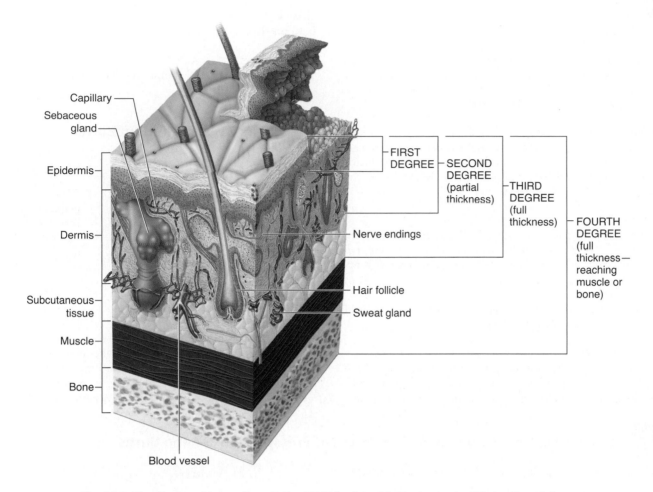

Capillary
Sebaceous gland
Epidermis
Dermis
Subcutaneous tissue
Muscle
Bone

Nerve endings
Hair follicle
Sweat gland
Blood vessel

FIRST DEGREE
SECOND DEGREE (partial thickness)
THIRD DEGREE (full thickness)
FOURTH DEGREE (full thickness—reaching muscle or bone)

• **Fig. 34.3** Classification of burns. (From Patton KT, Thibodeau GA. *The human body in health and disease*, ed 6, St Louis, 2014, Elsevier.)

Burn Prevention

Sunburn can be prevented by using sunscreen or sunblock and avoiding excess exposure to UV radiation. Chemical-related skin burns can be prevented by avoiding strong chemicals. "Stop, drop, and roll" should be the first actions if a person is on fire. A rug, blanket, or anything within reach can be used to smother flames. Care must be taken so that the individual does not inhale the smoke. Clothing must be carefully cut away so that skin is not pulled away. Blisters should not be opened because this will increase the chance for infection. All burned patients must receive appropriate tetanus prophylaxis.

Treatment of Burns

Treatment involves the administration of antibiotics, analgesics, and fluid replacement. Nonpharmacologic management includes monitoring cardiac output, tissue perfusion, urinary output, blood pressure and pulse, body weight, and renal function. Fluid balance is carefully monitored, as well as nutritional therapy (Box 34.2).

Silver Sulfadiazine

Silver sulfadiazine is the most frequently used topical agent for burns. It is used to prevent and treat infections in partial-thickness and full-thickness burns. The drug is bactericidal against

• **BOX 34.2** Management of Severe Burns

- Check for airway injury or impaired breathing. Airway injury is most likely to occur after facial burns or smoke inhalation in closed spaces.
- Remove overlying clothing and irrigate affected tissues. Avoid excessive cooling of the body.
- Pharmacologic therapy: antibiotics, intravenous analgesics, volume replenishment with crystalloid intravenous fluids to ensure adequate hydration.
- Gentle debridement of tissues followed by the application of nonadherent dressings, skin substitutes, topical antiseptics, or autografts, as dictated by circumstances.
- Nutritional and emotional support.

gram-positive and gram-negative organisms, but resistance has occasionally been reported.

Adverse Effects

Local skin reactions such as pain, burning, itching, and hypersensitivity are occasionally reported. Transient leukopenia occurs in 5% to 15% of patients, but there is no increased incidence of infectious complications.

Mafenide

Mafenide is an adjunctive antibacterial agent used for the treatment of first- and second-degree burns. It appears to act on bacterial cellular mechanisms. It interferes with bacterial folic acid synthesis through competitive inhibition of para-aminobenzoic acid. With topical application, mafenide is bacteriostatic against gram-positive and gram-negative bacteria.

Adverse Effects

Pain or a burning sensation after mafenide application is the most frequently reported adverse effect. Mafenide may cause alkaline diuresis, leading to acid-base abnormalities. It also inhibits epithelial regeneration (growth of new tissue).

Silver Nitrate

Silver nitrate is a broad-spectrum agent. It is bacteriostatic at a concentration of 5%. The effects of silver nitrate may result from silver ions readily combining with several biologically important chemical groups.

Adverse Effects

Silver nitrate is prepared with distilled water. The hypotonic solution may lead to electrolyte imbalance.

Povidone-Iodine

Povidone-iodine acts by destroying microbial protein and DNA. This drug has excellent in vitro antimicrobial activity but is inactivated by wound exudates. In vitro refers to a test that is done in glass or plastic vessels in the laboratory. More information about povidone-iodine is found in Chapter 33.

Adverse Effects

Systemic absorption of iodine results in renal and thyroid dysfunction.

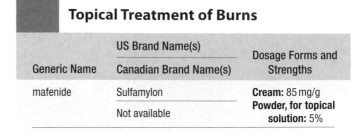

Topical Treatment of Burns

Generic Name	US Brand Name(s) / Canadian Brand Name(s)	Dosage Forms and Strengths
mafenide	Sulfamylon / Not available	**Cream:** 85 mg/g **Powder, for topical solution:** 5%
silver sulfadiazine[a]	Silvadene, Thermazene, SSD / Flamazine	**Cream:** 1%

Rehabilitation

During rehabilitation, individually fitted elastic garments are used to prevent hypertrophic scar formation, and joints are exercised to promote a full range of motion. Referrals for occupational therapy, psychological counseling, support groups, or social services are often necessary to assist the patient with life adjustments.

Summary of Drugs Used in the Treatment of Pressure Injuries and Burns

Generic Name	Brand Name	Usual Dose and Dosing Schedule	Warning Labels
Debriding Agents			
Collagenase	Santyl	Apply once daily (more if dressing becomes soiled)	DO NOT TOUCH THE TIP OF THE TUBE TO ANY SURFACE, INCLUDING A FINGER, THE WOUND, OR STERILE GAUZE PAD.
Topical Antibacterial Agents			
bacitracin	Generics	Apply 1–3 times daily for up to 7 days	NOT TO BE USED FOR LONGER THAN 1 WEEK UNLESS PRESCRIBED.
gentamicin[a]	Generics	**Topical:** Apply 3 or 4 times daily to affected area	REPORT ANY DIZZINESS OR SENSATIONS OF RINGING OR FULLNESS IN EARS.
mupirocin	Generics	Apply small amount to affected area 3 times a day for 7–14 days.	FOR TOPICAL USE ONLY. DISCONTINUE IF RASH, ITCHING, OR IRRITATION OCCURS.
silver sulfadiazine	Silvadene	Apply twice a day with a sterile-gloved hand; apply to thickness of 1/16 inch.	FOR EXTERNAL USE ONLY.
mafenide	Sulfamylon	Apply once or twice daily with a sterile-gloved hand; apply to thickness of 1/16 inch. The burned area should be covered with cream at all times	DISCONTINUE AND REPORT IMMEDIATELY IF RASH, BLISTERS, OR SWELLING APPEAR WHILE USING CREAM. FOR EXTERNAL USE ONLY.
silver nitrate	Generics	Apply a cotton applicator dipped in solution on the affected area 2 or 3 times/week for 2–3 weeks	DISCONTINUE IF REDNESS OR IRRITATION DEVELOPS.
Antiseptic Agents			
povidone-iodine	Betadine	Apply as needed for treatment and prevention of susceptible microbial infections	DO NOT SWALLOW. FOR EXTERNAL USE. AVOID CONTACT WITH THE EYES.

[a]Generic available.

Key Points

- Pressure injuries can be very mild, disappearing in a few hours after pressure is relieved, or very serious, extending into bone and internal organs.
- Pressure injuries form in areas exposed to continuous pressure, friction, or prolonged exposure to cold.
- The treatment for a pressure injury involves keeping the area clean and removing necrotic (dead) tissue, which can form a breeding ground for infection.
- Collagenase is used to promote debridement of necrotic tissue in dermal ulcers and severe burns.
- Fire, sun, electricity, chemicals, and radioactive agents can cause burns.
- The severity of a burn is determined by the depth and extent (percentage of body surface area [BSA]) of the lesion.
- One method of estimating the extent of BSA burned is called the rule of palms. It is based on the assumption that the palm size of a burn victim is approximately 1% of their total BSA.

- The rule of nines is another and more accurate method of determining the extent of a burn injury. With this method, the body is divided into 11 areas of 9%, with the area around the genitals, called the perineum, representing the additional 1% of BSA.
- Two common complications of burns are infection and dehydration.
- Silver sulfadiazine is the most frequently used topical agent for burns. It is thought to act via the inhibition of DNA replication and modification of the cell membrane and cell wall.
- Mafenide appears to act on bacterial cellular mechanisms. It interferes with bacterial folic acid synthesis through competitive inhibition of para-aminobenzoic acid.
- Silver nitrate is a broad-spectrum agent. It is bacteriostatic at a concentration of 5%.

Review Questions

1. Pressure sores typically occur in patients who are
   _____.
   a. confined to the bed
   b. chair-bound
   c. ambulatory
   d. a and b
2. The usual mechanism of forming a pressure injury is from
   _____.
   a. immobilization
   b. infection
   c. inflammation
   d. laceration
3. In stage _____ of a pressure injury, the wound has extended through all layers of the skin.
   a. 1
   b. 2
   c. 3
   d. 4
4. Frequent turning is optional to alleviate pressure on the wound and to promote healing.
   a. true
   b. false
5. The severity of a burn is determined by the _____ (percentage of body surface area) of the lesion.
   a. depth
   b. width
   c. extent
   d. a and c

6. The rule of nines is a more accurate method of determining the extent of a burn injury than the rule of palms.
   a. true
   b. false
7. Third-degree, or _____, burns are characterized by destruction of both the epidermis and dermis.
   a. partial-thickness
   b. full-thickness
   c. total thickness
   d. all of the above
8. Common complications of burns are _____ and _____.
   a. infection, dehydration
   b. infection, stroke
   c. dehydration, stroke
   d. stroke, shock
9. _____ is the most frequently used topical agent for burns.
   a. Gentamycin
   b. Silver sulfadiazine
   c. Bacitracin
   d. Mupirocin
10. The removal of necrotic skin and underlying tissue from a burn or pressure wound is termed _____.
    a. escharectomy
    b. escharotomy
    c. necrotomy
    d. ulcerectomy

Bibliography

Al Aboud AM, Manna B. *Wound pressure injury management*. Treasure Island, FL: StatPearls Publishing; 2023. Available from. https://www.ncbi.nlm.nih.gov/books/NBK532897/.

Carter DW. (2022). Burns. Retrieved January 14, 2023, from https://www.merckmanuals.com/en-ca/professional/injuries-poisoning/burns/burns.

Health Canada (2023). Drug Product Database. Retrieved January 14, 2023, from https://www.canada.ca/en/health-canada/services/drugs-health-products/drug-products/drug-product-database.html.

Norton L, Parslow N, Johnston D, et al. (2017). Best practice recommendations for the prevention and management of pressure injuries. In: Foundations of Best Practice for Skin and Wound Management. A supplement of Wound Care Canada. Retrieved January 14, 2023, from https://www.woundscanada.ca/docman/public/health-care-professional/bpr-workshop/172-bpr-prevention-and-management-of-pressure-injuries-2/file.

Thibodeau G, Patton K, eds. *Anatomy and physiology*. St Louis: Mosby; 2007.

U.S. Food and Drug Administration. (nd). Drugs@FDA: FDA Approved Drug Products. Retrieved January 14, 2023, from https://www.accessdata.fda.gov/scripts/cder/daf/index.cfm.

35

Treatment of Acne

LEARNING OBJECTIVES

1. Learn the terminology associated with acne.
2. Describe the types and causes of acne.
3. List and categorize medications used to treat acne.
4. Describe the mechanism of action for each class of drugs used to treat acne.
5. Identify significant drug look-alike and sound-alike issues.
6. Identify warning labels and precautionary messages associated with medications used to treat acne.

KEY TERMS

Acne Disorder resulting from the action of hormones and other substances on the skin's oil glands (sebaceous glands) and hair follicles.

Acne vulgaris Most common form of acne.

Blackhead Trapped sebum and bacteria partially open to the surface that turn black because of changes in sebum as it is exposed to air; also called an open comedone.

Comedone Enlarged and plugged hair follicles; the most characteristic sign of acne.

Cysts Deep, painful, pus-filled lesions that can cause scarring.

Keratolytic A peeling agent that causes the softening and shedding of the horny outer layer of the skin.

Milia Tiny little bumps that occur when normally sloughed skin cells become trapped in small pockets on the surface of the skin.

Nodule Large, painful, solid lesions that are lodged deep within the skin.

Papule Obstructed follicle that becomes inflamed.

Pustule Larger lesions that are more inflamed than papules and can be superficial or deep.

Whitehead Trapped sebum and bacteria that stay below the skin surface; may show up as tiny white spots, or they may be so small that they are invisible to the naked eye; also called a closed comedone.

Acne

Acne is a disorder that causes plugged pores and outbreaks of lesions, commonly called pimples. Acne lesions usually occur on the face, neck, back, chest, and shoulders (Fig. 35.1). Severe acne can lead to permanent scarring. It is a disease of the pilosebaceous units (PSUs). Found over most of the body, PSUs consist of sebaceous glands connected to canals called follicles that contain fine hairs (Fig. 35.2). These units are most numerous on the face, upper back, and chest. The sebaceous glands make sebum (an oily substance) that normally empties onto the skin surface through the opening of the follicle or pore.

When hair, sebum, and keratinocytes (the cells that line the follicle) fill the narrow follicle and produce a plug, it prevents sebum from reaching the surface of the skin through the pores. The mixture of oil and cells allows the bacteria *Propionibacterium acnes*, which normally live on the skin, to grow in the plugged follicles. These bacteria produce chemicals and enzymes and attract white blood cells that cause inflammation (swelling, redness, heat, and pain). When the wall of the plugged follicle breaks down, it spills sebum, shedding skin cells and bacteria into the nearby skin, leading to lesions or pimples.

Common acne, or *acne vulgaris*, occurs most frequently during adolescence because the rate of sebum secretion increases more than fivefold between 10 and 19 years of age. An estimated 80% of all people between the ages of 11 and 30 years have acne outbreaks at some point. For most people, acne tends to go away by the time they reach their 30s; however, some people in their 40s and 50s continue to experience this skin problem.

People with acne frequently have a variety of lesions. The basic acne lesion (*comedone*) is simply an enlarged and plugged hair follicle and is the most characteristic sign of acne. If the plugged follicle, or comedone, stays beneath the skin, it is called a closed comedone and produces a white bump called a *whitehead*. A comedone that reaches the surface of the skin and opens up is called an open comedone or -*blackhead* because it looks black on the skin's surface (Fig. 35.3). This black discoloration is caused by changes in sebum as it is exposed to air. It is not caused by dirt. Noninflammatory acne is characterized by whiteheads and blackheads.

Blackheads and whiteheads normally release their contents at the surface of the skin and then heal. When the follicle wall ruptures, inflammatory acne can ensue. This rupture can be caused by random occurrence or by picking or touching the skin. Inflammatory acne lesions include the following:

- *Papules*—inflamed lesions that usually appear as small pink bumps on the skin and can be tender to the touch.

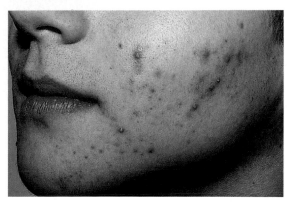

• **Fig. 35.1** Adult acne. (From Callen JP, Paller AS, Greer KE, Swinyer LF. *Color atlas of dermatology*, ed 2, Philadelphia, 2000, WB Saunders.)

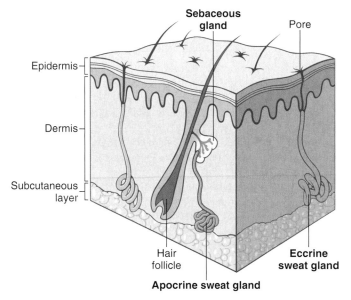

• **Fig. 35.2** Normal pilosebaceous unit. (From Chabner DE. *The language of medicine*, ed 10, St Louis, 2014, Elsevier.)

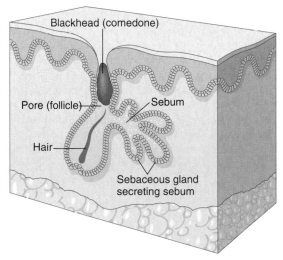

• **Fig. 35.3** Open comedone. (From Chabner DE. *The language of medicine*, ed 10, St Louis, 2014, Elsevier.)

- *Pustules* (pimples)—papules topped by white or yellow pus-filled lesions that may be red at the base. The pus-filled pimples result from secondary infections within or beneath the epidermis, often in a hair follicle or sweat pore.
- *Nodules*—large, painful, solid lesions that are lodged deep within the skin.
- *Cysts*—deep, painful, pus-filled lesions that can cause scarring.

Milia are tiny little bumps that occur when normally sloughed skin cells get trapped in small pockets on the surface of the skin. They are common in newborns across the nose and upper cheeks and can also be seen on adult skin. The bumps disappear as the surface is worn away and the dead skin is sloughed. In newborns, the bumps usually disappear within the first few weeks of life. Adult milia may persist indefinitely. Treatment is not indicated for children. Adults can have them removed by a physician for cosmetic reasons.

Causes of Acne

The exact cause of acne is unknown; however, it is believed to result from several related factors. One important factor is an increase in androgens (sex hormones). The hormones increase in boys and girls during puberty and cause the sebaceous glands to enlarge and make more sebum. Hormonal changes related to pregnancy or starting or stopping birth control pills can also cause acne.

Another factor is heredity or genetics. Researchers believe that the tendency to develop acne can be inherited from parents. For example, studies have shown that many school-age boys with acne have a family history of the disorder. Other risk factors for acne are the use of certain drugs, including androgens and lithium (Box 35.1), and the use of greasy cosmetics. They may alter the cells of the follicles and make them stick together, producing a plug. Other factors that make acne worse are shown in Box 35.2.

Myths About the Causes of Acne

There have been many theories concerning the causes of acne. Because adolescents commonly suffer from acne and indulge in fast food, junk food, and sweets, these food items are often blamed as the causes of acne. Not keeping one's skin clean is also blamed

---

• **BOX 35.1** **Medications That Trigger or Exacerbate Acne**

More Common
- Anabolic steroids (e.g., danazol, testosterone)
- Bromides
- Corticosteroids (e.g., prednisone)
- Corticotropin (H.P. Acthar)
- Isoniazid
- Lithium
- Phenytoin

Less Common
- Azathioprine
- Cyclosporine (Sandimmune, Neoral)
- Disulfiram
- Phenobarbital
- Quinidine
- Tetracycline
- Vitamins B₁, B₆, B₁₂, and D

• BOX 35.2   Factors That Can Worsen Acne

- Changing hormone levels in adolescent girls and adult women 2 to 7 days before their menstrual period starts
- Oil from skin products (moisturizers or cosmetics) or grease encountered in the work environment (e.g., a kitchen with fry vats)
- Pressure from sports helmets or equipment, backpacks, tight collars, or tight sports uniforms
- Environmental irritants (e.g., pollution, high humidity)
- Squeezing or picking at blemishes and hard scrubbing of the skin
- Stress

for causing blackheads, but that also is a myth. Although stress does not cause acne, it can make existing acne worse.

Treatment of Acne

The goals of treatment are to heal existing lesions, stop new lesions from forming, prevent scarring, and minimize the psychological stress and embarrassment. Drugs used to treat acne act by breaking down comedones (comedolytics), increasing cell turnover, destroying bacteria causing acne, and reducing hormones that increase acne.

Depending on the severity of the acne, one or more over-the-counter (OTC) or prescription topical medications may be applied. Combined therapy with oral and topical medicines may also be recommended. Mild acne can sometimes be controlled at home by gently washing the affected area(s) with warm water and a mild soap twice daily to remove dead skin cells and excess oil and then applying an acne product.

Treatment of Mild Acne With Over-the-Counter Medications

Topical OTC medicines are available in many forms, such as lotions, creams, washes, kits, scrubs, brushes and devices, gels, soaps, or pads. Treatment with OTC topical medicines may take up to 8 weeks before noticeable improvement can be seen. Common active ingredients found in OTC acne products are benzoyl peroxide (2.5% to 10%), salicylic acid (0.5% to 5%), α-hydroxy acids, and sulfur.

Once acne clears, treatment must be continued to prevent new lesions from forming. If the acne does not respond to at-home treatment, a dermatologist can assess the situation and determine an appropriate alternative therapy. In these cases, combination therapy of two or more treatments may be used. Combination therapy may include the use of a prescription topical antimicrobial agent or topical retinoid medication. These prescription topical products can be effective for clearing mild acne.

Antimicrobials

Benzoyl Peroxide

Mechanism of Action and Pharmacokinetics. Benzoyl peroxide is the most effective and widely used nonprescription medication currently available for the treatment of noninflammatory acne. It causes irritation and desquamation (skin peeling) that prevents closure of the pilosebaceous duct. Its irritant effects cause increased turnover of epithelial cells lining the follicular duct, which then increases sloughing and promotes resolution of the comedones. When benzoyl peroxide combines with proteins

in the comedones, oxygen is released. *P. acne* is anaerobic and is destroyed in the presence of oxygen. Approximately 5% of a topical dose is absorbed systemically.

Adverse Effects. The adverse effects are dryness and irritation of the skin. Benzoyl peroxide may also bleach clothing or hair that it comes in contact with.

Keratolytics

Salicylic Acid

Mechanism of Action and Pharmacokinetics. Salicylic acid is a mild comedolytic agent and surface keratolytic (peeling agent) that helps break down blackheads and whiteheads and cuts down the shedding of cells lining the hair follicles. In cleansing preparations, salicylic acid is considered an adjunctive treatment. Absorption of topically applied salicylates is variable and depends on the dosage formulation (range, 9% to 25%). The absorbed drug is 95% eliminated in urine, and treatment for 8 to 12 weeks is needed before improvement.

Adverse Effects. The adverse effects are burning, redness, and peeling of skin.

Sulfur-Resorcinol Combination

Mechanism of Action and Pharmacokinetics. Combinations of sulfur 3% to 8% with resorcinol 2%, which enhances the effects of the sulfur, are available without prescription. The combination is a keratolytic agent, fostering cell turnover and desquamation, and helping break down blackheads and whiteheads. Sulfur is a weak keratolytic and antibacterial agent. Resorcinol primarily acts as an adjuvant boosting the effectiveness of sulfur. Pharmacokinetic data for the sulfur-resorcinol combination (Acnomel) are unavailable.

Adverse Effects. The adverse effects are redness and peeling of skin. The odor of sulfur limits its use. Resorcinol may produce brown, scaly areas, which is reversible.

Treatment of Moderate to Moderately Severe Acne

In moderate to moderately severe acne, numerous whiteheads, blackheads, papules, and pustules appear to cover from 25% to 75% of the face and/or other affected area(s). Up to 100 comedones may be visible with 15 to 50 inflammatory lesions. Moderate to moderately severe acne usually requires the help of a dermatologist and combination therapy. Treatments used for moderate to moderately severe acne are as follows:

- Physical methods, such as comedone extraction or ultraviolet (UV) light therapy
- Oral antibiotics—help stop or slow the growth of bacteria and reduce inflammation
- Vitamin A derivatives (retinoids) unplug existing comedones, allowing other topical medicines, such as antibiotics, to enter the follicles; some may also help decrease the formation of comedones
- Prescription-strength topical keratolytic agents
- Oral contraceptives (OCs)

Antibiotics

Oral and topical antibiotics may be prescribed for the treatment of acne and are initial therapy for patients with moderate to severe inflammatory acne. Systemic antibiotics decrease *P. acnes* colonization and have intrinsic antiinflammatory effects. First-line oral antibiotics have included tetracycline, doxycycline, and minocycline. Clindamycin, sulfonamides, and erythromycin are less

Over-the-Counter Acne Products

Generic Name	US Brand Name(s) / Canadian Brand Name(s)	Dosage Forms and Strengths
benzoyl peroxide[a] (numerous OTC brands)	Clearasil Stubborn Acne, Clearasil Rapid Rescue, Differin Cleanser Daily Deep, Neutrogena On-The-Spot, Neutrogena Rapid Clear Stubborn Acne Medication Spot, Oxy Advanced Care, Oxy Rapid Spot Treatment, PanOxyl, PanOxyl Foaming Acne Wash, Persa-Gel-10, Proactiv, Zapzyt Acne Treatment Gel	**Cream**: 10% **Gel**: 2.5%, 5%, 10% **Lotion**: 2.5%, 5%, **Wash/Soap**: 3.5%, 4%, 5%, 10%
	Adasept BP Acne Gel, Benzac W Wash, Benzagel Acne Care Wash, Benzagel 5, Benzagel Spot-on Acne Gel, Clean & Clear Persagel 5, Clinique Acne Solutions, Eraser, Oxy Emergency Acne Cleanser, Panoxyl Acne Wash, PanOxyl Foaming Acne Wash, Proactiv	
resorcinol and sulfur	Acnomel Adult Acne, Rezamid	**Cream**: resorcinol 2% + sulfur 8%, resorcinol 2% + sulfur 5%
	Not available	
salicylic acid[a]	Cetaphil Gentle Clear, Clean & Clear Advantage Spot Treatment, Clearasil Daily Acne Cleansing Pads, Clearasil Rapid Rescue Deep Treatment Pads, Neutrogena Acne Wash Oil-Free, ZapZyt Acne Wash	**Cleanser**: 2% **Cream**: 2% **Cloths/Pads**: 1%, 2% **Gel**: 2% **Lotion**: 2%
	Clean and Clear Advantage Acne Spot treatment Clearasil Ultra Cleansing Cream Wash, Clearasil Deep Pore Cleansing Pads, Neutrogena Rapid Clear Spot Gel, Neutrogena Acne Stress Control, Oxy Deep Daily Cleansing Pads	

[a]Generic available.

commonly used for the treatment of acne. Because the resistance of *P. acne* to erythromycin has increased, it has become a second-line agent used when treatment with tetracycline antibiotics fails or is not tolerated. The mechanism of action and adverse effects produced by these antibiotics are described in Chapter 29.

Oral antibiotics must be taken for 6 to 8 weeks before results are evident, and treatment should be given for 6 months to prevent the development of microbial resistance. Oral antibiotics may be discontinued after inflammation has resolved; however, topical antibiotics may be continued for prophylaxis. Some patients may require long-term oral antibiotic therapy to control their acne and prevent scarring.

Topical antiinfective agents are used for the treatment of acne to reduce inflammation caused by bacteria rather than having a direct bactericidal effect. Topical antiinfective medications used for the treatment of acne are clindamycin, dapsone, and erythromycin.

Retinoids

Retinoids include vitamin A and its derivatives. Adapalene, tretinoin, and tazarotene are retinoids. Topical retinoids are effective in treating noninflammatory acne because they reduce the number of comedones, prevent comedone formation, and have mild antiinflammatory properties.

Adapalene

Mechanism of Action and Pharmacokinetics. Adapalene is a retinoid-type drug that affects the growth of skin cells and thereby reduces the formation of pimples. It is available for topical use only. Adapalene modulates cell differentiation and keratinization, which is responsible for the drug's ability to break down comedones. It

is also a potent antiinflammatory agent. The absorption, distribution, and metabolism of topically applied adapalene are unknown. Excretion appears to be primarily by the biliary route.

Adverse Effects. The adverse effects are irritation, redness, dryness, itching, peeling, and burning. It may also cause photoirritant reactions.

Tretinoin

Mechanism of Action and Pharmacokinetics. Tretinoin is a retinoid. It is used for the treatment of mild to moderate acne. Tretinoin increases cell turnover in the follicular wall and decreases the cohesiveness of cells, leading to the extrusion of comedones and inhibition of the formation of new comedones. The rapid turnover of cells prevents new pimples from forming. Tretinoin is administered topically and orally. The effects of topical administration appear approximately 2 to 3 weeks after initiation of therapy. When applied for cosmetic use to reduce wrinkles, the beneficial effects may take up to 6 months to be achieved. Tretinoin is well absorbed orally, but protein binding is greater than 95%. Tretinoin is metabolized by the cytochrome P450 hepatic enzyme system, and the drug appears to induce its own metabolism.

Adverse Effects. Common adverse effects of topical tretinoin are dry skin, peeling, itching, burning, stinging, redness, and photosensitivity.

Clindamycin-Tretinoin Combination

Mechanism of Action and Pharmacokinetics. Clindamycin and tretinoin are combined as a topical formulation for the treatment of acne. Clindamycin belongs to the lincomycin antibiotics class and works by slowing or stopping the growth of bacteria.

Topical clindamycin has minimal systemic absorption. Tretinoin is minimally absorbed after topical application.

Adverse Effects. Common adverse effects are redness, scaling, dryness, itching, burning, stinging, and sunburn.

Tazarotene

Mechanism of Action and Pharmacokinetics. Tazarotene is a retinoid prodrug that modulates the differentiation and proliferation of epithelial tissue and has some antiinflammatory and immunologic activity. Absorption is minimal when applied topically. It is metabolized rapidly via esterase hydrolysis in the skin to tazarotenic acid, an active metabolite. The topical half-life ($t_{1/2}$) of tazarotenic acid is approximately 18 hours.

Adverse Effects. Common adverse effects are itching, burning, stinging, redness, irritation, swelling, dryness of the skin, and pain.

Azelaic Acid

Mechanism of Action and Pharmacokinetics. Azelaic acid occurs naturally and is found in whole grains and animal products. It reduces redness and inflammatory papules and pustules associated with rosacea and acne. It works by killing the bacteria that infect pores and by decreasing the production of keratin, a natural substance that could lead to the development of acne. Approximately 4% of topically applied azelaic acid is absorbed systemically. Azelaic acid is mainly excreted unchanged in the urine; the half-life is approximately 12 hours after topical application.

Adverse Effects. Azelaic acid may cause slight stinging or burning, tingling, redness, and drying of the skin.

Drug Treatment for Moderate to Moderately Severe Acne

Generic Name	US Brand Name(s) Canadian Brand Name(s)	Dosage Forms and Strengths
adapalene[a]	Generics[b]	**Cream**: 0.1%
	Differin, Differin XP	**Gel**: 0.1%[b,c], 0.3%
		Lotion[c]: 0.1%
		Solution[c]: 0.1%
adapalene + benzoyl peroxide	Epiduo, Epiduo Forte	**Gel**: 0.1% adapalene + 2.5% benzoyl peroxide (Epiduo, Tactupump), 0.3% adapalene + 2.5% benzoyl peroxide (Epiduo Forte, Tactupump Forte)
	Tactupump, Tactupump Forte	
alitretinoin	Panretin	**Capsule (Toctino)**[d]: 10 mg, 30 mg
	Toctino	**Gel (Panretin)**[c]: 0.1%
azelaic acid[a]	Azelex, Finacea	**Cream (Azelex)**[c]: 20%
	Finacea	**Foam (Finacea)**[c]: 15%
		Gel (Finacea): 15%
benzoyl peroxide[a]	See earlier table for OTC acne products.	See earlier table for OTC acne products.
	See earlier table for OTC acne products.	
clindamycin (topical)[a]	Cleocin T, Clinda-derm, Clindagel, Clindets, Evoclin	**Foam**: 1%
		Gel: 1%
	Generics	**Lotion**: 1%
		Solution: 1%
		Swab: 1%
erythromycin base (topical)[a]	Erygel, Erythra-Derm	**Gel**: 2%
	Not available	**Solution, topical**[c]: 2%
benzoyl peroxide + erythromycin[a]	Benzamycin	**Gel**: benzoyl peroxide 5%, erythromycin 3%
	Benzamycin	
benzoyl peroxide + clindamycin[a]	Acanya, Benzaclin, Duac, Onexton	**Gel**: benzoyl peroxide 2.5% + clindamycin phosphate 1.2% (Acanya), benzoyl peroxide 3% + clindamycin 1% (Clindoxyl ADV), benzoyl peroxide 3.75% + clindamycin 1.2% (Onexton), benzoyl peroxide 5% + clindamycin phosphate 1.2% (Duac), benzoyl peroxide 5% + clindamycin phosphate 1% (Benzaclin, Clindoxyl)
	Benzaclin, Clindoxyl, Clindoxyl ADV	
dapsone[a,c]	Aczone	**Gel**: 5%, 7.5%
	Aczone	

Continued

Drug Treatment for Moderate to Moderately Severe Acne—cont'd

Generic Name	US Brand Name(s) / Canadian Brand Name(s)	Dosage Forms and Strengths
doxycycline hyclate[a]	Acticlate, Doryx, Oracea[e], Vibramycin, Doxycin, Doxytab, (Apprilon, Periostat)[e]	**Capsule:** 50 mg, 100 mg, 150 mg, 20 mg (Periostat), 40 mg (Oracea) **Tablet:** 20 mg, 75 mg, 100 mg, 150 mg **Tablet, delayed release:** 50 mg, 75 mg, 80 mg, 100 mg, 150 mg, 200 mg (Doryx), 60 mg, 120 mg (Doryx MPC)
doxycycline monohydrate[a]	Avidoxy, Monodox, Oracea / Not available	**Capsule:** 50 mg, 75 mg, 100 mg, 150 mg (Monodox) **Tablet (Avidoxy):** 100 mg
minocycline[a]	Amzeeq, Dynacin, Minocin, Minolira, Soladyn, Ximino / Generics	**Capsule (Dynacin, Minocin):** 50 mg, 75 mg[c], 100 mg **Capsule, extended release (Ximino)[c]:** 45 mg, 90 mg, 135 mg **Foam:** 1.5% (Zilxi), 4% (Amzeeq) **Tablet[c]:** 50 mg, 75 mg, 100 mg **Tablet ER[c]:** 55 mg, 65 mg, 80 mg, 105 mg, 115 mg (Solodyn), 105 mg, 135 mg (Minolira)
tetracycline[a]	Achromycin V / Generics	**Capsule:** 250 mg, 500 mg[c]
tazarotene[a]	Arazlo, Avage, Fabior, Tazorac / Arazlo, Tazorac	**Cream:** 0.05%, 0.1% **Foam (Fabior):** 0.1% **Gel:** 0.05%, 0.1% **Lotion:** 0.045%
tretinoin[a]	Altreno, Atralin, Avita, Renova, Retin-A, Retin-A Micro, Tretin-X / Retin-A, Retin-A Micro, Stieva-A, Vitamin A Acid	**Cream:** 0.01% (Stieva-A), 0.02% (Renova), 0.025% (Retin-A, Avita, Stieva-A), 0.05%, 0.1% (Avita, Retin-A, Stieva-A) **Gel:** 0.01%, 0.025% (Avita, Retin-A), 0.04%, 0.06%, 0.08%, 0.1% (Retin-A Micro), 0.05% (Atralin), 0.1% (Retin-A, Retin-A Micro) **Lotion:** 0.05% **Solution:** 0.05% (Retin A)
tretinoin + benzoyl peroxide	Twyneo / Not available	**Cream:** 0.1% tretinoin + 3% benzoyl peroxide
tretinoin + clindamycin[a]	Veltin, Ziana / Biacna	**Gel:** tretinoin 0.025% + clindamycin phosphate 1.2%

[a]Generic available.
[b]Over the counter.
[c]Available in the United States only.
[d]Available in Canada only.
[e]Indicated for treatment of periodontal disease or Lyme disease. See Chapter 29.
OTC, Over the counter.

Treatment of Severe Acne

Severe acne is characterized by deep cysts, inflammation, extensive damage to the skin, and scarring. Severe acne is characterized by more than 100 comedones, inflammatory lesions, and cysts. It requires an aggressive treatment regimen and should be treated by a dermatologist. Severe disfiguring forms of acne can require years of treatment, and individuals may experience one or more treatment failures. Almost every case of acne can be successfully treated. Treatment involves nonpharmaceutical methods and medications (isotretinoin, antibiotics, OCs). The pharmacology of OCs is described in Chapter 27.

Isotretinoin

For patients with severe inflammatory acne that does not improve with the medications discussed earlier, the physician may prescribe isotretinoin, a retinoid (vitamin A derivative). Isotretinoin is an oral drug that is usually taken once or twice daily with food for 15 to 20 weeks. Isotretinoin decreases the size and output of sebaceous glands and makes the cells that are sloughed off into the sebaceous glands less sticky and therefore less able to form comedones.

Adverse Reactions

Isotretinoin can produce fetal abnormalities. Women must use two separate, effective forms of birth control at the same time for 1 month before treatment begins, during the entire course of treatment, and for 1 full month after stopping the drug.

Other possible side effects of isotretinoin include dry eyes, mouth, lips, nose, or skin (very common), itching, nosebleeds, muscle aches, sensitivity to the sun, poor night vision, changes in mood, depression, suicidal thoughts, changes in the blood lipids (e.g., an increase in fat levels in the blood [triglycerides, cholesterol]), and changes in liver function. Blood tests to determine baseline liver function are taken before isotretinoin is started and periodically during treatment. Side effects usually cease after the medicine is stopped. Oral administration of isotretinoin may produce hyperglycemia.

> **❶ Tech Alert!**
>
> Isotretinoin must be dispensed in the manufacturer's original packaging with the warning label "Avoid Pregnancy."

FDA iPLEDGE Program for Isotretinoin

To make sure that women do not become pregnant while taking isotretinoin, the U.S. Food and Drug Administration (FDA) requires wholesalers, prescribers, pharmacies, and patients to participate in the iPLEDGE risk minimization program. Only prescribers registered and activated in iPLEDGE can prescribe isotretinoin, and only patients registered and qualified in iPLEDGE can be given isotretinoin.

See the following website for more details on the iPLEDGE program: https://www.ipledgeprogram.com.

Treatment for Severe Acne

Generic Name	US Brand Name(s) Canadian Brand Name(s)	Dosage Forms and Strengths
isotretinoin[a,b]	Absorica, Amnesteem, Claravis, Myorisan, Zenatane Accutane, Clarus, Epuris	**Capsule:** 10 mg, 20 mg, 30 mg, 40 mg (Amnesteem, Accutane, Clarus, Claravis, Epuris, Myorisan, Zenatane), 25 mg[b], 35 mg[b] (Absorica), 8 mg, 16 mg, 20 mg, 24 mg, 28 mg, 32 mg (Absorica LD)
oral antibiotics	See Chapter 29.	See Chapter 29.

[a]Generic available.
[b]Available in the United States only.

Treatment of Hormonally Influenced Acne in Women

In some women, acne is caused by an excess of androgen hormones. They may exhibit hirsutism (excessive growth of hair on the face or body), premenstrual acne flares, irregular menstrual cycles, and elevated blood levels of certain androgens. The physician may prescribe one of several drugs to treat women with this type of acne.

Oral Contraceptives

OCs help suppress androgens produced by the ovaries. Side effects are nausea, weight gain, menstrual spotting, and breast tenderness. OCs used to treat acne typically have estrogen and progestins with a low androgen level. OCs that produce low androgenic effects include drospirenone, desogestrel, and norgestimate. The choice of OC is typically based on tolerability.

Treatment of Hormonally Induced Acne in Women

Generic Name	US Brand Name(s) Canadian Brand Name(s)	Dosage Forms and Strengths
oral contraceptives[a]	See Chapter 27.	See Chapter 27.

[a]A complete listing of oral contraceptives is given in Chapter 27.

Nonpharmaceutical Treatment of Acne

Physicians may use other types of procedures in addition to drug therapy to treat patients with acne. For example, the physician may remove the patient's comedones during an office visit. Sometimes the physician will inject corticosteroids directly into lesions to help reduce the size and pain of inflamed cysts and nodules.

If scarring has occurred, dermabrasion (or microdermabrasion), which is a form of sanding down scars, is sometimes used. Another treatment option for deep scars caused by cystic acne is the transfer of fat from another part of the body to the scar. Alternatively, a synthetic filling material may be injected under the scar to improve its appearance.

TECHNICIAN'S CORNER

1. There are many OTC and prescription medications available for the treatment of acne. Make a list of prescription acne products that contain benzoyl peroxide.
2. What advice might be given to a teenager with acne about self-care?

Summary of Drugs Used for the Treatment of Acne

Generic Name	Brand Name	Usual Dose and Dosing Schedule	Warning Labels
Topical			
adapalene	Differin	Apply once daily at bedtime	FOR EXTERNAL USE ONLY—all. KEEP AWAY FROM EYES, EARS, AND MOUTH—azelaic acid, benzoyl peroxide + clindamycin, salicylic acid. BLEACHING AGENT; AVOID CONTACT WITH FABRIC AND HAIR—benzoyl peroxide. DO NOT USE IF PREGNANT—tazarotene, tretinoin. MAY CAUSE SENSITIVITY TO SUNLIGHT—tretinoin, tretinoin + clindamycin.
azelaic acid	Azelex	Apply and massage a thin film into affected area twice daily	
benzoyl peroxide	Various OTC and prescription brands and generics	**Cleansers:** Wash once or twice daily **Topical:** Apply sparingly once daily; increase to 2 or 3 times daily if needed	
benzoyl peroxide + clindamycin	BenzaClin, Duac	**BenzaClin:** Apply twice daily **Duac:** Apply once daily in the evening	
benzoyl peroxide + erythromycin	Benzamycin	Apply twice daily, morning and evening	
dapsone	Aczone	Apply a small amount twice daily	
resorcinol + sulfur	Acnomel	Apply a small amount to affected area as directed by physician	
salicylic acid	Clean and Clear Advantage Acne Spot treatment	**Cream, cloth, foam, liquid, gel:** Apply to skin once or twice daily and rinse thoroughly **Pads:** Apply to affected area 1–3 times daily **Wash:** Wash once daily	
tazarotene	Avage, Tazorac	Apply thin film once daily in the evening to the affected area	
tretinoin	Renova, Retin-A	Apply to acne lesions once daily before bedtime or on alternate days	
tretinoin + clindamycin	Ziana, Veltin	Apply to entire face every night at bedtime	
Systemic			
doxycycline	Vibramycin	50–100 mg twice daily or 40 mg (Oracea) once daily	AVOID PROLONGED SUNLIGHT—doxycycline, minocycline, isotretinoin. AVOID TAKING ANTACIDS, IRON, AND DAIRY PRODUCTS—minocycline. TAKE WITH FOOD—isotretinoin. AVOID PREGNANCY—doxycycline, minocycline, isotretinoin. AVOID USE OF VITAMIN A PRODUCTS—isotretinoin.
erythromycin	Various brands and generics	**Oral:** 250–500 mg twice daily	
isotretinoin	Accutane, Clarus, Clavaris	0.5–1 mg/kg/day PO given in two divided doses for 15–20 weeks	
minocycline	Solodyn ER	Take dose (1 mg/kg) once daily	
tetracycline	Generics	250–500 mg/dose every 6 h	

OTC, Over the counter; *PO*, by mouth/orally.

Key Points

- Acne is a disorder resulting from the action of hormones and other substances on the skin's oil glands (sebaceous glands) and hair follicles.
- Common acne, or acne vulgaris, occurs most frequently during adolescence as a result of overactive secretion by the sebaceous glands, accompanied by blockages and inflammation of their ducts.
- Pus-filled pimples, or pustules, that erupt on the skin are caused by secondary infections within or beneath the epidermis, often in a hair follicle or sweat pore.
- The goals of treatment for acne are to heal existing lesions, stop new lesions from forming, prevent scarring, and minimize the psychological stress and embarrassment caused by this disease.
- Benzoyl peroxide is the most effective and widely used nonprescription medication currently available for the treatment of noninflammatory acne.
- Salicylic acid is a mild comedolytic agent (keratolytic) that provides a milder, less effective alternative to the prescription agent tretinoin.
- Topical over-the-counter (OTC) medicines are available in many forms, such as gels, lotions, creams, soaps, and pads. In

some people, OTC acne medicines may cause side effects such as skin irritation, burning, or redness, which often get better or go away with continued use of the medicine.
- Adapalene is believed to affect the growth of skin cells and thereby reduce the formation of pimples.
- Azelaic acid works by killing the bacteria that infect pores and by decreasing the production of keratin, a natural substance that could lead to the development of acne.
- Tazarotene modulates the differentiation and proliferation of epithelial tissue and has some antiinflammatory and immunologic activity.
- Tretinoin increases cell turnover in the follicular wall and decreases the cohesiveness of cells.
- Severe acne is characterized by deep cysts, inflammation, extensive damage to the skin, and scarring. It requires an aggressive treatment regimen and should be treated by a dermatologist.
- For patients with severe inflammatory acne, a physician may prescribe isotretinoin, a retinoid (vitamin A derivative).
- Early treatment is the best way to prevent acne scars. Once scarring has occurred, dermabrasion may be used to treat irregular scars.

Review Questions

1. An enlarged and plugged hair follicle, the most characteristic sign of acne, is called a _____.
   a. milia
   b. pustule
   c. comedone
   d. papule
2. The warning label "Avoid Pregnancy" should be applied to prescription containers for _____.
   a. isotretinoin
   b. erythromycin
   c. salicylic acid
   d. benzoyl peroxide
3. _____ is the most effective and widely used nonprescription medication currently available for the treatment of noninflammatory acne.
   a. Salicylic acid
   b. Benzoyl peroxide
   c. Sulfur
   d. Doxycycline
4. At-home treatment for acne requires _____ to see improvement.
   a. 2 to 4 weeks
   b. 4 to 8 weeks
   c. 6 to 10 weeks
   d. 8 to 10 weeks
5. When acne is resistant to topical therapies, intravenous antibiotics may be used.
   a. true
   b. false

6. Which of the following oral antibiotics is less commonly used for the treatment of moderate to severe acne?
   a. Doxycycline
   b. Tetracycline
   c. Clindamycin
   d. Minocycline
7. _____ work(s) by killing the bacteria that infect pores and by decreasing the production of keratin, a natural substance that could lead to the development of acne.
   a. Azelaic acid
   b. Adapalene
   c. Benzoyl peroxide
   d. a and c
8. _____ is an effective medicine that can help prevent scarring.
   a. Tretinoin
   b. Isotretinoin
   c. Retinoin
   d. All of the above
9. Oral contraceptives are used to treat which type of acne?
   a. Mild
   b. Moderate
   c. Severe
   d. Hormonally induced
10. Which of the following drugs are used for treating hormonally influenced acne?
    a. Corticosteroids
    b. Antiandrogens
    c. Progestins
    d. All of the above

Bibliography

Decker A, Graber EM. Over-the-counter acne treatments: a review. *J Clin Aesthet Dermatol*. 2012;5(5):32–40.

Health Canada. (2023). Drug Product Database. Retrieved January 14, 2023, from https://www.canada.ca/en/health-canada/services/drugs-health-products/drug-products/drug-product-database.html.

Mayo Clinic Staff. (2018). Over-the-counter acne products: What works and why. Retrieved July 21, 2022, from https://www.mayo-clinic.org/diseases-conditions/acne/in-depth/acne-treatments/art-20045814?pg=2&p=1.

National Institute of Arthritis and Musculoskeletal and Skin Diseases. (2020). Acne. NIH Publication No. 15-4998. Retrieved January 17, 2020, from https://www.niams.nih.gov/health-topics/acne.

Repchinsky C. *Compendium of self-care products*. ed 2. Canadian Pharmacists Association; 2010:173–174.

Repchinsky C. *Patient self-care: helping your patients make therapeutic choices*. ed 2. Canadian Pharmacists Association; 2010:577–596.

Thibodeau G, Patton K. *Anatomy and physiology*. ed 6. St Louis: Mosby; 2007.

Titus S, Hodge J. Diagnosis and treatment of acne. *Am Fam Physician*. 2012;86(8):734–740.

U.S. Food and Drug Administration. (nd). Drugs@FDA: FDA Approved Drug Products. Retrieved January 14, 2023, from https://www.access-data.fda.gov/scripts/cder/daf/index.cfm.

Zaenglein AL, Pathy AL, Schlosser BJ, et al. Guidelines of care for the management of acne vulgaris. *J Am Acad Dermatol*. 2016;74:945–973.

36

Treatment of Atopic Dermatitis and Psoriasis

LEARNING OBJECTIVES

1. Learn the terminology associated with atopic dermatitis and psoriasis.
2. Describe the causes of atopic dermatitis and psoriasis.
3. List the symptoms of atopic dermatitis and psoriasis.
4. List and categorize medications used to treat atopic dermatitis and psoriasis.
5. Describe the mechanism of action for drugs used to treat atopic dermatitis and psoriasis.
6. Identify significant drug look-alike and sound-alike issues.
7. Identify warning labels and precautionary messages associated with medications used to treat atopic dermatitis and psoriasis.

KEY TERMS

Atopic dermatitis Chronic inflammatory disease of the skin.
Cutaneous Pertaining to the skin.
Dermatitis Inflammation of the skin.
Eczema General term used to describe several types of inflammation of the skin.
Phototherapy Treatment for atopic dermatitis that involves exposing the skin to ultraviolet A or B light waves.

Plaque psoriasis Most common form of psoriasis. It is characterized by raised, inflamed (red) lesions covered with a silvery white scale.
Psoriasis Chronic disease of the skin characterized by itchy red patches covered with silvery scales.

Overview

Eczema is a general term used to describe several types of inflammation of the skin. It is a common condition affecting millions of Americans and Canadians. There are several types of eczema—atopic dermatitis, allergic contact eczema, contact eczema, dyshidrotic eczema, neurodermatitis, nummular eczema, seborrheic eczema, and stasis dermatitis.

Atopic refers a group of diseases in which there is an inherited tendency to develop other allergic conditions. *Atopic dermatitis* is the most common form of eczema. Atopic dermatitis affects 20% of school-aged children and 10% of adults globally. It is a chronic disease of the skin that often develops in infancy and may continue throughout adulthood. It is a forerunner to asthma and food allergies. Up to 40% of individuals who have eczema (atopic dermatitis) also have allergies, asthma, and food allergies.

Unlike contact *dermatitis* (inflammation of the skin), in which symptoms appear after exposure to an allergen, the cause of atopic dermatitis is unknown. Atopic dermatitis is characterized by an autoimmune-mediated inflammatory response that produces abnormal changes in epidermal skin cells and a hyperactive dermal response to irritants. Common irritants are listed in Box 36.1.

Psoriasis is another autoimmune, chronic inflammatory condition of the skin. It affects 2% to 5% of the global population.

Psoriasis is a condition associated with the rapid turnover of skin cells. The normal rate of cell turnover is approximately 30 days, but the cell turnover rate may be as short as 3 to 4 days in people who have psoriasis.

Symptoms of Atopic Dermatitis and Psoriasis

Atopic dermatitis commonly produces symptoms of intense itching, redness (from scratching), skin irritation, and inflammation (Box 36.2). Eczematous patches may form that are flaky and crusting and may even ooze a clear fluid (Fig. 36.1). Individuals with psoriasis have thick silvery scaly patches; this is the most common type, known as *plaque psoriasis*. They may also have some redness and swelling. Itchy psoriatic patches may be found on the neck, elbows, genitals, scalp, hands, and feet.

Individuals with atopic dermatitis and psoriasis may experience periods when their symptoms worsen (exacerbation) and periods when they get better or go away completely (remission). It is not uncommon for eczema that has gone into remission in childhood to return with the onset of puberty. Factors that exacerbate symptoms of atopic dermatitis and psoriasis are as follows:
- Stress
- Contact with environmental pollutants and household cleaning products

- Food allergy (e.g., to eggs, peanuts, milk, fish, soy products, wheat)
- Wearing wool or clothing that rubs and irritates skin
- Factors that cause dry skin (e.g., low-humidity environments, not applying moisturizer, hot baths)
- Scratching

Scratching can break down the protective layer of the skin and increase the risk of developing secondary bacterial or viral infections.

Nonpharmaceutical Treatment of Atopic Dermatitis and Psoriasis

Nonpharmaceutical treatment for atopic dermatitis and other forms of eczema involves using skin care regimens that reduce irritation and avoiding allergens and known irritants (Box 36.3). Nonpharmaceutical treatment of psoriasis may also include the use of phototherapy. ***Phototherapy*** involves exposing the skin to ultraviolet (UV) A or B light waves. It may be used alone or in combination with drug therapy. Phototherapy is recommended only for those older than 12 years. Adverse reactions to the use of UV light therapy are premature aging of the skin and increased risk for skin cancer.

Dietary supplements and nutraceuticals have been promoted to benefit atopic dermatitis. They include probiotics, prebiotics, vitamin D, fish oil, evening primrose oil, borage seed oil, and Chinese herbal medicine. To date, only the combination of prebiotics and probiotics (symbiotics) has shown some benefit over placebo in randomized controlled trials. More studies are needed.

Pharmaceutical Treatment of Eczema and Psoriasis

The use of topical agents is a first-line treatment strategy for the treatment of atopic dermatitis, psoriasis, seborrhea, and other inflammatory skin conditions. Absorption of drugs across psoriatic skin is poor because thick, scaly plaques and dry skin reduce penetration of topically applied drugs. This may limit the effectiveness of topical treatments.

• BOX 36.1   Common Irritants

- Wool or synthetic fibers
- Soaps and detergents
- Perfumes and cosmetics
- Cleaning solvents, mineral oil, and chlorine
- Dust
- Sand

• BOX 36.2   Signs and Symptoms of Eczema

- Dry, rectangular scales on the skin
- Small rough bumps and papules on arms, legs, face
- Thickened, leathery patches of skin
- Inflammation around the corners of the mouth and face rash
- Darkened eyelids and skin around the eyes
- Extra skin fold under the eye
- Excess creases in the palms of the hands
- Hives (urticaria)
- Intense itching
- Redness

---

❶ Tech Alert!

The following drugs have look-alike/sound-alike issues:
fluocinolone and fluocinonide;
hydrocortisone, hydrocortisone butyrate, and hydrocortisone valerate;
betamethasone dipropionate and betamethasone valerate.

Corticosteroids

The use of topical corticosteroids continues to be a mainstay of therapy for the treatment of atopic dermatitis and psoriasis. The use of oral corticosteroids is reserved for severe symptoms.

• BOX 36.3   Recommended Skin Care for Persons with Eczema

- Avoid hot baths or showers
- Air-dry or gently pat skin dry after bathing (avoid vigorous rubbing)

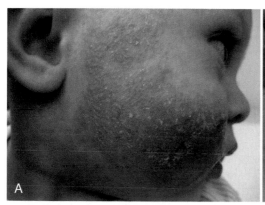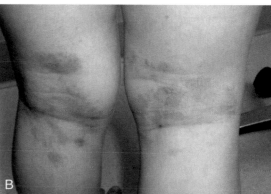

• **Fig. 36.1** Eczema. (A) Infantile phase. (B) Childhood phase. (A and B from Fitzpatrick JE, Morelli JG. *Dermatology secrets in color*, ed 3, Philadelphia, 2007, Mosby.)

• BOX 36.4   Potency Classification of Selected Topical Corticosteroids (Generic Names)

Class I: Super High Potency
- Clobetasol propionate
- Diflorasone diacetate

Class II: Super Potent
- Betamethasone dipropionate (optimized vehicle)
- Halobetasol propionate

Class III: Very Potent
- Amcinonide
- Desoximetasone
- Halcinonide
- Fluocinonide
- Mometasone furoate
- Diflorasone diacetate (cream)
- Triamcinolone (>0.5%)

Class IV: Potent
- Betamethasone dipropionate (regular vehicle)
- Flurandrenolide (ointment)
- Mometasone furoate

Class V: Medium Potency
- Beclomethasone
- Betamethasone valerate
- Diflucortolone valerate
- Fluocinolone acetonide
- Flurandrenolide (cream)
- Fluticasone propionate (cream)
- Hydrocortisone butyrate (cream)
- Hydrocortisone valerate (cream)
- Triamcinolone acetonide (>0.5%)

Class VI: Mild Potency
- Alclometasone dipropionate (cream, ointment)
- Desonide (cream)
- Prednicarbate

Class VII: Mildest Potency
- Dexamethasone
- Hydrocortisone base

Adapted from Raymond G, Houle M.-C. A review of corticosteroids for the treatment of psoriasis. *Skin Ther Lett* 2, 2007 (http://www.skintherapyletter.com/pharmacist-edition/corticosteroids-psoriasis-pharm/).

Topical corticosteroids are categorized into seven groups based on potency (Box 36.4). Class I agents (e.g., diflorasone diacetate) are superhigh potency. Class VII agents include hydrocortisone, which is mild enough for over-the-counter (OTC) use. The vehicle (base) in which the corticosteroid is suspended may influence the potency. For example, the betamethasone dipropionate augmented formula is formulated in a base that is superpotent (class II), whereas the same drug in a nonaugmented base is less potent (class IV). Higher potency corticosteroids have more adverse reactions. Only the mildest potency agents, such as hydrocortisone, should be used on the face.

Mechanism of Action and Pharmacokinetics

Topical corticosteroids possess antiinflammatory and immunosuppressive properties and produce vasoconstriction. They reduce the permeability of the cells to T lymphocytes and eosinophils, thereby decreasing the release of mediators of the inflammatory response (e.g., cytokines). They also reduce the number of inflammatory cells, which decreases redness, swelling, and inflammation.

Adverse Effects

Long-term use of topical corticosteroids can result in thinning of the skin, stretch marks (striae), spider veins, acne, milia, rosacea (enlarged blood vessels, especially on the nose), bruising, atrophy, lacerations, and poor wound healing when applied topically. Adverse reactions are more extensive when high-potency corticosteroids are used and they are applied to a large body surface area.

Topical Corticosteroids

Generic Name	US Brand Name(s) / Canadian Brand Name(s)	Dosage Forms and Strengths
alclometasone dipropionate[a]	Generics	**Cream:** 0.05%
	Not available	**Ointment:** 0.05%
amcinonide[a]	Generics	**Cream:** 0.1%
	Generics	**Lotion**[b]**:** 0.1% **Ointment**[b]**:** 0.1%
betamethasone dipropionate[a]	Diprolene, Sernivo	**Cream:** 0.05%
	Diprolene, Diprosone, Topilene, Topisone	**Gel, augmented:** 0.05%[b] **Lotion:** 0.05% **Lotion, augmented:** 0.05% **Ointment:** 0.05% **Ointment, augmented:** 0.05% **Spray, topical (Sernivo):** 0.05%

Continued

Topical Corticosteroids—cont'd

Generic Name	US Brand Name(s) / Canadian Brand Name(s)	Dosage Forms and Strengths
betamethasone valerate[a]	Beta-Val, Dermabet, Luxiq, Valnac	**Cream:** 0.05%[c], 0.1% **Lotion:** 0.05%[c], 0.1% **Ointment:** 0.05%[c], 0.1% **Topical foam (Luxiq):** 0.12%
	Betaderm	
clobetasol propionate[a]	Clobex, Cormax, Embeline, Impoyz, Olux, Olux-E	**Cream:** 0.025%[b], 0.05% **Foam (Olux, Olux-E):** 0.05% **Gel:** 0.05%[b] **Lotion:** 0.05% **Ointment:** 0.05% **Shampoo:** 0.05% **Spray:** 0.05% **Solution:** 0.05%
	Clobex, Dermovate	
clocortolone	Cloderm	**Cream:** 0.1%
	Not available	
desonide[a]	Desonate, Desowen, Verdeso	**Cream:** 0.05% **Foam (Verdeso)[b]:** 0.05% **Gel[b]:** 0.05% **Lotion[b]:** 0.05% **Ointment:** 0.05%
	Tridesilon	
desoximetasone[d]	Topicort	**Cream:** 0.05%, 0.25% (Topicort) **Gel:** 0.05% **Ointment:** 0.25%, 0.05%[b] **Spray[b]:** 0.25%
	Generics	
diflorasone diacetate[a]	Generics	**Cream:** 0.05% **Ointment:** 0.05%
	Not available	
fluocinolone acetonide[a,b]	Capex, DermaSmoothe/FS, Dermotic, Synalar	**Cream:** 0.01%, 0.025% **Oil, topical (Dermotic[c], DermaSmoothe/FS):** 0.01% **Ointment:** 0.025% **Shampoo (Capex):** 0.01% **Solution:** 0.01%
	DermaSmoothe/FS, Dermotic	
fluocinonide[a,b]	Lidex, Vanos	**Cream:** 0.05%, 0.1%[b] **Cream, emulsified (Lidemol):** 0.05% **Gel:** 0.05% **Ointment:** 0.05% **Solution:** 0.05%[b]
	Lidemol, Lidex, Lyderm, Tiamol	
flurandrenolide[a]	Cordran, Cordran SP, Cordran Tape	**Cream:** 0.025%, 0.05% **Lotion:** 0.05% **Ointment:** 0.05% **Tape:** 4 mcg/cm²
	Not available	
fluticasone propionate[a]	Generics	**Cream:** 0.05% **Lotion:** 0.05% **Ointment:** 0.005%
	Not available	
halcinonide[a]	Halog	**Cream:** 0.1% **Ointment:** 0.1% **Solution, topical:** 0.1%
	Not available	
halobetasol propionate[a,b]	Bryhali, Lexette, Ultravate	**Cream:** 0.05% **Foam (Lexette):** 0.05% **Lotion:** 0.01%, 0.05% **Ointment[d]:** 0.05%
	Bryhali, Ultravate	

Topical Corticosteroids—cont'd

Generic Name	US Brand Name(s)	Dosage Forms and Strengths
	Canadian Brand Name(s)	
hydrocortisone base[a] (only topical prescription trade names listed)	Ala-cort, Ala-Scalp, Stie-cort, Texacort	**Cream:** 1%, 2.5%
	Generics[d]	**Lotion:** 1%, 2%[b], 2.5%[b]
		Ointment: 1%
		Solution (Texacort): 2.5%
hydrocortisone acetate[a] (only prescription trade names listed)	Micort HC	**Cream:** 2.5%
	OTC only[d]	
hydrocortisone butyrate[a]	Locoid, Locoid Lipocream	**Cream:** 0.1%
	Not available	**Cream, lipocream:** 0.1%
		Lotion: 0.1%
		Ointment: 0.1%
		Solution: 0.1%
hydrocortisone probutate	Pandel	**Cream:** 0.1%
	Not available	
hydrocortisone valerate[a,b]	Generics	**Cream:** 0.2%
	Hydroval	**Ointment:** 0.2%
mometasone furoate[a]	Elocon	**Cream:** 0.1%
	Elocom	**Lotion:** 0.1%
		Ointment: 0.1%
prednicarbate[a,b]	Generics	**Cream, emollient:** 0.1%
	Dermatop	**Ointment:** 0.1%
triamcinolone acetonide[a]	Kenalog, Trianex, Triderm	**Cream:** 0.025%[b], 0.1%, 0.5%
	Aristocort C, Aristocort R, Triaderm	**Lotion**[b]**:** 0.025%, 0.1%
		Ointment: 0.05%[b], 0.1%
		Topical spray (Kenalog): 0.147 mg/g

[a]Generic available.
[b]Available in the United States only.
[c]Ear drops.
[d]Hydrocortisone topical 1% or less OTC in Canada.
OTC, Over the counter.

Immunomodulators: Calcineurin Inhibitors

Calcineurin inhibitors are immunomodulators. They control inflammation and reduce the immune system response to allergens. Pimecrolimus is indicated for the treatment of mild to moderate atopic dermatitis. It is approved for short-term and intermittent long-term therapy. Tacrolimus is approved for the treatment of moderate to severe atopic dermatitis that has failed to respond to corticosteroid treatment. Pimecrolimus and tacrolimus are not effective in treating plaque psoriasis.

Mechanism of Action and Pharmacokinetics

Pimecrolimus and tacrolimus inhibit T-cell activation and the production of cytokines, interleukins, and interferons that mediate the inflammatory response. Pharmacokinetic data on pimecrolimus are limited. Absorption through the skin is minimal and **cutaneous** metabolism is negligible. Pimecrolimus is marketed as a cream for topical application to affected areas. Tacrolimus ointment (Protopic) is used for the treatment of atopic dermatitis. Tacrolimus capsules and solution for injection (Avagraf

and Prograf) are used to reduce organ transplant rejection (see Chapter 32).

Adverse Effects

Common adverse reactions associated with topical application are local burning and itching of the skin. The US Food and Drug Administration (FDA) and Health Canada require manufacturers to include a boxed warning in the package insert, advising health care providers that pimecrolimus and tacrolimus may increase the risk for the development of lymphoma.

⊘ Tech Alert!

Prograf and PROzac have look-alike/sound-alike issues.

Vitamin D Analogs

Calcitriol is an active form of vitamin D_3. Calcipotriene is a synthetic analog of vitamin D. Its generic name is calcipotriol in

Calcineurin Inhibitors

Generic Name	US Brand Name(s) Canadian Brand Name(s)	Dosage Forms and Strengths[b]
pimecrolimus[a,b]	Elidel	**Cream:** 1%
	Elidel	
tacrolimus[a,b]	Protopic	**Ointment (Protoptic):** 0.03%, 0.1%
	Protopic	

[a]Generic available.
[b]Only topical dosage forms listed in table.

Canada. Calcitriol and calcipotriene (calcipotriol) are approved for the treatment of psoriasis. Signs of improvement can be seen in approximately 2 weeks after calcipotriene administration; however, maximum effects may take 4 to 8 weeks.

> ● *Tech Note!*
>
> Calcitriol capsules and oral solution (Rocaltrol) are used in the treatment of hypocalcemia caused by dialysis and vitamin D–resistant rickets.

Mechanism of Action and Pharmacokinetics

Calcipotriene (calcipotriol) inhibits the rapid and repeated production of new skin cells (proliferation). It inhibits the proliferation of T cells and the release of mediators of inflammation (e.g., cytokines, interleukins, interferons). The mechanism of action for topical calcitriol is unknown. When applied to skin with psoriasis, approximately 6% of the drug is absorbed. Absorption is slightly

less through intact skin (5%). Calcipotriene is rapidly metabolized to vitamin D_3 in the liver.

Adverse Effects

Most adverse reactions are localized to the site of application. Irritation and redness are common. When large areas of the body are covered with the drug, some systemic absorption may occur. Vitamin D plays an important role in calcium absorption. Calcipotriene (calcipotriol) can raise calcium levels in the blood and urine.

Furanocoumarins

The psoralens are a class of drugs that increase photosensitivity and are classified as furanocoumarins. Methoxsalen, the only drug in this class, is derived from a naturally occurring photoactive substance that is found in the seeds of the *Ammi majus* (Umbelliferae) plant. It is approved for the treatment of atopic dermatitis and psoriasis, along with UV light therapy. Methoxsalen and UV light work synergistically. Methoxsalen increases the skin's sensitivity to UV light, and UV light activates methoxsalen. Psoralen plus UVA light therapy is also known as PUVA.

> ● *Tech Note!*
>
> Methoxsalen solution for injection (UVADEX) is used for the treatment of cutaneous T-cell lymphoma (see Chapter 31).

Mechanism of Action and Pharmacokinetics

The action of methoxsalen on pyrimidine bases of the DNA molecule results in the suppression of DNA synthesis, which decreases cell replication and proliferation. DNA photo damage produces cutaneous immunosuppression by affecting leukocyte regulatory mechanisms. Psoralens may be administered orally, topically, or parenterally. Oxsoralen-Ultra should be taken with low-fat food

Vitamin D Analogs*

Generic Name	US Brand Name(s) Canadian Brand Name(s)	Dosage Forms and Strengths
calcipotriene[b] (calcipotriol in Canada)	Dovonex, Sorilux	**Cream**[b]: 0.005% **Foam (Sorilux)**[b]: 0.005%
	Dovonex	**Solution, scalp**[b]: 0.005% **Ointment:** 0.005%
calcipotriene + betamethasone dipropionate[a]calcipotriol + betamethasone dipropionate[a] (Canada)	Enstilar, Taclonex, Taclonex Scalp, Wynzora	**Cream (Wynzora):** 0.064% betamethasone + 0.005% calcipotriene **Foam (Enstilar):** 0.064% betamethasone + 0.005% calcipotriene (calcipotriol)
	Dovobet, Enstilar	**Gel (Dovobet):** 0.05% betamethasone + 0.005% calcipotriol **Ointment:** 0.05% betamethasone + 0.005% calcipotriol (Dovobet), 0.064% betamethasone + 0.005% calcipotriene (Taclonex) **Suspension (Taclonex):** 0.064% betamethasone + 0.005% calcipotriene
calcitriol	Vectical	**Ointment:** 3 mcg/g
	Silkis	

[a]Generic available.
[b]Generic is only available in the United States.
*Only topical dosage forms listed in table.

or milk. Methoxsalen is extensively metabolized in the liver, and 90% to 95% is eliminated in urine. The elimination half-life is approximately 2 hours.

Adverse Effects

Adverse reactions produced by oral methoxsalen therapy are photosensitivity, insomnia, headache, dizziness, leg cramps, itching, dry skin, nausea, and vomiting. Topical application can cause burning, blistering, and swelling at the site of application.

Furanocoumarins Used to Treat Psoriasis

Generic Name	US Brand Name(s) —— Canadian Brand Name(s)	Dosage Forms and Strengths
methoxsalen	Oxsoralen-Ultra —— Not available	**Capsule** (Oxsoralen-Ultra): 10 mg

Immunosuppressives and Immunomodulators

Atopic dermatitis is believed to be an autoimmune disease; therefore immune system modulation and immunosuppression can downregulate the body's response to allergens and other irritants. Cyclosporine and methotrexate are immunosuppressants used for the treatment of psoriasis. Both drugs are used to treat other conditions, such as cancer (Chapter 31), and methotrexate is also used to treat rheumatoid arthritis (Chapter 13). Cyclosporine is approved by the FDA for the short-term treatment of severe atopic dermatitis and psoriasis. Methotrexate is an antimetabolite that is indicated for the treatment of moderate to severe chronic psoriasis and psoriatic arthritis. Apremilast (Otezla) is approved for moderate to severe plaque psoriasis.

Etanercept, infliximab, and adalimumab are biologic agents that are indicated for the treatment of psoriasis. They are classified as tumor necrosis factor (TNF)-α inhibitors. TNF-α inhibitors are genetically engineered drugs that block the inflammatory process triggered by high concentrations of TNF. Psoriasis is a condition that is linked to high levels of TNF-α. TNF-α inhibitors decrease inflammation and epidermal thickness. Ixekizumab, secukinumab, and ustekinumab are interleukin inhibitors. Interleukins are proinflammatory substances that are released as part of the immune response. The biologic agents are approved for the treatment of moderate to severe plaque psoriasis.

Mechanism of Action and Pharmacokinetics

Cyclosporine selectively interferes with T-cell proliferation and interleukin production. The result is a decreased immune system response. Methotrexate also interferes with normal DNA synthesis. Apremilast improves psoriasis and thickening skin by reducing the release of substances that produce an inflammatory response. It is one of a few agents that is taken orally.

The absorption of modified cyclosporine (Neoral) is decreased by food. The absorption of methotrexate is dose-dependent. Absorption from the gastrointestinal tract occurs by active transport. Absorption decreases at higher doses. Food also delays absorption. Metabolism occurs in the liver, gut, and cells, and methotrexate is subject to first-pass metabolism. Because methotrexate is primarily eliminated in the kidney, high-dose therapy can cause high urine concentrations and crystalluria, leading to kidney damage. TNF-α inhibitors (e.g., etanercept) prevent cell lysis (destruction) and release of the substances that cause inflammation. Secukinumab and ixekizumab are monoclonal antibodies that work by inhibiting specific interleukins. The effectiveness of some of the biologic agents used in treating psoriasis (e.g., etanercept, infliximab, and adalimumab) may decrease over time. See Chapters 13 and 31 for additional pharmacokinetic information.

Adverse Effects

Cyclosporine and methotrexate may produce nausea and vomiting. Cyclosporine and methotrexate can cause kidney toxicity. Weight gain and hypertension are other side effects of cyclosporine therapy. Adverse reactions of etanercept are nausea, stomach pain, and headache. Adalimumab, etanercept, and infliximab are also associated with unspecified rashes and possible new-onset psoriasis. Immunosuppressive agents and immunomodulators can increase the risk of infections. Parenterally administered agents can cause redness and itching at the injection site. See Chapters 13 and 31 for a complete listing of adverse reactions.

> **Tech Note!**
> Folic acid is commonly prescribed to patients being treated with methotrexate.

Immunosuppressants and Immunomodulators

Generic Name	US Brand Name(s) —— Canadian Brand Name(s)	Dosage Forms and Strengths
cyclosporine[a]	Gengraf, Neoral —— Neoral	**Capsule, modified (Gengraf, Neoral):** 10 mg[b], 25 mg, 50 mg, 100 mg **Solution, oral, modified (Gengraf, Neoral):** 100 mg/mL (See Chapters 13 and 31 for additional dosage forms and brand names.)
Antimetabolites		
methotrexate[a]	Jylamvo —— Methotrexate	**Solution, oral (Jylamvo)[c]:** 2 mg/mL **Tablet:** 2.5 mg, 10 mg (See Chapters 13 and 31 for additional dosage forms and brand names.)

Continued

Immunosuppressants and Immunomodulators—cont'd

Generic Name	US Brand Name(s) / Canadian Brand Name(s)	Dosage Forms and Strengths
Immunomodulators (Biologic Agents)		
adalimumab	Humira	**Prefilled pen kit:** 40 mg/0.8 mL, 40 mg/0.4 mL[b]
	Humira	
adalimumab-aacf	Idacio	**Solution, subcutaneous for injection:** 40 mg/0.8 mL
	Idacio	
adalimumab-adbm	Cyltezo	**Solution, subcutaneous for injection:** 40 mg/0.8 mL
	Not available	
adalimumab-adaz	Hyrimoz	**Solution, subcutaneous for injection:** 40 mg/0.8 mL
	Hyrimoz	
adalimumab-afzb	Abrilada	**Prefilled pen kit:** 40 mg/0.8 mL, 40 mg/0.4 mL[b]
	Abrilada	
adalimumab-atto	Anjevita	**Solution, subcutaneous injection:** 20 mg/0.4 mL, 40 mg/0.8 mL (50 mg/mL)
	Amgevita	
adalimumab-aqvh	Yusimry	**Solution, subcutaneous for injection:** 40 mg/0.8 mL
	Yuflyma	
adalimumab-bwwd	Hadlima	**Solution, subcutaneous for injection:** 40 mg/0.8 mL
	Hadlima	
adalimumab-fkjp	Hulio	**Solution, subcutaneous for injection:** 20 mg/0.4 mL, 40 mg/0.8 mL[b]
	Hulio	
etanercept	Enbrel	**Injection, powder for reconstitution:** 25 mg/vial **Injection, solution:** 50 mg/(prefilled syringe)
	Enbrel	
etanercept	Not available	**Injection, solution:** 50 mg/(prefilled syringe)
	Brenzys	
etanercept-szzs	Elrezi	**Injection, solution:** 25 mg/0.5 mL[c], 50 mg/mL (prefilled syringe)
	Elrezi	
etanercept-ykro	Eticovo	**Injection, solution:** 25 mg/0.5 mL, 50 mg/mL (prefilled syringe)
	Not available	
infliximab	Remicade	**Injection, powder for reconstitution:** 100 mg/vial
	Remicade	
infliximab-abda	Renflexis	**Injection, powder for reconstitution:** 100 mg/vial
	Renflexis	
Infliximab-axxq	Avsola	**Injection, powder for reconstitution:** 100 mg/vial
	Avsola	
infliximab-dyyb	Inflectra	**Injection, powder for reconstitution:** 100 mg/vial
	Inflectra	
infliximab-qbtx	Xifi	**Injection, powder for reconstitution:** 100 mg/vial
	Not available	

Immunosuppressants and Immunomodulators—cont'd

Generic Name	US Brand Name(s) Canadian Brand Name(s)	Dosage Forms and Strengths
ixekizumab	Taltz	Solution, for injection: 80 mg/mL
	Taltz	
secukinumab	Cosentyx	Solution, for injection: 75 mg/0.5 mL[b], 150 mg/mL
	Cosentyx	
ustekinumab	Stelara	Solution, for injection: 45 mg/0.5 mL, 90 mg/mL, 5 mg/mL
	Stelara	
Miscellaneous		
apremilast[a]	Otezla	Tablets: 10 mg, 20 mg[c], 30 mg
	Otezla	

[a]Generic available.
[b]Available in Canada only.
[c]Available in the United States only.

Retinoids

Retinoid analogs are used to treat psoriasis. Acitretin is a synthetic retinoid, and tazarotene is a retinoid prodrug (see Chapter 35). Acitretin is used either as monotherapy or concurrently with phototherapy to increase its effectiveness.

Mechanism of Action and Pharmacokinetics

When acitretin binds to retinoic acid receptors, it modifies epithelial cell growth and differentiation. Tazarotene inhibits epidermal hyperproliferation in treated plaques. The absorption of tazarotene is minimal when applied topically. Metabolism occurs in the skin and results in the active metabolite tazarotenic acid. Tazarotenic acid is systemically absorbed and metabolized further. The half-life of tazarotenic acid is approximately 18 hours. A drug interaction with alcohol may convert acitretin to a new molecule that can take up to 3 years to fully eliminate from the body.

Adverse Reactions

Itching, burning, stinging, redness, and worsening of psoriasis occur in up to 30% of people using tazarotene. Up to 10% may experience eczema, contact dermatitis, fissures, and/or bleeding. Tazarotene is contraindicated in pregnancy, and a negative pregnancy test should be obtained before use. Acitretin use may produce hypervitaminosis A. In addition, up to 75% of people using acitretin develop cheilitis (inflammation of the lips), alopecia, and peeling skin. Redness, itching, dry skin, and a nail disorder may also occur.

Topical Phosphodiesterase 4 Inhibitors and Tyrosine Kinase Inhibitors

Phosphodiesterase, tyrosine kinase, and Janus kinase are enzymes that affect the cytokine inflammatory pathway. The phosphodiesterase 4 (PDE4) inhibitor crisaborole is used to treat mild to moderate atopic dermatitis. The tyrosine kinase inhibitor deucravacitinib is used to treat moderate to severe

Retinoids

Generic Name	US Brand Name(s) Canadian Brand Name(s)	Dosage Forms and Strengths
acitretin[a]	Generics	Capsule: 10 mg, 17.5 mg[b], 22.5 mg[b], 25 mg
	Soriatane	
tazarotene	Arazlo[c], Avage, Fabior, Tazorac	Cream: 0.05%, 0.1% Foam (Fabior): 0.1% Gel: 0.05%, 0.1% Lotion (Arazlo): 0.045%
	Arazlo[c], Tazorac	

[a]Generic available.
[b]Available in the United States only.
[c]For the treatment of acne.

Topical PDE4 and Tyrosine Kinase Inhibitors

Generic Name	US Brand Name(s) Canadian Brand Name(s)	Dosage Forms and Strengths
Topical PDE4 Inhibitors		
crisaborole	Eucrisa	Ointment: 2%
	Eucrisa	
Tyrosine Kinase Inhibitors		
deucravacitinib	Sotyktu	Tablet: 6 mg
	Not available	

plaque psoriasis. Crisaborole inhibits the enzyme PDE4, an enzyme that promotes the release of inflammatory cytokines. Crisaborole is currently the only drug in this class. The most common adverse reactions produced by crisaborole are pain, burning and stinging at the application site. Deucravacitinib disrupts signaling pathways that regulate cytokine inflammatory pathways. It is metabolized to an active metabolite by cytochrome P-450. Adverse reactions include increased risk of infection, headache, dizziness, muscle aches, nausea, vomiting, diarrhea, and abdominal pain. Deucravacitinib can reactivate dormant tuberculosis. Deucravacitinib is currently the only drug in this class.

TECHNICIAN'S CORNER

1. Because atopic dermatitis is allergy related, how can one prevent flareups from occurring?
2. How well do calamine lotion and oatmeal soap (both OTC products) work in decreasing the symptoms of atopic dermatitis?

Summary of Drugs Used for the Treatment of Eczema and Psoriasis

Generic Name	Brand Name	Usual Dose and Dosing Schedule	Warning Labels
Topical Corticosteroids			
alclometasone dipropionate[a]	Generics	**Cream or ointment:** Apply a thin film 2 or 3 times daily	FOR EXTERNAL USE.
amcinonide[a]	Generics	**All dosage forms:** Apply a thin film 2 or 3 times daily	FOR EXTERNAL USE.
betamethasone dipropionate[a]	Diprolene AF / Diprosone	**Cream, lotion, ointment:** Apply a thin film 2–4 times daily	FOR EXTERNAL USE.
betamethasone valerate[a]	Betaderm, Luxiq, Valisone	**Foam:** Apply twice a day **Cream, lotion, ointment:** Apply a thin film 2–4 times daily	FOR EXTERNAL USE. SHAKE WELL—foam, lotion.
clobetasol propionate[a]	Clobex, Olux	**All dosage forms:** Apply twice a day	SHAKE WELL—foam. FOR EXTERNAL USE.
desonide[a]	Desowen, Verdeso / Tridesilon	**Foam:** Apply twice a day **Cream, lotion, ointment:** Apply a thin film 2–4 times daily	FOR EXTERNAL USE. SHAKE WELL—foam.
desoximetasone[a]	Topicort	**Cream, gel, ointment:** Apply a thin film twice a day	FOR EXTERNAL USE.
diflorasone diacetate[a]	Generics	**Nonemollient dosage forms:** Apply a thin film 1–4 times daily **Emollient dosage forms:** Apply a thin film 1–3 times daily	FOR EXTERNAL USE.
fluocinolone acetonide[a]	Synalar / Derma-Smoothe/FS	**Cream, ointment, solution:** Apply a thin film 2–4 times daily **Oil:** Apply a thin film 3 times a day	FOR EXTERNAL USE.
halcinonide	Halog	**Cream, ointment, solution:** Apply a thin film 2–4 times daily	FOR EXTERNAL USE.
halobetasol propionate[a]	Ultravate	**Cream or ointment:** Apply a thin film once or twice daily	FOR EXTERNAL USE.
hydrocortisone, acetate[a]	Micort HC	**All dosage forms:** Apply 3 or 4 times daily	FOR EXTERNAL USE.
hydrocortisone butyrate[a]	Locoid	**All dosage forms:** Apply once or twice daily	FOR EXTERNAL USE.
hydrocortisone valerate[a]	Generics	**All dosage forms:** Apply 2–4 times daily	FOR EXTERNAL USE.
mometasone furoate[a]	Elocon	**Topical dosage forms:** Apply once daily	FOR EXTERNAL USE.
prednicarbate[a]	Dermatop	**Cream or ointment:** Apply a thin film twice daily	FOR EXTERNAL USE.
triamcinolone acetonide[a]	Generics	**Cream, lotion, ointment:** Apply a thin film 2–4 times daily	FOR EXTERNAL USE.
Calcineurin Inhibitors			
pimecrolimus	Elidel	**Atopic dermatitis:** Apply a thin layer twice a day	AVOID EXCESS EXPOSURE TO SUNLIGHT.
tacrilimus	Protopic	**Atopic dermatitis:** Apply a thin layer twice a day.	AVOID GRAPEFRUIT JUICE—capsule.

Summary of Drugs Used for the Treatment of Eczema and Psoriasis—cont'd

Generic Name	Brand Name	Usual Dose and Dosing Schedule	Warning Labels
Immunosuppressants			
cyclosporine	Neoral	**Psoriasis:** 1.25 mg/kg orally twice daily up to 4 mg/kg daily	TAKE WITH FOOD. AVOID PREGNANCY. AVOID ALCOHOL. SWALLOW WHOLE; DO NOT CRUSH OR CHEW.
methotrexate	Jylamvo	**Psoriasis:** 10–25 mg PO, IV, or IM given as a single weekly dose or 2.5–5 mg PO every 12 h for 3 doses every week	AVOID ALCOHOL. AVOID PROLONGED EXPOSURE TO SUNLIGHT. AVOID PREGNANCY. EXERCISE PRECAUTIONS FOR HANDLING, PREPARING, AND ADMINISTERING CYTOTOXIC DRUGS.
Vitamin D Analogs			
calcipotriene	Dovonex	**Psoriasis:** Apply a thin layer twice a day	FOR EXTERNAL USE. AVOID EXCESS EXPOSURE TO SUNLIGHT. AVOID FACE.
calcipotriene + betamethasone	Taclonex Dovobet Wynzora	**Psoriasis:** Apply a thin layer once daily for up to 8 weeks	
calcitriol	Vectical	**Mild to moderate psoriasis:** Apply twice a day	
Furanocoumarins			
methoxsalen	Oxsoralen-Ultra	**Psoriasis:** 1 cap 1.5–2 h before UVA therapy	TAKE WITH FOOD OR MILK. AVOID SUN EXPOSURE FOR 24 HOURS BEFORE AND 48 HOURS AFTER TREATMENT.
Immunomodulators			
adalimumab	Humira	**Chronic plaque psoriasis:** 80 mg subcutaneously in 2 injections on day 1, then 40 mg every other week	REFRIGERATE; DO NOT FREEZE— adalimumab, etanercept, infliximab, ixekizumab, secukinumab, ustekinumab. PROTECT FROM LIGHT—etanercept, ixekizumab, secukinumab, ustekinumab. GENTLY SWIRL RECONSTITUTED PRODUCT—infliximab. DO NOT SHAKE—infliximab, ixekizumab, secukinumab, ustekinumab. DISCARD ANY UNUSED PORTION— infliximab, ixekizumab, secukinumab, ustekinumab.
etanercept	Enbrel	**Psoriasis:** 50 mg subcutaneously weekly given as one 50-mg injection or as two 25-mg injections 3–4 days apart	
infliximab	Remicade	**Psoriasis:** 5 mg/kg IV given at week 0, 2, and 6 and repeated every 8 weeks thereafter	
ixekizumab	Taltz	Inject subcutaneously, 160 mg followed by 80 mg every 2 weeks on weeks 2, 4, 6, 8, 10, and 12; then 80 mg every 4 weeks	
secukinumab	Cosentyx	**Plaque psoriasis:** 300 mg by subcutaneous injection at weeks 0, 1, 2, 3, and 4 followed by 300 mg every 4 weeks	
ustekinumab	Stelara	**Plaque psoriasis (moderate to severe):** 100 kg or less—45 mg subcutaneously initially and at week 4; then 45 mg every 12 weeks Greater than 100 kg—90 mg subcutaneously initially and at week 4; then 90 mg every 12 weeks	
apremilast	Otezla	**Plaque psoriasis (moderate to severe):** Begin: 10 mg orally in AM; Day 2, 10 mg twice daily; Day 3, 10 mg in AM, 20 mg in PM; Day 4, 20 mg twice daily; Day 5, 20 mg in AM, 30 mg in PM Maintenance: Day 6 and thereafter, 30 mg orally twice daily	SWALLOW WHOLE; DO NOT CRUSH OR CHEW.

Continued

Summary of Drugs Used for the Treatment of Eczema and Psoriasis—cont'd

Generic Name	Brand Name	Usual Dose and Dosing Schedule	Warning Labels
Retinoids			
acitretin	Soriatane	**Recalcitrant psoriasis:** 25–50 mg PO once daily	TAKE WITH MAIN MEAL. AVOID ALCOHOL.
tazarotene	Tazorac	**Psoriasis:** Apply once daily, in the evening, to psoriatic lesions (max 12 weeks).	PROTECT SKIN FROM THE SUN. AVOID PREGNANCY.
Topical PDE4 Inhibitors			
crisaborole	Eucrisa	**Atopic dermatitis:** Apply twice daily to the affected area	FOR TOPICAL USE ONLY.
Tyrosine Kinase Inhibitors			
deucravacitinib	Sotyktu	**Plaque psoriasis:** Take 6 mg once daily	DO NOT CRUSH OR CHEW.

aGeneric available.

Key Points

- Atopic diseases are an autoimmune disorder.
- Atopic dermatitis is often referred to as eczema.
- Atopic dermatitis is a chronic disease of the skin that often develops in infancy and may continue throughout adulthood.
- Atopic dermatitis commonly produces symptoms of intense itching, redness (from scratching), skin irritation, and inflammation. Eczematous patches may form that are flaky, crusting, and may even ooze a clear fluid.
- Psoriasis is a condition associated with the rapid turnover of skin cells and is caused by hyperactivity of the T cells.
- Individuals with psoriasis have thick, silvery, scaly patches. They may also have some redness and swelling.
- Individuals with atopic dermatitis and psoriasis may experience periods when their symptoms worsen (exacerbation) and periods when they get better or go away completely (remission).
- Nonpharmaceutical treatment for eczema involves using skin care regimens that reduce irritation and avoiding allergens and irritants, and may include the use of phototherapy.
- Phototherapy involves exposing the skin to ultraviolet (UV) A or B light waves.
- UV light therapy may cause premature aging of the skin and increase the risk for skin cancer.
- The use of topical corticosteroids is a mainstay of therapy for the treatment of atopic dermatitis and psoriasis.
- Topical corticosteroids are categorized into seven groups based on potency.
- The vehicle (base) in which the corticosteroid is suspended may influence the potency.
- Higher potency corticosteroids cause more adverse reactions.
- Only the mildest potency agents, such as hydrocortisone, should be used on the face.
- Long-term use of topical corticosteroids can produce thinning of the skin, stretch marks (striae), spider veins, acne, milia, rosacea (enlarged blood vessels, especially on the nose), bruising, atrophy, lacerations, poor wound healing, and growth suppression (in children).
- Pimecrolimus and tacrolimus are calcineurin inhibitor immunomodulators that control inflammation and reduce the immune system response to allergens.
- Pimecrolimus is indicated for the treatment of mild to moderate eczema (atopic dermatitis).
- Tacrolimus is approved for the treatment of moderate to severe atopic dermatitis that has failed to respond to corticosteroid treatment.
- Calcipotriene is a synthetic analog of vitamin D. It is known as calcipotriol in Canada.
- Calcipotriene (calcipotriol) inhibits the rapid and repeated production of new skin cells and is used for the treatment of psoriasis.
- Calcitriol is an active form of vitamin D that is used topically for the treatment of psoriasis.
- Psoralens are a class of drugs that increase photosensitivity and are classified as furanocoumarins. Methoxsalen is the only drug in this class.
- Psoralens plus UVA therapy is also known as PUVA.
- Cyclosporine is approved by the FDA for the short-term treatment of severe atopic dermatitis and psoriasis. It decreases immune system hyperactivity.
- Methotrexate is an antimetabolite indicated for the treatment of moderate to severe chronic psoriasis and psoriatic arthritis.
- Methotrexate slows the rapid rate of skin cell turnover that occurs with eczema and psoriasis.
- The retinoids acitretin and tazarotene are used for the treatment of psoriasis.
- Adalimumab, etanercept, and infliximab are tumor necrosis factor-α inhibitors indicated for the treatment of plaque psoriasis.
- Ixekizumab, secukinumab, and ustekinumab are interleukin inhibitors that are approved for the treatment of moderate to severe plaque psoriasis. They block proinflammatory substances that are released as part of the immune response.
- Phosphodiesterase 4 (PDE4) inhibitors are used to treat mild to moderate atopic dermatitis.
- PDE4 inhibitors reduce inflammation by inhibiting the production of cytokines. Crisaborole (Eucrisa®) is the only drug in this class.
- Deucravacitinib (Sotyktu®) is a tyrosine kinase inhibitor that is used to treat moderate to severe plaque psoriasis.

Review Questions

1. A chronic disease of the skin characterized by itchy red patches covered with silvery scales is known as _____.
   - **a.** eczema
   - **b.** psoriasis
   - **c.** dermatitis
   - **d.** rosacea

2. All of the following treatments for psoriasis are applied topically, except _____.
   - **a.** Dovonex
   - **b.** Taclonex
   - **c.** Neoral
   - **d.** Eucrisa

3. When symptoms worsen, it is called _____, and periods when they get better or go away completely are called _____.
   - **a.** exacerbation, metastasis
   - **b.** exacerbation, remission
   - **c.** metastasis, inflammation
   - **d.** allergic, nonallergic

4. Phototherapy reduces the risk for skin cancer.
   - **a.** true
   - **b.** false

5. A mainstay of therapy for the treatment of eczema is the use of _____.
   - **a.** antibiotics
   - **b.** corticosteroids
   - **c.** antihistamines
   - **d.** none of the above

6. Pimecrolimus (Elidel) is indicated for the treatment of moderate to severe eczema.
   - **a.** true
   - **b.** false

7. All of the following treatments for psoriasis are administered by injection, except:
   - **a.** Humira
   - **b.** Soriatane
   - **c.** Enbrel
   - **d.** Remicade

8. All of the following products must be stored in the refrigerator, cxcept_____.
   - **a.** Stelara
   - **b.** Taltz
   - **c.** Cosentyx
   - **d.** Otezla

9. _____ is an antimetabolite indicated for the treatment of moderate to severe chronic psoriasis and psoriatic arthritis.
   - **a.** Anthralin
   - **b.** Cyclosporine
   - **c.** Methotrexate
   - **d.** Calcipotriene

10. Select the class VII corticosteroid that is safe for use on the face.
    - **a.** Hydrocortisone
    - **b.** Betamethasone
    - **c.** Clobetasol
    - **d.** Mometasone

Bibliography

Armstrong AW, Mehta MD, Schupp CW, et al. Psoriasis prevalence in adults in the United States. *JAMA Dermatol.* 2021;157(8):940–946.

Brown S. Molecular mechanisms in atopic eczema: insights gained from genetic studies. *J Pathol.* 2017;241:140–145.

GADA. (2022). Global Report on Atopic Dermatitis 2022. Retrieved February 16, 2023, from https://www.atopicdermatitisatlas.org/en/.

Health Canada. (2023). Drug Product Database. Retrieved February 16, 2023, from https://health-products.canada.ca/dpd-bdpp/index-eng.jsp.

Hoffman MB, Hill D, Feldman SR. Current challenges and emerging drug delivery strategies for the treatment of psoriasis. *Expert Opin Drug Deliv.* 2016;13(10):1461–1473.

Institute for Safe Medication Practices. (2016). FDA and ISMP Lists of Look-Alike Drug Names with Recommended Tall Man Letters. Retrieved December 29, 2022, from https://www.ismp.org/recommendations/tall-man-letters-list.

Institute for Safe Medication Practices. (2019). List of Confused Drugs. Retrieved December 29, 2022, from https://www.ismp.org/tools/confuseddrugnames.pdf.

Kalant H, Grant D, Mitchell J. *Principles of medical pharmacology,* ed 7. Toronto: Elsevier Canada; 2007:891–898.

Khandpur S, Sharma VK, Sumanth K. Topical immunomodulators in dermatology. *J Postgrad Med.* 2004;50:131–139.

Lance L, Lacy C, Armstrong L, et al. *Drug information handbook for the allied health professional,* ed 12. Hudson, OH: APhA Lexi-Comp; 2005.

Martin G. Novel therapies in plaque psoriasis: a review of tyrosine kinase 2 inhibitors. *Dermatol Ther (Heidelb).* 2023;13(2):417–435.

Martín-Santiago A, Puig S, Arumi D, Rebollo Laserna FJ. Safety profile and tolerability of topical phosphodiesterase 4 inhibitors for the treatment of atopic dermatitis: a systematic review and meta-analysis. *Curr Ther Res Clin Exp.* 2022;96:100679.

National Institute of Arthritis and Musculoskeletal and Skin Diseases. (2022). Atopic dermatitis. Retrieved February 16, 2023, from https://www.niams.nih.gov/health-topics/atopic-dermatitis.

National Institute of Arthritis and Musculoskeletal and Skin Diseases. (2020). Psoriasis. Retrieved February 16, 2023, from https://www.niams.nih.gov/health-topics/psoriasis.

Page C, Curtis M, Sutter M, et al. *Integrated pharmacology.* Philadelphia: Elsevier Mosby; 2005:506–508 512–514.

Raymond GP, Houle M-C. (2007). A Review of Corticosteroids for the Treatment of Psoriasis, Skin Therapy Letter–Pharmacist Edition 2. Retrieved February 16, 2023, from https://www.skintherapyletter.com/pharmacist-edition/corticosteroids-psoriasis-pharm/.

Sala M, Elaissari A, Fessi H. Advances in psoriasis physiopathology and treatments: up to date of mechanistic insights and perspectives of novel therapies based on innovative skin drug delivery systems (ISDDS). *J Control Release.* 2016;239:182–292.

Schlichte MJ, Vandersall A, Katta R. Diet and eczema: a review of dietary supplements for the treatment of atopic dermatitis. *Dermatol Pract Concept.* 2016;6(3):6.

Thomson RJ, Moshirfar M, Ronquillo Y. *Tyrosine kinase inhibitors.* Treasure Island (FL): StatPearls Publishing; 2022.

U.S. Food and Drug Administration. (nd). Drugs@FDA: FDA Approved Drug Products. Retrieved January 3, 2023, from https://www.accessdata.fda.gov/scripts/cder/daf/index.cfm.

Wawrzyniak P, Akdis CA, Finkelman FD, et al. Advances and highlights in mechanisms of allergic disease in 2015. *J Allergy Clin Immunol.* 2016;137:1681–1696.

Yang H, Wang J, Zhang X, et al. Application of topical phosphodiesterase 4 inhibitors in mild to moderate atopic dermatitis: a systematic review and meta-analysis. *JAMA Dermatol.* 2019;155(5):585–593.

37

Treatment of Lice and Scabies

LEARNING OBJECTIVES

1. Learn the terminology associated with lice and scabies.
2. Describe the epidemiology of lice and scabies infestation.
3. List the symptoms of lice and scabies infestation.
4. List prevention strategies.
5. List and categorize medications used to treat lice and scabies.
6. Describe the mechanism of action for drugs used to treat lice and scabies.
7. Identify warning labels and precautionary messages associated with medications used to treat lice and scabies.

KEY TERMS

Lice Group of parasites (*Pediculus humanus capitis, Pediculus humanus corporis, Pthirus pubis*) that can live on the body, scalp, or genital area of humans.
Nits Head lice eggs.
Nymph Baby louse.
Ovicidal Kills eggs.

Parasite Organism that benefits by living in, with, or on another organism.
Pediculicide Drug that kills lice.
Scabicide Drug that kills the scabies mite.
Scabies Parasitic infection caused by the mite *Sarcoptes scabiei*.

Epidemiology of Lice and Scabies Infestation

Lice and *scabies* infestations affect people worldwide without regard for social status or race. They are caused by parasites and are readily spread person to person. A *parasite* is an organism that benefits by living in, with, or on another organism (host), usually to the detriment of the host.

Lice

Head Lice

Head lice most commonly infest children aged 3 to 11 years and their families, but anyone can become infested (Fig. 37.1A and B). The parasite *Pediculus humanus capitis* is spread between individuals through head-to-head contact, as occurs during children's play and sports. Less commonly, transmission occurs by sharing personal items such as combs, brushes, hats, towels, scarves, pillows, and coats with someone who has head lice.

The life cycle of a head louse is approximately 4 to 6 weeks. The adult females lay eggs, also called *nits*, at the base of the hair shaft (see Fig. 37.1C) within 24 hours of mating. In approximately 7 days, the nits hatch and a nymph emerges. A *nymph* is a baby louse. The nymph becomes an adult in approximately 7 days and the adult lives for approximately 30 days.

Lice are parasites that feed on blood. This is why eggs are laid close to the base of the hair shaft and nits that are found within ¼ inch of the scalp are typically viable eggs. Newly hatched nymphs must be close to a blood source. Nit shells found farther than a fingertip away from the base of the scalp (2 to 5 cm) are likely

remains of an earlier infestation; treatment is not necessary. An adult louse can live for up to 3 days away from a human host. Head lice are a nuisance but are not a health risk.

> ● **Tech Note!**
>
> It is a myth that head lice infestation is caused by poor hygiene (lack of cleanliness).

> ● **Tech Note!**
>
> Head lice do not live on pets, there is no human-to-pet transmission, and pets need not be treated with pediculicides.

> ● **Tech Note!**
>
> Pharmacy technicians may have customers coming into the pharmacy asking about head lice treatments. Because these products are available over the counter (OTC), pharmacy technicians will be able to direct customers to the pharmacy shelves where available products are located.

Body Lice

Body lice infestations are caused by the parasite *Pediculus humanus corporis*. Infestations are a serious public health concern because body lice may cause epidemics of typhus and louse-borne relapsing

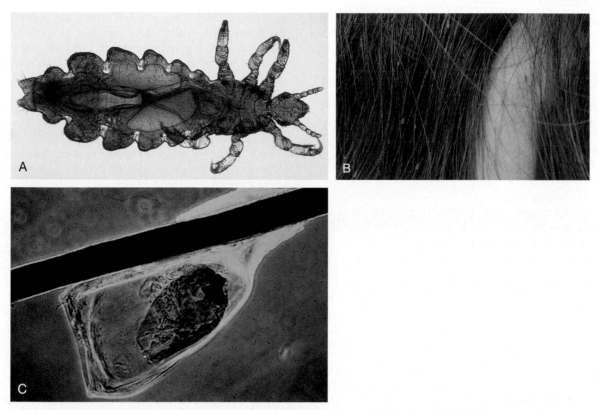

• **Fig. 37.1** (A) Adult head louse. (B) Head lice infestation. (C) Nit attached to hair shaft. ([A], Courtesy of Dr. Dennis D. Juranek, Centers for Disease Control and Prevention; [B], From Callen J, Greer K, Hood A, et al. *Color atlas of dermatology*, Philadelphia, 1993, WB Saunders; [C], from Kumar V, Abbas AK, Fausto M. *Robbins and Cotran pathologic basis of disease*, ed 7, Philadelphia, 2005, Saunders.)

fever. Body lice thrive in crowded environments with chronic poverty and unsanitary conditions, such as refugee camps, temporary housing from natural disasters, and prisons. In the United States and Canada, body lice infestations rarely occur except in populations without access to bathing facilities (e.g., homelessness).

Like head lice, body lice infestation is spread person to person through direct contact with a person who has body lice. Another mode of transmission is through shared bedding or clothes. Body lice can live in the seams of the clothing of infested individuals.

The life cycle of body lice is similar to that of head lice and begins with laying eggs. The nits hatch and nymphs mature to adults in 7 days. Adults can survive away from a human host for only 10 days.

Pubic Lice

Pubic lice, or "crabs," are sometimes classified as a sexually transmitted infection because they are usually spread through direct sexual contact (Fig. 37.2). Although the life cycle of pubic lice is the same as that of head lice, pubic lice and head lice are different species. Head lice do not inhabit the genitalia, and pubic lice do not live in the hair. Lice infestation in the pubic region is caused by the parasite *Pthirus pubis*.

> ● **Tech Note!**
>
> It is a myth that individuals can get pubic lice from sitting on a public toilet seat.

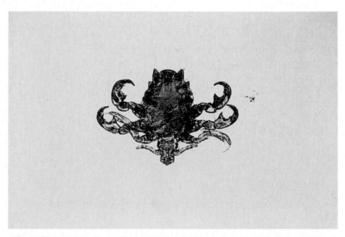

• **Fig. 37.2** Pubic lice. (From Mahon CR, Lehman DC, Manuselis G. *Textbook of diagnostic microbiology*, ed 3, St Louis, 2007, Saunders.)

Scabies

Scabies infestations are caused by a parasitic mite called *Sarcoptes scabiei*. The mite flourishes and spreads by person-to-person contact in environments in which the population density is high, such as hospitals, nursing homes, childcare facilities, and schools. Transmission occurs through close contact and sharing bedding, linen, clothing, or sexual relations. Infestations are common and can affect anyone.

The scabies mite burrows beneath the skin. Sites of infestation can be seen in the webbing between fingers and toes; skin folds of the breast, penis, and shoulder blades; and in the bends of the elbows, knees, and wrists. Like lice, *S. scabiei* feeds on blood and dies if away from a human host for longer than 48 to 72 hours. The adult mite can live for approximately 30 days.

Symptoms of Lice and Scabies Infestation and Prevention of Lice Reinfestation

Symptoms of lice and scabies infestation are listed in Box 37.1. Methods for the prevention of lice reinfestation are listed in Box 37.2.

> ### ● *Tech Note!*
>
> Shaving the head is not necessary to treat head lice!

Treatment of Head Lice, Pubic Lice, and Scabies

Head lice may be treated with nonprescription and prescription *pediculicides*. The Centers for Disease Control and Prevention (CDC) and Canadian Paediatric Society recommend that all family members with active infestations be treated. Treatment is more effective if a fine-toothed nit comb is used to remove eggs from the hair shaft. OTC and prescription agents are effective treatments for head lice and pubic lice. OTC products are more effective and have a lower risk of toxicity than lindane which has been

---

● BOX 37.1   Symptoms of Lice and Scabies Infestation

Head and Pubic Lice
- Itching
- Feeling of something moving in hair or genital area
- Sores (from scratching)

Body Lice
- Itching
- Rash
- Thickening and discoloration of skin

Scabies
- Intense itching
- Pimple-like rash

● BOX 37.2   Strategies to Prevent Reinfestation

- Treat all infested household members simultaneously.
- Use a nit comb to remove eggs. Use daily lice combing between pediculicidal treatments.
- Do not wash hair for 1 or 2 days after the treatment is rinsed from the hair.
- Vacuum the floor and furniture in an infested household.
- Wash clothing, linens, and bedding in hot water (130 °F [54°C]).
- Dry-clean clothing that is not washable.
- Place stuffed toys, clothing, and bedding that cannot be washed or dry-cleaned in a large plastic bag and seal the bag for 2 weeks.

---

discontinued. Drug resistance is a growing problem for OTC and prescription pediculicides, especially permethrin, because of the residue left after treatment. Yet, only one new pediculicide has been approved by the US Food and Drug Administration (FDA) in more than a decade (abametapir), and it has since been discontinued.

> ### ● *Tech Note!*
>
> There is no proof that lice sprays are any more effective than vacuuming. Lice transmission is via person-to-person contact; the risk of transmission by sitting on a piece of furniture is very low.

Pediculicides

Pediculicides that treat lice and/or scabies are crotamiton, dimethicone 100 cSt, isopropyl myristate and ivermectin, malathion, pyrethrins (plus piperonyl butoxide), permethrin, and spinosad. They are formulated in various dosage forms, such as shampoo, cream rinse, lotion, and household spray. Pyrethrins (plus piperonyl butoxide), permethrin, dimethicone 100 cSt, and isopropyl myristate are marketed for OTC use. Crotamiton is prescription access only in the United States.

Pyrethrins and Permethrin

Pyrethrins are naturally derived from the chrysanthemum flower. Their effectiveness is boosted by the addition of piperonyl butoxide, a petroleum distillate. Pyrethrins are indicated for the treatment of head lice, pubic lice, and body lice. Pyrethrins are not *ovicidal* (do not kill the eggs), so retreatment is necessary in 7 to 10 days to kill newly hatched nymphs. Permethrin is ovicidal.

Permethrin is a mixture of synthetic isomers of pyrethrins. It is more effective for the treatment of head lice but less effective against pubic lice. Studies have shown that 1% permethrin is less than 60% effective when used alone. The effectiveness was increased up to 87% when permethrin use was combined with nonpharmacologic methods such as combing the hair with a nit comb, using carrier oils (e.g., olive oil), and washing infected items. The low effectiveness is because of the high rate of resistance. Permethrin is also effective against the scabies mite.

Mechanism of Action and Pharmacokinetics
Pyrethrins and permethrin paralyze and kill. Their action is discontinued once the drug is washed off. Permethrin leaves a residue on the hair that can destroy eggs and newly hatched nymphs. Absorption of pyrethrins and permethrin through the skin is minimal. Both drugs are rapidly metabolized in the liver.

Adverse Effects
The most common adverse effects caused by topical application of pyrethrins are redness, itching and stinging, tingling, numbness and minor swelling.

> ### ● *Tech Note!*
>
> Permethrin is approved for use in children 3 months of age and older; however, the CDC recommends that manual removal of nits and lice in children younger than 2 years be tried first.

Pyrethrins and Permethrin

Generic Name	US Brand Name(s) / Canadian Brand Name(s)	Dosage Forms and Strengths	Prescription/OTC status
pyrethrins + piperonyl butoxide	ZAP Maximum Strength R&C Shampoo with Conditioner	**Shampoo:** pyrethrins 0.33% + piperonyl butoxide 3% (R&C), pyrethrins 0.33% + piperonyl butoxide 4% (ZAP)	OTC
permethrin[a]	Nix, RID Home Lice, Bedbug & Dust Mite Spray Kwellada-P Cream Rinse, Kwellada-P Lotion[b], Nix Cream Rinse, Nix Dermal Cream	**Cream rinse:** 1% **Lotion:** 1%, 5%[b] **Cream:** 5%	OTC

[a]Generic available.
[b]Available in Canada only.
OTC, Over the counter.

Noninsecticidal Products

Isopropyl myristate 50% plus ST-cyclomethicone 50% (Resultz®) is available in Canada for the OTC treatment of head lice. It is approved for use in children at least 4 years old. It is not available in the United States. Dimethicone 100 cSt (NYDA®) is another agent approved for use in children 2 years and older.

Mechanism of Action and Pharmacokinetics

Isopropyl myristate dissolves the louse exoskeleton, resulting in dehydration and death. It is not ovicidal, so nit removal and retreatment in 10 days are required. Dimethicone cSt 50% solution penetrates the louse respiratory system and gradually displaces oxygen, suffocating the parasite. It is effective against adult lice, larvae, and eggs.

Adverse Effects

Adverse effects caused by topical application of isopropyl myristate are redness, itching, and mild skin irritation. Adverse reactions reported with dimethicone were eye irritation (if the product entered the eyes), hair odor, and headache.

Ivermectin

Ivermectin has been used for more than 20 years worldwide as a treatment for filarial worm infections. It is also an effective head lice treatment. Ivermectin lotion 0.5% is approved for treatment of infested persons 6 months of age and older. It kills newly hatched lice but not the eggs. It is used as a single application on dry hair. A health care provider should be consulted before retreatment.

Mechanism of Action

Ivermectin is a member of the avermectin class of pediculicides that kill parasites. It increases the permeability of the cell membrane to chloride ions, causing hyperpolarization and paralysis of invertebrate nerve and muscle cells. Ivermectin does not readily cross the blood-brain barrier in humans.

Adverse Reactions and Precautions

The most common side effects are eye redness, burning of the skin, and dryness. Ivermectin should not be used in children weighing less than 15 kg or in pregnant women.

Malathion

Malathion is an organophosphate pesticide used in agriculture to control pests and medically to kill head lice and their eggs. It was withdrawn from the US market and then reintroduced in 1999 after labeling changes. It remains withdrawn from the market in Canada.

Mechanism of Action and Pharmacokinetics

Malathion is a prodrug that must be metabolized to its active metabolite malaoxon. It paralyzes the central nervous system of

Dimethicone and Isopropyl Myristate

Generic Name	US Brand Name(s) / Canadian Brand Name(s)	Dosage Forms and Strengths	Prescription/OTC status
Dimethicone 100 cSt	Not available		
	NYDA	**Solution:** 50%	OTC
isopropyl myristate + ST-cyclomethicone	Not available	**Solution:** 50%	OTC
	Resultz		

Ivermectin

Generic Name	US Brand Name(s) / Canadian Brand Name(s)	Dosage Forms and Strengths	Prescription/ OTC status
ivermectin	Sklice, Soolantra / Rosiver	**Cream (Rosiver, Scoolantra):** 1% **Lotion (Sklice):** 0.5%	**Prescription, OTC**

parasites by causing an accumulation of acetylcholine. The pharmacokinetics of malathion are dependent on the dose and route of exposure. Less than 10% of the applied dose is absorbed systemically. Absorption through the scalp of infants is greater, and the use of malathion is contraindicated in this age group. Safety in children less than 6 years old has not been established. The onset of action is 3 seconds to 1 hour. The elimination half-life ranges between 8 and 48 hours.

Adverse Effects

The most common adverse effects linked to malathion use are stinging, redness, minor swelling, itching, and tingling.

> ### ❶ Tech Alert!
> Malathion is flammable, and those using the product should stay away from open flames, hair dryers, curling irons, and lit cigarettes, cigars, and pipes.

Malathion

Generic Name	US Brand Name(s) / Canadian Brand Name(s)	Dosage Form and Strength	Prescription/ OTC status
malathion[a]	Generics / Not available	**Lotion:** 0.5%	**Prescription**

[a]Generic available.

Crotamiton

Crotamiton is a ***scabicide*** that can be used during pregnancy. Its mechanism of action is unknown. The pharmacokinetics and degree of systemic absorption of crotamiton after topical application have not been determined.

Adverse Effects

Crotamiton has few adverse reactions. Reactions are linked to drug allergy and include itchiness, minor swelling, and redness.

Crotamiton

Generic Name	US Brand Name(s) / Canadian Brand Name(s)	Dosage Forms and Strengths	Prescription/ OTC status
crotamiton	Eurax, Crotan / Eurax[a]	**Lotion:** 10%	**Prescription: United States**

[a]Product is dormant in Canada

Spinosad

Spinosad is a pediculicide indicated for the topical treatment of head lice infestations in patients 4 years of age and older. It is derived from *Saccharopolyspora spinosa*, a bacterium found in soil.

Mechanism of Action and Pharmacokinetics

Spinosad produces neuronal excitation in lice, resulting in hyperexcitation, paralysis, and death. The pharmacokinetics and degree of systemic absorption of spinosad after topical application have not been determined. Systemic exposure is not expected.

Spinosad

Generic Name	US Brand Name(s) / Canadian Brand Name(s)	Dosage Forms and Strengths	Prescription/OTC Status
spinosad	Natroba / Not available	**Topical suspension:** 0.9%	**Prescription**

Adverse Effects

Most common adverse reactions are application site redness (3%), redness and irritation of the eyes (2%), and application site irritation (1%).

> ### TECHNICIAN'S CORNER
> 1. Resistance to head lice treatments is a growing concern. Can drug resistance be limited? What are treatment options when drug resistance is encountered?
> 2. Why is it important to address the social determinants of health that give rise to body lice infestations?

Summary of Drugs Used for the Treatment of Lice and Scabies

Generic Name	Brand Name	Usual Dose and Dosing Schedule	Warning Labels
Over the Counter			
crotamiton	Eurax	Apply after bathing to the skin over the entire body from the chin to the toes. Repeat in 24 h. Bathe 48 h *after* second dose. Treatment may be repeated in 7–10 days if needed.	SHAKE WELL.
dimethicone 100 cSt	NYDA	Completely wet hair with spray. Leave on for 30 minutes. Use a lice comb to remove suffocated lice and nymphs. Let NYDA dry on hair for 8 h. Wash hair with regular shampoo. Repeat in 8–10 days.	DO NOT USE IN CHILDREN YOUNGER THAN 2 YEARS.
pyrethrins + piperonyl butoxide	R&C various	**Lice, shampoo, cream rinse:** Apply to dry hair. Saturate hair with product. Leave on for as long as instructed on product label. Rinse hair. Use nit comb to remove eggs. **Scabies, lotion, cream:** Apply after bathing to the skin over the entire body from the chin to the toes. Leave on overnight (or 8 h). Wash off. Repeat treatment in 7–10 days if needed.	SHAKE WELL (LOTION, CREAM RINSE)—all. DO NOT REWASH HAIR FOR 1–2 DAYS AFTER TREATMENT. SHAKE WELL. DO NOT USE IN CHILDREN YOUNGER THAN 2 MONTHS OLD.
permethrin	Kwellada, NIX	**Lice, cream rinse:** Apply to dry hair. Apply a sufficient amount of product to saturate the hair and scalp thoroughly. Let set for 10 min; then rinse hair with water and towel dry. Use lice comb to remove dead lice and nits. Retreat in 10 days.	
isopropyl myristate	Resultz	**Cream rinse:** Apply to dry hair. Apply a sufficient amount of product to saturate the hair and scalp thoroughly. Let set for 10 min; then rinse hair with water and towel dry. Use lice comb to remove dead lice and nits. Retreat in 10 days.	SHAKE WELL. DO NOT USE IN CHILDREN YOUNGER THAN 4 YEARS.
Prescription Only			
ivermectin	Sklice	Apply to dry hair. Saturate hair completely with product. Leave on for 10 min. Rinse hair. Use nit comb to remove eggs.	SHAKE WELL. WASH HANDS AFTER APPLYING.
malathion	Generics	Saturate hair with product. Leave on 8–12 h; then wash hair. Use nit comb to remove eggs.	FLAMMABLE; AVOID FLAMES.
spinosad	Natroba	Apply a sufficient amount of spinosad suspension to cover dry scalp and hair, up to one bottle (120 mL). Leave on for 10 min and then rinse thoroughly. If live lice are still seen 7 days after the first treatment, apply a second treatment.	WASH HANDS AFTER APPLYING.

Key Points

- Lice and scabies infestations affect people worldwide.
- Head lice, body lice, pubic lice, and scabies are spread through direct person-to-person contact.
- Lice and scabies infestations are caused by parasites.
- A parasite is an organism that benefits by living in, with, or on another organism (host), usually to the detriment of the host.
- Head lice infestation most commonly affects children aged 3 to 11 years and their families, but anyone can become infested.
- Head lice infestation is caused by the parasite *Pediculus humanus capitis*.
- Body lice infestations are caused by the parasite *Pediculus humanus corporis*.
- Body louse infestations are a serious public health concern because body lice may cause epidemics of typhus and louse-borne relapsing fever.
- Pubic lice, or "crabs," are sometimes classified as a sexually transmitted infection because they are most commonly spread through sexual contact.
- Lice infestation in the pubic region is caused by the parasite *Pthirus pubis*.
- Scabies infestations are common and are caused by a parasitic mite called *Sarcoptes scabiei*.
- The mite flourishes and spreads via person-to-person contact in environments in which the population density is high, such as hospitals, nursing homes, childcare facilities, and schools.
- Like lice, *S. scabiei* feeds on blood and dies if away from a human host for longer than 48 to 72 hours.
- Strategies to prevent lice and scabies reinfestation include the following: (1) treat all infested household members; (2) use a nit comb to remove eggs (lice); (3) wash clothing, linens, and bedding in hot water (130°F [54°C]); (4) dry-clean clothing that is not washable; and (5) place stuffed toys, clothing, and bedding that cannot be washed or dry-cleaned in a large plastic bag and seal the bag for 2 weeks.
- Head lice and pubic lice may be treated with nonprescription and prescription pediculicides.

- A pediculicide is a drug that kills lice.
- Drug resistance is a growing problem for over-the-counter and prescription pediculicides, especially permethrin, because of the residue left after treatment.
- Pyrethrins are indicated for the treatment of head lice, body lice, and pubic lice, whereas permethrin is approved only for the treatment of head lice.
- Permethrin is ovicidal (kills eggs).
- Dimethicone 100 cSt 50% is used to treat head lice. It works by asphyxiating the louse.

- Ivermectin is a prescription drug that is applied topically to treat head lice and orally to treat worm infections.
- Malathion is flammable; those using it should stay away from open flames, hair dryers, curling irons, and lit cigarettes, cigars, and pipes.
- Crotamiton is a scabicide that can be used during pregnancy.
- Spinosad is a pediculicide indicated for the topical treatment of head lice infestations in patients 4 years of age and older.

Review Questions

1. A _____ is an organism that benefits by living in, with, or on another organism (host), usually to the detriment of the host.
   a. parasite
   b. protozoan
   c. proteus
   d. bacterium

2. The life cycle of a head louse is approximately _____.
   a. 1 to 2 weeks
   b. 2 to 3 weeks
   c. 3 to 5 weeks
   d. 4 to 6 weeks

3. Select the topical pediculicide that is prescription only in the United States.
   a. Eurax
   b. Resultz
   c. NIX
   d. R&C shampoo

4. _____, or crabs, are sometimes classified as a sexually transmitted infection.
   a. Scabies
   b. Head lice
   c. Pubic lice
   d. Body lice

5. Select the pediculicide that is used to treat head lice that is marketed as an OTC product.
   a. Ivermectin
   b. Sklice
   c. Natroba
   d. NIX

6. _____ may be treated with nonprescription and prescription pediculicides.
   a. Scabies
   b. Head lice
   c. Pubic lice
   d. b and c

7. Pyrethrins are naturally derived from the _____ flower.
   a. passion
   b. chrysanthemum
   c. periwinkle
   d. cone

8. OTC head lice products that are available only in Canada are _____.
   a. Kwellada and NIX
   b. Sklice and Rosiver
   c. Eurax and Natroba
   d. Resultz and NYDA

9. Malathion, an organophosphate pesticide that is used to kill head lice and their eggs, is marketed in the United States and in Canada.
   a. true
   b. false

10. Crotamiton is a(n) _____ that can be used during pregnancy.
    a. scabicide
    b. pediculicide
    c. insecticide
    d. pesticide

Bibliography

Burgess I. Head lice: resistance and treatment options. *Pharm J*. 2016:297.

Centers for Disease Control and Prevention. (2019). Head Lice Treatment. Retrieved November 2, 2017, from https://www.cdc.gov/parasites/lice/head/treatment.html.

Centers for Disease Control and Prevention. (2019). Pubic Lice Treatment. Retrieved November 2, 2017, from https://www.cdc.gov/parasites/lice/pubic/treatment.html.

Centers for Disease Control and Prevention. (2018). Scabies Treatment. Retrieved November 2, 2017, from https://www.cdc.gov/parasites/scabies/treatment.html.

Centers for Disease Control and Prevention. Unintentional topical lindane ingestions—United States, 1998–2003. *MMWR Morb Mortal Wkly Rep*. 2005;54:533–535.

Cummings C, Finlay JC, MacDonald NE. Head lice infestations: a clinical update. *Paediatr Child Health*. 2018;23(1):e18–e24.

Health Canada. (2023). Drug Product Database. Retrieved January 14, 2023, from https://www.canada.ca/en/health-canada/services/drugs-health-products/drug-products/drug-product-database.html.

Salimi M, Saghafipour A, Firoozfar F, et al. Study on efficacy of 1% permethrin shampoo and some traditional physical treatment for head lice infestation. *Int J Prev Med*. 2021;12:1.

U.S. Food and Drug Administration. (nd). Drugs@FDA: FDA Approved Drug Products. Retrieved January 14, 2023, from https://www.accessdata.fda.gov/scripts/cder/daf/index.cfm.

Woods AD, Porter CL, Feldman SR. Abametapir for the treatment of head lice: a drug review. *Ann Pharmacother*. 2022;56(3):352–357.

APPENDICES: WORKBOOK EXERCISES

Appendix 1: Fundamentals of Pharmacology

TERMS AND DEFINITIONS

Match each term with the correct definition below.

A. Bioavailability
B. Biopharmaceuticals
C. Controlled substance
D. Dosage form
E. Dose
F. Dosing schedule
G. Drug
H. Drug delivery system
I. Enteral
J. Homeopathic medicines
K. Legend drug
L. Over-the-counter drug
M. Parenteral
N. Pharmacognosy
O. Pharmacology
P. Pharmacotherapy
Q. Toxicology

1. The study of the biological, biochemical features of drugs of plant and animal origins is called _____.
2. _____ is defined as the study of drugs and their interactions with living systems, including chemical and physical properties, toxicology, and therapeutics.
3. A(n) _____ is defined as a substance that is used to diagnose, treat, cure, prevent, or mitigate disease in humans or other animals.
4. A(n) _____ drug is administered orally, whereas a(n) _____ drug is administered by injection or infusion.
5. A(n) _____ may be obtained without a prescription, whereas _____ may be obtained only by prescription.
6. Medicines can be formulated into a different _____ (formulation) and a(n) _____ is designed to release a specific amount of drug.
7. A drug may be classified as a(n) _____ to restrict its possession because of its potential for abuse.
8. The term used to describe the use of drugs for the treatment of disease is _____.
9. The _____ is the frequency that the drug is administered (e.g., "four times a day").
10. Drugs produced by the process of bioengineering involving recombinant DNA technology are classified as _____.
11. _____ is the science dealing with the study of poisons.
12. The term used to describe the extent to which a drug reaches the site of action and is available to produce its effects is _____.
13. _____ are drugs that are administered in minute quantities and stimulate natural body healing systems.
14. If it is a(n) _____, then it is the amount for just one application or administration.

MULTIPLE CHOICE

1. All the following statements about pharmacy technicians who have a working knowledge of pharmacology are true *except*:
   A. Pharmacy technicians' work performance will be more accurate and efficient.
   B. Pharmacy technicians may be able to reduce dispensing errors.
   C. More time will be spent searching for drugs when pharmacy technicians have good brand/generic name recognition.
   D. The selection of appropriate warning labels (auxiliary labels) to place on prescription vials of dispensed medicines is made easier.
   E. Pharmacy technicians understand the importance of alerting the pharmacy to drug interactions, therapeutic duplication, and excessive dose alerts screened by the computer.
2. Which Greek physician is considered to be the "father of pharmacology"?
   A. Dioscorides
   B. Theophrastus
   C. Emperor Shen Nung
   D. Hippocrates
3. The stems -azepam and -azolam indicate that the drug is a(n) _____.
   A. H2 receptor antagonist
   B. calcium channel blocker
   C. corticosteroid
   D. nonsteroidal antiinflammatory drug (NSAID)
   E. benzodiazepine
4. Select the **false** statement regarding synthetic and naturally derived drugs.
   A. A naturally derived drug may be a chemical modification of a synthetic drug.
   B. A synthetic drug may be manufactured entirely from chemical ingredients unrelated to a natural drug.
   C. Plants have been collected, cultivated, and harvested for their healing properties and used in the treatment of illness.
   D. Natural drugs may be derived from plants, animals, or minerals.
5. Select the **true** statement.
   A. The official name of a drug is the brand name.

B. The proprietary name, or brand name, is assigned by the regulatory authority responsible for licensing the drug.

C. Factors considered when selecting a suitable proprietary name are whether (1) an existing drug has a look-alike or sound-alike name and (2) the generic name can be easily associated with the name of an active ingredient in the new drug.

D. The chemical name is the same as the generic name of the drug.

6. All the following statements about generic drugs are true *except*:

A. A generic drug contains the same active ingredient as the original manufacturer's drug.

B. A generic drug and its brand name equivalent have the same strength of the active ingredient and the same dosage form.

C. Generic drugs are more expensive than brand name drugs.

D. A generic drug may contain different inactive ingredients than the brand name product.

7. Which of the following is **true**?

A. Suspensions can be delivered orally, topically, or rectally.

B. Oral disintegrating tablets (ODTs) dissolve more slowly than sublingual tablets.

C. Capsules are solid dosage forms that contain the active ingredient only.

D. Delayed-action tablets are destroyed mostly in the stomach.

8. All the following statements about the preparation and administration of parenterally administered drugs are true *except*:

A. Aseptic technique must be used when preparing drugs for parenteral administration.

B. High doses of drugs administered intravenously (injected into a vein) must be injected rapidly to avoid destruction of red blood cells (hemolysis).

C. Drugs formulated for intramuscular administration (injected into a muscle) may produce a rapid onset or a slow onset of action.

D. Parenteral formulations may be administered intravenously, intramuscularly, or subcutaneously.

9. Select the drug formulation that has a slow onset of action and prolonged effects.

A. Inhalation (e.g., metered-dose inhaler)

B. Sublingual tablet (e.g., nitroglycerin)

C. Intramuscular depot injection (e.g., prolixin decanoate)

D. All the above

10. Medications can be formulated for injection into the _____.

A. vein

B. muscle

C. cerebrospinal fluid

D. joint

E. all the above

MATCHING

Match the US legislation with its intended effect.

A. Durham-Humphrey amendment

B. Kefauver-Harris amendment

C. Drug Price Competition and Patent Term Restoration Act (1984)

D. Pure Food and Drug Act (1906)

E. National Association of Provincial Regulatory Authority Schedule II

F. Controlled Substance Act (1970)

G. Combat Methamphetamine Epidemic Act (2005)

1. The _____ requires that all drugs be safe and effective before they are made available to the public.

2. The _____ is the first significant legislation passed to protect the public from harmful and ineffective drugs.

3. The _____ encouraged the creation of generic drugs.

4. The _____ established the distinction between legend drugs and over-the-counter drugs.

5. The _____ was passed to regulate over-the-counter sales of ephedrine, pseudoephedrine, and phenylpropanolamine.

6. The _____ regulates drugs that have a history of abuse.

7. Behind-the-counter drugs in Canada are classified as _____, allowing patients to receive the drug without a prescription but with the security of a pharmacist's intervention.

TRUE OR FALSE

1. _____ Egypt, Mesopotamia, India, and China have contributed to our body of knowledge of medicinals.

2. _____ A synthetic drug may be a chemical modification of a natural drug or manufactured entirely from chemical ingredients.

3. _____ The Drug Enforcement Agency regulates the new drug and investigational new drug process in the United States.

4. _____ The Health Products and Food Branch of Health Canada regulates the use of therapeutic drugs in Canada.

5. _____ The new drug application process includes preclinical research; clinical studies; phase 1, 2, and 3 trials; and postmarket safety studies.

6. _____ If a drug product contains multiple active ingredients, all official drug names must be listed on the medication label.

7. _____ In the United States, patent holders for new drugs are given up to 20 years' exclusive rights to manufacture and distribute the drugs.

8. _____ Generic drugs are often a cheaper option and must contain the same active and inactive ingredients as their brand name counterparts.

9. _____ A topically administered drug can produce a local effect only.

10. _____ Parenteral drugs with rapid onset of action are typically prepared in water-soluble solutions, and slow-onset, prolonged duration-of-action formulations are suspended in oil or other nonaqueous vehicles (solvents).

CASE STUDY

A 6-year-old child comes into the hospital with severe pain. The physician on duty chooses to prescribe fentanyl to reduce the pain.
1. Research the different available drug products for fentanyl. What are the advantages and disadvantages of each?

_____

_____

_____

_____

2. As you noticed from your research, fentanyl is unavailable as a conventional tablet. Why do you think this is so?

_____

_____

_____

_____

_____

For Critical Thinking, Research Activity, and answer key, please refer to Evolve.

Appendix 2: Principles of Pharmacology

TERMS AND DEFINITIONS

Match each term with the correct definition below.
A. Absorption
B. Biotransformation
C. Distribution
D. Duration of action
E. Diffusion
F. Electrolytes
G. Enzyme
H. First-pass effect
I. Half-life
J. Hydrophilic
K. Hydrophobic
L. Ionization
M. Lipid
N. Lipophilic
O. Metabolism
P. Metabolite
Q. Peak effect
R. Pharmacokinetics
S. Prodrug

1. Osmosis is an example of the process of _____, which is the passive movement of molecules across cell membranes from an area of high drug concentration to an area of lower drug concentration.
2. The cytochrome P-450 system consists of _____(s) capable of increasing the metabolism of drugs in the liver.
3. A product of metabolism, a(n) _____ may be an inactivated drug or active drug with equal or greater activity than the parent drug.
4. The length of time it takes for the plasma concentration of an administered drug to be reduced by half is known as the _____.
5. _____ is the chemical process involving the release of a proton (H^+). Ionized drug molecules may have a positive or negative charge.
6. Lipid-loving substances (_____) are _____ (water hating).
7. Small charged molecules involved with homeostasis are _____
8. A(n) _____ is a drug that is administered in an inactive form and metabolized in the body to an active form.
9. _____ drugs are water loving.

10. During the pharmacokinetic phase of _____, the drug undergoes _____, a process whereby the drug is converted to a more active, equally active, or inactive metabolite.
11. The first pharmacokinetic phase is _____, the process involving the movement of drug molecules from the site of administration into the circulatory system.
12. The _____ is the process whereby the liver metabolizes nearly all of a drug before it passes into the general circulation.
13. The maximum effect produced by a drug is known as the _____ and is achieved once the drug has reached its maximum concentration in the body.
14. _____ is the science dealing with the dynamic process a drug undergoes to produce its therapeutic effect.
15. A(n) _____ is a fatlike substance.
16. The process of movement of a drug from the circulatory system across barrier membranes to the site of drug action is called _____.
17. _____ is the time between the onset and discontinuation of drug action.

MULTIPLE CHOICE

1. Which of the following may be substituted for the brand name drug when authorized (i.e., follows product substitution laws)?
   A. Pharmaceutical alternative drug
   B. Pharmaceutical equivalent drug
   C. Bioequivalent drug
   D. Therapeutic alternative drug
2. Which of the following is *not* a pharmacokinetic phase?
   A. Disintegration
   B. Absorption
   C. Distribution
   D. Metabolism
   E. Elimination
3. The time it takes a drug to reach the concentration necessary to produce a therapeutic effect is the _____.
   A. site of action
   B. duration of action
   C. onset of action
   D. mechanism of action
4. The rate of absorption depends on the _____
   A. lipid solubility
   B. extent of ionization

C. surface area
D. all the above
E. none of the above
5. Which drug is most likely to cross the blood-brain barrier?
   A. A lipid-soluble drug
   B. A drug that is easily ionizable
   C. A hydrophilic drug
   D. A nonionized drug
   E. A and D
6. What factor would increase the bioavailability of a drug?
   A. Decreased drug absorption
   B. Increased first-pass effect
   C. Increased distribution of the drug
   D. Taking the drug orally rather than intravenously
7. Active drug transport _____.
   A. requires no energy
   B. can move a drug from a low to high concentration area
   C. is required to transport lipid-soluble drugs across the cell membrane
   D. is the method by which most drugs distribute throughout the body
8. The main organ for metabolism is the _____.
   A. kidney
   B. liver
   C. heart
   D. stomach
9. Metabolism of a drug can result in _____.
   A. converting a prodrug to its active form
   B. converting an active drug to an inactive metabolite
   C. converting an active drug to a more active metabolite
   D. all the above
   E. none of the above
10. Premature infants are especially sensitive to drugs because of all the following *except* _____.
    A. their kidneys are not well developed
    B. their drug-metabolizing capacity is limited
    C. their capacity for protein binding of drugs is excessive
    D. their lungs are not well developed

MATCHING

A. bioequivalent drug
B. pharmaceutical alternative
C. pharmaceutical equivalent
D. therapeutic alternative
   1. A _____ contains the same active ingredient as the brand name drug; however, the strength and dosage form may be different.
   2. A _____ shows no statistical differences in the rate and extent of absorption when it is administered in the same strength, dosage form, and route of administration as the brand name product.
   3. A _____ contains an identical amount of active ingredient as the brand name drug but may have different inactive ingredients or be manufactured in a different dosage form.
   4. A _____ contains different active ingredient(s) than the brand name drug yet produces the same desired therapeutic outcome.

MATCHING

A. Metabolism
B. Elimination

C. Hydrophilic
D. Lipophilic
   1. _____ Process of biotransformation taking place in the liver
   2. _____ Water loving
   3. _____ Process of drug removal from the body
   4. _____ Lipid loving

TRUE OR FALSE

1. _____ When taken orally, drugs must undergo disintegration and dissolution before absorption can take place.
2. _____ A synthetic drug may be a chemical modification of a natural drug or manufactured entirely from chemical ingredients.
3. _____ The first-pass effect describes why some drugs, if taken orally, would be inactivated before exerting an effect.
4. _____ Protein-bound drugs pass easily through capillary walls.
5. _____ Factors influencing metabolism are kidney function, disease, patient age, drug interactions, genetics, nutrition, and patient gender.
6. _____ When drugs are located in the basic solutions of the small intestine, it is the weakly acidic drugs that are absorbed more readily compared with weakly basic drugs.
7. _____ Drugs are absorbed across cell membranes via active and passive transport mechanisms.

CASE STUDY

A new patient at the pharmacy was prescribed clopidogrel to prevent a stroke. Clopidogrel is a substrate of the CYP450 2C19 enzyme and becomes inactive when metabolized.
1. Identify the changes in peak effect and duration of action if the patient was also taking amiodarone.
   _____
   _____
   _____
   _____
2. Identify the changes in peak effect and duration of action if the patient was also taking omeprazole.
   _____
   _____
   _____
   _____
   _____
3. Identify the changes in peak effect and duration of action if the patient was also taking phenobarbital, a barbiturate.
   _____
   _____
   _____
   _____
4. Clopidogrel is a prodrug. What does "prodrug" mean?
   _____
   _____
   _____
   _____
   _____

For Critical Thinking, Research Activity, and answer key, please refer to Evolve.

Appendix 3: Pharmacodynamics

TERMS AND DEFINITIONS

Match each term with the correct definition below.
A. Affinity
B. Agonist
C. Antagonist
D. Efficacy
E. Idiosyncratic reaction
F. Inverse agonist
G. Mechanism of action
H. Noncompetitive antagonist
I. Partial agonist
J. Pharmacodynamics
K. Pharmacotherapeutics
L. Potency
M. Receptor site
N. Therapeutic index

1. _____ is the study of drugs and their actions on a living organism.
2. An unexpected drug reaction is known as a(n) _____.
3. The use of drugs in the treatment of disease, _____, is the study of factors that influence the patient response to drugs.
4. The _____ is a ratio of the effective dose to the lethal dose.
5. _____ is the measure of a drug's effectiveness.
6. _____ is defined as the effective dose concentration.
7. _____ is defined as the attraction that the receptor site has for the drug.
8. The manner in which a drug produces its effect is the _____.
9. The drug that can turn "off" an activated receptor and turn "on" a receptor not currently active is known as a(n) _____.
10. A(n) _____ is a drug that binds to its receptor site and stimulates a cellular response.
11. A drug that binds to an alternative receptor site that prevents binding of an agonist is a(n) _____.
12. A binding drug that does not produce action is known as a(n) _____.
13. A(n) _____ behaves as an agonist under some conditions and acts as an antagonist under other conditions.
14. The location of drug-cell binding is known as the _____.

MULTIPLE CHOICE

1. Select the statement about drug-receptor binding that is **false**.
   A. The more similar a drug is to the shape of a receptor site, the greater is the affinity the receptor site has for the drug.
   B. Drug-receptor binding may enhance or inhibit normal biological processes.
   C. An agonist is a drug that binds to its receptor site and stimulates a cellular response.
   D. Antagonist binding turns off a receptor that was activated.
   E. Drug-receptor binding is like a "lock and key."
2. Individual variation in pharmacokinetic and pharmacologic responses may be caused by all the following *except* the patient's _____.
   A. weight and gender
   B. emotional state
   C. age
   D. disease state
   E. hair color
3. Patients who have been diagnosed with _____ tend to experience more severe adverse drug reactions.
   A. kidney disease
   B. liver disease
   C. lung disease
   D. all the above
4. Which drug is most potent?

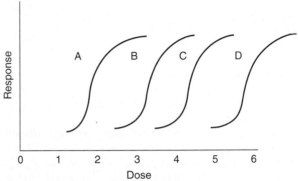

   A. Drug A
   B. Drug B
   C. Drug C
   D. Drug D
5. The basic requirement of a receptor is _____.
   A. recognition of molecules to bind and produce an effect in the cell
   B. that it fit only one drug
   C. that it is the place to deposit your genes
   D. none of the above
6. An elderly patient is likely to experience adverse drug reactions more frequently than an adolescent patient. Which factor primarily accounts for this?
   A. Drug clearance is more rapid in adolescents.
   B. Elderly patients are more likely to be taking multiple drugs than adolescent patients; therefore drug elimination is slower in elderly patients.
   C. Adolescent patients have increased blood flow to the gastrointestinal tract.
   D. Higher doses are given to geriatric patients.
7. Which statement about drug dependence is **false**?
   A. Drug dependence is an adverse reaction that is associated with antibiotics.
   B. When dependence develops, a patient must take increasing doses of a drug to get the desired effect.
   C. When dependence has developed, a patient must continue to take a drug to prevent withdrawal symptoms.
   D. All controlled drugs can produce dependence.
8. A drug that turns "off" a receptor that is normally activated is considered a(n) _____:
   A. competitive antagonist
   B. inverse agonist
   C. partial agonist
   D. none of the above

9. Mrs. Smith is picking up a new prescription for citalopram to treat depression. She thinks that "there's no way a small little pill is ever going to make me happy again." Based on this information, what factor is likely to affect her adherence to this medication?
   A. Dose schedule misunderstanding
   B. Ability to afford drug therapy
   C. Adverse drug reaction
   D. Perceived benefits of therapy

10. A pharmacy should report suspected adverse drug reactions to the _____.
   A. Drug Enforcement Agency (DEA)
   B. Food and Drug Administration (FDA)
   C. Centers for Disease Control and Prevention (CDC)
   D. board of pharmacy

MATCHING

A. teratogen
B. carcinogen
C. hepatotoxic drug
D. nephrotoxic drug

1. A _____ is able to produce a serious adverse reaction in the liver.
2. A _____ is able to produce a serious reaction in the kidney.
3. A _____ is able to produce harm to a developing fetus.
4. A _____ is able to stimulate the growth of cancers.

MATCHING

A. Ceiling effect
B. Potency
C. LD_{50}
D. Desensitization
E. ED_{50}

1. _____ Lethal dose for 50% of the population
2. _____ Maximum possible effect that could be produced
3. _____ Effective dose for 50% of the population
4. _____ Effective dose concentration
5. _____ Decreased drug response over time because of repeated exposure

TRUE OR FALSE

1. _____Drugs that are administered in very low doses yet produce a maximum effect have high efficacy.
2. _____A steep dose-response curve indicates that a large change in a drug dose is required to produce a big change in the drug response.
3. _____Safe drugs have a wide margin between the lethal dose and the effective dose.
4. _____Age, gender, disease, pregnancy, weight, and genetics are patient-related factors that influence the drug response.
5. _____The placebo effect demonstrates that only biological factors are responsible for the patient response to drugs.

6. _____Extended-release medications decrease patient adherence.
7. _____Patients may develop tolerance to the side effects of a drug without developing tolerance to its therapeutic effects.

CASE STUDY

An elderly patient comes into the pharmacy. When he is picking up his Benicar HCT to help lower his blood pressure, you notice that he should have been out of the medication 2 weeks ago. You ask him how his therapy has been going, and he responds by saying, "Not well. I've been keeping track of my blood pressure, and it's still high!"

1. Describe at least three potential reasons why this medication may not be working as intended for this patient.
   _____
   _____
   _____
   _____
   _____

2. Describe what you, along with the pharmacist's help, could do to resolve any potential adherence problems with the patient.
   _____
   _____
   _____
   _____

A few months later, the patient comes back to the pharmacy. According to his refill dates, you notice that his adherence to Benicar HCT has improved dramatically. You check his blood pressure journal and see that his most recent reading was 92/58, a level that is lower than desired. Upon further questioning, you also find out that he has liver disease. After consulting with the pharmacist, you understand that the current dose of Benicar HCT is too high.

3. Identify at least three physiologic factors that could explain why the patient's dose of Benicar is changing his blood pressure levels so drastically.
   _____
   _____
   _____
   _____
   _____

4. Benicar HCT has a relatively wide therapeutic index, so the patient was not harmed by the high dose. Explain the importance of proper adherence for lithium, warfarin, and other drugs that have narrow therapeutic indexes.
   _____
   _____
   _____
   _____

For Critical Thinking, Research Activity, and answer key, please refer to Evolve.

Appendix 4: Drug Interactions and Medication Errors

TERMS AND DEFINITIONS

Match each term with the correct definition below.

A. Additive effect
B. Antagonism
C. Drug-disease contraindication
D. Drug-drug interaction
E. Drug-food interaction
F. Medication error
G. Potentiation
H. Synergistic effects
I. Therapeutic duplication

1. An error made in the process of prescribing, preparing, dispensing, or administering drug therapy is called a(n) _____.

2. An altered drug response that occurs when a drug is administered with certain foods is called _____.

3. Interactions between two drugs may produce _____ that are greater than would be produced if either drug were administered alone.

4. _____ is the administration of two drugs that produce similar therapeutic effects and side effects.

5. _____ is a reaction that occurs when two or more drugs are administered at the same time.

6. When administration of the drug may worsen the patient's medical condition, a(n) _____ exists.

7. An increased drug effect, or _____, is produced when a second similar drug is added to therapy and the effects produced are greater than the effects produced by either drug alone.

8. _____ is a process by which one drug or food, acting at a separate site or via a different mechanism of action, increases the effect of another drug, yet produces no effect when administered alone.

9. A drug-drug interaction or drug-food interaction that decreases or blocks the effects of another drug is called _____.

MULTIPLE CHOICE

1. A drug interaction that can increase the risk for pregnancy may occur when _____ is(are) taken with oral contraceptives.
   A. birth control pills
   B. amoxicillin
   C. aspirin
   D. antihistamines
   E. ibuprofen

2. Which of the following fruits is implicated in food-drug interactions?
   A. Apple
   B. Pear
   C. Grapefruit
   D. Plum
   E. Grape

3. Which vitamin may be administered as an antidote for the drug warfarin?
   A. Vitamin A
   B. Vitamin B
   C. Vitamin C
   D. Vitamin D
   E. Vitamin K

4. Which way of writing the milligram (mg) strength of a drug can reduce medication errors?
   A. 1.0 mg
   B. 1 mg
   C. 1.00 mg
   D. 01 mg

5. Which is *not* a characteristic of an "aseptic attitude" when preparing parenteral medications?
   A. Handwashing
   B. Hood cleaning
   C. Dose calculating
   D. Proper technique
   E. Eating in the clean room

6. Pharmacy technicians may reduce medication errors by all the following *except* _____.
   A. always checking the original prescription against the prescription label and the NDC number (DIN number in Canada) on the stock bottle
   B. asking patients to spell sound-alike drugs when they call to request refills
   C. guessing what the medication might be when the handwriting on the prescription is difficult to read
   D. always placing a zero in front of the decimal point when calculating doses that are less than 1 mL or 1 mg.
   E. writing legibly

7. Medication errors can happen at all the following times *except* when _____.
   A. dispensing medication
   B. administering medication
   C. interpreting a written prescription
   D. writing a medication order
   E. all the above

8. Which statement about drug interactions is **false**?
   A. Drug interactions may be caused by induction or inhibition of metabolic enzymes.
   B. Interactions cannot be avoided by maintaining an up-to-date history of the patient's chronic and acute medical conditions.
   C. Interactions that involve competition for a common transport system in the kidney can affect the elimination of some drugs.
   D. Pharmacists and pharmacy technicians should screen all prescriptions for potential drug interactions before dispensing a medication.

9. When warfarin and _____ are administered together, excessive bleeding occurs.
   A. acetaminophen
   B. codeine
   C. penicillin
   D. aspirin

10. Which abbreviation can be found on the Joint Commission "Do Not Use" list?
    A. QD
    B. BID
    C. TID
    D. QID

MATCHING

A. "Chicken scratch"
B. "Sound-alike, look-alike" drug names
C. (ℨi)
D. NKDA
E. (ℨ)

1. _____ One dram
2. _____ Poor handwriting
3. _____ Ounce
4. _____ Zyprexa and Celexa
5. _____ No known drug allergies

MATCHING

A. Bagging error
B. Miscommunication
C. Improper medication preparation
D. Improper labeling
E. Product selection error

1. _____ Incorrect directions on the bottle
2. _____ Placing Jeni Smith's prescription together with Jenny Smith's prescription
3. _____ Dispensing Prozac when the prescription asked for Prilosec
4. _____ Mixing a sterile compound without washing your hands first
5. _____ Interpreting a hastily made voicemail incorrectly

TRUE OR FALSE

1. _____ The pharmacy should collect information about a patient's use of over-the-counter drugs and enter it into the patient profile.
2. _____ NKDA is an abbreviation commonly used in pharmacies that means the patient does not have drug allergies.
3. _____ Pharmacy technicians unfamiliar with apothecary symbols may confuse the symbols for ounce and dram.
4. _____ The more drugs that are administered to a patient, the less likely it is that interactions will occur.
5. _____ Coadministration of drugs and foods can affect absorption, distribution, metabolism, or elimination.
6. _____ The process by which a drug, or a food, increases the effects of another drug, yet does not produce any effects when administered alone, is called antagonism.
7. _____ Intravenous solutions of acids and bases are incompatible, and when the solutions are combined, solid particles (precipitates) form.
8. _____ Studies indicate that between 7% and 22% of adverse drug reactions are caused by drug-drug interactions.

9. _____ Medication errors can be made by both health care professionals and patients.
10. _____ Medication errors associated with prescribers are often a result of carelessness.

CASE STUDY

You work in a busy retail pharmacy located inside a grocery store, and the pharmacy manager has noticed a recent increase in the number of medication errors that are being made. Although these errors have been resolved before reaching the patient, the manager has decided to hold a team meeting to discuss error-prevention strategies.

1. Given the pharmacy location, what are at least three potential sources of distraction at this pharmacy? What can be done to reduce or eliminate those distractions?
   _____
   _____
   _____
   _____
   _____

2. You have personally noticed that a number of patients have mistakenly been given someone else's prescriptions. Describe two ways in which these errors occur and strategies to prevent each of them.
   _____
   _____
   _____
   _____
   _____

   A few months later, you apply for and accept a job inside a hospital pharmacy. You have little experience in this area of pharmacy, and you are nervous about making mistakes.

3. Compare the responsibilities of a retail pharmacy technician with those of a hospital pharmacy technician. What are the common sources of error in each setting?
   _____
   _____
   _____
   _____
   _____

4. What are the potential sources of distraction at this pharmacy? What can be done to reduce them in your workflow?
   _____
   _____
   _____
   _____

For Critical Thinking, Research Activity, and answer key, please refer to Evolve.

Appendix 5: Treatment of Anxiety

TERMS AND DEFINITIONS

Match each term with the correct definition below.

A. Anxiety
B. Anxiolytic
C. Drug dependence
D. Generalized anxiety disorder
E. Obsessive-compulsive disorder
F. Panic disorder
G. Phobia
H. Posttraumatic stress disorder
I. Tolerance

1. An irrational fear of things or situations, a(n) _____ produces symptoms of intense anxiety.
2. _____ is a condition associated with an inability to control or stop repeated unwanted thoughts or behaviors.
3. A stress disorder that develops in persons who have participated in, witnessed, or been a victim of a terrifying event is called a(n) _____.
4. When a person must take increasing doses of a drug to achieve the same effects as were achieved at previously lower doses, they have developed _____.
5. _____ is a condition that is associated with excessive worrying and tension that is experienced daily for more than 6 months.
6. Repeated episodes of a sudden onset of feelings of terror are associated with _____.
7. _____ is a condition associated with tension, apprehension, fear, or panic.
8. When a person taking a drug must continue to take the drug to avoid the onset of physical and/or psychological withdrawal symptoms, they have developed _____.
9. A(n) _____ is a drug used to treat anxiety.

MULTIPLE CHOICE

1. Anxiety disorders are *not* linked to _____ factors.
   A. environmental
   B. societal
   C. biological
   D. developmental
   E. socioeconomic
2. The following statements are true about benzodiazepines *except*:
   A. Abrupt discontinuation of those with short half-lives precipitates withdrawal symptoms quickly.
   B. Abrupt discontinuation of those with long half-lives leads to delayed withdrawal symptoms.
   C. Most benzodiazepines are C-IV, although some are C-III.
   D. Benzodiazepines are sometimes used in surgeries because they can cause the patient to "forget" about the procedure and have less anxiety about future operations.
3. Which of the following is *not* an accepted medical treatment for anxiety?
   A. Administration of anxiolytics
   B. Psychotherapy
   C. Cognitive-behavioral therapy
   D. Self-administration of alcohol
4. Select the **false** statement.
   A. Benzodiazepines may produce tolerance and dependence.
   B. Benzodiazepines may be long acting, intermediate acting, or short acting.
   C. Benzodiazepines may induce amnesia.
   D. Benzodiazepines close chloride ion (Cl^-) channels.
   E. Benzodiazepines bind to receptor sites on the $GABA_A$ complex.
5. All the following medications may be prescribed for anxiety *except* _____.
   A. selective serotonin reuptake inhibitors
   B. tricyclic antidepressants
   C. benzodiazepines
   D. opioids
6. Common physiologic symptoms of anxiety include _____.
   A. heart palpitations
   B. nausea
   C. decreased heart rate
   D. A and B
   E. all the above
7. A warning label that should be affixed to prescription vials for benzodiazepines is _____.
   A. AVOID PROLONGED EXPOSURE TO SUNLIGHT
   B. TAKE WITH LOTS OF WATER
   C. MAY BE HABIT FORMING
   D. AVOID ANTACIDS, DAIRY PRODUCTS, AND FE^{2+} PRODUCTS
8. Aside from anxiety, benzodiazepines can also be used for _____.
   A. insomnia
   B. muscle relaxation
   C. seizure disorders
   D. all the above
9. Which pair of drugs used to treat anxiety does *not* produce tolerance or dependence?
   A. Lorazepam and buspirone
   B. Buspirone and hydroxyzine HCl
   C. Hydroxyzine HCl and diazepam
   D. Diazepam and alprazolam

FILL IN THE BLANK: DRUG NAMES

1. What is the **brand name** for alprazolam? _____
2. What is the **generic name** for Effexor XR? _____
3. What is the **brand name** for clonazepam? _____
4. What is the **generic name** for Valium? _____
5. What is the **brand name** for lorazepam? _____
6. What is the **brand name** for escitalopram (United States)? _____
7. What is the **brand name** for buspirone? _____
8. What is the **generic name** for Cymbalta? _____
9. What is the **brand name** for paroxetine? _____

10. What is the **brand name** for hydroxyzine HCl? _____
11. What is the **generic name** for Prozac? _____
12. What is the **brand name** for sertraline? _____

MATCHING

Match each drug to its pharmacologic classification.
A. Benzodiazepines
B. Antidepressants
C. Miscellaneous (antihistamine)
D. Azapirones
E. β-Adrenergic antagonist
  1. _____ Clomipramine
  2. _____ BuSpar
  3. _____ Hydroxyzine HCl
  4. _____ Alprazolam
  5. _____ Propranolol

TRUE OR FALSE

1. _____ Anxiety disorders are the leading form of mental health illness.
2. _____ Treating obsessive-compulsive disorder (OCD) with antidepressants requires a lower dose and a shorter course of treatment when compared with treating depression.
3. _____ A drug classified as a controlled substance IV does not pose a risk for tolerance and dependence.
4. _____ Symptoms of anxiety are associated with hyperactivity of the autonomic nervous system.
5. _____ Most benzodiazepines bind to $GABA_A$ receptors. This interaction increases the affinity of GABA to its GABA receptors, opening more chloride ion channels in the process.
6. _____ Benzodiazepines can produce an amnesia that causes the person receiving the drug to "forget," reducing anxiety associated with future medical procedures.
7. _____ Some symptoms of serotonin syndrome include sedation, constipation, and decreased blood pressure.
8. _____ Propranolol may be administered to reduce palpitations caused by stage fright.

CASE STUDY

A patient was recently diagnosed with generalized anxiety disorder; she began to take alprazolam 4 weeks ago. Her doctor instructed her to use either one-half or one tablet as needed. During the past 2 weeks the patient has needed to use the whole tablet to relieve her anxiety symptoms. She says, "I really don't want to become addicted to these pills. I think I am going to stop taking them."
1. What is the difference between tolerance and dependence?
  _____
  _____
  _____
  _____
2. What are some withdrawal symptoms this patient could experience if she suddenly stopped taking her alprazolam?
  _____
  _____
  _____
  _____
  _____
3. List at least three other medications that the pharmacist could recommend to the patient's doctor to help treat anxiety disorder without producing tolerance and dependence.
  _____
  _____
  _____
  _____
  _____

The patient's doctor prescribes escitalopram, a selective serotonin reuptake inhibitor (SSRI), to help treat her generalized anxiety disorder.
4. How quickly should the patient expect this medication to work?
  _____
  _____
  _____
  _____
  _____

For Critical Thinking, Research Activity, and answer key, please refer to Evolve.

Appendix 6: Treatment of Depression

TERMS AND DEFINITIONS

Match each term with the correct definition below.
A. Adjunct
B. Bipolar disorder
C. Enuresis
D. Major depression
E. Monoamine oxidase
F. Serotonin syndrome

1. _____ is an enzyme that is responsible for degradation of certain neurotransmitters such as norepinephrine (NE), serotonin (5-HT), and dopamine (DA).
2. Bedwetting, or _____, is characterized by uncontrollable urination during sleep.
3. _____, a potentially life-threatening adverse drug reaction, is characterized by symptoms of confusion, agitation, tremors, and increased blood pressure.

4. A mental health illness associated with sudden swings in mood between depression and periods of insomnia, racing thoughts, and distractibility is _____.

5. _____ is a mental health illness associated with persistent feelings of sadness, emptiness, or hopelessness that persist for several weeks.

6. A drug is classified as _____ therapy when it is used to complement the effects of another drug.

MULTIPLE CHOICE

1. Clinical depression is caused by a _____.
   A. decrease in brain acetylcholine
   B. decrease in brain histamine
   C. decrease in brain serotonin, norepinephrine, and dopamine
   D. deficiency of certain neurotransmitters

2. Depression can have the following effects *except* _____.
   A. reduced self-esteem
   B. reduced concentration
   C. increased eating
   D. decreased sleeping
   E. all the above are effects of depression

3. Monoamine oxidase (MAO) inhibitors that are used to treat depression primarily interfere with which enzyme?
   A. MAO$_A$
   B. MAO$_B$
   C. MAO$_C$
   D. Both A and B

4. A blockade of cholinergic (muscarinic) receptors can lead to _____.
   A. dry mouth
   B. diarrhea
   C. increased focus
   D. weight gain

5. Symptoms of bipolar disorder are _____.
   A. racing thoughts
   B. distractibility
   C. increased goal-directed behavior
   D. insomnia
   E. all the above

6. What foods and beverages should be avoided by patients taking MAO inhibitors?
   A. Foods high in sodium
   B. Foods high in tyramine
   C. Foods low in sodium
   D. Foods low in tyramine

7. Which of the following medications may be prescribed for enuresis?
   A. Fluoxetine and olanzapine
   B. Phenelzine and trazodone
   C. Imipramine and nortriptyline
   D. Duloxetine and bupropion

8. What is the main mechanism of action of tricyclic antidepressants?
   A. 5-HT reuptake inhibitor
   B. NE reuptake inhibitor
   C. DA reuptake inhibitor
   D. A and B

9. Select the drug that is *not* used for the treatment of bipolar disorder.
   A. Lithium
   B. Paroxetine
   C. Carbamazepine
   D. Divalproex sodium
   E. Lamotrigine

FILL IN THE BLANK: DRUG NAMES

1. What is the *generic name* for Tofranil? _____
2. What is the *brand name* for desipramine? _____
3. What is a *brand name* for doxepin? _____
4. What is a *brand name* for trimipramine? _____
5. What is a *brand name* for nortriptyline? _____
6. What is the *generic name* for Lexapro (United States)? _____
7. What is the *brand name* for citalopram? _____
8. What is the *generic name* for Prozac? _____
9. What is the *generic name* for Luvox? _____
10. What is the *brand name* for paroxetine? _____
11. What is the *generic name* for Zoloft? _____
12. What is the *brand name* for phenelzine? _____
13. What is the *generic name* for Parnate? _____
14. What is the *brand name* for bupropion? _____
15. What is the *brand name* for mirtazapine? _____
16. What is the *generic name* for Desyrel? _____
17. What is the *brand name* for venlafaxine? _____
18. What is a *brand name* for lithium carbonate? _____
19. What is a *brand name* for carbamazepine? _____
20. What is the *generic name* for Lamictal? _____

MATCHING

Patient education is an essential component of therapeutics. Select the **best** warning label to apply to the prescription vial given to patients taking the drugs listed. An answer can be used more than once or not at all.
A. MAY DISCOLOR URINE
B. SWALLOW WHOLE; DO NOT CRUSH OR CHEW
C. AVOID PREGNANCY
D. AVOID TYRAMINE-CONTAINING FOODS
E. TAKE WITH FOOD
   1. _____ Nardil 15 mg
   2. _____ Effexor XR 75 mg
   3. _____ Wellbutrin 150 mg SR
   4. _____ Lithobid 300 mg
   5. _____ amitriptyline 10 mg

MATCHING

Match each drug to its pharmacologic classification.
A. tricyclic antidepressant (TCA)
B. selective serotonin reuptake inhibitor (SSRI)
C. monoamine oxidase inhibitor (MAOI)
D. serotonin-noradrenaline reuptake inhibitor (SNRI)
E. mood stabilizer/anticonvulsant
   1. _____ Prozac 20 mg
   2. _____ phenelzine 15 mg

3. _____ venlafaxine XR 75 mg
4. _____ imipramine HCl 10 mg
5. _____ carbamazepine ER 100 mg

MATCHING

Match each drug to its pharmacologic classification. An answer can be used more than once or not at all.

A. tricyclic antidepressant (TCA)
B. selective serotonin reuptake inhibitor (SSRI)
C. serotonin-noradrenaline reuptake inhibitor (SNRI)
D. noradrenaline-dopamine inhibitor (NA/DRI)
E. monoamine oxidase inhibitor (MAOI)
F. atypical antidepressant

1. _____ bupropion 150 mg SR
2. _____ desipramine 50 mg
3. _____ moclobemide 100 mg
4. _____ duloxetine DR 30 mg
5. _____ paroxetine 20 mg
6. _____ mirtazapine 15 mg

TRUE OR FALSE

1. _____Tricyclic antidepressants (TCAs) can increase cravings for sweets.
2. _____Prescriptions for large quantities of TCAs may be written for patients with depression who are believed to be suicidal.
3. _____Lithium has a narrow therapeutic index.
4. _____A hypertensive crisis is a fatal adverse reaction associated with TCAs.
5. _____Prescriptions for MAOIs should be dispensed with a list of tyramine-containing foods and a list of drugs to avoid.
6. _____Contents of Effexor XR capsules cannot be sprinkled onto food.
7. _____The endings *-tyline* and *-pramine* are commonly used for TCAs.
8. _____A common ending for SSRIs is *-oxetine*.
9. _____According to the biogenic amine theory, clinical depression results from an increase in monoamine neurotransmitters in the brain.

CASE STUDY

A patient comes to your pharmacy to drop off a prescription for amitriptyline. He says, "I'm not sure I want this filled. I haven't been feeling like myself for a few months. My doctor says I have depression, but starting medication for depression makes me feel like a failure. I should be able to deal with my feelings on my own."

1. Using your knowledge of the biogenic amine theory, describe the role neurotransmitters (norepinephrine, serotonin, and dopamine) have in depression.
_____
_____
_____

2. Describe the mechanism of action of amitriptyline.
_____
_____
_____
_____

Three months later, the patient returns to the pharmacy and says he has not been using his amitriptyline because he doesn't like the side effects. He is still feeling depressed and wants to know whether there is anything he can do to minimize side effects.

3. List common adverse effects associated with tricyclic antidepressants.
_____
_____
_____
_____

The pharmacist explains that all antidepressants are equally effective, and she recommends that the patient talk to his doctor about switching to an SSRI. The next week, the patient brings in a new prescription for sertraline.

4. No medication is without side effects. What adverse effects would the patient possibly experience with sertraline?
_____
_____
_____
_____

5. Serotonin syndrome is a rare but serious side effect associated with SSRIs. Describe the symptoms of serotonin syndrome.
_____
_____
_____
_____

For Critical Thinking, Research Activity, and answer key, please refer to Evolve.

Appendix 7: Treatment of Schizophrenia and Psychoses

TERMS AND DEFINITIONS

Match each term with the correct definition below.

A. Catatonia
B. Delusion
C. Extrapyramidal symptoms
D. Hallucination
E. Negative symptoms
F. Neuroleptic (antipsychotic)
G. Neuroleptic malignant syndrome
H. Positive symptoms
I. Postural hypotension
J. Pseudoparkinsonism
K. Psychosis
L. Schizophrenia
M. Tardive dyskinesia

1. A(n) _____ is a drug used to treat schizophrenia and psychoses.
2. Potentially fatal, _____ produces symptoms such as stupor, muscle rigidity, and high temperature.
3. Persons with schizophrenia may exhibit _____ such as hallucinations, delusions, or other unusual thoughts.
4. A(n) _____ is a mental state characterized by disorganized behavior and thought, delusions, hallucinations, and a loss of touch with reality.
5. _____ is a symptom of schizophrenia that is associated with unresponsiveness and immobility.
6. The administration of neuroleptics may cause _____, excessive muscle movement, and difficulty in walking.
7. The term for a sudden drop in blood pressure upon a change in posture is _____.
8. The administration of neuroleptics may produce _____, an adverse reaction that mimics Parkinson disease.
9. Persons with schizophrenia may have a(n) _____, which presents as irrational thoughts or false beliefs that do not change even when evidence is provided that beliefs are not valid.
10. The administration of neuroleptics may produce _____, an adverse reaction that causes involuntary thrusting of the tongue and changes in posture.
11. Persons with schizophrenia may exhibit _____, which present as a decreased ability to think, plan, or express emotion.
12. _____ is a type of psychosis characterized by delusions of thought, visual and/or auditory hallucinations, and speech disturbances.
13. Visions or voices that exist only in the mind and cannot be seen or heard by others are called a(n) _____.

MULTIPLE CHOICE

1. Neuroleptic malignant syndrome is characterized by symptoms of _____.
   A. hypothermia
   B. liver failure
   C. muscle rigidity
   D. B and C
2. Treatment for schizophrenia that involves dopamine blockade can produce _____.
   A. delusions
   B. neurolepsy
   C. psychosis
   D. pseudoparkinsonism
3. Paul Bunyan was institutionalized for schizophrenia. He was administered fluphenazine HCl, 2.5 mg IM every 6 hours, initially but has been switched to fluphenazine decanoate in preparation for discharge. Fluphenazine decanoate _____.
   A. is a slow-release preparation that is administered every 3 weeks
   B. should be dispensed with an oral syringe
   C. must be diluted in water or juice before administration
   D. is administered sublingually
4. Side effects of aripiprazole include _____.
   A. insomnia
   B. increased risk of death in patients with dementia
   C. hyperglycemia
   D. all the above
5. Patients receiving chlorpromazine oral concentrate, 100 mg/mL, should be given the following advice:
   A. MAY CAUSE DROWSINESS OR DIZZINESS
   B. AVOID ALCOHOL
   C. DILUTE WITH LIQUID BEFORE INGESTION
   D. AVOID PROLONGED EXPOSURE TO SUNLIGHT
   E. All the above
6. Dopamine antagonism in the _____ leads to symptoms of pseudoparkinsonism.
   A. nigrostriatal tract
   B. mesolimbic system
   C. substantia nigra
   D. hypothalamus
7. Which of the following statements about typical antipsychotics is true?
   A. Typical antipsychotics are much more clinically effective than atypical antipsychotics.
   B. Newer atypical antipsychotics are associated with less risk for extrapyramidal side effects.
   C. Medium-potency antipsychotics are associated with sedative and anticholinergic effects.

D. Atypical antipsychotics can only be given orally; they are prodrugs that must go through the first-pass effect in the liver to be effective.

8. Peripheral nervous system side effects of antipsychotics include _____.
   A. constipation
   B. sedation
   C. urinary retention
   D. A and C

9. Up to _____ of the people who are prescribed neuroleptics will experience adverse reactions.
   A. 20%
   B. 40%
   C. 60%
   D. 80%
   E. 100%

10. Clozapine use is restricted because this drug can produce a fatal drop in the _____.
    A. white blood cell level
    B. red blood cell level
    C. blood pressure
    D. pulse

FILL IN THE BLANK: DRUG NAMES

1. What is the *generic name* for Invega (United States)? _____
2. What is the *generic name* for Modecate (Canada)? _____
3. What is a *brand name* for olanzapine? _____
4. What is the *generic name* for Saphris? _____
5. What is the *generic name* for Abilify? _____
6. What is the *brand name* for lurasidone? _____
7. What is the *brand name* for fluphenazine? _____
8. What is a *brand name* for quetiapine? _____
9. What is the *generic name* for Clozaril (United States)? _____
10. What is the *generic name* for Fanapt? _____
11. What is the *generic name* for Loxitane (United States)? _____

MATCHING

Match each drug to its pharmacologic classification.
A. phenothiazines
B. benzisoxazoles
C. thioxanthenes
D. dibenzothiazepines
E. thienobenzodiazepines
   1. _____ Navane
   2. _____ clozapine
   3. _____ Seroquel
   4. _____ fluphenazine
   5. _____ Risperdal

TRUE OR FALSE

1. _____ Haloperidol and risperidone oral concentrates should not be mixed with coffee or tea.
2. _____ Patients, prescribers, and pharmacists must be enrolled in a registry to dispense clozapine.
3. _____ The dropper that comes packaged with oral concentrate may be interchanged with other droppers and dispensed with the medicine.
4. _____ The greater the affinity a neuroleptic drug has for dopamine (D_2) receptors, the less effective is the drug.
5. _____ Schizophrenia affects about 1% of the population worldwide. Symptoms typically begin in the early to mid-20s and may not develop until the early 30 s.
6. _____ Although dopamine is the most relevant neurotransmitter in schizophrenia, others play a role, including serotonin, cholecystokinin, and glutamate.
7. _____ Atypical antipsychotics have a strong affinity for dopamine receptors and often produce Parkinson disease–like symptoms.

CASE STUDY

John is a patient who has been coming to your pharmacy for many years. His facial expressions are flat, he doesn't show emotion, and he has a hard time interacting with pharmacy staff members. He will often talk to himself. A new technician comes to you, complains that John was rude to her, and asks you what is wrong with him. You explain that John has schizophrenia.

1. Distinguish the differences between negative and positive symptoms of schizophrenia. Give examples of each.
   _____
   _____
   _____
   _____
   _____

2. You receive a new prescription from John's doctor and in the notes he has written, "To treat extrapyramidal symptoms." What are extrapyramidal symptoms? Include examples.
   _____
   _____
   _____
   _____
   _____

3. John also has diabetes. List two medications that would be poor choices to treat John's schizophrenia because of their risk of causing hyperglycemia.
   _____
   _____

John is upset that he cannot refill one of his atypical antipsychotics because he forgot to go to his doctor's office to have his blood drawn. You explain to him that you must have the appropriate lab values to report to a special registry before you can dispense this medication.

4. Which medication is John trying to refill today?

_____

5. What value is being monitored by this lab work, and why is it important?

_____

_____

_____

_____

For Critical Thinking, Research Activity, and answer key, please refer to Evolve.

Appendix 8: Treatment of Alzheimer, Huntington, and Parkinson Disease

TERMS AND DEFINITIONS

Match each term with the correct definition below.
A. Acetylcholinesterase
B. Alzheimer disease
C. *ApoE4* allele
D. Bradykinesia
E. Cognitive function
F. Dementia
G. Huntington disease
H. Neurodegeneration
I. Neuroprotective
J. Parkinson disease
K. Plaques
L. Pseudoparkinsonism
M. Tangles

1. _____ is the progressive destruction of neurons.
2. The ability to take in information via the senses, process the details, commit the information to memory, and recall it when necessary is a(n) _____.
3. The enzyme that degrades the neurotransmitter acetylcholine is called _____.
4. The defective form of apolipoprotein E that is associated with Alzheimer disease is called the _____.
5. _____ are twisted fibers made up of tau that interfere with signal transmission.
6. A condition associated with memory loss is referred to as _____.
7. _____ is a drug-induced condition that resembles Parkinson disease.
8. The term used to describe slowness in initiating and carrying out voluntary movements is _____.
9. _____ and _____ are progressive disorders of the nervous system that impair muscle movement.
10. _____ is a neurodegenerative disease that causes memory loss and behavioral changes.
11. _____ agents protect nerve cells from damage.
12. Substances composed of beta-amyloid called _____ fill the spaces between neurons and interfere with the transmission of signals between neurons.

MULTIPLE CHOICE

1. What is Parkinson disease?
   A. A progressive and degenerative disease in newborns
   B. A drug-induced condition
   C. A disease resulting from a vitamin deficiency
   D. A progressive disorder of the nervous system
2. Entacapone and tolcapone are catechol-*O*-methyltransferase (COMT) inhibitors and boost the bioavailability of levodopa by _____.
   A. 10%
   B. 50%
   C. 0.5%
   D. 75%
3. Approximately _____ million people in the United States have Parkinson disease.
   A. 5
   B. 10
   C. 2
   D. 1
4. Which of the following statements is **false**?
   A. Sustained-release formulations of carbidopa/levodopa decrease bioavailability of the drug by 30% when compared with immediate-release formulations.
   B. The efficacy of levodopa remains fairly constant throughout the progression of Parkinson disease.
   C. COMT inhibitors are used as adjunctive therapy to increase levodopa bioavailability by as much as 50%.
   D. Side effects of carbidopa/levodopa therapy include hallucinations, nausea/vomiting, and hypotension.
5. All the following can be used to treat Parkinson disease *except* _____.
   A. Duodopa
   B. levodopa
   C. bromocriptine
   D. Miralax
6. Which adverse effect is *not* associated with anticholinergic drugs?
   A. Dry mouth
   B. Diarrhea
   C. Blurred vision

D. Constipation

E. Urinary retention

7. Huntington disease differs from Parkinson disease because _____.

   A. Huntington disease is a progressive and degenerative disease of neurons

   B. Huntington disease affects muscle movement, cognitive functions, and emotions

   C. Huntington disease is primarily treated with drugs that decrease excessive dopaminergic activity

   D. Huntington disease symptoms are caused by an imbalance between neurotransmitters (e.g., acetylcholine, dopamine, and GABA)

8. Parkinson disease is treated with _____.

   A. pharmaceuticals

   B. exercise

   C. nutritional support

   D. all the above

9. Huntington disease is primarily treated with drugs that decrease excessive _____ activity.

   A. cholinergic

   B. acetylcholinesterase

   C. dopaminergic

   D. norepinephrine

10. Which of the following drugs is indicated for the treatment of Huntington disease?

   A. Requip

   B. Xenazine

   C. Nitroman

   D. Haldol

FILL IN THE BLANK: DRUG NAMES

1. What is the **brand name** for amantadine? _____
2. What is the **brand name** for haloperidol? _____
3. What is the **generic name** for Stalevo (United States)? _____
4. What is a **brand name** for levodopa and carbidopa? _____
5. What is the **generic name** for Mirapex? _____
6. What is the **generic name** for Requip? _____
7. What is the **brand name** for levodopa and benserazide? _____
8. What is a **brand name** for benztropine? _____
9. What is the **generic name** for Lodosyn? _____
10. What is a **brand name** for tetrabenazine? _____

MATCHING

Match each drug to its pharmacologic classification or brand or generic name.

A. anticholinergic

B. dopamine agonist

C. tolcapone

D. MAO$_B$ inhibitor

E. levodopa

   1. _____ Azilect
   2. _____ trihexyphenidyl
   3. _____ Mirapex
   4. _____ dopamine precursor
   5. _____ COMT inhibitor

MATCHING

Patient education is an essential component of therapeutics. Select the **best** warning label to apply to the prescription vial given to patients taking the drugs listed.

A. AVOID FOODS HIGH IN TYRAMINE

B. SWALLOW WHOLE; DO NOT CRUSH

C. TAKE WITH FOOD

D. MAY DISCOLOR URINE

   1. _____ Mirapex ER 0.75 mg
   2. _____ selegiline 5 mg
   3. _____ galantamine 4 mg
   4. _____ Tasmar 100 mg

TRUE OR FALSE

1. _____ Bradykinesia will speed up voluntary movements.
2. _____ Parkinson disease is associated with other mental diseases, including depression and dementia.
3. _____ Cognitive functions are not involved in the ability to take in information via the senses, process the details, commit the information to memory, or recall the information when necessary.
4. _____ Huntington disease causes immobility, whereas Parkinson disease causes excessive movements.
5. _____ Carbidopa and benserazide are used only to reduce degradation of levodopa before it reaches the brain.

CASE STUDY

You are helping Susan at your pharmacy counter. Susan is a good customer of yours, and so is her mother, Mary. You tell Susan you have missed seeing Mary at the pharmacy lately. Susan explains that she has been taking care of Mary's medications because Mary has been getting more and more forgetful. "But that's all part of getting old, right?" Susan says.

1. List some characteristics that would be concerning for Alzheimer disease compared with normal aging.

   _____
   _____
   _____
   _____

2. List two risk factors for developing Alzheimer disease and at least three comorbid conditions that may speed the progression of the disease.

   _____
   _____
   _____
   _____
   _____

   A few months later, Susan returns to the pharmacy after Mary has a visit with her physician. She tells you that Mary has been diagnosed with Alzheimer disease. She gives you a prescription for donepezil.

3. Describe the mechanism of action of donepezil and the role acetylcholine plays in Alzheimer disease.

   _____
   _____
   _____
   _____
   _____

4. List some side effects Mary may experience after starting donepezil.

_____

_____

_____

_____

Susan tells the pharmacist she has been feeling very overwhelmed by her mother's new diagnosis. She is worried that she will also develop Alzheimer disease.

5. What are some nonpharmacologic measures Susan can take to reduce her risk for Alzheimer disease?

_____

_____

_____

_____

_____

For Critical Thinking, Research Activity, and answer key, please refer to Evolve.

Appendix 9: Treatment of Seizure Disorders

TERMS AND DEFINITIONS

Match each term with the correct definition below.

A. Anoxia
B. Aura
C. Complex focal seizures
D. Convulsions
E. Eclampsia
F. Epilepsy
G. Febrile seizure
H. Generalized seizures
I. Gingival hyperplasia
J. Hirsutism
K. Myoclonic seizure
L. Absence seizure
M. Seizure threshold
N. Simple focal seizures
O. Status epilepticus

1. The term that refers to a person's susceptibility to seizures is _____.
2. _____ is defined as a recurrent seizure disorder characterized by a sudden excessive, disorderly discharge of cerebral neurons.
3. The term used to describe excessive growth of body hair (especially in women) is _____.
4. A(n) _____ is associated with a sudden spike in body temperature.
5. _____ is a medical emergency brought on by repeated generalized seizures that can produce _____, a lack of oxygen to the brain.
6. _____ is/are characterized by a sudden contraction of muscles and is/are caused by seizures.
7. The term used to describe the condition in which gum tissue overgrows the teeth is _____.
8. A(n) _____ is an unusual sensation or auditory, visual, or olfactory hallucination that is experienced just before the onset of a seizure.
9. _____ is characterized by brief periods of unconsciousness and vacant stares.
10. _____ affect only one part of the brain and cause the person to experience unusual sensations or feelings.
11. _____ is/are a disorder that produces a blank stare, disorientation, repetitive actions, and memory loss.
12. _____ is a life-threatening condition that can develop in pregnant women.
13. _____ include tonic-clonic, myoclonic, and absence seizures.
14. A(n) _____ is a seizure that is characterized by jerking muscle movements and is caused by contraction of the major muscle groups.

MULTIPLE CHOICE

1. The World Health Organization estimates that _____ people worldwide have epilepsy.
   A. 2.2 million
   B. 5 million
   C. 50 million
   D. 1 billion
2. Seizures may be caused by all the following *except* _____.
   A. infection and high fevers
   B. anxiety and schizophrenia
   C. tumors and head trauma
   D. hypoglycemia and cerebrovascular disease
   E. drug and alcohol withdrawal
3. Sudden, excessive neuronal firing associated with seizures is inhibited by drugs that _____.
   A. inhibit dopamine synthesis and release
   B. delay the inflow of sodium ions and bind to T-type calcium channels
   C. inhibit serotonin reuptake
   D. inhibit acetylcholine
4. Which symptom is *not* associated with grand mal seizures?
   A. Convulsions
   B. Brief vacant stare
   C. Jerking movements
   D. Difficulty breathing
5. A grand mal seizure is also known as _____.
   A. a petit mal seizure
   B. a tonic-clonic seizure
   C. status epilepticus
   D. a febrile seizure
6. Joe Sherman is taking Lamictal 25-mg tablets. Which of the following warnings should he be given?
   A. MAY CAUSE DROWSINESS OR DIZZINESS
   B. AVOID ALCOHOL
   C. AVOID SUNLIGHT
   D. TAKE ON AN EMPTY STOMACH
   E. A and B

7. Which drug can be prescribed for seizures and neuropathic pain?
   A. Dilantin
   B. Neurontin
   C. Depakote
   D. Zarontin
8. June Schultz is taking Depakote 250-mg delayed-release tablets. Which of the following warnings should she be given?
   A. MAY CAUSE DROWSINESS OR DIZZINESS
   B. TAKE WITH FOOD
   C. SWALLOW WHOLE; DO NOT CRUSH OR CHEW
   D. AVOID ALCOHOL
   E. All the above
9. Pharmacy technicians should dispense the same manufacturer's formulation of _____ each time a prescription is filled, if possible.
   A. lamotrigine
   B. topiramate
   C. phenytoin
   D. levetiracetam

FILL IN THE BLANK: DRUG NAMES

1. What is the *generic name* for Dilantin? _____
2. What is the *generic name* for Depakote? _____
3. What is the *brand name* for fosphenytoin? _____
4. What is the *generic name* for Trileptal? _____
5. What is a *brand name* for carbamazepine? _____
6. What is a *brand name* for oxcarbazepine? _____
7. What is the *generic name* for Celontin? _____
8. What is the *brand name* for tiagabine? _____
9. What is the *generic name* for Lyrica (United States)? _____
10. What is the *generic name* for Sabril? _____
11. What is a *brand name* for ethosuximide? _____
12. What is the *brand name* for primidone? _____
13. What is the *generic name* for Valium? _____
14. What is the *brand name* for lacosamide? _____
15. What is a *brand name* for diazepam? _____
16. What is the *brand name* for levetiracetam? _____
17. What is the *generic name* for Topamax? _____
18. What is the *generic name* for Zonegran? _____

MATCHING

A. Characterized by brief periods of unconsciousness and vacant stares
B. Characterized by stiffened limbs, difficulty breathing, and jerking movements followed by disorientation and limpness
C. Medical emergency that results from repeated generalized seizures
D. Causes a person to experience unusual sensations or feelings
E. Characterized by jerking muscle movements and caused by contraction of major muscle groups
   1. _____ Myoclonic seizure
   2. _____ Status epilepticus
   3. _____ Simple focal seizure
   4. _____ Tonic-clonic seizure
   5. _____ Absence seizure

MATCHING

Patient education is an essential component of therapeutics. Select the **best** warning label to apply to the prescription vial given to patients taking the drugs listed.
A. AVOID ANTACIDS
B. MAY BE HABIT FORMING
C. SHAKE WELL; DISCARD WITHIN 30 DAYS OF RECONSTITUTION
D. AVOID ALCOHOL
   1. _____ Tegretol XR 200 mg
   2. _____ Sabril 500-mg suspension
   3. _____ phenytoin 50-mg chewable tablets
   4. _____ Lyrica 300 mg

MATCHING

Match each drug to its mechanism of action.
A. Modulates ion channels
B. Blocks the reuptake of GABA
C. Increases inhibitory effects of GABA
D. Inhibits the enzyme that inactivates GABA
E. Inhibits the excitatory neurotransmitter glutamate
   1. _____ Tegretol
   2. _____ vigabatrin
   3. _____ perampanel
   4. _____ Depakote
   5. _____ tiagabine

TRUE OR FALSE

1. _____Status epilepticus must be treated with intravenous medications.
2. _____Nearly 75% of all seizures have no known cause.
3. _____The aim of pharmaceutical treatment of seizures is to suppress seizure activity.
4. _____Carbamazepine should be protected from light and moisture.
5. _____Flashing or strobe lights, such as those used in fire alarm systems, can trigger a seizure in susceptible individuals with epilepsy.
6. _____Depakote sprinkles must be swallowed whole.
7. _____Most children who have febrile seizures will develop epilepsy.
8. _____Gabapentin produces its effects by binding to GABAA receptors.
9. _____There are only a few medications indicated to treat absence seizures.
10. _____One serious side effect of phenobarbital is respiratory depression.
11. _____Rectal diazepam may be used daily if needed.
12. _____People with epilepsy have abnormally high levels of excitatory neurotransmitters and low levels of inhibitory neurotransmitters.

CASE STUDY

Tyler is an adolescent male admitted to your hospital for seizures. His seizures are not characterized by convulsions or twitching, but instead he has been having episodes where he is unresponsive and staring off into space.

1. What type of seizures has Tyler been experiencing?

   _____

2. Describe the role that neurotransmitters, specifically GABA and glutamate, have in epilepsy.

   _____

   _____

   _____

   _____

Tyler has had numerous generalized seizures over a short period, and his doctors have determined he has progressed into status epilepticus. He has already been given IV diazepam, and now his doctor has ordered fosphenytoin.

3. Describe how fosphenytoin will be administered.

   _____

   _____

   _____

   _____

   _____

At discharge, Tyler's doctor would like to start him on a new medication to treat and prevent his seizures.

4. List three medications that are indicated for the type of seizure Tyler has been experiencing.

   _____

   _____

   _____

5. Tyler's doctor wrote a prescription for Depakote. Tyler expresses that he does not like swallowing large pills. What is a dosage form you could choose to dispense, and how would Tyler be instructed to use it?

   _____

   _____

   _____

   _____

   _____

For Critical Thinking, Research Activity, and answer key, please refer to Evolve.

Appendix 10: Treatment of Pain and Migraine Headache

TERMS AND DEFINITIONS

Match each term with the correct definition below.

A. Acute pain
B. Acupuncture
C. Analgesic
D. Arthritis
E. Biofeedback
F. Breakthrough pain
G. Cephalgia
H. Chronic pain
I. Cluster headache
J. Diabetic neuropathy
K. Dysphoria
L. Endorphins
M. Euphoria
N. Hyperalgesia
O. Inflammation
P. Migraine
Q. Neuropathic pain
R. Nociceptors
S. NSAID
T. Opiate naïve
U. Opioid
V. Patient-controlled analgesia
W. Plasticity
X. Shingles
Y. Substance P
Z. Trigeminal neuralgia

1. _____ are thin nerve fibers in skin, muscle, and other body tissues that carry pain signals.

2. _____ is a disorder that occurs in people with diabetes and causes numbness, pain, or tingling in the feet or legs.

3. A drug that reduces pain is called a(n) _____.

4. Naturally occurring or synthetically derived _____ analgesics have properties similar to those of morphine.

5. Sudden pain or _____ that results from injury or inflammation is usually self-limiting.

6. _____ is a response to tissue irritation or injury that is marked by signs of redness, swelling, heat, and pain.

7. _____ is a procedure that involves the application of needles to precise points on the body.

8. Pain that persists for a long period that is worsened by psychological factors and is resistant to many medical treatments is classified as _____.

9. _____ is a condition that is associated with joint pain.

10. Painful skin rash associated with _____ is caused by the reactivation of the herpes zoster virus.

11. The peptide that is involved in the production of pain sensations and that controls pain perception is called _____.

12. _____, enkephalins, and dynorphins are natural painkillers.

13. _____ is a painful condition that produces intense, stabbing pain in areas of the face innervated by branches of the trigeminal nerve.

14. _____ is a feeling of emotional and/or mental discomfort, restlessness, and depression and is the opposite of _____.

15. _____ involves relaxation techniques and the gaining of self-control over muscle tension, heart rate, and skin temperature.

16. The ability of the brain to restructure itself and adapt to injury is called _____.

17. A type of pain that is associated with nerve injury, called _____, may be caused by trauma, infection, or chronic diseases such as diabetes.

18. _____ is pain that occurs between scheduled doses of analgesics.

19. _____ is head pain.

20. _____ is intensely painful vascular headache that occurs in groups and produces pain on one side of the head.

21. _____ is heightened sensitivity to pain that can result from treatment of chronic pain with high-dose opioids.

22. A(n) _____ is a vascular headache that is often accompanied by nausea and visual disturbances.

23. _____ is the acronym for nonsteroidal antiinflammatory drug.

24. Buprenorphine will have an agonist effect in patients who are _____.

25. Using a device connected to a patient's IV line, the patient can push a button to deliver a dose of pain medication using _____.

MULTIPLE CHOICE

1. Duragesic patches should be replaced every _____ hours.
   A. 12
   B. 24
   C. 36
   D. 72

2. Buprenorphine tablets _____.
   A. may be prescribed by any licensed prescriber
   B. may be prescribed for the treatment of opioid dependence only by specially licensed and authorized prescribers
   C. are available in combination with naltrexone by the trade name Suboxone (United States)
   D. may cause excitation

3. If a patient has received too much Sublimaze in the operating room, which narcotic antagonist should be available to reverse respiratory depression?
   A. Diphenoxylate atropine
   B. Naltrexone
   C. Acetaminophen with codeine No. 4
   D. Naloxone

4. The μ-opioid receptor is known to cause which effects when activated?
   A. Decreased gastrointestinal (GI) motility
   B. Respiratory depression
   C. Physical dependence
   D. Analgesia
   E. All the above

5. Which of the following two agents might be used to treat opioid-dependent patients?
   A. Fentanyl and naltrexone
   B. Methadone and hydrocodone
   C. Stadol and oxycodone
   D. Suboxone and naltrexone

6. Migraine prophylaxis can be initiated _____.
   A. when a patient must use sumatriptan more than three times per week
   B. before trying acute agents such as Tylenol No. 3
   C. when a patient has six or more migraines per month
   D. in very few cases, as no drug has been shown to help

7. Select the statement that is **true**.
   A. Mixed opioids act like an agonist in patients who are currently taking meperidine.
   B. Naltrexone usually won't precipitate withdrawal symptoms when given to a patient who is dependent on opioids.
   C. Short-acting opioids are used for breakthrough pain.
   D. The use of fentanyl and hydrocodone is reserved for the management of drug dependence.

8. Which of these drugs is an opioid antagonist?
   A. Oxycodone
   B. Vicodin
   C. ReVia
   D. Dolophine

9. NSAIDs can cause all the following side effects *except* _____.
   A. decreased blood pressure
   B. GI ulcers
   C. fluid retention
   D. agranulocytosis

FILL IN THE BLANK: DRUG NAMES

1. What is the **brand name** for hydrocodone and ibuprofen? _____

2. What is the **generic name** for Tylenol with Codeine No. 4? _____

3. What is the **generic name** for Dilaudid? _____

4. What is the **generic name** for Suboxone? _____

5. What is the **brand name** for naproxen? _____

6. What is the **generic name** for Anexsia (United States)? _____

7. What is the **brand name** for indomethacin? _____

8. What are **brand names** for sustained-release morphine? _____ and _____

9. What is a **brand name** for meperidine? _____

10. What is the **generic name** for Toradol? _____

11. What is the **generic name** for Imitrex? _____

12. What is a **brand name** for buprenorphine? _____

13. What is the **brand name** for buprenorphine plus naloxone? _____

14. What is the **generic name** for Stadol? _____

15. What is the **brand name** for eletriptan? _____

MATCHING

Patient education is an essential component of therapeutics. Select the **best** warning label to apply to the prescription vial given to patients taking the drugs listed.

A. DO NOT EXCEED RECOMMENDED DOSAGE
B. DO NOT INJECT MORE THAN 2 DOSES IN 24 HOURS
C. AVOID ASPIRIN AND RELATED DRUGS

1. _____ Clinoril
2. _____ Maxalt
3. _____ Imitrex subcut

MATCHING

Match each drug to its pharmacologic classification.

A. Opioid agonist
B. Ergot alkaloids
C. Triptan
D. β-Blocker

1. _____ Duragesic
2. _____ DHE
3. _____ Frova
4. _____ Inderal

TRUE OR FALSE

1. _____ Opiate naïve means without knowledge or understanding of the use of painkillers.
2. _____ Duragesic patches should be dispensed with instructions on proper storage and disposal to prevent accidental poisoning.
3. _____ Patient-controlled analgesia increases the patient's anxiety associated with pain.
4. _____ Patient-controlled analgesia permits patients to control the frequency of administration of their dose of pain medications.
5. _____ Endorphins, enkephalins, and dynorphin are substances that are released by the body in response to painful stimuli and act as natural painkillers.
6. _____ Biofeedback and acupuncture are nonpharmacologic treatments for pain.
7. _____ The peptide that is involved in the production of pain sensations and that controls pain perception is called substance X.
8. _____ Celebrex is the only remaining COX-2 inhibitor marketed in the United States and Canada.

CASE STUDY

Dan is a 45-year-old male who fell from an 8-foot ladder while cleaning his gutters. He injured his back as a result of his fall. His doctor has prescribed meloxicam and hydrocodone/acetaminophen for his pain.

1. Explain why the doctor would choose meloxicam to treat Dan's pain. (Hint: What is the pharmacologic class of meloxicam?)
   _____
   _____
   _____
   _____
   _____

2. Describe the role of cytokines, prostaglandins, and other mediators of pain in inflammation.
   _____
   _____
   _____
   _____

One year later, you notice that Dan has been filling his hydrocodone/acetaminophen prescription more frequently than before. He explains to you that his low back pain has spread to pain in his legs and that he has needed to use more of his medication to control his pain.

3. Hydrocodone/acetaminophen is an opioid agonist. Describe the effects produced by μ-receptor activation by opioid agonists.
   _____
   _____
   _____
   _____
   _____

4. Compare and contrast tolerance and dependence.
   _____
   _____
   _____
   _____

5. Treating chronic pain requires a multimodal approach. Explain what this means, and list some nondrug therapies you could suggest to Dan to help manage his pain.
   _____
   _____
   _____
   _____

For Critical Thinking, Research Activity, and answer key, please refer to Evolve.

Appendix 11: Treatment of Sleep Disorders and Attention-Deficit/Hyperactivity Disorder

TERMS AND DEFINITIONS

Match each term with the correct definition below.

A. Hypnotic
B. Insomnia
C. Melatonin
D. Non–REM sleep
E. Rapid eye movement (REM) sleep
F. Rebound hypersomnia
G. Sedative
H. Stimulant

1. _____ is a hormone released by the pineal gland that regulates body temperature, helps regulate our circadian rhythm, and makes us feel drowsy.
2. _____, or excessive sleep, is an adverse effect associated with long-term use of drugs that depress REM and non–REM sleep.

3. A drug that increases activity in the brain is called a(n) _____ and can be used to treat attention-deficit/hyperactivity disorder (ADHD) and narcolepsy.

4. A(n) _____ is a drug that is used to treat _____, a condition characterized by difficulty in falling asleep and/or staying asleep.

5. A(n) _____ is a medication that causes relaxation and promotes drowsiness.

6. The stages of sleep are categorized as _____ and _____.

MULTIPLE CHOICE

1. Sleep deprivation is linked to all the following *except* _____.
   A. increased illness
   B. motor vehicle accidents
   C. increased mental agility
   D. lack of productivity

2. Patient GL has been diagnosed with narcolepsy and has been prescribed Provigil. GL is also taking Tylenol for headaches, Imitrex for migraines, Neurontin for nerve pain, and Sprintec for birth control. Of these four medications, which one has the most pressing interaction with Provigil?
   A. Tylenol
   B. Imitrex
   C. Neurontin
   D. Sprintec

3. Which of the following is *not* linked to insomnia?
   A. Sleep apnea
   B. Use of depressant drugs
   C. Consumption of caffeinated beverages and foods
   D. Use of stimulant drugs
   E. Chronic pain and illness

4. Select the advice that would *not* be a tip to prevent insomnia.
   A. Avoid stimulants close to bedtime.
   B. Adopt a regular sleeping schedule.
   C. Take daytime naps.
   D. Exercise.
   E. Do not lie in bed awake.

5. Prescription drugs used to treat insomnia are _____.
   A. benzodiazepine receptor agonists and benzodiazepines
   B. decongestants and analgesics
   C. NSAIDs and antibiotics
   D. barbiturates and decongestants

6. Homer Street calls the pharmacy to renew his "sleeping pill." His profile shows he has recently taken the drugs listed below. Which drug is the "sleeping pill"?
   A. Buspirone
   B. Alprazolam
   C. Triazolam
   D. Fluoxetine

7. The pharmacist reminds Mr. Street to avoid concurrent use of _____ when he takes his "sleeping pill."
   A. ASA
   B. antacids
   C. APAP
   D. alcohol

8. Pharmaceutical treatment of ADHD is achieved with the administration of all the following *except* _____.
   A. temazepam
   B. methylphenidate
   C. Adderall
   D. Concerta

9. A patient comes into the pharmacy complaining of recent insomnia. What is something he can try before beginning pharmacologic treatment?
   A. Have a small snack before bed to avoid going to bed hungry.
   B. If he can't fall asleep quickly, he should simply lie in bed until he can.
   C. Exercise 1 to 2 hours before bedtime.
   D. Drink a cup of coffee with dinner.

10. Which warning label should not be affixed to prescription vials for Adderall XR?
    A. TAKE WITH FOOD
    B. MAY BE HABIT FORMING
    C. SWALLOW WHOLE; DO NOT CRUSH OR CHEW
    D. MAY CAUSE DROWSINESS

FILL IN THE BLANK: DRUG NAMES

1. What is the **brand name** for doxepin? _____
2. What is the **generic name** for Unisom? _____
3. What is a **brand name** for armodafinil? _____
4. What is the **generic name** for Dalmane? _____
5. What is the **generic name** for Restoril? _____
6. What is the **generic name** for Halcion? _____
7. What is the **generic name** for Lunesta (United States)? _____
8. What is the **generic name** for Sonata (United States) and Starnoc (Canada)? _____
9. What is the **generic name** for Ambien (United States)? _____
10. What is the **generic name** for Imovane (Canada)? _____
11. What is the **brand name** for amphetamine plus dextroamphetamine? _____
12. What is the **generic name** for Provigil (United States)? _____
13. What is the **brand name** for dextroamphetamine? _____
14. What are **brand names** for methylphenidate? _____
15. What is the **brand name** for atomoxetine? _____

MATCHING

Match each drug to its pharmacologic classification.
A. melatonin agonist
B. benzodiazepine
C. amphetamine
D. nonamphetamine stimulant
   1. _____ Strattera
   2. _____ Vyvanse
   3. _____ Halcion
   4. _____ Ramelteon

TRUE OR FALSE

1. _____Rapid-eye-movement sleep is the stage of sleep where dreaming occurs.
2. _____Pharmacologic treatment for insomnia is recommended for long-term therapy.
3. _____Our normal sleep-wake cycle is linked to changes in sunlight.

4. _____Melatonin and valerian root are natural remedies that have proven effectiveness for promoting sleep.
5. _____Benzodiazepines provide an effective treatment option for patients with narcolepsy.

CASE STUDY

A patient comes into the pharmacy with a new prescription for zolpidem IR 10 mg. It's obvious that the patient is very drowsy and lethargic, and upon reviewing her chart, you notice that she's been taking this medication for 2 months with good adherence. When at the register, the patient says, "Maybe I shouldn't be taking this medication. I mean, it's clearly not working, I've only gotten four or five good nights of sleep since taking it! What other pills can I take to help me sleep?"

1. Before discussing other pharmacotherapy options, what are some questions you can ask this patient to assess her sleep hygiene? Write at least three questions.

_____
_____
_____

2. The patient is worried about becoming dependent upon zolpidem. What are some medications for insomnia that are not controlled substances (in the United States)? What side effects might she experience with these medications?

_____
_____

_____
_____
_____

A few months later, the patient comes back to the pharmacy to thank you for your advice regarding the treatment of insomnia. She is no longer taking zolpidem. She is pregnant and beginning to worry about her child getting ADHD.

3. What advice can you give this patient to reduce the risk of ADHD in her child?

_____
_____
_____
_____
_____

4. Would you tell her that following your advice listed above would eliminate any risk of her child getting ADHD? Why or why not?

_____
_____
_____
_____
_____

For Critical Thinking, Research Activity, and answer key, please refer to Evolve.

Appendix 12: Neuromuscular Blockade and Muscle Spasms

TERMS AND DEFINITIONS

Match each term with the correct definition below.

A. Acetylcholinesterase
B. Amyotrophic lateral sclerosis
C. Anaphylactic shock
D. Botulinum toxin
E. Central-acting muscle relaxants
F. Cerebral palsy
G. Clonus
H. Depolarizing neuromuscular blockers
I. Endotracheal intubation
J. End plate
K. Multiple sclerosis
L. Neuromuscular junction
M. Nondepolarizing competitive blockers
N. Peripheral-acting muscle relaxants
O. Sarcomere
P. Soleplate
Q. Spasticity
R. Tetanus

1. The space between the motor neuron end plate and the muscle sole plate that neurotransmitters must cross is called the _____.
2. _____ is the process of inserting a tube down into the trachea, or windpipe, to facilitate mechanical ventilation.
3. _____ is a condition that causes increased muscle tone and exaggerated motion.
4. Drugs that compete with acetylcholine for binding sites are called _____.
5. _____ is an autoimmune disorder characterized by the progressive destruction of the body's nerves.
6. A projection extending off the end of a motor neuron is called a(n) _____ and is where the neurotransmitter acetylcholine is released.
7. _____ block nerve transmission between the motor end plate and skeletal muscle receptors.
8. The portion of the membrane of muscle cells that receives messages transmitted by motor neurons is called the _____.
9. The fatal condition _____ is characterized by continuous muscle spasm and is also known as "lockjaw."
10. Drugs that produce relaxation of muscles by central nervous system depression, blocking nerve transmission between the spinal cord and muscles, are called _____.
11. A poison produced by the bacterium *Clostridium botulinum*, _____, causes muscle paralysis.
12. An acute, life-threatening allergic reaction is also known as _____.
13. _____ produce sustained depolarization by causing acetylcholine receptor sites to convert to an inactive state.
14. An enzyme that degrades acetylcholine and reverses acetylcholine-induced depolarization is called _____.

15. _____ is more commonly known as Lou Gehrig's disease.
16. _____ is a neurologic disorder that affects muscle movement and coordination.
17. The _____ is the contracting unit of muscle fibers.
18. Involuntary rhythmic muscle contraction, called _____, causes the feet and wrists to involuntarily flex and relax.

MULTIPLE CHOICE

1. Depolarizing neuromuscular blockers produce sustained depolarization by causing _____ receptor sites to convert to an inactive state.
   A. norepinephrine
   B. dopamine
   C. GABA
   D. acetylcholine
2. Which symptom is *not* associated with anaphylactic shock?
   A. Peripheral vasodilation
   B. Bradycardia
   C. Bronchospasm
   D. Laryngeal edema
   E. Airway obstruction
3. Neuromuscular blocking drugs are classified as "_____" by the Interdisciplinary Safe Medication Use Expert Committee of the United States Pharmacopoeia.
   A. dangerous
   B. high alert
   C. low alert
   D. use with caution
4. Select the drug that reverses the effects of neuromuscular blocking agents.
   A. Vecuronium
   B. Rocuronium
   C. Neostigmine
   D. Mivacurium
   E. Pancuronium
5. According to the Interdisciplinary Safe Medication Use Expert Committee of the United States Pharmacopoeia, the warning label _____ should always be placed on dispensed neuromuscular blocking drugs.
   A. KEEP IN REFRIGERATOR
   B. WARNING: PARALYZING AGENT
   C. WARNING: ALLERGIC REACTIONS POSSIBLE
   D. FOR ONE-TIME USE ONLY
6. Which of the following is true about the use of neuromuscular blocking agents?
   A. Neuromuscular blocking drugs are delivered parenterally because of poor absorption when taken orally.
   B. Neuromuscular blockers are generally safe and do not require any extra precautions for safety.
   C. They are commonly used when patients have an acute anxiety attack.
   D. None of the above are true.
7. Botox injections can cause all the following adverse reactions *except* _____.
   A. droopy eyelid muscles
   B. headache
   C. muscle weakness
   D. drowsiness
   E. flulike syndrome
8. Which drug is used for the treatment of muscle strain?
   A. Carisoprodol
   B. Diazepam
   C. Dantrolene
   D. Baclofen
9. Which of the muscle relaxants listed can discolor urine?
   A. Diazepam
   B. Chlorzoxazone
   C. Methocarbamol
   D. B and C

FILL IN THE BLANK: DRUG NAMES

1. What is the **brand name** for succinylcholine? _____
2. What is the **generic name** for Botox? _____
3. What is the **generic name** for Nimbex? _____
4. What is the **generic name** for Dantrium? _____
5. What is the **brand name** for rocuronium? _____
6. What is the **generic name** for Zanaflex? _____
7. What is the **brand name** for pyridostigmine? _____

MATCHING

Match each drug to its pharmacologic classification.
A. Depolarizing neuromuscular blocker
B. Nondepolarizing neuromuscular blocker
C. Neuromuscular blockade reversal agent
   1. Succinylcholine _____
   2. Onabotulinumtoxin A _____
   3. Pyridostigmine _____

TRUE OR FALSE

1. _____Acetylcholinesterase is an enzyme that reverses acetylcholine-induced depolarization by degrading acetylcholine.
2. _____Botox is known to cause side effects such as droopy eyelids, headache, nausea, and muscle weakness.
3. _____The onset of action of neuromuscular blocking drugs is slow (1–2 hours) and the duration of action is long (12–24 hours).
4. _____The endings *-curonium* and *-curium* are commonly used for nondepolarizing neuromuscular blockers.
5. _____Look-alike packaging is a problem that can be attributed to drug manufacturers as well as to pharmacies dispensing drugs.
6. _____Skeletal muscle relaxants should be used along with nonpharmaceutical therapies such as rest, exercise, cryotherapy, and physical therapy.
7. _____There are five phases in the development of spasticity.

CASE STUDY

You are working in a small hospital as a pharmacy technician. The number of surgeries and intubations at the hospital is increasing, so the pharmacy manager decides to start carrying more neuromuscular blockers in the pharmacy. To keep things organized, the manager wants to store all the neuromuscular blockers on a single shelf.

1. What advice can you offer the pharmacy manager about the proper storage of neuromuscular blocking agents? Provide at least three examples.

   _____

   _____

   _____

   _____

2. As a pharmacy technician, what are some key administration pieces of information to remember when you are dispensing a neuromuscular blocking agent?

   _____

   _____

   _____

   _____

For Critical Thinking, Research Activity, and answer key, please refer to Evolve.

Appendix 13: Treatment of Gout, Osteoarthritis, and Rheumatoid Arthritis

TERMS AND DEFINITIONS

Match each term with the correct definition below.

A. Arthritis
B. Autoimmune disease
C. Autoantibody
D. Gout
E. Hyperuricemia
F. Rheumatoid arthritis
G. Rheumatoid factor
H. Synovium
I. Tumor necrosis factor
J. Urates
K. Uricosuric

1. The immunoglobulin (antibody) _____ is present in many people who have _____, a chronic disease characterized by inflammation of the joints.
2. _____ is a condition characterized by increased levels of urates in the blood.
3. A disease that occurs when the immune system turns against the parts of the body it is designed to protect is called a(n) _____.
4. _____ is an inflammatory condition that produces joint pain.
5. The _____ is a thin layer of tissue that lines the joint space.
6. The term used to describe an abnormal antibody that attacks healthy cells and tissues is _____.
7. _____ is a disease characterized by joint deposits of urate crystals.
8. The inflammatory cytokine found in the synovial fluid of rheumatoid arthritis patients is called _____.
9. A drug that increases the body's clearance of urates is referred to as _____.
10. _____ is/are the product of purine metabolism.

MULTIPLE CHOICE

1. Hyperuricemia is associated with all the following conditions *except* _____.
   A. coronary heart disease and stroke
   B. diabetes and insulin resistance
   C. rheumatoid arthritis
   D. kidney disease
   E. hypertension
2. Which of the following is a joint commonly affected by gout?
   A. Big toe
   B. Ankle
   C. Knee
   D. Wrist
   E. All the above
3. Which drug blocks the final enzymatic step in the production of uric acid?
   A. Colchicine
   B. Probenecid
   C. Allopurinol
   D. Hydrochlorothiazide
   E. Celecoxib
4. Which foods and beverages are most likely to increase the risk of a gout attack?
   A. Seafood such as anchovies, herring, mussels, or trout
   B. Seafood such as crab, lobster, oysters, or shrimp
   C. Meats such as beef, duck, chicken, or pork
   D. Dairy such as skim milk and cheese
5. Select the warning label that should *not* be applied to prescriptions for cyclosporine oral solution.
   A. DO NOT REFRIGERATE
   B. PROTECT FROM LIGHT
   C. DILUTE SOLUTION AND USE IMMEDIATELY
   D. REFRIGERATE; DO NOT FREEZE
6. Cyclosporine parenteral solution is stable for _____ hours in normal saline glass bottles.
   A. 6
   B. 9
   C. 12
   D. 24
7. Which of the following statements regarding the progression of rheumatoid arthritis is false?
   A. Swelling, pain, and stiffness begin in phase 1, when the synovium becomes inflamed.
   B. In phase 2, rapid cell death causes the synovium to become thinner.

C. Pain and disability increase in phase 3 as enzymes digest bone and cartilage.

D. Rheumatoid arthritis can cause other symptoms such as fatigue, weakness, muscle pain, decreased appetite, and depression.

8. Which of the following is **not** an adverse effect of glucocorticoids?
   A. Hypoglycemia
   B. Insomnia
   C. Weight gain
   D. Euphoria

9. Select the **true** statement.
   A. Biological response modifiers stimulate the release of cells that mobilize to fight what the body believes is a harmful invasion.
   B. Biological response modifiers interfere with the activity of cytokines, leukocytes, B cells, and T cells.
   C. Selective COX-2 inhibitors decrease the risk for cardiovascular toxicity and gastrointestinal ulceration.
   D. Tumor necrosis factor-α inhibitors are produced by the body and block the inflammatory process.

10. Gold compounds are used in the treatment of _____.
    A. rheumatoid arthritis
    B. multiple sclerosis
    C. myositis
    D. systemic lupus erythematosus

11. Which drug is *not* used for the treatment of rheumatoid arthritis?
    A. Remicade
    B. Gold salts
    C. Leflunomide
    D. Dantrolene
    E. Penicillamine

FILL IN THE BLANK: DRUG NAMES

1. What is the *brand name* for colchicine? _____
2. What is the *generic name* for Krystexxa? _____
3. What is the *brand name* for febuxostat? _____
4. What is a *brand name* for prednisolone? _____
5. What is the *generic name* for Cortef? _____
6. What is a *brand name* for celecoxib? _____
7. What is the *generic name* for Medrol? _____
8. What is the *brand name* for hydroxychloroquine? _____
9. What is the *generic name* for Imuran? _____
10. What is a *brand name* for etanercept? _____
11. What is the *generic name* for Sandimmune and Neoral? _____
12. What is a *brand name* for adalimumab? _____
13. What is the *brand name* for infliximab? _____
14. What is the *brand name* for anakinra? _____
15. What is the *brand name* for leflunomide? _____
16. What is a *brand name* for auranofin? _____
17. What is the *generic name* for Cuprimine and Depen? _____

MATCHING

Patient education is an essential component of therapeutics. Select the **best** warning label to apply to the prescription vial given to patients taking the drugs listed.

A. TAKE ON AN EMPTY STOMACH
B. AVOID GRAPEFRUIT JUICE
C. AVOID ASPIRIN
D. AVOID PROLONGED EXPOSURE TO SUNLIGHT
E. MAY CAUSE DIZZINESS OR DROWSINESS

1. _____ Cyclosporine oral solution
2. _____ Allopurinol
3. _____ Probenecid
4. _____ Hydroxychloroquine
5. _____ Penicillamine

TRUE OR FALSE

1. _____ Probenecid and allopurinol should be taken on an empty stomach.
2. _____ Colchicine is a uricosuric.
3. _____ Osteoarthritis is the most common of all arthritic conditions.
4. _____ The presence of rheumatoid factor in a patient is a definitive sign that the patient has rheumatoid arthritis.
5. _____ The reconstituted solution of azathioprine must be shaken vigorously.
6. _____ The pharmacy should try to dispense the same manufacturer's product of cyclosporine each time the prescription is refilled.
7. _____ Rheumatoid arthritis is far more common in men than in women.
8. _____ Celecoxib is the only selective COX-2 inhibitor still available for use in the United States and Canada.

CASE STUDY

A familiar patient at the retail pharmacy where you work has been recently diagnosed with rheumatoid arthritis. She states that the doctor did not give her much information on her new disease; the doctor simply handed her a few new prescriptions and told her to schedule another appointment in 3 months. The patient is confused and asks for your help in her treatment for this disease.

1. In simple terms, describe the effects that rheumatoid arthritis has on the body. What is the difference between rheumatoid arthritis and arthritis?

   _____
   _____
   _____

2. The doctor gave the patient prescriptions for celecoxib, methotrexate, and Humira. How do each of these medications help in the treatment of rheumatoid arthritis? What is the onset of action for each of these three medications?

   _____
   _____
   _____
   _____

For Critical Thinking, Research Activity, and answer key, please refer to Evolve.

Appendix 14: Treatment of Osteoporosis and Paget Disease of the Bone

TERMS AND DEFINITIONS

Match each term with the correct definition below.

A. Bone mineral density
B. Bone resorption
C. Osteoblasts
D. Osteoclasts
E. Osteoporosis
F. Remodeling

1. _____ is a chronic, progressive disease of bone characterized by loss of bone density and increased risk for fractures.
2. The _____ test measures the degree of bone loss.
3. The term used to describe the process of continual turnover of bone is _____.
4. The process by which bone is broken down to mineral ions (calcium) is called _____.
5. _____ are cells responsible for bone formation, deposition, and mineralization of the collagen matrix of bone.
6. The cells responsible for bone resorption are called _____.

MULTIPLE CHOICE

1. The lifetime risk for fractures in women with osteoporosis is _____.
   A. 1 in 3
   B. 1 in 4
   C. 1 in 10
   D. 1 in 100
2. In a person with osteoporosis, a fragility fracture may occur when the person _____.
   A. falls
   B. coughs
   C. sneezes
   D. is in a car accident
   E. B and C
3. The percentage of total body calcium located in the skeleton is _____.
   A. 10%
   B. 50%
   C. 75%
   D. 99%
   E. 100%
4. Which hormone is *not* involved in the regulation of serum calcium levels?
   A. Parathyroid hormone
   B. Glucagon
   C. Calcitonin
   D. Vitamin D
5. _____ is a condition with the potential to cause secondary osteoporosis.
   A. Hypothyroidism
   B. Rheumatoid arthritis
   C. Inflammatory bowel disease
   D. All the above
6. Which drug must be taken on an empty stomach at least 30 minutes before the first meal or beverage of the day?
   A. Calcium
   B. Evista
   C. Fosamax
   D. Estrace
7. Patients taking Didronel and Actonel must sit upright or stand for at least _____ minutes after dosing to avoid possible esophageal ulceration.
   A. 30
   B. 60
   C. 90
   D. 120
8. What is the difference between calcium carbonate and calcium citrate supplements?
   A. Carbonate should be taken on an empty stomach, and citrate may be taken with or without food.
   B. Carbonate should be taken on a full stomach, and citrate may be taken with or without food.
   C. Carbonate provides the greatest amount of elemental calcium per tablet.
   D. B and C
9. The use of teriparatide, a genetically engineered form of human parathyroid hormone and the only drug currently available in this category, is limited because of risks for _____.
   A. fractures
   B. osteosarcoma
   C. pituitary tumors
   D. all the above

FILL IN THE BLANK: DRUG NAMES

1. What is a **brand name** for pamidronate? _____
2. What is the **generic name** for Actonel? _____
3. What is a **brand name** for alendronate? _____
4. What is the **brand name** for etidronate? _____
5. What is the **generic name** for Zometa? _____
6. What is the **brand name** for raloxifene? _____
7. What is the **generic name** for Fosamax Plus D (United States)? _____
8. What is a **brand name**(s) for denosumab? _____
9. What is the **generic name** for Boniva? _____
10. What is the **generic name** for Climara? _____
11. What is the **brand name** for conjugated estrogens? _____
12. What is the **generic name** for Premphase and Prempro? _____
13. What is the **generic name** for Climara Pro? _____
14. What is the **generic name** for Ogen? _____
15. What is the **generic name** for Forteo (United States)? _____

MATCHING

Patient education is an essential component of therapeutics. Select the **best** warning label to apply to the prescription vial given to patients taking the drugs listed.

A. ROTATE SITE OF APPLICATION
B. STORE IN MANUFACTURER'S SEALED FOIL POUCH
C. TAKE WITH FOOD
D. TAKE 30 MINUTES BEFORE THE FIRST MEAL OF THE DAY
E. TAKE WITH OR WITHOUT FOOD
F. TAKE 1 HOUR BEFORE THE FIRST MEAL OF THE DAY

1. _____ Actonel
2. _____ Climara
3. _____ Premarin
4. _____ CombiPatch
5. _____ Boniva
6. _____ Evista

MATCHING

Match each drug to its pharmacologic classification.

A. Monoclonal antibody
B. Bisphosphonate
C. Selective estrogen receptor modulator
D. Estrogen replacement
E. Anabolic agent

1. _____ Premarin
2. _____ Evista
3. _____ Forteo
4. _____ Fosamax
5. _____ Prolia

TRUE OR FALSE

1. _____ Denosumab binds to RANKL, resulting in an inhibition of osteoblast activation.
2. _____ Unlike Forteo, bisphosphonates cannot increase bone remodeling. They can only prevent further bone degradation.
3. _____ Some studies show that selective estrogen receptor modulators may increase the risk of esophageal cancer.
4. _____ If a patient is prescribed levothyroxine, it is important to avoid calcium tablets within 30 minutes of taking the levothyroxine.
5. _____ Although Paget disease of the bone and osteoporosis have different pathologies, they are treated similarly.
6. _____ Non–weight-bearing exercise such as swimming will help keep bones strong.

CASE STUDY

A 77-year-old female patient comes into the hospital with a broken wrist secondary to a fall. After a bone mineral density test, the doctor diagnoses the patient with osteoporosis. The pharmacist has assigned you to do a medication reconciliation on this patient.

1. Name at least five medications and five disease states that may be contributing to this patient's recently diagnosed condition.

_____
_____
_____
_____

2. Based on the patient's age, how much calcium does she need per day? What are three to five good sources of calcium that the patient may be able to add to her diet?

_____
_____
_____
_____

3. In your conversation with the patient, she tells you that she gets most of her exercise from swimming. Would you recommend any additional form of exercise for this patient? If so, what exercises would you recommend?

_____
_____
_____

4. Research strategies to reduce falls in the patient's home using the following resource: https://www.ncoa.org/caregivers/health/prevention/falls-prevention. Recommend three prevention steps she can take to prevent future falls.

_____
_____
_____
_____

For Critical Thinking, Research Activity, and answer key, please refer to Evolve.

Appendix 15: Treatment of Diseases of the Eye

TERMS AND DEFINITIONS

Match each term with the correct definition below.

A. Angle-closure glaucoma
B. Aqueous humor
C. Blepharitis
D. Conjunctivitis
E. Cytomegalovirus retinitis

F. Dry eye disease
G. Herpes simplex keratitis
H. Herpes zoster ophthalmicus
I. Intraocular pressure
J. Iritis
K. Keratitis
L. Open-angle glaucoma
M. Peripheral vision
N. Photopsia
O. Stye
P. Uveitis
Q. Vitreous floaters

1. _____ is a disorder characterized by elevated pressure in the eye; it can lead to permanent blindness.
2. Particles that float in the vitreous and appear as spots or spiders are referred to as _____.
3. _____ is a disease of the eye that results in the formation of scales on the eyelids and eyelashes.
4. _____ is a herpes virus infection of the eye characterized by excessive tearing, decreased vision, a gritty feeling in the eye, and pain when looking at bright light.
5. _____ is a condition associated with flashes of light.
6. The fluid that is made in the front part of the eye is called _____.
7. Inflammation of the iris is referred to as _____.
8. _____ is sometimes called "side vision."
9. Blindness may occur as a result of _____, a painful herpes virus infection of the eye that causes a rash or sores around the eyes.
10. A(n) _____ is a painful lump located on the eyelid margin caused by a self-limiting infection of the oil glands of the eyelid.
11. _____ is the pressure in the eye.
12. _____ is a condition that results from a lack of tears, whether as a result of lower production or faster evaporation.
13. _____ is characterized by a sudden increase in intraocular pressure caused by obstruction of the drainage portal between the cornea and the iris (angle).
14. _____, or more commonly known as pink eye, is a common ailment that produces itching and burning of the eye.
15. _____ is an opportunistic infection of the eye that occurs in patients who have HIV/AIDS or who take immunosuppressive drugs.
16. A severe infection of the cornea that may be caused by bacteria or fungi is called _____.
17. _____ is a serious eye condition that produces inflammation of the uvea and can cause scarring of the eye and blindness if untreated.

MULTIPLE CHOICE

1. _____ is usually the first area of vision to be lost with glaucoma.
   A. Peripheral vision
   B. Near vision
   C. Far vision
   D. Central vision
2. Carbonic anhydrase inhibitors may cause allergic reactions in people who have allergies to _____ antiinfective agents.
   A. penicillin
   B. tetracycline
   C. sulfonamide
   D. macrolide
3. Adverse effects of α-agonists include _____.
   A. dry eyes
   B. decreased night vision
   C. blurred vision
   D. all the above
4. The mechanism of action for drugs used in the treatment of glaucoma is _____.
   A. to increase the formation of aqueous humor
   B. to decrease the formation of aqueous humor
   C. to promote the drainage of aqueous humor
   D. to decrease the drainage of aqueous humor
   E. B and C
5. All the following drug classifications decrease formation of the aqueous humor *except* _____.
   A. β-blockers
   B. prostaglandin analogs
   C. α-adrenergic agonists
   D. carbonic anhydrase inhibitors
6. Which carbonic anhydrase inhibitor is administered orally?
   A. Acetazolamide
   B. Brinzolamide
   C. Trusopt
   D. Cosopt

7. Most ophthalmic drugs used for the treatment of glaucoma require contact lens wearers to wait at least _____ before reinserting their contact lenses.
   A. 5 minutes
   B. 10 minutes
   C. 15 minutes
   D. 30 minutes
8. Carbonic anhydrase inhibitors often share the suffix _____.
   A. *-prost*
   B. *-zolamide*
   C. *-olol*
   D. *-onidine*

FILL IN THE BLANK: DRUG NAMES

1. What is a ***brand name*** for betaxolol? _____
2. What is the ***generic name*** for Betagan? _____
3. What is a ***brand name*** for timolol maleate? _____
4. What is the ***generic name*** for Iopidine? _____
5. What is the ***generic name*** for Diamox? _____
6. What is the ***brand name*** for dorzolamide? _____
7. What is the ***generic name*** for Azopt? _____
8. What is the ***generic name*** for Alphagan? _____
9. What is the ***generic name*** for Combigan? _____
10. What is the ***brand name*** for dorzolamide and timolol? _____
11. What is the ***generic name*** for Isopto Carbachol? _____
12. What is the ***brand name*** for bimatoprost? _____
13. What is the ***generic name*** for DuoTrav PQ? _____
14. What is the ***brand name*** for latanoprost? _____
15. What is the ***generic name*** for Phospholine Iodide (United States)? _____

MATCHING

Match each drug to its pharmacologic classification.
A. α-Adrenergic agonist
B. Cholinergic agonist
C. Prostaglandin analog
D. Carbonic anhydrase inhibitor
E. β-Adrenergic antagonist
   1. _____ Timoptic
   2. _____ Alphagan
   3. _____ Dorzolamide
   4. _____ Latanoprost
   5. _____ Pilocarpine

TRUE OR FALSE

1. _____ Children born with congenital glaucoma often have cloudy eyes, light sensitivity, and excessive tearing.
2. _____ The ending *-zolamide* is commonly used for carbonic anhydrase inhibitors.
3. _____ Prostaglandin analogs constrict the trabecular meshwork.
4. _____ Glaucoma is the leading cause of blindness worldwide.
5. _____ The risk for glaucoma decreases with age.
6. _____ Open-angle glaucoma is more common than angle-closure glaucoma.
7. _____ Miotics are drugs that dilate the pupil.
8. _____ Iritis is a condition associated with inflammation of the cornea.
9. _____ Conjunctivitis (pink eye) may be caused by a virus or bacteria.

CASE STUDY

You work at a retail store with a primarily elderly population. The pharmacists you work with have been noticing a recent increase in the number of patients requiring glaucoma treatment, and you want to provide a pamphlet to patients that would explain their condition and treatment. They ask you to help create the pamphlet.

1. How would you describe open-angle and angle-closure glaucoma? Remember to use patient-friendly language to explain these conditions.
   _____
   _____
   _____

2. Write a concise one- to two-sentence description for each class of medication currently used to treat glaucoma. What are three medications that are within each of these classes?
   _____
   _____
   _____
   _____

3. What other images or information would you use in this pamphlet? Explain why you chose them.
   _____
   _____
   _____
   _____

For Critical Thinking, Research Activity, and answer key, please refer to Evolve.

Appendix 16: Treatment of Disorders of the Ear

TERMS AND DEFINITIONS

Match each term with the correct definition below.

A. Cerumen
B. Equilibrium
C. Labyrinth
D. Ménière disease
E. Otitis
F. Otitis externa
G. Otitis media
H. Tinnitus
I. Tympanic membrane
J. Vertigo

1. The waxlike substance secreted by modified sweat glands in the ear is called _____.
2. _____, the feeling of spinning in space, is a symptom of _____, a chronic inner ear disease associated with intermittent buildup of fluid in the inner ear.
3. _____ is inflammation of the ear canal.
4. The _____, a bony structure in the inner ear, is involved in maintaining _____, or balance.
5. Symptoms of _____ are intermittent or continuous whistling, crackling, squeaking, or ringing in the ears.
6. _____ is inflammation of the ear.
7. _____ is known as the eardrum.
8. _____ is typically caused by a viral or bacterial infection and observed clinically as inflammation of the middle ear.

MULTIPLE CHOICE

1. Select the **false** statement.
   A. Hearing loss can be caused by otosclerosis, autoimmune disease, or sudden sensorineural hearing loss.
   B. Otosclerosis may cause hearing loss and tinnitus.
   C. Otosclerosis is a disorder that causes destruction of bone in the ear.
   D. Otosclerosis is also called Ménière disease.
2. Drugs that may cause tinnitus are _____.
   A. aspirin and alcohol
   B. diphenhydramine and scopolamine
   C. diazepam and triazolam
   D. methocarbamol and cyclobenzaprine
3. Which of the following conditions is *not* linked to vertigo?
   A. Ménière disease
   B. Benign paroxysmal positional vertigo
   C. Gout
   D. Head trauma
   E. Infection
4. Symptoms of vertigo include all the following *except* _____.
   A. dizziness
   B. nausea
   C. muscle weakness
   D. blurred vision
   E. disorientation
5. Meclizine should be used with caution in _____.
   A. patients with prostate disease
   B. patients with asthma
   C. lactating women
   D. A, B, and C
6. Which is *not* a property of cerumen?
   A. Antiviral
   B. Bactericidal
   C. Water repellent
   D. Lubricant
7. Carbamide peroxide 6.5% is the only approved agent for _____ removal.
   A. cerumen (ear wax)
   B. water or fluid
   C. bacteria
   D. foreign material
8. What is the difference between water-clogged ears and swimmer's ear?
   A. Only swimmer's ear is caused by excessive fluid in the ear.
   B. Only swimmer's ear can cause an earache.
   C. Only swimmer's ear produces inflammation and infection.
   D. Only swimmer's ear is treated with alcohol or vinegar.

FILL IN THE BLANK: DRUG NAMES

1. What is the **generic name** for Serc (Canada)? _____
2. What is the **brand name** for dimenhydrinate? _____
3. What is the **generic name** for Transderm Scop (United States) and Transderm V (Canada)? _____
4. What is the **generic name** for Auralgan? _____
5. What is the **generic name** for Auro-Dri Ear Drying Aid? _____
6. What is the **generic name** for Debrox and Murine Ear Wax Removal System? _____

MATCHING

Match the drug to its correct classification.

A. Analgesic
B. Cerumenolytic
C. Anticholinergic
D. Drying agent

1. _____ Scopolamine
2. _____ Antipyrine and benzocaine
3. _____ Isopropyl alcohol and glycerin
4. _____ Carbamide peroxide

TRUE OR FALSE

1. _____ Otitis externa is an infection of the middle ear.
2. _____ The tympanic membrane is commonly known as the eardrum.
3. _____ One scopolamine patch prevents motion sickness for up to 5 days.
4. _____ A commonly used ending for local anesthetics is *-caine*.
5. _____ Our perception of balance and movement is a function of input from the eye, inner ear, and sense receptors on the skin and skeleton.
6. _____ When the ear is inflamed, otic solutions that contain alcohol can cause stinging.

CASE STUDY

A regular patient comes into your pharmacy to pick up a refill. As you help her at the register, she mentions that she will be going on a cruise for the first time in a month and is worried about motion sickness.

1. Provide two or three nonpharmacologic recommendations that would help this patient prevent motion sickness.
   _____
   _____
   _____

2. What are three over-the-counter medications that this patient could take to prevent motion sickness? How do they work?
   _____
   _____
   _____

One month later, the patient comes into the pharmacy to thank you for your advice and to tell you about her trip. She states that she did a lot of swimming and seems to still have some fluid in her ear. She asks for your advice.

3. How would you differentiate water-clogged ear from swimmer's ear in this patient?
   _____
   _____
   _____
   _____

4. Assuming that that she has water-clogged ear, what are two over-the-counter treatments available for this patient? How do they work?
   _____
   _____
   _____
   _____

For Critical Thinking, Research Activity, and answer key, please refer to Evolve.

Appendix 17: Treatment of Angina

TERMS AND DEFINITIONS

Match each term with the correct definition below.

A. Angina pectoris
B. Arteriosclerosis
C. Atheromas
D. Atherosclerosis
E. Coronary artery disease
F. Embolus
G. Hyperlipidemia
H. Ischemia
I. Ischemic heart disease
J. Myocardial infarction
K. Necrosis
L. Thrombus
M. Vasospasms

1. _____is a condition that occurs when the arteries that supply blood to the heart muscle become hardened and narrowed.
2. Myocardial _____is a deficient blood supply to the heart.
3. _____are hardened plaques that have formed within an artery.
4. An ischemic heart disease, _____ is characterized by a severe squeezing or pressure-like thoracic pain brought on by exertion or stress.
5. _____ is the term used to describe cell death and may be caused by lack of blood and oxygen to an affected area.
6. _____ is a condition in which there is an increased concentration of cholesterol and triglycerides in the blood.
7. A stationary blood clot is called a(n) _____.
8. _____ is any condition in which heart muscle is damaged or works inefficiently because of an absence or relative deficiency of its blood supply.
9. _____ is a process in which plaques containing cholesterol, lipid material, and lipophages are formed within arteries.
10. Symptoms of angina may be caused by _____ that constrict blood vessels and reduce the flow of blood and oxygen.
11. _____ is a condition in which artery walls thicken and lose their elasticity.
12. A(n) _____ is a moving clot.
13. _____ is also referred to as a "heart attack"; it results in heart muscle tissue death and is caused by the occlusion of a coronary artery.

MULTIPLE CHOICE

1. Risk factors for angina include all the following *except* _____.
   A. smoking
   B. a diet high in cholesterol and salt
   C. excessive alcohol consumption
   D. mild exercise
   E. obesity
2. All the following drugs are used in the treatment of angina *except* _____.
   A. nitrates
   B. diuretics
   C. β-blocking drugs
   D. calcium channel blockers

3. A woman was awakened in the middle of the night with severe chest pain. Her physician prescribed sublingual nitroglycerin. Which of the following adverse reactions is associated with sublingual nitroglycerin?
   A. Flushing of the skin
   B. Headache
   C. Stinging under the tongue
   D. A, B, and C
4. Which of the following is *not* considered a true type of angina?
   A. Stable angina
   B. Unstable angina
   C. Variant angina
   D. Microvascular angina
   E. None of the above
5. Patients using nitroglycerin transdermal patches should be advised to _____.
   A. wear the patch for 24 hours each day
   B. apply a patch at the onset of symptoms of angina
   C. rotate the sites on the skin to prevent skin irritation
   D. apply the patch directly over the heart
6. Which drug may be taken concurrently with nitroglycerin?
   A. Viagra
   B. Cialis
   C. Tenormin
   D. Levitra
7. Which nitrate dosage form is used only to treat acute angina?
   A. Nitroglycerin patch
   B. Isosorbide dinitrate tablets, IR
   C. Nitroglycerin injection
   D. Nitroglycerin ointment
8. Which statement about β-adrenergic blockers is **false**?
   A. β-Adrenergic blockers reduce the heart's demand for oxygen.
   B. β-Adrenergic blockers decrease the frequency and severity of stable angina.
   C. β-Adrenergic blockers increase the heart's demand for oxygen.
   D. β-Adrenergic blockers are contraindicated in patients with asthma and diabetes.
9. How do calcium channel blockers help in the treatment of angina?
   A. They decrease heart rate.
   B. They decrease the strength of heart contractions.
   C. They reduce vasospasms and cause vasodilation.
   D. All the above

FILL IN THE BLANK: DRUG NAMES

1. What is a **brand name** for isosorbide mononitrate? _____
2. What is the **generic name** for Dilatrate-SR (United States)? _____
3. What is a **brand name** for nitroglycerin patches? _____
4. What is a **brand name** for nitroglycerin SL? _____
5. What is the **brand name** for atenolol? _____
6. What is the **brand name** for amlodipine plus atorvastatin? _____
7. What is a **brand name** for propranolol? _____

8. What is the **generic name** for Corgard (United States)? _____
9. What is the **brand name** for amlodipine? _____
10. What is the **generic name** for Cardizem and Tiazac? _____
11. What is the **generic name** for Procardia (United States) and Adalat? _____
12. What is the **generic name** for Calan? _____

MATCHING

Patient education is an essential component of therapeutics. Select the best warning label to apply to the prescription vial given to patients taking the drugs listed.
A. STORE IN ORIGINAL CONTAINER
B. SWALLOW WHOLE; DO NOT CRUSH OR CHEW
C. TAKE WITH FOOD
D. HOLD SPRAY IN MOUTH AT LEAST 10 SECONDS BEFORE SWALLOWING
E. TAKE ON AN EMPTY STOMACH
   1. _____ Isordil 10 mg
   2. _____ Metoprolol tartrate
   3. _____ Nitrolingual
   4. _____ Nitroglycerin 0.4 mg SL
   5. _____ Toprol XL 100 mg

MATCHING

Match the nitroglycerin dosage form with its therapeutic use.
A. Used for relief of acute anginal attacks
B. Used for prevention of anginal attacks
   1. _____ Nitroglycerin SL
   2. _____ Nitroglycerin patch
   3. _____ Nitroglycerin capsule
   4. _____ Nitroglycerin spray
   5. _____ Nitroglycerin ointment

MATCHING

Match each drug to its pharmacologic classification.
A. Nitrate
B. β-Blocker
C. Calcium channel blocker
   1. _____ Tenormin
   2. _____ Imdur
   3. _____ Verapamil

TRUE OR FALSE

1. _____ Atherosclerosis is sometimes called "hardening of the arteries."
2. _____ Nitroglycerin should always be dispensed without a safety cap for easy access.
3. _____ Patients who experience angina will have only symptoms of tightness and pain near their heart.
4. _____ Calcium channel blockers are used in the treatment of stable, variable, and unstable angina.
5. _____ Unstable angina may occur at rest.

6. _____When using transdermal nitrates, it is important to have a 10- to 12-hour nitrate-free period each day.

7. _____β-Blockers are widely used in patients with angina and asthma because they treat both diseases simultaneously.

CASE STUDY

Dylan is a new patient in your community pharmacy who was recently diagnosed with stable angina. He has started a few new medications and comes to you for help and advice. You talk to him first about lifestyle modifications. After questioning him, you discover that Dylan walks his dog twice a day for exercise and eats a large dinner every day.

1. What lifestyle modifications would you recommend to Dylan? Provide at least three specific and sustainable modifications for this patient.

   _____
   _____
   _____

2. Dylan was given metoprolol succinate as one of his new prescriptions. After reviewing his profile, you see that his asthma has been well controlled since he was a child. How would you warn Dylan about this potential drug-disease interaction?

   _____
   _____
   _____
   _____

3. Dylan was also prescribed Nitrostat, and the prescription states to "use as directed." How should Dylan take this medication? When should he take it? When should he or another person call 911?

   _____
   _____
   _____

A few months later, Dylan comes back to the pharmacy. He states that he has been taking his new medications and that his lifestyle adjustments are going well. He is at the pharmacy to fill a new prescription, Levitra, for his erectile dysfunction.

4. Would you fill this medication? Why or why not?

   _____
   _____
   _____
   _____

For Critical Thinking, Research Activity, and answer key, please refer to Evolve.

Appendix 18: Treatment of Hypertension

TERMS AND DEFINITIONS

Match each term with the correct definition below.
A. Aldosterone
B. Angiotensin II
C. Angiotensin-converting enzyme
D. Cardiac output
E. Diastolic blood pressure
F. Diuretic
G. Hyperkalemia
H. Hypertension
I. Isolated systolic hypertension
J. Metabolic syndrome
K. Orthostatic hypotension
L. Elevated or prehypertension
M. Peripheral vascular resistance
N. Renin–aldosterone–angiotensin system
O. Systolic blood pressure

1. A potent vasoconstrictor, _____ is produced when the renin–aldosterone–angiotensin system (RAAS) is activated.
2. The_____ is defined as the volume of blood ejected from the left ventricle in 1 minute.
3. _____ is defined as resistance to the flow of blood in peripheral arterial vessels that is associated with blood vessel diameter, vessel length, and blood viscosity.
4. _____ is the measure of blood pressure when the heart is at rest.
5. _____ is a hormone that promotes sodium and fluid reabsorption.
6. The term for elevated diastolic or systolic blood pressure is _____.
7. _____ is the measure of the pressure when the heart's ventricles are contracting.
8. A sudden drop in blood pressure that occurs when arising from lying down or sitting to standing is called _____.
9. The term for excessive serum potassium levels is _____.
10. _____ is the name of the enzyme that catalyzes the conversion of angiotensin I to angiotensin II.
11. _____ is defined as systolic blood pressure ranging between 120 and 129 mm Hg and diastolic blood pressure less than 80 mm Hg.
12. The_____ is activated when there is a drop in renal blood flow that increases blood volume, blood flow to the kidney, vasoconstriction, and blood pressure.
13. _____ is a drug that produces diuresis (urination).
14. _____ is the elevated systolic blood pressure only. Diastolic blood pressure is within the normal range.
15. _____ is an important risk factor of hypertension that promotes the development of atherosclerosis and cardiovascular disease.

MULTIPLE CHOICE

1. Side effects associated with metolazone include _____.
   A. hypokalemia
   B. hypernatremia
   C. hyperglycemia
   D. A and C
2. What is guanfacine's mechanism of action?
   A. Relax smooth muscle and decrease peripheral vascular resistance
   B. Relax smooth muscle and reduce urethral resistance
   C. Inhibit the conversion of angiotensin I to angiotensin II
   D. Increase fluid loss and decrease vasoconstriction
3. Which of the following effects of calcium channel blockers is responsible for reducing blood pressure?
   A. Increased force of cardiac contractions leading to increased cardiac output
   B. Relaxation of blood vessels (decreased peripheral resistance)
   C. Decreased renal blood flow
   D. Increased heart rate
4. Patients who are taking which medication(s) should be advised to avoid salt substitutes?
   A. Bisoprolol
   B. Chlorthalidone
   C. Spironolactone
   D. Ramipril
   E. C and D
5. Stage 1 hypertension is classified as systolic blood pressure ranges between _____.
   A. 130 to 139 mm Hg systolic and 80 to 89 mm Hg diastolic
   B. 100 to 120 mm Hg systolic and 70 to 80 mm Hg diastolic
   C. 120 to 129 mm Hg systolic and less than 80 mm Hg diastolic
   D. 140 mm Hg systolic and 90 mm Hg diastolic
6. All the following are classifications for diuretics *except* _____.
   A. thiazides
   B. loop
   C. calcium sparing
   D. potassium sparing
7. Pharmacy technicians should apply the warning label _____ to prescription vials containing potassium-sparing diuretics.
   A. MAY BE ADVISABLE TO EAT BANANAS OR DRINK ORANGE JUICE
   B. AVOID SALT SUBSTITUTES
   C. MAY CAUSE DROWSINESS
   D. TAKE WITH LOTS OF WATER
8. Select the **false** statement about angiotensin-converting enzyme (ACE) inhibitors.
   A. ACE inhibitors lower blood pressure by blocking the action of angiotensin-converting enzyme.
   B. Dry cough is a common side effect of ACE inhibitors.
   C. ACE inhibitors produce potassium loss.
   D. ACE inhibitors are contraindicated in pregnancy because they can interfere with fetal development of the kidneys.
9. Select the **false** statement about β-blockers.
   A. β-Blockers lower blood pressure by increasing heart rate.
   B. β-Blockers decrease peripheral resistance.
   C. β-Blockers used in the treatment of hypertension may be selective (b1) or nonselective (b1, b2).
   D. β-Blockers should be used with caution in patients with asthma and diabetes.
10. Select the pair of angiotensin II antagonists.
    A. Coreg and Trandate
    B. Prinivil and Vasotec
    C. Inderal and Tenormin
    D. Cozaar and Diovan

FILL IN THE BLANK: Drug Names

1. What is the **brand name** for hydrochlorothiazide (HCTZ)? _____
2. What is the **generic name** for Accupril? _____
3. What is the **brand name** for irbesartan? _____
4. What is the **generic name** for Tenex? _____
5. What is the **brand name** for benazepril? _____
6. What is the **generic name** for Vasotec? _____
7. What are two **brand names** for lisinopril? _____
8. What is the **generic name** for Micardis HCT? _____
9. What are two **brand names** for lisinopril plus hydrochlorothiazide? _____
10. What is the **generic name** for Cozaar? _____
11. What is the **brand name** for doxazosin? _____
12. What is the **generic name** for Hyzaar? _____
13. What is the **brand name** for valsartan plus hydrochlorothiazide? _____

MATCHING

Match each drug to its pharmacologic classification.
A. Thiazide diuretic
B. Nonselective β-blocker
C. Angiotensin II antagonist
D. Selective β-blocker
E. Aldosterone receptor blocker

1. _____ Spironolactone 25 mg
2. _____ Propranolol 10 mg
3. _____ Acebutolol 200 mg
4. _____ Eprosartan 600 mg
5. _____ Indapamide 1.25 mg

MATCHING

Match each drug to its pharmacologic classification.
A. Thiazide diuretic
B. ACE inhibitor
C. Angiotensin II antagonist
D. β-Blocker
E. Loop diuretic

1. _____ Bisoprolol 10 mg
2. _____ Vasotec 2.5 mg
3. _____ Furosemide 40 mg
4. _____ Chlorthalidone 50 mg
5. _____ Atacand 4 mg

MATCHING

Match each drug to its pharmacologic classification.
A. Potassium-sparing diuretic
B. Combined α- and β-blocker
C. a1-Antagonists

D. Direct renin inhibitor
E. β-Blocker
  1. _____ Tekturna 150 mg
  2. _____ Carvedilol 6.25 mg
  3. _____ Nadolol 40 mg
  4. _____ Triamterene plus HCTZ 37.5 mg/75 mg
  5. _____ Doxazosin 1 mg

MATCHING

Patient education is an essential component of therapeutics. Select the **best** warning label to apply to the prescription vial given to patients taking the drugs listed.
A. MAY BE ADVISABLE TO EAT BANANAS OR DRINK ORANGE JUICE
B. TAKE WITH FOOD
C. MAY CAUSE A DRY COUGH
D. DON'T CRUSH OR CHEW
E. AVOID PROLONGED EXPOSURE TO SUNLIGHT
  1. _____ Inderal LA 120 mg
  2. _____ Amiloride plus HCTZ
  3. _____ Captopril 12.5 mg
  4. _____ Bumetanide 1 mg
  5. _____ Spironolactone 25 mg

MATCHING

Patient education is an essential component of therapeutics. Select the **best** warning label to apply to the prescription vial given to patients taking the drugs listed.
A. ROTATE SITE OF APPLICATION
B. AVOID PREGNANCY
C. MAY BE ADVISABLE TO EAT BANANAS OR DRINK ORANGE JUICE
D. AVOID SALT SUBSTITUTES AND POTASSIUM-RICH DIETS
E. DON'T CRUSH OR CHEW
  1. _____ Metoprolol SR 100 mg
  2. _____ Clonidine 0.1 mg patch
  3. _____ Ramipril 10 mg
  4. _____ Valsartan
  5. _____ Furosemide 20 mg

TRUE OR FALSE

1. _____ Complications of untreated hypertension include stroke, myocardial infarction, and kidney damage.
2. _____ It is dangerous to the mother and fetus to treat hypertension with any medication.
3. _____ Diuretics, especially loop diuretics, should not be taken at night to avoid nocturia.
4. _____ Sites for blood pressure control are the kidneys, heart, blood vessels, and lungs.
5. _____ When peripheral vascular resistance increases, blood pressure increases.
6. _____ High blood pressure is associated with obesity, excess dietary sodium intake, physical inactivity, and poor diet.
7. _____ Hydralazine is recommended for hypertensive emergencies (parenteral use) and is safe for use in pregnant women.

CASE STUDY

Mary is a patient who uses your pharmacy regularly, and you know that she is recently pregnant. She comes into your pharmacy today to get her blood pressure checked. After having her sit for 5 minutes, you read her blood pressure at 146/93. You wait and check after another 5 minutes with similar results. You tell Mary that her blood pressure reading is high.

1. According to this measurement, Mary is in which stage of hypertension?
  _____
  _____
  _____
  _____

2. Should Mary seek additional medical attention for her blood pressure? Why or why not?
  _____
  _____
  _____
  _____

Two weeks later, Mary comes back with new prescriptions for lisinopril and hydrochlorothiazide.

3. Should the pharmacist fill both of these medications for Mary? Why or why not? (Hint: Look up the pregnancy category for these medications.)
  _____
  _____
  _____

4. What lifestyle modifications can Mary make to reduce her blood pressure? Describe at least three specific and sustainable steps she can take.
  _____
  _____
  _____
  _____

For Critical Thinking, Research Activity, and answer key, please refer to Evolve.

Appendix 19: Treatment of Heart Disease and Stroke

TERMS AND DEFINITIONS

Match each term with the correct definition below.

A. Anticoagulant
B. Antiplatelet drug
C. Antithrombotic
D. Atherosclerosis
E. Atherothrombosis
F. Cardiac glycosides
G. Cholesterol
H. Ejection fraction
I. Heart failure
J. Hemostasis
K. High-density lipoprotein (HDL)
L. Hyperlipidemia
M. Myocardial infarction
N. Ischemia
O. Low-density lipoprotein (LDL)
P. Natriuretic peptides
Q. Partial thromboplastin time (PTT)
R. Platelets
S. Plaque
T. Positive inotropic effect
U. Prothrombin time (PT)
V. Thrombolytic
W. Tissue plasminogen activator (TPA)
X. Transient ischemic attack (TIA)
Y. Triglycerides

1. A(n) _____ is a drug that prevents accumulation of platelets, thereby blocking an important step in the clot formation process.
2. _____ are metabolized to very-low-density lipoproteins (VLDLs) and are a form of energy storage found in fat tissue muscle.
3. Hormones that play a role in cardiac physiology and homeostasis are called _____.
4. _____ is a test given to determine effectiveness of heparin, while _____ is a test given to determine the effectiveness of warfarin.
5. A drug that inhibits clot formation by reducing the action of thrombin is called _____.
6. "Bad cholesterol" is known as _____, and "good cholesterol" is known as _____.
7. _____ is a condition characterized by excess fatty substances in the blood.
8. The formation of _____, or fatty cholesterol deposits, contributes to worsening atherosclerosis.
9. A(n) _____ occurs when there is a sudden loss of blood supply to a certain area, such as the heart or the brain, resulting in cell death.
10. A disease in which the heart cannot pump enough blood to meet the body's metabolic needs is known as _____.
11. A(n) _____ is considered a stroke that lasts for only a few minutes.
12. A naturally occurring thrombolytic substance is called _____.
13. _____ are found in the blood and play an active role in the coagulation process.
14. When the force of myocardial contractions has increased, that is considered a(n) _____.
15. _____ is a disease characterized by the buildup of lipids and plaque inside artery walls. This buildup impedes blood flow and oxygen.
16. The heart is said to have a low _____ if it pumps only a small amount of blood from the ventricles with each heartbeat.
17. The process of stopping blood flow is called _____.
18. _____ is/are a class of medications that has the ability to alter cardiovascular function.
19. The reduction of blood supplied to tissues that is typically caused by blood vessel obstruction resulting from atherosclerosis, stenosis, or plaque is called _____.
20. Excess _____ can cause atherosclerosis, but this naturally occurring substance is also needed to synthesize vitamin D.
21. A class of drugs that is used to dissolve existing blood clots is known as _____.
22. _____ is the formation of a clot inside an artery.
23. A class of medication that is used to prevent clot formation and prolong coagulation is known as _____.

MULTIPLE CHOICE

1. Which of the following statement(s) about digoxin is/are **true**?
   A. It increases heart rate.
   B. It decreases exercise tolerance.
   C. It increases the force of myocardial contractions.
   D. A and C
2. Regarding compensatory mechanisms that are "switched on" when the heart function fails, which of the following is **false**?
   A. The renin–aldosterone–angiotensin system (RAAS) is activated to increase blood volume.
   B. The RAAS is activated to increase cardiac output.
   C. Natriuretic peptides are released to promote vasoconstriction.
   D. Natriuretic peptides are released to promote sodium and water elimination by the kidneys.
3. All the following drugs are used in the treatment of heart failure *except*_____.
   A. angiotensin II receptor antagonists
   B. "statins"
   C. vasodilators
   D. nonsteroidal antiinflammatory drugs (NSAIDs)
4. Modifiable heart attack and stroke risk factors include _____.
   A. diet
   B. smoking
   C. alcohol consumption
   D. B and C
   E. all the above
5. _____ typically causes hemorrhagic strokes.
   A. An embolism
   B. An aneurysm
   C. Atherosclerosis
   D. Ischemia
6. Select the class of drug that is not used in the treatment of myocardial infarction or stroke.
   A. Anticoagulants
   B. Antiplatelets

C. Angiotensin-converting enzyme (ACE) inhibitors
D. Antihyperlipidemics
E. Thrombolytics

7. Which of the following nonprescription drugs and supplements can enhance the effect of antiplatelet medications?
A. NSAIDs
B. Garlic
C. Fish oil
D. All the above

8. Which of the following antiplatelet drugs must be administered parenterally?
A. Aspirin
B. Abciximab
C. Clopidogrel
D. Dipyridamole
E. Ticlopidine

9. The antidote for warfarin overdose is _____, whereas the heparin overdose antidote is _____.
A. vitamin D; protamine zinc
B. vitamin D; protamine sulfate
C. vitamin K; Digibind
D. Digibind; vitamin K
E. vitamin K; protamine sulfate

10. Which drug class do prescribers prefer for pregnant women with hyperlipidemia?
A. Statins
B. Bile acid sequestrants
C. Fibric acid derivatives
D. Nicotinic acid derivatives

FILL IN THE BLANK: DRUG NAMES

1. What is the *generic name* for Plavix? _____
2. What is the *brand name* for dipyridamole? _____
3. What is the *generic name* for Ticlid? _____
4. What is the *generic name* for Coumadin? _____
5. What is the *brand name* for dalteparin? _____
6. What is the *generic name* for Lovenox? _____
7. What is a *brand name* for heparin sodium? _____
8. What is the *generic name* for Innohep? _____
9. What is the *brand name* for alteplase? _____
10. What is the *generic name* for Lipitor? _____
11. What is the *brand name* for pravastatin? _____
12. What is the *generic name* for Crestor? _____
13. What is the *generic name* for Vytorin? _____
14. What is the *brand name* for niacin plus lovastatin? _____
15. What is the *brand name* for colestipol? _____
16. What is the *brand name* for chlorothiazide? _____
17. What is the *generic name* for Bumex (United States) and Burinex (Canada)? _____
18. What is the *generic name* for Aldactone? _____
19. What is the *generic name* for Zebeta (United States) and Monocor (Canada)? _____
20. What is the *brand name* for benazepril? _____
21. What is the *generic name* for Cozaar? _____
22. What is the *generic name* for Apresoline? _____
23. What is the *brand name* for isosorbide dinitrate? _____

MATCHING

Match each drug to its pharmacologic classification. Each class may be used more than once.
A. Thiazide diuretic
B. ACE inhibitor
C. Angiotensin II antagonist
D. Combined α- and β-blocker
E. Vasodilator

1. _____ Carvedilol
2. _____ Candesartan
3. _____ Hydralazine
4. _____ Indapamide
5. _____ Chlorthalidone
6. _____ Benazepril

MATCHING

Match each drug to its pharmacologic classification. Each class may be used more than once.
A. Antiplatelet
B. Thrombolytic
C. Antihyperlipidemic
D. Anticoagulant

1. _____ Lovenox
2. _____ Reteplase
3. _____ Livalo
4. _____ Clopidogrel
5. _____ Eptifibatide
6. _____ Ticlopidine
7. _____ Alteplase
8. _____ Fondaparinux
9. _____ Lescol
10. _____ Cholestyramine
11. _____ Aggrastat
12. _____ Tricor
13. _____ Warfarin
14. _____ Lovastatin
15. _____ Aspirin
16. _____ Pradaxa

MATCHING

Patient education is an essential component of therapeutics. Select the best warning label to apply to the prescription vial given to patients taking the drugs listed.
A. AVOID PREGNANCY
B. STORE IN ORIGINAL CONTAINER
C. TAKE ON AN EMPTY STOMACH
D. AVOID ALCOHOL

1. _____ Gemfibrozil
2. _____ Niaspan
3. _____ Warfarin
4. _____ Pradaxa

TRUE OR FALSE

1. _____Prothrombin time test is also known as international normalized ratio (INR) test.
2. _____Symptoms of a myocardial infarction last 1 to 5 minutes and may be relieved by rest.
3. _____Stroke symptoms may include confusion, facial numbness, and lost balance.
4. _____Diseases that can increase the risk for stroke and myocardial infarction include anxiety, hypotension, and stomach ulcers.
5. _____Anticoagulants and antiplatelets can dissolve existing clots.
6. _____All antithrombotic medications increase bleeding risk.
7. _____Niacin can decrease VLDL synthesis and increase HDL.
8. _____Fibric acid derivatives might cause myositis and rhabdomyolysis, two life-threatening side effects.
9. _____There are four heart failure stages, and stage I is the most severe.
10. _____Food can increase the absorption of digoxin.
11. _____Heart failure can affect the left side, the right side, or both sides of the heart at the same time.
12. _____Hydralazine reduces peripheral resistance and has been shown to indirectly increase positive inotropic effect on the heart.

CASE STUDY

Victor is a 57-year-old pharmacy patient. He is in great shape with a physically demanding job, but he eats a diet high in salt and saturated fat. He binges on alcohol on the weekends, and he takes high doses of naproxen and hydrocodone/APAP for back pain. His other medical conditions include hypertension, hyperlipidemia, prediabetes, and PTSD. He used to smoke but quit 5 years ago. He refuses to take medications for his chronic conditions because he does not believe he needs them.

1. What lifestyle modifications should Victor use to reduce his chances of developing heart failure? Or a myocardial infarction/stroke?
   _____
   _____
   _____
   _____

2. Of the two medications Victor takes, which is of most concern as regards a heart attack or stroke? Explain your reasoning.
   _____
   _____
   _____
   _____

3. Which class of heart failure does Victor seem to be in currently? Explain your reasoning.
   _____
   _____
   _____
   _____

A few years later, Victor comes back to the pharmacy with his son. After retiring from his job, Victor gained weight; he relied on his son to push his wheelchair. Victor's son explains that his father had a heart attack 6 months ago, which put Victor into stage II heart failure. Now, the doctors say he has progressed to stage III. Victor's son hands you a prescription for digoxin.

4. Is digoxin a proper treatment option for Victor at this time? (Hint: Refer to Table 19.3 in your textbook.)
   _____
   _____
   _____
   _____

5. What other medications should Victor be taking for his class III heart failure?
   _____
   _____
   _____
   _____

For Critical Thinking, Research Activity, and answer key, please refer to Evolve.

Appendix 20: Treatment of Arrhythmia

TERMS AND DEFINITIONS

Match each term with the correct definition below.
A. Atrial fibrillation
B. Atrial flutter
C. Automaticity
D. Depolarization
E. Ectopic
F. Electrical cardioversion
G. Refractory period
H. Repolarization
I. Supraventricular tachycardia
J. Ventricular fibrillation
K. Ventricular tachycardia

1. The _____ is the time between contractions that it takes for repolarization to occur.
2. During _____, the atria beat between 300 and 400 beats/min, and contractions are uncoordinated.
3. The period when the heart is recharging and preparing for another contraction is called _____.
4. A(n) _____ beat is a heartbeat that occurs outside of the normal pacemaker locations.

5. Persons who have a(n) _____ have a heart rate of 160 to 350 beats/min and contractions of the atrium exceed the number in the ventricles.
6. The term used to describe spontaneous contraction of heart muscle cells is _____.
7. _____ is the process of applying an electrical shock to the heart with a defibrillator.
8. An arrhythmia that produces heartbeats up to 600 beats/min and uncoordinated contractions is _____.
9. _____ occurs in a region above the ventricles and produces a heart rate up to 200 beats/min.
10. _____ causes the ventricles to beat faster than 200 beats/min.
11. _____ is the process where the heart muscle conducts an electrical impulse, causing a contraction.

MULTIPLE CHOICE

1. The process where the heart muscle conducts an electrical impulse causing a contraction is called _____.
   A. repolarization
   B. depolarization
   C. automaticity
   D. refractory period
2. Which disease requires the most immediate medical attention?
   A. Atrial flutter
   B. Atrial fibrillation
   C. Supraventricular tachycardia
   D. Ventricular tachycardia
   E. Ventricular fibrillation
3. Supraventricular tachycardia is an arrhythmia that originates in an area _____ the ventricles.
   A. below
   B. above
   C. within
4. Select the nonmodifiable risk factor for arrhythmia.
   A. Obesity
   B. Age
   C. Smoking
   D. Excessive alcohol consumption
   E. Stimulant use
5. Which of the following is *not* a disease risk factor for arrhythmia?
   A. Coronary heart disease (CHD) and stroke
   B. Diabetes
   C. Thyroid disease
   D. Obstructive sleep apnea
   E. Epilepsy
6. Which of the following is true about digoxin?
   A. It is a class III antiarrhythmic.
   B. It is not approved for the treatment of atrial fibrillation in the United States.
   C. It can be administered orally or intravenously.
   D. Its therapeutic index is high.
7. Which medication class significantly reduces first-time atrial fibrillation risk in hypertensive patients?
   A. Angiotensin-converting enzyme (ACE) inhibitors
   B. Angiotensin type II receptor blockers
   C. Thiazide diuretics
   D. A and B

8. Tinnitus is a sign of _____ toxicity.
   A. amiodarone
   B. procainamide
   C. mexiletine
   D. quinidine
9. Which class I antiarrhythmic drug must be administered parenterally?
   A. Procainamide
   B. Lidocaine
   C. Tocainide
   D. Propafenone
10. Persons taking amiodarone may experience all the following adverse effects *except* _____.
    A. constipation
    B. photosensitivity
    C. skin discoloration
    D. visual disturbances
    E. corneal deposits

FILL IN THE BLANK: DRUG NAMES

1. What is the **brand name** for flecainide? _____
2. What is the **generic name** for Norpace (United States) and Rythmodan (Canada)? _____
3. What is a **brand name** for propafenone? _____
4. What is the **brand name** for dofetilide? _____
5. What is the **brand name** for acebutolol? _____
6. What is the **generic name** for Corvert? _____
7. What is the **brand name** for esmolol? _____
8. What is the **generic name** for Xylocard (Canada)? _____
9. What is the **brand name** for propranolol? _____
10. What is a **brand name** for amiodarone? _____
11. What is the **generic name** for Betapace (United States)? _____
12. What is the **generic name** for Isoptin SR? _____

MATCHING

Patient education is an essential component of therapeutics. Select the **best** warning label to apply to the prescription vial given to patients taking the drugs listed.
A. DILUTE ORAL CONCENTRATE
B. AVOID PROLONGED EXPOSURE TO SUNLIGHT
C. TAKE WITH FOOD
D. TAKE ON AN EMPTY STOMACH
E. PROTECT FROM MOISTURE
   1. _____ Dofetilide
   2. _____ Mexiletine
   3. _____ Procainamide
   4. _____ Propranolol
   5. _____ Amiodarone

MATCHING

Match each drug to its pharmacologic classification.
A. Class Ia
B. Ca^{2+} channel blockade
C. K^+ channel blockade
D. Class Ic

E. Class Ib
  1. _____ Amiodarone
  2. _____ Lidocaine
  3. _____ Flecainide
  4. _____ Disopyramide
  5. _____ Verapamil

TRUE OR FALSE

1. _____Class I antiarrhythmic agents can produce local anesthesia.
2. _____β-Blockers are the only drug class for the primary management of ventricular arrhythmias.
3. _____Nonmodifiable risk factors for atrial fibrillation include age, emotional stress, gender, and bradycardia.
4. _____Atrial flutter treatments include the antiarrhythmic medications quinidine gluconate and esmolol.
5. _____Calcium channel blockers can cause headache, flushing, and peripheral edema.

CASE STUDY

Brady is a 63-year-old man and a regular pharmacy patient. He eats well, exercises often, and is without chronic conditions. He has never smoked but drinks a few beers weekly. Today he walks in with a new prescription for valsartan. Brady tells you the doctor prescribed him the medication for stroke prevention to keep his heart from "beating weird."
1. What condition is Brady's physician trying to prevent? How does that condition relate to having a stroke?
   _____
   _____
   _____
   _____

2. How does valsartan help prevent this condition?
   _____
   _____
   _____

A few months later, Brady returns with a new prescription for amiodarone. He says that he got an infection that brought him to the hospital, and the physical stress from the infection caused an arrhythmia. He asks you for advice on his new medication.
3. What class of antiarrhythmic agents is amiodarone in? How does amiodarone work to treat arrhythmias?
   _____
   _____
   _____
   _____

4. What side effects should you warn Brady of before starting this medication?
   _____
   _____
   _____
   _____

5. You want to warn Brady that all antiarrhythmic drugs can cause other arrhythmias. How would you say this to Brady so that he understands the risk, yet remains compliant with the medication?
   _____
   _____
   _____
   _____

For Critical Thinking, Research Activity, and answer key, please refer to Evolve.

Appendix 21: Treatment of Gastroesophageal Reflux Disease, Laryngopharyngeal Reflux, and Peptic Ulcer Disease

TERMS AND DEFINITIONS

Match each term with the correct definition below.
A. Duodenal ulcer
B. Gastric ulcer
C. Gastroesophageal reflux
D. Gastroesophageal reflux disease (GERD)
E. Hiatal hernia
F. Laryngopharyngeal reflux (LPR)
G. Lower esophageal sphincter
H. Peptic ulcer disease (PUD)
I. Peristalsis
J. Reflux
K. Ulcer
L. Upper esophageal sphincter
  1. _____ is a motility disorder associated with impaired peristalsis.
  2. The condition in which the lower esophageal sphincter shifts above the diaphragm is _____.

3. _____ is a forceful wave of contractions in the esophagus that moves food and liquids from the mouth to the stomach.
4. _____ is a condition in which stomach contents may flow upward into the esophagus to produce heartburn.
5. Backflow or _____ of gastric contents into the esophagus or laryngopharyngeal region is responsible for symptoms of PUD and GERD.
6. _____ is a term that is used to describe ulcers that are located in either the duodenum or stomach.
7. The _____ separates the esophagus and the stomach.
8. An ulcer that is located in the upper portion of the small intestine or duodenum is called a(n) _____.
9. The _____ separates the pharynx and esophagus.
10. A(n) _____ is an open wound or sore.
11. _____ is a condition in which gastric contents reflux into the larynx and pharynx.
12. A(n) _____ is an ulcer that is located in the stomach.

MULTIPLE CHOICE

1. Which of the following is *not* a lifestyle factor that worsens GERD?
   A. Coffee consumption
   B. Cigarette smoking
   C. Alcohol consumption
   D. Chewing gum
2. If left untreated, GERD may increase the risk for development of _____.
   A. stomach cancer
   B. asthma
   C. hemorrhage
   D. all the above
3. All the following may be used in the treatment of PUD *except* _____.
   A. cimetidine
   B. aluminum hydroxide gel
   C. sucralfate
   D. methylprednisolone
   E. lansoprazole
4. A patient taking an antacid preparation develops constipation. What combination of ingredients in antacids is likely to cause this side effect?
   A. Magnesium hydroxide gel plus simethicone
   B. Magaldrate plus simethicone
   C. Aluminum hydroxide plus calcium carbonate
   D. Aluminum hydroxide plus magnesium hydroxide gel
5. Chronic cough and excessive phlegm or saliva are hallmark symptoms of _____.
   A. PUD
   B. LPR
   C. NSAID-induced ulcer
   D. GERD
6. Which treatment for GERD is a proton pump inhibitor?
   A. Tagamet
   B. Axid
   C. Pepcid
   D. Nexium
7. The leading cause of PUD is _____.
   A. *Helicobacter pylori* infection
   B. stress
   C. drug therapy
   D. spicy foods
8. Ulcer formation is a possible adverse reaction of all of the following drugs *except* _____.
   A. aspirin
   B. lansoprazole
   C. NSAIDs
   D. prednisone
9. What is the mechanism of action of domperidone?
   A. Neutralizes stomach acid and decreases pepsin secretion
   B. Increases peristalsis by stimulating acetylcholine release
   C. Stimulates the production of protective mucus and stomach bicarbonate
   D. Increases peristalsis by blocking peripheral dopamine receptors
10. Which drug promotes healing of ulcers and acts like a "Band-Aid"?
    A. cimetidine
    B. sucralfate
    C. esomeprazole
    D. misoprostol

FILL IN THE BLANK: Drug Names

1. What is the **brand name** for famotidine? _____
2. What is the **generic name** for Tagamet (United States)? _____
3. What is a **brand name** for nizatidine? _____
4. What is the **generic name** for Metozolv ODT and Reglan? _____
5. What is the **generic name** for Prevacid? _____
6. What is the **generic name** for Prilosec (United States) and Losec (Canada)? _____
7. What is the **brand name** for famotidine + calcium carbonate + magnesium hydroxide?
8. _____
9. What is the **generic name** for Protonix (United States) and Pantoloc (Canada)?
10. _____
11. What is the **generic name** for Vimovo? _____
12. What is the **generic name** for Aciphex (United States) and Pariet (Canada)? _____
13. What is the **generic name** for Reglan (United States)? _____ `
14. What is the **brand name** for dexlansoprazole? _____

MATCHING

Patient education is an essential component of therapeutics. Select the **best** warning label to apply to the prescription vial given to patients taking the drugs listed.
A. TAKE 30 MINUTES BEFORE A MEAL
B. TAKE 60 MINUTES BEFORE A MEAL
C. SHAKE WELL AND DISCARD AFTER 30 DAYS
D. MAY CAUSE DROWSINESS
E. AVOID PREGNANCY

1. _____ Misoprostol 100 mcg
2. _____ Prevacid 30 mg
3. _____ Pepcid 40 mg/5 mL
4. _____ Metoclopramide 10 mg
5. _____ Nexium 20 mg

TRUE OR FALSE

1. _____ Ranitidine binds to both H_1 and H_2 receptors equally.
2. _____ The use of antacids such as aluminum hydroxide and calcium carbonate has fallen out of favor with better over-the-counter options for PUD and GERD.
3. _____ Misoprostol blocks drug absorption, including H_2 receptor antagonists, proton pump inhibitors (PPIs), and some antibiotics.
4. _____ The main use of antacids is to provide a protective coating to the stomach lining.
5. _____ Stress and spicy foods can cause ulcers.
6. _____ Prescribers always combine antibiotics with gastric acid–reducing drugs to fight *H. pylori* infection.
7. _____ PPIs have the common ending -*prazole*.

CASE STUDY

Mark walks into your community pharmacy today. He is a healthy 72-year-old man with no chronic diseases. He tells you that he has been feeling increasing chest pain, especially after dinner. You gather that he gets this feeling after eating a large dinner and that the pain comes with belching and bloating. He does not smoke, but he does have a glass or two of wine a few nights weekly with dinner. When asked about the types of meals he eats, he says that he has been trying out new restaurants around town with his wife. He asks you what he can do about the pain.

1. Out of GERD, LPR, and PUD, which condition do you think he has? Why?
2. What lifestyle risk factors does Mark have for his disease?

3. What lifestyle modifications would you have Mark implement?
4. What would be the best choice for Mark to address his symptoms: an antacid, an H$_2$ receptor antagonist, or a PPI? Why?

For Critical Thinking, Research Activity, and answer key, please refer to Evolve.

Appendix 22: Treatment of Irritable Bowel Syndrome, Ulcerative Colitis, and Crohn's Disease

TERMS AND DEFINITIONS

Match each term with the correct definition below.
A. Antidiarrheals
B. Constipation
C. Crohn's disease
D. Diarrhea
E. Gastroenteritis
F. Inflammatory bowel disease (IBD)
G. Irritable bowel syndrome (IBS)
H. Laxatives

1. _____ is an infection in the gastrointestinal (GI) tract that can cause postinfection IBS.
2. Constipation is treated with _____ , medicines that induce evacuation of the bowel.
3. _____ are used to reduce abnormally frequent passage of loose and watery stools.
4. _____ is a condition characterized by chronic abdominal distress, resulting in frequent diarrhea or constipation.
5. A person who has _____ has inflammation of the intestine, and _____ may produce inflammation anywhere along the GI tract.
6. _____ is abnormally delayed or infrequent passage of dry, hardened feces.
7. Abnormally frequent passage of loose and watery stools is known as _____

MULTIPLE CHOICE

1. Which of the following gastrointestinal conditions is *not* characterized by inflammation?
   A. IBD
   B. Ulcerative colitis
   C. IBS
   D. Crohn's disease
2. Select the **false** statement.
   A. Ulcerative colitis and Crohn's disease are inflammatory bowel diseases.
   B. IBS may be associated with abnormally low levels of the neurotransmitter norepinephrine.
   C. In ulcerative colitis and Crohn's disease, the body's immune system recognizes the bacteria that normally inhabit the GI tract as harmful invaders and releases anti–tumor necrosis factor (TNF).

   D. Ulcerative colitis produces inflammation in the upper layers of the lining of the small intestine and colon.
   E. Lifestyle modification can reduce symptoms of IBS, ulcerative colitis, and Crohn's disease.
3. Which drug(s) may be prescribed only by physicians enrolled in a drug-specific prescribing program?
   A. Sulfasalazine
   B. Alosetron
   C. Tegaserod
   D. Fiber supplements
   E. Loperamide
4. Which of the following lifestyle modifications would help reduce symptoms for a patient with Crohn's disease?
   A. Limit carbonated beverages
   B. Eat small meals
   C. Reduce daily water intake
   D. A and B
   E. All the above
5. Ulcerative colitis can affect which of the following locations?
   A. Colon
   B. Small intestine
   C. Mouth
   D. All the above
6. Which statement about glucocorticosteroid use for the treatment of Crohn's disease is **false**?
   A. Glucocorticosteroids decrease inflammation.
   B. Glucocorticosteroids increase inflammation.
   C. Glucocorticosteroids are immunosuppressants.
   D. Glucocorticosteroids reduce flareups.
7. Which drug *does not* induce remission of Crohn's disease?
   A. Azathioprine
   B. Infliximab
   C. 6-Mercaptopurine
   D. Methotrexate
   E. Olsalazine

FILL IN THE BLANK: Drug Names

1. What is the ***generic name*** for Lotronex (United States)? _____
2. What is the ***brand name*** for diphenoxylate plus atropine? _____
3. What is the ***generic name*** for Atreza (United States)? _____

4. What is the *generic name* for Bentyl (United States) and Bentylol (Canada)? _____
5. What is the *brand name* for balsalazide? _____
6. What is the *brand name* for mesalamine (United States) and mesalazine (Canada)?
7. _____
8. What is the *brand name* for natalizumab? _____
9. What is the *generic name* for Azulfidine (United States) and Salazopyrin (Canada)? _____
10. What is the *brand name* for olsalazine? _____
11. What is the *generic name* for Cortifoam? _____
12. What is the *generic name* for Amitiza? _____
13. What is the *brand name* for polycarbophil? _____
14. What is the *brand name* for methylprednisolone? _____
15. What is the *generic name* for Imuran? _____
16. What is the *brand name* for 6-mercaptopurine? _____
17. What is a *brand name* for infliximab? _____

MATCHING

Match each drug to its therapeutic classification.
A. Serotonin receptor antagonist
B. Immunosuppressant
C. Immunomodulator
D. Corticosteroid
1. _____ Hydrocortisone enema
2. _____ Alosetron 1 mg tab
3. _____ Methotrexate 2.5 mg tab
4. _____ Infliximab 100 mg

MATCHING

Match each drug to its therapeutic classification.
A. Immunosuppressant
B. Anticholinergic
C. Bulk-forming laxative
D. Antidiarrheal
E. Aminosalicylate
1. _____ Mesalamine 250 mg ER cap
2. _____ Loperamide 2 mg
3. _____ Imuran 50 mg tab
4. _____ Dicyclomine 20 mg tab
5. _____ Equalactin 625 mg

TRUE OR FALSE

1. _____ Crohn's disease produces inflammation and damage only in the colon.
2. _____ Ulcerative colitis and Crohn's disease are both associated with low levels of serotonin.
3. _____ One potentially serious side effect of immunomodulators is that they can reactivate dormant infections such as tuberculosis.
4. _____ IBS may be associated with abnormally low levels of the neurotransmitter serotonin.
5. _____ Toxic megacolon is a life-threatening adverse effect of alosetron.
6. _____ All commercially available aminosalicylates (5-ASA) are formulated as delayed-release products.
7. _____ Ulcerative colitis most commonly occurs between the ages of 30 and 50 years.

CASE STUDY

Lucy comes into your pharmacy today with a new prescription for lubiprostone. After being asked about her new condition, she states that she has been recently diagnosed with IBS. She doesn't understand how she could get the disease because she is 32 years old and in relatively good health. She is interested in hearing more about IBS because her doctor didn't explain it in detail.

1. How would you explain her recent diagnosis of IBS? What is IBS and at what age do patients tend to see symptoms?
_____
_____
_____
_____

2. How will lubiprostone help with her IBS? What side effects can the medication have?
_____
_____
_____
_____

3. What lifestyle modifications can Lucy make to reduce her IBS symptoms?
_____
_____
_____
_____

4. After a few months, Lucy comes back to the pharmacy complaining that the lubiprostone isn't helping much. She asks for your advice.
_____
_____
_____

5. What other options does Lucy have if she has predominantly diarrhea? What about if she has predominantly constipation?
_____
_____
_____
_____

For Critical Thinking, Research Activity, and answer key, please refer to Evolve.

Appendix 23: Treatment of Asthma and Chronic Obstructive Pulmonary Disease

TERMS AND DEFINITIONS

Match each term with the correct definition below.

A. Allergic asthma
B. Asthma
C. Bronchodilator
D. Chronic obstructive pulmonary disease (COPD)
E. Forced expiratory volume
F. Metered-dose inhaler (MDI)
G. Nebulizer
H. Peak flow meter
I. Spacer
J. Spirometry

1. Two tests that measure volume of air are _____ and _____.

2. _____ is a progressive disease of the airways that produces gradual loss of pulmonary function.

3. _____ is typically defined as a chronic disease that affects the airways, producing irritation, inflammation, and difficulty breathing; however, symptoms of _____ occur upon exposure to environmental allergens.

4. Whereas corticosteroids are used in the treatment of asthma to reduce inflammation and swelling of airways, a(n) _____ will relax tightened airway muscles.

5. A device that creates an inhalable mist out of a liquid solution is called a(n) _____.

6. The _____ is a handheld device that is used to measure the volume of air exhaled and how fast the air is moved out.

7. A(n) _____ is a device that delivers a specific amount of inhaled medication. A(n) _____ can be attached to the device to facilitate drug delivery into the lungs rather than the back of the throat.

MULTIPLE CHOICE

1. Symptoms of asthma include all the following *except* _____.
   A. coughing
   B. wheezing
   C. sneezing
   D. shortness of breath
   E. chest tightness

2. _____ may serve as a trigger for an asthma attack.
   A. Warm, moist air
   B. Strenuous exercise
   C. Crying or laughing
   D. All the above

3. Treatment of COPD involves the administration of _____.
   A. bronchodilators
   B. glucocorticosteroids
   C. antibiotics when infections are present
   D. oxygen
   E. all the above

4. Which of the following drugs is *not* a "reliever" medicine prescribed for the treatment of acute symptoms of asthma?
   A. Albuterol (or salbutamol)
   B. Levalbuterol
   C. Beclomethasone
   D. Terbutaline
   E. Ipratropium bromide

5. Select the **false** statement.
   A. Long-acting β_2-agonists (LABAs) are approved monotherapy for asthma and COPD.
   B. Excess short-acting β_2-agonist (SABA) use indicates poor disease management in asthma patients.
   C. Glucocorticoids reduce lung inflammation; they don't help with bronchoconstriction.
   D. Xanthine derivatives similar to caffeine have multiple mechanisms of action to help manage asthma symptomology.

6. Which of the following classes of drugs is *not* a "controller" medicine, prescribed to prevent symptoms of asthma?
   A. LABAs
   B. SABAs
   C. Inhaled corticosteroids
   D. Leukotriene modifiers
   E. Mast cell stabilizers

7. Select the **false** statement.
   A. Leukotriene modifiers are administered to patients with mild asthma to reduce inflammation.
   B. Leukotriene modifiers inhibit the release of proinflammatory substances.
   C. The packet of montelukast granules may be opened and premixed hours in advance for convenience.
   D. Montelukast granules may be mixed in food.

FILL IN THE BLANK: Drug Names

1. What is the *generic name* for Ventolin? _____
2. What is the *generic name* for Xopenex (United States)? _____
3. What is the *generic name* for Atrovent HFA? _____
4. What is the *brand name* for ciclesonide? _____
5. What is the *brand name* for albuterol plus ipratropium bromide? _____
6. What is the *brand name* for fenoterol hydrobromide plus ipratropium bromide? _____
7. What is the *generic name* for Foradil? _____
8. What is the *generic name* for Serevent Diskus? _____
9. What is the *generic name* for Qvar? _____
10. What is the *brand name* for budesonide? _____
11. What is the *brand name* for fluticasone? _____

12. What is the *generic name* for Advair Diskus? _____
13. What is the *brand name* for formoterol plus budesonide? _____
14. What is the *generic name* for Singulair? _____
15. What is the *generic name* for Accolate? _____
16. What is the *generic name* for Zyflo CR (United States)? _____
17. What is a *brand name* for theophylline? _____
18. What is a *brand name* for omalizumab? _____

MATCHING

Patient education is an essential component of therapeutics. Select the **best** warning label to apply to the prescription vial given to patients taking the drugs listed.
A. TAKE ON AN EMPTY STOMACH
B. SWALLOW WHOLE; DON'T CRUSH OR CHEW
C. REFRIGERATE; DO NOT FREEZE
D. DO NOT SWALLOW CAPSULES (FOR INHALATION ONLY)
   1. _____ Omalizumab
   2. _____ Spiriva inhaler
   3. _____ Accolate
   4. _____ Zileuton

MATCHING

Match each drug to its therapeutic classification.
A. Short-acting β_2-adrenergic agonists
B. Long-acting β_2-adrenergic agonists
C. Inhaled corticosteroids
D. Anticholinergic
E. Leukotriene modifiers
   1. _____ Pulmicort
   2. _____ Spiriva
   3. _____ Metaproterenol
   4. _____ Salmeterol
   5. _____ Zafirlukast

TRUE OR FALSE

1. _____ An MDI canister will float to the top of a jar of water when the contents are full.

2. _____ Long-acting β_2-adrenergic agonists (e.g., salmeterol) have been associated with an increased risk of severe asthma exacerbations and asthma-related death.
3. _____ A common ending for leukotriene modifiers is *-lukast*.
4. _____ A common ending for xanthine derivatives is *-phylline*.
5. _____ Xolair is for mild to moderate asthma monotherapy.
6. _____ Asthma symptoms cannot be managed with lifestyle modification only.
7. _____ Asthma is the most common chronic childhood disease.
8. _____ Research shows that COPD is primarily hereditary and not affected by environmental factors.
9. _____ The use of orally inhaled corticosteroids may cause thrush (a "yeast" infection).

CASE STUDY

Carly is a patient at your retail pharmacy. She is a 27-year-old mother who has a 4-year-old son, Robert. Carly has asthma that is well controlled with Singulair plus a Ventolin inhaler for exercising. Recently she noticed Robert coughing often, especially when he's laughing and running with his preschool friends. She also noticed that his coughing gets worse when winter and spring begin. The coughing fits happen about twice a week, but Carly is concerned and asks for your advice. What signs and symptoms does Robert have? What asthma classification would you give him and why?
1. Do you think Robert's asthma is related to Carly's? Why or why not?
2. What lifestyle modifications would you recommend for Carly and her son?
   One week later, Carly and Robert come back to the pharmacy with a prescription for ProAir for Robert. Carly is concerned that the doctor didn't prescribe him Ventolin like her.
3. What can you tell Carly about the similarities and differences between Ventolin and ProAir?
4. Considering Robert's age, would you recommend a spacer with his rescue inhaler? Why or why not?

For Critical Thinking, Research Activity, and answer key, please refer to Evolve.

Appendix 24: Treatment of Allergies

TERMS AND DEFINITIONS

Match each term with the correct definition below.

A. Allergen
B. Allergic rhinitis
C. Allergy
D. Anaphylaxis
E. Angioedema
F. Histamine
G. Immunoglobulin E
H. Leukotriene
I. Mast cells
J. Urticaria
K. Wheal

1. A(n) _____ is a hypersensitivity reaction by the immune system upon exposure to a(n) _____.
2. Persons who have _____ experience seasonal or perennial nasal swelling and a runny nose.
3. _____ is a life-threatening allergic reaction.
4. The medical term for a raised blister-like area on the skin caused by allergic reaction is _____.
5. An allergic response begins with the release of _____, granule-containing cells found in tissue.
6. _____ may be life threatening if swelling involves the mucous membranes and the viscera.
7. _____ is an organic nitrogen compound involved in local immune responses as well as regulating physiologic function in the gut and acting as a neurotransmitter.
8. _____ is known as hives.
9. _____ is a proinflammatory mediator released as part of the allergic, inflammatory response.
10. _____ is an antibody that *is* associated with allergies.

MULTIPLE CHOICE

1. Symptoms of seasonal allergic rhinitis (SAR) include all the following *except* _____.
   A. runny nose
   B. rash
   C. itching nose
   D. stuffy nose
2. Decongestant overuse for allergic conjunctivitis can lead to _____.
   A. rebound nasal congestion
   B. an allergic reaction
   C. rebound eye redness
   D. excessive facial angioedema
3. Which of the following is a common allergen?
   A. Cat dander
   B. Dust
   C. Mold
   D. Pollen
   E. All the above
4. Pharmacy technicians are at risk for developing latex allergy. Symptoms of latex allergy include all the following *except* _____.
   A. sneezing
   B. itchy eyes
   C. scratchy throat
   D. hives
   E. blurred vision
5. Drugs used to treat allergic symptoms include all the following *except* _____.
   A. fexofenadine
   B. Rhinocort AQ
   C. cromolyn
   D. pseudoephedrine
   E. Nasacort
6. Cromolyn sodium _____.
   A. is a leukotriene receptor antagonist
   B. should begin 1 week before contact with allergens
   C. is available without a prescription
   D. B and C
   E. all the above
7. Steps to protect oneself from latex exposure and allergy in the workplace include _____.
   A. selecting nonlatex gloves when possible
   B. using powder-free latex gloves with reduced protein content
   C. avoiding oil-based hand creams and lotions when wearing latex gloves
   D. washing hands with a mild soap and drying thoroughly after removing latex gloves
   E. all the above

FILL IN THE BLANK: Drug Names

1. What are **brand names** for desloratadine? _____
2. What is the **generic name** for Allegra? _____
3. What is the **brand name** for fluticasone furoate? _____
4. What is the **generic name** for Xyzal? _____
5. What is a **brand name** for clemastine? _____
6. What is the **generic name** for Flonase? _____
7. What is the **generic name** for Nasacort AQ? _____
8. What is the **brand name** for cromolyn sodium? _____

MATCHING

Patient education is an essential component of therapeutics. Select the **best** warning label to apply to the prescription vial given to patients taking the drugs listed.
A. SWALLOW WHOLE; DON'T CRUSH OR CHEW
B. PROTECT FROM MOISTURE
C. SHAKE WELL
D. MAY CAUSE DROWSINESS

1. _____ Diphenhydramine
2. _____ Allegra 24 hour
3. _____ Loratadine disintegrating tabs
4. _____ Flonase

MATCHING

Match each drug to its therapeutic classification.
A. Antihistamine
B. Mast cell stabilizer
C. Glucocorticosteroid
D. H_1 antagonist

1. _____ Cromolyn sodium

2. _____ Beclomethasone
3. _____ Desloratadine
4. _____ Astelin

TRUE OR FALSE

1. _____The immune system treats the allergen as an invader and produces antibodies to the substance.
2. _____The production of allergen-specific IgE antibodies and T-cell responses directed against allergens develop after age 7 years.
3. _____Antihistamines are not for children under 10.
4. _____Pharmacy technicians are at risk for developing latex allergy.
5. _____Exposure to pets early in life may reduce asthma and allergy risk.
6. _____The use of intranasal corticosteroids may cause nosebleeds and a sore throat.
7. _____Diphenhydramine is used to treat allergy symptoms and insomnia.

CASE STUDY

You are newly hired to a hospital pharmacy. You are learning to mix common IV solutions with sterile technique. At day's end, you take off your latex gloves and notice that your hands are red and very itchy. You also notice that your breathing has become heavy despite a lack of physically strenuous activity.

1. What symptoms of a latex allergy are you experiencing?
   _____
   _____
   _____
   _____
2. Knowing that you have a latex allergy, what steps can you take to protect yourself from latex exposure at work? Provide at least four steps.
   _____
   _____
   _____
   _____
3. What common hospital products contain latex and therefore should be avoided if possible?
   _____
   _____
   _____
4. What items outside the hospital contain latex? Write down at least three examples.
   _____
   _____
   _____
   _____

For Critical Thinking, Research Activity, and answer key, please refer to Evolve.

Appendix 25: Treatment of Thyroid Disorders

TERMS AND DEFINITIONS

Match each term with the correct definition below.
A. Graves disease
B. Hashimoto disease
C. Hyperthyroidism
D. Hypothyroidism
E. Thyroid-releasing factor
F. Thyroid-stimulating hormone (TSH)
G. Tetraiodothyronine (T$_4$)
H. Triiodothyronine (T$_3$)

1. A hormone released by the pituitary gland that stimulates the thyroid gland to produce and release thyroid hormones is _____.
2. _____ is a hormone released by the hypothalamus that stimulates the pituitary gland to release TSH.
3. Hormones released by the thyroid gland are _____ and _____.
4. _____, a condition in which there is an excessive production of thyroid hormones, is also called _____.
5. _____, a condition in which there is an insufficient production of thyroid hormones, is also called _____.

MULTIPLE CHOICE

1. All the following may be used in the treatment of hyperthyroidism except _____.
   A. methimazole
   B. levothyroxine
   C. propylthiouracil
   D. radioactive iodine
2. What warning label should be applied to a prescription for methimazole 5 mg tab?
   A. AVOID PREGNANCY
   B. AVOID FERROUS PRODUCTS OR MULTIPLE VITAMINS WITHIN 4 HOURS OF DOSE
   C. AVOID ALCOHOL
   D. SWALLOW WHOLE; DO NOT CRUSH OR CHEW
   E. AVOID PROLONGED EXPOSURE TO SUNLIGHT
3. What warning label should be applied to a prescription for levothyroxine 0.05 mg tab?
   A. AVOID PREGNANCY
   B. AVOID FERROUS PRODUCTS OR MULTIPLE VITAMINS WITHIN 4 HOURS OF DOSE
   C. AVOID ALCOHOL
   D. SWALLOW WHOLE; DO NOT CRUSH OR CHEW
   E. AVOID PROLONGED EXPOSURE TO SUNLIGHT
4. Hormones secreted by the thyroid gland are _____.
   A. tetraiodothyronine (T$_4$)
   B. triiodothyronine (T$_3$)
   C. calcitonin
   D. all the above
5. Select the **false** statement.
   A. When thyroid antibodies are present, autoimmune thyroid disease is diagnosed.

B. Low-dose radioactive iodine (^{131}I) is administered to measure the amount of radioactivity taken up by the thyroid gland.

C. High-dose ^{131}I is administered to treat hyperthyroidism.

D. Graves disease is an autoimmune disease that causes hypothyroidism.

E. The full effects of ^{131}I therapy are achieved after 2 to 3 months in most people.

6. Which of the following statements is true?
A. It takes 2 to 4 weeks of propylthiouracil therapy before maximum effects are achieved.
B. Radioactive iodine can cause a hypothyroid state in rare cases, resulting in lifelong thyroid replacement therapy.
C. Patients with other autoimmune diseases have higher risks of developing a thyroid disease.
D. Hashimoto disease is an autoimmune disorder that causes hyperthyroidism.
E. The most common treatment for hypothyroidism is T_3 replacement therapy.

FILL IN THE BLANK: DRUG NAMES

1. What is the *generic name* for Cytomel and Triostat?
   _____

2. What are some *brand names* for levothyroxine? _____

3. What is the *generic name* for Tapazole? _____

MATCHING

Match each drug to its pharmacologic classification.
A. Thioamides
B. Synthetic T_3
C. Synthetic T_4
   1. _____ Cytomel 50 mcg
   2. _____ Methimazole 5 mg
   3. _____ Levothyroxine 0.2 mg

TRUE OR FALSE

1. _____Hyperthyroidism and hypothyroidism are more prevalent in women than in men.

2. _____Liothyronine (T_3) and levothyroxine (T_4) have similar onset and duration of therapy.

3. _____Children with chronically low levels of thyroid hormones will have no negative effects on growth and development.

4. _____Cigarette smoking increases the risk for developing thyroid-related eye disease.

5. _____A low TSH level signals hypothyroidism.

6. _____Free T_4 index (FT4I) or FT4 levels are high when hyperthyroidism is present.

7. _____A serious side effect of propylthiouracil and methimazole is agranulocytosis, especially at higher doses.

CASE STUDY

Mark is a 58-year-old male who frequently visits your pharmacy. He has been coming into the pharmacy in full winter gear despite an outdoor temperature around 70°F. You've noticed a slower speech and swollen face and hands. The pharmacist notices as well and talks to Mark about his symptoms.

1. Do you think Mark has hypothyroidism or hyperthyroidism? Explain.
   _____
   _____
   _____
   _____

2. Your pharmacist has convinced Mark to see a physician. What tests could the physician use to confirm or deny Mark's diagnosis?
   _____
   _____
   _____
   _____

Mark returns 1 month later with a prescription for Synthroid 100 mcg. His physician diagnosed him with hypothyroidism. His doctor also suggested he purchase a multivitamin, since he hasn't been eating very well lately.

3. What should you tell Mark about the combination of Synthroid and the multivitamin?
   _____
   _____
   _____
   _____

A few months later, Mark comes into the pharmacy again to request a refill of his Synthroid. He tells you that this new prescription is working great and that he has more energy than ever. You notice that Mark cannot sit still for more than a few seconds. He is talking faster than ever, and it seems that he has lost a considerable amount of weight since the last time you've seen him.

4. What do you think is the cause of Mark's restlessness and weight loss? What can be done to reduce these symptoms?
   _____
   _____
   _____
   _____

For Critical Thinking, Research Activity, and answer key, please refer to Evolve.

Appendix 26: Treatment of Diabetes Mellitus

TERMS AND DEFINITIONS

Match each term with the correct definition below.
A. Diabetes mellitus
B. Fasting blood glucose
C. Gestational diabetes
D. Hemoglobin A_{1c}
E. Hyperglycemia
F. Hypoglycemia
G. Insulin resistance
H. Prediabetes

I. Type 1 diabetes
J. Type 2 diabetes
   1. Diabetes mellitus produces _____ (elevated blood glucose levels).
   2. An adverse effect to sulfonylurea drugs is _____ (decreased blood glucose levels).
   3. _____ is a condition of impaired fasting glucose (IFG) and impaired glucose tolerance (IGT) in which the body consistently has high normal glucose levels.
   4. _____ may be caused by the hormones of pregnancy or a shortage of insulin.
   5. Whereas a person with _____ produces little or no insulin, _____ is a condition in which the pancreas produces a sufficient amount of insulin but insulin receptors lack sensitivity to the insulin produced.
   6. A precursor to type 2 diabetes, known as _____, is a condition in which the body does not respond to insulin.
   7. A(n) _____ test is taken after a person has not eaten for 8 to 12 hours.
   8. _____ is a chronic condition in which the body is unable to convert food into energy.
   9. The _____ blood test measures a person's average blood glucose level over a period of weeks or months.

MULTIPLE CHOICE

1. Which of the following is a symptom of hypoglycemia?
    A. Frequent urination
    B. Confusion and difficulty concentrating
    C. Sweating
    D. B and C
    E. All the above
2. Select the **false** statement.
    A. Insulin is released by the β cells in the islets of Langerhans.
    B. Insulin is administered only for the treatment of type 1 diabetes.
    C. Insulin lowers blood glucose levels.
    D. Insulin may be administered by IV infusion, insulin pump, subcutaneous injection, and inhalation therapy.
3. Select the **true** statement.
    A. Prediabetes causes IFG and IGT.
    B. In type 1 diabetes, the immune system attacks and destroys the β cells in the pancreas, so insufficient amounts of insulin are produced.
    C. In type 2 diabetes, the pancreas usually produces sufficient amounts of insulin but is unable to use the insulin effectively.
    D. Gestational diabetes may be caused by the hormones of pregnancy or a shortage of insulin.
    E. All the above are true.
4. Elevated glucose levels may be measured by _____.
    A. urine glucose testing
    B. blood glucose monitoring
    C. hemoglobin A_{1c} (HbA_{1c}) test
    D. all the above
5. All the following agents stimulate insulin secretion from β cells in the pancreas except _____.
    A. meglitinides
    B. miglitol
    C. sulfonylureas

6. All the following agents are administered orally to treat type 2 diabetes except _____.
    A. glimepiride
    B. insulin
    C. miglitol
    D. sitagliptin
    E. metformin
7. Which of the following nonpharmacologic approaches is *not* recommended in patients with diabetes?
    A. Getting 150 minutes of exercise weekly
    B. Eating a diet high in low-glycemic foods
    C. Stopping smoking
    D. Consuming multiple alcoholic drinks per day
8. Which pair of insulin products would be appropriate for basal-bolus administration?
    A. Lantus and Levemir
    B. Humalog and Humulin N
    C. NovoLog and Humalog
    D. Humulin N and Lantus
9. The mechanism of action of metformin includes the following *except* _____.
    A. decreasing the degradation of glucagon-like peptide 1 (GLP-1)
    B. decreasing hepatic gluconeogenesis
    C. increasing glucose transport across cell membranes
    D. increasing peripheral glucose uptake in skeletal muscles and adipose tissue

FILL IN THE BLANK: Drug Names

1. What is the *generic name* for Humalog? _____
2. What is the *brand name* for insulin glargine? _____
3. What is the *brand name* for glyburide? _____
4. What is the *generic name* for Amaryl? _____
5. What is the *generic name* for Glucophage? _____
6. What are the *brand names* for acarbose? _____
7. What is the *generic name* for Victoza? _____
8. What is the *brand name* for repaglinide? _____
9. What is the *generic name* for Actos? _____
10. What is the *generic name* for Avandia? _____
11. What is the *brand name* for metformin and sitagliptin? _____
12. What is the *generic name* for Januvia (United States)? _____
13. What is the *generic name* for Tradjenta? _____
14. What is the *brand name* for pramlintide? _____

MATCHING

Match each drug to its pharmacologic classification.
A. Thiazolidinediones
B. Meglitinides
C. α-Glucosidase inhibitors
D. Glucagon-like peptide receptor agonist
E. Sulfonylureas
   1. _____ Amaryl 2 mg
   2. _____ Acarbose 50 mg
   3. _____ Rosiglitazone 2 mg
   4. _____ Nateglinide 120 mg
   5. _____ Bydureon 2 mg

MATCHING

Patient education is an essential component of therapeutics. Select the **best** warning label to apply to the prescription vial given to patients taking the drugs listed.

A. REFRIGERATE; DO NOT FREEZE
B. TAKE WITH THE FIRST BITE OF A MEAL
C. AVOID ALCOHOL

1. _____ Pioglitazone
2. _____ Acarbose
3. _____ Humalog

TRUE OR FALSE

1. _____ A common ending for thiazolidinediones is *-glitazone*.
2. _____ Extended-release dosage forms of metformin are substitutable.
3. _____ Pramlintide can be mixed with other injectables, including insulin.
4. _____ Insulin can be used to treat type 1 and type 2 diabetes mellitus but not gestational diabetes.
5. _____ Conventional and micronized dosage forms of glyburide are not substitutable.
6. _____ Bromocriptine is a cholesterol-lowering agent approved by the Food and Drug Administration for the management of type 2 diabetes mellitus.
7. _____ Alcohol, aspirin, and decongestants can all affect blood sugar.

CASE STUDY

Lexie is a 17-year-old female recently diagnosed with type 1 diabetes. She comes into your pharmacy with a prescription for three vials of insulin detemir. She seems extremely worried and nervous at the drop-off counter. Lexie tells you that her physician gave her a lot of information about her new disease, but she's not sure that she can properly handle it.

1. What type of insulin is insulin detemir? When is its onset of action? When should it be administered to minimize the risk of nighttime hypoglycemia?
   _____
   _____
   _____

2. What other products does Lexie need to properly manage her insulin therapy? Does Lexie need a prescription for these products?
   _____
   _____
   _____

3. After acquiring the necessary products, the pharmacist counsels Lexie and eases her worries. At the end of their conversation, the pharmacist recommends that Lexie keep a pack of glucose tablets in her purse at all times. Why would the pharmacist tell her to do this?
   _____
   _____
   _____

For Critical Thinking, Research Activity, and answer key, please refer to Evolve.

Appendix 27: Drugs That Affect the Reproductive System

FILL IN THE BLANK

Match each term with the correct definition below.

A. Amenorrhea
B. Atrophic vaginitis
C. Abnormal uterine bleeding
D. Dysmenorrhea
E. Endometriosis
F. Hypogonadism
G. Hysterectomy
H. Infertility
I. Menopause
J. Menorrhagia
K. Pelvic inflammatory disease
L. Polycystic ovary disease
M. Premenstrual dysphoric disorder
N. Premenstrual syndrome
O. Supraovulation
P. Toxic shock syndrome

1. _____ is excessive menstrual bleeding; the opposite is _____, the absence of normal menstruation.
2. The medical term for surgical removal of the uterus is _____.
3. _____ and _____ are related conditions that have symptoms such as depression, anxiety, or irritability and are linked to the menstrual cycle.
4. _____ is an inability to achieve pregnancy during 1 year or more of unprotected intercourse.
5. _____ is a condition in which functioning endometrial tissue is located outside the uterus. The condition may cause _____ (difficult or painful menstruation).
6. _____ is a condition in which there is an inadequate production of sex hormones.
7. The definition of _____ is the termination of menstrual cycles.
8. _____ is irregular or excessive uterine bleeding that results from either a structural problem or hormonal imbalance.
9. _____ is a rare disorder caused by certain Staphylococcus aureus strains; the disorder is seen in women using tampons.
10. _____ is the simultaneous rupture of multiple mature follicles.
11. Postmenopausal thinning and dryness of the vaginal epithelium related to decreased estrogen levels is known as _____.

12. _____ is a condition that is characterized by ovaries twice the normal size that are studded with fluid-filled cysts.

13. _____ is an infection of the uterus, fallopian tubes, and adjacent pelvic structures that is not associated with pregnancy or surgery.

MULTIPLE CHOICE

1. Which of the following is *not* an effective method of birth control?
   A. Foam and condom
   B. Diaphragm and spermicide
   C. Withdrawal
   D. Oral contraceptives
   E. IUD

2. The diaphragm must be inserted sometime before sexual intercourse and should remain in the vagina for _____ after a man's last ejaculation.
   A. 1 to 2 hours
   B. 3 to 4 hours
   C. 5 to 6 hours
   D. 6 to 8 hours

3. Which of the following methods of contraception can prevent sexually transmitted infections such as HIV and syphilis?
   A. Oral contraceptives
   B. IUD
   C. Diaphragm
   D. Condoms

4. Emergency contraceptives (Plan B) must be taken _____ of unprotected intercourse.
   A. within 1 to 2 hours
   B. within 3 to 6 hours
   C. within 24 hours
   D. within 72 hours
   E. within 1 week

5. How do oral contraceptives help prevent pregnancies?
   A. They decrease the number of sperm excreted during ejaculation.
   B. They provide a physical barrier to prevent ovulation.
   C. They kill sperm within the vagina.
   D. They inhibit FSH and LH, preventing ovulation.

6. What condition(s) is/are treated with selective serotonin reuptake inhibitors (SSRIs)?
   A. Atrophic vaginitis
   B. Premenstrual syndrome
   C. Premenstrual dysphoric disorder
   D. B and C
   E. All the above

FILL IN THE BLANK: Drug Names

1. What is the **brand name** for copper-releasing IUD? _____

2. What is the generic name for Aviane (United States) and Min-Ovral (Canada)? _____

3. What is the **brand name** for medroxyprogesterone acetate? _____

4. What is the **generic name** for Plan B? _____

5. What is the **brand name** for cetrorelix? _____

6. What is the **generic name** for Ovidrel? _____

7. What is a **brand name** for esterified estrogen? _____

8. What is the **brand name** for conjugated estrogens + medroxyprogesterone? _____

9. What is the **generic name** for Androderm? _____

10. What is the **brand name** for goserelin? _____

11. What is the **generic name** for Synarel? _____

12. What are **brand names** for leuprolide? _____

MATCHING

Match each drug to its pharmacologic family.
A. Estrogen
B. Selective serotonin reuptake inhibitor modulator (SERM)
C. Gonadotropin-releasing hormone agonist
D. Androgen agonist
   1. _____ Lupron 3.75 mg
   2. _____ Brisdelle 7.5 mg
   3. _____ Fluoxymesterone 10 mg tab
   4. _____ Estrace 2 mg

MATCHING

Match each drug to its therapeutic use.
A. Infertility
B. Endometriosis
C. Hypogonadism
D. Oral contraceptive
E. Hormone replacement therapy
   1. _____ Danazol 100 mg
   2. _____ FemHRT
   3. _____ Clomiphene 50 mg
   4. _____ Yasmin
   5. _____ Testosterone

TRUE OR FALSE

1. _____ A common ending of androgen agonists is *-sterone*.
2. _____ Testosterone patches are *not* substitutable.
3. _____ Symptoms of menopause may include hot flashes, vaginal dryness, mood swings, and decreased sexual drive.
4. _____ Vivelle and Vivelle-Dot patches are substitutable.
5. _____ Androgen agonists are safe, easy-to-use medications that cause only mild side effects.

CASE STUDY

Morgan is a 15-year-old female who walks up to your pharmacy counter with a notebook in her hands. She says that she is required to research types of birth control for both males and females as homework for her sex education class. She asks for your help in completing this project.

1. Provide at least one advantage and one disadvantage for the following types of birth control methods:
   Abstinence
   Condoms
   Diaphragms
   IUDs

Oral contraceptives   _____
Transdermal patch   _____
Vaginal ring   _____
_____   _____
_____
_____

2. She chose to do a research paper for the class because she is concerned that she might have either PMS or something else called PMDD. Provide at least two similarities and two differences between these conditions.

For Critical Thinking, Research Activity, and answer key, please refer to Evolve.

Appendix 28: Treatment of Prostate Disease and Erectile Dysfunction

TERMS AND DEFINITIONS

Match each term with the correct definition below.
A. Benign prostatic hyperplasia (BPH)
B. Erectile dysfunction
C. Incontinence
D. Prostate gland
E. Prostate-specific antigen (PSA)
F. Prostate-specific antigen test
G. Urinary frequency

1. _____ is defined as the persistent inability to achieve or maintain an erection sufficient for satisfactory sexual intercourse.
2. The _____ examines the blood to measure the percentage of PSA that is unbound.
3. _____ is a protein that is elevated in men who have prostate cancer, infection, or inflammation of the prostate gland and BPH.
4. BPH and infections may produce _____, the need to urinate more often than normal.
5. Prostatitis is inflammation of the _____.
6. _____ is a loss of bladder or bowel control.
7. _____ is a noncancerous growth of cells in the prostate gland.

MULTIPLE CHOICE

1. _____ is prescribed for BPH and male pattern baldness.
   A. Finasteride
   B. Dutasteride
   C. Progesterone
   D. Testosterone
2. Adverse reactions for phosphodiesterase type 5 (PDE5) inhibitors include _____.
   A. sudden hearing loss
   B. nasal congestion
   C. diarrhea
   D. B and C
   E. all the above
3. The therapeutic effects of 5α-reductase inhibitors may take _____ months to be achieved.
   A. 1 to 2
   B. 3 to 6
   C. 6 to 12
   D. 12 to 18

4. The pharmacist should advise males taking finasteride and dutasteride _____.
   A. to use barrier contraceptives such as condoms
   B. that pregnant women and women of childbearing age should avoid contact with broken or crushed tablets
   C. may decrease desire for sex
   D. may cause erectile dysfunction
   E. all the above
5. Which factor is *not* a cause of erectile dysfunction?
   A. Lifestyle
   B. Heredity
   C. Psychological
   D. Physiological
   E. Neurological
6. Select the **false** statement about drugs used for the treatment of erectile dysfunction.
   A. Sildenafil, tadalafil, and vardenafil are classified as PDE5 inhibitors.
   B. Cialis constricts smooth muscle and decreases the blood supply to the blood vessels that control penile engorgement.
   C. Sildenafil, tadalafil, and vardenafil are contraindicated in patients taking nitroglycerin.
   D. Alprostadil must be inserted into the urethra or by intracavernosal injection.

FILL IN THE BLANK: Drug Names

1. What is the **generic name** for Uroxatral (United States) and Xatral (Canada)? _____
2. What is the **brand name** for doxazosin? _____
3. What is the **generic name** for Jalyn? _____
4. What is the **generic name** for Rapaflo? _____
5. What is the **brand name** for dutasteride? _____
6. What is the **generic name** for Proscar? _____
7. What are **brand names** for sildenafil? _____
8. What is the **generic name** for Cialis? _____
9. What is the **generic name** for Levitra? _____
10. What are **brand names** for avanafil? _____

MATCHING

Patient education is an essential component of therapeutics. Select the **best** warning label to apply to the prescription vial given to patients taking the drugs listed.
A. DO NOT DRINK ALCOHOL TO EXCESS

B. TAKE WITH MEAL
C. AVOID CONTACT WITH PREGNANT WOMEN
D. REFRIGERATE; DON'T FREEZE
1. _____ Silodosin
2. _____ Proscar
3. _____ Cialis
4. _____ Alprostadil inserts

MATCHING

Match each drug to its therapeutic classification.
A. α₁-Adrenergic antagonists
B. 5α-Reductase inhibitors
C. Phosphodiesterase-type 5 inhibitors
D. Prostaglandins
1. _____ Dutasteride
2. _____ Tadalafil
3. _____ Terazosin
4. _____ Alprostadil

TRUE OR FALSE

1. _____Saw palmetto may reduce urinary BPH symptoms, but prostate cancer must be ruled out before starting therapy.
2. _____A high PSA level is a sign of BPH only.
3. _____Aggressive treatment for BPH is recommended when patients are asymptomatic or symptoms do not produce much discomfort.
4. _____A common ending for 5α-reductase inhibitors is -steride.
5. _____5α-Reductase inhibitors commonly cause cardiovascular-related side effects that include reflex tachycardia and postural hypertension.
6. _____A common ending for α₁-adrenergic antagonists is -zosin.
7. _____Chronic diseases such as hyperlipidemia and depression can cause erectile dysfunction.

CASE STUDY

David is a 68-year-old male who is a familiar patient at your retail pharmacy. David comes in with a new prescription for finasteride and his recent lab results. He says that he just had a digital rectal examination (DRE) and a PSA test. On this form, you also see his free PSA count. Here is the summary of the sheet:
DRE: indicates enlarged prostate
PSA: elevated, but within normal limits
Free PSA: elevated, but within normal limits
David is still confused after his tests and examination, so he asks for your help.
1. Explain to David what each of his three results means.
_____
_____
_____
2. Why did the doctor prescribe finasteride and not an α-1 antagonist?
_____
_____
_____
3. What other condition is finasteride used for? Would you tell David about it? Why or why not?
_____
_____
_____
_____
4. What potential side effects should you inform David about?
_____
_____
_____
_____

For Critical Thinking, Research Activity, and answer key, please refer to Evolve.

Appendix 29: Treatment of Bacterial Infections

TERMS AND DEFINITIONS

Match each term with the correct definition below.
A. Antibiotic
B. Antimicrobial
C. Bactericidal
D. Bacteriostatic
E. Broad-spectrum antibiotic
F. Microbial resistance
1. Whereas antiinfective agents that can destroy bacteria are _____, antiinfective agents that are _____ inhibit bacterial proliferation.
2. A natural substance produced by one organism that can destroy or inhibit the growth of bacteria is called a(n) _____.
3. The term used to describe the process of bacteria developing mechanisms to overcome the bactericidal effects of an antibiotic is _____.
4. A(n) _____ is a substance capable of destroying or inhibiting the growth of a microorganisms.
5. An antimicrobial that can destroy a wide range of bacteria is a(n) _____.

MATCHING

A. *ceph-* or *cef-*
B. *sulf-*
C. *-thromycin*
D. *-cycline*

E. *-cillin*

F. *-floxacin*

1. A common suffix for the fluoroquinolone family of antiinfectives is _____
2. A common prefix for the cephalosporin family of antiinfectives is _____
3. A common suffix for the macrolide family of antiinfectives is _____
4. A common suffix for the penicillin family of antiinfectives is _____
5. A common prefix for the sulfonamide family of antiinfectives is _____
6. A common suffix for the tetracycline family of antiinfectives is _____

MULTIPLE CHOICE

1. Select the **false** statement.
   A. Poverty, malnutrition, and lack of clean water increase the risk for infectious disease.
   B. Poor sanitation and inadequate housing increase the risk for infectious disease.
   C. Infectious disease is no longer a leading cause of morbidity and mortality globally.
   D. Antibiotics have played a key role in improving the survival of individuals with bacterial infections.
2. Select the **false** statement about microbial resistance.
   A. It can result in new "super bugs" that are resistant to currently available antiinfective agents.
   B. It cannot be transferred to other bacteria.
   C. It can be caused by failure to complete the full course of therapy.
   D. It can be caused by inappropriate prescribing.
3. Which of the following antibiotics is a glycopeptide?
   E. Isoniazid
   F. Metronidazole
   G. Telavancin
   H. Vancomycin
4. β-Lactam antibiotics target the bacterial cell wall. All the following drugs are β-lactam antibiotics *except* _____.
   A. penicillins
   B. erythromycin
   C. cephalosporins
   D. carbapenems
   E. monobactams
5. Some penicillins (e.g., penicillin G and ampicillin) lack stability in gastric acids, which is why most are administered _____.
   A. on an empty stomach
   B. with food
   C. with a full meal
   D. sublingually
6. Select the **false** statement.
   A. Cephalosporins may be classified as first, second, third, fourth, and fifth generation.
   B. Clarithromycin is a key ingredient in treatment regimens for peptic ulcer disease caused by the bacteria *Helicobacter pylori*.
   C. Gastrointestinal upset is a common adverse reaction that occurs with erythromycin.
   D. Sulfonamides may be used to treat AIDS-related pneumonia (*Pneumocystis carinii*).

FILL IN THE BLANK: Drug Names

1. What is the **brand name** for cephalexin? _____
2. What is the **generic name** for Suprax? _____
3. What are **brand names** for linezolid? _____
4. What is the **generic name** for Levaquin? _____
5. What is the **brand name** for clarithromycin? _____
6. What is the **generic name** for Flagyl? _____
7. What is a **brand name** for minocycline? _____
8. What is the **generic name** for Vibativ? _____
9. What is a **brand name** for sulfamethoxazole + trimethoprim? _____
10. What is the **generic name** for Bactroban? _____
11. What is the **generic name** for Cleocin? _____
12. What is a **brand name** for piperacillin-tazobactam? _____

MATCHING

Match each drug to its pharmacologic family.
A. Tetracycline family
B. Sulfonamide family
C. Oxazolidinone family
D. Aminoglycoside family
E. Carbapenem family

1. _____ Tobramycin 0.3% OS
2. _____ Linezolid 2 mg/mL
3. _____ Merrem 500 mg powder
4. _____ Minocin 100 mg cap
5. _____ Sulfadiazine cream 1%

MATCHING

Match each drug to its therapeutic use.
A. Acne rosacea
B. Tuberculosis
C. Bacterial meningitis
D. Pseudomembranous colitis
E. Impetigo

1. _____ Isoniazid 300 mg
2. _____ Bactroban 2% ointment
3. _____ Metronidazole 1% topical gel
4. _____ Clindamycin 150 mg cap
5. _____ Chloramphenicol 1 g powder

MATCHING

Match the cephalosporin to its correct generation. Answers may be used more than once.
A. First generation
B. Second generation
C. Third generation
D. Fourth generation

1. _____ Cefpodoxime
2. _____ Ceftriaxone
3. _____ Cefepime
4. _____ Cefazolin
5. _____ Cefaclor
6. _____ Cefuroxime

TRUE OR FALSE

1. _____The warning label TAKE WITH LOTS OF WATER is applied to prescription vials for sulfonamides.
2. _____Oral and parenteral fluoroquinolones are contraindicated in pregnant women and people older than 16 to 18 years.
3. _____Persons who are allergic to penicillin may also be allergic to cephalosporins.
4. _____Tetracyclines are contraindicated in pregnancy and small children because they can weaken fetal bone, retard bone growth, weaken tooth enamel, and stain teeth.
5. _____The milligram strength of clavulanic acid is the same for all strengths and dosage forms of Augmentin (United States) and Clavulin (Canada).
6. _____Macrolides and penicillins may decrease the effectiveness of oral contraceptives.

CASE STUDY

Jerry walks into the pharmacy with his 9-year-old daughter Lilly. You have seen them many times before, and it doesn't take long to notice that Lilly isn't feeling very well. She coughs frequently and blows her nose often. Jerry hands you a prescription for Zithromax tablets.

1. What is the normal dosing for Zithromax? Include dose, frequency, and duration.
2. What side effects might Lilly experience when taking this medicine?
3. What would you ask Lilly before filling the prescription? (Hint: Lilly is 9 years old, and the prescription is for tablets.)
4. If Lilly feels better after 2 days, should she stop taking the medication? Why or why not?

For Critical Thinking, Research Activity, and answer key, please refer to Evolve.

Appendix 30: Treatment of Viral Infections

TERMS AND DEFINITIONS

Match each term with the correct definition below.
A. AIDS
B. Antiretroviral
C. Antiviral resistance
D. CD4 T lymphocyte
E. Cross-resistance
F. Highly active antiretroviral therapy (HAART)
G. Oncovirus
H. Virion
I. Virustatic
J. Virus
   1. The infectious particles of a virus are called _____
   2. A virus may develop _____, an ability to overcome the suppressive action of an antiviral agent.
   3. A(n) _____ antiviral agent can suppress viral proliferation.
   4. _____ is a type of white blood cell that fights infection.
   5. _____ is the most severe form of HIV infection.
   6. A(n) _____ is an intracellular parasite that consists of a DNA and RNA core surrounded by a protein coat and sometimes an outer covering of lipoprotein.
   7. A virus may develop _____, resistance to multiple drugs in a particular drug classification.
   8. A(n) _____ is a medication that inhibits the replication of retroviruses.
   9. _____ is a combination of three or more antiretroviral medications taken in a regimen.
   10. _____ is a virus that is an etiologic agent in a cancer.

MATCHING

A. *-cyclovir* and *-ciclovir*
B. *-navir*
C. *-mantadine*
D. *-amivir*
   1. A common ending for antivirals that inhibit viral uncoating is _____.
   2. A common ending for antivirals used for the treatment of herpes virus infections is _____
   3. A common ending for protease inhibitors is _____.
   4. A common ending for neuraminidase inhibitors is _____.

MULTIPLE CHOICE

1. HIV-infected patients are diagnosed with AIDS when their CD4 cell count falls below _____ or if they develop an AIDS-defining illness.
   A. 200 cells/mm³
   B. 300 cells/mm³
   C. 400 cells/mm³
   D. 600 cells/mm³
2. Highly active antiretroviral therapy (HAART) is a treatment regimen for the treatment of HIV/AIDS that consists of _____.
   A. one antiretroviral drug
   B. one or two antiretroviral drugs
   C. two or three antiretroviral drugs
   D. three or more antiretroviral drugs
3. The risk of perinatal mother-to-child transmission of HIV may be reduced by the administration of a dose of _____ to the mother during delivery and to the baby upon birth or zidovudine only.
   A. zidovudine + nevirapine
   B. abacavir + zidovudine
   C. tenofovir + zidovudine
   D. Sustiva + zidovudine
4. A virus that is linked to cervical cancer is _____.
   A. cold sores
   B. human papillomavirus (HPV)

C. HIV

D. herpes zoster

5. The nucleoside/nucleotide reverse transcriptase inhibitor (NRTI) that may be administered as monotherapy for the prevention of mother-to-child transmission (PMTCT) of HIV is _____.

A. zidovudine

B. ganciclovir

C. emtricitabine

D. Sustiva

6. Select the **false** statement.

A. Antivirals are effective only against a specific virus.

B. Antibiotics are effective against viral infections.

C. Viruses continually mutate, making it difficult to develop a vaccine to prevent virus infection.

D. Antivirals inhibit virus-specific steps in the replication cycle.

7. Which drug is *not* prescribed for the treatment of cytomegalovirus retinitis?

A. Cidofovir

B. Saquinavir

C. Foscarnet

D. Ganciclovir

8. The steps in the HIV life cycle are _____.

A. binding, fusion, and uncoating

B. reverse transcription and integration

C. genome replication and protein synthesis

D. protein cleavage, assembly, and virus release

E. all the above

9. Nevirapine is associated with fatal _____ toxicity, and the Food and Drug Administration has required changes in the package labeling to warn of this adverse effect.

A. kidney

B. heart

C. liver

D. thyroid

FILL IN THE BLANK: DRUG NAMES

1. What is the **brand name** for peramivir? _____

2. What is the **generic name** for Flumadine (United States)? _____

3. What is the **generic name** for Tamiflu? _____

4. What is the **brand name** for zanamivir? _____

5. What is the **generic name** for Pegasys? _____

6. What is the **generic name** for PEG-Intron (United States)? _____

7. What is the **generic name** for Famvir? _____

8. What is the **generic name** for Foscavir (United States)? _____

9. What is the **generic name** for Denavir? _____

10. What is the **generic name** for Viroptic? _____

11. What is the **brand name** for valacyclovir? _____

12. What is the **generic name** for Virazole? _____

13. What is the **generic name** for Ziagen? _____

14. What is the **brand name** for didanosine? _____

15. What is the **generic name** for Emtriva? _____

16. What is the **brand name** for stavudine? _____

17. What is the **brand name** for emtricitabine + tenofovir DF? _____

18. What is the **generic name** for Truvada? _____

19. What is the **generic name** for Trizivir? _____

20. What is the **brand name** for delavirdine? _____

21. What is the **brand name** for lamivudine + zidovudine? _____

22. What is the **brand name** for efavirenz? _____

23. What is the **brand name** for efavirenz + emtricitabine + tenofovir? _____

24. What is the **brand name** for atazanavir? _____

25. What is the **generic name** for Prezista? _____

26. What is the **brand name** for indinavir? _____

27. What is the **generic name** for Lexiva (United States) and Telzir (Canada)? _____

28. What is the **generic name** for Viracept? _____

29. What is the **brand name** for saquinavir? _____

30. What is the **brand name** for lopinavir + ritonavir? _____

MATCHING

Match each drug to its pharmacologic family.

A. Inhibitor of viral uncoating

B. Neuraminidase inhibitor

C. Interferon

D. Inhibition of DNA replication

1. _____ Valcyte

2. _____ Relenza

3. _____ Intron-A

4. _____ Amantadine

MATCHING

Match each drug to its therapeutic use.

A. Herpes

B. Influenza

C. Hepatitis C

D. Respiratory syncytial virus (RSV)

E. Cytomegalovirus (CMV)

1. _____ Peginterferon alfa-2b

2. _____ Tamiflu

3. _____ Virazole

4. _____ Cytovene

5. _____ Penciclovir

MATCHING

Match each drug to its pharmacologic family. Each answer may be used more than once.

A. NRTIs

B. Non–nucleoside reverse transcriptase inhibitors (NNRTIs)

C. Protease inhibitor

D. Fusion inhibitor

E. CCR5 antagonist

F. Integrase inhibitor

1. _____ Nevirapine

2. _____ Fuzeon

3. _____ Norvir

4. _____ Lamivudine

5. _____ Rilpivirine

6. _____ Zerit

7. _____ Selzentry

8. _____ Saquinavir

9. _____ Raltegravir

10. _____ Kaletra

TRUE OR FALSE

1. _____ Cross-resistance to similar antiviral medications can occur, such as with lamivudine and emtricitabine.
2. _____ Neuraminidase inhibitors are not effective against influenza B.
3. _____ In combination with other agents, ribavirin can treat hepatitis C. Alone it can be used for RSV.
4. _____ HAART requires strict adherence to every medication for a patient's lifetime.

CASE STUDY

Henry comes to your pharmacy with a new prescription. He says, "My doctor gave me this prescription for Valtrex for my genital herpes." He has a few questions about this new medication. He asks you these questions.

1. "How does this medication work to treat my condition?"
   _____
   _____
   _____

2. "What are the side effects from taking this medication?"
   _____
   _____
   _____
   _____

3. "What can I do to limit the chance of spreading this to my significant other?" (Hint: Use the Internet to find more information about this topic. Suggested website: https://www.cdc.gov/std/herpes/stdfact-herpes.htm.)
   _____
   _____
   _____

As Henry leaves, another customer tells you she overheard your conversation with Henry. She's confused because she takes the same medication (Valtrex), but her doctor said to take it for cold sores. She asks you, "Did my doctor lie to me? Do I actually have genital herpes?"

4. What would you say to this patient to help ease her fears?
   _____
   _____
   _____

5. Assuming the same dose, would Valtrex have the same side effects in Jane as in Henry? Why or why not?
   _____
   _____
   _____
   _____

For Critical Thinking, Research Activity, and answer key, please refer to Evolve.

Appendix 31: Treatment of Cancers

TERMS AND DEFINITIONS

Match each term with the correct definition below.

A. Benign
B. Cancer
C. Chemotherapy
D. Complementary and alternative medicine (CAM)
E. Malignant
F. Mammogram
G. Melanoma
H. Metastasis
I. Neoplasm
J. Oncovirus
K. Polyp
L. Prostate-specific antigen (PSA) test
M. Radiation therapy
N. Stage
O. Stem cell
P. Tumor marker

1. A tumor that is not cancerous is _____ and does not spread to surrounding tissues or other parts of the body.
2. _____ is a type of cell from which other types of cells can form.
3. A(n) _____ is a screening examination to detect breast cancer.
4. The spread of cancer from one part of the body to another is called _____.
5. _____ is the extent of a cancer within the body. Staging is based on the size of the tumor, whether lymph nodes contain cancer, and whether the disease has spread from the original site to other parts of the body.
6. _____ is a test that measures level of free PSA, a protein produced by the prostate gland. Levels are elevated in men who have prostate cancer, infection, or inflammation of the prostate gland and benign prostatic hyperplasia (BPH).
7. Cancerous tumors that can invade and destroy nearby tissue and spread to other parts of the body are considered to be _____.
8. Treatment with drugs that kill cancer is known as _____.
9. _____ is a term for diseases in which abnormal cells divide without control.
10. _____ is a virus that is an etiologic agent in a cancer.
11. Treatments that may include dietary supplements, herbal preparations, acupuncture, massage, magnet therapy, spiritual healing, and meditation are known as _____.
12. _____ is a growth that protrudes from a mucous membrane.
13. A substance sometimes found in the blood, other body fluids, or tissues that may signal the presence of a certain type of cancer is known as a(n) _____.

14. _____ uses high-energy radiation from x-rays, gamma rays, neutrons, and other sources to kill cancer cells and shrink tumors.

15. _____ is a form of skin cancer that arises in melanocytes, the cells that produce pigment.

16. _____ is another word for tumor.

MULTIPLE CHOICE

1. Which of the following is a test to screen for colorectal cancer?
   A. PSA
   B. Pap
   C. Fecal occult blood test (FOBT)
   D. Mammogram

2. Which of the following cancers is *not* linked to increased risk because of family history?
   A. Breast
   B. Stomach
   C. Colon
   D. Skin

3. Cancers are categorized by stage. Staging is based on all the following *except* _____.
   A. size of the tumor
   B. lymph node involvement
   C. metastasis
   D. length of time cancer has been present

4. Which source of ionizing radiation is *not* used for treatment of cancers?
   A. X-rays
   B. Gamma rays
   C. Neutrons
   D. UV light

5. A cancer that arises in the cells that produce pigment in the skin is called _____.
   A. melanoma
   B. lymphoma
   C. leukemia

6. Which treatment would *not* be classified as CAM?
   A. Dietary supplements and herbal preparations
   B. Acupuncture and massage
   C. Magnet therapy
   D. Chemotherapy
   E. Spiritual healing and meditation

7. A warning label that is commonly affixed to most prescriptions for orally administered chemotherapeutic agents for women is _____.
   A. AVOID PREGNANCY
   B. TAKE WITH LOTS OF WATER
   C. SHAKE WELL
   D. AVOID PROLONGED SUNLIGHT

8. Select the **false** statement about lung cancer.
   A. Lung cancer is the most common form of cancer.
   B. A history of smoking tobacco is nearly always the cause of small cell lung cancer.
   C. Lung cancer is classified as small cell lung cancer and non–small cell lung cancer.
   D. Antineoplastic agents used to treat lung cancer are effective against both forms of the disease.

9. Which drug is *not* approved for the treatment of breast cancer?
   A. Tamoxifen
   B. Hydroxyurea
   C. Taxol
   D. Femara

10. Which of the following is *not* a common side effect of methotrexate?
    A. Increased appetite
    B. Hair loss
    C. Nausea
    D. Increased risk of infection

FILL IN THE BLANK: DRUG NAMES

1. What is the **brand name** for fulvestrant? _____
2. What is the **generic name** for Soltamox (United States) and Nolvadex-D (Canada)? _____
3. What is a **brand name** for exemestane? _____
4. What is the **generic name** for Fareston (United States)? _____
5. What is the **generic name** for Arimidex? _____
6. What is the **generic name** for Femara? _____
7. What is the **brand name** for goserelin? _____
8. What is the **generic name** for Megace? _____
9. What is the **generic name** for Cytoxan? _____
10. What is the **generic name** for Taxotere? _____
11. What is the **generic name** for Taxol? _____
12. What is the **brand name** for vinorelbine? _____
13. What is the **generic name** for Adriamycin? _____
14. What is the **generic name** for Ellence (United States) and Pharmorubicin PFS (Canada)? _____
15. What is the **brand name** for everolimus? _____
16. What is the **generic name** for Camptosar? _____
17. What is the **brand name** for erlotinib? _____
18. What is the **generic name** for Eloxatin? _____
19. What is the **generic name** for Xeloda? _____
20. What is the **generic name** for Keytruda? _____
21. What is the **brand name** for fludarabine? _____
22. What is the **brand name** for bevacizumab? _____
23. What is the **generic name** for Gemzar? _____
24. What is the **brand name** for pemetrexed? _____
25. What is the **generic name** for Purinethol? _____
26. What is the **generic name** for Emcyt? _____
27. What is the **generic name** for Cosmegen? _____
28. What is the **generic name** for Tykerb? _____

MATCHING

Match each drug to its pharmacologic classification.
A. Aromatase inhibitors
B. Taxanes
C. Anthracyclines
D. Topoisomerase inhibitors
E. Vinca alkaloid
F. Microtubule inhibitor

1. _____ Vincristine
2. _____ Teniposide
3. _____ Anastrozole
4. _____ Paclitaxel
5. _____ Doxorubicin
6. _____ Eribulin

MATCHING

Match each drug to its pharmacologic classification.
A. Aromatase inhibitors
B. Taxanes
C. Anthracyclines

D. Topoisomerase inhibitors
E. Platinum compounds
F. Kinase inhibitors
  1. _____ -poside and -tecan
  2. _____ -trozole
  3. _____ -platin
  4. _____ -rubicin
  5. _____ -taxel
  6. _____ -tinib

TRUE OR FALSE

1. _____ Melanoma is the most treatable form of skin cancer.
2. _____ Cancerous tumors are benign.
3. _____ Specific cancers are named according to the site where the cancerous growth begins and the type of cells involved.
4. _____ A woman who has never been pregnant is at a decreased risk of breast cancer.
5. _____ Radon is a radioactive gas that, if inhaled in sufficient quantity, can lead to lung cancer.
6. _____ A polyp is a growth that forms on the torso.
7. _____ A lymphoma is a cancer that begins in cells of the skin.
8. _____ Metastasis is the spread of cancer from one part of the body to another.
9. _____ Implant radiation is also known as brachytherapy.
10. _____ Selective estrogen receptor modulators (SERMs) are indicated only for use in postmenopausal women.
11. _____ Doxorubicin and doxorubicin liposomal are not substitutable.
12. _____ Kinase inhibitors block signaling pathways required for tumor growth.

CASE STUDY

Joan is a 62-year-old female recently screened with a mammogram. Her doctor said her results may be a bit concerning and wants to run more tests. Joan has a sister who was diagnosed with breast cancer a few years back. Joan lives at home with her husband, has three children, and does not have a history of smoking or drinking.

1. Using information from Joan's history, what risk factors does she have for developing breast cancer?
  _____
  _____
  _____

2. List at least five factors that influence a patient's treatment options, including three that are specific to breast cancer.
  _____
  _____
  _____
  _____

Following a biopsy and other tests, the doctor has determined that the lump seen on Joan's mammogram is a malignant tumor. The cancer has not yet metastasized to other parts of Joan's body. She and her doctor decide to start with anastrozole and trastuzumab.

3. Using your knowledge of these medications, explain what you know about the tumor's affinity for estrogen receptors and the expression of human epidermal growth factor receptor 2 (HER2).
  _____
  _____
  _____
  _____

4. Describe the mechanism of action of anastrozole.
  _____
  _____
  _____

For Critical Thinking, Research Activity, and answer key, please refer to Evolve.

Appendix 32: Vaccines and Immunomodulators

TERMS AND DEFINITIONS

Match each term with the correct definition below.
A. Antigen
B. Cold chain
C. Conjugate vaccine
D. Immunomodulator
E. Immunosuppressant
F. Immunization
G. Inactivated killed vaccine
H. Live attenuated vaccine
I. Toxoid vaccine
J. Vaccine
  1. A(n) _____ is a substance that prevents disease by taking advantage of your body's ability to make antibodies and release "killer" cells to disease.
2. The _____ is a set of safe handling practices that ensure vaccines and immunologic agents requiring refrigeration are maintained at a required temperature.
3. A(n) _____ links antigens or toxoids to polysaccharide or sugar molecules that certain bacteria use as a protective device to disguise themselves.
4. A drug that inhibits cell proliferation is known as a(n) _____.
5. A vaccine that stimulates the immune system to produce antibodies to a specific toxin that causes illness is called a(n) _____ .
6. A(n) _____ is a deliberate, artificial exposure to disease to produce acquired immunity.
7. _____ is a living but weakened version of a disease.
8. _____ is a chemical agent that modifies the immune response or the functioning of the immune system.

9. A substance, usually a protein fragment, that causes an immune response is a(n) _____.
10. _____ provides less immunity than live vaccines but has fewer risks for vaccine-induced disease.

MULTIPLE CHOICE

1. Which of the following is **true** regarding inactivated killed vaccines?
   A. Inactivated killed vaccines can mutate to a virulent virus strain.
   B. Booster shots are usually needed for continued immunity.
   C. Inactivated killed vaccines produce greater immunity than live attenuated vaccines.
   D. The measles, mumps, and rubella (MMR) vaccine is an inactivated killed vaccine example.
2. Which of the following is **true** about the influenza vaccine?
   A. Flu vaccines are reformulated annually based on predictions of the virus epidemiologists believe will be most virulent.
   B. Influenza vaccine comes in an inactivated killed vaccine and a live attenuated vaccine form.
   C. The influenza vaccine is for those 6 months of age and older.
   D. All the above.
3. Select the **false** statement. Each time the cold chain is disrupted, _____.
   A. the effectiveness of the vaccine is reduced
   B. the loss of potency is cumulative
   C. the vaccine potency is unaffected
   D. the shelf life of the vaccine is reduced
4. Cold chain protocols for drugs should be established for all the following *except* _____.
   A. receiving
   B. stocking
   C. storage
   D. transport
   E. administration
5. Which of the following reliably indicates the cold chain was broken during shipment?
   A. Thawed freezer packs
   B. Visible clumps after vaccine shaking
   C. A color change
   D. None of the above
6. Which of the following monoclonal antibody immunomodulators is used to prevent kidney transplant rejection?
   A. Adalimumab
   B. Basiliximab
   C. Certolizumab
   D. Daclizumab
7. Whereas vaccines boost the immune response, immunopharmacologic drugs such as cyclosporine _____.
   A. suppress cells of the immune system
   B. boost cells of the immune system
   C. have no effect on cells of the immune system
8. Cyclosporine _____.
   A. is derived from a bacterium
   B. suppresses rejection of organ transplants
   C. suppresses interferon-α
   D. has product formulations that are substitutable
9. Which drug is for mild to moderate chronic atopic dermatitis?
   A. Basiliximab
   B. Glatiramer

C. Tacrolimus
D. Temsirolimus

FILL IN THE BLANK: DRUG NAMES

1. What is the **brand name** for Hib conjugate vaccine? _____
2. What is the **generic name** for Boostrix and Adacel? _____
3. What is the **generic name** for Havrix? _____
4. What are the **brand names** for meningococcal group B conjugate vaccine? _____
5. What is the **generic name** for Engerix-B and Recombivax? _____
6. What is the **brand name** for pneumococcal 13-valent conjugate vaccine? _____
7. What is the **generic name** for Varivax? _____
8. What is the **brand name** for pneumococcal polysaccharide 23-polyvalent vaccine? _____
9. What is the **generic name** for RabAvert? _____
10. What is the **generic name** for Sandimmune and Neoral? _____
11. What is the **brand name** for sirolimus? _____
12. What is the **generic name** for Prograf and Protopic? _____
13. What is the **generic name** for Gammagard? _____
14. What is the **generic name** for CellCept? _____
15. What is the **brand name** for basiliximab? _____
16. What is the **generic name** for Thymoglobulin? _____
17. What is the **brand name** for daclizumab? _____
18. What is the **generic name** for WinRho SDF? _____

MATCHING

Patient education is an essential component of therapeutics. Select the **best** warning label to apply to the prescription vial given to patients taking the drugs listed.
A. TAKE ON AN EMPTY STOMACH
B. REFRIGERATE; DISCARD WITHIN 30 DAYS OF OPENING
C. SWALLOW CAPSULES WHOLE; DON'T CRUSH OR CHEW
D. PROTECT FROM LIGHT
   1. _____ Rh$_o$[D] immune globulin
   2. _____ Cyclosporine caps
   3. _____ Sirolimus
   4. _____ Prograf

TRUE OR FALSE

1. _____A live attenuated vaccine can mutate to a virulent form of the disease.
2. _____Cyclosporine oral liquid *nonmodified* (Sandimmune) is substitutable with cyclosporine oral liquid *modified* (Neoral, Gengraf).
3. _____A common ending for monoclonal antibody immunomodulators is -*mab*.
4. _____Dry powders are more sensitive to degradation. Therefore they are more likely to be affected by a breach in the cold chain than solutions.
5. _____Rh$_o$[D] immune globulin is administered to pregnant women who are Rh(−) to prevent erythroblastosis fetalis.

6. _____There is research currently being conducted on genetically engineered food as a delivery form for vaccines.

CASE STUDY

Cheryl has recently had a kidney transplant and brings new prescriptions to your pharmacy for prednisone, tacrolimus, and mycophenolate mofetil.

1. How should you educate Cheryl on tacrolimus and mycophenolate mofetil, especially with regard to meals?

   _____

   _____

   _____

2. Describe the mechanisms of action of tacrolimus and mycophenolate mofetil.

   _____

   _____

   _____

   _____

3. Immunosuppressant medications put patients at increased risk of infection. List some infections that Cheryl might have in the future.

   _____

   _____

   _____

Imagine that Cheryl's doctors chose belatacept (Nulojix) instead of tacrolimus to prevent transplant organ rejection.

4. Patients taking belatacept should not receive live attenuated vaccines. List at least four vaccines that would be contraindicated for Cheryl.

   _____

   _____

   _____

   _____

For Critical Thinking, Research Activity, and answer key, please refer to Evolve.

Appendix 33: Treatment of Fungal Infections

TERMS AND DEFINITIONS

Match each term with the correct definition below.

A. Antifungal
B. *Candida*
C. Fungus (*pl.* fungi)
D. Mycosis
E. Onychomycosis
F. Ringworm
G. Vulvovaginal candidiasis

1. The general term for fungal infection is _____.
2. _____ is a fungal infection involving the fingernails or toenails.
3. A drug used to treat a fungal infection is called a(n) _____.
4. Another name for _____ is yeast vaginitis.
5. A(n) _____ is an organism similar to plants but lacking chlorophyll and capable of producing mycotic (fungal) infections.
6. Although its common name is "yeast," _____ is a type of fungus.
7. _____ is a group of tinea infections involving the body or scalp.

MULTIPLE CHOICE

1. Which condition cannot be treated over the counter (OTC)?
   A. Tinea pedis
   B. Onychomycosis
   C. Vulvovaginal candidiasis
   D. Jock itch
2. Which statement about ringworm is **false**?
   A. Infections are caused by a roundworm.
   B. Infections have a characteristic ringlike shape.
   C. Infections may be spread person to person.
   D. Infections may be spread animal to person.

3. Tinea capitis is a fungal infection located on the _____.
   A. torso
   B. fingernails
   C. scalp
   D. groin
4. Which of the following is *not* a mechanism of action of antifungal agents?
   A. Inhibiting antimetabolite activity
   B. Inhibiting fungal cell wall synthesis
   C. Fungal cell membrane destruction
   D. Interfering with nucleic acid synthesis
5. Select the drug that should *not* be taken concurrently with posaconazole.
   A. Sertraline
   B. Nitroglycerin SL
   C. Cimetidine
   D. Sucralfate
6. Common vaginal yeast infection risk factors include _____.
   A. broad-spectrum antibiotics, oral contraceptives, or hormone replacement therapy
   B. corticosteroids
   C. tight-fitting clothing and synthetic underwear
   D. all the above
7. Which recommendation will *not* decrease the risk for recurrent athlete's foot infections?
   A. Keep feet clean and dry.
   B. Avoid walking barefoot across the floor of public facilities.
   C. Wear nylon socks.
   D. Use antifungal powders.
8. Select the antifungal drug that can be obtained without a prescription.
   A. Diflucan
   B. Sporanox
   C. Clotrimazole
   D. Posaconazole

9. Which antifungal should you take on an empty stomach?
   A. Itraconazole
   B. Voriconazole
   C. Terbinafine
   D. Griseofulvin
10. Select the antifungal that is indicated for prevention of athlete's foot.
    A. Tolnaftate
    B. Nystatin
    C. Terbinafine
    D. Griseofulvin
    E. Miconazole

FILL IN THE BLANK: DRUG NAMES

1. What is the **brand name** for fluconazole? _____
2. What is the **generic name** for Lotrimin (United States) and Canesten (Canada)? _____
3. What is the **brand name** for itraconazole? _____
4. What is the **generic name** for Spectazole (United States)? _____
5. What is the **brand name** for oxiconazole (United States)? _____
6. What is the **generic name** for Nizoral? _____
7. What is the **brand name** for voriconazole? _____
8. What is the **generic name** for Monistat? _____
9. What is a **brand name** for nystatin? _____
10. What is the **generic name** for Noxafil (United States) and Posanol (Canada)? _____
11. What is the **brand name** for naftifine? _____
12. What is the **generic name** for Exelderm (United States)? _____
13. What is the **brand name** for tolnaftate? _____
14. What is the **generic name** for Terazol? _____
15. What is the **brand name** for caspofungin? _____
16. What is the **generic name** for Vagistat? _____
17. What are **brand names** for ciclopirox? _____
18. What is the **generic name** for Mentax (United States)? _____
19. What is the **generic name** for Gris-PEG? _____
20. What is the **generic name** for Lamisil? _____
21. What are **brand names** for undecylenic acid? _____
22. What is the **generic name** for Fungizone (Canada)? _____
23. What is the **generic name** for Natacyn? _____
24. What is the **brand name** for anidulafungin (United States)? _____
25. What is the **generic name** for Mycamine (United States)? _____
26. What is the **generic name** for Betadine? _____

MATCHING

Match the fungal infection to its location.
A. Tinea cruris
B. Tinea corporis
C. Tinea unguium
D. Thrush
E. Tinea capitis
   1. _____ Mouth
   2. _____ Scalp
   3. _____ Groin
   4. _____ Nails
   5. _____ Body

MATCHING

Match the antifungal to its pharmacologic class.
A. Allylamine
B. Echinocandin
C. Imidazole
D. Polyene
E. Thiocarbamate
F. Triazole
   1. _____ Voriconazole
   2. _____ Miconazole
   3. _____ Amphotericin B
   4. _____ Terbinafine
   5. _____ Micafungin
   6. _____ Tolnaftate

TRUE OR FALSE

1. _____ Tinea unguium is also known as onychomycosis.
2. _____ Griseofulvin is an orally administered drug used to treat onychomycosis.
3. _____ Echinocandins are formulated only for parenteral use.
4. _____ A common ending for allylamine antifungals is -fungin.
5. _____ Most fungal infections of the skin are caused by a group of fungi called dermatophytes.
6. _____ Women who take broad-spectrum antibiotics may develop a yeast infection.
7. _____ Diflucan is OTC in the United States.
8. _____ Nystatin, natamycin, and amphotericin B are all derived from the fungi-like bacteria.
9. _____ Griseofulvin should be taken with a high fat content meal.
10. _____ *Candida* thrives in cool, dry areas.
11. _____ Frequently removing and replacing artificial nails increases susceptibility to nail fungal infections.

CASE STUDY

Brian comes to the pharmacy counter looking for a product to treat a rash on his foot. After asking a few questions, the pharmacist sees that the skin between Brian's toes is flaking, blistered, and red. Brian says it itches and burns. This started a couple of weeks ago after Brian began to take a kickboxing gym class, and the symptoms have become worse over the last few days. He says he has been showering at the gym before going home.

1. What infection does Brian probably have? Is this something that can be treated with OTC medications, or should the pharmacist refer Brian to his doctor?
   _____
   _____
   _____
   _____

2. List at least three topical creams available OTC (brand and generic names) the pharmacist can recommend to Brian.
   _____
   _____
   _____
   _____

3. How did Brian most likely acquire this infection? List at least five things Brian can do to prevent getting this infection again.

_____

_____

_____

A few months later, Brian returns. He did not follow your advice for good foot hygiene. Now his toenails are thick, yellow, and crumbly. He asks, "Can I use the stuff I got last time" to treat his nails.

4. Can he treat this toenail fungal infection with OTC medications, or should the pharmacist refer Brian to his doctor?

_____

_____

_____

_____

For Critical Thinking, Research Activity, and answer key, please refer to Evolve.

Appendix 34: Treatment of Pressure Injuries and Burns

TERMS AND DEFINITIONS

Match each term with the correct definition below.
A. Blister
B. Debridement
C. Pressure injury
D. Dehiscent wound
E. Eschar
F. First-degree burn
G. Fourth-degree burn
H. Full-thickness burn
I. Partial-thickness burns
J. Rule of palms
K. Rule of nines
L. Second-degree burn
M. Third-degree burn

1. A(n) _____ involves underlying muscles, fasciae, or bone.
2. _____ is blackened necrotic tissue of a pressure injury.
3. A "bedsore" is a type of _____.
4. A burn that involves deep epidermal layers and causes damage to the upper layers of dermis is called a(n) _____.
5. An injured area in which fluid collects below or within the epidermis as a result of a burn is called a(n) _____.
6. A(n) _____ causes minor discomfort and reddening of the skin.
7. A burn that is characterized by destruction of the epidermis and dermis is called a(n) _____.
8. First- and second-degree burns are also known as _____; in contrast, a third-degree burn is known as a(n) _____.
9. _____ is a surgical removal of foreign material and dead tissue from a wound to prevent infection and promote healing.
10. _____ is a formula for estimating the percentage of adult body surface covered by burns; it divides the body into 11 areas, each representing 9% of the body surface area.
11. _____ is a rule for estimating the extent of a burn surface area in which the palm size of the victim is about 1% of total body surface area.

12. A(n) _____ is a wound that has reopened after it has been surgically closed.

MULTIPLE CHOICE

1. Which advice is *not* given to a person who has caught on fire?
   A. Stop
   B. Drop
   C. Roll
   D. Run
2. One formula for estimating the percentage of adult body surface covered by burns is called the _____.
   A. Rule of fives
   B. Rule of sevens
   C. Rule of nines
   D. Rule of 12s
3. A third-degree burn _____.
   A. involves deep epidermal layers and causes damage to the upper layers of the dermis
   B. is characterized by destruction of the epidermis and dermis
   C. causes minor discomfort and reddening of the skin
   D. involves underlying muscles or bone
4. Which of the following is **false** about pressure injuries?
   A. Pressure injuries are "bedsores."
   B. To prevent these injuries, you should reposition an immobilized patient every 2 hours.
   C. The scale for assessing a patient's risk for developing pressure injuries runs from 1 to 4, with 4 representing the highest risk.
   D. Pressure injuries tend to form near bones close to the skin.
5. Which answer correctly characterizes wound severity staging?
   A. Stage 1: Wounds extend through skin involving underlying muscle, tendons, and bone.
   B. Stage 2: Wounds have blisters and an exposed dermis.
   C. Stage 3: Infection is not a concern.
   D. Stage 4: Skin is unbroken from a superficial wound.
6. Debridement of dead tissue is accomplished by applying all the following *except* _____.
   A. collagenase
   B. hydrocortisone
   C. papain and urea
   D. Granulex

7. The most used topical medicine for the treatment of burns is _____.
   A. erythromycin ointment
   B. silver sulfadiazine cream
   C. butter
   D. hydrocortisone cream
8. Which is a potential burn complication?
   A. Scarring
   B. Bone and joint problems
   C. Pneumonia
   D. Infection
   E. All the above
9. The most common adverse effect of mafenide is _____.
   A. itchiness
   B. burning
   C. coldness
   D. dry skin

FILL IN THE BLANK: DRUG NAMES

1. What is a **brand name** for bacitracin? _____
2. What is the **generic name** for Santyl? _____
3. What is the **generic name** for Polysporin? _____
4. What are the **brand names** for mupirocin? _____
5. What is the **generic name** for Silvadene (United States) and Flamazine (Canada)? _____
6. What is the **brand name** for mafenide? _____
7. What is the **generic name** for Betadine? _____

TRUE OR FALSE

1. _____According to the rule of palms, a burn victim's palm size is equivalent to about 5% of total body surface area.
2. _____There are three categories of burns (first, second, and third degree).
3. _____An alternative name for first- and second-degree burns is partial-thickness burns.
4. _____In treating pressure injuries, one should remove necrotic tissue from the wound.
5. _____Two common complications of burns are infection and edema.
6. _____Fourth-degree burns result in a patient insensitive to pain just after injury.

CASE STUDY

Gene is an elderly male living at home with diabetes. He's independent, but his daughter comes into your pharmacy looking for a product to help a sore on Gene's hip. Gene's health has declined over the last few months. He is not very mobile and spends most days in his recliner. He has also not been eating well as of late. You ask Gene's daughter to take a picture of the sore, and she brings it to you. You see a nickel-sized broken blister surrounded by redness on his hip.

1. What stage characterizes Gene's wound? Should the pharmacist instruct the daughter to seek medical assistance immediately, or can this be treated at home?
   _____
   _____
   _____

2. The goal of care is to cover, protect, and clean the area. List at least four dressing types that would be appropriate to cover and protect Gene's wound.
   _____
   _____
   _____

3. What other measures can Gene and his daughter take to heal his wound and to prevent further pressure injuries?
   _____
   _____
   _____

4. What is the biggest concern with Stage 3 and 4 wounds?
   _____
   _____
   _____

5. List three different products a wound care specialist could choose for debridement to slough off necrotic tissue from the pressure injury.
   _____
   _____
   _____
   _____

For Critical Thinking, Research Activity, and answer key, please refer to Evolve.

Appendix 35: Treatment of Acne

TERMS AND DEFINITIONS

Match each term with the correct definition below.
A. Acne
B. Acne vulgaris
C. Blackhead
D. Comedones
E. Cysts
F. Keratolytic
G. Milia
H. Nodule
I. Papule
J. Pustule
K. Whitehead

1. A(n) _____ agent is a peeling agent.

2. A(n) _____ is a large, inflamed lesion and may be superficial or deep.

3. _____ is a condition that occurs as a result of the action of hormones and other substances on the skin's oil glands and hair follicles.

4. A(n) _____ contains sebum and bacteria that have become trapped in the hair follicle and move to the surface.

5. An obstructed follicle that becomes inflamed is called a(n) _____.

6. _____ are tiny little bumps that occur when normally sloughed skin cells get trapped in small pockets on the surface of the skin.

7. A pimple that contains trapped sebum and bacteria and stays below the skin surface is called a(n) _____.

8. _____ are deep, painful pus-filled lesions that can cause scarring.

9. The most characteristic sign of acne is enlarged, plugged hair follicles or _____.

10. A large, painful solid lesion lodged deep in the skin is called a(n) _____.

11. _____ is the most common form of acne.

MULTIPLE CHOICE

1. Factors that make acne worse include all the following *except* _____.
   A. changing hormone levels in adolescence
   B. grease encountered in the work environment
   C. cosmetics
   D. chocolate
   E. stress

2. Drugs that can cause acne include all the following *except* _____.
   A. lithium
   B. penicillin
   C. prednisone
   D. phenytoin

3. What is the goal of acne treatment?
   A. Heal existing lesions
   B. Stop new lesion formation
   C. Prevent scarring
   D. Reduce psychological stress
   E. All the above

4. Acne is treated with the administration of all the following *except* _____.
   A. antibiotics
   B. keratolytics
   C. topical corticosteroids
   D. oral contraceptives

5. Which statement about isotretinoin is **false**?
   A. Women taking isotretinoin must use birth control for 1 month before treatment, throughout the duration of treatment, and for 1 month after stopping treatment.
   B. Isotretinoin is taken once or twice daily, orally, with food.
   C. Baseline kidney function tests are taken before starting treatment.
   D. Isotretinoin decreases the size and output of sebaceous glands.

6. In the United States, prescribers, pharmacies, and patients are required to register in the Food and Drug Administration iPLEDGE program as a condition for use of _____ to minimize risks of birth defects.

A. minocycline
B. erythromycin
C. isotretinoin
D. tetracycline

7. Which topical medication is the most effective and widely used nonprescription medication available for noninflammatory acne?
   A. Clindamycin gel
   B. Erythromycin solution
   C. Tazarotene
   D. Benzoyl peroxide

8. _____ works by killing the bacteria that infect pores.
   A. Tazarotene
   B. Azelaic acid
   C. Adapalene
   D. Tretinoin

9. Which oral antibiotic is a first-line therapy for *Propionibacterium acnes* (*P. acnes*)?
   A. Doxycycline
   B. Erythromycin
   C. Clindamycin
   D. Amoxicillin

FILL IN THE BLANK: DRUG NAMES

1. What are the **brand names** for doxycycline hyclate? _____

2. What is the **generic name** for PanOxyl? _____

3. What is the **generic name** for Epiduo? _____

4. What is the **brand name** for adapalene? _____

5. What is the **generic name** for Aczone? _____

6. What is the **generic name** for Azelex (United States) and Finacea (Canada)? _____

7. What is the **brand name** for benzoyl peroxide and erythromycin? _____

8. What is the **brand name** for alitretinoin? _____

9. What is the **brand name** for tazarotene? _____

10. What is the **generic name** for Benzaclin? _____

11. What is the **generic name** for Accutane? _____

12. What is the **generic name** for Minocin? _____

13. What is the **generic name** for Renova and Retin-A? _____

14. What is the **generic name** for Ziana (United States)? _____

MATCHING

Patient education is an essential component of therapeutics. Select the **best** warning label to apply to the prescription vial given to patients taking the drugs listed.

A. AVOID PREGNANCY
B. BLEACHING AGENT—AVOID CONTACT WITH FABRIC AND HAIR
C. MAY CAUSE SENSITIVITY TO SUNLIGHT
D. AVOID TAKING ANTACIDS, IRON, AND DAIRY PRODUCTS

1. _____ Retin-A 0.025%
2. _____ Minocycline 100 mg
3. _____ Benzoyl peroxide 10%
4. _____ Accutane 20 mg

TRUE OR FALSE

1. _____Pilosebaceous units consist of a sebaceous gland connected to a hair follicle.
2. _____A blackhead is a closed comedone.
3. _____Acne vulgaris occurs most frequently in the adolescent years.
4. _____Benzoyl peroxide may cause dry skin and redness.
5. _____Blackheads appear black because of changes in sebum as it is exposed to air.
6. _____*Propionibacterium* is a bacterium that causes acne.
7. _____Milia are a serious skin condition in newborns that should be treated with medications.
8. _____It often takes 6 to 8 weeks before oral antibiotics show evidence of improving acne.

CASE STUDY

A teenage girl and her mother approach a pharmacy checkout counter. The girl looks embarrassed as the mother says they are looking for acne treatment. The mother says, "I told her to stop eating junk food, but her breakouts are getting worse."

1. Is junk food contributing to acne? List at least four factors that can worsen acne.

_____

_____

2. Describe the four different types of inflammatory acne lesions associated with breakouts.

_____

_____

_____

After examining the girl's condition, the pharmacist determines that she has mild acne. He recommends that she gently wash her face twice daily with warm water and a mild soap. He then takes her to the acne area in the over-the-counter section to help her select a medication to treat and prevent future breakouts. There are many options, but the pharmacist explains that they all contain the same active ingredient.

3. Which is the most effective and widely used nonprescription medication for acne?

_____

_____

_____

4. Describe the mechanism of action of benzoyl peroxide.

_____

_____

_____

5. What is an important point the pharmacist should tell the mother and daughter about products containing benzoyl peroxide?

_____

_____

_____

_____

For Critical Thinking, Research Activity, and answer key, please refer to Evolve.

Appendix 36: Treatment of Atopic Dermatitis and Psoriasis

TERMS AND DEFINITIONS

Match each term with the correct definition below.
A. Atopic dermatitis
B. Cutaneous
C. Dermatitis
D. Eczema
E. Phototherapy
F. Psoriasis
G. Plaque psoriasis

1. The term used to describe inflammation of the skin is _____.
2. _____ is a treatment for atopic dermatitis that involves exposing the skin to ultraviolet A or B light waves.
3. A chronic disease of the skin, _____ is characterized by itchy red patches covered with silvery scales.
4. _____is a chronic inflammatory condition that affects the skin.
5. A general term used to describe several types of inflammation of the skin is _____.
6. _____ is a term that means pertaining to the skin.
7. _____ is the most common form of psoriasis.

MULTIPLE CHOICE

1. Irritants that aggravate the skin of persons with atopic dermatitis are _____.
   A. cotton and silk
   B. perfumes and cosmetics
   C. rice and potatoes
   D. cleaning solvents and detergents
   E. B and D
2. Psoriatic patches are typically found in all the regions except _____.
   A. neck
   B. face
   C. elbows
   D. genitals
   E. hands and feet
3. Which advice would not be given to a person with eczema?
   A. Avoid wearing wool or clothing that feels "scratchy."
   B. Increase humidity in the household environment.
   C. Apply moisturizers and lotion to the skin.
   D. Take hot baths.

4. Of the following, the most potent corticosteroid classification is _____.
   A. class I
   B. class II
   C. class III
   D. class IV
   E. class V
5. Select the corticosteroid that is in the least potent category.
   A. Clobetasol
   B. Betamethasone dipropionate (optimized)
   C. Hydrocortisone base cream
   D. Halobetasol propionate
   E. Fluocinonide
6. Which of the following adverse effects is not linked to topical use of corticosteroids?
   A. Thinning of the skin
   B. Cushing syndrome
   C. Stretch marks (striae)
   D. Spider veins
   E. Acne
7. Select the drug that is indicated for the treatment of severe psoriasis and arthritis.
   A. Cyclosporine
   B. Azathioprine
   C. Methotrexate
   D. Calcipotriene
8. Which of the following correctly describes the mechanism of action of topical corticosteroids?
   A. Corticosteroids decrease redness, swelling, and inflammation by reducing the number of inflammatory cells.
   B. Corticosteroids increase cell permeability to T lymphocytes and eosinophils.
   C. Corticosteroids increase cytokine release.
   D. Topical corticosteroids cause vasodilation.
9. The Food and Drug Administration and Health Canada require manufacturers to include a Black Box warning in the package insert for _____, describing the increased risks for cancer.
   A. Dermatop-E and Dovonex
   B. Cutivate and Ultravate
   C. Methotrexate and Enbrel
   D. Pimecrolimus and tacrolimus
10. Dovonex is a synthetic analog of _____.
    A. vitamin A
    B. vitamin B
    C. vitamin C
    D. vitamin D

FILL IN THE BLANK: DRUG NAMES

1. What is a **brand name** for betamethasone dipropionate? _____
2. What is the **generic name** for Soriatane? _____
3. What is the **generic name** for Luxiq (United States) and Valisone-G (Canada)? _____
4. What is the **brand name** for desoximetasone? _____
5. What is the **generic name** for ApexiCon E? _____
6. What are **brand names** for fluocinolone acetonide? _____
7. What is the **generic name** for Clobex? _____
8. What is the **brand name** for fluticasone? _____

9. What is the **generic name** for DesOwen (United States)? _____
10. What is the **brand name** for halcinonide? _____
11. What is the **generic name** for Tazorac? _____
12. What is the **brand name** for halobetasol? _____
13. What is the **brand name** for clocortolone? _____
14. What is the **brand name** for hydrocortisone valerate (Canada)? _____
15. What is the **generic name** for Lidex? _____
16. What is the **brand name** for prednicarbate? _____
17. What is the **generic name** for Cordran? _____
18. What is the **brand name** for pimecrolimus? _____
19. What is the **generic name** for Locoid (United States)? _____
20. What is the **brand name** for tacrolimus? _____
21. What is the **generic name** for Elocon (United States) and Elocom (Canada)? _____
22. What is the **brand name** for calcipotriene (United States) and calcipotriol (Canada)? _____
23. What is the **generic name** for Vectical (United States) and Silkis (Canada)? _____
24. What are **brand names** for methoxsalen? _____
25. What is the **generic name** for Taclonex (United States) and Dovobet (Canada)? _____
26. What are **brand names** for infliximab? _____
27. What is the **generic name** for Neoral? _____
28. What is the **brand name** for etanercept? _____
29. What is the **generic name** for Stelara? _____
30. What is the **generic name** for Otezla? _____

MATCHING

Match each drug to its pharmacologic classification.
A. Furanocoumarins
B. Corticosteroid
C. Vitamin D analog
D. Calcineurin inhibitor
E. Immunosuppressants
   1. _____ Dovonex
   2. _____ Methotrexate
   3. _____ Mometasone
   4. _____ Elidel
   5. _____ Oxsoralen-Ultra

MATCHING

Patient education is an essential component of therapeutics. Select the **best** warning label to apply to the prescription container given to patients taking the drugs listed.
A. AVOID PROLONGED EXPOSURE TO SUNLIGHT
B. REFRIGERATE; DO NOT FREEZE
C. SWALLOW WHOLE; DON'T CRUSH OR CHEW
D. AVOID CONTACT WITH FACE
E. AVOID SUN EXPOSURE FOR 24 HOURS BEFORE AND 48 HOURS AFTER TREATMENT
   1. _____ Elidel
   2. _____ Methoxsalen
   3. _____ Apremilast
   4. _____ Enbrel
   5. _____ Taclonex

TRUE OR FALSE

1. _____Stress and dry skin may aggravate psoriasis.
2. _____It is uncommon for eczema that has gone into remission in childhood to return with the onset of puberty.
3. _____Corticosteroids are categorized into five potency categories.
4. _____Topical corticosteroids possess antiinflammatory and immunosuppressive properties.
5. _____Phototherapy involves exposing the skin to ultraviolet A, B, and C light waves.
6. _____The vehicle (base) in which the corticosteroid is suspended has no influence on potency.
7. _____Eczema is a specific type of atopic dermatitis.
8. _____Phototherapy can prematurely age skin and increase patients' skin cancer risk.
9. _____Atopic dermatitis is believed to be an autoimmune disease.
10. _____Elidel and Protopic are topical agents for plaque psoriasis.

CASE STUDY

Martha is a pharmacy patient who comes to the counter and asks for "the creams for my skin condition." You notice that Martha has thick, silvery, scaly patches on her hands and elbows. You examine her medication profile and fill her prescriptions for betamethasone cream and Dovonex cream.

1. Using your understanding of Martha's medications and symptoms, what kind of skin condition do you think she has?
   _____
   _____

_____
2. List at least four factors that can exacerbate symptoms of atopic dermatitis and psoriasis.
   _____
   _____
   _____
   _____

Next month, Martha returns to the pharmacy after a visit with her dermatologist. She hands you a Humira prescription.

3. Adalimumab (Humira) is a biologic monoclonal antibody. What is the target of adalimumab?
   _____
   _____
   _____

4. List some adverse effects associated with adalimumab.
   _____
   _____
   _____

5. Identify another biologic agent with the same target that Martha's doctor could have selected to treat her condition.
   _____
   _____
   _____
   _____

_____
For Critical Thinking, Research Activity, and answer key, please refer Evolve.

Appendix 37: Treatment of Lice and Scabies

TERMS AND DEFINITIONS

Match each term with the correct definition below.
A. Lice
B. Nits
C. Nymph
D. Ovicidal
E. Parasite
F. Pediculicide
G. Scabies
H. Scabicide

1. An organism that benefits by living in, with, or on another organism is called a(n) _____.
2. A(n) _____ is a drug that kills _____, a parasitic mite that causes infection.
3. A drug that is _____ is able to kill the eggs of lice.
4. Another name for head lice eggs is _____.
5. A drug that kills lice is called a(n) _____.
6. _____ are a group of parasites that can live on the body, scalp, or genital area of humans.
7. The term used to describe a baby louse is _____.

MULTIPLE CHOICE

1. Which parasite is *not* a louse?
   A. *Pediculus humanus capitis*
   B. *Sarcoptes scabiei*
   C. *Pediculus humanus corporis*
   D. *Pthirus pubis*
2. _____ is a parasitic infection classified as a sexually transmitted infection (STI).
   A. *Pediculus humanus capitis*
   B. Scabies
   C. *Pediculus humanus corporis*
   D. *Pthirus pubis*
3. Pharmacy technicians should apply the warning label _____ to prescription vials containing lindane shampoo.
   A. SHAKE WELL
   B. DILUTE BEFORE USE
   C. FOR EXTERNAL USE ONLY
   D. APPLY SPARINGLY
4. Which warning should be given to persons receiving a prescription for malathion?
   A. AVOID OPEN FLAMES (e.g., LIT CIGARETTES, CIGARS, AND PIPES)
   B. MAY STAIN CLOTHING AND HAIR
   C. MAY BLEACH CLOTHING AND HAIR
   D. DILUTE BEFORE USE

5. Select the drug for which the Food and Drug Administration requires manufacturers to place a Black Box warning in the package insert.
   A. Lindane
   B. Permethrins
   C. Pyrethrins
   D. Crotamiton

6. Lindane is _____.
   A. nephrotoxic
   B. neurotoxic
   C. hepatotoxic
   D. ototoxic

7. Spinosad works by _____.
   A. paralyzing the parasites' central nervous system with an acetylcholine accumulation
   B. dissolving the exoskeleton of a louse
   C. asphyxiating lice
   D. producing neuronal excitation in lice, resulting in paralysis and death

8. Which of the following statements about body lice is **false**?
   A. Body lice infestations are caused by the parasite *Pediculus humanus corporis*.
   B. Adult body lice can survive away from a human host for 30 days.
   C. Body lice infestations are a serious public health concern.
   D. Body lice may cause epidemics of typhus and louse-borne relapsing fever.

9. In which environmental conditions do scabies thrive?
   A. Dense populations such as in prisons and nursing homes
   B. Warm environment
   C. Moist environment
   D. Arid environment
   E. Scarcely populated environment

10. Strategies to prevent lice reinfestation include all the following *except* _____.
    A. treat all household members.
    B. wash clothing, linens, and bedding in hot water.
    C. throw away toys, clothing, and bedding that cannot be washed.
    D. use a nit comb to remove eggs.

FILL IN THE BLANK: DRUG NAMES

1. What is the *generic name* for Ovide (United States)? _____

2. What is the *brand name* for crotamiton? _____

3. What is the *generic name* for Elimite Cream and Nix? _____

4. What is the *generic name* for RID (United States) and R&C (Canada)? _____

5. What is the *brand name* for benzyl alcohol? _____

6. What is the *generic name* for Sklice? _____

7. What is the *generic name* for Natroba? _____

TRUE OR FALSE

1. _____Treatment of head lice requires shaving the head.
2. _____Malathion was withdrawn from the market in Canada but is still available in the United States.
3. _____Head lice most commonly affect children aged 3 to 11 years.
4. _____Head lice infestation is caused by poor hygiene.
5. _____Individuals *cannot* get pubic lice from sitting on public toilet seats.

6. _____Permethrin is approved for the treatment of head lice, body lice, and pubic lice.
7. _____Permethrin is ovicidal (kills eggs), but pyrethrins are not.
8. _____Ivermectin is safe to use in pregnant women.
9. _____Permethrins and pyrethrins may be obtained only by prescription.
10. _____Lindane is a first-line therapy for treating scabies.

CASE STUDY

Lisa is a mother to two young children. She comes to your pharmacy counter in a panic because there is a lice outbreak at her children's daycare center. She is on her way home from work and has not had a chance to determine whether her children have an active case, but she wants to pick up a product to treat all her family members.

1. What are two options for treating lice that are available over the counter in the United States?
   _____
   _____
   _____

2. Lisa chooses to purchase Nix. What are two important points that would help Lisa most effectively treat and remove the lice?
   _____
   _____
   _____
   _____

3. In addition to treating all family members, list five strategies to help prevent lice reinfestation in Lisa's home.
   _____
   _____
   _____
   _____

Lisa returns to your pharmacy 3 weeks later. She is upset because she treated all her family members with Nix and followed all the pharmacist's instructions, but she found a louse and several nits in her daughter's hair. She heard from a friend that there is a problem with "super lice."

4. Explain the problem of drug resistance in relationship to pediculicides.
   _____
   _____
   _____
   _____

Lisa returns from her pediatrician's office with a prescription for Sklice 0.5% solution.

5. Lisa's daughter is 6 years old and weighs 44 lbs. Is Sklice safe to use for Lisa's daughter?
   _____
   _____
   _____

6. Describe the mechanism of action of ivermectin.
   _____
   _____
   _____

For Critical Thinking, Research Activity, and answer key, please refer to Evolve.

Glossary

Absorption Process involving movement of drug molecules from the site of administration into the circulatory system.

Acetylcholinesterase Enzyme that degrades acetylcholine and reverses acetylcholine-induced depolarization.

Acne vulgaris Most common form of acne.

Acne Disorder resulting from the action of hormones and other substances on the skin's oil glands (sebaceous glands) and hair follicles.

Acupuncture Nonpharmacologic treatment for pain that involves the application of needles to precise points on the body.

Acute pain Sudden pain that results from injury or inflammation; usually self-limiting.

Additive effect Increased drug effect produced when a second similar drug is added to therapy that is greater than the effects produced by either drug alone.

Adenosine triphosphate Nucleotide that supplies the energy required for muscle contraction.

Adjunct Drug used to complement the effects of another drug.

Affinity Attraction that the receptor site has for the drug.

Agonist Drug that binds to its receptor site and stimulates a cellular response.

AIDS (acquired immunodeficiency syndrome) Most severe form of human immunodeficiency virus (HIV) infection. HIV-infected patients are diagnosed with AIDS when their CD4 cell count falls below 200 cells/mm³ or they develop an AIDS-defining illness (an illness that is very unusual in someone who is not HIV-positive).

Aldosterone Hormone that promotes sodium and fluid reabsorption.

Allergen Substance that produces an allergic reaction.

Allergic asthma Asthma symptoms induced by a hypersensitivity reaction caused by overexpression of immunoglobulin E antibodies on exposure to environmental allergens.

Allergic conjunctivitis Inflammation of the tissue lining the eyelids caused by the reaction to an allergy-causing substance.

Allergic rhinitis Seasonal condition characterized by inflammation and swelling of the nasal passageways (rhinitis) accompanied by a runny nose (rhinorrhea).

Allergy Hypersensitivity reaction by the immune system on exposure to an allergen.

Alzheimer disease Neurodegenerative disease that causes memory loss and behavioral changes.

Amenorrhea Absence of normal menstruation.

Amyotrophic lateral sclerosis Degenerative disease that causes muscle wasting and muscle weakness; also known as Lou Gehrig disease.

Analgesic Drug that reduces pain.

Anaphylactic shock Acute, life-threatening allergic reaction that produces peripheral vasodilation.

Anaphylaxis Life-threatening allergic reaction.

Aneurysm Weakened spot of the artery wall that has stretched or burst, filling the area with blood.

Angina pectoris Symptomatic manifestation of ischemic heart disease characterized by a severe squeezing or pressure-like chest pain; brought on by exertion or stress.

Angioedema Allergic skin disease characterized by patches of circumscribed swelling involving the skin and its subcutaneous layers, the mucous membranes, and sometimes the viscera.

Angiotensin-converting enzyme Enzyme that catalyzes the conversion of angiotensin I to angiotensin II.

Angiotensin II Potent vasoconstrictor that is produced when the renin–aldosterone–angiotensin system is activated.

Angle-closure glaucoma Sudden increase in intraocular pressure caused by obstruction of the drainage portal between the cornea and iris (angle); can rapidly progress to blindness.

Anion Negatively charged particle.

Anoxia Absence of oxygen supply to cells that results in cell damage or death.

Antagonism Drug-drug interaction or drug-food interaction that causes decreased effects (e.g., when a pharmacologic antagonist is administered to block the effect of another drug).

Antagonist Drug that binds to the receptor site and does not produce an action. An antagonist prevents another drug or natural body chemical from binding and activating the receptor site.

Antibiotic Naturally occurring substance produced by a microorganism or semisynthetic substance derived from a microorganism capable of destroying or inhibiting the growth of another microorganism.

Anticoagulant Drug that prolongs coagulation time and is used to prevent clot formation.

Antidiarrheal Drug that prevents or relieves diarrhea.

Antifungal Drug used to treat a fungal infection.

Antigen Substance, usually a protein fragment, that causes an immune response.

Antimicrobial Substance capable of destroying or inhibiting the growth of a microorganism.

Antimicrobial resistance Ability of bacteria to overcome the bactericidal or bacteriostatic effects of an antiinfective agent. Resistance traits are encoded on bacterial genes and can be transferred to other bacteria.

Antinuclear antibody Autoantibody or abnormal antibody that attacks the nucleus of normal cells.

Antiplatelet drug Drug that prevents accumulation of platelets, thereby blocking an important step in the clot formation process.

Antiretroviral Medication that interferes with the replication of retroviruses (e.g., HIV is a retrovirus).

Antithrombotic Drug that inhibits clot formation by reducing the coagulation action of the blood protein thrombin.

Antiviral resistance Ability of a virus to overcome the suppressive action of antiviral agents.

Antiviral Medication that is able to inhibit viral replication.

Anxiety Condition associated with tension, apprehension, fear, or panic.

Anxiolytic Drug used to treat anxiety.

ApoE4 allele Defective form of apolipoprotein E associated with Alzheimer disease.

Aqueous humor Portion of anterior cavity that lies in front of the lens and is filled with a clear watery liquid.

Arterial plaque Hardened lipid streak within an artery formed by deposits of cholesterol, lipid material, and lipophages.

Arteriosclerosis Loss of elasticity (hardening) of the arteries. Thickening and loss of elasticity of arterial walls; sometimes called hardening of the arteries.

Arthritis Condition that is associated with joint pain.

Asthma Chronic disease that affects the airways and causes irritation, inflammation, and difficulty breathing.

Atheromas Hard plaque formed within an artery.

Atherosclerosis Process in which plaques (atheromas) containing cholesterol, lipid material, and lipophages are formed within arteries, impeding the flow of blood and oxygen.

Atherothrombosis Formation of a blood clot in an artery.

Atopic dermatitis Chronic inflammatory disease of the skin.

Atrial fibrillation Rapid and uncoordinated contractions during which the heart may beat from 300 to 400 beats/min.

Atrial flutter Irregular heart beat in which contractions in the atrium exceed the number of contractions in the ventricle. The heart rate is from 160 to 350 beats/min.

Atrophic vaginitis Postmenopausal thinning and dryness of the vaginal epithelium related to decreased estrogen levels.

Aura Unusual sensation and/or auditory, visual, or olfactory hallucination experienced just before the onset of a seizure.

Autoantibody Abnormal antibody that attacks healthy cells and tissue.

Autoimmune disease Disease that occurs when the immune system turns against the parts of the body it is designed to protect.

Automaticity Spontaneous depolarization (contraction) of heart cells.

Autonomic nervous system (ANS) Division of nervous system that controls involuntary body functions; consists of sympathetic and parasympathetic divisions.

Bactericidal Able to destroy bacteria.

Bacteriostatic Able to inhibit bacterial proliferation; host defense mechanisms destroy the bacteria.

Benign prostatic hyperplasia Noncancerous growth of cells in the prostate gland.

Benign Tumor that is not cancerous and does not spread to surrounding tissues or other parts of the body.

Bicarbonate Substance used as a buffer to maintain the normal levels of acidity (pH) in blood and other fluids in the body.

Bioavailability Fraction of administered drug dose that enters the systemic circulation and is available to produce a drug effect.

Bioequivalent drug Drug that shows no statistical differences in the rate and extent of absorption when it is administered in the same strength, dosage form, and route of administration as the brand name product.

Biofeedback Nonpharmacologic treatment for pain that involves relaxation techniques and gaining self-control over muscle tension, heart rate, and skin temperature.

Biopharmaceutical Pharmaceutical derived from biological sources (e.g., proteins, gene sequences) and manufactured using biotechnology methods such as recombinant DNA technology.

Biotransformation Process of drug metabolism in the body that transforms a drug to a more active, equally active, or inactive metabolite.

Bipolar disorder Mental illness associated with sudden swings in mood between depression and periods of mania, racing thoughts, distractibility, and increased goal-directed behavior.

Blackhead (open comedone) Trapped sebum and bacteria partially open to the surface that turn black due to changes in sebum as it is exposed to air.

Blepharitis Chronic disease of the eye that produces distinctive flaky scales that form on the eyelids and eyelashes.

Blister Collection of fluid below or within the epidermis.

Bone mineral density test Test carried out to measure the degree of bone loss.

Bone resorption Process during which bone is broken down into mineral ions (e.g., calcium).

Botulinum toxin Toxin produced by the bacterium *Clostridium botulinum* that causes muscle paralysis.

Bradykinesia Slowness in initiating and carrying out voluntary movements.

Breakthrough pain Pain that occurs in between scheduled doses of analgesics.

Broad-spectrum antibiotic Antimicrobial capable of destroying a wide range of bacteria.

Bronchodilator Drug that relaxes tightened airway muscles and improves air flow through the airways.

Cancer Term for diseases in which abnormal cells divide without control. Specific cancers are named according to the site where the cancerous growth begins.

Candida Type of fungus; also called yeast.

Cardiac output Volume of blood ejected from the left ventricle in 1 minute.

Cardioglycosides Class of drugs, generally derived from the foxglove plant, that can alter cardiovascular function. Digitalis is representative of this class of drugs.

Cardiomyopathy Heart disease that causes abnormal enlargement of the heart.

Catatonia Symptom of schizophrenia associated with unresponsiveness and immobility.

CD4 T lymphocyte White blood cell that fights infection.

Central nervous system (CNS) Consists of the brain and spinal cord.

Central-acting muscle relaxant Drug that produces relaxation of muscles through central nervous system depression blocking nerve transmission between the spinal cord and muscles.

Cephalgia Head pain.

Cerebral palsy Neurologic disorder that affects muscle movement and coordination.

Cerumen Waxlike substance secreted by modified sweat glands in the ear.

Chemotherapy Treatment with drugs that kill cancer.

Cholesterol Naturally occurring waxy substance produced by the liver and found in foods that maintain cell membranes; needed for vitamin D production. Excess cholesterol can cause atherosclerosis.

Chronic obstructive pulmonary disease Progressive disease of the airways that produces gradual loss of pulmonary function.

Chronic pain Pain that persists for a long period that is worsened by psychological factors and is resistant to many medical treatments.

Circadian rhythms Biological changes that occur according to time cycles.

Clonus Involuntary rhythmic muscle contraction that causes the feet and wrists to flex and relax involuntarily.

Cluster headache Intensely painful vascular headache that occurs in groups and produces pain on one side of the head.

Cognitive function Ability to take in information via the senses, process the details, commit the information to memory, and recall it when necessary.

Cold chain Set of safe handling practices that ensure that vaccines and immunologic agents requiring refrigeration are maintained at the required temperature from the time of manufacture until the time of administration to patients.

Colloids Proteins or other large molecules that remain suspended in the blood for a long period and are too large to cross membranes.

Colonoscopy Examination of the colon for signs of inflammation and damage; performed by inserting a thin tube with a small light and camera at the end (i.e., endoscope) into the anus.

Comedone Enlarged and plugged hair follicle; the most characteristic sign of acne.

Complementary and alternative medicine (CAM) Treatments that may include dietary supplements, herbal preparations, acupuncture, massage, magnet therapy, spiritual healing, and meditation.

Complex focal seizure Seizure disorder that produces a blank stare, disorientation, repetitive actions, and memory loss.

Computed tomography (CT) Diagnostic examination in which a series of detailed pictures are taken of areas inside the body; created by a computer linked to an x-ray machine.

Condom Thin, flexible, penile sheath made of synthetic or natural material that is placed over the penis; used to prevent pregnancy and some sexually transmitted infections.

Conduction impairment Blocking of air waves as they are conducted through the external and middle ears to the sensory receptors of the inner ear.

Conjugate vaccine Vaccine that links antigens or toxoids to polysaccharide or sugar molecules; used by certain bacteria as a protective device to disguise themselves.

Conjunctivitis (pink eye) Common, self-limiting ailment that causes itching, burning, and teary outflow.

Constipation Abnormally delayed or infrequent passage of dry hardened feces.

Controlled substance Drug whose possession and distribution is restricted because of its potential for abuse as determined by federal or state law. Controlled substances are placed in schedules according to their abuse potential and effects if abused.

Convulsions Sudden contraction of muscles caused by seizures.

Cornea Clear part of the eye located in front of the iris.

Coronary artery disease Condition that occurs when the arteries that supply blood to the heart muscle become hardened and narrowed.

Crohn's disease Irritable bowel disease that produces inflammation and damage anywhere along the gastrointestinal tract.

Cross-resistance Development of resistance to one drug in a particular class that results in resistance to other drugs in that class.

Crystalloid Intravenous solution that contains electrolytes in concentrations similar to those of plasma.

Cutaneous Pertaining to the skin.

Cyclooxygenase-2 inhibitor Analgesic antiinflammatory drug that preferentially blocks cyclooxygenase-2, an enzyme that produces prostaglandin, which is a substance involved in mediating pain.

Cysts End products of pustules or nodules.

Cytomegalovirus retinitis Viral opportunistic infection of the eye that can cause pain and blindness.

Debridement Surgical removal of foreign material and dead tissue from a wound to prevent infection and promote healing.

Decubitus ulcer Pressure sore or "bed sore."

Dehiscent wound A wound that has reopened after it has been closed surgically.

Delusion Irrational thoughts or false beliefs that dominate a person's behavior and viewpoint and do not change, even when evidence is provided that these beliefs are not valid.

Dementia Condition associated with loss of memory and cognition.

Deoxyribonucleic acid (DNA) DNA is the repository of hereditary characteristics; it is a nucleic acid that contains the genetic blueprint.

Depolarization Process during which the heart muscle conducts an electrical impulse, causing a contraction.

Depolarizing neuromuscular blocker Drug that acts as an agonist at acetylcholine receptor sites and produces sustained depolarization, causing the receptors to convert to an inactive state.

Dermatitis Inflammation of the skin.

Desquamation Shedding of the outer layers of the skin.

Diabetes mellitus Chronic condition in which the body is unable to use glucose (sugar) as energy effectively.

Diabetic neuropathy Nerve disorder caused by uncontrolled diabetes. It leads to pain or a loss of feeling in the toes, feet, legs, hands, and/or arms.

Diaphragm Rubber or plastic cup that fits over the cervix; used for contraception.

Diarrhea Abnormally frequent passage of loose and watery stools.

Diastolic blood pressure Blood pressure measured when the heart is at rest (diastole).

Diffusion Passive movement of molecules across cell membranes from an area of high drug concentration to an area of lower concentration.

Digestion Complete process of altering the physical and chemical composition of ingested food materials so they can be absorbed and used by the body's cells.

Digital rectal examination Screening examination involving palpation of the prostate gland; conducted by insertion of a gloved lubricated finger into the rectum.

Disinhibition Opposite of inhibited.

Distribution Process of movement of the drug from the circulatory system across barrier membrane(s) to the site of drug action.

Diuretic Drug that produces diuresis (urination).

Dosage form Drug formulation (e.g., capsule, tablet, solution).

Dose Amount of a drug required for one application or administration.

Dosing schedule How frequently a drug dose is administered (e.g., "four times a day").

Double-contrast barium enema Diagnostic test to examine the colon and rectum in which an individual is administered a barium-containing enema and then radiographs are taken.

Drug delivery system Dosage form or device designed to release a specific amount of drug.

Drug dependence Occurs when a person taking a drug does not continue to take it and suffers from physical or psychological withdrawal symptoms, or both.

Drug resistance testing Laboratory test to determine whether an individual's HIV strain is resistant to any anti-HIV medications.

Drug Substance used to diagnose, treat, cure, prevent, or mitigate disease in humans or other animals.

Drug-disease contraindication No rationale for drug use; drug administration should be avoided because it may worsen the patient's medical condition.

Drug-drug interaction Reaction that occurs when two or more drugs are administered at the same time.

Drug-food interaction Altered drug response that occurs when a drug is administered with certain foods.

Dry eye disease Occurs when the eye does not produce tears properly, or when the tears are not of the correct consistency and evaporate too quickly.

Duodenal ulcer Ulcer located in the upper portion of the small intestine or duodenum.

Duration of action Time between the onset of drug action and discontinuation of drug action.

Dysfunctional uterine bleeding Irregular or excessive uterine bleeding that results from a structural problem or hormonal imbalance.

Dysmenorrhea Difficult or painful menstruation.

Dysphoria Feeling of emotional or mental discomfort, restlessness, and depression; the opposite of euphoria.

Eclampsia Life-threatening condition that can develop in pregnant women that causes high blood pressure and seizures.

Ectopic Occurring in an abnormal location.

Eczema General term used to describe several types of inflammation of the skin.

Efficacy Measure of a drug's effectiveness.

Ejaculation Release of semen from the penis during orgasm.

Ejection fraction Percentage of blood ejected from the left ventricle with each heartbeat.

Electrical cardioversion Process of applying an electrical shock to the heart with a defibrillator to convert the heart to a normal rhythm.

Electrolytes Small charged molecules essential for homeostasis that play an important role in body chemistry.

Elimination Process that results in the removal of drug from the body.

Embolic stroke Stroke caused by an emboli obstructing the flow of blood through an artery.

Embolus Moving blood clot.

Endometriosis Presence of functioning endometrial tissue outside the uterus.

Endorphins, enkephalins, and dynorphin Substances released by the body in response to painful stimuli that act as natural painkillers.

Endoscope Thin flexible tube with a small video camera and light attached to one end.

Endoscopy Test used to look for ulcers inside the stomach and small intestine using an endoscope.

Endotracheal intubation Process of inserting a tube into the trachea or windpipe to facilitate mechanical ventilation.

Endplate Projection extending off the end of a motor neuron where the neurotransmitter acetylcholine is released.

Enteral Refers to a drug dosage form that is administered orally.

Enuresis Bedwetting or uncontrollable urination during sleep.

Enzyme Protein capable of causing a chemical reaction. Enzymes are involved in the metabolism of some drugs.

Epilepsy Recurrent seizure disorder characterized by a sudden, excessive, disorderly discharge of cerebral neurons.

Equilibrium Steadiness or balance accompanied by a sense of knowing where the body is in relationship to surroundings.

Erectile dysfunction Persistent inability to achieve and/or maintain an erection sufficient for satisfactory sexual intercourse.

Erythrocytes Red blood cells.

Erythropoiesis Formation of red blood cells.

Eschar Blackened necrotic tissue of a decubitus ulcer or pressure sore.

Escharotomy Removal of necrotic skin and underlying tissue.

Euphoria State of intense happiness or well-being; the opposite of dysphoria.

Exacerbation Aggravation of symptoms or increase in the severity of the disease.

Extrapyramidal symptoms Excessive muscle movement (motor activity) associated with the use of neuroleptics; includes muscular rigidity, tremor, bradykinesia (slow movement), and difficulty in walking.

Fasting blood glucose Blood glucose level after a person has not eaten for 8 to 12 hours (usually overnight).

Febrile seizure Seizure associated with a sudden spike in body temperature.

Fecal occult blood test (FOBT) Test to check for blood in stool.

Fertility Being fertile; able to reproduce.

First-degree burn Minor discomfort and reddening of the skin.

First-pass effect Process whereby only a fraction of an orally administered drug reaches the systemic circulation because much of the drug is metabolized in the liver to an inactive metabolite before entering the general circulation.

Fistula Ulcer that tunnels from the site of origin to surrounding tissues.

Fontanels Soft spots found in a baby's skull.

Forced expiratory volume (FEV) The maximum volume of air that can be breathed out in 1 second; also called forced vital capacity.

Fourth-degree burn Burn that involves underlying muscles, fasciae, or bone.

Full-thickness burn Third degree burn in which the epidermis and dermis are destroyed.

Fungus (pl., fungi) Organism similar to a plant but lacking chlorophyll; capable of producing mycotic (fungal) infection.

Fusarium keratitis Rare fungal infection that occurs in soft contact lens wearers; can result in blindness.

Gastric ulcer Ulcer located in the stomach.

Gastroenteritis Inflammation of the lining membrane of the stomach and intestines.

Gastroesophageal reflux disease (GERD) Motility disorder associated with impaired peristalsis that results in the backflow of gastric contents into the esophagus.

Generalized anxiety disorder Condition associated with excessive worrying and tension that is experienced daily for more than 6 months.

Generalized seizures Seizures that spread across both cerebral hemispheres; include tonic-clonic seizures.

Gestational diabetes Diabetes that may be caused by the hormones of pregnancy or a shortage of insulin.

Gingival hyperplasia Excess growth of gum tissue that could grow over the teeth.

Glial cells Cells that form the blood-brain barrier and support function of the neurons.

Gout Disease associated with deposits of urate crystals in the joints that produces inflammation; caused by hyperuricemia.

Graves disease Autoimmune disorder that causes hyperthyroidism.

Gynecomastia Painful breast enlargement in men.

Half-life ($t_{1/2}$) Length of time it takes for the plasma concentration of an administered drug to be reduced by 50%.

Hallucination Visions or voices that exist only in a person's mind and cannot be seen or heard by others.

Hashimoto disease Autoimmune disorder that causes hypothyroidism.

Heart failure Clinical syndrome in which the heart is unable to pump blood at a rate necessary to meet the body's metabolic needs.

Helminthes Group of parasitic worms that can cause eye infection and blindness.

Hemoglobin A1c test Blood test that measures a person's average blood glucose level over a period of 2 to 3 months.

Hemoglobin Red pigment made up of iron atoms; transports oxygen and carbon dioxide in the body.

Hemorrhagic stroke Sudden bleeding into or around the brain.

Hemostasis Process of stopping the flow of blood.

Hepatoxicity Serious adverse reaction that occurs in the liver.

Herpes simplex keratitis Painful eye infection caused by a herpesvirus that can lead to blindness.

Herpes zoster ophthalmicus Painful eye infection caused by a herpesvirus that can lead to blindness.

Hiatal hernia Condition in which the lower esophageal sphincter shifts above the diaphragm.

High-density lipoprotein Lipoprotein that transports cholesterol, triglycerides, and other lipids from blood to body tissues; known as good cholesterol.

Highly active antiretroviral therapy (HAART) Combination of three or more antiretroviral medications taken in a regimen.

Hirsutism Excessive hair growth in women.

Histamine Organic nitrogen compound involved in local immune responses; has a regulating physiologic function in the gut and acts as a neurotransmitter.

Homeopathic medicine Medical field in which drugs are administered in minute quantities to stimulate natural body healing systems.

Host Individual infected with a virus.

Huntington disease Progressive and degenerative disease of neurons that affects muscle movement, cognitive functions, and emotions.

Hydrophilic Having a strong affinity for water; water-loving; able to dissolve in and absorb water.

Hydrophobic Lacking an affinity for water; water-hating; resistant to wetting.

Hyperalgesia Heightened sensitivity to pain that can result from treatment of chronic pain with high-dose opioids.

Hyperglycemia Condition of elevated blood glucose levels.

Hyperkalemia Condition in which the serum potassium level is higher than 5.5 mEq/L.

Hyperlipidemia Increased concentration of cholesterol and triglycerides in the blood associated with the development of atherosclerosis.

Hyperopia Farsightedness.

Hyperplasia Abnormal increase in the number of cells in an organ or tissue.

Hypertension High blood pressure; elevated diastolic or systolic blood pressure, or both.

Hyperthyroidism Condition in which there is an excessive production of thyroid hormones.

Hyperuricemia Condition in which urate levels build up in the blood.

Hypnotic Drug that induces sleep.

Hypoglycemia Low blood glucose levels.

Hypogonadism Inadequate production of sex hormones.

Hypothyroidism Condition in which there is insufficient production of thyroid hormones.

Hysterectomy Surgical removal of the uterus.

Idiosyncratic reaction Unexpected drug reaction.

Immunization Deliberate artificial exposure to disease to produce acquired immunity.

Immunoglobulin E Antibody associated with allergies.

Immunomodulator Chemical agent that modifies the immune response or functioning of the immune system.

Immunosuppressant Drug that inhibits proliferation of the cells of the immune system; also known as an immunopharmacologic agent.

Implant radiation Procedure, also known as brachytherapy, in which radioactive material sealed in needles, seeds, wires, or catheters is placed directly into or near a tumor in the body.

Inactivated killed vaccine Killed vaccine; provides less immunity than live vaccines but has fewer risks for vaccine-induced disease.

Incontinence Loss of bladder or bowel control.

Infarction Sudden loss of blood supply to an area that results in cell death. A myocardial infarction (MI) is known as a heart attack. A cerebral infarction is also known as a stroke.

Infertility Inability to achieve pregnancy during 1 year or more of unprotected intercourse.

Inflammation Response to tissue irritation or injury marked by signs of redness, swelling, heat, and pain.

Inflammatory bowel disease (IBD) Chronic disorder of the gastrointestinal tract characterized by inflammation of the intestines; results in abdominal cramping and persistent diarrhea.

Insomnia Condition characterized by difficulty falling asleep, staying asleep, or both.

Insulin resistance Condition in which the body does not respond to insulin; contributes to the development of type 2 diabetes.

Interferon Antiviral protein that enhances T cell recognition of antigens (interferon-γ) and produces immune system suppression (interferon-α, interferon-β).

Intraocular pressure Inner pressure of the eye. Normal intraocular pressure ranges from 12 to 22 mm Hg.

Intrauterine device (IUD) Device inserted in the uterus to prevent pregnancy.

Inverse agonist Drug that has affinity and activity at the receptor site. The drug can turn off a receptor that is activated or turn on a receptor that is not currently active.

Ionization Chemical process involving the gain or release of a proton (H^+). Ionized drug molecules may have a positive or negative charge.

Ionizing radiation Type of high-frequency radiation produced by x-ray procedures, radioactive substances, and ultraviolet (UV) light that can lead to health risks, including cancer, at certain doses.

Iris Colored part of the eye that can expand or contract to allow the correct amount of light to enter the eye.

Iritis Condition associated with inflammation of the iris.

Irritable bowel syndrome Condition that causes abdominal distress and erratic movement of the contents of the large bowel resulting in diarrhea and/or constipation.

Ischemia Reduction of blood supplied to tissues; typically caused by blood vessel obstruction due to atherosclerosis, stenosis, or plaque.

Ischemic heart disease Any condition in which heart muscle is damaged or works inefficiently because of an absence or relative deficiency of its blood supply.

Ischemic stroke Ischemia in the brain.

Isolated systolic hypertension Condition involving only elevated systolic blood pressure. Diastolic blood pressure is within the normal range.

Kallman syndrome Congenital disorder that causes hypogonadism and loss of the sense of smell.

Keratitis Severe infection of the cornea that may be caused by bacteria or fungi.

Keratolytic Pertains to keratolysis, the softening and shedding of the horny outer layer of the skin. A keratolytic agent is a peeling agent.

Klinefelter syndrome A chromosomal disorder in males. People with this condition are born with at least one extra X chromosome.

Labyrinth Bony structure in the inner ear consisting of three parts (vestibule, cochlea, and semicircular canals) involved in balance.

β-Lactamase Enzyme secreted by some microbes that can destroy β-lactam antibiotics.

Laryngopharyngeal reflux Reflux of gastric contents into the larynx and pharynx.

Laxative Medicine that induces evacuation of the bowel.

Legend drugs Drugs required by state or federal law to be dispensed by a prescription only. Prescriptions must be written for a legitimate medical condition and issued by a practitioner authorized to prescribe.

Leukemia Cancer that starts in blood-forming tissue such as the bone marrow.

Leukocytes White blood cells (WBCs).

Leukocytosis Abnormally high WBC count.

Leukopenia Abnormally low WBC count.

Leukotriene Proinflammatory mediator released as part of the allergic inflammatory response. Leukotrienes also trigger contractions in the smooth muscles of airways.

Lice Group of parasites (*Pediculus humanus capitis, Pediculus humanus corporis, Pthirus pubis*) that can live on the body, scalp, or genital area of humans.

Lipid Fatlike substance.

Lipophilic Having an affinity for lipids; lipid-loving.

Lipoprotein Small globules of cholesterol covered by a layer of protein.

Live attenuated vaccine Living, but weakened, version of an invader that does not cause disease in nonimmunocompromised individuals (nonvirulent).

Low-density lipoprotein Compound consisting of a lipid and protein that carries most of the total cholesterol in the blood and deposits the excess along the inside of arterial walls; also known as bad cholesterol.

Lower esophageal sphincter Sphincter separating the esophagus and stomach.

Lower motor neurons Neurons that branch out from the spinal cord to the muscles and tissues of the body.

Lymphoma Cancer that begins in cells of the immune system.

Major depression Mental illness associated with persistent feelings of sadness, emptiness, or hopelessness that lasts for several weeks.

Malignant Cancerous tumors that can invade and destroy nearby tissue and spread to other parts of the body.

Mammography Screening examination to detect breast cancer in which a radiograph is taken of the breast.

Mast cells Granule-containing cells found in connective tissue. They contain many granules rich in histamine, which are released during allergic reactions.

Mastication Chewing.

Materia medica Medicinal materials.

Mechanism of action Manner in which a drug produces its effect.

Medication error Error made in the process of prescribing, preparing, dispensing, or administering drug therapy.

Melanoma Form of skin cancer that arises in melanocytes, the cells that produce pigment.

Melatonin Hormone released by the pineal gland that makes a person feel drowsy.

Ménière disease Chronic inner ear disease associated with intermittent buildup of fluid in the inner ear that causes hearing loss and vertigo.

Menopause Termination of menstrual cycles; an event usually marked by the passage of at least 1 year without menstruation.

Menorrhagia Excessive menstrual bleeding.

Metabolic syndrome Important risk factor of hypertension that promotes the development of atherosclerosis and cardiovascular disease.

Metabolism Biochemical process involving transformation of active drugs to a compound that can be easily eliminated, or the conversion of prodrugs to active drugs.

Metabolite Product of drug metabolism. Metabolites may be inactivated drugs or active drugs with equal or greater activity than the parent drug.

Metastasis Spread of cancer from one part of the body to another.

Metered-dose inhaler Device used for delivering a dose of inhaled medication. A solution or powder is delivered as a mist and inhaled.

Microvilli Brushlike border of each villus in the small intestine; increases the surface area for absorption.

Migraine Vascular headache that is often accompanied by nausea and visual disturbances.

Milia Tiny little bumps that occur when normally sloughed skin cells get trapped in small pockets on the surface of the skin.

Mitral valve stenosis Disease of the mitral valve involving the buildup of plaquelike material around the valve.

Monoamine oxidase Enzyme found in the liver, intestine, and terminal neurons; responsible for degradation of monoamine neurotransmitters and dietary amines.

Mother to child transmission Transmission of a substance or virus (e.g., HIV from an HIV-infected mother) to her baby during pregnancy or delivery, or through breast milk (also called perinatal transmission).

Motor neuron Neuron that connects to the sarcolemma to form a neuromuscular junction.

Multiple sclerosis Autoimmune disease that causes progressive damage to nerves resulting in spasticity, pain, mood changes, and other physical symptoms.

Myasthenia gravis Autoimmune disease in which the immune system attacks the muscle cells at the neuromuscular junction and is characterized by muscle weakness.

Mycosis General term for a fungal infection.

Myelin Fatty covering that insulates nerve cells in the brain and spinal cord.

Myocardial infarction Condition that results in heart muscle tissue death; caused by the occlusion (blockage) of a coronary artery; also referred to as a heart attack.

Myoclonic seizure Seizure characterized by jerking muscle movements; caused by contraction of major muscle groups.

Myopia Nearsightedness.

Myositis Autoimmune disease that causes chronic inflammation of the muscles.

Natriuretic peptides Hormones that play a role in cardiac homeostasis.

Nebulizer Device that creates a mist out of a liquid inhalant solution, making drug delivery easier.

Necrosis Cell death that may be caused by lack of blood and oxygen to the affected area(s).

Negative symptoms Spasticity symptoms, which may indicate schizophrenia, that can produce muscle weakness, decreased endurance, and reduction in the ability to make voluntary muscle movements.

Neoplasm Tumor.

Nephrotoxicity Serious adverse effect that occurs in the kidneys.

Neurodegeneration Destruction of nerve cells.

Neurodegenerative disease Disorder that results in progressive destruction of neurons.

Neuroleptic malignant syndrome Potentially fatal reaction to administration of neuroleptics. Symptoms include stupor, muscle rigidity, and high temperature.

Neuroleptic Drug used to treat schizophrenia and psychoses.

Neuromuscular junction Space between motor neuron endplate and muscle sole plate that neurotransmitters must cross.

Neuron Functional unit of the nervous system, which includes the cell body, dendrites, axon, and terminals.

Neuropathic pain Type of pain associated with nerve injury caused by trauma, infection, or chronic diseases such as diabetes.

Neuroprotective Protects nerve cells from damage.

Neurotransmitter Protein that transmits nerve signals from one neuron to another.

Nigrostriatal pathway Pathway located in the substantia nigra that stimulates and inhibits movement.

Nits Head lice eggs.

Nociceptors Thin nerve fibers in the skin, muscle, and other body tissues that carry pain signals.

Nocturia Nighttime urination.

Nodule Ruptured pustules that form abscesses.

Noncompetitive antagonist Drug that binds to an alternative receptor site that prevents the agonist from binding to and producing its desired action.

Nondepolarizing competitive blockers Drugs that compete with acetylcholine for binding sites.

Non-rapid eye movement (REM) sleep Stages 1 through 4 of the sleep cycle.

NSAID Nonsteroidal antiinflammatory drug.

Nymph Baby louse.

Obsessive-compulsive disorder Condition associated with the inability to control or stop repeated unwanted thoughts or behaviors.

Oncovirus Virus that is a causative agent in a cancer.

Onset of action Time it takes for drug action to begin.

Onychomycosis Fungal infection involving the fingernails or toenails; also known as tinea unguium.

Open-angle glaucoma Disorder characterized by elevated pressure in the eye that can lead to permanent blindness.

Opiate-naïve Refers to a person who has no current exposure to opioids.

Opioid Naturally occurring or synthetically derived analgesic with properties similar to those of morphine.

Optic nerve Bundle of nerve fibers located in the back of the eye that connects the retina to the brain.

Orthostatic hypotension Sudden drop in blood pressure that occurs when arising from lying down or sitting to standing.

Osmosis Movement of water across a semipermeable membrane from an area of higher concentration to an area of lower concentration.

Osteoblast Cell responsible for bone formation, deposition, and mineralization of the collagen matrix of bone.

Osteoclast Cell responsible for bone resorption.

Osteolysis Dissolution or degradation of bone.

Osteopenia Decrease in bone mineral density that places people at increased risk of developing osteoporosis.

Osteoporosis Chronic progressive disease of bone characterized by loss of bone density and bone strength; results in increased risk for fractures.

Otitis Inflammation of the ear.

Otitis externa Inflammation of the ear canal or external ear.

Otitis media Infection of the middle ear; typically caused by viral or bacterial infection.

Otoliths Calcium carbonate crystals found in the utricle and saccule of the inner ear.

Otorrhea Discharge coming from the external auditory canal or inside the canal.

Otosclerosis Hardening of the bones of the middle ear.

Ototoxicity Damage or toxicity to the ear or eighth cranial nerve (associated with hearing).

Over-the-counter (OTC) drugs Drugs that can be obtained without a prescription.

Ovicidal Able to destroy eggs.

Panic disorder Condition associated with repeated sudden onset of feelings of terror.

Pap test (Pap smear) Screening test in which cells from the cervix are examined to detect cancer and changes that may lead to cancer.

Papule Obstructed follicle that becomes inflamed.

Parasite Organism that benefits by living in, with, or on another organism.

Parasympathetic nervous system Division of the autonomic nervous system (ANS) that functions during restful situations; the "rest and digest" part of the ANS.

Parenteral Refers to a drug dosage form administered by injection or infusion.

Parkinson disease Progressive disorder of the nervous system involving degeneration of dopaminergic neurons and causing impaired muscle movement.

Partial agonist Drug that behaves like an agonist under some conditions and acts like an antagonist under different conditions.

Partial thromboplastin time Blood test that determines the effectiveness of heparin in reducing antithrombotic activity; measures how long it takes for blood to clot.

Partial-thickness burns First- and second-degree burns.

Pathophysiology Study of structural and functional changes produced by disease.

PCA Patient-controlled analgesia.

Peak effect Maximum drug effect produced by a given dose of drug after the drug has reached its maximum concentration in the body.

Peak flow meter Handheld device used to measure the volume of air exhaled and how rapidly the air is moved out.

Pediculicide Drug that kills lice.

Pelvic inflammatory disease Infection of the uterus, fallopian tubes, and adjacent pelvic structures that is not associated with pregnancy or surgery.

Peptic ulcer disease Term used to describe ulcers located in the duodenum or stomach.

Peripheral nervous system (PNS) Division of the nervous system outside the brain and spinal cord.

Peripheral vascular resistance Resistance to the flow of blood in peripheral arterial vessels that is associated with blood vessel diameter, vessel length, and blood viscosity.

Peripheral vision Sometimes called side vision, this is usually the first area of vision to be lost with glaucoma.

Peripheral-acting muscle relaxants Drugs that block nerve transmission between the motor endplate and skeletal muscle receptors.

Peristalsis Forceful wave of contractions in the esophagus that moves food and liquids from the mouth to the stomach.

Petit mal seizure Absence seizure in which the person experiences a brief period of unconsciousness and stares vacantly into space.

Pharmaceutical alternative Drug that contains the same active ingredient as the brand name drug; however, the strength and dosage form may be different.

Pharmaceutical equivalent Drug that contains identical amount of active ingredient as a brand name drug but may have different inactive ingredients, be manufactured in a different dosage form, and exhibit different rates of absorption.

Pharmacodynamics Study of drugs and their actions on a living organism.

Pharmacognosy Science dealing with the biologic and biochemical features of natural drugs and their constituents. It is the study of drugs of plant or animal origin.

Pharmacokinetics Science dealing with what the body does to a drug; includes the study of absorption, distribution, metabolism, and elimination.

Pharmacology Study of drugs and their interactions with living systems, including chemical and physical properties, toxicology, and therapeutics.

Pharmacotherapeutics Use of drugs in the treatment of disease. It is the study of factors that influence patient response to drugs.

Pharmacotherapy Use of drugs in the treatment of disease.

Phenylketonuria Disease marked by failure to metabolize the amino acid phenylalanine to tyrosine; results in severe neurologic deficits in infancy if untreated.

Phobia Irrational fear of things or situations that produce symptoms of intense anxiety.

Phosphodiesterase type 5 inhibitor Drug used to relax smooth muscle and blood vessels that supply the corpus cavernosum and control penile engorgement.

Photopsia Condition similar to floaters; associated with flashes of light.

Phototherapy Treatment for atopic dermatitis that involves exposing the skin to ultraviolet A or B light waves.

Pilosebaceous units (PSUs) These consist of a sebaceous gland connected to a canal, called a follicle; contain fine hairs.

Plaque psoriasis Most common form of psoriasis characterized by raised inflamed (red) lesions covered with a silvery white scale.

Plaque Fatty cholesterol deposits; patchy areas of inflammation and demyelination that disrupt nerve signals between the brain and the rest of the body.

Plasticity Ability of the brain to restructure itself and adapt to injury.

Platelets Structures found in the blood involved in the coagulation process.

Polycystic ovary disease Condition characterized by ovaries twice the normal size that contain fluid-filled cysts.

Polymyositis Form of myositis that affects multiple muscles, particularly the muscles closest to the trunk.

Polyp Growth that protrudes from a mucous membrane.

Positive inotropic effect Increase in the force of myocardial contractions.

Positive symptoms Hallucinations, delusions, or other unusual thoughts or perceptions that are symptoms of schizophrenia; also, spasticity symptoms that cause muscle spasms and hyperexcitable reflexes.

Positron emission tomography (PET) Diagnostic examination used to detect cancer cells in the body in which a small amount of radioactive glucose (sugar) is injected into a vein and a scanner is used to make detailed, computerized pictures of areas inside the body where the glucose is used.

Postprandial After eating.

Posttraumatic stress disorder Stress disorder that develops in persons who have participated in, witnessed, or been a victim of a terrifying event.

Postural hypotension Drop in blood pressure caused by a change in posture.

Potency Measure of the amount of drug required to produce a response. It is the effective dose concentration.

Potentiation Process whereby one drug, acting at a separate site or via a different mechanism of action, increases the effect of another drug but produces no effect when administered alone. Food can also potentiate the effects of a drug.

Prediabetes Condition of impaired fasting glucose and impaired glucose tolerance in which the body consistently has elevated glucose levels.

Pregnancy Condition of having a developing embryo or fetus in the body after successful conception.

Prehypertension Systolic blood pressure ranging between 120 and 139 mm Hg and diastolic blood pressure ranging between 80 and 89 mm Hg.

Premenstrual dysphoric disorder Disorder characterized by symptoms such as depression, anxiety, hopelessness, sad feelings, and self-depreciation.

Premenstrual syndrome Condition involving a group of symptoms (e.g., headache, irritability, depression, fatigue, sleep changes, weight gain) that occur before the start of the menstrual cycle.

Pressure injury Pressure sore or "bedsore."

Primary tumor Original tumor or initial tumor.

Prodrug Drug administered in an inactive form that is metabolized in the body to an active form.

Prolactinoma Pituitary tumor that produces an excessive amount of prolactin.

Prostate gland Gland in the male reproductive system just below the bladder, surrounding the urethra.

Prostate-specific antigen (PSA) Protein produced by the prostate gland. Levels are elevated in men who have prostate cancer, infection or inflammation of the prostate gland, or benign prostate hyperplasia.

Prostate-specific antigen (PSA) test Blood test to measure PSA. A free PSA test result reports the percentage of PSA that is not attached to another chemical compared with the total amount in a man's blood. Free PSA is linked to benign prostate hyperplasia but not to cancer.

Prostatitis Inflammation of the prostate gland.

Prothrombin time Test given to determine the effectiveness of warfarin in reducing clotting time.

Pseudoparkinsonism Adverse reaction to the administration of neuroleptics; characterized by symptoms mimicking those of Parkinson disease.

Psoriasis Chronic disease of the skin characterized by itchy red patches covered with silvery scales.

Psychosis Mental state characterized by disorganized behavior and thought, delusions, hallucinations, and loss of touch with reality.

Purine One of two nitrogen-containing bases found in DNA and RNA. Purine bases are metabolized.

Pustule Larger lesions that are more inflamed than papules; can be superficial or deep.

Radiation therapy Use of high-energy radiation from x-rays, gamma rays, neutrons, and other sources to kill cancer cells and shrink tumors.

Radioactive iodine uptake Test using radioactive iodine to screen for thyroid disease.

Radionuclide scan Diagnostic test in which an individual is administered a small amount of radioactive material. A scanner is used to take pictures of the internal parts of the body to detect where the radiation concentrates.

Radon Radioactive gas that if inhaled in sufficient quantity can lead to lung cancer.

Rapid eye movement (REM) sleep Stage of sleep when dreaming occurs.

Rebound hypersomnia Condition associated with excessive sleep that follows long-term insomnia or the use of drugs that depress REM and non-REM sleep.

Receptor site Location of drug-cell binding.

Reflux Backflow of gastric contents into the esophageal or laryngopharyngeal region.

Refractory period Time between contractions that it takes for repolarization to occur.

Remission Lessening in severity or abatement of symptoms.

Remodeling Process of continual turnover of bone.

Renin–aldosterone–angiotensin system System that is activated when there is a drop in renal blood flow. Activation increases blood volume, blood flow to the kidneys, vasoconstriction, and blood pressure.

Repolarization Period of time when the heart is recharging and preparing for another contraction.

Rh factor Antigen present in the red blood cells of Rh-positive individuals.

Rhabdomyolysis Breakdown of muscle fibers and release of muscle fiber contents into the circulation.

Rheumatoid arthritis Chronic disease characterized by inflammation and remodeling of the joints.

Rheumatoid factor Immunoglobulin (antibody) present in many people who have rheumatoid arthritis.

Ribonucleic acid (RNA) Nucleic acid involved in protein synthesis that carries and transfers genetic information and assembles proteins.

Ringworm Group of tinea infections involving the body or scalp that have a characteristic ringlike shape. Ringworm is spread by person to person and animal to person contact.

Rule of nines Formula for estimating the percentage of adult body surface covered by burns; divides the body into 11 areas, each representing 9% of the total body surface area.

Rule of palms Rule for determining the extent of a burn surface area. A palm size of a burn victim is about 1% of the total body surface area.

Saccule Saclike inner ear structure that senses vertical motion of the head.

Salpingitis Inflammation of the fallopian tube, usually as a result of a sexually transmitted infection.

Sarcomere Basic contractile unit of the muscle cell.

Sarcoplasmic reticulum (SR) Networks of tubules and sacs contained in muscle cells.

Scabicide Drug that kills the scabies mite.

Scabies Parasitic infection caused by the mite *Sarcoptes scabiei.*

Schizophrenia Type of psychosis characterized by delusions of thought, visual or auditory hallucinations (or both), and speech disturbances. Paranoid schizophrenia is characterized by delusions of persecution.

Second-degree burn Burn that involves deep epidermal layers and causes damage to the upper layers of the dermis.

Sedative Drug that causes relaxation and promotes drowsiness.

Seizure threshold Measure of a person's susceptibility to seizures.

Semen Fluid containing sperm and secretions from glands of the male reproductive tract.

Serotonin syndrome Potentially life-threatening adverse drug reaction that produces symptoms of confusion, agitation, diarrhea, tremors, and increased blood pressure; caused by excessive serotonin.

Shingles Recurring and painful skin rash caused by the herpes zoster virus.

Simple focal seizures Seizure that affects only one part of the brain; causes the person to experience unusual sensations or feelings.

Sinus cavity Mucus-lined, air-filled space found in the frontal bone (frontal sinuses), sphenoid, ethmoid, maxillae (paranasal sinuses), and middle and inner ear (mastoid sinuses).

Soleplate Portion of the membrane of muscle cells that receives messages transmitted by motor neurons.

Somatic nervous system Division of the nervous system that carries information to the somatic effectors or skeletal muscles.

Sonogram Computer image of internal organs and tissues produced by ultrasound.

Spacer Device attached to the end of a metered-dose inhaler that facilitates drug delivery into the lungs (rather than to the back of the throat).

Spasticity Motor disorder that causes increased muscle tone, exaggerated tendon jerks, and hyperexcitable muscles.

Spirometry Test that measures the volume of air that is expired (blown out of the lungs) after taking a deep breath and how rapidly the volume of air is expired.

Stage Refers to the extent of a cancer within the body. Staging is based on the size of the tumor, whether lymph nodes contain cancer, and whether the disease has spread from the original site to other parts of the body (metastasis).

Status epilepticus Medical emergency brought on by repeated generalized seizures that can deprive the brain of oxygen.

Stem cell Type of cell from which other types of cells develop; for example, blood cells develop from blood-forming stem cells.

Stem cell transplantation Procedure used to replace cells that were destroyed by cancer treatment.

Stimulant Drug that increases activity in the brain and is used to treat ADHD and narcolepsy.

Stroke volume Equal to the volume of blood ejected by the left ventricle during each cardiac contraction minus the volume of blood in the ventricle at the end of systole.

Stye Painful lump located on the eyelid margin caused by an acute self-limiting infection of the oil glands of the eyelid.

Substance P Peptide involved in the production of pain sensations; controls pain perception.

Substantia nigra Part of the basal ganglia containing clusters of dopamine-producing neurons.

Supraovulation Simultaneous rupture of multiple mature follicles.

Supraventricular tachycardia Heart rate up to 200 beats/min that originates in an area above the ventricles.

Sympathetic nervous system Division of the ANS that functions during stressful situations; fight-or-flight part of the ANS.

Synapse Gap between neurons where nerve information is transmitted from one neuron to another.

Synarthrosis Immovable joint (skull).

Synergistic effect Drug-drug or drug-food interaction that produces an effect greater than the effect that would be produced if either drug were administered alone.

Synovium Thin layer of tissue that lines the joint space.

Systemic lupus erythematosus (SLE) Autoimmune disease that affects almost all body systems.

Systolic blood pressure Measure of the pressure when the heart's ventricles are contracting (systole).

Tangles Twisted fibers made up of clumps of a protein called tau that interfere with nerve signal transmission.

Tardive dyskinesia Inappropriate postures of the neck, trunk, and limbs accompanied by involuntary thrusting of the tongue.

Tear deficiency Also known as dry eyes.

Tetanus Potentially fatal condition characterized by a continuous muscle spasm caused by exposure to the nerve toxin produced by the bacterium *Clostridium tetani*. It is also known as lockjaw.

Tetraiodothyronine (T$_4$) Most abundant thyroid hormone; contains four atoms of iodine; also known as thyroxine.

Tetraiodothyronine test Test to measure the level of free circulating thyroid hormone.

Therapeutic alternative Drug that contains different active ingredient(s) than the brand name drug but produces the same desired therapeutic outcome.

Therapeutic duplication Administration of two drugs that produce similar effects and side effects.

Therapeutic index (TI) Ratio of the effective dose to the lethal dose.

Third-degree burn Burn characterized by destruction of the epidermis and dermis.

Thrombocytes Platelets.

Thrombocytopenia Condition that results from a deficiency in the platelet count.

Thrombolytic Drug used to dissolve blood clots.

Thrombosis Formation of a blood clot.

Thrombotic stroke Stroke caused by thrombosis.

Thrombus Stationary blood clot.

Thyroid antibody test Diagnostic test used to measure levels of thyroid antibodies; diagnostic for autoimmune thyroid disease.

Thyroid-releasing factor Hormone released by the hypothalamus that stimulates the pituitary gland to release thyroid-stimulating hormone.

Thyroid-stimulating hormone (TSH) Hormone released by the pituitary gland that stimulates the thyroid gland to produce and release thyroid hormones.

Thyroid-stimulating hormone test Diagnostic test used to measure the level of TSH in the blood; low level signals hyperthyroidism.

Tinnitus Intermittent or continuous whistling, crackling, squeaking, or ringing noise in the ears.

Tissue plasminogen activator Naturally occurring thrombolytic substance.

Tolerance Increasing doses of a drug are required to achieve the same effects as were achieved previously at lower doses.

Tonic-clonic (grand mal) seizure Generalized seizure that causes stiffening of the limbs, difficulty breathing, and jerking movements; is followed by disorientation and limbs that become limp.

Tonometry Use of a device to measure the pressure in the eye.

Toxic megacolon Life-threatening condition characterized by a very inflated colon, abdominal distention, and sometimes fever, abdominal pain, or shock.

Toxic shock syndrome Rare disorder caused by certain *Staphylococcus aureus* strains that occurs in women using tampons.

Toxicology Science dealing with the study of poisons.

Toxoid vaccine Vaccine that stimulates the immune system to produce antibodies to a specific toxin that causes illness.

Trabecular meshwork Small openings around the outer edge of the iris that form meshlike drainage canals surrounding the iris; sometimes referred to as the canal of Schlemm.

Transient ischemic attack (TIA) Stroke that typically lasts for a few minutes; also known as a ministroke.

Trigeminal neuralgia Painful condition that produces intense stabbing pain in areas of the face innervated by branches of the trigeminal nerve.

Triglycerides Storage form of energy found in fat tissue muscle; metabolize to very low-density lipoproteins.

Triiodothyronine (T$_3$) Hormone secreted by the thyroid gland; contains three atoms of iodine.

Tumor marker Substance sometimes found in the blood, other body fluids, or tissues that may signal the presence of a certain type of cancer; for example, a high level of PSA is a signal for possible prostate cancer.

Tumor necrosis factor (TNF) Inflammatory cytokine released as part of the immune response; found in the synovial fluid of people with rheumatoid arthritis.

Tumor Abnormal mass of tissue that results from excessive cell division. Tumors may be benign (not cancerous) or malignant (cancerous).

Turner syndrome Congenital endocrine disorder caused by failure of the ovaries to respond to pituitary hormone (gonadotropin) stimulation.

Tympanic membrane Eardrum.

Type 1 diabetes Autoimmune disease that results in high blood glucose levels. Pancreatic β-cells are destroyed and insufficient amounts of insulin are produced.

Type 2 diabetes Condition that results in high blood glucose levels. People with type 2 diabetes have insulin resistance.

Ulcer Open wound or sore.

Ulcerative colitis Irritable bowel disease that results in inflammation, ulcers, and damage to the colon.

Upper esophageal sphincter Sphincter separating the pharynx and esophagus. It relaxes to permit passage of food and liquids during swallowing, prevent air from entering the esophagus during breathing, and prevent gastric secretions from entering the pharynx.

Upper motor neurons Neurons that carry messages from the brain down to the spinal cord.

Urate Product of purine metabolism. Urate crystals may accumulate in joints and produce inflammation and pain.

Uricosuric Drug that increases the renal clearance of urates.

Urinalysis Microscopic and chemical examination of a fresh urine sample.

Urinary frequency Need to urinate more often than is normal.

Urticaria Hives.

Uveitis Serious eye condition that produces inflammation of the uvea; can cause scarring of the eye and blindness if untreated.

Vaccine Substance that prevents disease by taking advantage of the body's ability to make antibodies and prime killer cells to fight disease.

Vaginitis Inflammation of the vagina.

Vasospasm Spasms that constrict blood vessels and reduce the flow of blood and oxygen.

Ventricular fibrillation Life-threatening arrhythmia during which the heart beats up to 600 beats/min.

Ventricular tachycardia Condition in which ventricles beat faster than 200 beats/min.

Vertigo Feeling of spinning in space (dizziness and loss of balance).

Viral load Amount of materials from the virus that get released into the blood when HIV reproduces.

Virion Infectious particles of a virus.

Virostatic Able to suppress viral proliferation.

Virus Intracellular parasite that consists of a DNA and RNA core surrounded by a protein coat and sometimes an outer covering of lipoprotein.

Vitreous floaters Particles that float in the vitreous and cast shadows on the retina; these appear as spots, cobwebs, or spiders.

Vulvovaginal candidiasis Yeast vaginitis.

Wheal Raised blister-like area on the skin.

Whitehead (closed comedone) Trapped sebum and bacteria that stay below the skin surface; may show up as tiny white spots or may be so small that they are invisible to the naked eye.

Index

Page numbers followed by "*f*" indicate figures, "*t*" indicate tables, and "*b*" indicate boxes.

A

Abacavir, 405, 405*t*–406*t*, 411*t*–413*t*
Abacavir + lamivudine, 405*t*–406*t*, 411*t*–413*t*
Abacavir + lamivudine + zidovudine, 405*t*–40 6*t*, 411*t*–413*t*
Abaloparatide, 171*t*, 172*t*–173*t*, 173–174
Abatacept, 160, 161*t*, 162*t*–163*t*
Abciximab, 243, 246*t*, 252*t*–256*t*
Abemaciclib, 421–422, 422*t*, 433*t*–439*t*
Abiraterone, 425, 425*t*, 433*t*–439*t*
Abnormal uterine bleeding, 356
AbobotulinumtoxinA, 143*t*
Absence seizures. *See* Petit mal seizures
Absorption
　blood flow on, 20
　factors influencing, 19–20
　pH and, 19–20
　surface area and, 20, 21*f*
　tissue thickness on, 20
Acarbose, 335*t*, 341*t*–344*t*
Acebutolol
　for arrhythmia, 262*t*, 263*t*–265*t*
　for hypertension, 224*t*, 230*t*–234*t*
ACE inhibitors. *See* Angiotensin-converting enzyme (ACE) inhibitors
Acetaminophen, 24, 111*b*, 148*t*–149*t*
　for migraine headaches, 122*t*
　for muscle strain, 148*t*–149*t*
　for pain, 107*t*–109*t*, 112*t*–113*t*, 113*t*–115*t*
Acetazolamide, 186–187, 187*t*, 189*t*–190*t*
Acetic acid, 198*t*
Acetic acid solution, 198*t*
Acetylcholine (ACh)
　neuromuscular blockade and, 141
　opioid antidiarrheals and, 281
　Parkinson disease and, 84–86, 85*f*
Acetylcholinesterase (AChE)
　inhibitors of, 187
　　for Alzheimer's disease, 82, 84*t*
　neuromuscular blockade and, 142
ACh. *See* Acetylcholine
AChE. *See* Acetylcholinesterase
Acitretin, 499, 500*t*–502*t*
Acne, 481–490, 482*t*
　causes of, 482–483, 483*b*
　definition of, 481
　treatment of, 483–489, 488*t*
　　hormonally influenced acne, 487–489, 487*t*
　　mild acne, 483
　　moderate to moderately severe acne, 483–486, 485*t*–486*t*
　　nonpharmaceutical, 487–489
　　severe acne, 486–487, 487*t*
Acne vulgaris, 481
Acquired immunodeficiency syndrome (AIDS), 167, 404
　HAART for, 396, 405

Acquired immunodeficiency syndrome (AIDS) (*Continued*)
　treatment of, 404–413, 411*t*–413*t*
　　pharmacological, 405–413
Acrophobia, 49
Activated partial thromboplastin time (aPTT) test, 243
Active transport, 19
Acupuncture, for pain, 116–117
Acute nonlymphocytic leukemia (ANLL), 32
Acute pain, 103–104
Acyclovir, 400, 401*t*, 401*t*–403*t*
Acyclovir + hydrocortisone, 401*t*
Adalimumab, 160–164, 161*t*, 162*t*–163*t*, 285, 285*t*, 286*t*–287*t*, 452*t*, 454*t*–455*t*, 497, 497*t*–499*t*, 500*t*–502*t*
Adalimumab-aacf, 497*t*–499*t*
Adalimumab-adaz, 497*t*–499*t*
Adalimumab-adbm, 497*t*–499*t*
Adalimumab-afzb, 497*t*–499*t*
Adalimumab-aqvh, 497*t*–499*t*
Adalimumab-atto, 497*t*–499*t*
Adalimumab-bwwd, 497*t*–499*t*
Adamantanes, 396–397, 396*b*, 397*t*
Adapalene, 485*t*–486*t*, 488*t*
Additive effects, 38
Adefovir, 398, 398*b*, 399*t*, 401*t*–403*t*
ADHD. *See* Attention-deficit hyperactivity disorder
Adjunct, 58
Ado-trastuzumab, 433*t*–439*t*
α₁-Adrenergic antagonists, 366, 366*b*, 367*t*
β₂-Adrenergic agonists
　anticholinergics and, 302*t*–305*t*
　inhaled corticosteroids and, 302*t*–305*t*
　long-acting, for asthma, 293–296, 295*b*, 295*t*, 296*t*–297*t*, 301*t*, 302*t*–305*t*
　short-acting, for asthma, 294, 295*t*, 302*t*–305*t*
Aducanumab (Aduhelm), 82–83, 84*t*, 85*t*
Aduhelm (aducanumab), 82–83, 84*t*, 85*t*
Adverse drug reactions (ADRs)32, 32*b*, 33*b*, 39. *See also specific drugs*
　GI tract and, 38*f*
　reporting, 33–35
Adverse Event Reporting System (AERS), 33
Afatinib, 425, 426*t*, 433*t*–439*t*
Affinity, 28
Age
　calcium and, 168*t*
　cancer and, 417
　on metabolism, 23
　myocardial infarction and, 239
　pharmacotherapeutics and, 31
　stroke and, 239
Agonists, 29, 29*f*, 29*t*. *See also specific agonists*
　opioid, 105, 107*t*–109*t*, 112*t*–113*t*

α₂-Agonists, central-acting, 228, 228*b*, 228*t*
Agoraphobia, 49
AIDS. *See* Acquired immunodeficiency syndrome
Alafenamide, 399*t*
Albendazole, 183
Albumin, 22
Albuterol, 293–294, 295*t*, 302*t*–305*t*
Alclometasone dipropionate, 493*b*, 493*t*–495*t*, 500*t*–502*t*
Alcohol, 37, 39*t*
　blood glucose levels and, 328*b*
　cancer and, 417
　drug interactions and, 39*t*
Aldosterone, 215
Aldosterone antagonists, 240, 242, 252*t*–256*t*
Aldosterone receptor antagonists, 217–218, 219*t*, 230*t*–234*t*
Alendronate, 169, 169*t*, 172*t*–173*t*
Alfuzosin, 366, 367*t*, 368*t*
Alginates, 274–275
Alginic acid, 275*t*
Aliskiren, 228–235, 229*t*, 230*t*–234*t*
Alitretinoin, 485*t*–486*t*
Alkylating agents, 431–432, 432*b*, 432*t*
Allergens, 308
　occupational, 309
Allergic asthma, 299
Allergic conjunctivitis, 309, 312*t*
Allergic rhinitis, 309, 312*t*
Allergies, 308
　drug, 31
　immunotherapy for, 313–315
　management of, 309–315, 309*b*
　sequence of, 308
　symptoms of, 308*b*, 309, 309*b*
　triggers of, 308
Allopurinol, 153–154, 154*t*, 155*t*
　dosage for, 155*t*
Allylamines, 463–465, 465*t*, 468*t*–470*t*
Almotriptan, 119*t*, 120*t*, 121*t*
Alogliptin, 337*t*, 341*t*–344*t*
Alogliptin + metformin, 337*t*, 341*t*–344*t*
Alogliptin + pioglitazone, 337*t*, 341*t*–344*t*
Alosetron, 280, 280*b*, 280*t*, 286*t*–287*t*
Alpelisib, 422*t*, 433*t*–439*t*
Alpha-adrenergic agonists, 186, 187*t*
Alpha₁-adrenergic antagonists (α₁-blockers), 223, 225*f*, 225*t*, 230*t*–234*t*
Alpha blocker, 366, 367*t*, 368*t*
Alpha-lipoic acid, 340
Alprazolam, 50*t*, 51*b*, 53*t*–54*t*
Alprostadil, 370–371, 371*t*, 372*t*
ALS. *See* Amyotrophic lateral sclerosis
Alteplase (t-PA), 247, 248*t*, 252*t*–256*t*
Aluminum hydroxide, 275*t*
Alzheimer's disease, 81–84
　drug treatment for, 82–83, 84*t*